Andrea M. Pievaroli
Roberto Properzi
J. Brad Case
Francesco Collivignarelli

Laparoscopy and Thoracoscopy in the dog and cat

Foreword
David Twedt

edra
PUBLISHING

Laparoscopy and Thoracoscopy in the dog and cat
A. Pievaroli, R. Properzi, J. Brad Case, F. Collivignarelli

ISBN: 978-19-57260-77-8
eISBN: 978-19-57260-84-6

Book Publishing Manager: Costanza Smeraldi, Edra S.p.A.
Project Manager: Elisa Bechi, Edra S.p.A
Paper, Printing and Binding Manager: Paolo Ficicchia, Edra S.p.A.
Cover: Ursula Giusti, Edra S.p.A.
Copyediting: Jorge Viejo Adiego, Grupo Asís Biomedia, Zaragoza, Spain (chapters 1–28, 32–35, 46–59); Mercedes González Fernández de Castro, Science & Health Publications (chapters 29–31, 36–45)
Layout: Marian Izaguerri Casado, Nieves Marín Ortiz, Grupo Asís Biomedia, Zaragoza, Spain

Edra Publishing US LLC
3309 Northlake Boulevard, Suite 203
Palm Beach Gardens, FL, 33403
EIN: 844113980
info@edrapublishing.com
www.edrapublishing.com

edra
PUBLISHING

Printed in Italy by Printer Trento S.r.l., Trento–June 2023

EDITORS

Andrea M. Pievaroli graduated in 1992 from the Università degli Studi in Milan. Since 1993 he has worked in Rome in a private referral clinic, mainly dealing with soft tissue surgery, minimally invasive surgery, and orthopedics. He spent periods at Michigan State University College of Veterinary Medicine, Texas A&M University College of Veterinary Medicine, and the Animal Medical Center (NY, USA). Since 2000 he is particularly experienced in minimally invasive endoscopic surgery (laparoscopy and thoracoscopy), cystoscopy, and other endoscopic techniques. He is an instructor for minimally invasive endoscopic courses and has presented at international congresses and events. He is a member and liaison of VES (Veterinary Endoscopy Society) and secretary of SICMIV (Italian Society of Veterinary Mini-Invasive Surgery).

Roberto Properzi is the author of several scientific articles, mainly in the surgical field. He has presented numerous dissertations at specialized international conferences organized by VES, SICV, SIOVET, SICEV, SLEV, ASAEE, and EVENDOC. He participated in four courses in Cáceres (Spain) at the CCMIJU (Jesús Usón Minimally Invasive Surgery Center), in 2009 and 2011 as a student, in 2018 and 2022 as an instructor. He was a lecturer in the master of surgery in 2021-2022 at the Faculty of Veterinary Medicine of Teramo (Italy). He is mainly focused on orthopedic and minimally invasive surgery and is particularly keen on laparoscopy, thoracoscopy, and arthroscopy. He is an associate member of the following organizations: VES, ASAEE, EVENDOC, MINIMAL, SIOVET, SICV, SICMIV, SITOV, ESVOT, SLEV, and SICEV. His hobbies are both the mountain, where he practices ski mountaineering, and the sea, where he sets sail with his motorboat.

J. Brad Case is a professor of Small Animal Minimally Invasive and Soft Tissue Surgery at the University of Florida. He obtained his DVM degree from the University of California, Davis. He did an internship in medicine and surgery at Texas A&M University. He then went on to complete a surgery residency and master's degree at Colorado State University. He has been a surgeon at the University of Florida since 2011. During this time, he has trained multiple surgery residents and minimally invasive surgery fellows. He has developed a vascular interventional service after training with University of Florida interventional radiologists. His translational research has been funded by the NIH and the Society of Thoracic Surgeons and has led to the development of devices and procedures intended for use in humans with cardiovascular disease.

Francesco Collivignarelli graduated from the University of Perugia (Italy) and has a master's degree in oncology and oncologic surgery at the University of Pisa and a PhD from the University of Teramo. He did an internship in soft tissue surgery at the University of Bristol with Prof. Peter Holt (ECVS). After that, he gained a fellowship in oncologic surgery at University of Torino (Italy) under the supervision of Prof. Paolo Buracco (ECVS). He is the coauthor and collaborator of the book *Advances in Small Animal Care* vol. 1 (Elsevier, 2020) and the author and coauthor of many scientific studies and papers. He is often invited as guest speaker at international meetings. Since 2020 he has been a contract professor in the master of small animal surgery and a lecturer in the master of diagnostic image at the University of Teramo. Currently, he is a surgeon at the University of Teramo Teaching Hospital and at AniCura Policlinico Roma Sud. His fields of interest are sentinel lymph node, minimally invasive surgery, oncologic surgery, cardiovascular surgery, and oromaxillofacial oncologic surgery. He is the secretary of AIVPA and SICEV. He is also a professional CCR diver.

CONTRIBUTORS

Antoine Adam, DVM
Swissvetgroup SA & Vetmidi SA, Lausanne, Switzerland

Giovanni Allevi, DVM, PhD
Ospedale Veterinario Città di Bergamo, Bergamo, Italy

Agnieszka Antończyk, DVM, PhD
Faculty of Veterinary Medicine, Department and Clinic of Surgery, Wroclaw University of Environmental and Life Sciences, Wroclaw, Poland

Massimo Barilli, DVM
Metatron centro veterinario olistico, Bologna, Italy

Deborah De Bastiani, DVM
Clinica Veterinaria Gran Sasso, Milan, Italy

Maurici Batalla, DVM
Maurici Batalla Veterinaris, Vilanova i la Geltrú, Spain

Joshua G. Becker, DVM
Guardian Veterinary Specialists, Brewster, NY, USA

Lucie Bonneau, DVM, MSc
Centre Hospitalier Vétérinaire des Cordeliers, Meaux, France

Luciano Borghetti, DVM
AniCura Clinica Veterinaria Apuana, Carrara, Italy

Elisa Bortolami, DVM, PhD, DECVAA, MRCVS
Clinica Veterinaria San Marco, Veggiano, Italy

Paolo Boschi, DVM
Ortovet Veterinary Orthopedic Service, Parma, Italy

Fausto Brandão, DVM, MSc, VEaMIS
Karl Storz SE & Co., H. V. Atlântico, Mafra, Portugal

Michael Brückner, DVM, DECVS, MRCVS, EBVS
AWAKE Djursjukhus, Stockholm, Sweden

Floryne O. Buishand, DVM, PhD, DECVS, FHEA, MRCVS
The Royal Veterinary College, University of London, London, UK

Roberto Bussadori, DVM, MSc, Phd
Clinica Veterinaria Gran Sasso, Milan, Italy

J. D. Carrillo, DVM, PhD, DACVSMR
CEU, San Pablo CEU University Foundation, Madrid, Spain

Diego. L. Casas García, DVM, PhD, VEaMIS
Centro Veterinario de Mínima Invasión Canarias, Las Palmas de Gran Canaria, Spain

Flavia Catanzaro, DVM
AniCura Policlinico Veterinario Roma Sud S.r.l., Rome, Italy

Leonardo Cavaliere, DVM, PhD
AniCura Clinica Veterinaria CMV Varese, Varese, Italy

Christopher J. Chamness, DVM
Karl Storz SE & Co. KG, Tuttlingen, Germany

Alexander Chernov, DM, DVM, PhD
Veterinary Clinic Endovet, VESK, Kurgan, Russia

Filippo Cinti, DVM, PhD, GPCert (SASTS), DECVS, MRCVS
Clinica Veterinaria San Marco, Veggiano, Italy

Fabien Collard, DVM, DECVS
Freelance surgeon, Rousson, France

William Culp, VMD, DACVS
School of Veterinary Medicine, University of California, Davis, CA, USA

Boris Dalpozzo, DVM, PhD
Clinica Veterinaria dell'Orologio, Sasso Marconi, Bologna, Italy

Bastien Dekerle, DVM, DECVS
AzurVeT, Saint-Laurent-du-Var, France

Giulia Dolce, DVM, MSc
AniCura Policlinico Veterinario Roma Sud S.r.l., Rome, Italy

David Durán-Rey, DVM, MSc, PhD
Centro de Cirugía de Mínima Invasión Jesús Usón, Cáceres, Spain

Stanisław Dzimira, DVM, PhD
Faculty of Veterinary Medicine, Department of Pathology, Wroclaw University of Environmental and Life Sciences, Wroclaw, Poland

Giacomo Federici, DVM
Clinica Veterinaria Ponente, Genoa, Italy

Luca Formaggini, DVM, MRCVS, GPcert SASTS
Clinica Veterinaria Lago Maggiore, Dormelletto, Italy

Boel A. Fransson, DVM, PhD, DACVS, ACVS Founding Fellow MIS
College of Veterinary Medicine, Washington State University, Pullman, WA, USA

Lynetta J. Freeman, DVM, MS, MBA
College of Veterinary Medicine, Purdue University, West Lafayette, IN, USA

Justin Ganjei, DVM, DACVS-SA
Veterinary Referral Associates, Vienna, VA, USA

David García Rubio, DVM, VEaMIS, Acre. AVEPA Tej. Blandos
Hospital Veterinario AniCura San Fermín, Pamplona, Spain

Roberto Giaconella, DVM
Clinica Veterinaria Giaconella, Rome, Italy

Veronica Giaconella, DVM
Clinica Veterinaria Giaconella, Rome, Italy

Erin Gibson, DVM, DACVS
School of Veterinary Medicine, University of California, Davis, CA, USA

Manuel Ramón González Portillo, DVM
Centro de Cirugía de Mínima Invasión Jesús Usón, Cáceres, Spain

Jorge Gutiérrez del Sol, DVM, MSc
VETMI, Cirugía Veterinaria de Mínima Invasión, Cáceres, Spain

Hiroo Kanai, DVM, PhD
Kanai Veterinary Surgery, Himeji, Japan

Constantin Vasile Ifteme, DVM
Veterinary Hospital for Endoscopy and Minimally Invasive Surgery, Vet Endoscopy Training Center, Bucharest, Romania

Ikuya Ehara, DVM
St. Luke's Animal Medical Center, Toyonaka, Osaka, Japan

Francesca Izzo, DVM, MSc, GPCert (SAS)
AniCura Clinica Veterinaria Apuana, Carrara, Italy

Ivan Jevtic, DVM
IVAVET Veterinary Clinic, Belgrade, Serbia

Łukasz Juźwiak, DVM, PhD
Faculty of Veterinary Medicine, Department and Clinic of Surgery, Wroclaw University of Environmental and Life Sciences, Wroclaw, Poland

Zdzisław Kiełbowicz, DVM, PhD
Faculty of Veterinary Medicine, Department and Clinic of Surgery, Wroclaw University of Environmental and Life Sciences, Wroclaw, Poland

J. Kirpensteijn, DVM, PhD, DACVS, DECVS
Hill's Pet Nutrition, Topeka, KS, USA

Kumiko Ishigaki, DVM, PhD
Laboratory of Veterinary Surgery, Department of Veterinary Medicine, College of Bioresource Sciences, Nihon University, Fujisawa, Kanagawa, Japan

P. A. Kuznetsov, DVM
Veterinary clinic Medvet, Moscow, Russian Federation

Luca Lacitignola, DVM, PhD
Dipartimento di Medicina di Precisione e Rigenerativa (DiMePRe-j), Università degli Studi di Bari Aldo Moro, Bari, Italy

Stéphane Libermann, DVM, DESV
Centre Hospitalier Vétérinaire des Cordeliers, Meaux, France

Felipe Lillo-Araya, DVM, DICM, PhD
School of Veterinary Medicine, Faculty of Life Sciences, Andrés Bello University, Viña del Mar, Chile

Bartłomiej Liszka, DVM, PhD
Faculty of Veterinary Medicine, Department and Clinic of Surgery, Wroclaw University of Environmental and Life Sciences, Wroclaw, Poland

Isabel López-Agudelo, DVM
Centro de Cirugía de Mínima Invasión Jesús Usón, Cáceres, Spain

Marco Augusto Machado Silva, DVM
Department of Veterinary Medicine, School of Veterinary and Zootechnics, Federal University of Goiás, Goiânia, Goiás State, Brazil

Alessandra Malavasi, DVM, MSc
Freelance anesthetist, Chiavari, Italy

Mathieu Manassero, DVM, MSc, PhD, DECVS
École Nationale Vétérinaire d'Alfort, Maisons-Alfort, France

Francisco Martínez Gomariz, DVM, PhD, VEaMIS
Faculty of Veterinary Medicine, University of Murcia, Murcia, Spain

Philipp D. Mayhew, BVM&S, MRCVS, DACVS
School of Veterinary Medicine, University of California, Davis, CA, USA

Ming Ju Huang, DVM, MS
Mercy Animal Medical Center, Kaohsiung, Taiwan

Francesca Molinari, DVM
Galeavet, Genoa, Italy

Eric Monnet, DVM, PhD, DACVS, DECVS
Department of Small Animal General Surgery, Colorado State University, Fort Collins, CO, USA

Motoki Kondo, DVM, PhD
Small Animal Endoscopic Surgery Center, Apple Tree Animal Hospital, Aichi, Japan

S. A. van Nimwegen, DVM, PhD, DECVS
Faculty of Veterinary Medicine, Utrecht University, Utrecht, the Netherlands

P. V. Osichkin, DVM
Department of RUDN ATI Veterinary Medicine, RUDN University, Moscow, Russian Federation

Robson Pasquale, DVM, MSc
Oncovet, Centro de Tratamento do Câncer em Animais, Curitiba, Brazil

Dariusz Patkowski, MD, PhD
Pediatric Surgery and Urology Department, Wroclaw Medical University, Wroclaw, Poland

Francisco. J. Pérez Duarte, DVM, PhD
VETMI, Cirugía Veterinaria de Mínima Invasión, Cáceres, Spain

Edoardo Poggi, DVM, GPCert (SASTS), PGCert VEaMIS
AniCura Clinica Veterinaria Apuana, Carrara, Italy

Przemysław Prządka, DVM, PhD
Faculty of Veterinary Medicine, Department and Clinic of Surgery, Wroclaw University of Environmental and Life Science, Wroclaw, Poland

Jeffrey J. Runge, DVM, DACVS, ACVS Founding Fellow MIS
Guardian Veterinary Specialists, Brewster, NY, USA

C. Sanchez, DVM
Veterinary Medical Center Oregon Zoo, Portland, OR, USA

Miguel Ángel Sánchez Hurtado, DVM, PhD
VETMI, Cirugía Veterinaria de Mínima Invasión, Cáceres, Spain

Francisco Miguel Sánchez-Margallo, DVM, PhD
Centro de Cirugía de Mínima Invasión Jesús Usón, Cáceres, Spain

Valery F. Scharf, DVM, MS, DACVS
College of Veterinary Medicine, North Carolina State University, Raleigh, NC, USA

Ameet Singh, DVM, DVSc, DACVS-SA
Ontario Veterinary College, University of Guelph, Guelph, Canada

Enrico Sponza, DVM, MSc Onc
Oncology Galeavet S.r.l, Genoa, Italy

Jung-Hsien Sun, DVM
Veterinarians facility, Fresno, CA, USA

Christopher B. Thomson, DVM, DACVS-SA
Veterinary Specialty Hospital – North County, San Marcos, CA, USA

Beau B. Toskich, MD
Mayo Clinic, Jacksonville, FL, USA

Joanna Tunikowska, DVM, PhD
Faculty of Veterinary Medicine, Department and Clinic of Surgery, Wroclaw University of Environmental and Life Sciences, Wroclaw, Poland

David Twedt, DVM, DACVIM
Small Animal Internal Medicine, Colorado State University, Fort Collins, CO, USA

Maurício Veloso Brun, DVM, MSc, PhD, Post-PhD
Department of Small Animal Clinical Sciences, Universidade Federal de Santa Maria, Santa Maria, Brazil

Samuele Venuta, DVM
Freelance anesthetist, Genoa, Italy

Emanuela Vitali, DVM
Clinica Veterinaria Giaconella, Rome, Italy

L. R. Wang, DVM, MS
Mercy Animal Medical Center, Kaohsiung, Taiwan

Yi Fu Chang
Mercy Animal Medical Center, Kaohsiung, Taiwan

FOREWORD

The beginnings of veterinary minimally invasive surgery dates back almost 50 years to my mentor Jerry Johnson. Jerry was an internist on staff at the Animal Medical Center, a large veterinary teaching hospital, in New York City. He and I would regularly visit the gastroenterology section of a large human hospital in New York to learn things we could take back and apply to our veterinary patients. We were able to watch a "new" laparoscopic diagnostic procedure used to collect liver biopsies and marveled at this groundbreaking technique. We felt this could be performed in our patients supplanting the need for abdominal surgery. Lacking funds at the time to purchase a human laparoscope we modified the procedure by using a rigid sigmoidoscope (a 20 mm diameter rigid tube with a light source); placing it through the abdominal wall and using room air for insufflation we were able to view the liver and direct a biopsy needle for sample collection. Likely these were the first true clinical diagnostic procedures performed in dogs. Several years later we were able to purchase an operating laparoscope, a cannula and biopsy forceps. Laparoscopy then became our primary means of abdominal organ biopsy, and we published results of 75 laparoscopic liver biopsies in 1977. In those early days, veterinary laparoscopy was primarily performed by internists, as surgeons preferred the traditional surgical approach. Fast forward ahead 10 years when human surgeons began performing routine laparoscopic cholecystectomies. Shortly thereafter that, the pendulum began to shift in veterinary laparoscopy from only a diagnostic tool to performing basic surgical procedures. In 1993 laparoscopic vasectomy was first described and in the early 2000s laparoscopic-assisted gastropexy and laparoscopic ovariectomy were reported. Thus began an exponential growth in minimally invasive surgery in veterinary medicine as surgeons and private practitioners alike began performing more and more laparoscopic and thoracoscopic procedures. The advantages of endoscopic surgery became obvious and surgical textbooks devoted sections to minimally invasive surgical techniques. Later, stand-alone minimally invasive surgery textbooks evolved.

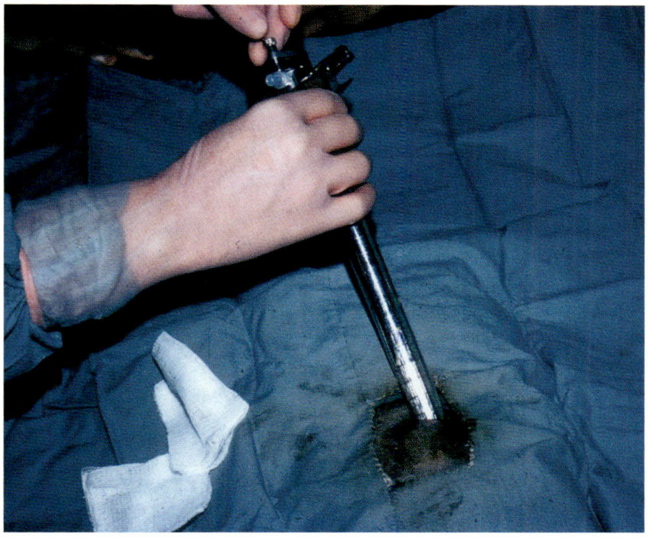

The first liver biopsies were obtained using a human sigmoidoscope that was placed through the abdominal wall by a small surgical incision to view the liver and direct a biopsy needle to collect tissue.

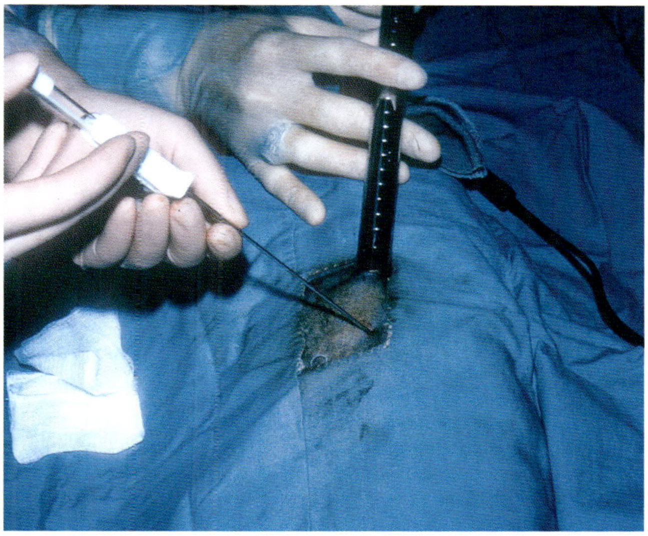

A human 10 mm operating laparoscope was used to view the liver and by passing a cup-type biopsy forceps through the laparoscope channel liver tissue was collected.

One becomes competent in minimally invasive surgery through knowledge and experience. Experience occurs by learning basic surgical principles and by practicing them as much as possible. Knowledge comes from textbooks such as the one in front of you. It is my pleasure to introduce the text *Laparoscopy and Thoracoscopy in the dog and cat*. This textbook is both unique and quite different from other books in veterinary minimal invasive surgery. It hosts an impressive list of authors from around the world having a wealth of endoscopic experience. Each chapter includes a detailed description of a surgical procedure with illustrations showing operating room layout and portal placement, a list of instruments required for the procedure and a guide to postoperative management. Each chapter also includes a table that reviews key takeaway points. The book also contains a large number of high-quality pictures and many video clips that demonstrate important aspects of the various procedures. Most chapters also include a series of clinical cases in which the minimally invasive procedure was performed. Some of the cases include new techniques performed by the authors but have yet to be described in the literature. This is not a textbook that should sit in your library, but rather it should be placed next to the surgery suite for quick consultation by you and your assistants prior to a procedure. This book captures the current state of the art of veterinary minimally invasive surgery and includes all known procedures currently performed. This book is a must for both the practitioner and the specialist.

I personally enjoyed reading many of the chapters and came away with a slight smile on my face. The smile is from how far we have come in the technology, the procedures we perform and advancements we have made for our clinical patients. I look forward to seeing where we will go in the future. Enjoy the book.

David C. Twedt, DVM, DACVIM
Professor Emeritus
Colorado State University
Fort Collins, CO, USA

INTRODUCTION

The large-scale introduction of minimally invasive laparoscopic and thoracoscopic surgery in human medicine dates back to the early 1980s. With the development of miniaturized cameras and increasingly technologically advanced endoscopic instruments, the advantages and the potential of this branch of surgery became immediately clear to everyone. This procedure started to expand so quickly that nowadays it has become the preferred technique for many surgical procedures.

Since then, it has not been long before laparoscopy and thoracoscopy started to be employed also in veterinary medicine, especially in dogs, cats, and horses. These techniques are now widely used worldwide and appreciated by pet owners themselves, who recognize their undoubted advantages in terms of reduced invasiveness and faster postoperative recovery.

This book was born from the authors' idea to produce a comprehensive, up-to-date, practical text which could be used even just before entering the operating room. The result is a text that describes in detail the minimally invasive surgical procedures currently recognized in dogs and cats and includes the experience of many colleagues worldwide, who suggest original procedures not yet described in the literature.

Our aim was to produce a reference text that could be of valuable help to both the neophyte, the new graduate whose future is in their own hands, and the experienced surgeon.

This volume consists of specific chapters, written with the support of internationally renowned coauthors, which describe in detail every single step of laparoscopic and thoracoscopic surgical procedures. Some chapters are enriched by clinical cases authored by eminent colleagues from all over the world who shared their personal experience and insights with the aim of helping surgeons facing difficult cases. The text is accompanied by illustrations showing the precise layout of the operating room and the arrangement of portals for each procedure, and by endoscopic images and videos.

A special thanks goes to our colleagues who collaborated in the volume. Without their passion for this subject, and without their commitment to this project, this book would not have been possible.

We would also like to thank our beloved pets, and therefore their families, for literally putting a part of their hearts in our hands.

A word of thanks also goes to Edra for believing in our project and for following us and supporting our vision until publication.

Lastly, special praise to the readers for placing your trust in our work. We wish this book lives up to your expectations.

Andrea M. Pievaroli
Roberto Properzi
J. Brad Case
Francesco Collivignarelli

TABLE OF CONTENTS

Section III. THORACOSCOPY 533

Endoscopic ports

T1, port for telescope
T2, port for right hand
T3, port for left hand

Section I

GENERAL PRINCIPLES

LEARNING FROM THE PAST

Everything in surgery is complicated until one learns to do it well, then it is easy.

R. E. Condon

1 HISTORY OF VETERINARY MINIMALLY INVASIVE SURGERY

Lynetta J. Freeman

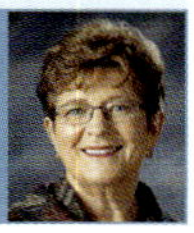

The evolution of minimally invasive surgery (MIS) in animals has followed its counterpart in the human field. Although internists and researchers were the first to utilize laparoscopy in animals, Dr. Tim McCarthy, a veterinary surgeon in private practice, began using flexible and rigid laparoscopy in clinical patients in the early 1980s, started to perform arthroscopy in 1983, and published on application of thoracoscopy in 1990. In the author's opinion, the modern techniques in veterinary MIS developed because animal studies were initially conducted to explore, develop, and validate devices and procedures for application in human surgery. Animals were also used to educate surgeons to perform procedures using new instrumentation. New devices became available and were utilized, and the skills and techniques in human surgery were then learned and applied to performing MIS in animals.

In 1981, Dr. David Twedt demonstrated laparoscopy and laparoscopic liver biopsy in dogs at Colorado State University. During the author's residency at Washington State University, (1984–1987), Dr. Myron Person, a pioneer in canine shoulder and stifle arthroscopy, was performing early procedures. These two individuals built the foundation for the author in MIS. After joining Ethicon in 1989, she spent the next 15 years performing research on surgical pharmaceuticals, suture materials, stapling equipment, and products for MIS in people. This chapter will explore behind the scenes at Ethicon and Ethicon Endo-Surgery in the 1990s and discuss the subsequent impact on MIS in animals.

The technological stage for laparoscopy was set by the French gynecologist Raoul Palmer, in the 1940s and 1950s, and was further developed by the German gynecologist and instrument maker Kurt Semm from the 1960s through the 1980s. In 1966, the medical equipment maker Karl Storz released a laparoscope that integrated a new fiber optic technology for better illumination of the visual field. By the 1980s, laparoscopy was mostly being performed by gynecologists. In 1983, Semm began performing laparoscopic appendectomies, and in 1986, the German surgeon Erich Muhe reported using a 3 mm scope to laparoscopically remove a patient's gallbladder. Rather than accolades, both Semm and Muhe were criticized and censored by their skeptic peers. In 1987, the French surgeon Phillipe Mouret performed the first laparoscopic gallbladder removal but did not promote it further. Two US surgeons, J. Barry McKernan and William B. Saye, attended a lecture by Semm on his experience in performing laparoscopic appendectomy and thought "why not a cholecystectomy?" Unaware of the previous work by Mouret, they pioneered laparoscopic appendectomy by general surgeons in May 1988. Then in June 1988, they performed their first human laparoscopic cholecystectomy with no complications, swift recovery, and minimal scarring. Dr. Eddie J. Reddick and Dr. Douglas O. Olson and their colleagues in Nashville, Tennessee, performed five laparoscopic cholecystectomy procedures and then began widespread promotion of laser-assisted laparoscopic cholecystectomy.

Against this backdrop, interest in MIS was propelled by the introduction of laparoscopic cholecystectomy at the 1989 American College of Surgeons meeting. At that meeting, the United States Surgical Corporation (USSC) introduced a laparoscopic clip applier and Karl Storz demonstrated video equipment that vastly enhanced the efficiency of laparoscopic surgery. Videos of the procedure fueled interest among general surgeons and equipment manufacturers. Following this, the Wall Street Journal and the New York Times published articles that attracted national media attention, causing patients to demand the less invasive surgery. In the following 3 years, laparoscopic cholecystectomy became the gold standard and over 80% of US cholecystectomy procedures were being performed laparoscopically. Instrument manufacturers developed video systems, automatic insufflators, scopes, disposable trocars, clip appliers, staplers, and handheld instruments to enable the procedures to be performed. Although the new ways of performing existing procedures were met with skepticism, even the conservative academic centers started to embrace the technology, and laparoscopy expanded to other procedure areas such as hernia repair, colectomy, gastroesophageal reflux disease, urology, hysterectomy, and video-assisted thoracic surgery. Over the next few years, virtually every abdominal operation was performed and perfected by laparoscopic technique including splenectomy, adrenalectomy, Roux-en-Y gastric bypass, pancreaticoduodenectomy, radical prostatectomy, and aortofemoral bypass, and surgeons started to perform thoracic procedures with video-assisted techniques. The lack of training in MIS among thoracic and general surgeons, urologists, and cardiologists was overcome by educational courses offered by instrument makers. These courses included live laboratories on pigs, and many were held at veterinary schools and research labs, spreading interest and knowledge of MIS to the veterinary community.

BEAGLE OVARIOHYSTERECTOMY MODEL

Disposable trocars and pretied sutures were the first products developed by engineers and scientists at Ethicon. Intracorporeal and extracorporeal knot tying was being used for laparoscopic tubal ligation and early appendectomy procedures. The first products were chromic gut sutures attached to a straight needle with a plastic push rod. Using them required the surgeon to tie an external Roeder knot and use the rod to push it to the application site. Beginning in 1989, the proprietary polymers Vicryl (polyglactin 910) and PDS (polydioxanone) were used by Ethicon to make pretied suture loops. To evaluate these new knots and ensure their security in tissue, the author and her colleagues developed a technique for performing laparoscopic ovariohysterectomy in Beagle dogs. At that time, there were few automatic insufflators, rudimentary video systems, a limited number of reusable trocars, and only basic instruments such as reusable grasping forceps and scissors. Through much trial, they learned to place five trocars, introduce a pretied suture loop, pass grasping forceps through the loop and grasp the ovarian pedicle. They placed a second grasping forceps on the distal pedicle, transected with scissors between the two forceps, and tightened the loop over the proximal ovarian pedicle. The process was repeated to place another loop on the distal pedicle and uterine body, before cutting and removing the uterus through one of the port sites. The first procedures took more than 2 hours and subcutaneous emphysema was a common complication. With practice, the procedure time was reduced, and monitoring of abdominal insufflation was improved so that subcutaneous emphysema was less prevalent. The author and her colleagues went on to evaluate PDS and Vicryl pretied loop ligatures in the model. This Beagle ovariohysterectomy was presented as a poster session, using a VHS tape to demonstrate the procedure, at the 1991 ACVS meeting in San Francisco. Veterinarians would comment "why in the world would anyone want to do that? I can spay a dog in half an hour!" The results of our study were never published because the procedure was considered too difficult for the general practitioner and, at that time, the equipment was not readily available to veterinarians. Despite this, and the skepticism towards clinical application, the team persisted!

OPEN APPROACH TO THE ABDOMEN

Rather than using a Veress needle for access, the open approach to the abdomen, developed by Dr. Harrith Hasson in 1971, was taught to the author's team by Dr. McKernan. He believed the open approach was safer than using a Veress needle for initial insufflation. Because they had seen splenic trauma from using a Veress needle in the dog, they quickly adopted the Hasson approach.

TROCAR AND CLIP APPLIER TESTING

In the early days, reusable stainless steel trocars with very sharp tips were available, but considered not ideal, so trocars with safety shields were developed to make it safer to enter the abdominal cavity. The dog's abdominal wall is much thinner than the human abdominal wall, so pigs became the animal model for trocar development and testing, for teaching laparoscopic cholecystectomy, and developing most other procedures. Dr. Lucy Senter conducted the early studies of trocars. Dr. Ron Kolata, over his 30-plus-year career with Johnson & Johnson, became a world authority in the design and development of trocars (**Fig. 1**). Early challenges included developing gaskets that would not tear or dislodge, utilizing reducing caps to allow 5 and 10 mm instrument exchanges, developing various safety shield mechanisms, and developing means to secure the trocar sleeve in the body wall. Dr. Kolata assisted in the design and testing of numerous improvements to trocars and holds several patents for medical device development. Ultimately, one of his

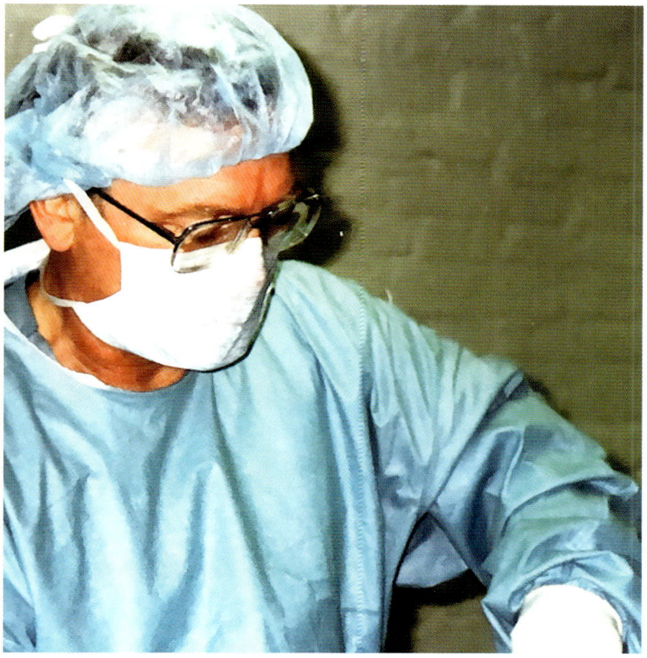

FIGURE 1. Dr. Ron Kolata is preparing to perform laparoscopic ovariohysterectomy on a lion at the Audubon Zoo in New Orleans.

most significant contributions was the optical trocar that allowed visualized entry into the abdominal cavity using a laparoscope inserted through the trocar.

Clip appliers were essential for ligation of the cystic duct and artery in human laparoscopic cholecystectomy. The earliest clip appliers were reusable and involved applying one clip at a time to the operative site. Some of the challenges were to develop a clip applier that could be inserted through a 10 mm trocar without tearing the trocar gasket and deliver the clip to the site without dropping it out of the applier. The author spent many hours testing various clips and appliers, and the engineers ultimately developed a clip applier that could fire multiple clips without removing the device to be reloaded.

EXPANSION OF PRECLINICAL RESEARCH AND DEVELOPMENT

In 1991, about 35 engineers, marketing, and the preclinical veterinarians from Somerville, New Jersey, relocated to Cincinnati and joined with the mechanical stapling company. Plans were made to build an institute for research and training that included a 20-table teaching lab and a vivarium to house pigs used in educational courses. While the building was being constructed, this group leased space in the basement of a hospital, where they continued to work in developing and testing disposable laparoscopic instruments. The group was led by Dr. Doug Sheffield and Dr. David Stoloff. Dr. Suzanne Thompson, Dr. Ron Kolata, Dr. Laura Gallagher, Dr. Ray Rudd, and later, Dr. Mike Clem and Dr. Jill Sackman, all ACVS diplomates or residency-trained veterinary surgeons, were hired to conduct preclinical research and development for both open and minimally invasive surgery. Each of them, including the author, with their knowledge of anatomy, physiology, and surgery, became a specialist in a procedure area and worked with engineers and thought leaders throughout the world to develop the devices and procedures that were being used in human surgery (**Fig. 2**).

Dr. Laura Gallagher performed studies with cryptorchid dogs to evaluate the Endobag specimen retrieval bags for safe removal of tissue without dropping it into the abdomen or contaminating the body wall. Her work was presented as an abstract at the ACVS meeting in 1992. Dr. Gallagher made significant contributions in the area of video-assisted thoracic surgical procedures. She worked with Dr. Rob McKenna and other thought leaders in human surgery to understand the special nuances of video-assisted thoracic surgery that included one-lung ventilation, trocar positioning for procedures, and techniques for performing a pericardial window, lung biopsy with Endoloops, thymectomy, and pleurodesis. She presented her technique for partial pericardiectomy in dogs at the 1992 ACVS meeting in Miami, Florida. Dr. Gallagher contributed to the development of numerous instruments for thoracic surgery including a rigid thoracic trocar with a solid obturator, a flexible trocar that could be cut to length, and the expandable obturator for intercostal insertion to protect the intercostal nerve, artery, and veins. Dr. Gallagher played a pivotal role in the development and refinement of the harmonic scalpel with all its nuances and end effectors. This device and its further enhancements became essential technology in precise dissection and tissue coagulation. Dr. Gallagher conducted studies to compare the ultrasonic technology to other modalities used for cutting and coagulation in many tissues, including its use for thyroidectomy and tonsillectomy.

Dr. Suzanne Thompson supported general surgery. She helped develop techniques for inguinal hernia repair, including the development of a staple applier used to secure mesh in the inguinal region. Using pigs with congenital inguinal hernia, Dr. Thompson evaluated and developed techniques for preperitoneal hernia repair using balloon dissectors to open the potential space between the peritoneum and internal rectus sheath.

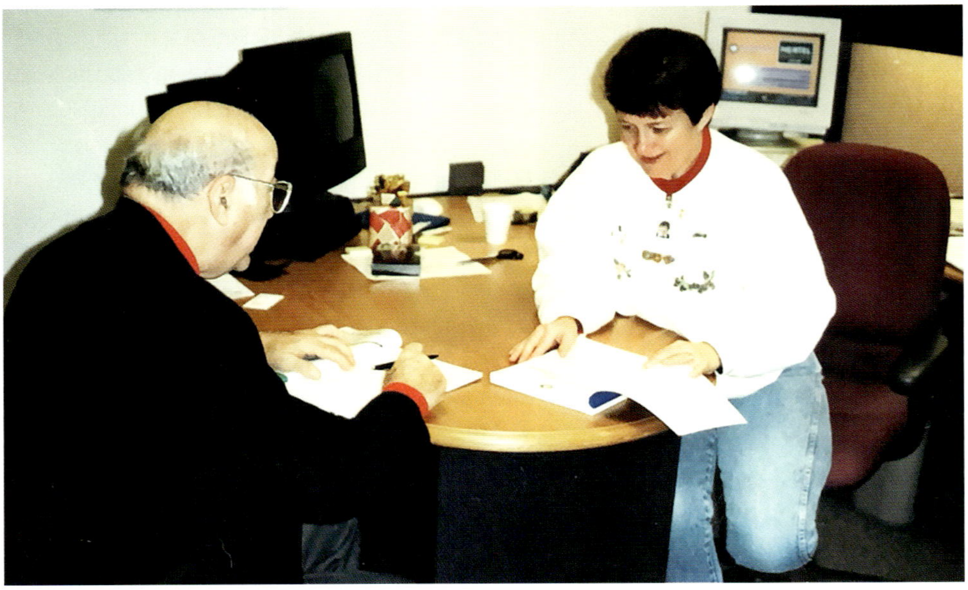

FIGURE 2. Dr. Jordan Phillips, past president of the American Association of Gynecologic Laparoscopists (AAGL), and Dr. Lynetta Freeman are discussing recent publications in surgery. In 1971, Dr. Phillips and ten charter members founded the AAGL. An early adopter of the laparoscopic surgical technique, Dr. Phillips was a visionary who imagined an infinite future for gynecologic surgery.

Dr. Thompson also participated in the development and testing of laparoscopic staplers. The initial metal stapler was 25 mm in diameter, delivered four rows of staples, and required a huge stainless steel trocar for insertion. Its design was based on an open stapler, and it required two hands to hold and fire the stapler. Over time, the diameter of the staplers was reduced, and the mechanisms were refined so that it placed six rows of staples and could be used with one hand. Dr. Thompson developed a technique for performing a stapled gastropexy in dogs that involved creating a tunnel in the submucosa and abdominal wall, inserting one fork of the stapler in each, firing the device to staple the stomach to the body wall, and closing the common opening with a hernia stapler. Her work was presented at the 1992 ACVS meeting. Having a device that could simultaneously join tissue and cut between the middle rows of staples greatly expanded the number and variety of procedures that could be performed. Laparoscopic intestinal resection and anastomosis in dogs was performed and reported at the 1992 ACVS meeting. Dr. Ray Rudd worked with human urologists to develop techniques for laparoscopic correction of vesicoureteral reflux. Dr. David Stoloff developed special expertise in laparoscopic suturing. He worked with surgeons in the human field including Dr. Zoltan Szabo, Dr. Alfred Cuchieri, and Dr. Howard Topel in developing a self-righting needle holder, various types of laparoscopic suture and needle combinations, and the techniques for performing and teaching intracorporeal and extracorporeal knot tying. The novel studies and significant contributions of each veterinarian are too numerous to list here.

EARLY KNOWLEDGE DISSEMINATION

The author and her colleagues were passionate about sharing knowledge with others. They invited veterinary thought leaders to participate with them in research projects. Dr. Clarence Rawlings (**Fig. 3**) visited their research facility several times to assist them in developing new techniques and to share his techniques for laparoscopic assisted surgery. From these visits, he and they developed a vision about what MIS could mean for veterinary medicine. Ethicon sponsored courses at the ACVS meetings in 1993 and 1995. Drs. Freeman, Thompson, Kolata, and Gallagher gave lectures and assisted in teaching live animal laboratories. Dr. Gallagher and Dr. Eric Monnet worked together on thoracoscopic techniques. The team collaborated with other veterinarians, such as Dr. Audrey Remedios and Dr James Ferguson at Western College of Veterinary Medicine, University of Saskatchewan, Dr Ralph Henderson at Auburn University, and others supporting MIS educational courses at other institutions to share knowledge and research ideas. Dr. Chris Chamness and his colleagues at Karl Storz Veterinary Endoscopy supported early courses by providing video systems at each workstation for the animal labs.

In 1999, Mosby published *Veterinary Endosurgery*, a textbook written mostly by the author and her colleagues with contributions from two large animal surgeons, Dr. Dean Hendrickson and Dr. Steven Trostle, and from Dr. Tim McCarthy and Dr. Robert Cook. This book was an introduction to veterinary

MIS and described techniques that they had performed in the research lab and the work of others performing surgery on animal models, but these procedures were not widely adopted in clinical patients until much later. The book did little to immediately advance the clinical experience, rather it laid a foundation for MIS in veterinary medicine.

EARLY CLINICAL APPLICATION

Pioneers such as Dr. David Twedt, Dr. Eric Monnet, Dr. Gilles Dupre, and Dr. Tim McCarthy continued to perform laparoscopy in small animals throughout this time. The next advance in veterinary MIS was made by Dr. Clarence Rawlings. He developed and reported on a series of laparoscopic-assisted procedures including prophylactic gastropexy (2001), cryptorchid castration (2004), cystoscopy (2003), cystopexy (2002), and feeding tube placement (2002). Dr. Rawlings was a gifted teacher and these techniques allowed procedures to be performed without advanced (expensive) devices and without the need for intracorporeal suturing. Laparoscopic-assisted techniques allowed a balance between the advantages of improved patient recovery with small incisions and the need for visualization and were readily embraced by veterinary surgeons and general practitioners. Dr. Philipp Mayhew, Dr. Jolle Kirpensteijn, Dr. MaryAnn Radlinsky and many others made important contributions to advancing clinical techniques.

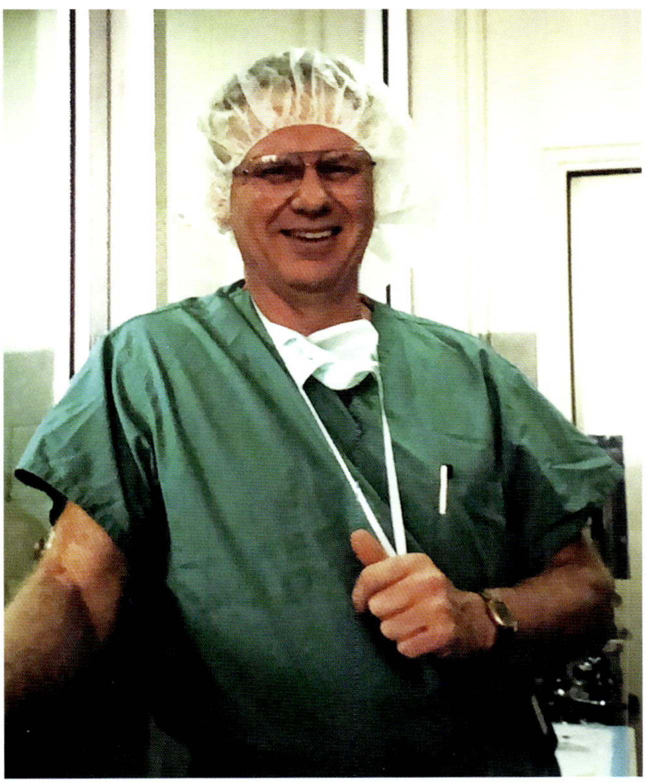

FIGURE 3. Dr. Clarence Rawlings, a pioneer in veterinary minimally invasive surgery.

VETERINARY ENDOSCOPY SOCIETY

To disseminate knowledge about MIS in veterinary medicine, Dr. Eric Monnet and Dr. Dave Twedt had the vision to form the Veterinary Endoscopy Society (VES) in 2003. Unlike other groups, the VES was a cross-functional group of individuals from large animal, orthopedics, internal medicine, research, surgery, academia, and private practice that shared a genuine passion for MIS. Bringing together veterinarians with a broad spectrum of experience has fostered innovation in adoption of new technology and refinement in techniques. Over the years, there has been a progression from single case reports or research studies to multicenter trials organized by members of the VES. Special editions of *Veterinary Surgery* focused on MIS have been published. Now, the VES is sponsoring research projects for residents in MIS. Two other notable contributions from the VES, driven by Dr. Monet, were the inclusion of MIS in residency training for surgery residents in 2009 and the formation of the ACVS Founding Fellow program in Minimally Invasive Surgery in 2017, which paved the way for postgraduate fellowship programs in MIS.

ADVANCES IN EDUCATION

Dr. Boel Fransson and her research group at Washington State University have driven the development of the training models to assess and validate laparoscopic training methods. The textbook *Small Animal Laparoscopy and Thoracoscopy*, authored by Dr. Boel Fransson and Dr. Philipp Mayhew, was published by Wiley Blackwell in 2015 and in 2022. Worldwide adoption of MIS is now occurring, and participation in the VES is global, with contribution from Central and South America, several European countries, Australia, Japan, and other Asian countries. Dr. Chris Chamness and his colleagues at Karl Storz Veterinary Endoscopy and Dr. John Huhn and his colleagues at the USSC and later Covidien (now Medtronic) were staunch supporters of MIS in animals, and they are largely responsible for supporting the global dissemination of these techniques. They provided support to the VES, and developed instruments at price points specifically for veterinarians, and have sponsored numerous courses to train veterinarians.

NATURAL ORIFICE TRANSLUMINAL ENDOSCOPIC SURGERY (NOTES)

In the 2000s, natural orifice surgery arose as a joining of interventional flexible endoscopy and surgery. Initially, flexible endoscopes were used to create a hole in the stomach to access the retroperitoneum to drain retroperitoneal pancreatic abscesses. Anthony Kalloo and the team from Johns Hopkins Hospital in Baltimore, Maryland, reported on the first NOTES procedures being performed in a survival study in pigs. Drs. Rao and Reddy from Hyderabad, India, reported on the first human transgastric NOTES appendectomy in 2002. In 2005, leaders in laparoscopy and gastrointestinal endoscopy met and formed the Natural Orifice Surgery Consortium for Assessment and Research (NOSCAR), a collaborative effort between the American Society for Gastrointestinal Endoscopy (ASGE) and the Society of American Gastrointestinal and Endoscopic Surgeons (SAGES). The group identified potential barriers to the development of NOTES and proposed the research and safety studies that had to be performed before clinical evaluation could occur.

In 2006, in collaboration with gastroenterologists at Indiana School of Medicine, the author received a NOSCAR research grant to study transgastric access to the abdominal cavity in dogs for performing an ovariectomy. Over the next several years, the author's group developed and refined techniques for transgastric surgery in dogs, mapped the learning curve, and demonstrated that these procedures could be performed under conscious sedation. They also performed NOTES gastropexy and conducted a clinical study in Collie dogs. Although the transgastric access was technically successful in dogs, it was tedious and did not translate to clinical practice because there was no good means to close the gastrotomy incision.

In 2007, the first report of transvaginal hybrid NOTES cholecystectomy was published. Transvaginal surgery was considered the best platform for NOTES, which allowed surgeons to use a standard rigid laparoscope to approach intra-abdominal organs in a way that more resembled standard laparoscopy. At Purdue University, Drs. Tim Lescun, Karin Pader, and the author developed a technique to perform transvaginal ovariectomy in mares and published the work in 2011. Transvaginal hybrid and totally transvaginal approaches to ovariectomy and ovariohysterectomy have been described and compared in dogs by Dr. Mauricio Brun in Brazil, and transvaginal ovariectomy has been performed in 66 dogs and reported in 2019 by Arntz.

SINGLE-INCISION LAPAROSCOPIC SURGERY

Single-incision laparoscopic surgery arose out of the desire to perform a simpler NOTES procedure. This technique provides the benefit of single access and improved visualization through a single incision and provides an avenue for large tissue removal. This technique has been adopted and used for numerous procedures including laparoscopic ovariectomy, gastropexy, and laparoscopic-assisted procedures in animals.

FUTURE OF MINIMALLY INVASIVE SURGERY IN ANIMALS

Although veterinary MIS followed human surgery initially, expansion is now underway into more complex procedures. Veterinary MIS is being used at an increasing number of general veterinary practices, and laparoscopic spays are routinely being performed. This book chapter has reflected on 30 years since the first laparoscopic ovariohysterectomies were performed. Progress in the field of MIS in veterinary medicine will assuredly continue far into the future.

SUGGESTED READINGS

2 LOW-IMPACT SURGERY
A 360° point of view on minimal invasiveness

Luca Formaggini

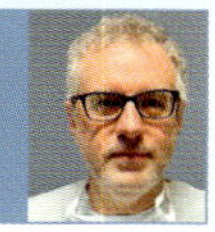

It is well established that any surgical procedure can lead, to a greater or lesser extent depending on the type and site of intervention, to a series of alterations in homeostasis, both inflammatory and neuroendocrine, which in turn influence the metabolic response of the patient in the postoperative period (**Fig. 1**). Therefore, we have to ask ourselves if modifying *only* the surgical technique and talking about minimally invasive "surgery" is sufficient to improve the quality of recovery, or if, with more farsightedness, it would be better to focus on a much broader concept of minimally invasive "therapy". This concept can become more obvious when the clinician realizes that the pattern of complications after surgery is always multimodal rather than unimodal (**Fig. 2**).

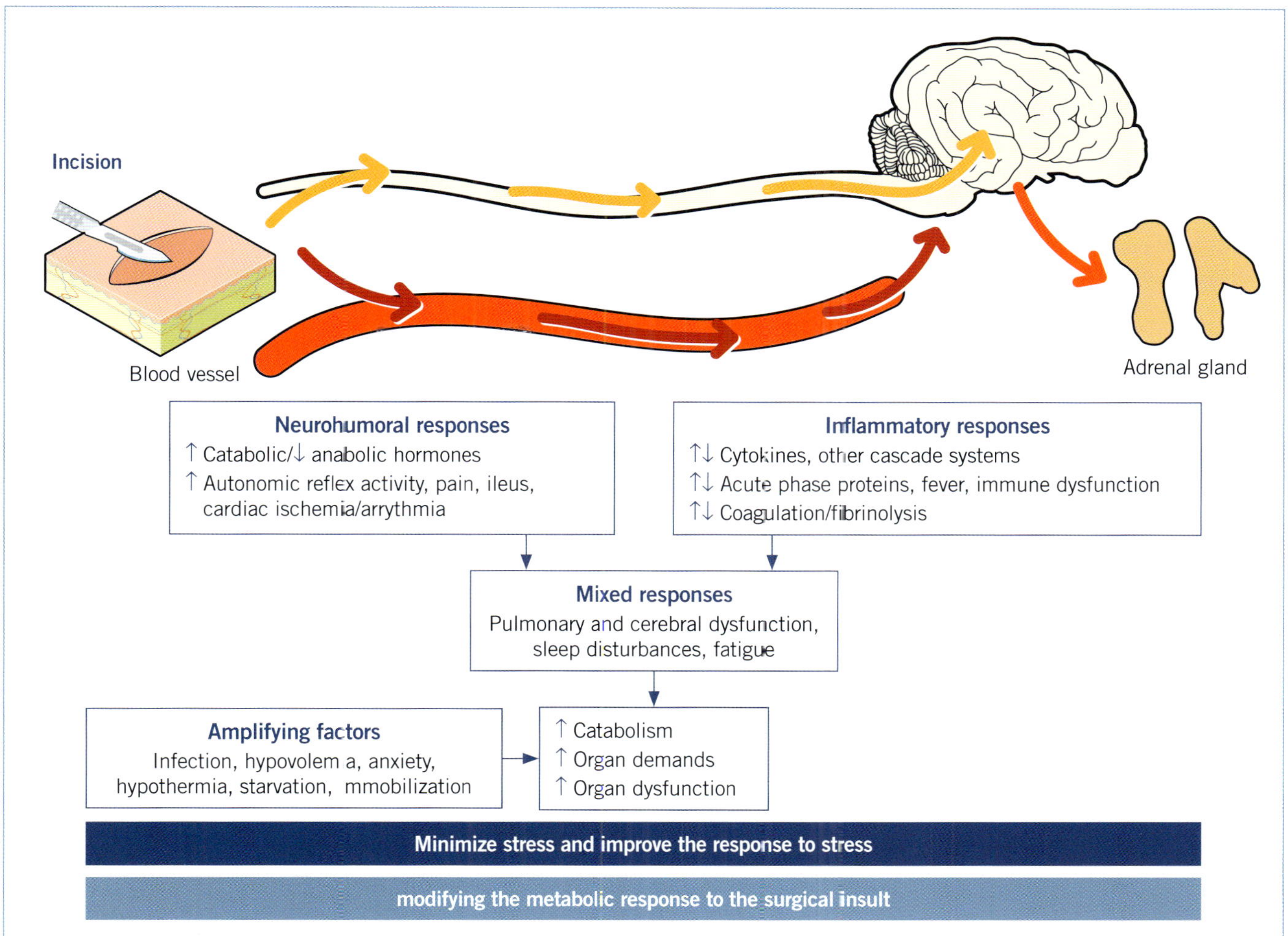

FIGURE 1. Mediators and modulators of the catabolic responses after an operation. Modified from H. Kehlet and D. W. Wilmore, Multimodal strategies to improve surgical outcome, *Am J Surg*, 2002.

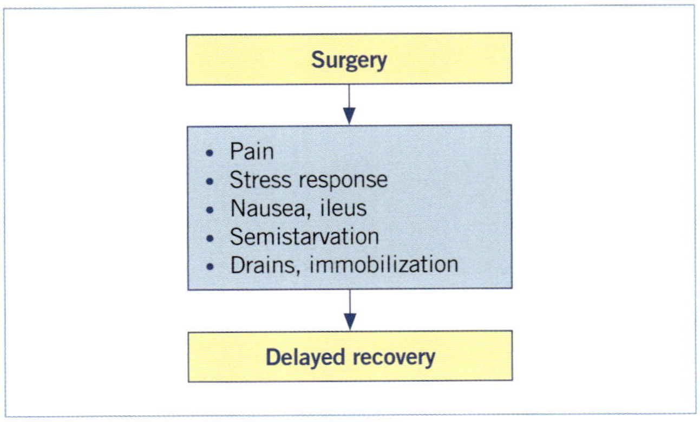

FIGURE 2. The multimodal nature of postoperative complications. Modified from D. W. Wilmore and H. Kehlet, Management of patients in fast track surgery, *BMJ*, 2001.

In this regard, the practice of fast-track surgery took hold in human medicine between the late 1990s and the early 2000s. Fast-track surgery is a protocol that provides an application of different techniques of management of patients that undergo elective surgery in order to promote the best recovery and their discharge in the shortest possible time. The term *fast-track surgery* was later changed to *enhanced (early) recovery after surgery* (ERAS), a name that better reflects the purpose for which all these care activities are implemented (quality of recovery rather than speed of discharge). The author prefers to use the term *low-impact surgery* (LIS), an expression that, in his opinion, better reflects the situation of veterinary surgery; our patients, due to a series of factors that are out of the scope of this book, have a tendency to early mobility and, often because of a lack of adequate hospitalization, to early discharge. However, this does not mean that the principles listed below can be contravened.

Among others, the main points on which LIS is based are:

- epidural or regional anesthesia
- minimally invasive surgical technique
- excellent pain control
- aggressive postoperative rehabilitation (early feeding and rapid mobilization).

The combination of these approaches improves the body's response to surgical stress and reduces organ dysfunction (**Fig. 3**).

In veterinary medicine there is still no evidence that the application of the LIS protocol has a real positive impact on postoperative care; however, its concepts are so logical as to make this road at least viable pending confirmation.

It is a common, and otherwise correct, concept to use the term *minimally invasive surgery* as a synonym for laparoscopic and thoracoscopic procedures; therefore, it seems consequential to apply these techniques as the first choice in case of surgical diseases and, in particular, within the LIS protocol. Although this is obviously true, their use can be limited by several factors, from the economic ones to those of the learning curve, which, for complex procedures, is quite long. Another limiting factor is the individual predisposition of the surgeon to switch to a technique that presupposes an excellent ability of hand–eye coordination and a habit of working in 2D instead of 3D.

However, there are other techniques and expedients that can make the surgery less impactful on the patient. In fact, within the surgical procedure itself, in addition to incision length and organ manipulation—which can determine ileus and postoperative inflammation and pain—we must also take into account other factors and ask ourselves whether an excessive duration of surgery and anesthesia is minimally invasive, just as prolonged fasting in the perioperative period and the excessive use of opiates, which can cause ileus and nausea, are certainly not.

The surgical techniques we know today can be grouped into different and broad categories, more specifically open surgery, laparo/thoracoscopic surgery, video-assisted surgery,

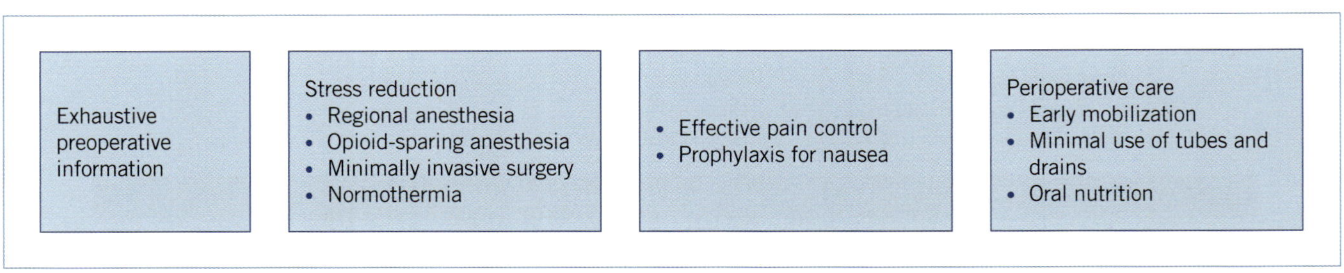

FIGURE 3. Example of minimal interventions for improvement in recovery quality. Modified from D. W. Wilmore and H. Kehlet, Management of patients in fast track surgery, *BMJ*, 2001.

hand-assisted surgery, and robotic surgery. Neglecting robotic surgery, not yet widespread in veterinary medicine, video-assisted surgery and hand-assisted surgery are surely less invasive than open surgery (smaller incisions) and more invasive than laparo/thoracoscopic surgery, but faster, probably with a shorter duration of anesthesia, and maintaining tactile sensation. However, it is possible to make open surgery less invasive by using, for example, radial atraumatic retractors to enlarge incisions (**Figs. 4 and 5**). This type of retractor maintains moisture at the incision site, allows visualization of the incision margins, allows for maximal exposure with a minimal incision size, and provides exposure without the trauma associated with prolonged point retraction. In some studies, they have been shown to reduce complications from surgical site infection and possibly even tumor seeding. These retractors have versatility (open and video-assisted surgery), facilitate specimen removal, have potential for hand-assisted surgery, and are cost effective.

This is only one of the factors on which it is possible to act to make surgery more tolerable. The gentleness in the manipulation of organs and tissues combined with an adequate management of the perioperative period could certainly further improve the quality of postoperative recovery even after open surgery.

To summarize, it would be better to emphasize the multimodal approach to the surgical patient and the need to adapt the therapy to the individual needs, the surgeon's skills, and the owner's budget, without losing sight of all the concepts of LIS. All this, as a consequence, promotes the fast recovery of the patient.

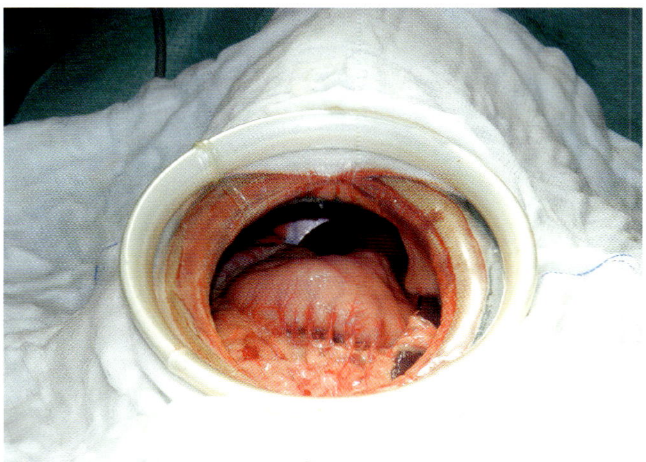

FIGURE 4. Use of a radial atraumatic wound retractor in open abdominal surgery.

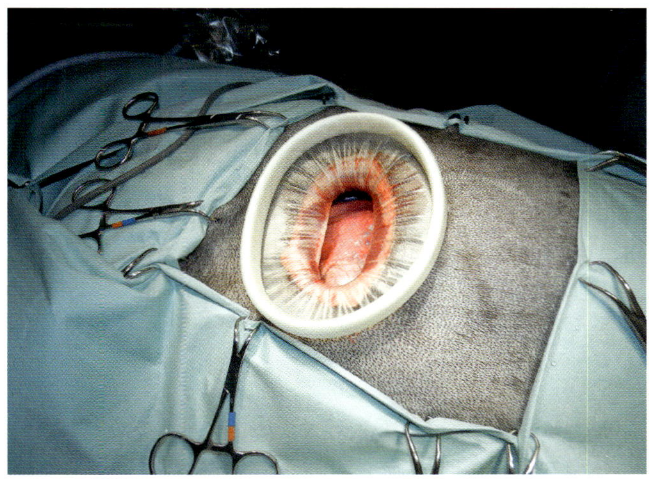

FIGURE 5. Use of a radial atraumatic wound retractor in open thoracic surgery.

SUGGESTED READINGS

3 EQUIPMENT FOR MINIMALLY INVASIVE SURGERY

Fausto Brandão, Christopher J. Chamness

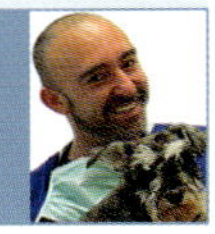

Minimally invasive procedures, especially laparoscopy and thoracoscopy, are now considered the gold standard approach for many surgical conditions. Over the last decade, the rapid dissemination of knowledge and the growing number of practitioners performing minimally invasive surgery (MIS) has led to the widespread introduction of the latest human medicine technologies into the veterinary field.

Most advanced imaging modalities, electrosurgical devices, instrumentation, and accessories are now routinely used in small animal minimally invasive procedures, combined with the trend to incorporate modern operating rooms.

This chapter is practical and aims to familiarize the veterinary surgeon with the latest technologies in small animal laparoscopic imaging systems, instrumentation, and accessory devices.

IMAGING SYSTEMS

Modern MIS operating rooms include a modular system, mostly set on a mobile cart (trolley) or ceiling booms. These systems correspond largely to full high-definition (HD) technologies (1980×1200 pixels), and recently to ultra-HD (UHD) or 4K. Regardless of the type of imaging system, they all include several standard components which are presented below.

Compact systems with full HD technologies are also available, but they are usually a better option for smaller or multidisciplinary operating rooms (**Fig. 1**).

LIGHT SOURCES

LED light sources are the standard technology currently recommended for MIS. The bulbs last up to 30,000 working hours and produce a very white light of around 6000 to 6400 kelvins. Proper LED illumination facilitates a natural coloration of tissues, with optimal brightness. Dedicated compact light sources are affordable and can be used with all types of rigid and some flexible endoscopes (**Fig. 2**). They lack air insufflation, necessary for other types of endoscopic procedures (e.g., gastrointestinal endoscopy). It is desirable to work at low power settings, since more light output does not necessarily lead to greater illumination due to the auto exposure feature of most cameras. Higher light output and brightness may lead to more reflection or "white-out" of the tissues. This overexposure of a portion of the image may result in a reduction in brightness of the rest of the image, thus

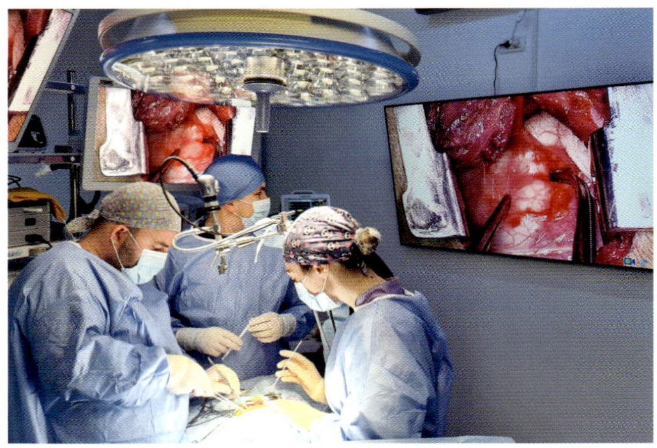

FIGURE 1. Modern small animal operating room with ceiling booms and a 4K imaging system (Rubina 4K, Karl Storz SE & Co. KG). Image courtesy of Dr. Constantine Ifteme, Bucharest, Romania.

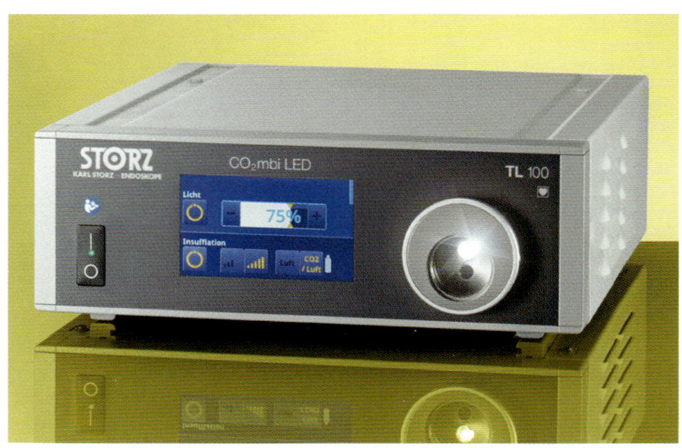

FIGURE 2. All-purpose LED light source CO_2mbi LED. Image courtesy of Karl Storz SE & Co. KG.

sometimes darkening the surgical background. To minimize this effect, some camera control unit (CCU) systems feature a digital enhancement mode (e.g., Clara, Image1 S, Karl Storz) to lighten the secondary surgical field. This results in optimal lighting balance for the primary and secondary surgical planes.

State-of-the-art light sources include various lighting modalities such as near-infrared (NIR) emission and fluorescence modalities (indocyanine green, ICG), or other customized filters. Most LED light sources are "silent" and produce minimal thermal heat. However, side or back panel grids are present in some units, which must be surrounded by enough clearance to allow air circulation for cooling.

LIGHT TRANSMITTING CABLES

Most laparoscopic and thoracoscopic procedures are performed under white light from regular LED light sources. The light cables have hundreds of fiber-optic bundles that transmit the light from the light source to the rigid scope attachment. Under special modalities such as fluorescence imaging, cables might contain special transmitting fluid. Standard recommendations for the light cables include an extended working length of 300 cm for better ergonomics, especially when working far away from the imaging system, such as in large-breed dogs, or when using specific table positions (e.g., Trendelenburg, Fowler). In small animal MIS, a 3.5 mm diameter light cable is recommended for scopes up to 6 mm. If 10 mm scopes are used, a 4.8 mm diameter light cable should be used.

Reprocessing of these components includes hygiene with appropriate enzymatic soap and disinfectants. Sterilization procedures might include high-level disinfectants, hydrogen peroxide, or autoclave sterilization. Sterile cover sleeves are often preferred since they do not stress the cables with excessive cleaning, while maintaining complete sterility. Light cables should be properly set in trays for sterilization and stored in a loosely coiled position to avoid fiber breakage.

After a long period of use, fibers degrade, thus reducing the ability to transmit light. Fiber integrity can be assessed by holding one end of the cable to a window or artificial light while looking at the other end for gray or black spots where light would normally be transmitted. If a light cable loses over 20% of its fibers, the practitioner should consider replacing it to ensure the surgical field receives enough illumination.

CAMERA CONTROL UNITS AND CAMERA HEADS

The CCU is considered the heart of the imaging system; this component defines the final quality of the image displayed. Full HD corresponds to 1980×1200 pixels, which is currently considered the standard in small animal MIS. Camera heads and CCUs should match and have the same technology level regardless of the system used. Complementary metal-oxide semiconductor (CMOS) is the current state-of-the-art imaging chip technology, and a single-chip camera is considered suitable for most common procedures, as it is now capable of producing HD images. Their affordability, lightweight body, and ergonomic design make these cameras the go-to choice for most practitioners (**Fig. 3**). Since they are not autoclavable, it is highly desirable to work with disposable cover sleeves

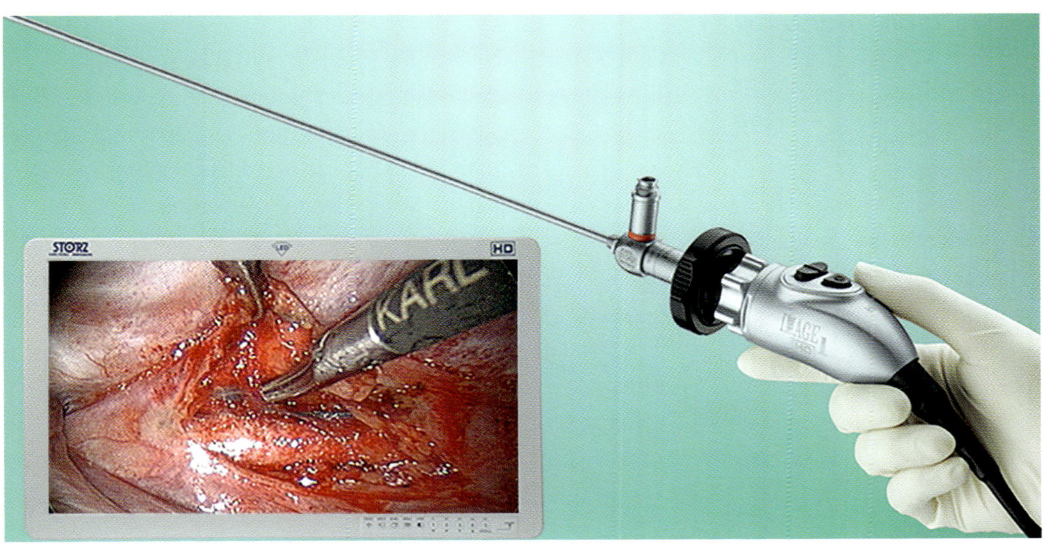

FIGURE 3. Single-chip CMOS full HD camera head HX. Image courtesy of Karl Storz SE & Co. KG.

to maintain optimal sterility throughout the procedure. Such sleeves also offer the advantage of reduced reprocessing time, by maintaining the absolute cleanliness of the components, and enable the cameras' ongoing use.

Modern veterinary camera heads are equipped with programmable buttons which can be set for the most common tasks such as white balance, image capture, video recording, and the activation of digital modes for image enhancement. When combined with an adequate CCU, this allows for image and video capture in full HD format during procedures. As a result, this sometimes eliminates the need for a dedicated image recording unit, which is recommended for publishing, training purposes, and surgical reports.

Fluorescence-guided surgical procedures have become more popular and establish a new option for several surgical interventions. Special camera heads and CCUs are required for fluorescence applications since they include filter settings which are capable of wavelength detection for special light emission.

NIR/ICG is the most commonly used fluorescence technology in small animal MIS. It might greatly improve tissue differentiation in procedures such as cholecystectomy, sentinel lymph node resection, liver lobectomy, abdominal and thoracic tumor assessment, thoracic duct ligation, and cisterna chyli ablation.

In some instances, this technology might be difficult to access due to cost as well as ICG dye availability and licensing. Fluorescence imaging modalities also include filters and digital enhancement that can guide surgeons through color mapping that correlates with fluorescence intensity (e.g., fluorescence intensity mapping, Rubina, Karl Storz). This increases the practitioner's perception of fluorescent dye differences in the tissues and vascularization, since subtle changes might not be detected with standard fluorescence blue light emission. The result is an increase in accuracy of the surgical approach and procedure.

INSUFFLATORS

Insufflators are an essential element of MIS equipment during laparoscopic surgery, allowing for the creation and maintenance of the working space through an automated process of carbon dioxide (CO_2) insufflation into the patient.

Medical CO_2 is supplied in a pressurized tank and delivered to the insufflation unit through a high-pressure hose. It is important to understand that modern insufflators include an internal pressure reducer device which enables the unit to be directly connected to the pressurized tank or pipe system.

A bacterial filter should be placed between the unit and the patient insufflation tube to prevent contamination from the gas tank to the patient or from the patient to the insufflator. This filter also protects the unit from being permanently damaged if any fluid is accidentally aspirated back into the insufflator.

For routine use in small animal laparoscopic and thoracoscopic surgery, 20 L/min is considered sufficient, although modern high-performance 40 or 50 L/min units provide additional gas warming, reducing the possibility of hypothermia when larger volumes of gas are consumed in complex procedures.

DOCUMENTATION UNITS

Dedicated recording units are of great use, since they can combine recording ability and data management of patients and provide integration with the imaging network. However, in practice, most modern full HD CCUs are provided with at least one USB connection that can be used as an external recording transfer platform for customers' ease. It should be considered that despite the CCU's built-in recording capability, file size compression might occur when data is transferred to a USB drive, thus affecting its original format. Documentation units are normally connected to the CCU by means of HDMI or DVI pin connecting cables, which allow the acquisition of surgical images and videos at optimal quality.

Integrated operating room software platforms might also enable the capture of other imaging modalities and the ability to combine those files with the patient's endoscopic data.

SURGICAL MONITORS

LED monitors are now the standard choice for surgery, thanks to their light weight and image performance. Moreover, their high resolution results in the display of true tissue colors. Large-format screens from 24″ to 50″ are considered optimal. Furthermore, depending on imaging technology, certain sizes might be necessary. For example, with 4K (UHD) monitors, a minimum size of 32″ is required, and no image degradation is observed even when displayed on a 50″ screen.

The current recommendation in MIS suites is to have at least two medical screens, 27″ and 32″, located in front of the main and assistant surgeons, respectively, resulting in better performance and ergonomics. Ideally, ceiling-mounted screens with a dedicated arm rack optimize logistics for every surgical procedure. Large-format screens, such as 32″ or more, are noticeably heavier, requiring sophisticated integrated ceiling systems that might be cost-prohibitive for a standard veterinary facility.

It is critical that medical-grade screens be used. Although newer LED TV screens or high-performance monitors are advertised to be of optimal quality, medical-grade monitors yield superior performance and image sharpness. These monitors are also licensed for every signal output required for surgical quality (common smart TV screens are not capable of reproducing all output signals). Although a significant difference in cost is inevitable, the ultimate result will pay off in the long term.

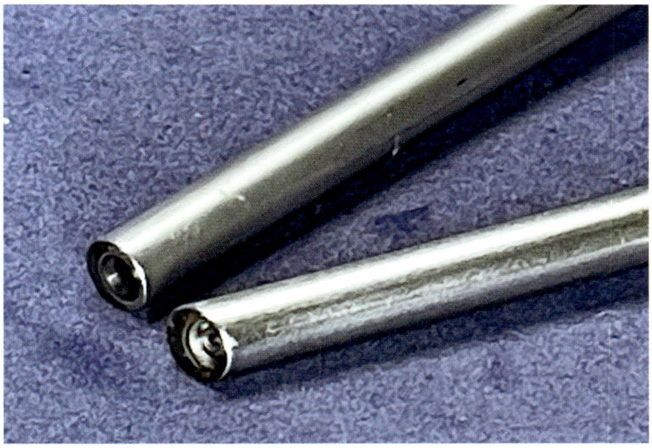

FIGURE 4. Rigid 5 mm telescopes: 0° (top) and 30° (bottom).

INSTRUMENTATION

Instruments for laparoscopy and thoracoscopy are highly diverse and range from miniature instruments (2.0–3.5 mm) to regular (5 mm) or larger and stronger instruments (10 mm). It is recommended that practitioners start with a standard 5 mm instrument set and gradually upgrade it as additional approaches and techniques are required. Regular miniature laparoscopic instruments, 3 mm in diameter, are optimal for feline patients and small/toy breed dogs, and this is considered the second most important set for a surgeon to acquire, after a regular 5 mm set.

RIGID SCOPES

The standard small animal laparoscope is 5 mm×29 cm×30°. The use of straight forward 0° rigid scopes is recommended for surgeons at the initial stages of surgical proficiency. However, for advanced surgical levels or procedures, they offer limited visibility when tighter spaces need to be accessed. It is advisable for an evolving surgeon to have both 0° and 30° laparoscopes (**Fig. 4**). On the one hand, a 0° laparoscope offers optimal visual access in specific approaches, such as the subxiphoidal transdiaphragmatic approach in thoracoscopy for animals in dorsal recumbency. In this case, a Ternamian threaded trocar is inserted at the cranial aspect of the abdomen and rotated clockwise in the cranial direction until the diaphragm is surpassed. This allows the procedure to be monitored with the scope inside the trocar until it reaches the inner surface of the thoracic cavity. On the other hand, a 30° laparoscope is generally preferred for visual inspection of the thoracic cavity, since less space is often present between the rib cage and the lung surface during regular two-lung ventilation.

Hopkins rigid telescopes provide a sharper, brighter, and more magnified image over standard-construction laparoscopes, since rod lenses are considered superior by far.

Variable-angle laparoscopes are also available in 4 and 10 mm versions. The latter can rotate from a 0° to a 120° retroflexed view. These scopes might present some advantages, especially when performing thorough examinations in the thorax, such as in pericardioscopy. However, since these scopes have been introduced just recently, their use is still limited, and few scientific publications in veterinary medicine offer clear evidence.

PALPATION PROBES, GRASPERS, AND DISSECTORS

This group of instruments represents the foundation of a laparoscopic surgical set, since they offer the ability to palpate, move, grasp, and hold tissue. Palpation probes consist of an atraumatic metal shaft often with 10 mm marks, so that the surgeon can measure the size of lesions or use them as references for distances inside the cavities. Most palpation probes are available in 3 and 5 mm diameters (**Fig. 5**). The 3 mm version is part of the miniature set, while the 5 mm one is the most used instrument for palpating lesions and performing small organic retractions.

The standard set should also include a minimum of four grasping instruments: a Maryland curved grasping and dissecting forceps, a 90° right-angled dissector, an atraumatic Babcock grasper, and a Mouret or Rothenberg bowel grasper (**Fig. 6**).

The Maryland grasper and dissector is mostly used for precise dissection, since its curved tip facilitates separation of fascial planes and careful dissection in delicate areas. The tip grasping capability offered by this instrument allows for delicate manipulation of smaller structures in perivascular areas.

The 90° right-angled forceps is particularly helpful when dissecting around ducts and vessels, since it allows the passage of the instrument tip behind the back plane of the structure. It is commonly used in combination with another dissector, such as the curved or straight Maryland dissector (**Fig. 7**).

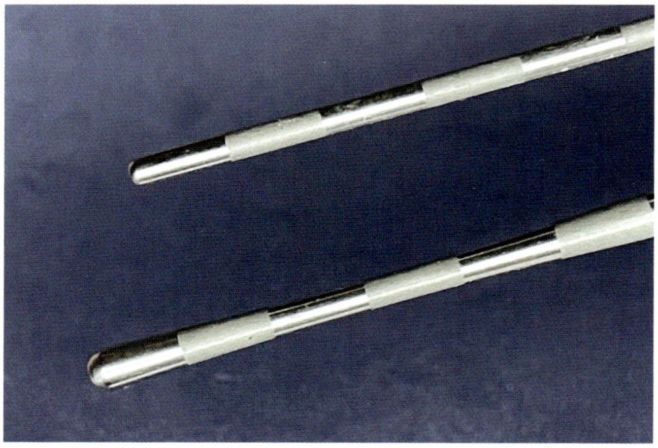

FIGURE 5. Detail of the atraumatic tips of a 3 mm (top) and a 5 mm (bottom) laparoscopic palpation probe.

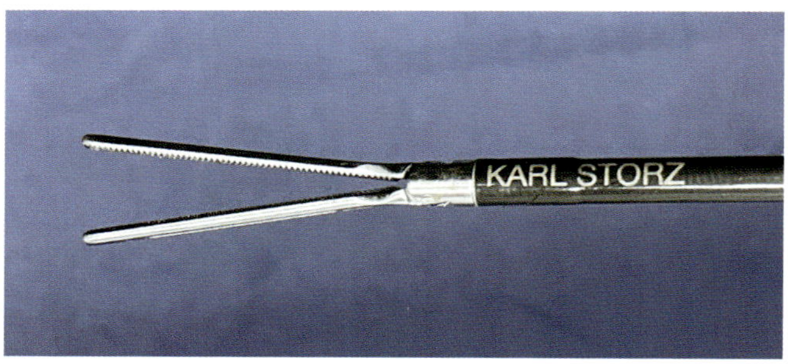

FIGURE 6. Rothenberg atraumatic grasper.

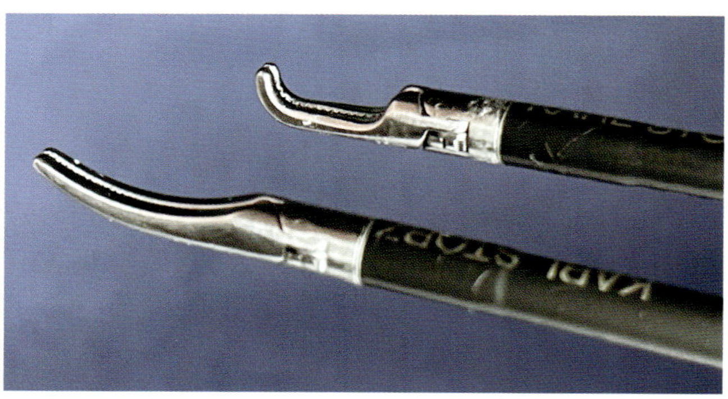

FIGURE 7. 90° right-angled dissector (top) and curved Maryland dissector (bottom).

Babcock graspers exist with sharp teeth or a serrated atraumatic tip. The most common is the serrated atraumatic due to its greater versatility. Atraumatic grasping and manipulation of the small intestine, colon, bladder, and other major structures can be safely performed with this instrument. However, the sharp-toothed Babcock grasper can yield specific advantages in some procedures, such as laparoscopic extraction of ovaries, testis, and other small portions of tissue that might require a strong and solid grasp when traversing the abdominal wall without the help of a low-friction wound retraction device.

Mouret, Rothenberg, or Croce-Olmi graspers are preferably used in parenchymatous organs that require very delicate and atraumatic handling. The common features of these instruments are a rounded and elongated working insert tip, combined with a smooth grooved surface that holds the tissue. The choice is based on the surgeon's preference or experience with a given procedure. For example, Croce-Olmi graspers are commonly used for grasping organs trapped within body wall hernias, while bowel or Mouret graspers are used for the intestines, lungs, and other organs.

SCISSORS

Laparoscopic scissors commonly used in MIS procedures include monopolar and bipolar connector pins, with several tip types, such as conical, micro scissors, Metzenbaum, hook scissors, and supercut. Most scissors include general features such as rotatable shafts and curved jaws.

BIOPSY FORCEPS

There are three main types of biopsy forceps: oval cups, spoons, and punches. In small animal laparoscopic and thoracoscopic procedures, two main types are routinely used:

- Oval cup biopsy forceps. It is mostly utilized in parenchymatous organs such as the liver, prostate, and spleen (**Fig. 8**).
- Punch biopsy forceps. Due to its jaw mechanism, it is most appropriate for performing biopsies in the peritoneal wall, pancreas, pleura, lymph nodes, and/or some mediastinal masses or structures.

It should be noted that the cutting edges might become dull over time and degrade the quality of harvested tissue samples, thus permanent maintenance and replacement when cutting becomes difficult are required.

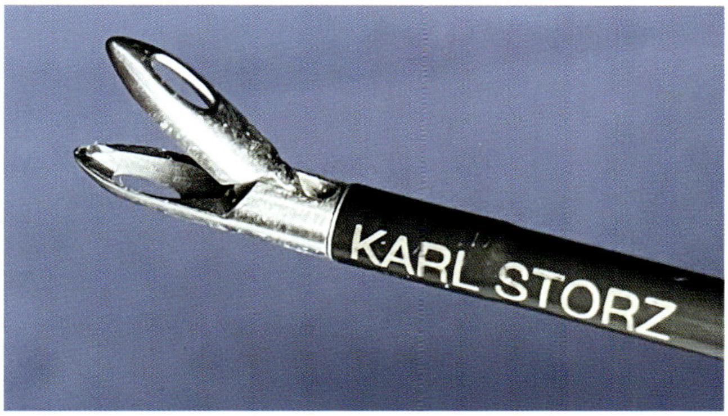

FIGURE 8. Oval cup biopsy forceps.

TISSUE SEPARATORS AND RETRACTORS

Organic retraction is useful in more complex surgeries, especially when working in surgical planes underneath other structures or when suspension becomes critical. There are three main types of retractors, and the selection depends on the surgery being performed. Cuschieri retractors consist of a main shaft that can be bent into a circular shape upon rotation of a knob in the instrument handle. These are the strongest retractors used in laparoscopy and might be especially useful, for example, when lifting a large part of the liver parenchyma. Fan retractors are the most popular amongst veterinary surgeons, but one must exercise caution when using them, since the tip of the fan blades might induce trauma if forced into tissues (**Fig. 9**). Some surgeons prefer rubber-coated fan retractors, which are obviously single-use instruments. However, if proper care is observed, they offer great versatility in both abdominal and thoracic MIS.

Single-blade retractors might also be of use; however, given their limited retraction capabilities, they are not considered a priority in standard instrument sets.

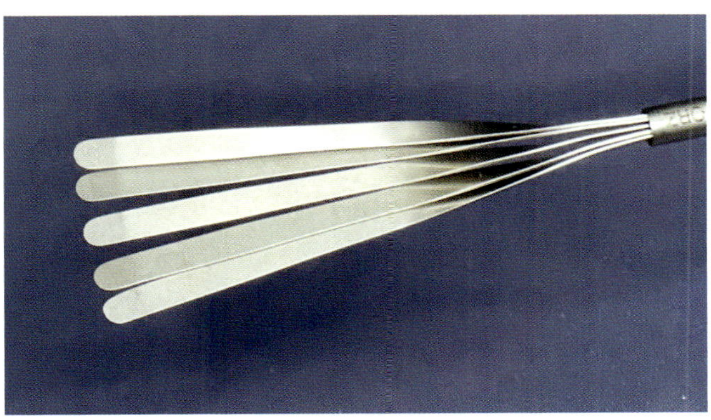

FIGURE 9. 5 mm fan retractor.

NEEDLE HOLDERS, KNOT TIERS, AND CLIP APPLICATORS

When considering tissue healing, mechanical tissue restoration includes intracorporeal and extracorporeal suturing as well as clip application.

Although traditionally considered a difficult task, intracorporeal suturing has become a routine practice for many intermediate to advanced veterinary surgeons. When acquiring needle holders, a few features should be considered: handle design, length and diameter of the shaft, and tip design (see below). High-quality stainless steel construction with a tungsten carbide flat tip is always desirable, as it does not crush the suture material, which would substantially reduce its intrinsic biomechanical properties. Some instruments are presented as self-positioning needle holders, but they have a curved cup tip that crushes the suture string and might weaken or break the suture.

Needle holder handles are available in several shapes. Straight handles are the first choice for novice surgeons. Pistol-grip handles are more ergonomic, enhancing suturing speed and reducing wrist effort (**Fig. 10**). It is essential that the release mechanism be positioned opposite the thumb so that minimal maneuvering is required to open and close the needle holder.

Needle holder tips can vary greatly in shape, from Parrot to Flamingo to standard jaws. Standard left, right, or straight tips might be considered the first choice for most surgeons, but when performing intracorporeal sutures, different types of needle holders can be combined to aid the task in smaller or narrower spaces (**Fig. 11**). In intermediate to advanced procedures, it is recommended that surgeons have a minimum set of two additional needle holders.

The shaft length and diameter of the needle holder varies according to the size of the patient and set. When considering a miniature set, a 3 mm instrument is required, whereas in standard procedures a 5 mm needle holder is more commonly used.

When performing extracorporeal knot tying, either atraumatic dissectors or knot tiers are routinely used to push the suture knots. Knot tiers consist of a metal shaft with a semiopen distal tip that conducts the suture string for an easy push and secure tying (**Fig. 12**). They are used when the required strength surpasses the surgeon's ability to tighten the knots using a standard instrument and needle holder. Extracorporeal suturing has been demonstrated to be secure and versatile for several applications where tight spaces restrict instrument triangulation and freedom of movement. Pretied suture loops are also available (see below).

Clip applicators come in reusable or disposable versions. Reusable clip applicators provide advantages such as autoclave sterilization and reduced consumable cost, limited to sterile clip cartridges. Semiautomatic disposable clip applicators come as precharged devices with a variable number of sterile clips (10–20 clips) and offer the advantage of clip application without the need to remove the instrument to charge each clip individually. These clips are commonly built in titanium for MRI compatibility, but there are also sterile plastic clips with a self-locking mechanism that activates once they are compressed around the tissues. The choice depends on the surgeon's preference, on the procedure, and often on local availability.

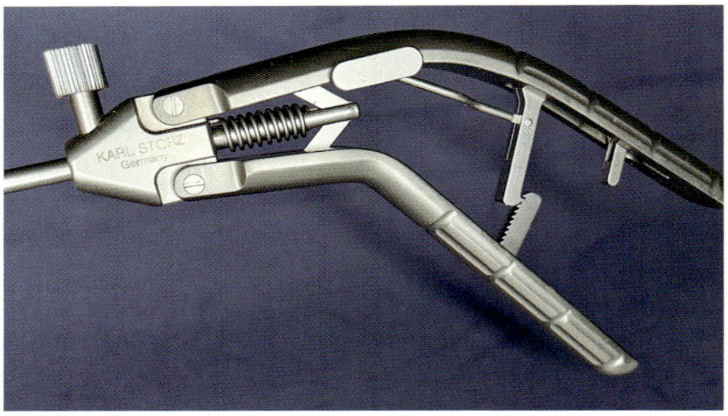

FIGURE 10. Pistol-grip ergonomic handle in a standard straight 5 mm laparoscopic needle holder.

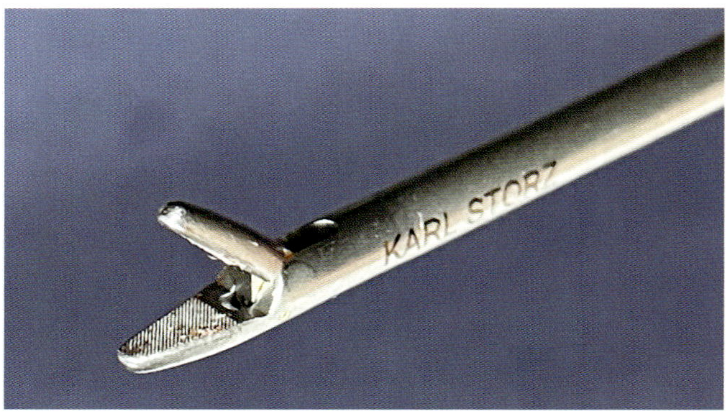

FIGURE 11. Detail of a needle holder tungsten carbide standard straight jaws.

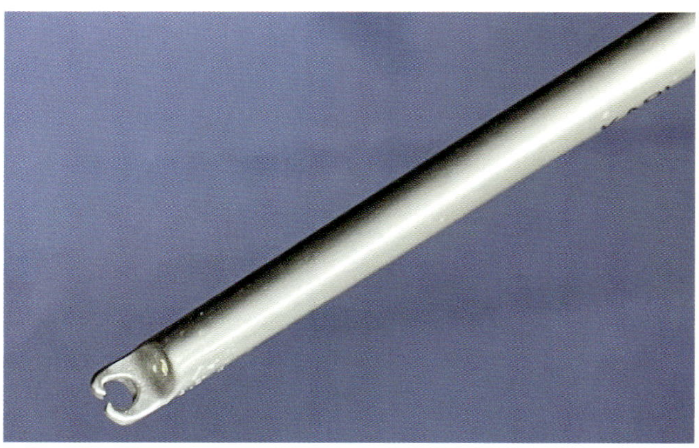
FIGURE 12. 5 mm knot tier for extracorporeal suturing or knot tying.

COAGULATION ELECTRODES AND SUCTION TUBES

If minimal coagulation is required during MIS procedures, monopolar electrosurgery is often adequate. Energy is conducted through a monopolar connector pin present in different types of instruments including dedicated electrodes. The most common coagulation electrodes feature a metal right-angled tip or hook that can perform coagulation and delicate dissection. Hook coagulation electrodes are preferred because they minimize trauma and provide precise separation of tissues without bleeding. Laparoscopic electrodes are available in various lengths (20–43 cm) and diameters (2.5–5 mm) (**Fig. 13**).

Irrigation and suctioning are frequently performed for lavage and rinsing and for fluid or blood aspiration to keep the operating field clean. Irrigation instruments can be connected to a fluid bag (gravity) or to an irrigation pump. Pressure bags are often used to minimize the cost of a dedicated irrigation unit, whereas a standard surgical aspiration unit or vacuum system is connected to the suction post of the instrument to permit fluid evacuation.

Some suction tubes also have coagulation capabilities if an electrode is present on their tip, allowing for both tasks without the need to exchange the instruments through the ports.

Standard care recommendations should be observed with monopolar energy use. The neutral plate contact area should be clipped, and contact gel applied. Insulated bedding is required to minimize accidental contact and short circuit with the metal tabletop, which can lead to electrical burns.

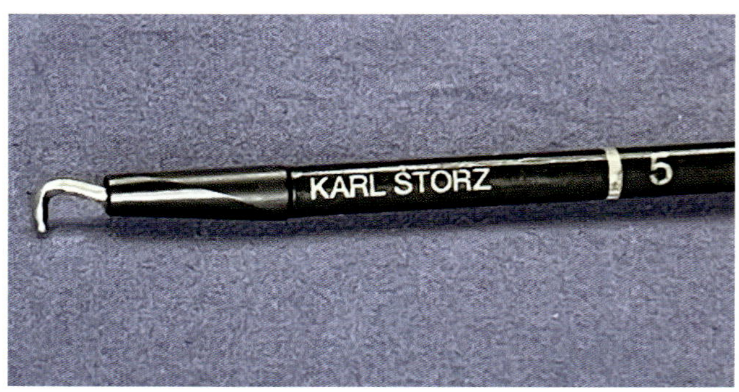

FIGURE 13. Standard hook monopolar coagulating electrode.

BIPOLAR COAGULATION INSTRUMENTS

Standard bipolar electrosurgery is one of the most useful coagulation methods to minimize surgical bleeding. Dedicated bipolar instruments are available in various shapes, and most comprise a double-jaw insulated tip and a connection to the electrosurgical unit via a bipolar cord. Activation is generally performed with a double foot switch pedal, for cutting and coagulation modes. Kelli and Clermont-Ferrand models are among the most preferred.

Caution should be observed when using bipolar coagulation to avoid contact and thermal spread to surrounding tissues, which can result in accidental burns with catastrophic consequences.

TROCARS, PORTALS, AND VERESS NEEDLES

The choice of approach to the abdominal or thoracic cavity is critical and might differ based on the selected technique and surgeon's preference. Trocars and accessories are explained below. Capnoperitoneum and abdominal entry techniques are addressed elsewhere in this book.

The most common techniques for entry in the abdomen are Veress needle insufflation and the modified Hasson technique.

The Veress needle has a spring-loaded mechanism that allows entrance into the abdomen and subsequent filling with CO_2 until the desired working pressure is achieved. The needle can be inserted either into the linea alba or in a paramedian location; in addition, intercostal access has also been described in the literature. The major advantages of using the Veress needle technique are its simplicity and ease of use. However, disadvantages include possible minor perforation-induced trauma to the liver or spleen, and major complications can occur if the stomach, bowel, or gallbladder are pierced.

The standard Veress needle for small animal laparoscopy is 10 cm long with a diameter of 2.1 mm, although other lengths are also available. The needle includes a Luer connection so that the insufflation tube connects the needle to the insufflator, allowing CO_2 passage into the patient.

Following surgical procedures and prior to sterilization, the needle should be completely disassembled to ensure thorough cleaning, since blood released from traversing the abdominal wall often enters the lumen of the needle. If not completely cleaned, biofilm and contamination can occur.

The modified Hasson technique has become the most popular trocar insertion technique among veterinary MIS surgeons. Current preferences include lightweight and threaded cannulas, smooth or sharp obturators, and self-screwing trocars, such as the Ternamian Endotip (**Fig. 14**).

Standard trocars are 6 mm in diameter, allowing for passage of 5 mm instruments, and are available in various lengths (6–10.5 cm). Ternamian threaded trocars are made of surgical stainless steel and enable the surgeon to directly see trocar entry while rotating the device through the abdominal or thoracic wall by means of a telescope inside. Lightweight alloy trocars are placed in the body cavity by performing a small incision with a number 11 scalpel blade, which is bluntly enlarged using a small mosquito or hemostatic forceps. Both trocar types are completely reusable, and when the rubber sealing valves become defective, they can be easily replaced to maintain optimal functionality. Blunt obturators are recommended over sharp ones since they substantially diminish iatrogenic tissue trauma if accidentally driven into an organ (**Fig. 15**). A side-port Luer connector is frequently included in most

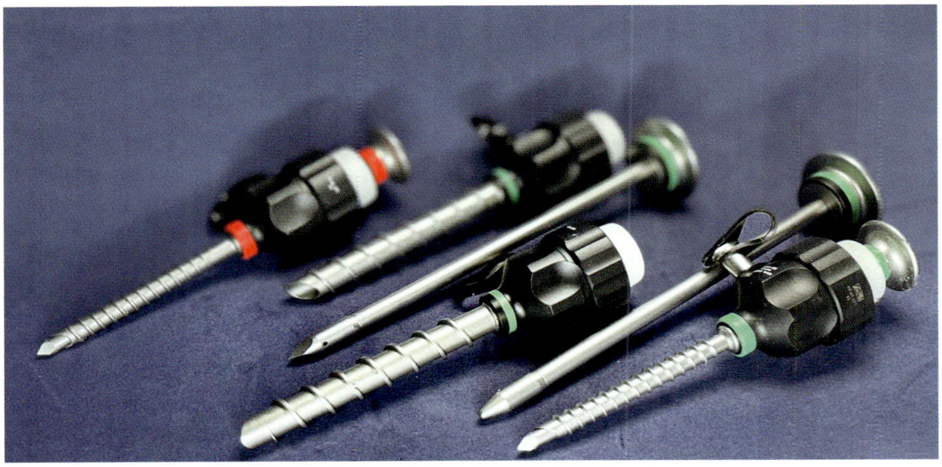

FIGURE 14. 3.5, 3.9, and 6 mm threaded trocars.

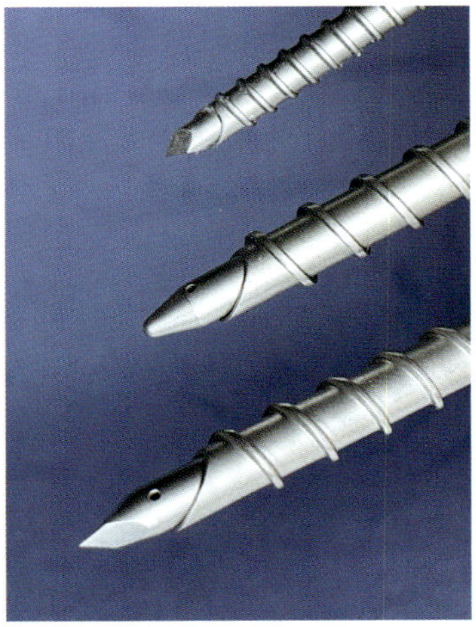

FIGURE 15. Detail of pyramidal and blunt obturators for 3.9 and 6.0 mm threaded trocars.

trocars, allowing for gas insufflation, especially for laparoscopic surgery.

For thoracic MIS, shorter soft rubber trocars are also available, and preferred by some surgeons. They are considered disposable components, although reprocessing and effective sterilization has already been addressed in the peer-reviewed veterinary literature.

ELECTROSURGERY UNITS AND VESSEL-SEALING TECHNOLOGY

Electrosurgery is a critical component of successful advanced MIS. Since achieving perfect hemostasis is necessary to effectively maintain surgical field cleanliness and technique effectiveness, various modalities of electric current are often used in MIS procedures.

Monopolar energy is the simplest form of electrosurgery and effectively facilitates coagulation and cutting procedures. To establish the voltaic arch, a neutral plate is placed under the patient and connected to the electrosurgical unit, while an active electrode cable is connected from the unit to the standard laparoscopic instrument, insulated for monopolar use. Parameters are set at the main unit and activation is achieved with a foot switch pedal. Since electric current passes from the tip of the instrument to the neutral plate, through the patient's body, proper care should be observed to avoid contact with tissue or uninsulated areas and accidental electric burns.

Bipolar energy is preferred when major coagulation is necessary. The voltaic arch is limited to the space between the instrument tips, thus enhancing the safety and efficacy of the process. A dedicated bipolar instrument is attached to the main unit with a bipolar cable. It is suggested that monopolar and bipolar cables be 300 cm long to allow for better ergonomics while performing MIS, since the equipment is generally placed on a trolley or boom-arm distant from the surgical field.

Since tissue fusion devices have become more available across the veterinary profession, they are now the standard choice for advanced electrosurgery in laparoscopy and thoracoscopy. Examples include vessel sealers and harmonic scalpels (ultrasonic energy).

Advanced bipolar electrosurgical units generally comprise vessel-sealing technology. An instrument connected to the main unit with an integrated cable delivers pulsed energy, while its sensors are responsible for impedance feedback. Using an algorithm, this information is processed in the main unit and the energy cycle is adjusted and stopped when resistance indicates total tissue desiccation and sealing. Often referred to as smart technology, audible feedback is provided by some units when sealing has been successfully achieved.

The ultrasonic energy tissue fusion modality is also extremely useful, as no electric current is delivered to the tissue. This technology consists of a specific physical process known as cavitation, which is a hybrid form of vaporization that facilitates dissection. It enables cutting, desiccation, and protein coagulation. This method brings some advantages for thoracoscopy, and especially lung lobe dissection, since it does not interfere with cardiac conduction.

ACCESSORY DEVICES

Auxiliary devices are of great value while performing ligation and separation. Clip applicators have already been described above. Linear, curved, or circular staplers and suture loops very often comprise useful tools in MIS.

Pretied loops or handmade sliding knots are routinely used for simple procedures, such as lung biopsy, or even ligation of small vascularized structures, such as ovarian pedicles. They come as individual single-use products, mostly in a 5 mm plastic applicator. Suture materials vary according to the procedure, but the most common types are absorbable braided and nonabsorbable monofilament.

Most mechanical staplers deliver several rows of intercalated clips (3–6) and are available in several lengths and clip sizes. Modern staplers can deliver small 2.0 mm clips and were successfully tested and reported for performing lung lobectomies in small- to medium-breed dogs. However, most MIS veterinary surgeons often use vascular staplers with cartridges delivering 3.5 mm clips. A 4.8 mm clip stapler can also be used for partial resection of parenchymatous organs. The stapler is often 10 mm in diameter and requires a 12–15 mm trocar to enter the cavity. Cartridge length generally varies between 30 and 65 mm, but some brands offer devices up to 80 mm in length.

SURGICAL TABLES AND RACKS

Since MIS has replaced several standard surgical procedures as the gold standard technique, the need for updating preexisting operating rooms and building new ones has become routine in facility planning. A dedicated MIS operating room requires enough space to accommodate all imaging systems and combine them with other imaging modalities such as interventional radiology and interventional endoscopy. The increasing number of devices used for electrosurgery, surgical aspirators, and lasers has added an additional need for platforms to combine all units ergonomically while maintaining functionality and floor cleanliness. Surgical racks and ceiling booms are now often implemented in the standard design of modern MIS veterinary operating rooms (**Fig. 16**).

Surgical tables should provide such features as radiotransparency for concurrent use of fluoroscopy, Trendelenburg and Fowler tilting capability, lateral tilt capability, and automated height regulation for ease of patient repositioning during the procedure. Surgical tables should also ideally have a warming system to keep the patient's body temperature within the physiological range. Heated-air circulation mattresses are recommended, as they are the most efficient heating method for veterinary patients regardless of their size.

Surgical lamps are now provided with LED technology as the standard and should include MIS/Endo modes emitting green illumination for surgeon's eye comfort during surgical procedures. Double-plate illumination is mostly preferred because it diminishes the shadowing effect.

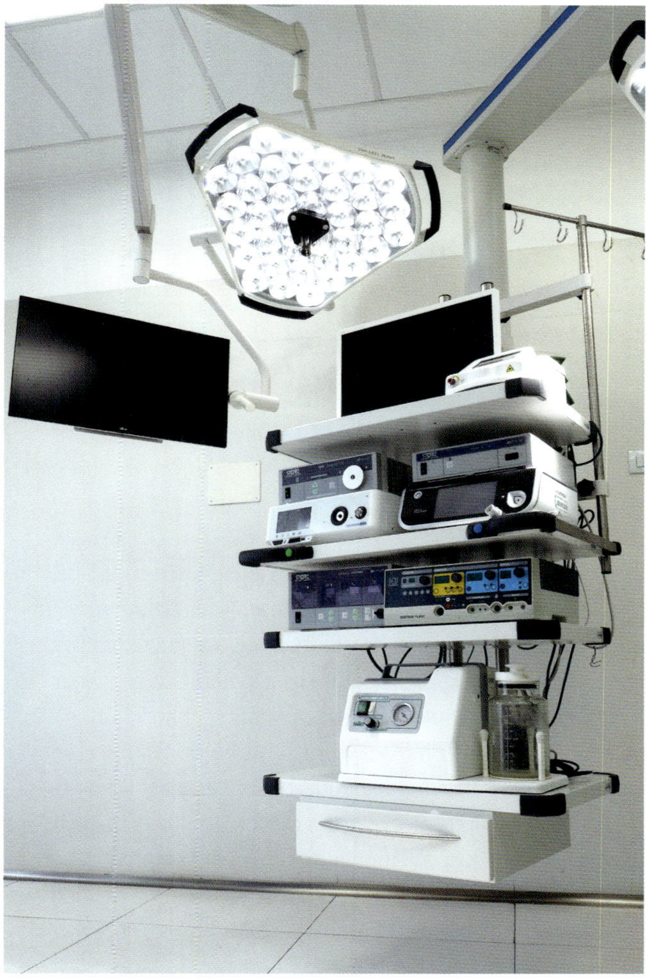

FIGURE 16. Movable surgical racks on ceiling-mounted booms allow for the ergonomic combination of units while maintaining functionality and floor cleanliness.

OTHER ACCESSORY UNITS AND DEVICES FOR LAPAROSCOPY AND THORACOSCOPY

As veterinary MIS has become an important part of the surgical routine in small animal surgery, the availability of disposable accessories and devices has increased, enabling professionals to pursue safer and faster procedures. The current complexity of surgeries performed in small animal MIS is also the result of the accessibility of veterinary professionals to advanced instrumentation, units, and devices, so as to enable tasks that could only be performed with open surgery or very advanced skills (e.g., tissue stapling).

In the sections below, an overview of some routinely used units and devices is discussed to familiarize prospective MIS surgeons with progressive tasks and skills.

VESSEL-SEALING INSTRUMENTS

As already mentioned above, vessel sealers have become the standard technology utilized in veterinary surgery. Tissue fusion is now a familiar term for practitioners, but some differences in the devices still exist and might influence surgeons' preference (**Fig. 17**).

Since electrosurgical technology does not differ greatly between units, a few critical aspects of accessory instrumentation make some devices more commonly chosen for certain applications. Length, diameter, and working tip type represent the criteria for a rational choice in the surgical routine.

For most applications, a length of 35–37 cm is considered standard. When dealing with smaller patients (<10 kg), a working length of 20–22 cm is suggested for ease of triangulation and improved ergonomic instrument maneuvering. For abdominal procedures in large-breed dogs (>45 kg), a 43 cm long instrument might be considered to access deeper structures.

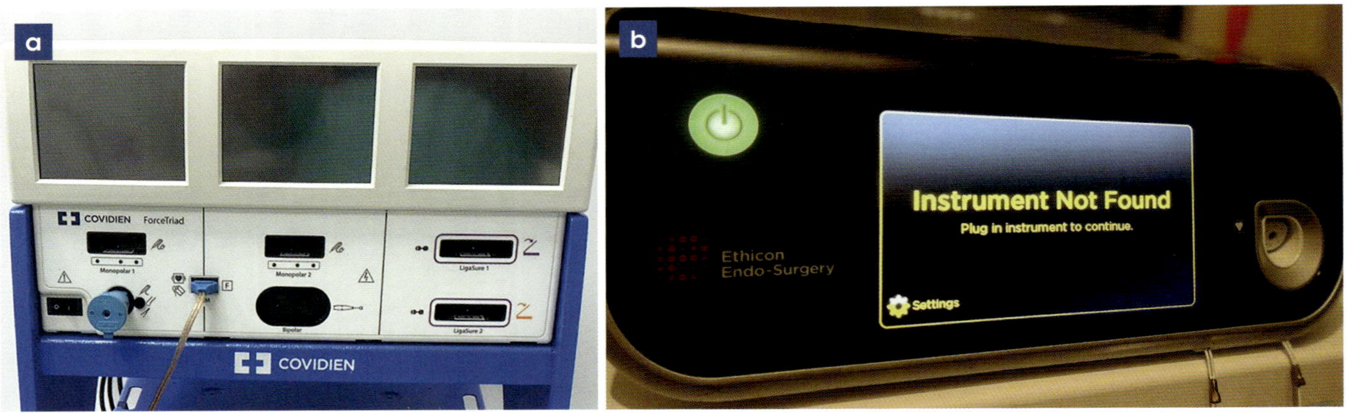

FIGURE 17. a) Ligasure ForceTriad. Complete electrosurgical unit providing monopolar, bipolar, and vessel-sealing energy technologies. Image courtesy of Dr. Constantine Ifteme, Bucharest, Romania. b) Enseal Gen11, Ethicon. Electrosurgery unit combining bipolar vessel-sealing and ultrasonic (Harmonic) energy technologies.

Ideally, for cats and toy breed dogs, instrument diameter should be 3 mm, but these are rarely available, except for human pediatric surgery, due to the increased cost of units and instrumentation (e.g., JustRight 3 mm Vessel Sealer, Bolder Surgical). That said, standard instrumentation commercially available for small animal MIS is 5 mm in diameter. 10 mm diameter instrumentation can also be found but is rarely used.

The working tip is probably the most critical aspect to choose one instrument over another. It determines the surgeon's ability to safely perform a task in a specific organ within a defined surgical plane.

When dissecting the tissue planes, a thin smooth-tipped dissector is preferred, so a straight or curved Maryland instrument is the usual choice (**Fig. 18**). In some instances, a longer straight tip might be preferred (e.g., LigaSure Dolphin Tip).

For routine procedures such as splenectomy, ovariectomy, or cryptorchidectomy a simple straight or curved vessel sealer blade is routinely used, thus minimizing instrumentation costs (e.g., Enseal Trio) (**Fig. 19**).

The newer generation instrument recently released by Ethicon, the Enseal X1 curved jaw tissue sealer, is highly promising; performance tests demonstrate more tissue grasping and sealing compared to other similar instrumentation from other brands. This instrument is provided with a unique 24 mm long jaw, a cut length of 21.8 mm, and 13.4 mm aperture, which are distinctive features in the current market.

The length considerations observed above also apply to ultrasonic vessel-sealing instruments, although instrument tips remain similar for all market options.

A unique combined bipolar and ultrasonic vessel sealer is also available (Thunderbeat, Olympus). Although not often used due to its high cost, this system presents the advantage of combining increased and safe bipolar coagulation with precise and fast dissection, offered by ultrasonic energy. Bipolar, ultrasonic,

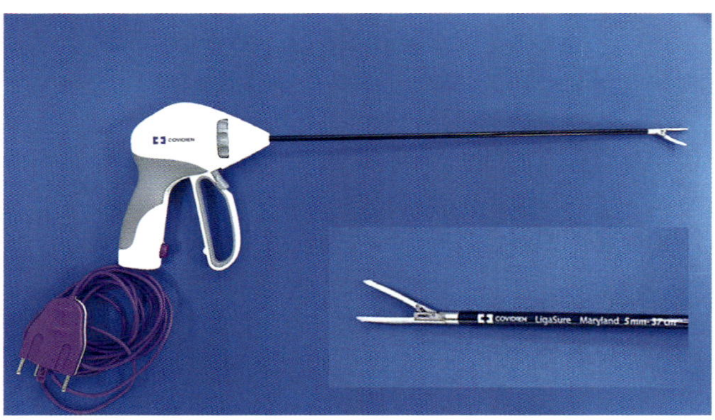

FIGURE 18. LigaSure curved Maryland instrument. Image courtesy of Dr. Constantine Ifteme, Bucharest, Romania.

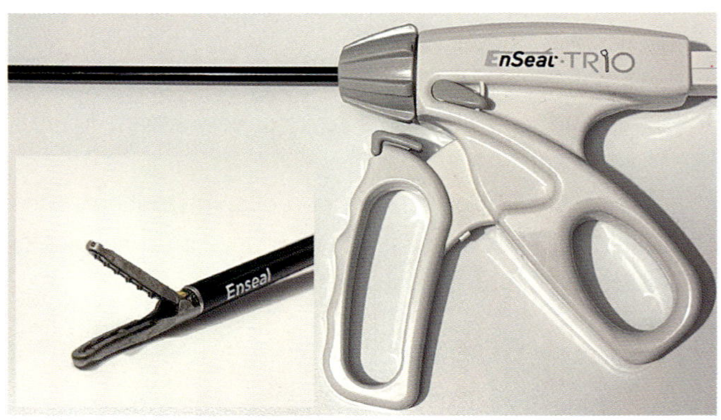

FIGURE 19. Enseal Trio 5 mm curved blade vessel-sealing instrument.

or hybrid energy forms can be used with the same instrument, resulting in better performance without the need for instrument exchange through the trocars.

WOUND RETRACTION DEVICES

Port-site metastasis is a major concern while performing neoplastic tissue extraction. To protect the surgical wound during organ extraction, and to perform video-assisted surgery techniques (uniportal), plastic wound retraction devices provide an atraumatic circumferential effect, minimizing tissue trauma and devascularization. This results in increased working field as well as enhanced exposure and visualization. Several diameters, ranging from 2 to 17 cm, are available from different commercial companies. This device generally consists of a hollow plastic channel with two plastic rings at each edge. It is placed with gentle pressure at its lower ring, through a small incision. By rolling down the external ring, progressive circumferential distraction is achieved (**Figs. 20 and 21**).

Wound retraction devices have become popular for uniportal video-assisted thoracoscopic surgery and some uniportal laparoscopic-assisted techniques such as splenectomy or ovariohysterectomy.

EXTRACTION BAGS

Surgical wounds and incisions can be quite small in MIS. Therefore, organ or tissue extraction might be challenging or present risk of contamination, extravasation, or metastasis. MIS-dedicated extraction bags are available in different models and shapes, with a wide volume range from 50 up to 1500 mL. Generally speaking, this device is passed into the body cavity through a 10 mm accessory, thus requiring a 12 or 13 mm trocar. In small animal MIS, procedures such as cholecystectomy (**Fig. 22**), adrenalectomy, cranial mediastinal mass extraction, or sentinel lymph node removal have made retrieval devices increasingly popular throughout the veterinary community.

IRRIGATION AND SUCTION PUMPS

With the increasing complexity of minimally invasive procedures, lavage and suction have become mandatory tasks for technical safety and accuracy. Regular surgical aspirators or vacuum systems can be used for surgical aspiration, but a combined unit enabling both irrigation and suction is ideal (**Fig. 23**). Such units provide pressure-controlled irrigation and suction by using a double tubing system and a trumpet valve-operated cannula. Advantages include ease and accuracy of operation, since both actions occur at the designated point of the surgical field, enhancing its visualization. If fluid or blood obscure the surgical site, fast assessment and cleaning is possible with this system.

Aspiration cannulas are available in sterilizable and disposable versions for the surgeon's ease and preference. Although representing an increased initial cost, sterilizable models allow

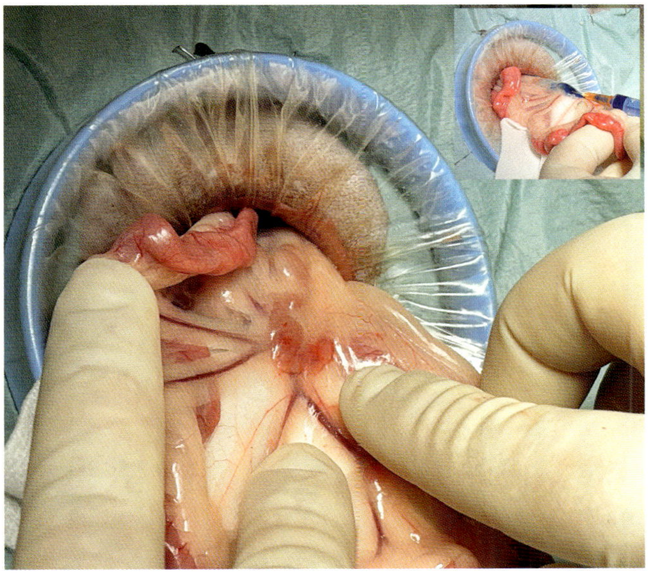

FIGURE 20. SurgiSleeve (Covidien) wound retraction device used for identification and expose of an ileocolic lymph node for methylene blue injection for thoracoscopic thoracic duct ligation.

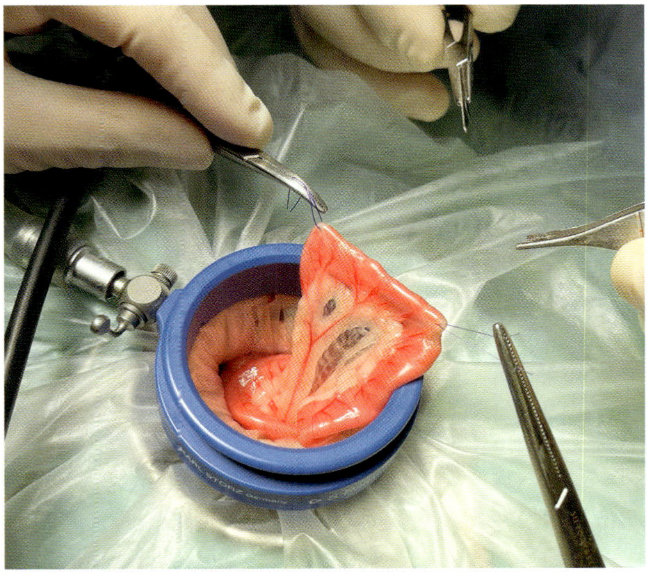

FIGURE 21. V-drape system including a wound retraction ring with plastic surgical drape used in a single-port multiorgan laparoscopic-assisted biopsy procedure (S-Port, Karl Storz).

a fast return on investment, since these cannulas are everyday use tools.

Provided with sterilizable bottles, suction and irrigation units offer a huge potential for thoracoscopy and laparoscopy (**Figs. 24 and 25**).

SINGLE-USE DISSECTORS

When delicate dissection or tissue separation is required in laparoscopic and thoracoscopic surgery, single-use swab dissectors (that mimic open surgery cotton tip applicators) are recommended. Although small cotton gauze pads can be cut to small bits and used with a straight or curved Maryland dissector, dedicated cotton swabs affixed to a 5 mm shaft are commercially available (e.g., Endo Peanut, Covidien). These devices allow for an atraumatic and blunt dissection in delicate soft tissues and aid in controlling minor intraoperative bleeding. They are of great use in procedures such as thoracic duct ligation, cranial mediastinal mass removal, and adrenalectomy.

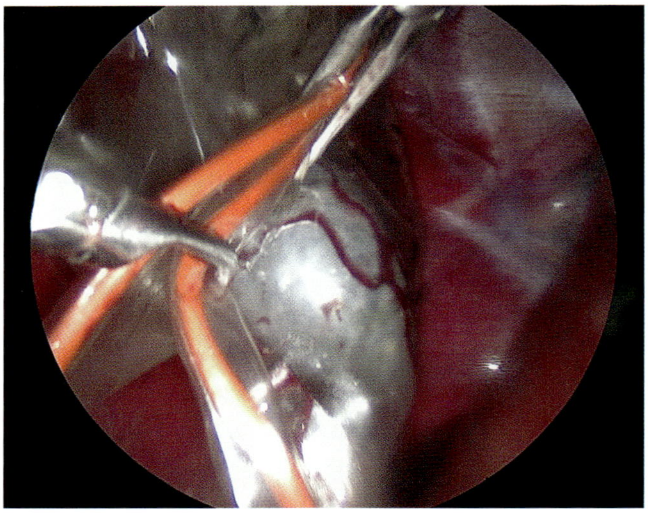

FIGURE 22. Extraction bag used in laparoscopic cholecystectomy.

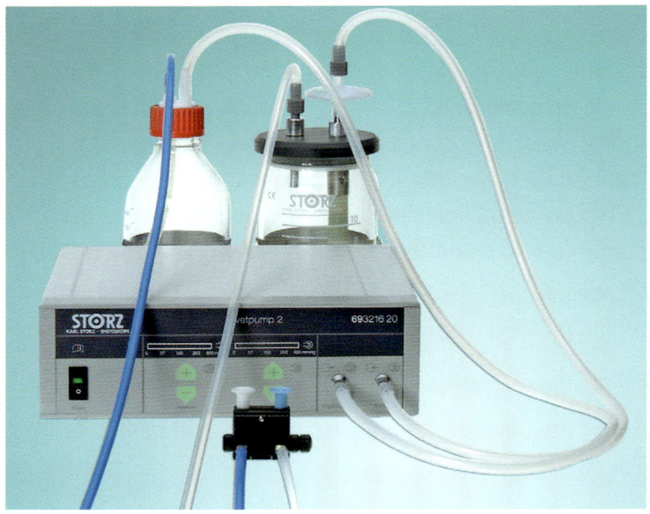

FIGURE 23. Combined aspiration/suction pressure-controlled device Vetpump 2. Image courtesy of Karl Storz SE & Co. KG.

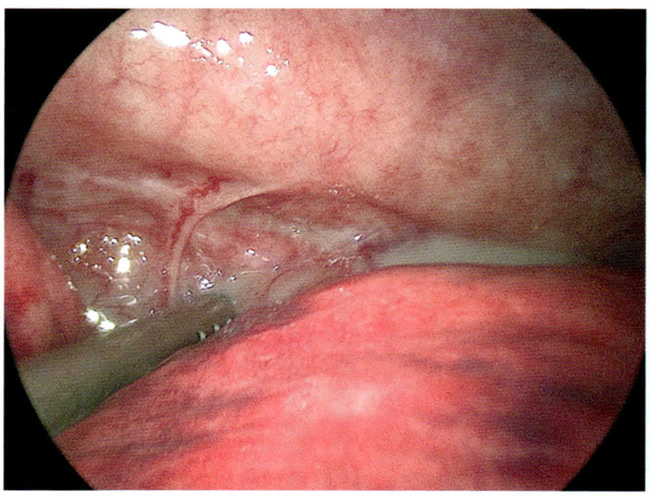

FIGURE 24. Chylothorax aspiration with a 5 mm sterilizable aspiration/irrigation cannula.

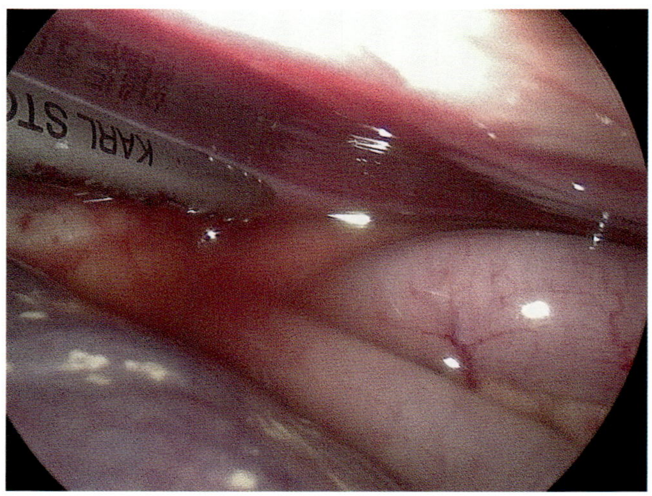

FIGURE 25. Laparoscopic fluid aspiration with a 5 mm sterilizable aspiration/irrigation cannula.

Quick reference guide for small animal laparoscopic and thoracoscopic surgery equipment and instrumentation

For the novice and intermediate veterinary surgeon, a quick reference choice guide for units and instrumentation is suggested below. It represents the authors' suggestions and preferences, so other individual preferences should be considered as well.

Basic to intermediate imaging system	
Monitor	24″, 27″, with DVI or HDMI input
CCU	Full HD (1920×1080)*
Camera head	Full HD*
Light source	LED (insufflation capability required to operate with videogastroscopes)
Documentation unit	Required for true full HD recording USB output might compress image signal
Light cable	3.5 mm×300 cm

*Ensure CCU and camera head compatibility.

Intermediate to advanced imaging system	
Monitor	24″, 27″ (or 32″)* A minimum of two monitors is suggested
CCU	Full HD (1920×1080) or 4K (3840×2160)**
Camera head	Full HD or 4K**
Light source	LED for standard applications Dedicated LED fluorescence light source for NIR/ICG applications Xenon might be required for specific filter fluorescence applications
Documentation unit	Required for full HD and 4K recording
Light cable	3.5 mm×300 cm (standard applications) 3.5 mm×230 cm (dedicated fluorescence applications)

*32″ or bigger dedicated sizes are required for 4K outputs.
**Ensure CCU and camera head compatibility.

Basic 5 mm laparoscopic/thoracoscopic set	
Rigid scope	5 mm×29 cm×30°
Instruments	1× Laparoscopic palpation probe 1× Curved Maryland dissector 1× Atraumatic Babcock grasping forceps 1× Curved conical scissors 1× Biopsy cup forceps
Trocars	3× 6 mm lightweight threaded trocars, or alternative combinations: ■ 2× 6 mm lightweight trocars+1× 6 mm Ternamian Endotip ■ 3× 6 mm Ternamian Endotip trocars Disposable short-profile rubber trocars might be used

Quick reference guide for small animal laparoscopic and thoracoscopic surgery equipment and instrumentation

Intermediate- to advanced-level additional 5 mm instruments for laparoscopy and thoracoscopy	
Rigid scopes	5 mm × 29 cm × 30° + 5 mm × 29 cm × 0° 0° distal angle tip is suggested for transdiaphragmatic subxiphoidal approach
Additional instruments	1× Right-angled (90°) dissector 1–2× Laparoscopic needle holder (curved and/or straight jaws) 1× Rothenberg grasper 1× Croce-Olmi grasper 1× Hook scissors 1× Biopsy punch forceps 1× Aspiration/irrigation tube 1× Coagulation hook electrode 1× Knot pusher
Trocars	Single-port system Additional 6 mm lightweight trocars Dedicated short-profile trocars for thoracoscopy

Additional miniature laparoscopic set	
Additional miniature laparoscopic instruments	1× 3 mm curved dissector 1× 3 mm right-angled dissector 1× 3 mm biopsy cup forceps 1× 3 mm curved conical scissors 1× 3 mm atraumatic grasper 1× 3 mm laparoscopic needle holder 1× 3 mm laparoscopic palpation probe 1× 3 mm coagulation hook electrode 1× 3.5 mm aspiration/irrigation tube
Miniature laparoscopic trocars	1× 3.9 mm threaded trocar 2–3× 3.5 mm threaded trocars

Other common accessories	
Sterile sleeves	13 cm diameter × 240 cm long are suggested to easily accommodate camera head or light cable
Vessel sealers	5 mm × 35–37 cm bipolar vessel-sealing instrument (curved tip) Consider having 24 cm long for small patients and 43 cm long for large/giant-breed dogs
Ultrasonic scalpel	5 mm × 36 cm instrument Consider having 20 cm long for small patients Dedicated cable is required or integrated cable instrument
Wound retraction devices	Consider having at least two sizes available covering 4–14 cm diameter
Extraction bags	50–250 mL are often used
Titanium clips	5 mm and 10 mm (disposable multiclip applicators) 10 mm sterilizable clip applicator + clip charges
Staplers	2.0 mm or 3.5 mm clips (vascular) Lengths of 30–65 mm are often used Roticulating stapling devices preferred due to increased ergonomics
Barbed sutures	4/0, 3/0 and 2/0 are often used for small animal MIS 3/8 circle needles 16–19 mm are suggested Suggested suture length of 15 cm Long absorption (180 days)

SUGGESTED READINGS

4 OPERATING ROOM AND HYGIENE MEASURES

Roberto Properzi, Francesco Collivignarelli

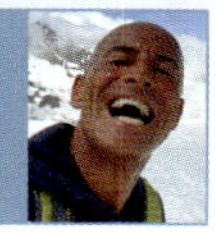

Currently, there are no guidelines for operating room setup and hygiene in veterinary medicine; therefore, human medicine guidelines are used.

CONSIDERATIONS FOR A MINIMALLY INVASIVE OPERATING ROOM

Operating rooms specialized for minimally invasive procedures should be provided with at least two towers, one dedicated to anesthesia and one to minimally invasive surgery (**Fig. 1**), and there should be enough space to move the surgical equipment around the operating table.

Hybrid operating rooms, in which both interventional radiology and endoscopy can be performed, are recommended.

BASIC ERGONOMIC CONSIDERATIONS

Correct monitor positioning is often underestimated. It is crucial for the surgeon to have a posture that is as neutral as possible. Monitors positioned too high up can create muscle pain in the head and neck and consequently decrease attention during surgery. Having a comfortable position improves surgery. Ideally, two or three monitors are placed on booms or on equipment towers. It has been shown that the preferred viewing angle for video displays is between 10° and 25° below the line of sight.

Another important consideration about the surgeon's ergonomics is the handle design of the instruments for minimally invasive surgery. It has been demonstrated that correct wrist positioning, secondary to an adequate instrument design, improves surgeon's performance, optimizing surgical times and decreasing the risk of musculoskeletal disorders in the surgeon.

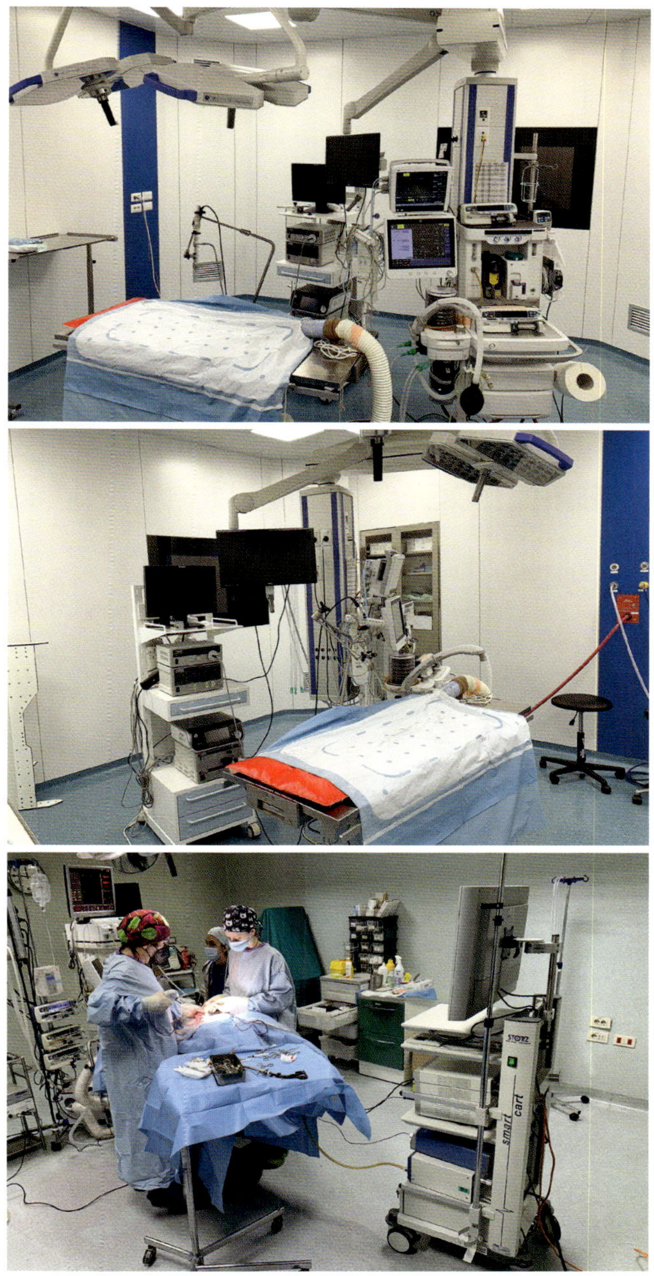

FIGURE 1. Operating room equipped with an anesthesia tower and a minimally invasive surgery tower.

OPERATING ROOM CHECKLIST

At the beginning of a surgical session, a checklist of surgical equipment needed should be used.

- Check the light source.
- Turn on the insufflator and check the filling status of the working cylinder and the availability of a reserve cylinder.
- Verify the correct functioning of the camera and monitor.
- Check the correct functioning of the electric tools.
- Check the availability of every surgical tool eventually needed in case of conversion to open surgery.
- Confirm the availability of other disposables necessary (e.g., staplers, graspers, trocars, surgical loops).

PREPARATION FOR OPEN SURGERY

All tools that could be possibly needed to convert to open surgery must be available. They must be sterile and ready for use at any time.

HYBRID ROOMS

Multipurpose rooms for minimally invasive surgery require fluoroscopy equipment (C-arm), either a floor-wheeled or ceiling boom suspended unit. In human hospitals, complex hybrid rooms also contain interventional CT or MRI units for intraoperative imaging, navigation, and reconstruction.

HYGIENE MEASURES

For the adequate implementation of hygiene measures it is necessary to start from a careful planning of the design of the operating room, which must meet requirements such as to allow the correct positioning of the necessary equipment with the possibility for the staff to move freely without impediments inside the operating room.

All the instruments must be subjected to sterilization and/or sanitization processes. In this regard, it is important that all the instrumentation is certified to be able to undergo these treatments.

The operating room must be cleaned after each surgery and sanitized at the end of the surgical session.

As for the instruments that could be used in the surgical session, it is advisable to follow a checklist of the operations necessary for the correct maintenance of hygiene measures.

- Emptying, cleaning, and removal of bins and containers for paper and waste collection.
- Sweeping of floors.
- Dusting of surfaces and furnishings.
- Cleaning and disinfection of surfaces.
- Cleaning and disinfection of furnishings.
- Manual washing and disinfection of floors.
- Mechanical washing of floors.
- Cleaning of radiators, air conditioners, air vents, rolling shutters, blinds, vertical slat blinds, and shutters.
- Washing of light points.
- Cleaning of windows and fixtures.
- Washing of washable walls.
- Dewaxing and waxing of floors.
- Maintenance of unwaxed floors.
- Renovation of marble floor (crystallization).
- Removal of cobwebs and vacuuming of ceilings.
- Cleaning in case of accidental contamination with organic material.

The meticulous adherence to the scheduled procedures listed above considerably reduces the risk of nosocomial infections whose eradication often requires complete stamping out (all empty, all full).

CLEANING OF HANDS

A variety of methods for surgical hand preparation are available (**Fig. 2**):

- Aqueous solutions containing either povidone-iodine (PVP) or chlorhexidine gluconate (CHX) have been standard for many decades.
- Alcohol-based hand rubs have also been described for surgical hand preparation for more than a century (**Fig. 3**).

To comply with current medical standards, the veterinary community should aim at introducing alcohol-based hand rub solutions in presurgical and hygienic surgical hand disinfection protocols.

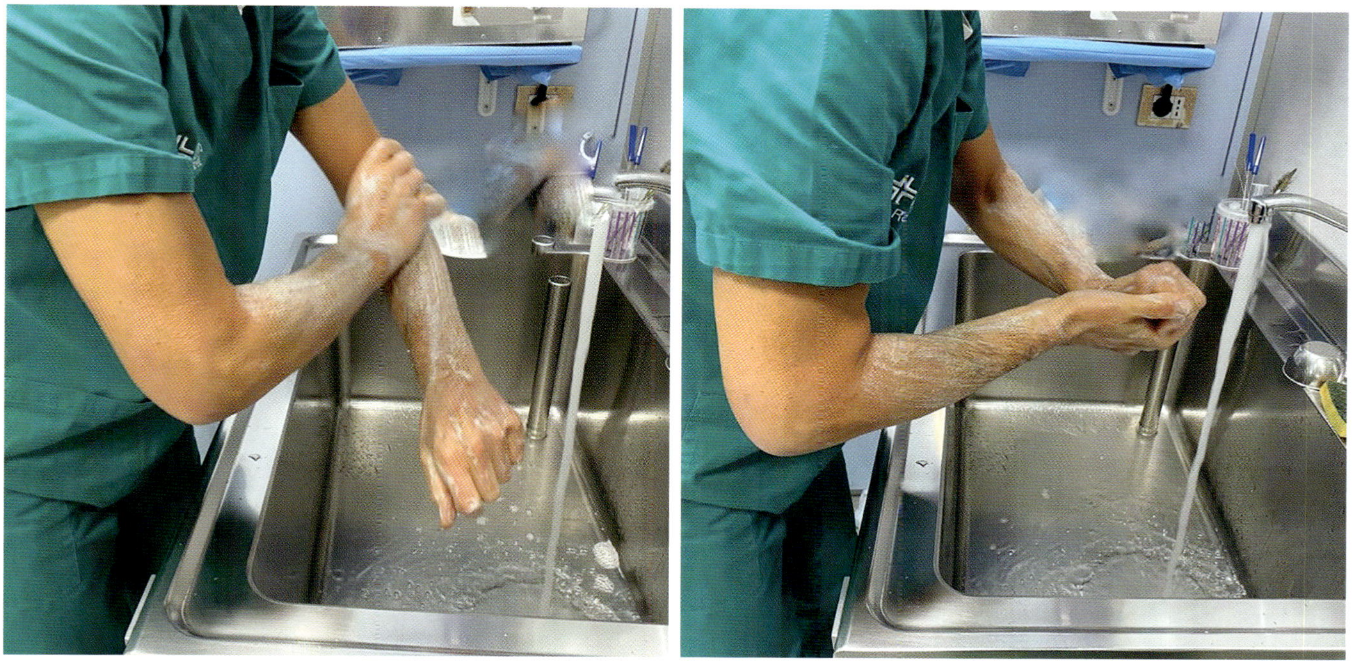

FIGURE 2. Hand washing with soap and water, including the forearm up to the elbow.

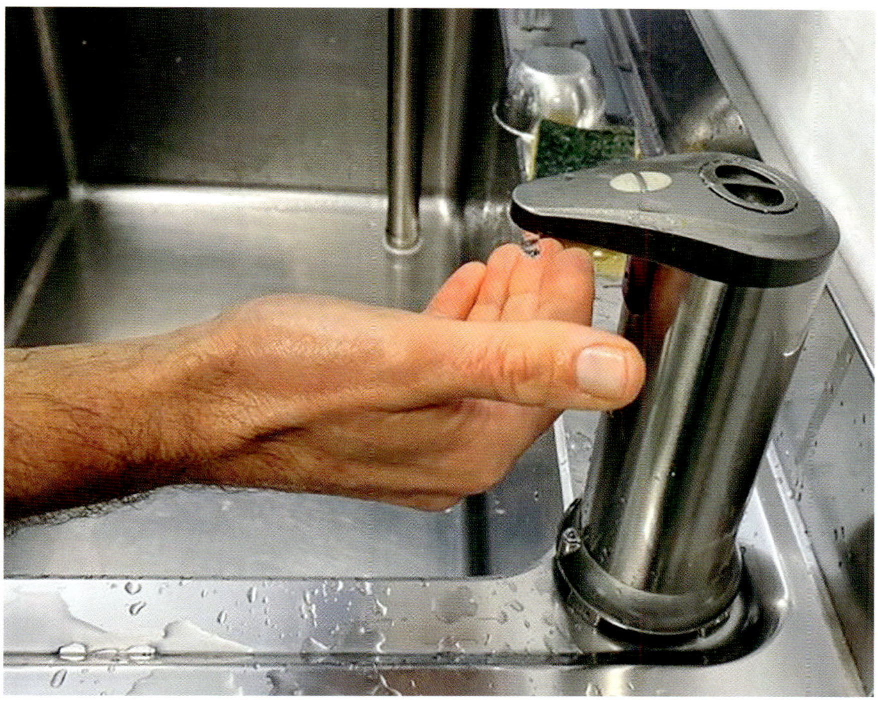

FIGURE 3. Alcohol-based hand rub application following hand washing with soap and water.

SUGGESTED READINGS

5 ERGONOMICS IN LAPAROSCOPY AND THORACOSCOPY

Andrea M. Pievaroli

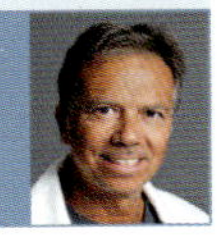

Ergonomics, in the medical field, can be considered an anthropocentric scientific discipline aimed at the design and manufacture of products and workplaces that are safe and more easily usable by healthcare personnel. The term *ergonomics* derives from the ancient Greek words *ergon*, meaning work, and *nomos*, meaning natural laws or arrangement. Generally, it can also be identified as *human factors engineering*, reflecting the definition of "fitting the job to the worker". In human medicine, this science has especially established itself in some areas of surgery where there has been greater technological development, such as cardiac surgery, interventional radiology, orthopedics, and minimally invasive surgery (laparoscopy and thoracoscopy).

The traditional figure of the surgeon, as identified in the collective imagination, is characterized by an intellectual preparation, creative skills, motor skills, an ability to manage emergencies, and a high physical resistance in an efficient work context. All these requirements, in combination with the technological evolution necessary for the execution of some surgical procedures, have led to a more in-depth analysis in this area to propose a more suitable ergonomic method useful for the surgeon.

Minimally invasive surgery, specifically laparoscopy and thoracoscopy, offers undoubted advantages for the patient but may require, compared to traditional open surgery, a different type of care for the surgeon who performs it. The limitation of movements, the inability to touch the organs with one's hands, the indirect view of the operating field, the required fixed posture, and a higher level of attention and concentration are factors that determine greater physical and mental stress for the surgeon. For this reason, the interaction with instruments, surgical devices, and the operating room layout has now become critical to avoid fatigue and human errors. In minimally invasive surgery ergonomics is extremely important, because physical and mental reserves are worn down much more quickly, even when performing simple tasks, as they become more stressful and fatiguing (**Fig. 1**).

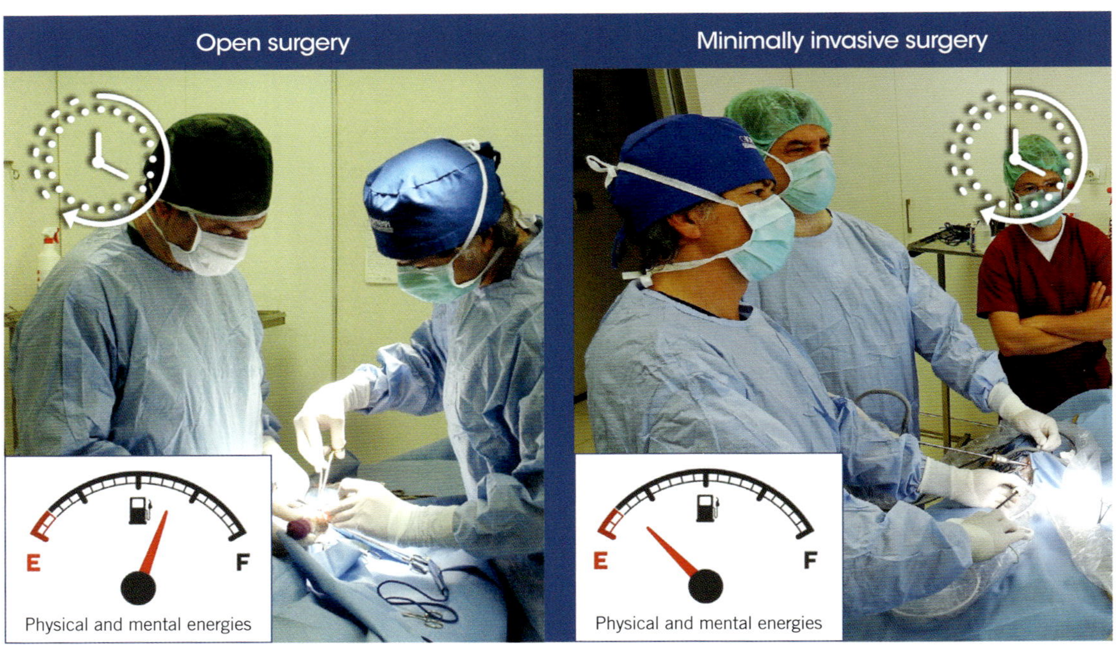

FIGURE 1. In a minimally invasive surgical procedure, physical and mental reserves are worn down much more quickly compared to open surgery.

DOMAINS OF ERGONOMICS

Three domains of ergonomics can be recognized, which are closely connected to each other (**Fig. 2**). Each has a different weight and value, depending on the type of surgery to be performed, the professional skills of the team, the environmental organization, and the technological complexity available. The interaction between these domains must ensure a unitary ergonomic project, aimed at ensuring comfort and safety for all those who are part of it at that time.

PHYSICAL ERGONOMICS

It deals with the compatibility between the anatomical, biomechanical, and anthropometric characteristics of the surgeon and their staff and the static and dynamic parameters of the operating room and the instruments to be used: layout of the operating room, posture, manipulation of instruments, health, and safety.

PERCEPTIVE–COGNITIVE ERGONOMICS

It studies human–machine–environment interactions in which cognitive and emotional factors come into play, linked to the dynamics of perception, learning, memorization, problem-solving, and the activation of motor responses by humans in the interaction with the system. In the operating room, the surgeon perceives stimuli and understands signals from the technology at their disposal and, consequently, activates the controls and carries out the adjustment of the systems in relation to the ability to evaluate the mental workload and decision-making.

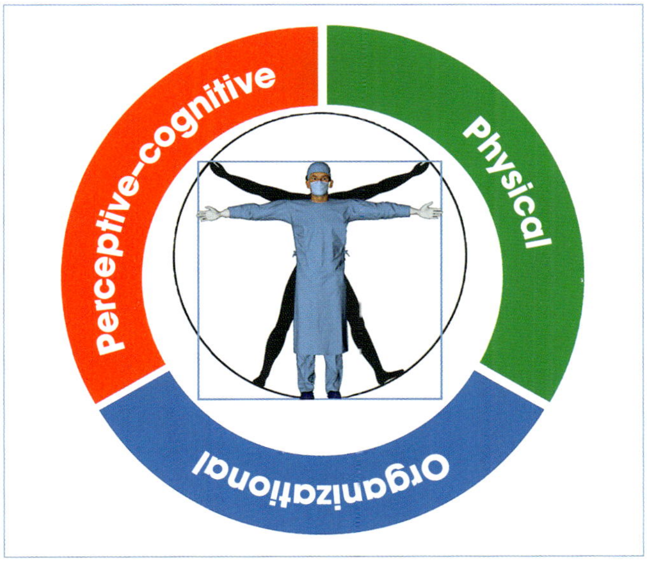

FIGURE 2. The three domains of ergonomics.

ORGANIZATIONAL ERGONOMICS

It refers to the so-called work design and deals with human–organization interaction. The preparation and execution times of the work, the times and rhythms of the activity to be carried out, the communication with the people involved, the management of team resources, and the optimization of technical processes are taken into consideration.

OPERATING ROOM SETUP

The overall room layout is important for the efficiency of the surgery and safety of the patient. The size of a room used for minimally invasive surgery should be larger than that of a typical room used for open surgery. It must be equipped with an efficient environmental temperature control system and a ventilation system with filters to purify the air. The surgeon and their staff must have the necessary space to move freely around the operating table during the steps of the surgery. In addition, large multilevel wheeled carts are used to accommodate the various medical devices needed for laparoscopy and thoracoscopy. These endoscopic carts must be able to be moved without hindrance to various positions in the operating room, depending on the type of procedure to be performed. They have the disadvantage of being bulky and requiring multiple power cables from the wall to the cart that flow on the floor, as well as numerous cables and tubes connecting the cart to the surgical area. This discomfort can be improved by adopting suspended solutions, such as movable ceiling-mounted booms or wall-mounted storage areas which reduces the number of cables on the floor.

During laparoscopy or thoracoscopy, surgeons face multiple physical issues that directly expose them to the risk of developing musculoskeletal disorders. The type of operating table, the arrangement of the various trolleys and instruments in the operating room, and the design of the surgical instruments are fundamental ergonomic factors because they affect the comfort of those who use them and the result of the procedure.

FACTORS LINKED TO MUSCULOSKELETAL DISORDERS

To minimize the risk of musculoskeletal injuries for the operator, it is essential that they assume a correct posture while performing the surgery. The surgeon's neck and back should be maintained in a comfortable and upright position, facing the monitor.

During a laparoscopic or thoracoscopic procedure factors like static body posture, repetitive upper extremity movements, limited range of movements of the instruments, bidimensional vision, and duration of work lead to physical stress, with more than 15% of surgeons reporting frequent back pain and stiffness following laparoscopic operations. To minimize these disorders, the surgeon has to take minibreaks, relax the muscles, and rest their mind, by releasing the handle from the surgical instruments and looking away from the monitor.

MALE VERSUS FEMALE SURGEONS

The height of the surgeon and the size of their hands can affect the onset of upper extremity discomfort and musculoskeletal disorders. A 2004 study showed that female surgeons are significantly more likely to seek treatment for hand injuries, hand paresthesias, and temporary compression neuropathies of the fingers (**Fig. 3**) associated with shoulder discomfort. Surgeons with smaller hands have greater difficulty in using laparoscopic instruments, in particular laparoscopic staplers, than those with medium to large hands (P <0.001). Instrument handle design was reported as a cause of physical complaints in up to 83% of respondents, with reports of pressure areas (36%), neurapraxia (26%), and uncomfortable posture (57%). Manufacturers should consider different sizes of laparoscopic handles to better match the instrument to the user.

SURGEON EXPERIENCE

Electromyography has been used to analyze the surgeon's postural muscle activity during laparoscopic surgery using different instrument handles (**Fig. 4**). Surface electromyography has

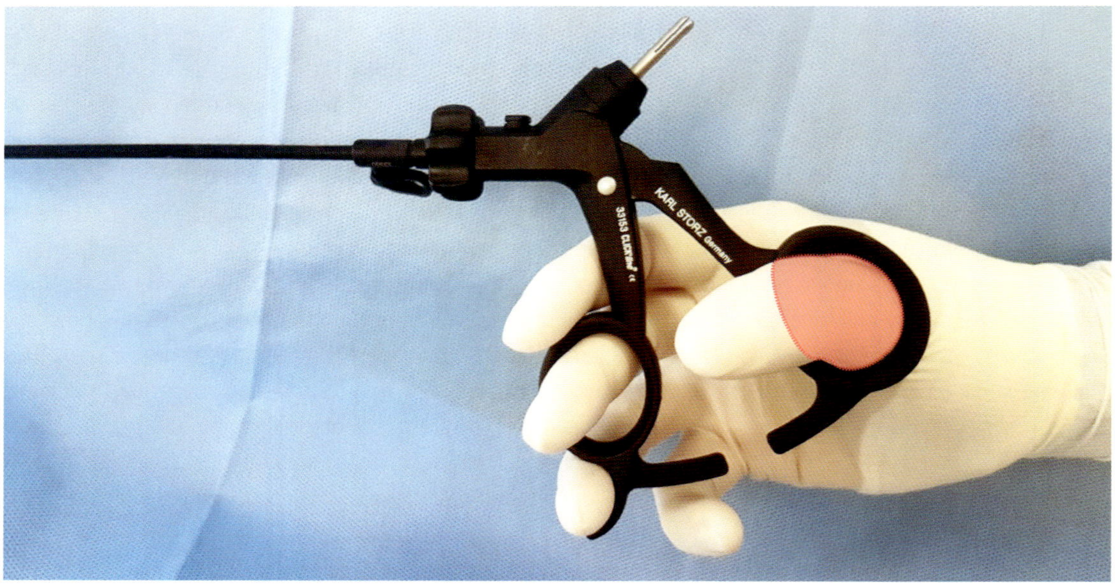

FIGURE 3. Area of thumb compression neuropathy (pink area).

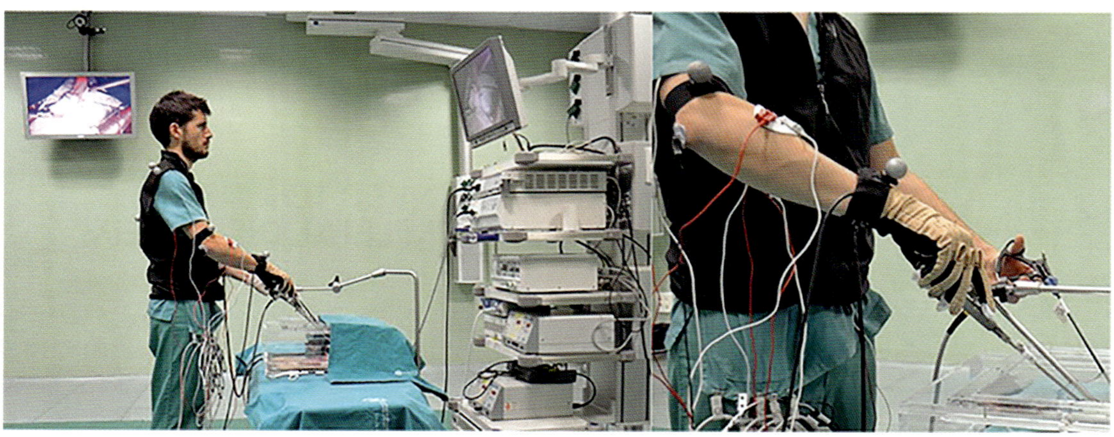

FIGURE 4. Electromyography and data acquisition glove to analyze the surgeon's postural muscle activity during laparoscopic surgery simulation using different instrument handles. Images reproduced with permission of Centro de Cirugía de Mínima Invasión Jesús Usón, Cáceres (Spain).

demonstrated that assistants exhibit maximal voluntary contraction of the biceps, triceps, trapezius forearm flexors, and forearm extensors muscle groups compared to primary surgeons and are therefore more likely to experience ergonomic stress. On the contrary, as reported in similar studies, surgeons with a higher degree of laparoscopic experience exhibited a lower level of muscle activity and, consequently, were less affected by ergonomic stress.

OPERATING TABLE AND PATIENT HEIGHT

The operating table is very important in minimally invasive surgery, especially in veterinary medicine because there is a large difference in size between patients. The table must allow a wide range of movement to adjust the height of the top, and it must be able to tilt in the Trendelenburg and reverse Trendelenburg positions and also laterally to the right and left. It is preferable if the table is equipped with a remote-controlled motorized system to carry out these movements and to facilitate its adaptations during the surgical phases (**Fig. 5**). Ergonomically, laparoscopic instrument handles must be slightly below the level of the surgeon's elbows, so the table should be adjusted for this purpose, taking into consideration that the angle between the lower and upper arm should be between 90° and 120° (**Fig. 6**).

PATIENT POSITIONING

The concept of ergonomics and safety in the operating room must also concern the patient, the main subject around whom the entire surgical act revolves. Before scrubbing, special attention must be paid to patient positioning and stabilization. The choice of recumbency must take into account the duration of the surgical procedure, guaranteeing a comfortable positioning on padded cushions and evaluating the complications on any pressure points.

Depending on the surgery to be performed, it is often necessary to tilt the surgical table to facilitate the movement of the organs. In addition to verifying that the patient has been properly secured to the table, it is important to monitor physiological parameters during excessive table tilts, including prolonged head-down position (Trendelenburg position).

MONITOR POSITION

The quality and the position of the monitor are critical for relieving fatigue and reducing discomfort in the surgeon's neck and back. With the introduction in the operating room of the first monitors in the 1980s, various studies were conducted to determine the optimal position with respect to the surgeon.

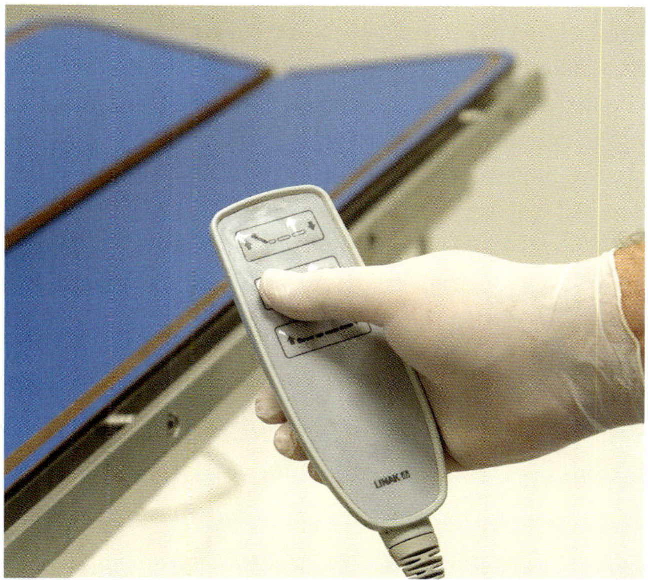

FIGURE 5. A remote control is preferable for making adjustments to the operating table.

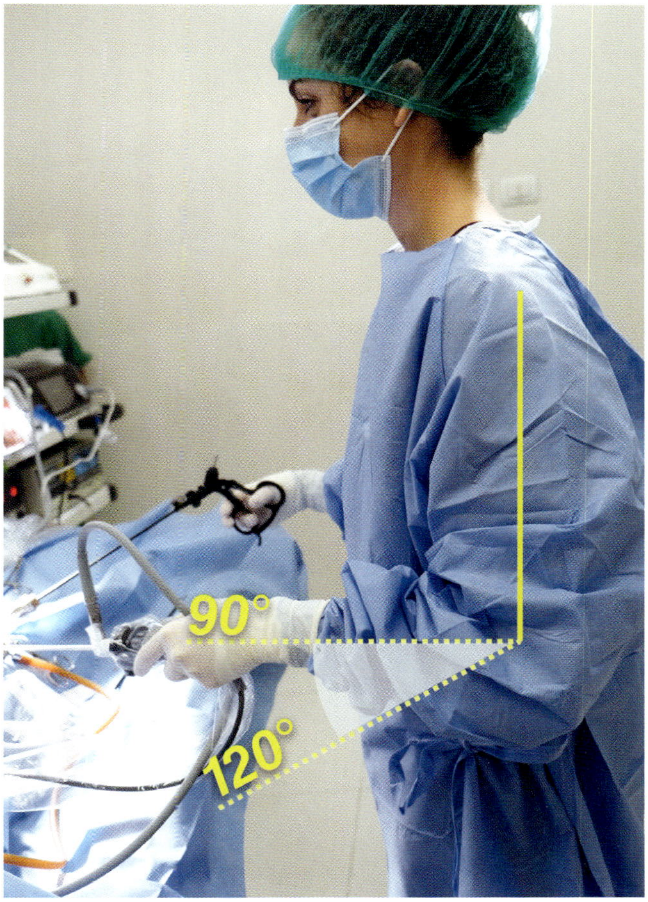

FIGURE 6. The angle between the surgeon's lower and upper arm should be between 90° and 120°.

Eyestrain is influenced by monitor distance, vertical angle, and lateral position. The neutral position of the human eye is oriented at an angle of 15° downwards, with a focal length of 0.8 m and an average convergence distance of 1 m. These studies demonstrated the importance of positioning the monitor directly in front of the surgeon at a distance of 0.8–1.2 m, and 15°–40° below the surgeon's eye level to get the maximum comfort (**Fig. 7**). With large and ultra-high-definition screens, the distance may be greater. It is preferable to have the monitor in the surgeons' direct line of sight, in line with their forearm–instrument motor axis, to avoid lateral rotation of the head. To orient the monitor in the ideal position for the surgeon, the best solution is to have flat screens installed on ceiling-mounted booms. This way, the surgeon can, using sterile handles, independently position the monitor according to their needs (**Fig. 8**).

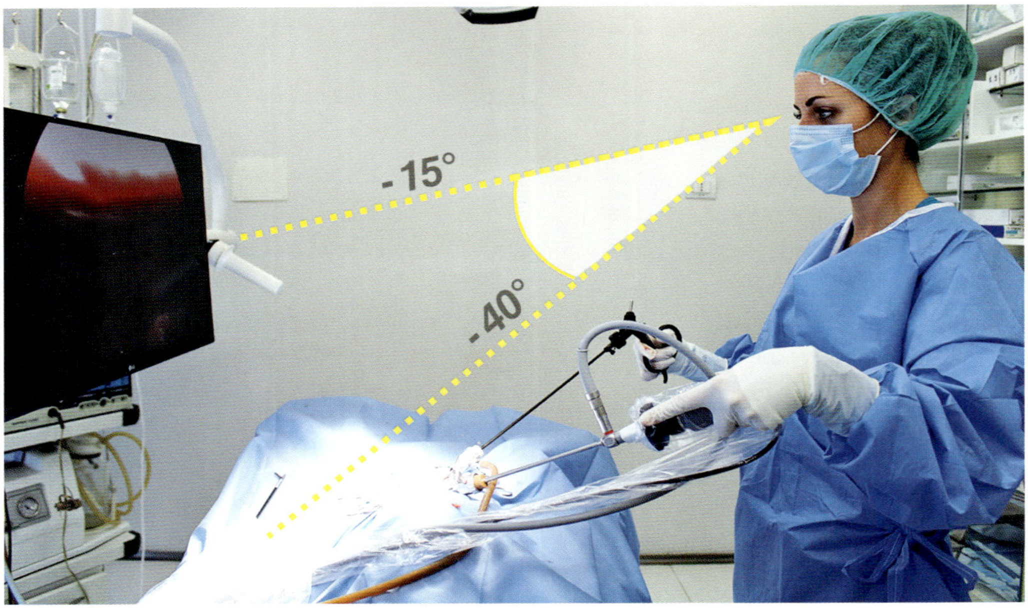

FIGURE 7. Position of the monitor in front of the surgeon, at 15°–40° below eye level.

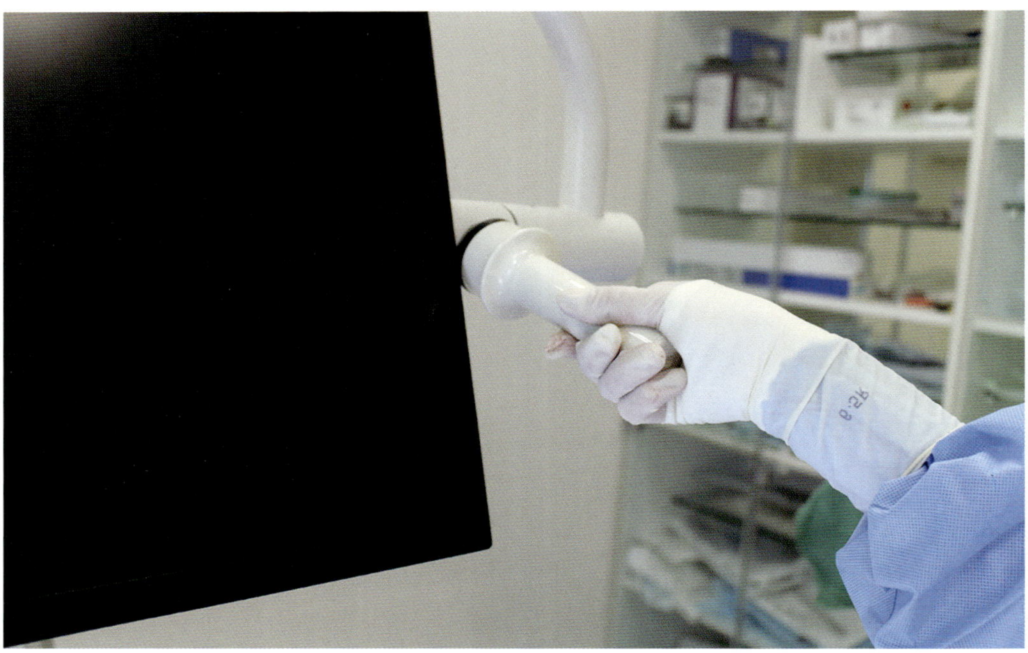

FIGURE 8. Sterile handle to orient a monitor installed on ceiling-mounted booms.

FOOT PEDALS

Most electronic instruments for electrocauterization, such as sealing devices, harmonic scalpels, and bipolar devices, can be activated by switches on the handpiece. However, in some cases, surgeons prefer to use foot pedals to activate these medical devices or for other purposes (e.g., to raise and lower the operating table or start/stop a recording session of the surgery images). In these cases, foot pedals should be within a natural, easy-to-reach position near the foot and aligned in the same direction as the instruments, toward the target. They should have tactile properties to be activated without twisting the body or leg and without the need to look, especially in the dark.

INSTRUMENT DESIGN

The success of a laparoscopic or thoracoscopy procedure depends not only on the experience of the surgeon but also on the quality and design of the surgical instruments. The conception of surgical instruments has changed in the last 20 years, enhancing the pistol grip handle with a round, rotating shaft and a single- or double-action grasping tip. The improvement of these characteristics has positively influenced the position of surgeon's arms, hands, and fingers, which is highly dependent on the design of surgical instruments. A 2018 study demonstrated that laparoscopic instruments require 3–5 times the muscle contraction force of open instruments, due to a 3–6 times less efficient transfer of energy. The surgeon needs to squeeze harder, bend their wrists more, and hold their arms higher when using laparoscopic instruments compared to open instruments, producing substantial hand and shoulder fatigue during laparoscopic surgery. Modern laparoscopic instruments should help to minimize wrist flexion and rotation and ulnar deviation, keeping both arms at the sides of the body, and avoiding pressure points on the hands and fingers. Some handles incorporate a locking or ratchet mechanism that will maintain the force to relieve muscle tension. **Table 1** lists the most important ergonomic and functional characteristics to be considered when choosing an instrument for minimally invasive surgery.

PORTAL POSITIONING

Portal placement for laparoscopic and thoracoscopic procedures are dictated by standard configurations or by the surgeon's preferences based on individual experience. The anatomic point of insertion of the trocars must be identified following the principles of the minimally invasive technique. Usually, they are placed in a triangular fashion to facilitate smooth instrument manipulation along with a more natural visualization of the target field. This is termed *triangulation*. When two portals are placed, they create a plane, and the angle between the two endoscopic instruments is called *angle of triangulation* (**Fig. 9**). Having the portals positioned correctly allows the surgeon to work in ergonomic conditions without suffering from musculoskeletal disorders and with less mental stress and frustration. Inadequate or incorrect portal positioning can make it difficult to carry out the surgery and may compromise its success.

TABLE 1. Most important ergonomic and functional characteristics of instruments for minimally invasive surgery

Instrument	Characteristics
Handle	Rounded, smooth, and broad-surfaced contours to avoid pressure points and finger entrapment.
Internal mechanism	Smooth, precise, and allowing good tactile feedback from the tip of the instrument to the handle.
Easy access for fingers	Easy and intuitive access for the fingers to any additional controls that govern shaft rotation, jaw locking, or electrocautery or suction activation
Electrical insulation	Sturdy insulation of the instrument shaft all the way to the base of the jaws to avoid stray electrocautery injury during use.
Electrocautery pin connector	It keeps the electrocautery cable out of the way of the surgeon's hand during use of the instrument.
Stapler and clip applier	Broad, smooth pistol-type handle that permits the surgeon to use a power grasp hand position.

Source: Berguer R. Ergonomics in laparoscopic surgery. In: *The SAGES Manual of Perioperative Care in Minimally Invasive Surgery.* Springer-Verlag New York; 2006.

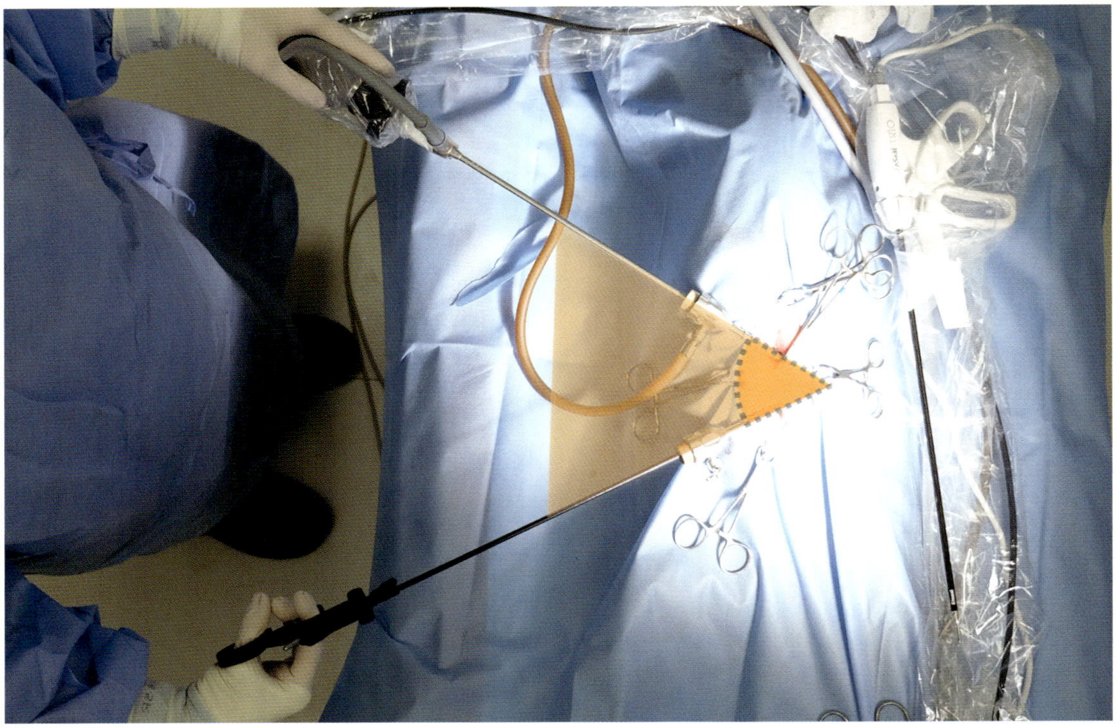

FIGURE 9. The angle between the two endoscopic instruments is called angle of triangulation.

Key points

- Use a large operating room with integrated and movable ceiling-mounted booms storage systems.
- When using floor-based equipment carts, be sure they cannot get in the way of the surgical team and can be easily moved when needed.
- Adjust the operating table height so that the instrument handles are at elbow height, the angle between the lower and upper arm being 90°–120°.
- Apply the concept of ergonomics and safety to the patient positioned on the operating table as well.
- Choose instruments with comfortable and efficient handles that minimize wrist flexion and rotation and ulnar deviation.
- Position the monitor directly in front of the primary surgeon, 15°–40° below the line of sight. If the surgical assistant is on the opposite side of the table, use a secondary monitor placed in front of them (with the same criteria).
- If foot pedals are used, place them near the foot in an easy-to-reach position, aligned in the same direction as the instruments.
- Follow the principles of the minimally invasive technique to choose the points of insertion of the trocars in a triangular fashion toward the target field.
- During complex and difficult procedures, physical and mental reserves wear out much more quickly, even when performing simple tasks.

SUGGESTED READINGS

6 PRINCIPLES OF TRIANGULATION IN LAPAROSCOPY AND THORACOSCOPY

Andrea M. Pievaroli

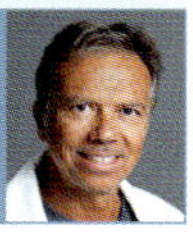

Laparoscopic and thoracoscopic procedures are called minimally invasive because they use a limited access to approach the operative field. Instruments and telescopes are passed into the body cavity through cannulas (trocars), which are inserted into specific points of the body wall. These access routes are called ports or portals. For each surgical procedure, specific port placement layouts are indicated to perform the surgery in the most ergonomic way (**Fig. 1**). The exact location of the trocars is important because laparoscopy and thoracoscopy carry a set of mechanical and visual constraints in the execution that could lead to surgeon discomfort and reduced performance, which were thoroughly discussed in Chapter 5. These constraints are the restrictions that the surgeon encounters while using endoscopic instruments to manipulate tissues through the ports which are placed in a fixed position for the duration of the surgical procedure (**Table 1**).

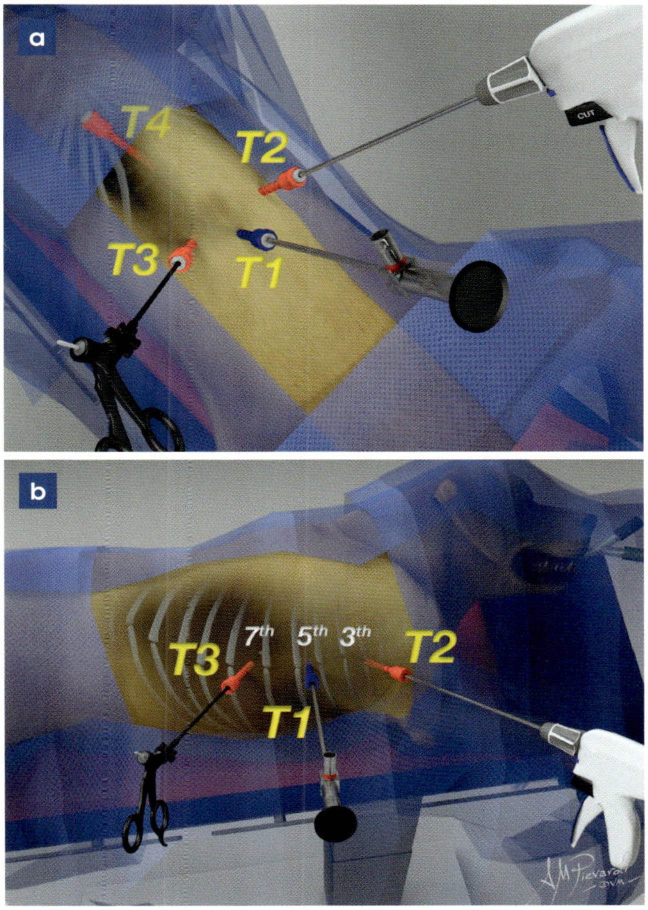

FIGURE 1. Examples of port placement. a) Laparoscopic procedure. b) Thoracoscopic procedure.

TABLE 1. Mechanical and visual restrictions in laparoscopy and thoracoscopy

Mechanical restrictions	Visual restrictions
■ Limited number of degrees of freedom ■ Port positions ■ Length and size of endoscopic instruments ■ Indirect tactile feedback ■ Available working space ■ Tissue retrieval concerns	■ Bidimensional vision (only in 2D systems) ■ Quality of telescope, camera, and monitor ■ Absence of shadows ■ Size of endoscopic field of view ■ Dirty lens ■ Port location ■ Relationship (angles) between instruments

MECHANICAL CONSTRAINTS

In laparoscopy and thoracoscopy, there are four degrees of freedom (DOFs) of movements: three in independent directions and a rotation around one axis (**Fig. 2**).

- Side-to-side movement along the x-axis.
- Up and down movement along the y-axis.
- In and out movement along the z-axis.
- Rotational movement around the z-axis.

The combinations of DOFs generate movements of the endoscopic instruments. This limited number of DOFs makes handling of tissues during endoscopy more difficult and challenging than during conventional open surgery, in which several dozen DOFs of movement have been identified.

Another important limitation is indirect tactile feedback from the instrument's tip. Even if endoscopic instruments are designed to reproduce the same instruments used in open surgery, more skills and time are required to acquire the coordination and sensitivity to use them. This feeling in the surgeon's hands is markedly diminished due to the length of endoscopic instruments and the friction between the instruments and the cannulas. It is more difficult to identify the nature and consistency of tissues, and the surgeon must pay more attention not to damage the tissues due to excessive manipulation of the instruments.

Shaft length and diameter affect its effectiveness. The longer the shaft, the more hand tremors are exaggerated, especially in a magnified endoscopic field. Shorter instruments are easier to manipulate, especially the thin 3 mm set designed for pediatric surgery; in veterinary surgery, they are used for very small patients (dogs and cats <3-4 kg). The stem must not be too long, because it would have fewer mechanical advantages. Furthermore, the use of an instrument that is too long compared to the patient's size will result in a large external arc of arm movement by the surgeon.

Tissue retrieval from the abdominal or thoracic cavity must also be considered among the mechanical restrictions. The advantages of minimally invasive surgery must be preserved as much as possible until the end of the procedure. The length of the abdominal wall incision at the level of one of the trocars will depend on the size of the tissue or organ to be removed. The tissue could be reduced in size to be extracted using specific retrieval bags or applying a circular wound retractor; this also reduces the risk of dissemination of neoplastic cells in the abdomen or along the port access.

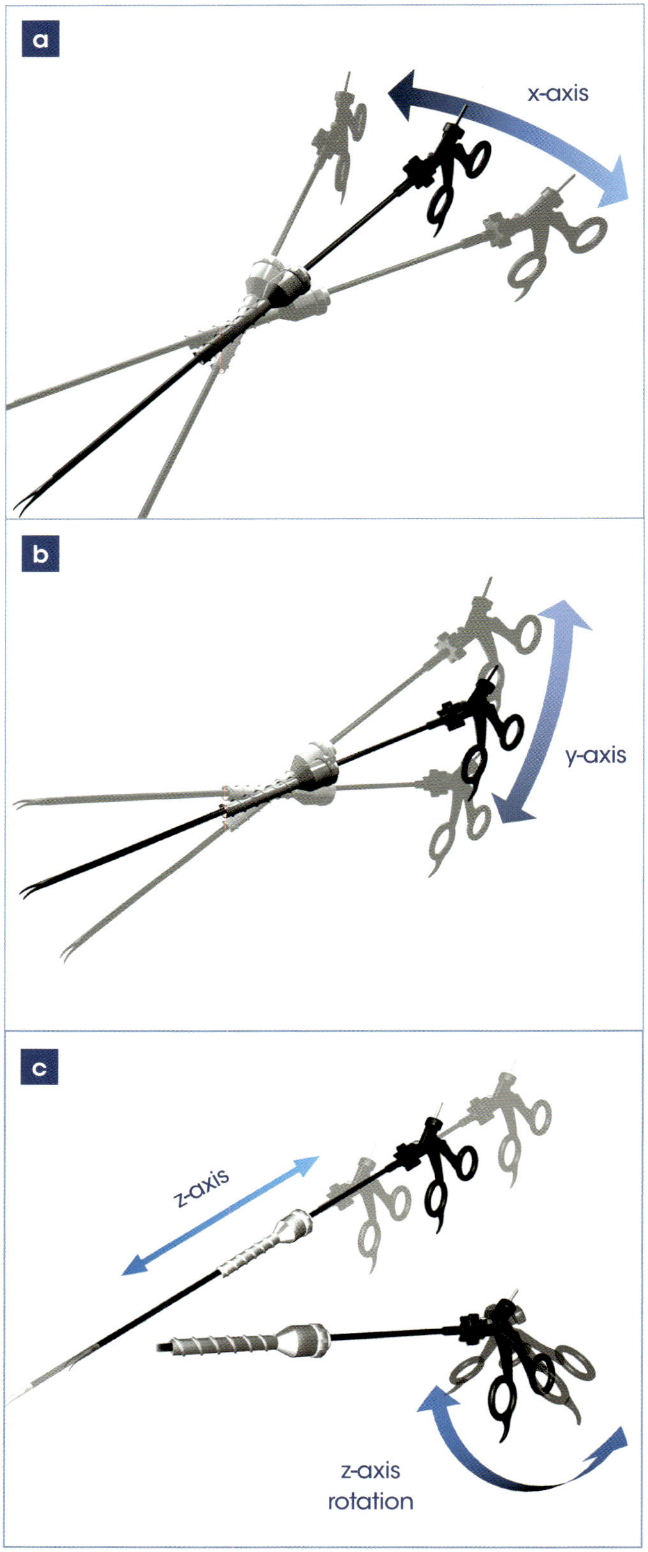

FIGURE 2. The four DOFs of movement with endoscopic instruments. a) Side-to-side movement along the x-axis. b) Up and down movement along the y-axis. c) In and out movement and rotation along the z-axis.

VISUAL RESTRICTIONS

In minimally invasive surgery, the surgeon does not have a direct vision of the operative field, and instead they use an image display system to perform the surgery. The consequent visual limitations depend on some factors such as the quality of the telescope, camera, and monitor and the ability to keep the tip lens clean during the procedure. A reduced field of view associated with poor image quality can lead to a degraded task performance in endoscopic surgery compared to direct vision, also increasing the risks for the patient.

Even if 3D vision technology is available, especially in human surgery, in most cases the visualization of the operating field is on a 2D screen. The surgeon must therefore sustain greater mental and physical processing to reconstruct 3D anatomy from the 2D image on the screen, which more likely leads to fatigue, inaccuracy, and errors. Moreover, rigid endoscopes have a coaxial alignment of the lens system and the illuminating optical light fibers. This design feature does not allow shadows to form in the operating field, further accentuating the problem of the absence of depth of field in the 2D vision.

Another visual restriction is the size of the endoscope. The smaller the telescope, the smaller the size of the field of view and the amount of light that can be transmitted to illuminate the operating field. The size also determines the working distance from the target. It has been demonstrated that the optimal distance between the telescope and the target should be 75–150 mm. At this distance from the objective lens, the field of view is sufficient to triangulate instruments without clashing and to operate more comfortably. However, this is not always possible in very small dogs or cats or when the working space is very limited.

As already described in Chapter 5, correct positioning of the monitor relative to the surgeon is important. The screen must be directly in front of the surgeon at a distance of 0.8–1.2 m and 15°–40° below the surgeon's eye level to achieve the maximum comfort. The basic principle of the best possible alignment between surgeon, telescope, operative field, and monitor should be respected (**Fig. 3**). Finally, the triangulation rules must be applied to ensure the appropriate relationship (angle) between the endoscopic instruments and the operative field.

Port nomenclature

The following abbreviations will be used to refer to the individual ports:

- T1: port for the telescope.
- T2: port for the endoscopic instrument operated by the surgeon's right hand.
- T3: port for the endoscopic instrument operated by the surgeon's left hand.
- T4, etc.: ports for additional tools.

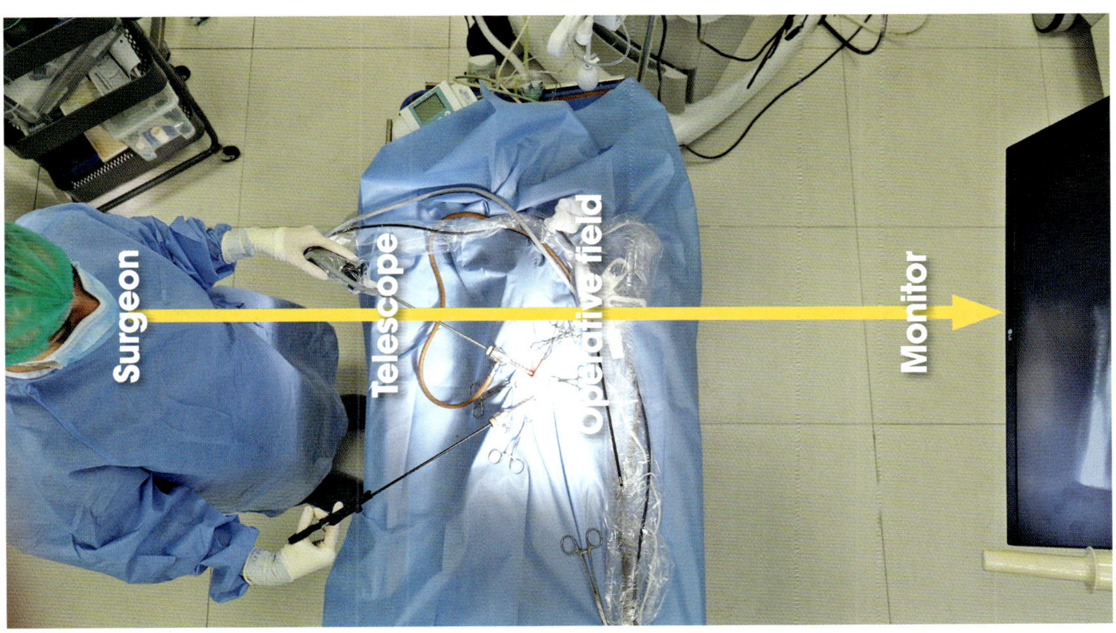

FIGURE 3. The basic principle of the best possible alignment between surgeon, telescope, operative field, and monitor should be respected.

OPTIMAL POSITION OF THE RIGID ENDOSCOPE (T1)

Rigid endoscopes have a direction of view, the optical axis. This can coincide with the physical axis of the endoscope or form a specific angle with it, generally 30° or 45°. The choice of an endoscope with a specific angle of view is made by the surgeon according to the needs and the procedure to be performed. The angle between the optical axis of the endoscope and the plane of the target is referred to as the optical axis-to-target view (OATV) angle (**Fig. 4**). Optimum task performance is obtained with an OATV angle approximating 90°. In practice, smaller angles, up to 45°, can also be used, but with a reduction in image fidelity (**Fig. 5**). The optimum OATV angle is determined by two main factors: the exact location of the optical port and the direction of view of the endoscope. The direction of view of the endoscope (0°, 30°, or 45°) has no significant effect on the execution time or the quality of task performance when the OATV angle is about 90°. Oblique-viewing endoscopes may at the beginning be more difficult and unnatural to use, but in practice they have more advantages because they provide more visual information and allow visualization from different angles by rotating the endoscope.

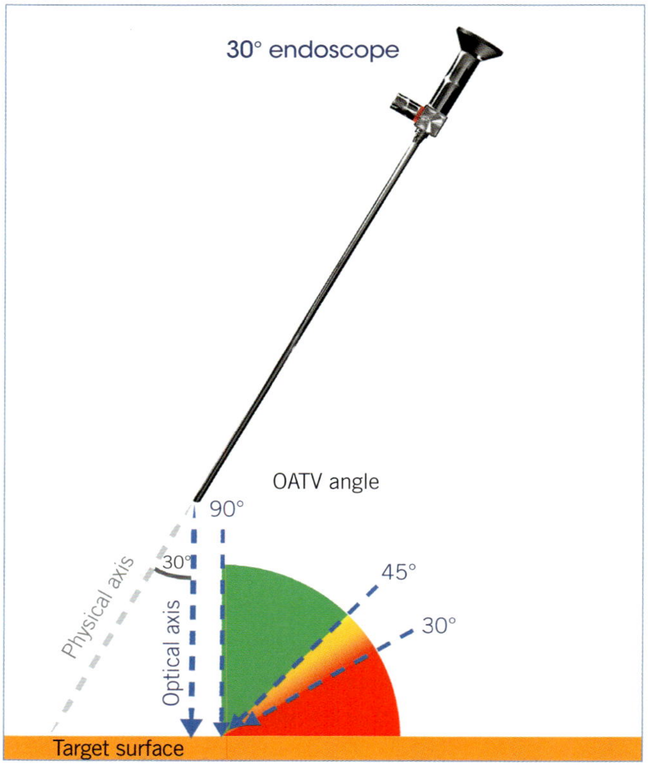

FIGURE 5. The best range of view is achieved with an OATV angle of 90°. Values up to 45° are acceptable. Values below 30° are not recommended because the vision is excessively tangential.

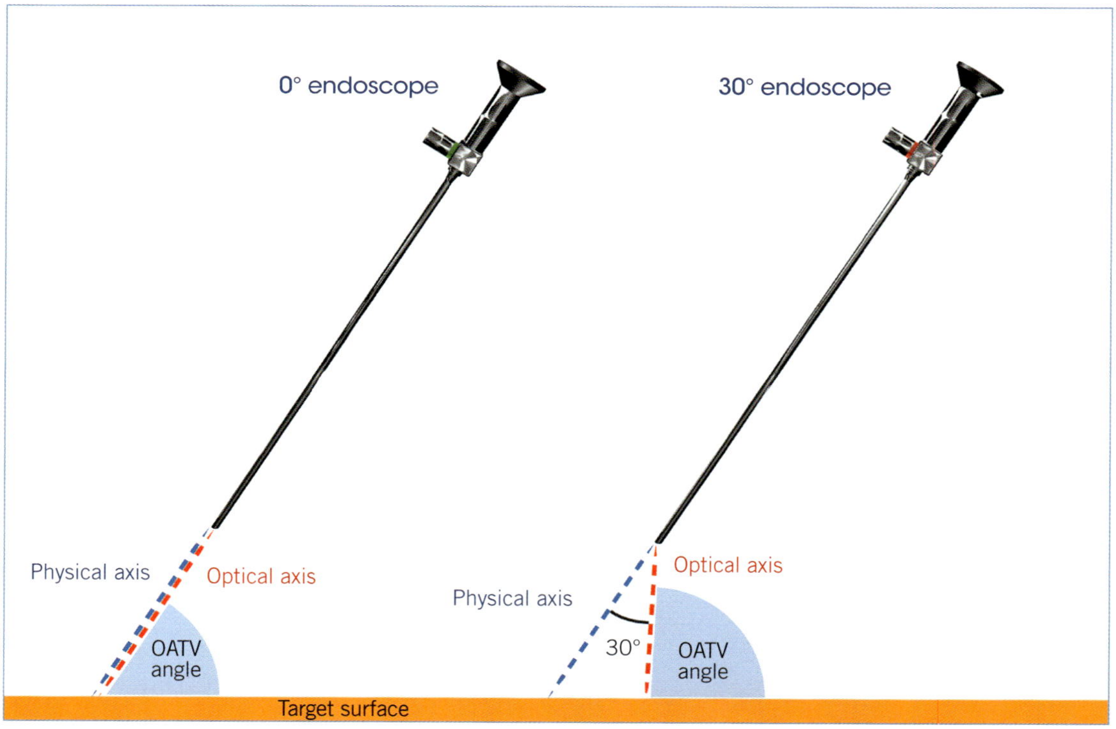

FIGURE 4. OATV angle of the endoscope. In the 0° endoscope, the physical axis coincides with the direction of view. In the 30° endoscope, an angle of 30° is formed between the axis and the direction of view, and the OATV angle is larger.

OPTIMAL POSITION OF OPERATIVE INSTRUMENTS (T2, T3)

Correct positioning of the instrument trocars is essential to maximize surgery efficiency and quality. The ideal position should respect the principles of ergonomics, with the arms close to the body and an elbow angle between 90° and 120°. As a general rule, the ports should all be oriented in the same direction to achieve a more natural manipulation of the instruments (first-order paradoxical movement). In this case, the displayed image of the instrument tip will move in the same direction as the actual tip (**Fig. 6**). On the contrary, the surgeon should avoid operating in the reverse alignment condition, as manipulation becomes difficult due to the paradoxical movements of the instrument tips. In this configuration, the instruments are aligned against the opposite direction of the camera, and the displayed image of the instrument tip will move in a direction opposite to that of the actual tip (second-order paradoxical movement); the up and down movements, however, remain in first-order paradox (**Fig. 7**). Surgeons should anyway be trained

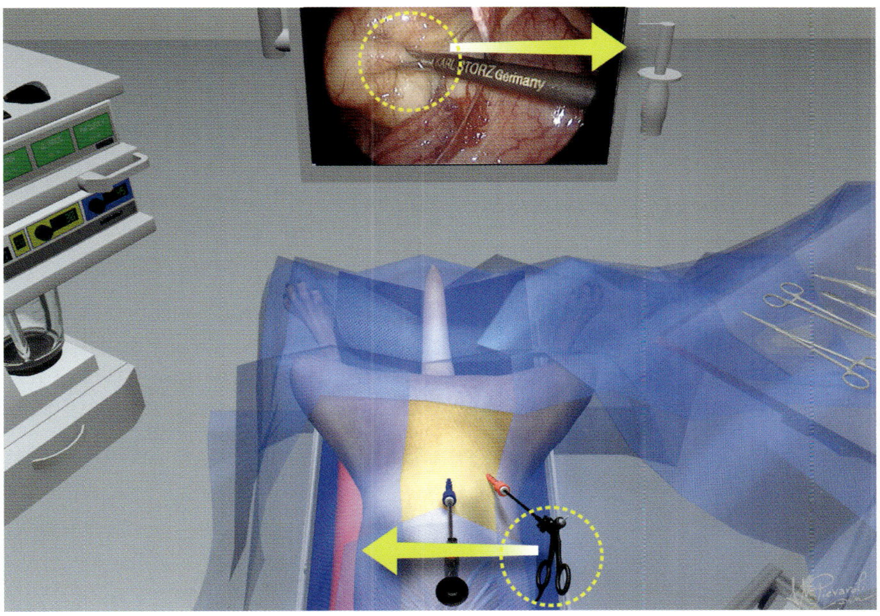

FIGURE 6. First-order paradoxical movement. The displayed image of the instrument tip moves in the same direction as the actual tip.

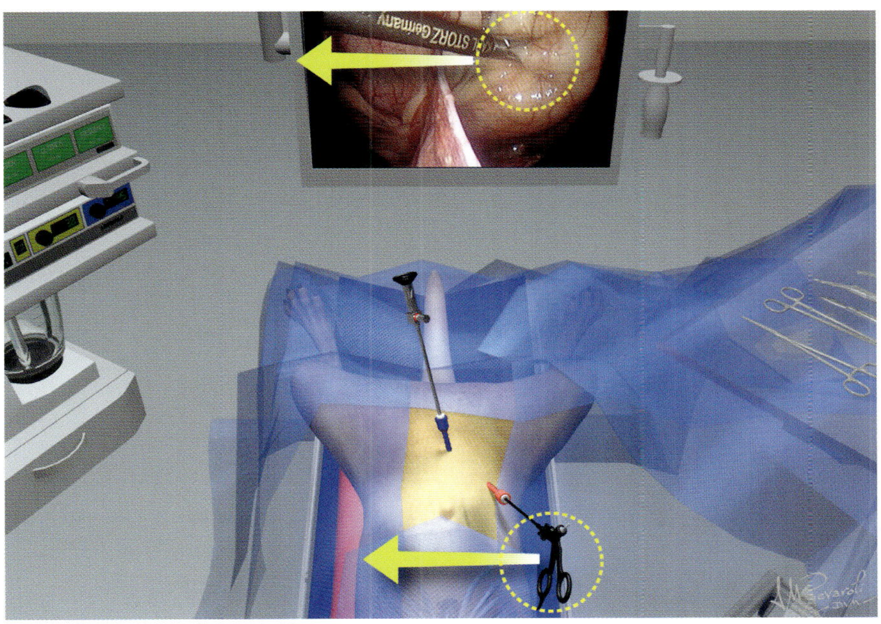

FIGURE 7. Second-order paradoxical movement. The displayed image of the instrument tip moves in a direction opposite to the actual tip. Up and down movements remain in first-order paradox.

to operate looking at an inverted mirror image because, in some particular conditions of the procedure, it could be necessary to change the position of the ports, switch the instruments with each other, or move to the other side of the operating table.

MANIPULATION ANGLE

The operating trocars (T2, T3) are positioned laterally to the optic trocar (T1) to reproduce the optimal relationship between the eyes and the hands of the surgeon. The distance between the two hands of the surgeon depends on the distance between T2 and T3. This distance affects the manipulation angle, defined as the angle between the two instruments (active and assisting). The maximal efficiency and quality performance of manipulating tissues, resecting tissues, and intracorporeal knotting are obtained with a manipulation angle ranging from 45° to 75°, with the ideal being 60°. Manipulation angles below 30° or above 90° are accompanied by increased difficulty and degraded performance (**Fig. 8**).

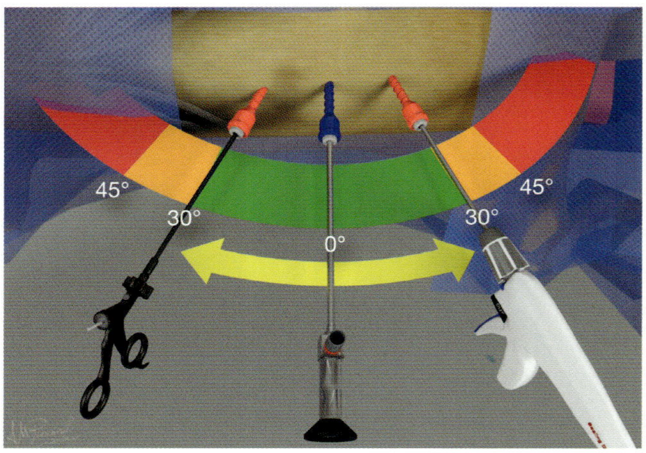

FIGURE 8. The manipulation angle of the working instruments should ideally be around 60°.

AZIMUTH ANGLE

The angle formed between the telescope axis and the operating instruments is called the azimuth angle. Improved task efficiency is achieved with equal rather than wide unequal azimuth angles on either side of the optical port (**Fig. 9**). In practice, however, it is not always possible to obtain the same azimuth angle, sometimes for anatomical reasons. If there is a large difference between the azimuth angles of the two working instruments, better performance can be achieved with an off-axis endoscopic viewing from the nondominant side (**Fig. 10**).

ELEVATION ANGLE

The elevation angle is the angle that the operating instruments form with the horizontal plane. This angle should range from 30° to 60° to manipulate the instruments comfortably. Values lower than 30° determine a too tangential position towards the target, while values greater than 60° determine a too vertical position (**Fig. 11**). A rule of thumb to ensure adequate task efficiency is that the elevation angle should be equal to the manipulation angle. In this case, the execution time and quality performance are optimal for dissecting tissues or knotting (**Fig. 12**).

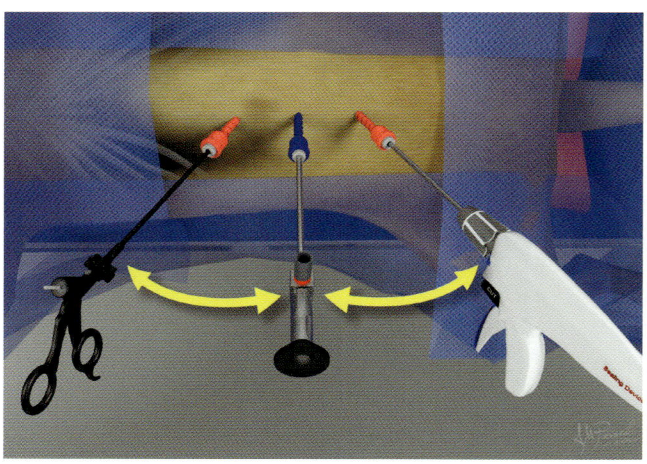

FIGURE 9. Azimuth angles between the telescope and working instruments. Ideally, they should be equal on both sides.

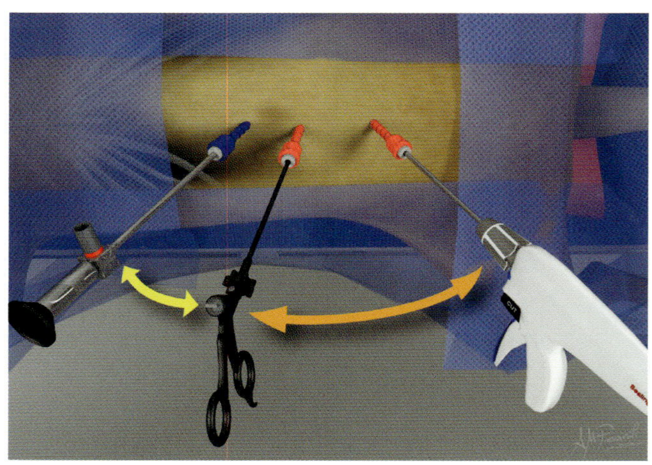

FIGURE 10. Off-axis viewing in case of wide azimuth angle inequality. Note that the telescope is placed in a lateral port and the working instrument is placed in the optical port.

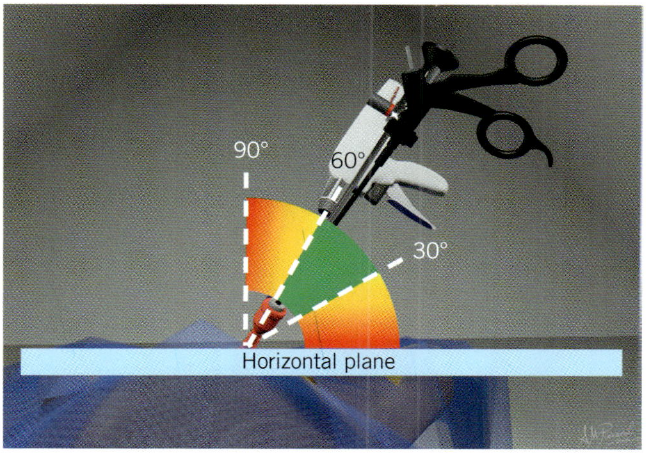

FIGURE 11. The elevation angle should range from 30° to 60°.

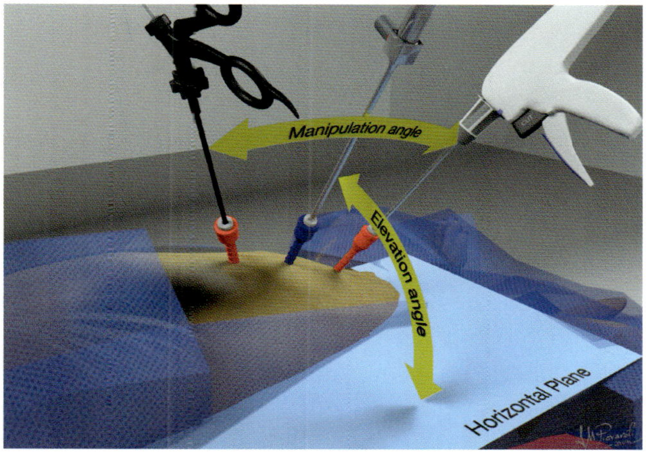

FIGURE 12. The best performance is achieved when the elevation angle is equal to the manipulation angle.

RELATIONSHIP BETWEEN THE ENDOSCOPE AND THE WORKING INSTRUMENTS

OPTICAL AXIS-TO-INSTRUMENT PLANE (OAIP) ANGLE

The OAIP angle is the angle between the optical axis of the endoscope and the instruments' plane. It determines how the instruments appear to enter the operative field and can be positive or negative depending on the most forward or rearward position of the working ports (T2, T3) with respect to the endoscope (T1) (**Fig. 13**). When the optical axis is above the instrumental plane, the instruments appear to enter the field from the lower sides of the monitor. Conversely, when the optical axis is below the instrumental plane, the instruments appear to enter the field from the upper sides of the monitor (**Fig. 14**). Best performance is obtained with a configuration of the endoscope viewing from above or the same plane as the instruments. An excessively backward or advanced position does not respect the principles of triangulation (**Fig. 15**). Generally, the rear position is used when the distance of the operating field is quite variable.

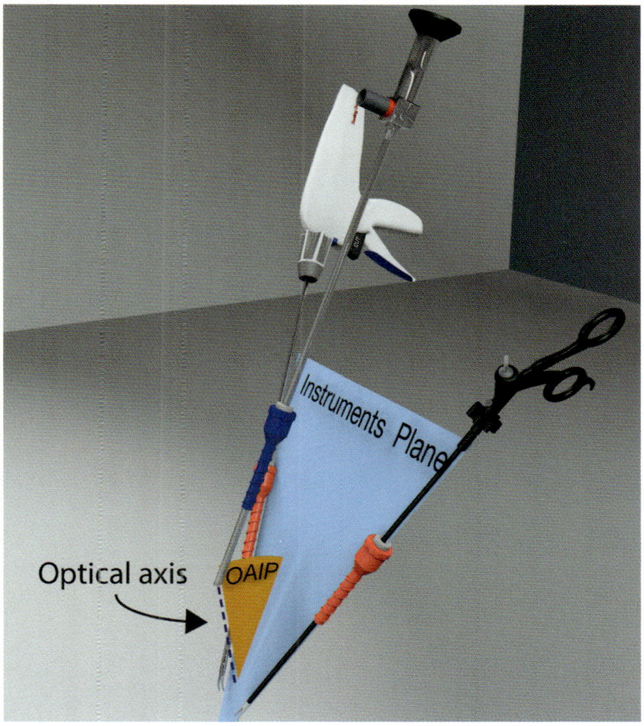

FIGURE 13. OAIP angle.

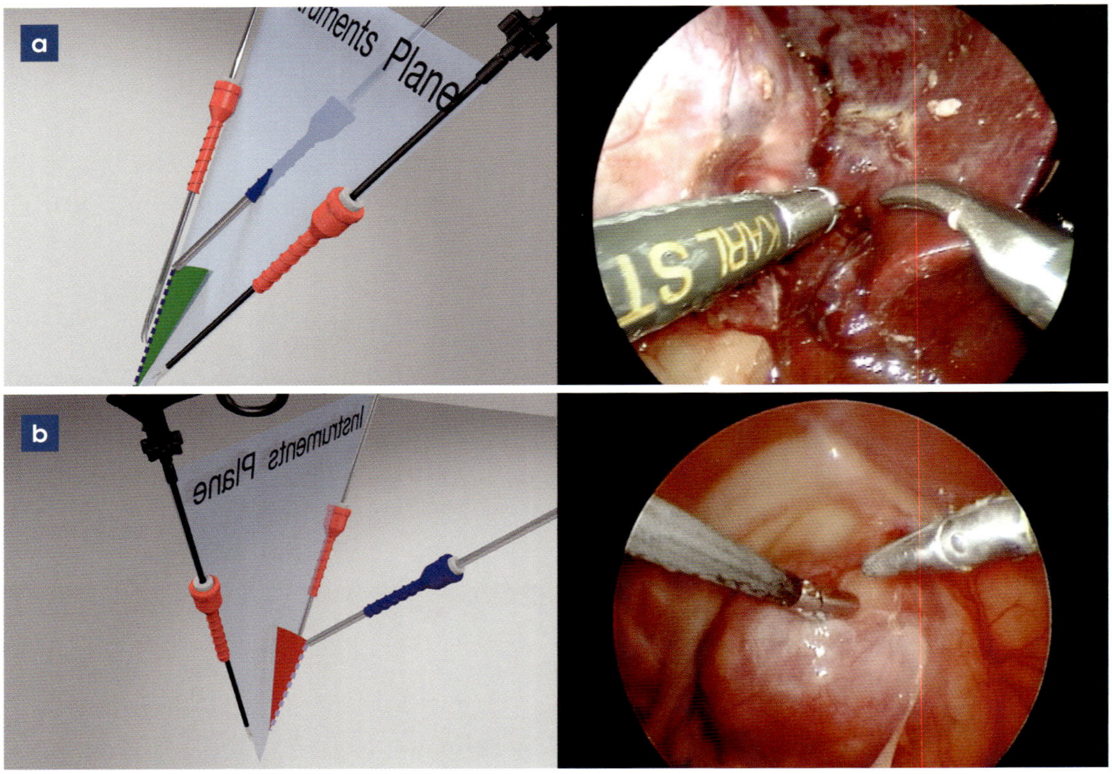

FIGURE 14. The OAIP angle determines the display of the instruments on the monitor. a) Ideally, the OAIP angle should be positive (green), as it is more natural. b) A negative OAIP angle (red) is counterintuitive.

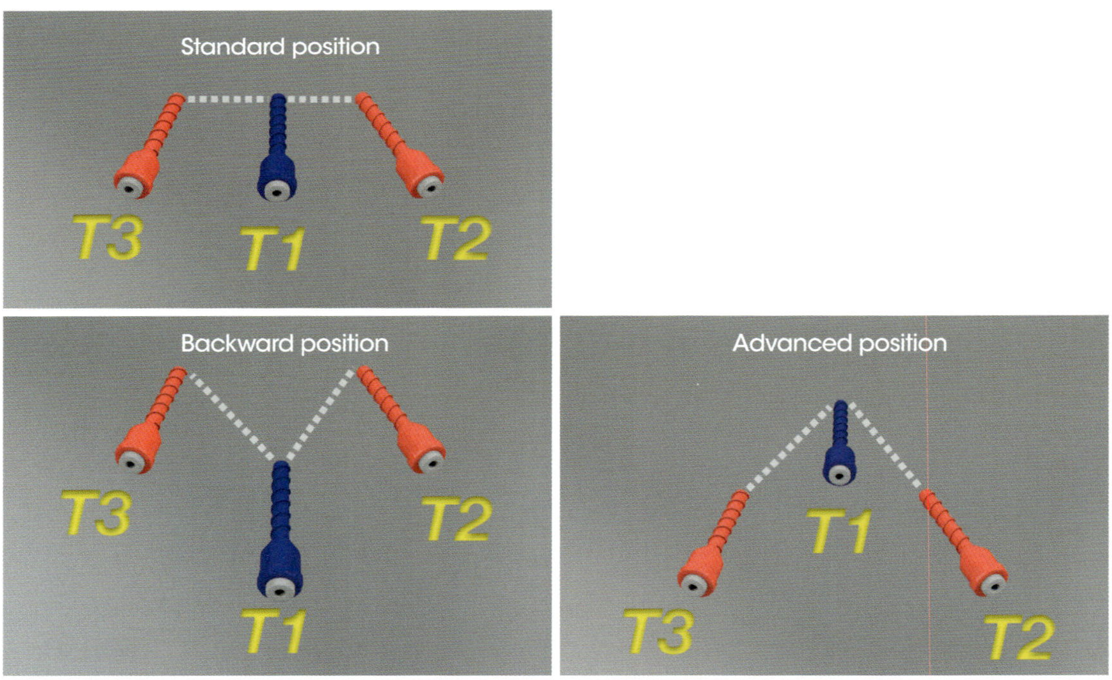

FIGURE 15. Optimal relationship between the endoscope and the working ports.

SUGGESTED READINGS

7 SINGLE-INCISION (SINGLE-PORT) LAPAROSCOPIC TECHNIQUE

Jeffrey J. Runge, Joshua G. Becker

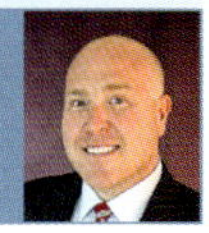

Benefits

- Reduced surgical time
- Decreased intraoperative complications
- Decreased postoperative pain
- Reduced incisional morbidity (e.g., splenic laceration)
- Incisional utility (i.e., common/consistent point of entry, improving familiarity of the approach and potentially reducing risks of complication)
- Increased owner satisfaction

Challenges

- A single surgical point of entry results in reduced working space, limited field of view, decreased exposure, altered principles of triangulation, and increased potential for instrument collision
- Although standard instruments can be used for single-port surgery, specific single-incision laparoscopic instruments and devices have been developed for this platform
- A learning curve is present

Single-incision laparoscopic surgery (SILS) is an operative platform that, as the name implies, enables laparoscopic surgery to be performed through a single surgical incision site. The nomenclature used throughout the published literature varies and can be confusing to follow, although the principle remains constant. Terms used to describe this platform include, but are not limited to, single-port surgery, reduced-port surgery, laparoendoscopic single-site surgery, and single-incision laparoscopic surgery.

The goal of the single-port operative platform is to further minimize minimally invasive surgery by reducing the overall number of laparoscopic ports needed to successfully execute a procedure. This operative approach has been described for both thoracic and abdominal procedures within the veterinary literature. Introduced in Philadelphia in 2008 by Curcillo et al., the platform was originally described for human abdominal procedures and later termed single-port access surgery. Curcillo's translational cross-pollinating collaboration with Runge et al. enabled the early adoption of the single-port access technique in small animal veterinary patients. This began the early introduction of many other veterinary single-port procedures globally.

There is a growing trend for human literature to illustrate the potential benefits of single-port over multiport laparoscopy, and in the last 10 years veterinary literature has been suggestive of the same, although this technology is still developing and further studies are needed to fully understand the potential benefits of the platforms. This chapter details the general approaches of single-port surgery and discusses techniques and preferred equipment for various operative procedures currently available.

Single-port procedures described in the literature

- Ovariectomy
- Ovariohysterectomy
- Cryptorchidectomy
- Intestinal surgery
- Organ biopsy
- Adrenalectomy
- Splenectomy
- Artificial urethral sphincter placement
- Gastropexy
- Cholecystectomy
- Ureteronephrectomy

The first use of separate instruments and ports through a single incision was described in 1997 by Navarra et al., when they published "One-wound laparoscopic cholecystectomy". A modification of that technique was done by Curcillo in 2008.

PRINCIPLES OF SINGLE-PORT SURGERY

The location of the incision, which becomes the single entry point for the operative procedure, is paramount. It needs to allow the surgeon to see the region of interest, allow for safe dissection, provide adequate working space for the instruments, enable tissue extraction, and ultimately safely and properly execute the operative procedure. This location often coincides with the region where multiport laparoscopic ports would be placed; however, it should be fluid and based on the surgeon's needs, the patient's size, and the requirements of the procedure. Although triangulation is a core concept in conventional multiport laparoscopy, this principle is significantly altered in single-port surgery, as having a single point of entry inherently negates the traditional principles of instrument triangulation. The close proximity of the instruments and optics reduces the surgical working space both intra-abdominally and extra-abdominally. This increases the technical complexity when compared to multiport procedures due to the deviation from traditional triangulation, a compromised field of view, decreased exposure, and frequent instrument collision. To overcome these challenges in single-port laparoscopy, angled optical telescopes and articulating instruments are used. This novel arrangement of both the optics and instruments creates more internal and external working space, effectively allowing for sufficient triangulation to occur. Although standard instrumentation can be used for single-port surgery, novel single-port instruments and entry devices have been proven to be superior for successful procedures.

INSTRUMENTATION

In order to mitigate the technical difficulties associated with triangulation and the use of using standard rigid instrumentation in single-port surgery, bent and articulating instruments have been developed. Nevertheless, single-port surgery is absolutely feasible using standard rigid instrumentation, and there is an extensive body of literature discussing this in both human and veterinary medicine. A wide variety of articulating and prebent laparoscopic instruments have been developed and are marketed specifically for the single-port platform. Bent or coaxial deviating instruments are fixed and specifically offset from the straight axis of a standard instrument in order to improve internal and external working spaces. This curved design provides acceptable intracorporeal triangulation and good ergonomic positioning of the hands. Articulating instruments have a design that mimics the movements of a surgeon's wrist and have a distal tip that can deflect relative to their shaft, offering seven degrees of freedom of movement (**Fig. 1**). Many of these instruments also offer axial 360° rotation for tip orientation similar to that of conventional rigid instruments. All of the articulating instruments can be introduced in both single-port devices and conventional rigid trocar–cannula assemblies. The double prebent instruments are intended to mimic triangulation via a curve at both ends of the instrument, leading to antipodal directions of the tips and handles when the instruments are held in parallel. The double-bent instruments can only be used with soft, flexible, or specifically designed entry devices for bent instruments because the bends in these instruments prevent their introduction into a rigid trocar–cannula assembly.

OPTICS

With the close proximity of the scopes and instruments in single-port surgery, adjustments are required to avoid instrument and optic interference; this is most easily accomplished through the use of an angled scope. The most common scope used for single-port laparoscopy in veterinary medicine is one with a 30° angle. To further reduce the external clashing of instruments with the light cable, a right-angle adaptor for the light cable can be used (**Fig. 2**). Recently, advanced laparoscopes geared specifically for single-port surgery have emerged, including a

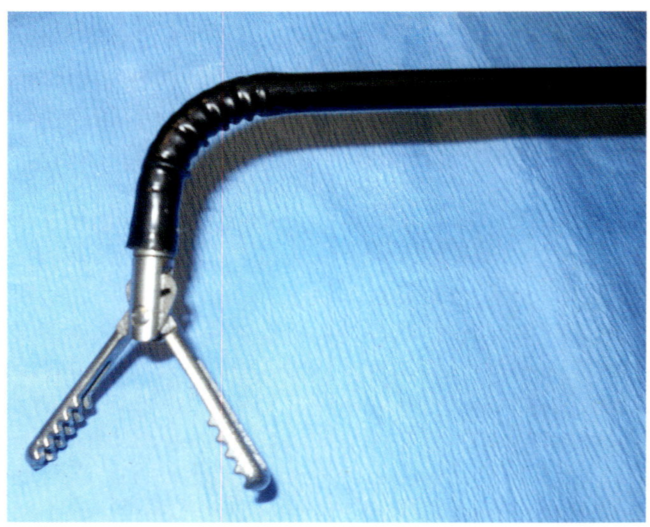

FIGURE 1. Articulating instrument (SILS Clinch).

traditional fixed-rod design that contains a rotating lens at the distal end (EndoCAMeleon, Karl Storz Endoscopy), or alternatively a design that uses the "chip on the tip" concept by placing an image processor at the distal tip of an articulating laparoscope (EndoEye, Olympus; Idealeye Stryker, Kalamazoo, MI). In veterinary single-port surgery, it has been shown that using either a 30° telescope or an advanced deflecting optic enables the telescope's camera head and tip to be directed away from the other instruments during the procedure, improving working space while simultaneously maintaining excellent visualization.

SINGLE-PORT ACCESS METHODS

SINGLE-PORT ACCESS

A single skin incision (most commonly at the umbilicus) enables separate individual fascial incisions to be made with traditional trocar–cannula assemblies through the abdominal wall (**Fig. 8**). Single-port access has also been adapted for paramedian, transvaginal, and retroperitoneal approaches. A recent systematic review assessing complications related to laparoscopic access found that complications were 11.7 times more likely with a paramedian approach compared to a ventral midline approach.

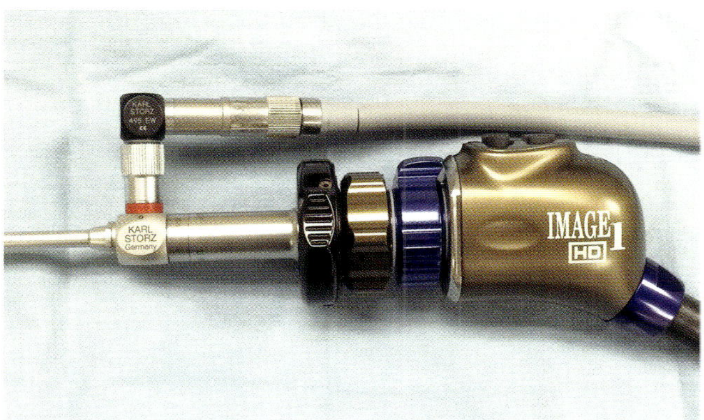

FIGURE 2. A right-angle adaptor placed onto the connection between the light cable and telescope can reduce interference between the light cable and instruments during single-port surgery.

COMMERCIALLY AVAILABLE SINGLE-PORT DEVICES

Commercially available single-port access devices have been specifically manufactured for single-port surgery and are intended to be inserted through a single full-thickness abdominal incision. They can have multiple 5 to 12 mm access channels to enable an array of instrumentation to enter into the abdominal cavity. Commonly, the SILS port is utilized in veterinary single-port procedures.

OPERATIVE LAPAROSCOPY AND ADVANCED OPERATIVE LAPAROSCOPY

This method utilizes a traditional simple operative laparoscope with a 5 mm working channel through which instruments can be passed (**Fig. 3**). Advanced laparoscopy includes a triangulating operating platform, such as the Spider surgical system (TransEnterix Surgical, Durham, NC), which provides the surgeon with multiple independent flexible arms that can be extended through a rigid operating laparoscope shaft. Purists do not consider operating laparoscopy under the same family as single-port laparoscopy.

EQUIPMENT-SPECIFIC ACCESS METHODS

The devices and equipment used for single-port surgery can be broadly classified as follows:

A. Specifically manufactured devices for single-port surgery

B. Standard instruments and trocar–cannula assemblies used for conventional laparoscopy inserted through one skin incision

C. Innovative adoptions of existing equipment not primarily intended for laparoscopy

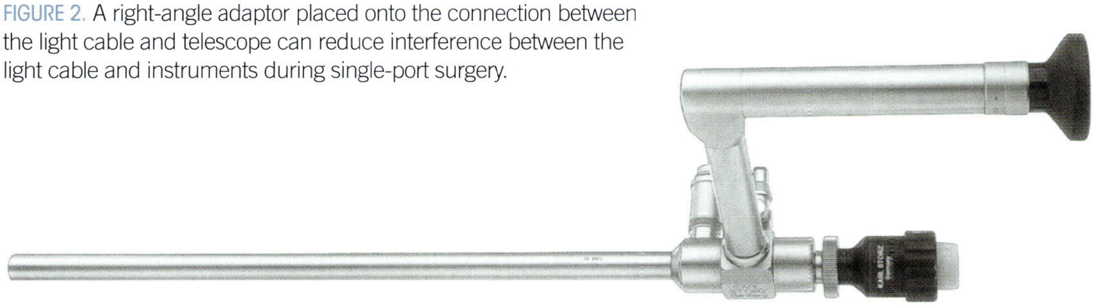

FIGURE 3. This operating laparoscope (Karl Storz Endoscopy, Goleta, CA) incorporates a 5 mm working channel through which 5 mm rigid instrumentation can be passed. Image courtesy of Karl Storz GmbH & Co. KG.

A INSERTION TECHNIQUES FOR SPECIFICALLY MANUFACTURED SINGLE-PORT DEVICES

Device

GelPOINT Access System (Applied Medical, Rancho Santa Margarita, CA) (**Fig. 4**)

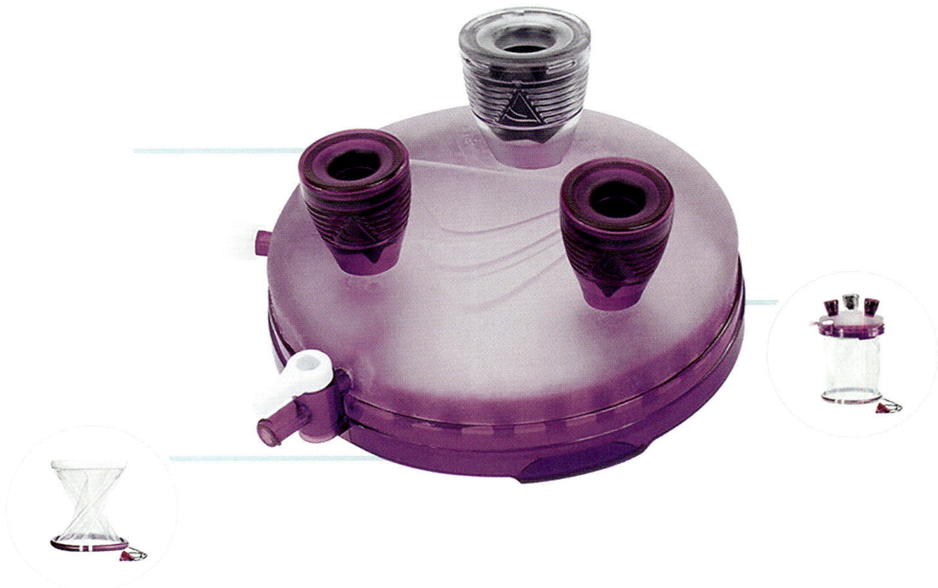

FIGURE 4. GelPOINT Access System. Image courtesy of Applied Medical Resources Corporation.

PROCEDURE

- A 2 to 7 cm minilaparotomy incision is created in advance for insertion of the port.
- This single-port device consists of a wound retractor, GelSeal cap, and four 5 to 10 mm cannulas. The wound retractor portion of this port provides 360° atraumatic retraction of an abdominal incision 2 to 7 cm in length.
- The wound retractor portion is required to be inserted initially by passing the inner flexible ring through the abdominal incision.
- The outer ring is then rolled until it reaches the incision, causing radial retraction.
- The cannulas are inserted through the GelSeal cap, and the GelSeal cap is then fitted to the outer ring of the wound retractor.
- The insufflator tubing is then attached, and the abdomen is insufflated to 8 to 10 mmHg with carbon dioxide using a pressure-regulating mechanical insufflator.

Key points

- The wound retractor sleeve is able to accommodate the widest range of body wall thicknesses compared with other single-port devices.
- The wound retractor portion can accommodate a 7 cm incision, which allows for large tissue removal.
- The GelSeal cap can be removed and reattached repeatedly during the procedure without compromising the ability to reinsufflate the abdomen.

Device

SILS Port (Covidien) (**Figs. 5 and 6**)

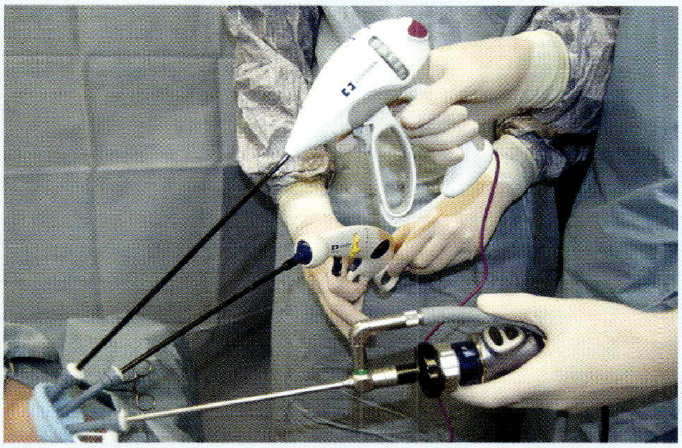

FIGURE 5. The SILS Port (Medtronic, Mansfield, MA) allows the placement of three cannulas and has a separate carbon dioxide insufflation port.

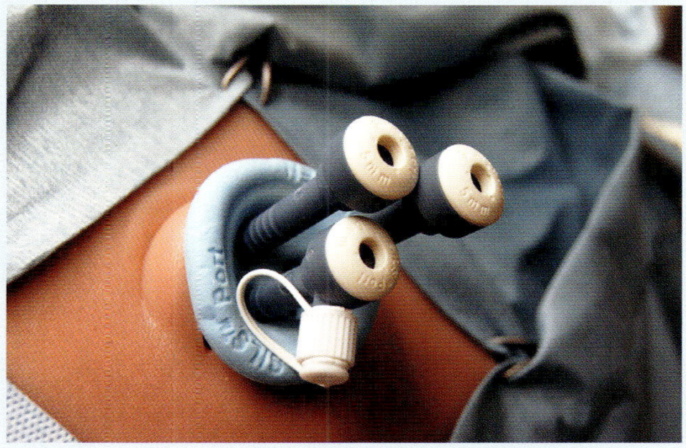

FIGURE 6. With the SILS Port (Medtronic, Mansfield, MA), it is recommended to stagger the cannulas to minimize interference.

PROCEDURE

- A 2 to 3 cm minilaparotomy is created in advance for insertion of the port.
- A small amount of sterile lubricant is applied to the soft base of the single-port device before insertion.
- The port is inserted into the abdominal incision by clamping two curved Rochester Carmalt forceps at the base in a staggered fashion. Varying techniques have been described for insertion into the incision: it can be performed without abdominal wall countertraction or with a form of countertraction such as grasping the fascial edges with two large rat-toothed tissue forceps, Army-Navy retractors, or stay sutures. Regardless of traction, the tips of the Rochester Carmalt forceps are directed into the incision in a cranial direction toward the diaphragm or away from any underlying viscera.
- When the base is seeded within the incision, the clamps are released to allow the bottom portion of the port to expand and fit snugly within the incision.
- Three 5 mm cannulas (supplied with the port) are then inserted into the three inner cylinders with the aid of a 5 mm blunt obturator. The SILS port is also supplied with a 12 to 15 mm trocar–cannula assembly to allow for larger instruments to be inserted with two other 5 mm cannulas. The heights of the cannulas are staggered to minimize cannula contact (**Fig. 6**).
- Insufflator tubing is then attached, and the abdomen is insufflated to 8 to 10 mmHg with carbon dioxide using a pressure-regulating mechanical insufflator.

Key points

- The multitrocar port can be positioned to have the three 5 mm cannulas at the 12, 4, and 8 o'clock positions relative to the surgical site, although any arrangement is possible.
- There is relative ease of insertion and reinsertion during a procedure.
- Fits snugly within the incision, preventing loss of pneumoperitoneum.
- Despite being sold as single-use instruments, it is not uncommon to reuse various minimally invasive surgery devices in veterinary medicine due to economic reasons. Multiple studies have been conducted to test the reusability of SILS devices. Results indicate that the ports can be decontaminated and sterilized by ethylene oxide and hydrogen peroxide vapor for repeated use. In one study, the foam component was found to have positive light growth after eight uses. The reuse of SILS ports appears to carry a low risk of infection to the patient; however, the mechanical stability of the ports after reuse has yet to be widely tested.

Device

TriPort System (Olympus) (**Fig. 7**)

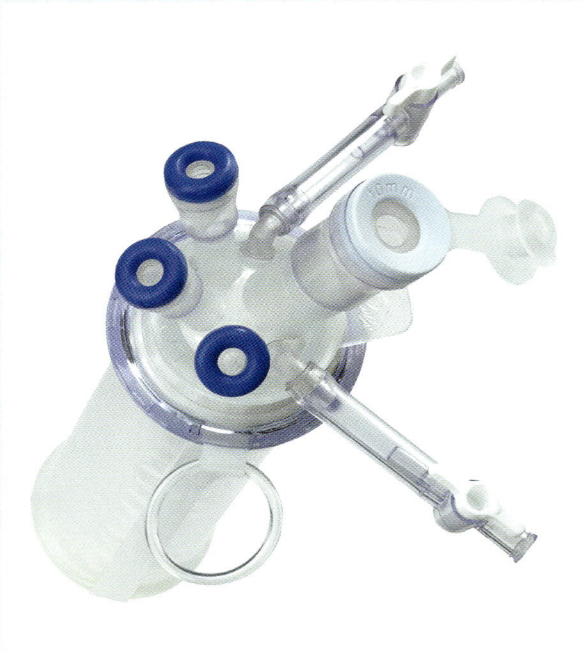

FIGURE 7. TriPort System. Image courtesy of Olympus America.

PROCEDURE

- A 1.5 to 2 cm minilaparotomy is created in advance for insertion of the port.
- This single-port device is inserted into the abdominal incision by directing the internal ring of the wound retractor through the incision. A small amount of sterile lubricant can be applied to the inner retractor ring to aid in the insertion.
- The inner ring is released from the supplied introducer within the incision to the abdominal cavity.
- The ring is then adjusted to sit just on the inside of the incision.
- The transparent sleeve attached to the inner ring is pulled up and away from the patient while the outer ring is simultaneously pushed down toward the incision.
- The inner and outer rings are firmly pushed together while the plastic sleeve is pulled to ensure the rings are tight against the abdominal wall.
- The excess transparent plastic sleeve is cut, allowing 1 to 2 cm of excess to be folded into the incision.
- The soft plastic trocar cap is then firmly fitted to the outer ring.
- The insufflator tubing is then attached, and the abdomen is insufflated to 8 to 10 mmHg with carbon dioxide using a pressure-regulating mechanical insufflator.

Key points

- The wound retractor sleeve is able to accommodate a wide range of body wall thicknesses, up to 10 cm.
- The soft outer cap can be removed and reattached repeatedly during the procedure to allow for tissue extraction without compromising the ability to reinsufflate the abdomen.

B INSERTION TECHNIQUE OF STANDARD TROCARS FOR SINGLE-PORT ENTRY (FIG. 8)

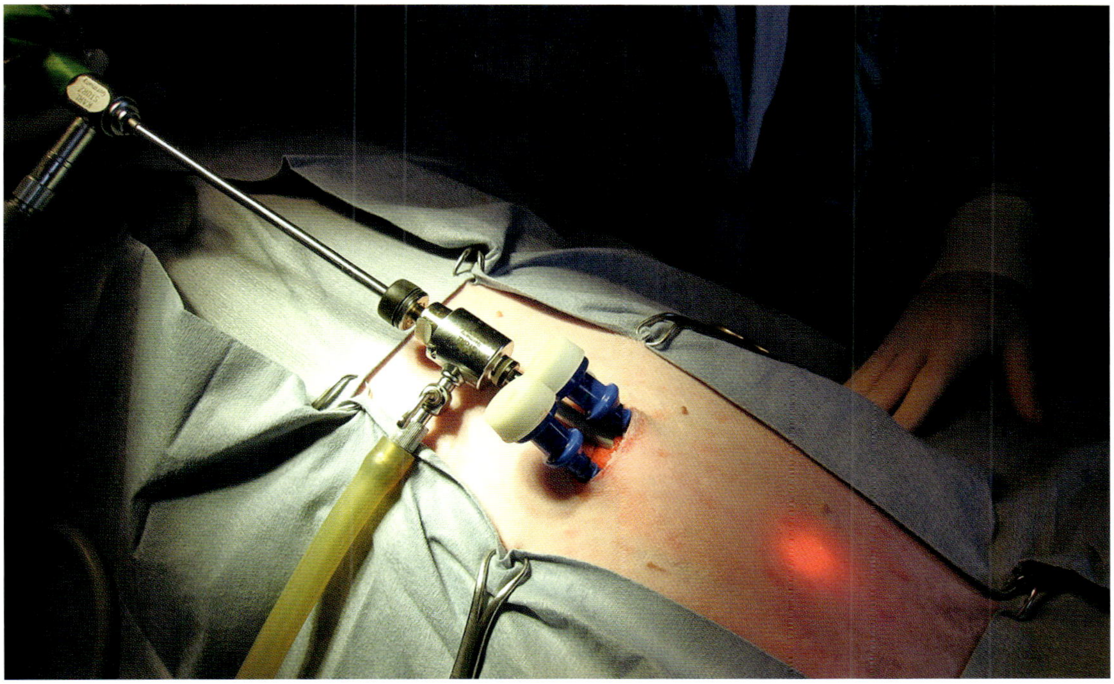

FIGURE 8. Single-port access laparoscopy performed by the passage of three separate cannulas through one skin incision but separate fascial incisions.

PROCEDURE

- A 1.5 to 2 cm skin incision is made on the ventral midline in the region of the umbilicus.
- Using the modified Hasson abdominal access technique a 5 mm blunt laparoscopic low-profile trocar–cannula assembly is inserted into the abdomen.
- The abdomen is insufflated using a pressure-regulating mechanical insufflator to an intra-abdominal pressure between 9 and 12 mmHg.
- After a brief abdominal exploration with a 30° telescope, two additional very-low-profile 5 mm trocar–cannula assemblies are inserted in a triangular pattern adjacent to the initial port.
- For the second and third low-profile trocar–cannula insertions, the abdomen is partially deflated to approximately 6 to 8 mmHg to facilitate mobilization of the skin and soft tissue associated with the initial skin incision and to enable a small soft tissue flap to be created, which allows for tunneling of the ports adjacent to the initial trocar.
- Using minimal blunt dissection, a tunnel is undermined 1 to 2 cm laterally and caudally on either side of the initial 5 mm trocar–cannula assembly using a Kelly hemostat.
- Through these tunneled paths, the two low-profile trocar–cannula assemblies are inserted through the abdominal wall into the peritoneal cavity using the sharp trocars under optical visualization.
- The three trocars are arranged in a deliberate triangular arrangement that causes the skin to stretch in a lateral direction. Via a sing 2 cm skin incision, this arrangement enables each low-profile cannula to enter the abdomen through separate fascial openings.

Key points

- Existing standard metal and reusable trocar–cannula assemblies can be used, avoiding the cost associated with purchasing disposable equipment.

C INNOVATIVE ADAPTATIONS OF EXISTING EQUIPMENT

Device

Wound retractor with latex glove and finger ports (**Fig. 9**)

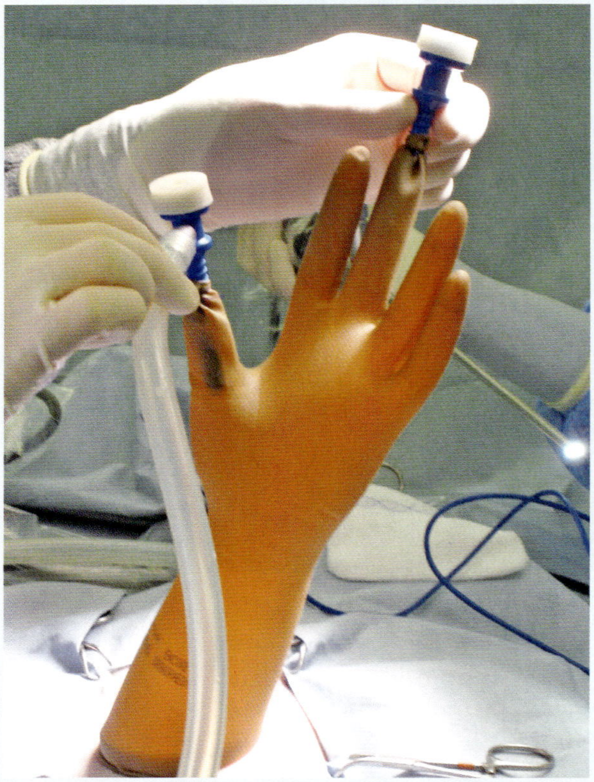

FIGURE 9. A wound retractor with latex glove and finger ports can be used as an inexpensive single-port device.

PROCEDURE

- A 2 to 3 cm minilaparotomy incision is created in advance for insertion of the port.
- The inner ring of a 360° atraumatic wound retraction device (Alexis Wound Retractor, Applied Medical; or SurgiSleeve Wound Protector, Covidien) is first inserted through the minilaparotomy incision (**Fig. 10**).
- The outer ring of the wound retractor is rolled until it reaches the level of the skin, causing the retractor sheath to be pulled taut.
- The tips of the fingers of a sterile latex glove are cut to just allow a 5 to 10 mm trocar–cannula assembly to be inserted.
- Suture or rubber bands created from strips cut from the surgical glove finger are tied securely around the trocar–cannula assembly at the junction of the latex fingertip and the port.
- The wrist portion of the glove is then stretched over the external ring of the wound retractor.
- The insufflator tubing is attached to any of the finger port Luer-lock fittings, and then insufflation of carbon dioxide to an intra-abdominal pressure of 8 to 10 mmHg is performed using a pressure-regulating mechanical insufflator.

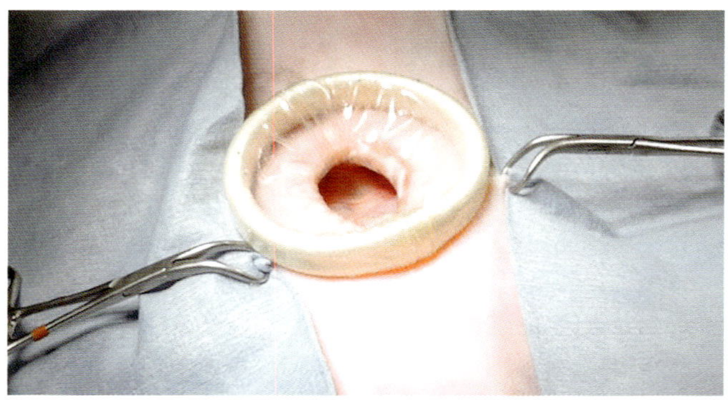

FIGURE 10. This wound retractor (Alexis, Applied Medical, Rancho Santa Margarita, CA) provides a protected retracted access incision through which organs can be exteriorized.

Key points

- All five glove fingers can be used as ports of entry if necessary.
- This technique has been recently published for use in dogs undergoing ovariohysterectomy.

SUGGESTED READINGS

8 LAPAROSCOPIC INTRACORPOREAL AND EXTRACORPOREAL SUTURING

M. A. Sánchez Hurtado, J. Gutiérrez del Sol, F. J. Pérez Duarte

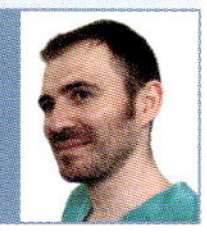

In veterinary medicine, laparoscopic and thoracoscopic surgery have evolved from the performance of basic diagnostic procedures to others involving more demanding maneuvers. Unlike in conventional surgery, laparoscopic suturing (LS) and knot tying are skills that cannot be extrapolated directly, which is why they can be frustrating, time-consuming, and associated with a long learning curve. Although LS virtually replicates the steps of traditional suturing, there are some specific differences due to the inherent limits of the method. This chapter aims to provide veterinarians with general and thorough ideas and recommendations from a practical point of view, as there is no single procedure that will suffice for every case due to the different port placement sites, types of instruments and knots (intracorporeal vs. extracorporeal), and devices (commercial systems vs. traditional suture thread). On the other hand, the concept of repeated and standardized practice with simulators or experimental animal models is the most accepted methodology to reduce the learning curve.

As in human medicine, veterinarians have combined efforts to implement and standardize LS for the benefit of our patients. Hence, we can observe the evolution of sentences of references on laparoscopic gastropexy from "Gastropexy sutures were placed, tied, and knotted extracorporeally to simplify the procedure and avoid laparoscopic suturing which can be time-consuming" or "In our study, extra- and intracorporeal suturing tasks were excluded because these skills are still relatively infrequently performed in clinical small animal surgery. Therefore, we believed that they would not represent the clinical surgical experience of our study participants" to others available in 2009 and 2010 in which intracorporeal suturing is already discussed in veterinary simulation papers or standardized for pure laparoscopic gastropexy with barbed suture.

Finally, it should be pointed out that, depending on the source consulted, there are numerous types of knots, tips and tricks for their configuration, unstandardized terminology, and port and instrument combinations. This is why this chapter cannot discuss all of them and, instead, it compiles the authors' personal experience in LS and other commonly described recommendations found in the vast bibliography.

The pioneers in developing and improving laparoscopic suturing instruments and methods were Semm et al. and Clarke et al. in the 1970s. In veterinary medicine, laparoscopic knot tying seems to have been described first in the mid-1990s by Ragle et al. in horses.

Clinical applications of LS in veterinary medicine are constantly evolving. **Table 1** lists some procedures using LS that have been described in the literature.

TABLE 1. Described surgical procedures involving laparoscopic suturing

Thoracoscopy	Laparoscopy
■ Thoracic duct ligation ■ Peritoneopericardial diaphragmatic hernia ■ Retraction suture for ligamentum arteriosum elevation prior to clipping or bipolar sealing ■ Repair of small pulmonary air leaks and bleedings ■ Repair of small local defects in esophagus or trachea	■ Ovarian pedicle and uterine horn ligation (spay) ■ Colopexy, gastropexy, cystopexy, and colposuspension ■ Cystotomy closure for uroliths ■ Ureterotomy and ureteral reimplantation ■ Gastrotomy and enterotomy closure ■ Artificial urinary sphincter (AUS) fixation ■ Duct and vascular pedicle ligation either with extracorporeal or intracorporeal suturing: cystic duct, ureter, renal artery and vein, orchidectomy, biopsies (pancreas, intestine) ■ Duct and vascular pedicle retraction suture for elevation prior to clipping or bipolar sealing ■ Inguinal ring closure for small hernia repair ■ Transanal minimally invasive surgery (TAMIS) for polyp removal

ERGONOMICS

Unlike in conventional suturing, laparoscopic intracorporeal suturing (LIS) and laparoscopic extracorporeal suturing (LES) are greatly influenced by factors intrinsic and extrinsic to the surgeon. Especially in LIS, it is important that the operating table permits the change of position, the arrangement of the modules of the laparoscopic tower, the placement of the trocars, and a choreographed knotting technique. The surgeon's position should be as ergonomic as possible; otherwise, fatigue can lead to increased surgical times and mistakes, as well as musculoskeletal injuries in all the surgical team. The table should be at an appropriate height, and the surgeon should adopt a comfortable general posture for the different angles of the elbow, wrist, and neck. The variability in patient size and intraoperative maneuvers makes it desirable that the operating table has an up/down and a tilting rotation/lateralization system or, alternatively, that the surgeon and assistant use any step or footrest to achieve the optimal position. Likewise, it is recommended that the main monitor be in front of the surgeon at eye level. The most natural and ergonomic way to perform LS and to avoid paradoxical movements is to aim for an aligned frontal, coaxial arrangement, in which the surgeon and assistant, the trocars, the suturing space in the operating field, and the monitor form a straight line. This is also known as SCOPe alignment (surgeon, camera, organ, and picture). It is also recommended that the assistant be provided with an auxiliary monitor under the same conditions.

Setting an adequate number and position of the trocars will lead to a comfortable handling of tissues, placement of the needle and thread, and passage of the needle through the tissue and final knotting. In addition, adequate training of the surgical team in simulation is essential in order to efficiently perform all the suturing steps. Good triangulation of the trocars is desirable. For this, the scope should be placed in the center, with the trocars for the instruments contralateral, that is, on each side of the central trocar (**Fig. 1a**). Depending on the surgeon, the trocars can form a U shape, a semicircle, a triangle, or a line, but the visualization port should always be in the center and the instrument ports on each side. The linear configuration is a comfortable trocar placement used in veterinary medicine, for example, during the typical three-trocar midline arrangement for genitourinary laparoscopy.

The effective working area of the instruments is known as target organ or home base (**Fig. 1b**). To work comfortably, in many procedures the optical port is placed about 10 cm from the home base, and the two working ports are placed in the same 10 cm circumferential arc on either side of the optical port. This allows an ideal angle of manipulation of the working instruments of around 60°–90°. The azimuth angle (between the telescope and the working instrument) should ideally be equal on both sides (30°–45°). If necessary, additional assistant ports can be placed on the same arc. Also, ideally 50% of the needle holder shaft should be inside the patient.

The distance between the working ports should be chosen according to the intracorporeal length of the instruments to create an appropriate angle to the home base. If the intracorporeal instrument length is short or if there is too much distance between the working ports, there would be an obtuse angle between the instruments, which makes maneuvering technically difficult. This situation can be seen in the case of continuous sutures, such as those used in pure laparoscopic gastropexy. If the distance has not been properly calculated, as the suture progresses toward the trocars, the maneuvers can become difficult to perform. Therefore, a greater, but not excessive, separation between the working ports is preferable whenever possible, as this will result in a greater intracorporeal instrument path.

On the other hand, depending on the procedure and the target organ, there may be noncoaxial, ipsilateral, or sectorization variants (**Fig. 1c**), in which the optic is placed laterally to the working trocars and lateral to the home base. As there is no triangulation in these cases, LIS is more complicated. Thus, noncoaxial/ipsilateral configurations can be found more frequently in cases of extracorporeal looped lung or pancreatic biopsies, or for the introduction of staplers or retrieval bags when only one 10 or 12 mm port is available. Although LIS is not required in these cases, at certain times it may be necessary to introduce the optic laterally to the working trocars to facilitate optimal ergonomic manipulation.

LIS is facilitated when the surgeon's posture is ergonomically correct. This is achieved when the angle between the arm and the forearm is 90°–120°. It should be taken into account that sometimes the trocars and instruments can be elevated or lowered because of the patient's size, the abdominal wall distension due to the pneumoperitoneum, and the Trendelenburg and reversed Trendelenburg positions, thereby preventing such ideal angle.

INSTRUMENTS AND EQUIPMENT

The instruments can range from the standard 5, 10, or 12 mm to a smaller of about 3 mm (needlescopic).

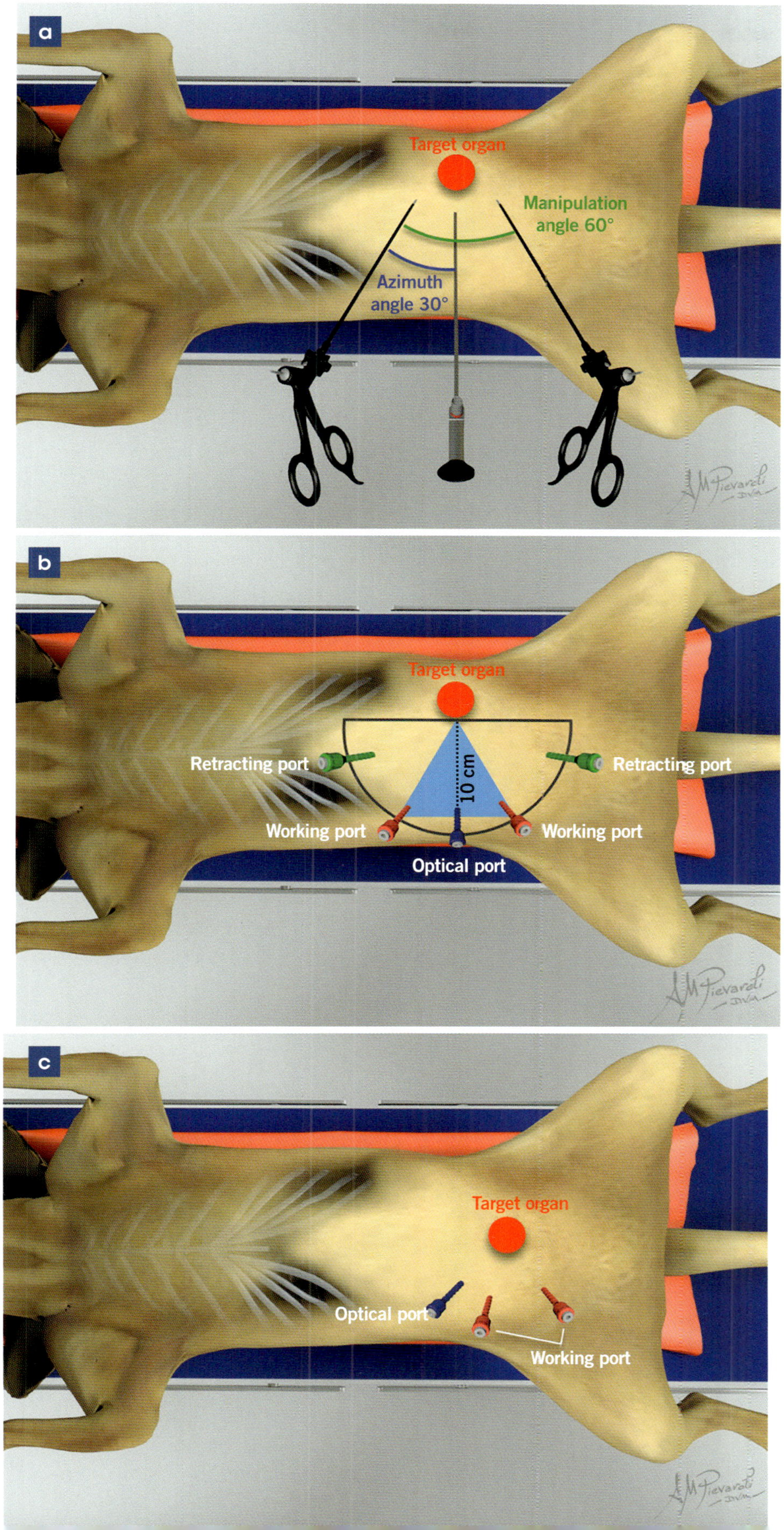

FIGURE 1. Optimal angles for contralateral a) three-port and b) five-port triangulation. c) Ipsilateral sectorization.

TROCARS (FIG. 2)

Needles are more easily inserted and withdrawn through 10–12 mm trocars. Therefore, if possible, it is recommended to use 10–12 mm ports with reducer systems or those with a special valve that also allows 5 mm instruments. Thus, it is easier to pass the needle through, and this larger port is normally the one used for the optic. Also, the size of the needle is important concerning the trocar diameter and its type of valves for the needle not to remain impacted inside either the cannula or the valves.

In veterinary medicine, good fixation of the trocar cannula is key to avoid constant leaks and emphysema, since the abdominal and thoracic walls of animals offer less resistance than those of people, as can be seen in the references taken from human pediatrics. In our field, as in human pediatrics, low-weight and low-profile trocars (nonbulky head) are preferred. Therefore, it is likely that reusable and smooth-walled trocars may need to be fixed to the wall with stitches, although there are wall-threaded reusable trocars that provide a very good fixation and a very secure twist-in insertion method. Finally, there are special designs that allow stable fixation of the trocar core sheath at the desired point, avoiding unnecessary movements during the operation. In particular, some disposable trocars have an inflatable balloon (Hasson trocar) or a ring anchor in the cannula itself.

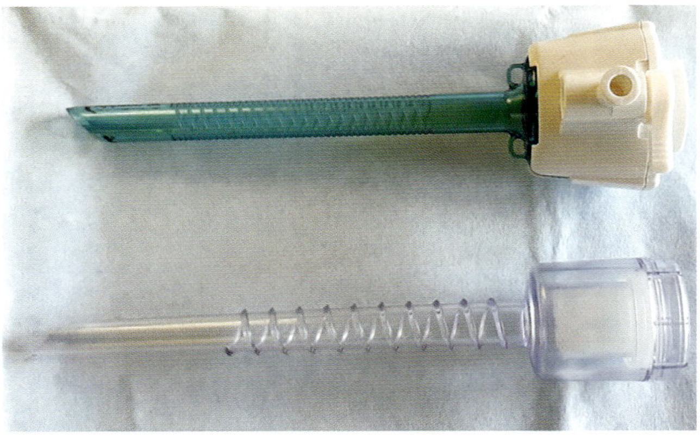

FIGURE 2. Trocars: single-use, low-profile threaded 5 mm.

NEEDLE HOLDERS (FIG. 3)

Needle holders (NHs), or needle drivers, are the most important instruments for LS because they carry out the entire process of needle transportation and tie the intracorporeal knot. An ideal NH should be ergonomic and light, with a stable needle grip, a firm handle grip, and a friendly ratchet locking mechanism. Different designs of the handle (curved, straight), the location of the opening and closing ratchet (central, right, left), and the action and curvature of the jaws (straight or curved, single or double) are available. Some NHs are capable of straightening the needle, but they only allow a fixed angle of impact on the tissue to be sutured of 90°.

An additional NH in the contralateral nondominant hand (NDH) will help the NH of the dominant hand (DH) to complete the suturing procedure, allowing stable control of the needle.

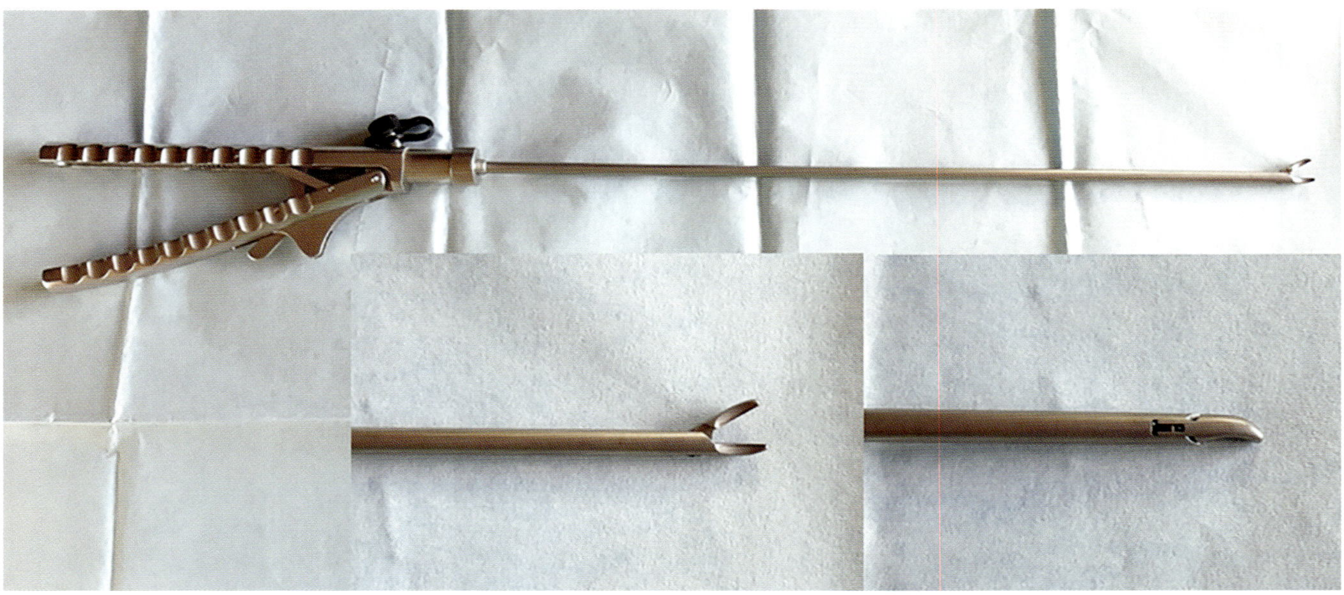

FIGURE 3. Needle holder: straight handle and curved tip (left-hand instrument).

Flat atraumatic jaws are preferred for securing grasping of sutures and tissues.

The authors remark that the orientation of the jaws of curved laparoscopic NHs plays a key role in LS. Although a straight tip is more versatile, to be used for right- and left-handed stitches, a curved tip allows for a better visualization while grasping the needle and facilitates loop creation. Both tips of a right- or left-handed curved NH must point medially (a right-handed NH tip points to the left, and a left-handed NH tip points to the right).

KNOT PUSHERS (FIG. 4)

A knot pusher is an instrument used to push down a previously tied extracorporeal knot through the trocar cannula into the abdominal cavity. There are different knot pushers depending on the type of knot they advance: simple half hitches stacked upon each other or compound knots like the Roeder knot. Alternatively, Babcock forceps, a NH, or atraumatic forceps can also be used.

The most commonly used knot pusher devices have an elongated body and a straight or curved tip, with a groove along the length of the tip (open loop or closed jaw/push rod). Other knot pushers have grooves in both jaws, like the Babcock forceps, but they work on the same principle as the rod type.

DISSECTORS AND GRASPING FORCEPS (FIG. 5)

Dissectors or grasping forceps may be used when an assistant NH is not required in the contralateral NDH. Traditionally, a dissector, either curved (Maryland type) or straight, is usually used, as its fine tip and rotating system facilitate the delicate grasping of the thread and the knotting maneuver. It is also possible to use grasping forceps (fenestrated or not), which should be as atraumatic as possible so as not to damage the thread. Its jaws should ideally be single hinged and without groove marks that are likely to entrap the suture. Also, when possible, any ancillary double-action instrument with exposed hinges should be avoided in LS. The authors do not recommend the use of right-angled (90°) dissectors for LIS, as they are only efficient at the extreme point of the jaws and may lead to too many inefficient attempts to grasp the thread and needle.

SCISSORS (FIG. 6)

The most commonly used scissors are those with a straight or curved Metzenbaum blade. Ideally, the scissors used to cut the suture material should not be the same as those used for dissection, because they lose cutting performance.

VISUALIZATION AND IMAGING SYSTEMS

The two-dimensionality of the image obtained from most laparoscopic imaging systems results in a lack of depth perception. Besides, fine movements using long handled instruments, limitations in the working field, and limited visualization make LS and knot tying difficult tasks. With sufficient training, it is possible to perform high-quality suturing on any standard 2D laparoscopic tower with a home monitor. But the higher the image quality, the

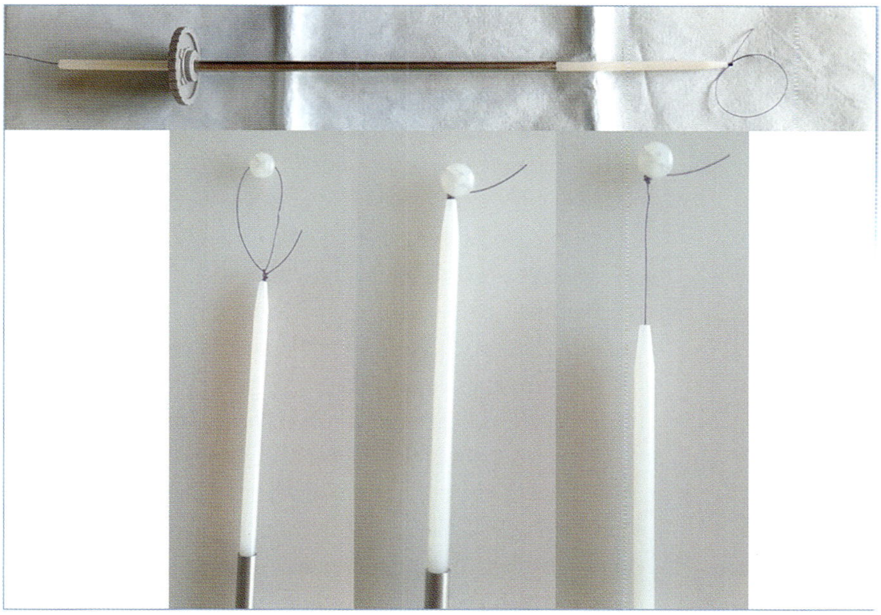

FIGURE 4. Knot pusher: closed tip with a self-made Roeder knot.

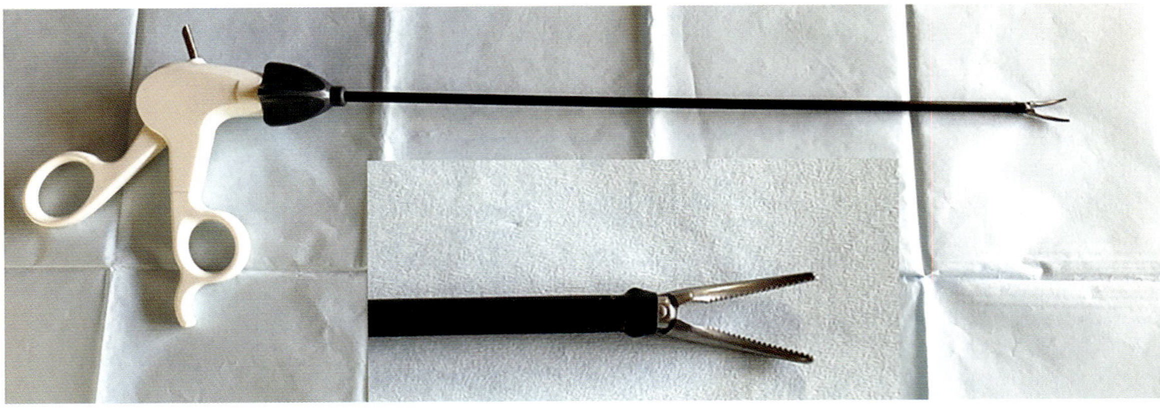

FIGURE 5. Maryland type (curved jaws) laparoscopic dissector.

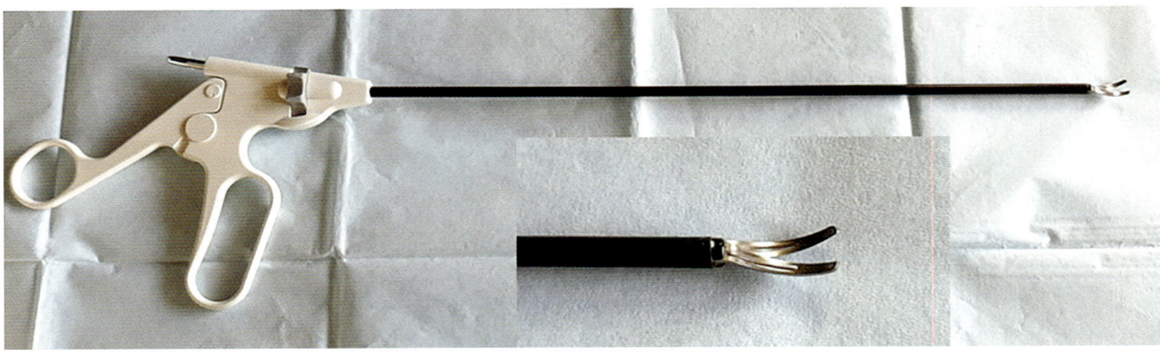

FIGURE 6. Laparoscopic scissors with long and curved jaws.

better the structures will be differentiated; and the sharper the image, the more confident the surgical team will feel.

Recently, vision systems have evolved to 3D cameras and HD, 2K, or 4K monitors, which greatly facilitate suturing. In veterinary medicine, a randomized controlled trial of 3D vs. 2D imaging systems for pure laparoscopic gastropexy concluded that these systems do not seem to improve surgical duration, surgical complications, or the surgeon's mental or physical workload. In the authors' experience, the quality provided by HD, 2K, or 4K systems may be sufficient to achieve optimal image quality without resorting to 3D systems.

The authors recommend the use of 5 mm optics, with an angle of 30° or over 0°, because they are versatile for different patient sizes and provide a better perspective in enclosed spaces, such as thoracoscopy or gastropexy.

TRAINING IN LAPAROSCOPIC SUTURING

There is no generally accepted model of minimally invasive surgery (MIS) training, and there are various combinations of teaching and assessment tools (simulation vs. clinical environment). In any case, training is based on the use of simulators, which have been incorporated into different curricula. LS requires constant learning based on repetitive maneuvers until adequate competence of these skills is acquired. In the initial stages, these competencies must be learned outside the operating room and away from the live patient, and they can be acquired through structured curricula, such as the Veterinary Assessment of Laparoscopic Skills (VALS), or through various formal training courses in different learning centers and universities. All combine basic and advanced modules, and LS is usually included in the latter. Training on low-fidelity homemade simulators is possible, as this has been shown to have comparable efficacy to training on commercial simulators. Advanced technical skills such as LS can be practiced on simulators with inanimate models (inorganic or organic) or on more realistic models, such as experimental live animals or cadavers.

The traditional learning model of conventional surgical education cannot be applied for MIS, least of all LS. This is where simulation plays a vital role. It is important to realize that simulation can go beyond mere repetitive trained skills, because it also permits the evaluation of surgical performance as a whole.

Live experimental animal models have a comparable anatomy and provide the opportunity to replicate real-life intraoperative complications. They are, of course, expensive and restricted by ethical protocols and require the technical involvement of anesthesiologists and qualified veterinary staff. Simulators can be physical (box trainer), which are the most affordable, or based on virtual reality, but both are equally well suited for teaching and assessing.

In any case, a hypothetical ideal learning model would be divided into the following steps:

1. Theoretical knowledge of the MIS approach, instruments, and equipment.
2. Deliberate practice on simulation models.
3. Deliberate practice on live anesthetized animal models or cadavers.
4. Tutoring by experts using remote videoconferencing systems and face-to-face mentorship in a clinical setting.

SUTURE MATERIALS

The surgeon must decide beforehand which type of suture is appropriate for each tissue in each surgical situation, since LS replicates the same methodology used in conventional surgery. On the other hand, there are differences in the laparoscopic approach with respect to the conventional approach in terms of exposure of the surgical field, handling of the suture threads, needle placement and angle of entry, and force applied to the knot and to the tissues because of the working distance, among others. For example, monofilament sutures are more difficult to handle and more prone to breakage if not handled delicately, and more care is required when locking the knot, since they tend to loosen (low coefficient of friction) compared to multifilament material. The coefficient of friction of suture materials has a direct impact on knot security. The authors recommend that in the initial stages of LS learning, for example in simulator practice, a suture material with low memory, easy handling, and low stiffness (higher coefficient of friction), as well as less tendency for the knot to loosen, should be used. Ideally, this suture should have a gauge of 2-0 and a 17–22 mm long semicircular round-bodied needle with an atraumatic tip (taper or blunt, no cutting edge). In general clinical practice, semicircular surgical needles with a round body, a conical tip, and a length that varies according to the tissue to be sutured are almost exclusively used.

Suture length is of paramount importance, because the surgeon must calculate the minimum length necessary for each suture pattern. Excessively short sutures are not recommended, whereas sutures that are too long will lead to frustration. In general, a 12–15 cm thread is sufficient for an intracorporeal single stitch (LIS), no more than 20 cm is needed for an intracorporeal running suture (LIS), and ideally a 90 cm thread should be used for extracorporeal knot tying (LES).

Surgical needles are available in different shapes: straight, ½ curve (Endoski needle), ½ circle, ¼ circle, 3/8 circle, 5/8 circle, or J-shaped. They may be distinguished by their tip (rounded, conical, diamond) and body (circular, oval, triangular, lancet, hexagonal).

There are no universal rules about the ideal choice of suture for LS, although it is recommended to use the same type of suture as in open surgery. In general, 2-0 or 3-0 sutures with a round-bodied (taper cut) needle may be applied to tissues of firm consistency (muscular and fascial closure or thicker tissues), and 3-0, 4-0, or 5-0 sutures are used for fine suturing. The ideal needle size can range from 18 to 20 mm.

Of special mention are transparietal straight surgical needles, which can be used to suspend organs such as the stomach, gallbladder, intestine, ovaries and uterus, bladder, or intra-abdominal testicles in order to improve exposure of the operative field.

TYPES AND PATTERNS OF LAPAROSCOPIC SUTURING

LS, both LIS and LES, may well be the qualitative differentiating factor between a MIS surgeon who performs basic procedures and one who wants to progress to a more advanced level. Some authors consider LS the workhorse of laparoscopy due to its versatility, because it is the qualitative leap from performing diagnostic and ablative laparoscopy to carrying out reconstructive laparoscopy, and it can be a tedious and frustrating process if not practiced properly. For example, in veterinary studies using simulators, 18 repetitions have been established as the average number required to reach proficiency in LIS. Other clinical studies in small animals comparing LIS and LES ligation concluded that, after adequate training, both knotting techniques were safe and effective for ligation of the ovarian pedicle and uterine horn in dogs via three-trocar laparoscopic oophorectomy through the ventral midline. The mean time was around 18 minutes for each ovary with LIS, and about 15 minutes with LES.

Thus, there is no room for self-deception: training time, effort, and skills are required to achieve mastery of LS. There are also intraoperative differences between procedures in which standard simple stitches are applied in a comfortable postural position (e.g., ovarian pedicle ligation, gastrotomy) and others that require suturing with more changes in needle position and in a more uncomfortable position (e.g., inguinal hernia, gastropexy).

Generally speaking, there are two categories of laparoscopic knots: intracorporeal (LIS) and extracorporeal (LES). Intracorporeal knots are made entirely inside the body cavity by using laparoscopic instruments. Extracorporeal knots are created after retrieving both ends of suture outside the laparoscopic ports, and they are usually cinched down by means of a laparoscopic knot pusher. Laparoscopic knots can be subdivided as well according to the method used for tying: flat knots (e.g., square, surgeon's knot) and sliding knots (e.g., Roeder knot, intracorporeal slip-square).

Although there is thorough research that compares the biomechanics of different types of open and laparoscopic knots, it can be summarized that, after proper training, laparoscopic square knots are as secure as open square knots, and there is no substantive difference in the security of these knots tied intracorporeally or extracorporeally. Nonetheless, surgeons should know certain particularities of the knots they are going to use (e.g., sliding or not, locking or not).

Regardless of the type of knot, suture patterns in LS have certain particularities, such as less tactile feedback, less freedom of movements, and more technical skill requirements compared to open knotting. There are two suture patterns: simple interrupted and continuous (running). For the former, if optimized and taking advantage of the standard 12–15 cm thread length, two or three simple stitches can be performed, whereas a longer thread is required for the latter. The initial and termination knotting steps of continuous LS can be accomplished in several ways:

- By performing standard LIS with a NH and an assistant NH or with a NH and a dissector (e.g., surgeon's knot or square knot).
- By creating a starting slip knot or a preformed loop at the distal end of the suture (after piercing the tissues with the needle, the needle is pulled through the preformed loop; the thread is then tied and the loop works as a closure system).
- By using special clipping devices at the beginning and end of the suture line.

Key points

- The ideal knot is characterized by being:
  - Safe: ensuring maximum strength between tissue edges with the smallest bulk.
  - Quick and easy to tie: easily drawn and configured (shaped). Especially in slip knots, easy to run down.
  - Efficient: to avoid inefficacious maneuvers and too tight knots. That is, the simplest and sufficiently secure knots are preferred, such as the square knot or the surgeon's knot.
- Surgeons should be familiar and proficient with at least one knot for LIS and another for LES, and within this group, with at least one compound sliding knot and one noncompound (static) knot, to adapt knot configuration according to the different intraoperative scenarios.

LAPAROSCOPIC INTRACORPOREAL SUTURING

Concerning LS, LIS is the most familiar to most surgeons due to its similarity to knotting with conventional instruments. LIS can be performed with a NH in the DH and another NH in the NDH, or with a NH in the DH and a grasping forceps or dissector in the NDH. The ideal and versatile NH, suitable for most situations, is as follows: 5 mm in diameter, with a straight axial handle and a noncurved tip. In the practical situation of a pure laparoscopic gastropexy, this type of NH could be interchanged between both hands in each of the passages of the stomach and abdominal wall.

NEEDLE INSERTION

There are several ways to insert the needle into the working cavity. The most common is to hold the thread with the NH about 2 cm from the base of the needle. 10 mm trocars allow entry of a wide range of needles, but if 5 mm trocars are used, the curvature of the needle may be slightly flattened outside the patient.

The total length of the thread to be manipulated must fit the size of the abdominal cavity (the smaller the cavity, the shorter the suture); therefore, in case of an intracorporeal stitch, the length of the thread may range from 7 to 12 cm approximately. Thread length influences needle entry in such a way that sometimes, when the needle has been introduced into the cavity, there may be thread remaining inside the trocar cannula. This can be avoided if the NH grasps both the free end of the thread and the thread close to the needle at the same time, reducing the length of the thread by half (**Fig. 7**).

An alternative option without using a trocar is to insert the needle under direct visualization through the scope to see how the needle and all the thread pass transparietally, through the abdominal or thoracic wall.

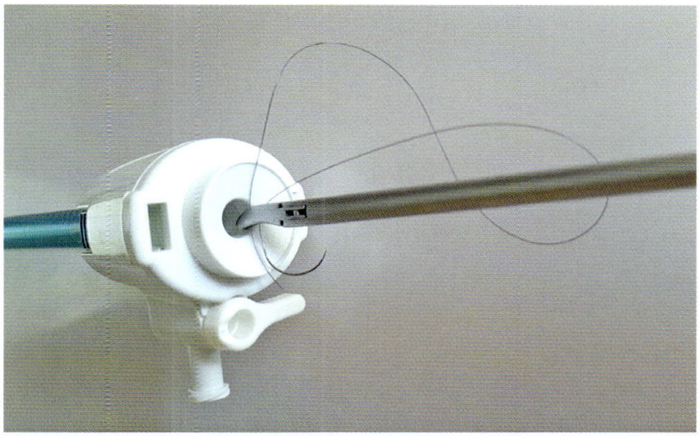

FIGURE 7. Routine maneuver for safe introduction of the needle into the body cavity.

NEEDLE POSITIONING

As already mentioned, LIS has been described with the use two NHs, one in the DH and another in the NDH, although an assistant grasping forceps (generally, a curved or straight Maryland dissector or fenestrated forceps) can also be used in the NDH. The surgeon uses the DH to pass the needle with the NH, and the NDH assists in placing the needle and holding the thread and tissues.

The ideal angle of separation between the assisting instrument in the NDH and the NH in the DH is 60°–90°. In human medicine, the optimal distance between the trocars is 12 cm for anastomosis suturing. In veterinary medicine, if the patient is very small or the surgical field has a narrow working space or home base (e.g., thoracoscopy, single-incision laparoscopy, laparoscopy of the pelvis or esophageal hiatus, transanal minimally invasive surgery), the distance may be reduced to 5–7 cm. In these cases, LIS may be more challenging than LES.

Once the needle is inside the working space, it is essential that the assistant and the main surgeon keep the combination of needle, thread, and instrument as centered as possible on the monitor screen at all times (working on the sides of the monitor should be avoided). In addition, visualizing the home base (the virtual area where the knot is placed) is very helpful while performing these maneuvers.

Together with knotting, needle placement is perhaps one of the stages that requires the most training time. This step must be a simple, elegant, and efficient "pirouette" maneuver to place the needle held in the NH in the correct position. For this, while the NDH instrument grasps the needle tip and the thread is grasped with the NH in the DH, the needle is pirouetted until proper alignment is achieved and grasped with the DH instrument. The authors encourage repetitive practice of this step to avoid inefficient time and unnecessary transfer of the needle between instruments during clinical situations.

There is no universally efficient needle position for all surgical situations. However, especially when using standard 2D imaging equipment, it is very useful to distinguish four basic or neutral needle positions (**Fig. 8**; **Table 2**). Although any entry angle can be virtually achieved with these four positions, they are designed for a neutral position of 90° of the needle with respect to the NH shaft. These positions are not fixed and may undergo modifications depending on the desired needle entry angle into the tissue.

In general, most stitches can be performed in the neutral positions 1 and 3 ("smiling") with the right and left DH, respectively. As apprenticeship of these maneuvers progresses, ambidexterity should be encouraged in order to be able to respond to different surgical situations.

For a right-handed surgeon, a right to left stitch is usually performed with the needle in position 1. For this, the "wake up the needle" maneuver is quick to learn (**Fig. 9**). First, the NH in the right hand pulls the thread close to the needle and, using the needle's own weight, the needle is placed on a surface as flat as possible (e.g., body cavity floor, intestinal loops, stomach, bladder, lung) and in a position as close as possible to the smiling position 1. Then, with the NH slightly open, the needle is carefully held by its most proximal third (close to the needle base), and the wake up the needle effect is achieved: the needle lifts up by itself and is placed in the most neutral position, with an ideal angle of 90° between the NH and the needle.

Another technique, more versatile, is to place the needle in the air with both hands, through the pirouette maneuver (**Fig. 10**). Regardless of whether the stitch will be performed with the right hand (positions 1 and 2) or left hand (positions 3 and 4), it is useful to divide the needle into two halves, so that during the pirouette maneuver the left half of the needle is held by the left-hand instrument and the right half of the needle is held by the right-hand instrument, without crossing them. First, the NH in the right hand holds the suture thread about 2 cm from the needle, while the instrument in the left hand (another NH or a dissector) holds the needle near its tip and oriented to the left.

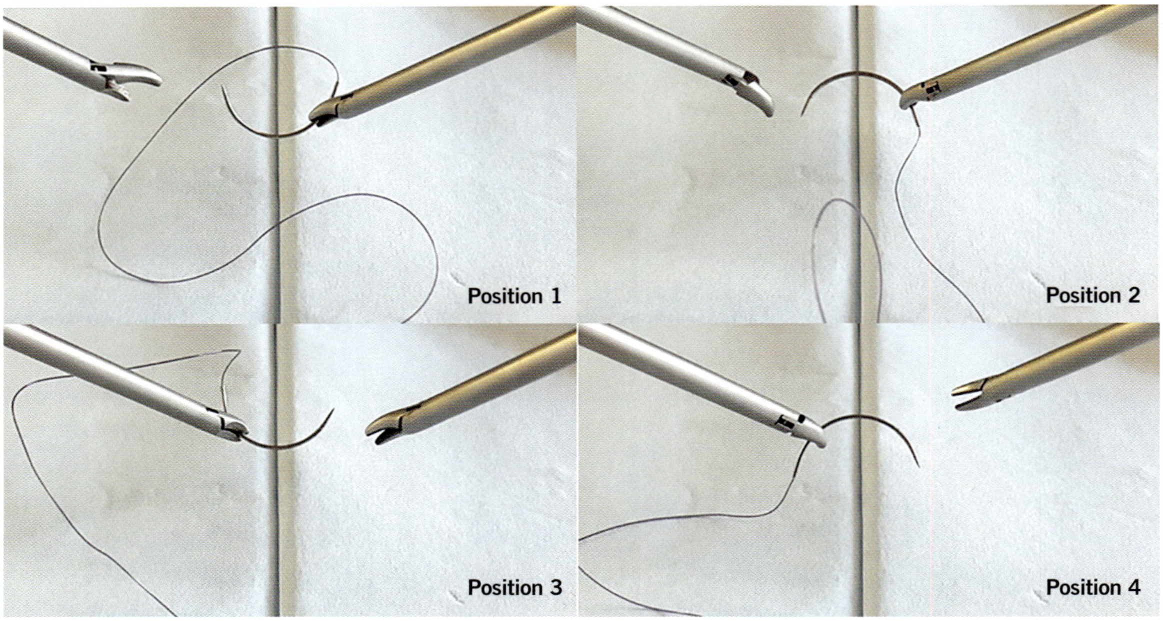

FIGURE 8. The four basic or neutral positions of the needle to pierce any tissue.

The needle must now be "straightened" before the NH can immobilize it in the optimal position (smiling). This is achieved through pirouette maneuvers, which are figuratively cited as needle dance, hair pulling maneuver, grinding coffee maneuver, or flag maneuver. For this, the NH continues to hold the suture thread about 2 cm from the needle base and performs up–down and forward–backward twisting movements. On the other side, the left hand also performs fine rotational movements to facilitate needle positioning. When the needle is straightened with the left-hand instrument in position 1, the NH grasps the needle, slowly approaching it until the needle is held in its most basal

TABLE 2. Needle and needle holder orientations for any of the four basic positions

Position	Characteristics
1	NH in the right hand drives the needle in a "smiling" (concave) position, with its tip pointing to the left.
2	NH in the right hand drives the needle in a "sad" (convex) position, with its tip pointing to the left.
3	NH in the left hand drives the needle in a "smiling" (concave) position, with its tip pointing to the right.
4	NH in the left hand drives the needle in a "sad" (convex) position, with its tip pointing to the right.

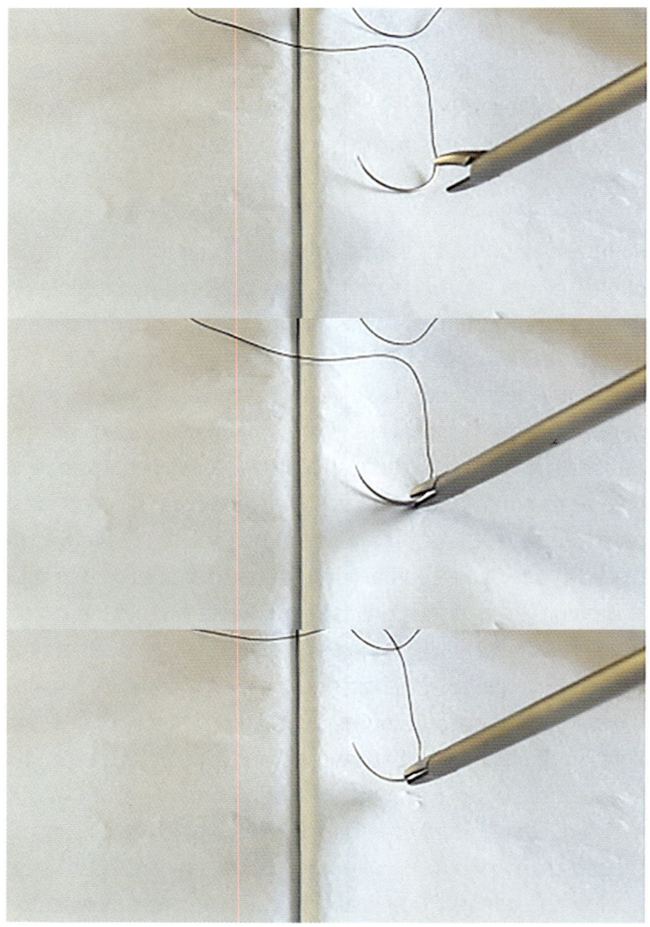

FIGURE 9. "Wake up the needle" maneuver to fix the needle in position 1.

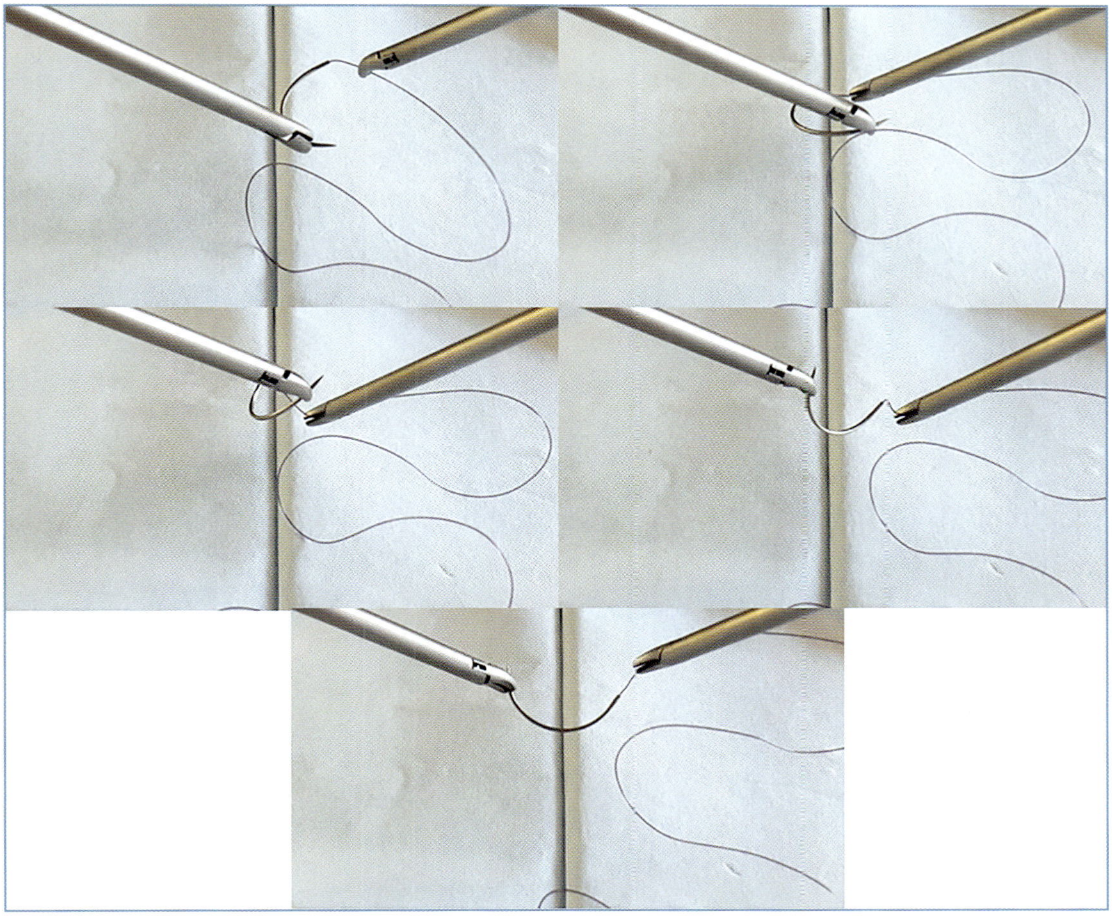

FIGURE 10. Pirouette maneuver to fix the needle in position 1.

third and trying not to displace the needle while approaching. The tip of the NH is the active part that should always be used to pick up the needle; otherwise, as in open surgery, if the needle is grasped with the base of the jaws of the NH, accuracy will be lost in the passages through the tissue. As mentioned earlier, the angle of the needle with respect to the NH should be of about 90° for a standard stitch, although this is the step in which the angle can be fine-tuned and readjusted, reaching 120°–135°.

Passing through the tissue layers with low trauma involves the needle approaching the tissue at a right angle. For that, the tissue resistance, needle tip, needle body, grasping point, and direction of force should be assembled on the same axis. The direction of the force of the needle tip and NH must be identical, but opposite to the tissue resistance; otherwise, the needle will be deflected within the instrument jaws (**Fig. 11**). In LS, as in microsurgical suturing, needle deflection is avoided by practicing needle placement at the desired angle, in addition to performing gentle rotational movements of the wrist or fingers (avoiding wide movements of the whole arm).

When the needle is placed in the position of passage through the tissue, it is recommended to fictitiously check in the air the correct passage of the needle. This is known as the cross-verification maneuver and consists of replicating the wrist rotation maneuver and the passage of the needle near the incision and thus verifying if the angle is correct or if the needle will be deflected (**Fig. 11**).

After the cross-verification maneuver, the left-hand instrument lifts the right edge of the incision, so that the ideal plane in which the NH enters, with respect to the incision line and the tissue, is as parallel as possible, in order to exert an effective rotation of the wrist on the needle (**Fig. 12**). The needle passes perpendicularly through the tissue, from the outside to the inside of the incision, and is held again at its tip by the left-hand instrument. The needle is repositioned close to the incision line, without moving away from the home base, so as not to leave too much loose thread in between. The needle is then passed from the inside to the outside, with the same angulation as before and with a fine rotational movement.

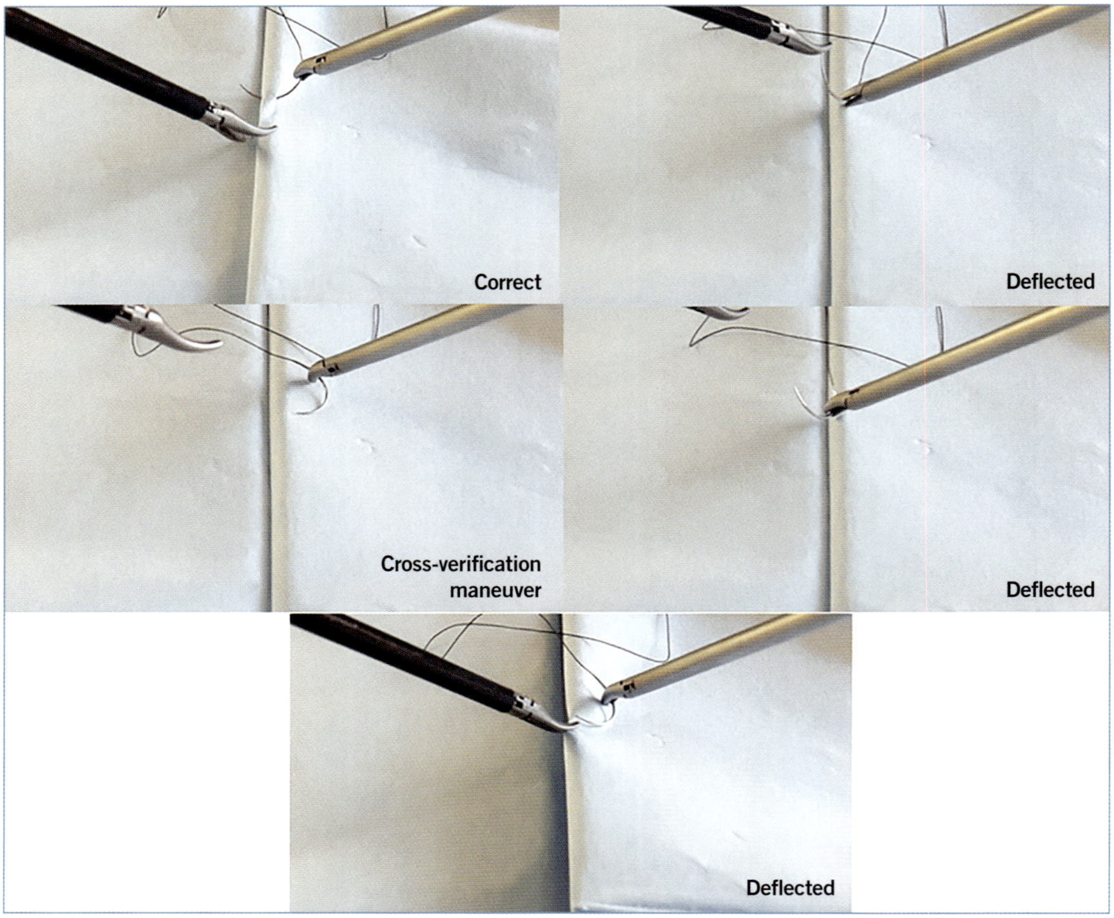

FIGURE 11. Needle deflection while holding the needle leads to an inefficient tissue entry point.

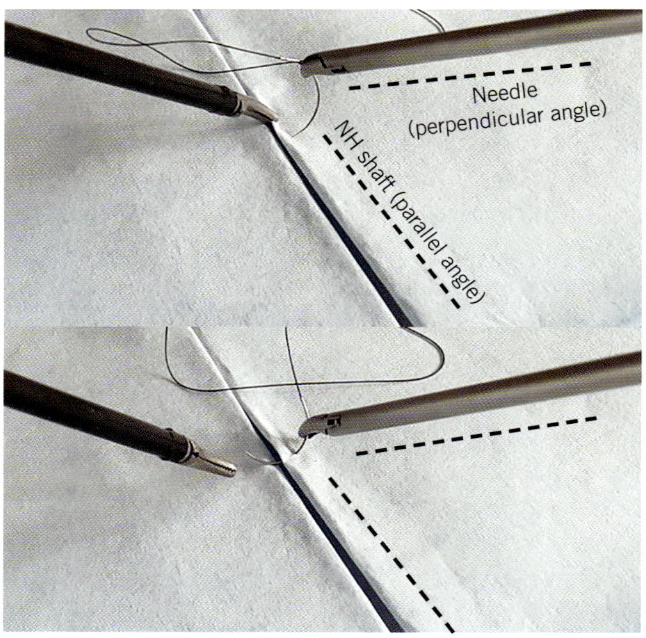

FIGURE 12. Relation of angles between the needle, the needle holder (NH), and the incision for an ideal perfect stitch.

The tip of the needle is pulled out of the tissue again, but without excessive traction, so that it always remains in the field of view and does not damage any adjacent structures.

All these maneuvers and recommendations are intended to comply with the ideal theory of the perfect stitch. Even so, laparoscopy does not always allow these postulates to be fulfilled, since factors like the working distances due to patient size, the setting of the trocars, or whether the incision line is horizontal or vertical influence LS.

PASSING THE NEEDLE THROUGH THE TISSUE

The ideal and most orthodox option is to undertake the maneuver in two stages or passages (**Fig. 13**). This way, the entry and exit point at the edges of the incision can be observed in detail. First, the NDH should securely and firmly, but gently, pull the first edge of the incision. This makes it easier for the NH to advance the needle through the tissue (from the outside to the inside) at the entry point. The needle is then grasped by the

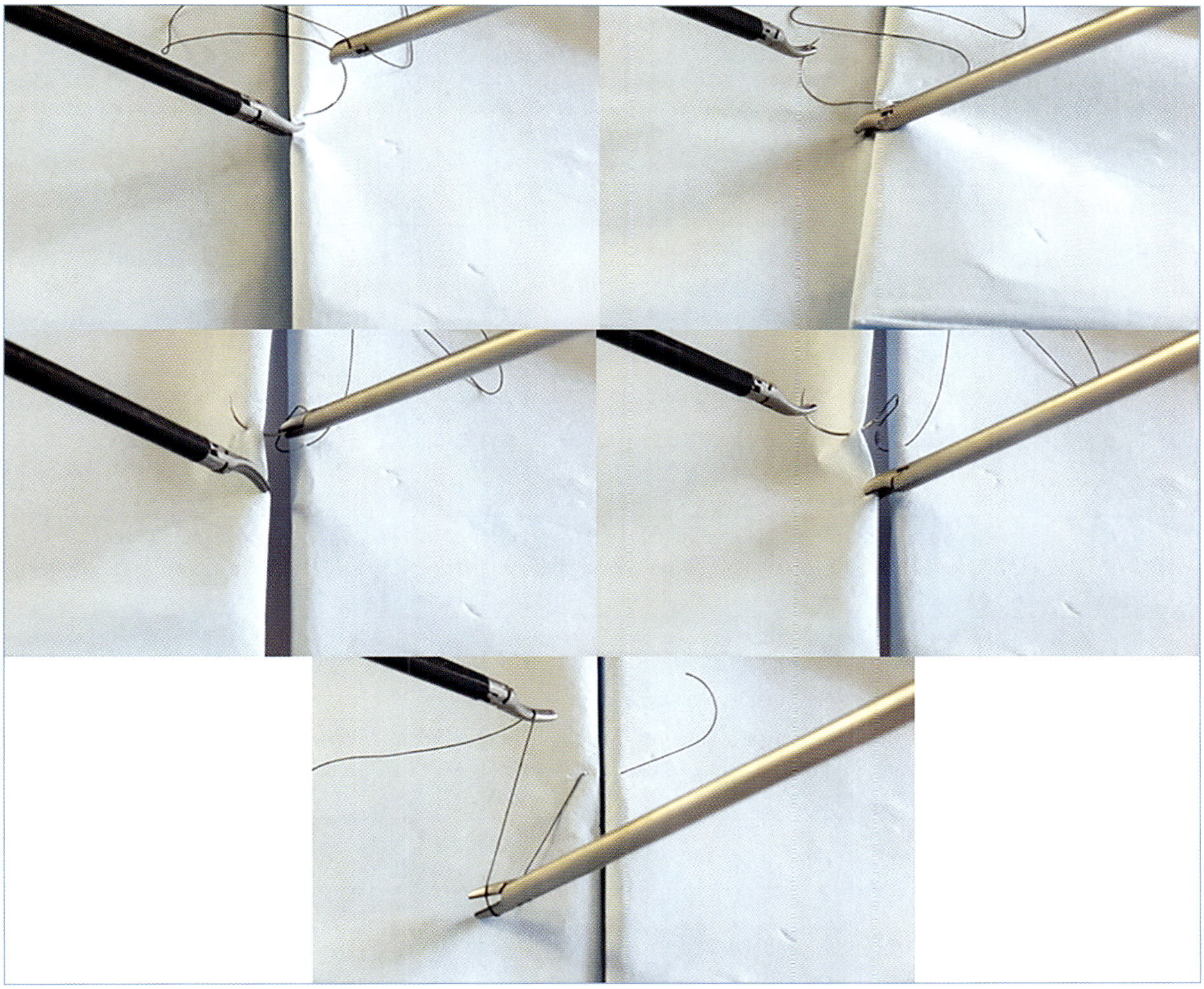

FIGURE 13. Passing of the needle and thread through the edges of the incision, entry point (outside–inside) and exit point (inside–outside).

NDH and withdrawn from the tissue to reposition it back on the NH, and the same maneuvers are reproduced (from the inside to the outside). Another option that requires less time and fewer accessory maneuvers is to pass the needle from the entry point to the exit point in a single move, without having to release the needle.

KNOTTING

The choice of suture material is a factor to be taken into account, both in learning and in practice. Given the stiffness (memory) of monofilament suture materials (polydioxanone, polyglecaprone, polygluconate, polyamide, polypropylene), performing the loop is usually less demanding, but they are stiffer than multifilament sutures and more effort is usually required to place the needle in the correct position. The handling characteristics of multifilament materials (polyglycolic acid, polyglactin, lactomer, silk, polyester) are optimal for needle placement, but more unfolding maneuvers are required due to their low stiffness.

The type of material is important when finalizing the suture and cutting the excess thread ends. In monofilament sutures (low friction), a greater distance should be left when finishing the knot, as they have a greater tendency to unravel.

It should be noted that knotting terminology is almost endless, as it comes from different day-to-day situations. There are two types of knots, ornamental and utility. Surgical knots fall into the latter group, and **Table 3** shows a selection of those that, in the authors' opinion, have the greatest practical application.

A proverb says that the devil is in the details. The peculiarities of minimally invasive surgical approaches correspond highly to this quote, even more so in the case of LS. According to Dr. Alfred Cuschieri and Dr. Zoltan Szabo, pioneers in the study of LS, theoretically there are only two possibilities of tying a basic flat square knot correctly, the overwrap and the underwrap.

TABLE 3. Surgical knots: Nomenclature and definitions	
Nomenclature	**Definition**
Monomanual and bimanual	■ Monomanual (LIS): Only the DH makes the turns. ■ Bimanual (LIS): Both hands collaborate alternatively for each turn.
Suture limb, tail, or strand	After any suture is passed through tissue, two limbs (tails, posts) are created to tie the knot.
Turn, wrap, or loop	Number of twists in a given throw (under or over).
Throw	Each of the knot's steps or layers (e.g., a simple square knot is formed by two throws, with each throw having one turn in reverse directions).
Reverse throw or turn	Refers to alternating underhand with overhand and vice versa.
Knot	A knot is composed of two or more throws. Knots are divided into two main groups: flat knots and sliding knots.
Effective knot	Possesses the attributes of both knot security (the effectiveness of a knot to resist slippage when load is applied) and loop security (the ability of a knot to maintain a tight suture loop as a knot is tied).
Flat knot	Also known as symmetrical or square knot (basic square or reef knot, granny knot, surgeon's knot) because the coefficient of friction is equally distributed between the two tails of the suture, and each tail of the suture enters and leaves the knot in an opposite direction.
Sliding (slip) knot	Also known as asymmetrical knot because the coefficient of friction is not equally distributed and each suture tail enters and leaves the throw in the same direction. In sliding knots, the PL is held fixed, under tension, while the NPL makes the loop and slides around it.
Capsizing the knot	Changing a symmetrical flat knot's geometry under asymmetrical stress (e.g., a simple-turn or double-turn overhand throw may be changed to a sliding knot configuration if more tension is applied in one tail than the other).
Post, standing, fixed, or passive limb (PL)	The straight suture limb under the most tension.
Half-hitch or half knot	One simple turn around the PL (in sliding knots).
Double half knot	Two consecutive simple turns. The two turns of a double half knot, either under- or overhand, are not yet a complete safe knot!
Nonpost, loop, wrapping, working, or active limb (NPL)	The free portion of the suture limb that wraps around the PL.
Post switching or reversing the knot	Also known as flipping the knot. It means alternating the PL for each successive loop that is thrown. The alternation does not refer to the direction of the subsequent loops, which may be underhand–underhand, overhand–overhand, or combined, as in the case of the three reversed half hitches on alternating posts (3-RHAP).
Flyping the knot	In LES, the term *proximal* means the suture limb near the surgeon's position and *distal* refers to the suture limb near the tissue. Therefore, knot geometry may completely suffer a "turning outside in" deformation process if the knot is flyped, that is, configured by changing the sequence of turns of the NPL around the PL, either proximal to distal or distal to proximal.
Noncompound (static) sliding slip knot	The knot is built by a sequence of consecutive stacked half hitches or by performing a square/surgeon's knot.
Compound sliding slip knot	The knot is completed outside before being pushed with the knot pusher. These knots have more than one half hitch of the NPL around the PL (i.e., any sliding knot other than a half hitch).
Nonlocking sliding knot	Throwing additional loops on top of the sliding knot after it is seated. It can be easily ensured by performing the additional three reversed half hitches on alternating posts (3-RHAP).
Locking sliding knot	With a one-way ratchet effect or self-locking effect. Changing the sliding knot into a nonsliding knot after it is seated. Even if these knots are self-locking by definition, it has been shown that additional half hitches increase loop security.

They also reported as many as 29 incorrect possibilities (incorrect crossing of instruments, poor thread arrangement, or undesired results due to violation of surgical principles). Research by Medina M. identified similar possibilities and concluded that poor instrumentation, improper port placement, and the limitations of a 2D video monitor are well-known causes of difficulties in learning LIS. However, if the apprentice is not aware of the number of the possibilities to err while performing a basic flat square knot in LIS, they will inevitably end up practicing randomly and confusing the technique.

The most accepted types of knotting used in LIS are the square knot and the surgeon's knot (**Fig. 14**), and they are composed of throws of simple or double turns, either overhand or underhand. Depending on the direction of the turns, the knot can become a granny knot, a tumble sliding knot, or a locking knot, among others (**Fig. 14**), but there are as many as exist in conventional surgery, as LIS reproduces a technique already used in traditional surgery (**Table 4**). The square knot and the surgeon's knot normally used in laparoscopy should always be flat on the tissue to avoid overlapping, thus providing a greater chance of healing. Therefore, when the knot is formed by equally pulling the two ends of the thread, a hypothetical midline will divide the flat knot into two equal parts.

A flat knot is the final configuration, but the prior knotting maneuvers can be referred to as single-handed monomanual (Rosser method) or two-handed bimanual (Szabo method). The Szabo technique involves more shifting maneuvers of the thread and needle to tie the knot, with more tendency to deploy a horizontal plane of the thread, and it tends to be less dependent on the swage (rigid tail) of the needle or a vertical positioning of the thread. On the contrary, in the Rosser technique, only the DH ties the knot around the thread in a vertical position on the

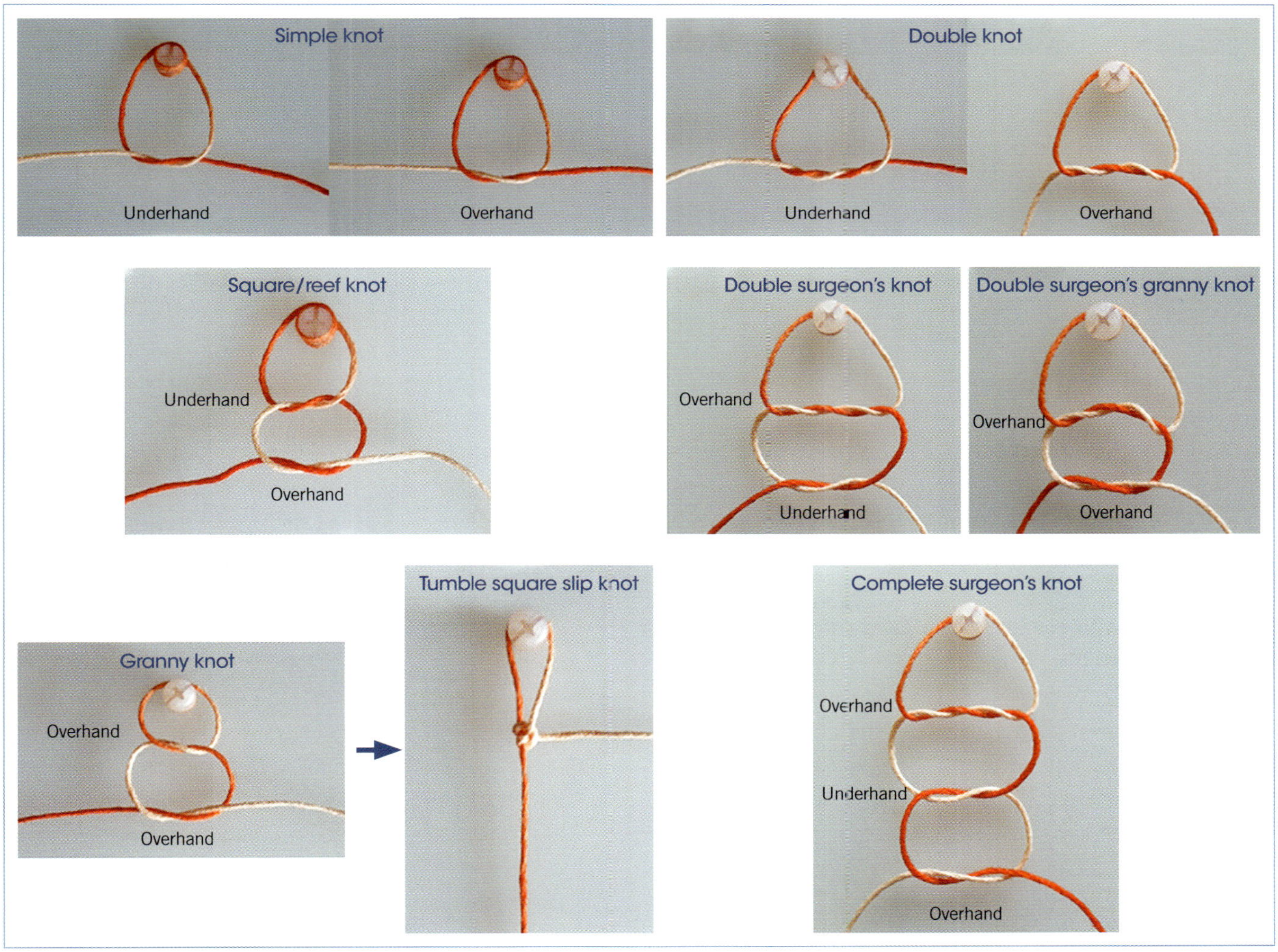

FIGURE 14. Knots frequently used in LS.

TABLE 4. Knots used in laparoscopic intracorporeal suturing

Most frequently used knots
■ Surgeon's knot ■ Square (reef) knot and tumble square/slip knot ■ Dundee jamming anchor knot and Aberdeen/Cuschieri termination knot: intracorporeal mixed knot for continuous suturing (the anchoring loop is preformed extracorporeally)
Other knots
■ Suturing in laparoendoscopic single-site surgery (LESS) ■ Sling suture ■ Heaving line knot: intracorporeal mixed knot for continuous suturing (the starting knot is preformed extracorporeally) ■ Purse string suture line

screen or around the swage of the needle, also with a vertical direction on the screen. Few needle transfers between instruments are required in this method.

From now on, a simplified numerical formula will be used to easily identify the number of turns in each throw of a knot. It should be noted that such simplified formula does not specify the direction of each turn (clockwise or counterclockwise, overhand or underhand) or if they are made with the DH or the NDH. For example, the basic knot is represented as 1:1, meaning that it has two throws with only one turn in each throw.

Single interrupted sutures

Surgeon's knot

The surgeon's knot is ideally suited for approximation of tissues under mild or moderate tension. It may be summarized as 2:1:1, that is, a double wrap on the first throw, followed by two opposing, alternating single throws.

Surgeon's knot with dominant right hand only (monomanual or Rosser method) (Fig. 15):

- Once inside the abdominal/thoracic cavity, the needle can be placed on a viscera in such a way that the surgeon can easily grasp it in a standard position 1 ("smiling"/concave position and the tip pointing to the left). Another option is to grasp the thread with the NH about 1 cm away from the needle and suspend the needle in the air like a puppet. The needle is then grasped near its tip with the left-hand instrument, before grasping it at the distal third with the tip of the NH, perpendicular to the axis of the NH.
- After closing the NH firmly by locking the ratchet system, the left-hand instrument takes the right edge of the incision to begin the stitch at the entry point (from outside to inside). The needle is introduced perpendicular to the axis of the incision by twisting the wrist, never pulling the NH (otherwise, the needle will turn). When the needle protrudes through the tissue, constant pressure of the NH on the tissue is maintained, and the needle is grasped with the left-hand instrument. The NH ratchet system is then released to allow the left-hand instrument to remove the needle completely from the first edge of the incision (again, only by twisting, not pulling). During this last maneuver, the NH must not be quiescent; it can be used, via opposite action on the tissue, to avoid tissue tears. The same movements are repeated in the other edge of the incision (from inside to outside).
- Once the needle has completed passage through the exit point at the second edge of the incision, the thread is first pulled with the left-hand instrument and then either alternatively with both hands or only with the left-hand instrument and applying a fixing opposite action on the tissue with the NH. The suture is pulled through enough that an adequate distal end (short tail of ≈3 cm) is left on the right side of the incision. Before knotting, the surgeon should make sure that the short tail is on the right side of the screen and the long tail and needle are on the left side (toward the bottom of the screen).
- To facilitate the first double half knot, it is key that the long tail be grasped with the tip of the left-hand instrument with sufficient thread distance (closer to the needle than to the incision). At this point, the long tail is pulled gently with the NH and straightened. This, known as the thread's horizon, is used to form a reverse C to avoid the particular lack of stiffness of braided sutures, and it will keep the thread near the left-hand instrument as rectilinear as possible (rising the bight) and, preferably, pointing toward the top right of the screen.
- With the left-hand instrument near the incision (home base), the tip of the NH is rotated clockwise around the thread to make a double loop (two half knots) near the tip of the left-hand instrument. As if using knitting needles, movements should be gentle and smooth, without sudden changes of the speed of the instruments. At this point, there are alternative methods for faster and easier creation of single or double turns, and for any type of knot. They are normally applied in clinical situations with lack of maneuverability or

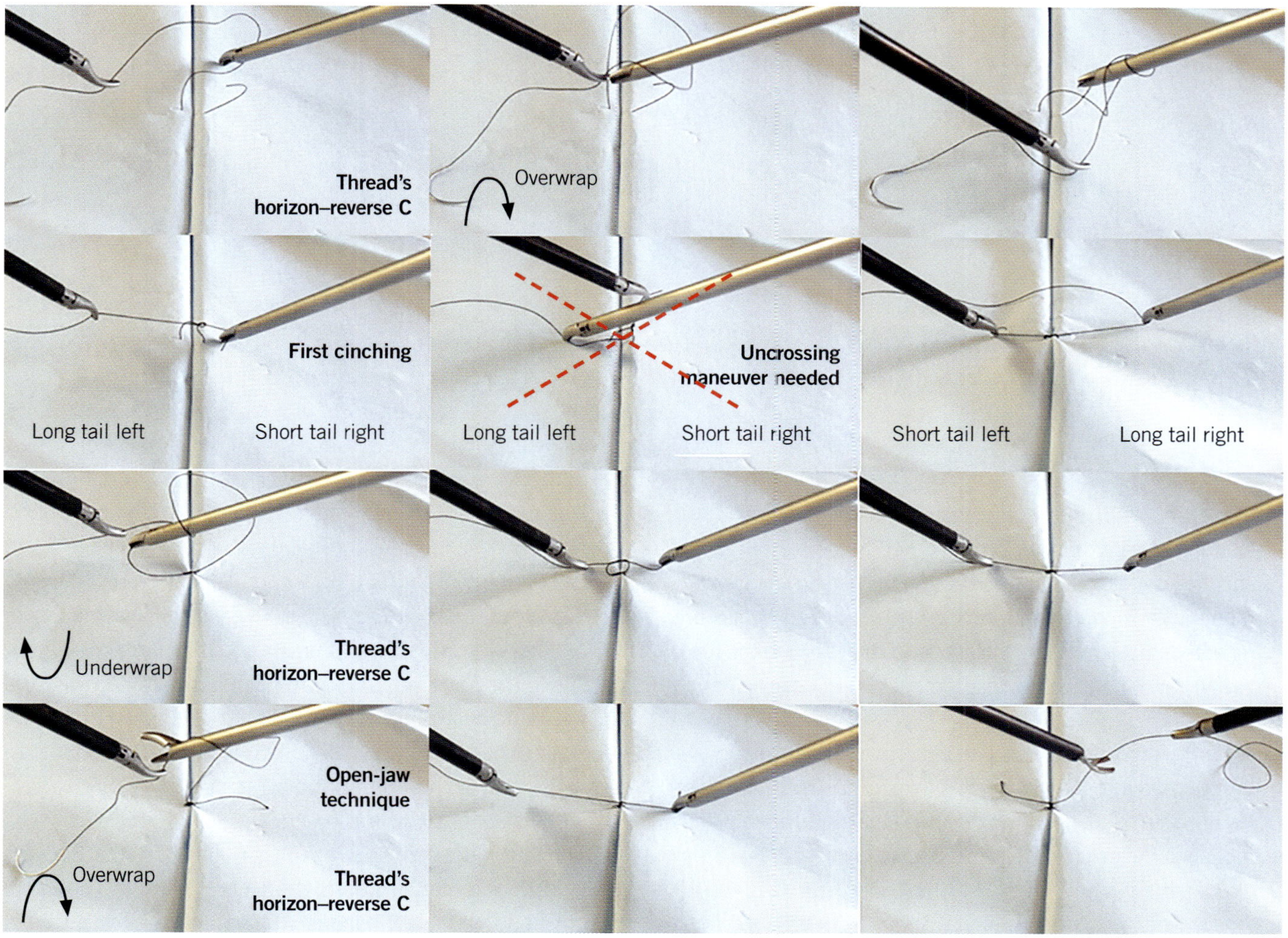

FIGURE 15. Surgeon's knot with dominant right hand only (monomanual or Rosser method). Note the thread's horizon–reverse C, the uncrossing maneuver, and the open-jaw technique for aiding knotting.

when the long tail is shorter than usual. The surgeon may opt for the open-jaw rule (or Romeo's gladiator rule) or for the needle rule (**Fig. 16**), in which the needle is held with the left-hand instrument and the NH creates quick overwraps or underwraps around the rigid base of the needle (swage).

- Once the first double wind is made, the two instruments uniformly move to the right side to make the NH jaws grab the short tail. The thread is then gently pulled with the left-hand instrument, without moving the NH holding the short tail, until the double loop goes beyond the tip of the NH. The surgeon should make sure that the resulting double knot is not twisted, but perfectly aligned (flat) over the incision. Consequently, uncrossing the instruments is needed in the monomanual method. For this, after cinching the double turn of the first throw, the surgeon must release both suture tails to realign the thread and create a flat knot. Both tails are then grasped (long tail with the NH, short tail with the left-hand instrument) close to the knot and pulled firmly to produce a firm knot without displacing the short tail, which should remain the same length (≈3 cm).
- After leaving the long tail (with the needle) on the left side of the screen, but near the incision (home base), it is grasped with the left-hand instrument at about 8 cm away from the first double knot placed on the incision. If the long tail is grabbed very close to the double knot, the knot is more likely to loosen and circular movements are impaired. A new thread's horizon and reverse C must be made; otherwise, taking further single or double winds over or under the NH will be uncomfortable. After this, the tip of the NH is gently rotated counterclockwise around the thread, without moving

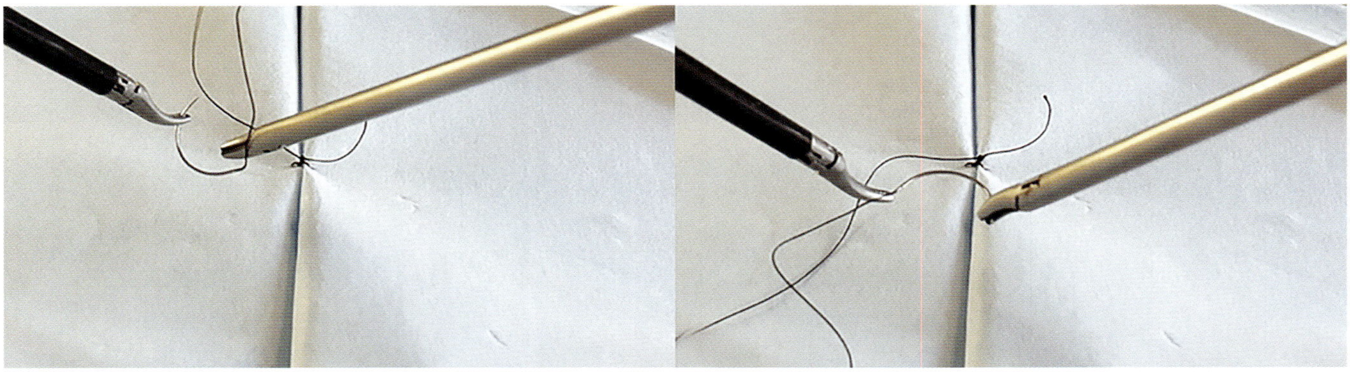

FIGURE 16. Needle rule technique for aiding knotting.

the left-hand instrument, to make a single loop. The two instruments are then uniformly moved to the right side, the short tail is grasped with the NH, and the same pulling movements with the left-hand instrument described earlier are repeated, that is, pulling until the loop goes beyond the tip of the NH and making sure that the knot is perfectly tightened and aligned.

- A standard surgeon's knot has been made (double and single opposite turns), but at least a third loop is recommended to increase knot security. For this, the first maneuver is repeated, but in this case a clockwise rotation to create a single loop is sufficient.
- Finally, both tails are trimmed at about 1 cm from the knot. The resulting stitch must exert correct and balanced pressure on the tissue: strong enough to prevent leaks, but loose enough to prevent ischemia.
- Additional single stitches are performed exactly the same way, equidistant from each other, symmetrically including the same amount of tissue on both sides of the incision, and perpendicular to the incision. The result must be a homogeneous, balanced, and harmonious closure.

Surgeon's knot alternating both hands (bimanual or Szabo method) (Fig. 17): This type of knot tying is one of the most commonly used in the scientific literature. Moreover, the authors recommend learning it because the use of both hands in each of the loops increases the surgeon's ambidexterity skills, which are essential in LS. It can be performed indistinctly with two NHs or with a NH in the DH and a grasping forceps or dissector in the NDH.

- In this case, unlike in the Rosser method, the remaining long tail with the needle is kept on the right side of the incision (right part of the screen), near the short tail of ≈3 cm. Before knotting, the thread is grasped with the right-hand NH and pulled to lengthen it and to create a C-shaped figure (laying the bight). If the right hand is kept prone (counterclockwise), the thread lays horizontal (flat) against the tissue, and the creation of the C-shaped loop is facilitated.
- Two turns (overwraps) are made over the thread with the left-hand instrument while the right-hand NH remains static. The short tail is picked up with the left-hand instrument, and both hands cinch symmetrically the first (double) flat knot.
- For the opposing second (simple) flat knot, the long tail is moved to the left side of the incision, and the thread is grasped with the left-hand instrument to create, this time, a reverse C-shaped figure. A single turn (overwrap) is made with the NH while the left-hand instrument remains static. The resulting single flat knot is cinched symmetrically.
- Finally, another C-shaped figure with a subsequent overwrap is made for the opposing third (simple) flat knot, as described for the first knot.

Square (reef) knot

The square knot is an adaptation of the one tied using the classic microsurgical technique and is especially indicated for the approximation of tissues under tension (e.g., edematous tissue, hiatal hernia, pyloroplasty). It can be made in two ways, resulting in either an intracorporeal nonsliding square knot (1:1 or 1:1:1) or an intracorporeal sliding square knot (tumble square slip knot) (1:1:capsizing:1). In both, the first simple hitch is always followed by an opposite single hitch; the first sets the tension on the tissue, whereas the second secures the knot. The square knot should not be confused with the granny knot, in which the first and second half hitches are made in the same direction.

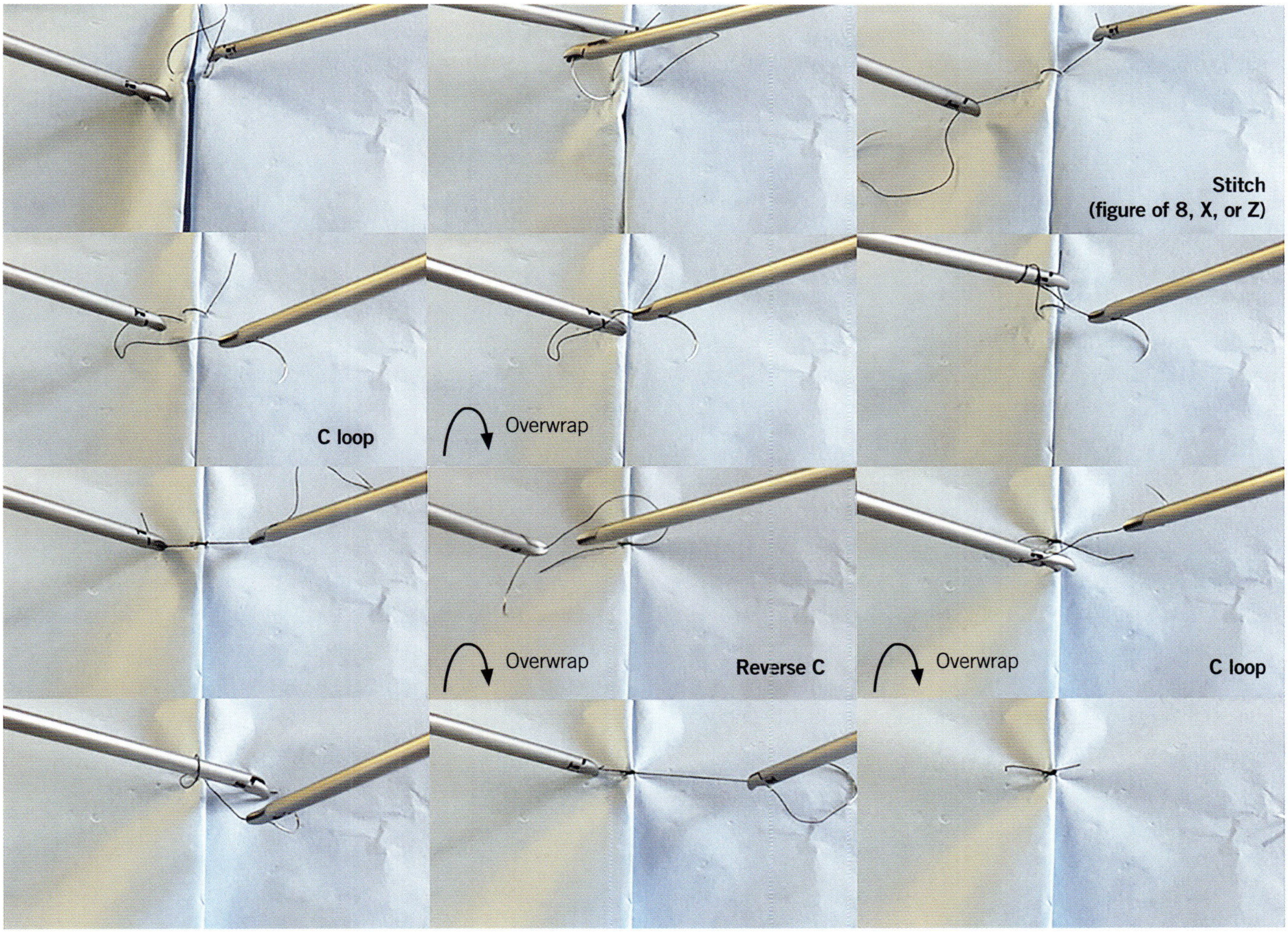

FIGURE 17. Surgeon's knot alternating both hands (bimanual or Szabo method) for a stitch of two passages in figure of 8, X, or Z. Note the C-shaped loops (laying the bight) and reverse C. Uncrossing the instruments is not needed.

Intracorporeal tumble square slip knot:

- The first flat knot (a single overwrap on the first throw) is followed by a second flat knot (a single overwrap in the opposing direction, with the opposing hand).
- The resulting square knot is converted into a tumble square slip knot by capsizing to a sliding configuration.
- After tissue approximation, the knot is reconverted to a locking configuration, and a final third flat knot may be added (single overwrap in the opposing direction, as in the first flat knot).

The intracorporeal tumble square slip knot is a useful alternative resource to tackle complicated situations when the first two turns of the surgeon's knot are not achievable (loose).

Square knot with dominant right hand only (monomanual or Rosser method): The technique is very similar to that used for tying the classic intracorporeal surgeon's knot.

- After passing the needle through the tissue, the thread is pulled almost all the way through, leaving a short tail of only 1–2 cm. The long tail is grasped with the left-hand instrument to make a thread's horizon and reverse C. The NH holding the long tail close to the needle is then twisted clockwise to form an overwrap single loop around the tip of the left-hand instrument. After moving both instruments simultaneously to the right side and grasping the short tail with the NH, the long tail is stretched in the opposite direction to that of the NH, so that the single loop advances and forms the first simple flat knot that brings the edges of the incision closer. Keep in mind that uncrossing the instruments is needed in the first single turn of the monomanual method, after cinching the first single turn; that is, the surgeon must release both tails to realign (uncrossing) the thread to create a flat knot.

- The same procedure is repeated counterclockwise and underwrap to produce a second flat (locking) knot.
- At least a third flat knot is recommended in the opposite direction to the previous one (as for the first loop) to reinforce the whole knot.

Square knot alternating both hands (bimanual or Szabo method) (Fig. 18): Tying this knot requires the same methodology as described for the surgeon's knot alternating both hands.

- For the first (simple) flat knot, the long tail is brought from the left side to the right side of the field, near the short tail. A C-shaped loop is formed with the long tail, keeping the NH prone (counterclockwise) so that the C-shaped loop lays horizontal (flat) against the tissue (laying the bight). While holding the long tail with the NH, the C-shaped loop is turned over with the left-hand instrument, and both instruments are moved to wrap the long tail once over the left-hand instrument. The short tail on the right side is then grasped with the left-hand instrument, moving both instruments simultaneously. The tails are gently and confidently pulled in opposite directions, and parallel to the tissue, to tighten the first (simple) flat knot.
- For the opposing second (simple) flat knot, the short tail remains on the left side of the field, and the surgeon brings the long tail toward the left side to create a reversed C-shaped loop configuration, that is, a mirror image of the first knot. The long tail is grasped with the tip of the left-hand instrument (laying the bight), and the thread is wrapped once over the instrument using the NH, making another single turn. With both instruments on the left side of the incision, the short tail is grasped with the NH to perform the same maneuver as before, tightening the second (simple) flat knot. Again, with the bimanual method there is no need to uncross the threads or to cross the instruments in the surgical field to tighten any of the knots. In contrast to the monomanual method, after cinching the first single turn (or double turn for a surgeon's knot), the knot is not flat yet. Thus, the surgeon must release both threads to realign them and create a flat knot.

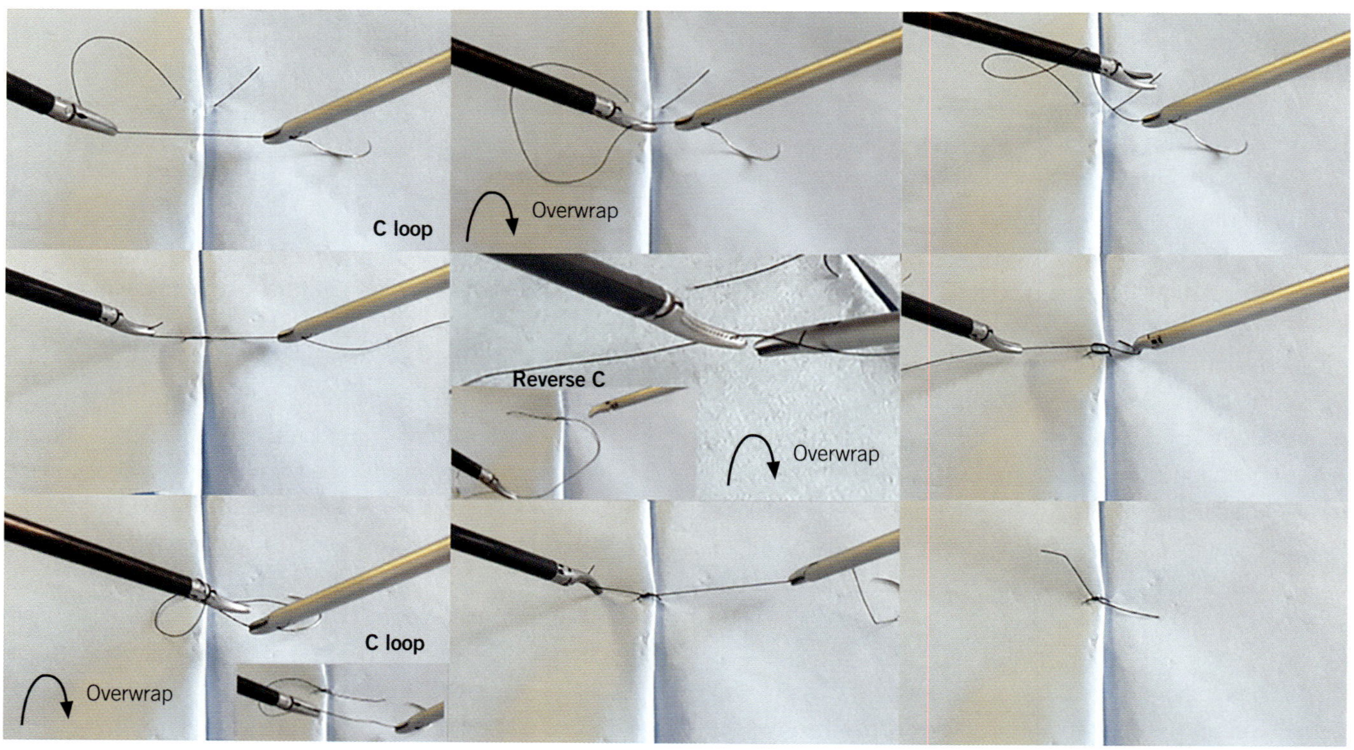

FIGURE 18. Square knot alternating both hands (bimanual or Szabo method). Note the C-shaped loops (laying the bight) and the reverse C, without the need of uncrossing instruments.

Repositioning the knot (converting a square knot into a tumble square slip knot) (Fig. 19): At this point, the simple square knot is changed to a slip configuration by repositioning (capsizing) it; that is, the (locking) square knot converts into a sliding configuration.

- The knot should be mentally divided into a left side and a right side. In case of a right to left needle passage, the left side of the thread is straightened before applying the unlocking traction that will create the slip configuration. This is achieved by grasping the suture loop (the portion of thread between the tissue exit point and the knot) with the left-hand instrument. The long tail is grasped with the NH, keeping the thread straightened on the ipsilateral left side.
- After the unlocking traction, the knot is converted into the slipping configuration when a sudden snapping is detected. If successful, the shape of the knot changes from an infinity sign (∞) to a double eyelet or pretzel.
- The knot is then ready to slide. While the NH maintains the tension of the long tail, the left-hand instrument pushes the knot down ("milking" the knot like a knot pusher) closer to the tissue until gentle approximation is achieved.
- The knot is reconverted to its locking flat square configuration by changing the traction sides. Then, with the left-hand instrument holding the standing part (long tail) on the left side and the NH grasping the short tail, both instruments pull in opposite directions and parallel to the tissue (as for the first and second square knots). To prevent slipping, an opposing third flat knot with a C-shaped loop is recommended (in the same manner as the first flat knot). Finally, the suture tails are cut.

Running continuous sutures (for right-handed surgeons)

The starting knot is tied following the same steps as those described for LIS knotting (usually a surgeon's knot or a square knot), except that a longer thread is needed to complete the whole suture line. In addition, the starting knot may be a preformed slipping noose loop or the very used Dundee jamming slip knot (**Fig. 20**), or a preformed stopper knot (heaving line knot). In either case, the progression of the continuous suture will be facilitated if a second surgeon holds the tension of the suture line after every passage by pulling up with an atraumatic

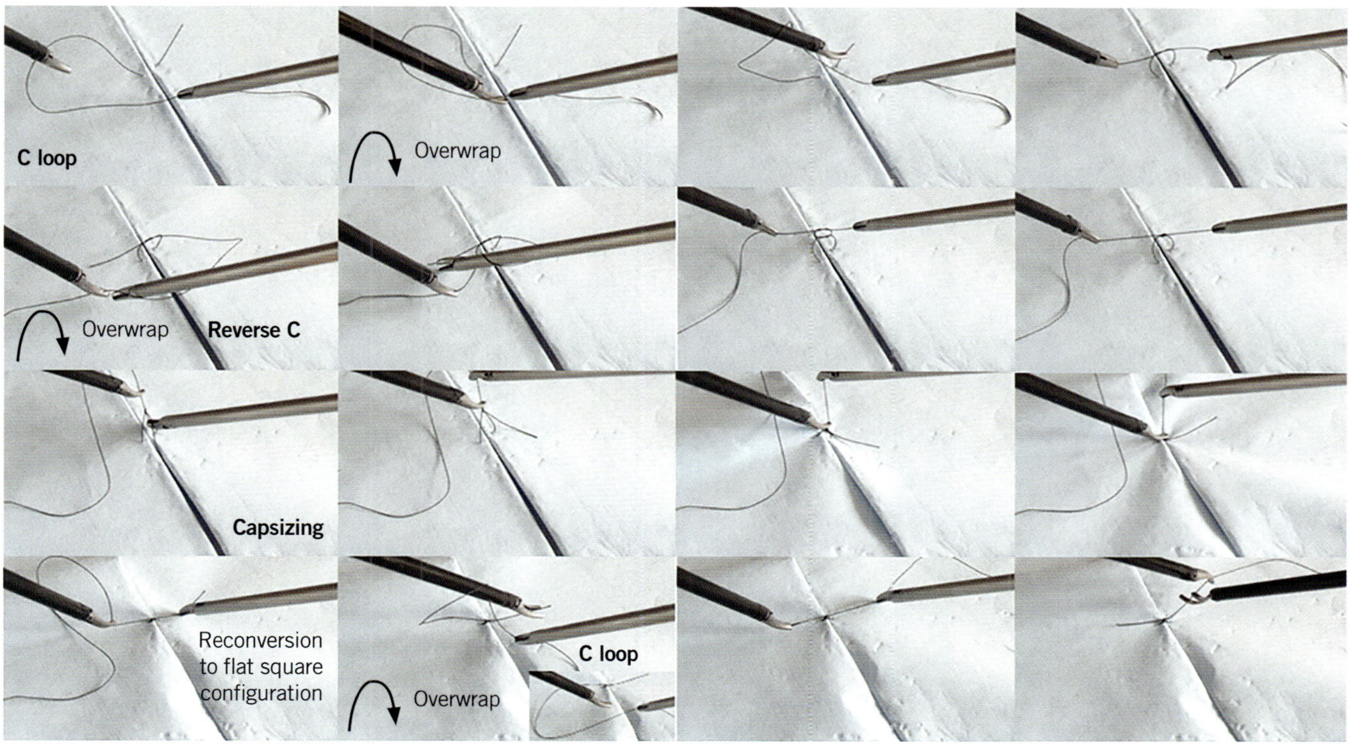

FIGURE 19. Square knot alternating both hands (bimanual or Szabo method). Converting a square knot to a tumble square slip knot by repositioning/capsizing the knot.

forceps. The first surgeon positions the needle correctly, as described before. After every needle passage, the first surgeon, either alone or with the help of the second surgeon, must ensure good tension of the suture line (pulled up about 3 cm from the tissue line). This facilitates consecutive passages of the needle. The same pattern is repeated until enough length (ideally ≥7 cm) of the long tail remains to tie the termination knot. Before tying the termination knot, the surgeon must ensure a firm tension is kept along the entire length of the suture; if this is not the case, the traction should be corrected to avoid leaks.

Termination knots for completion of the running suture can be the three-legged tie (**Fig. 21**) with a typical surgeon's knot or square knot, as for open surgery, by leaving a termination

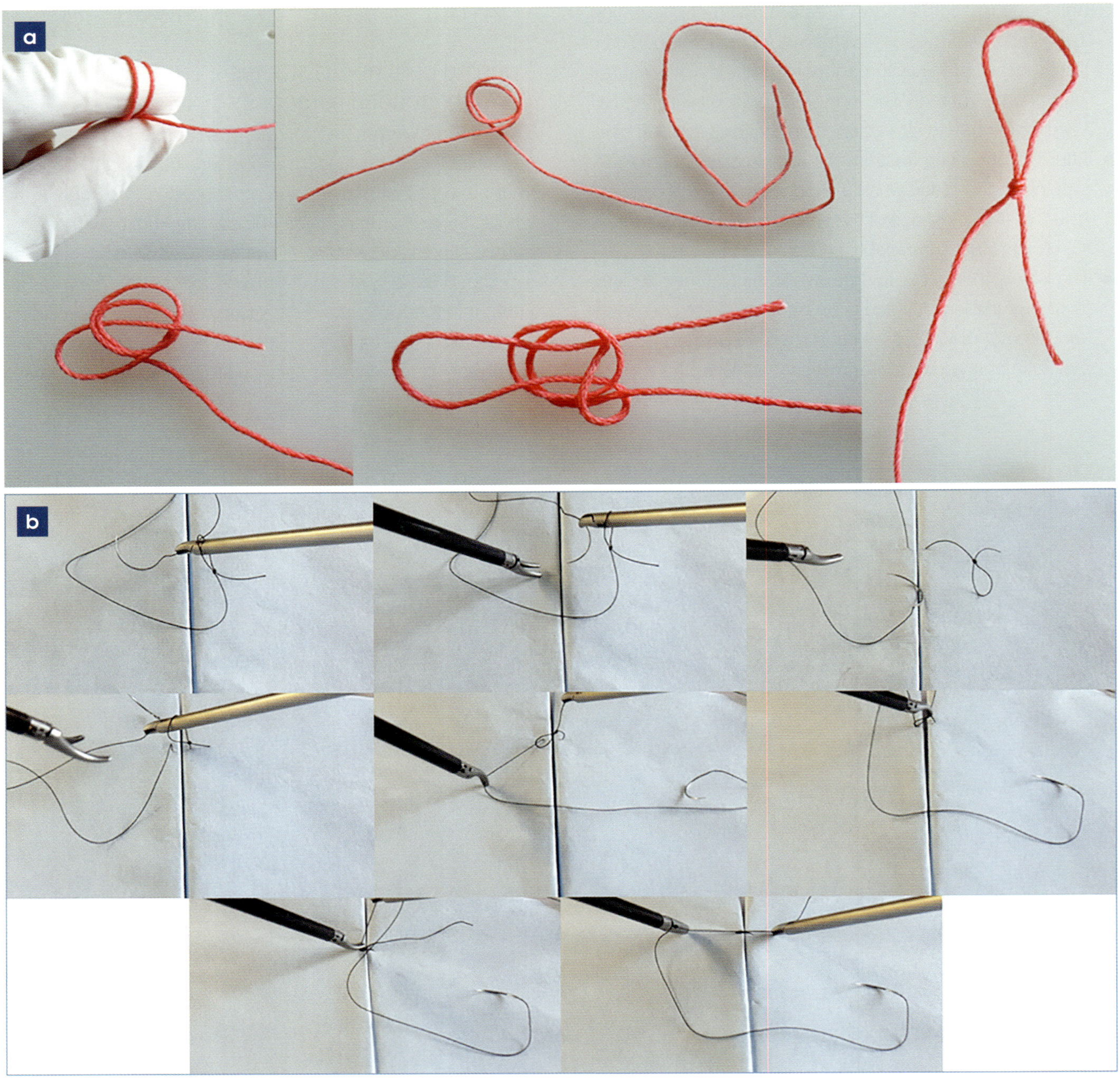

FIGURE 20. Starting Dundee jamming anchor knot. a) Extracorporeal creation of the loop. b) Loop anchoring to the incision.

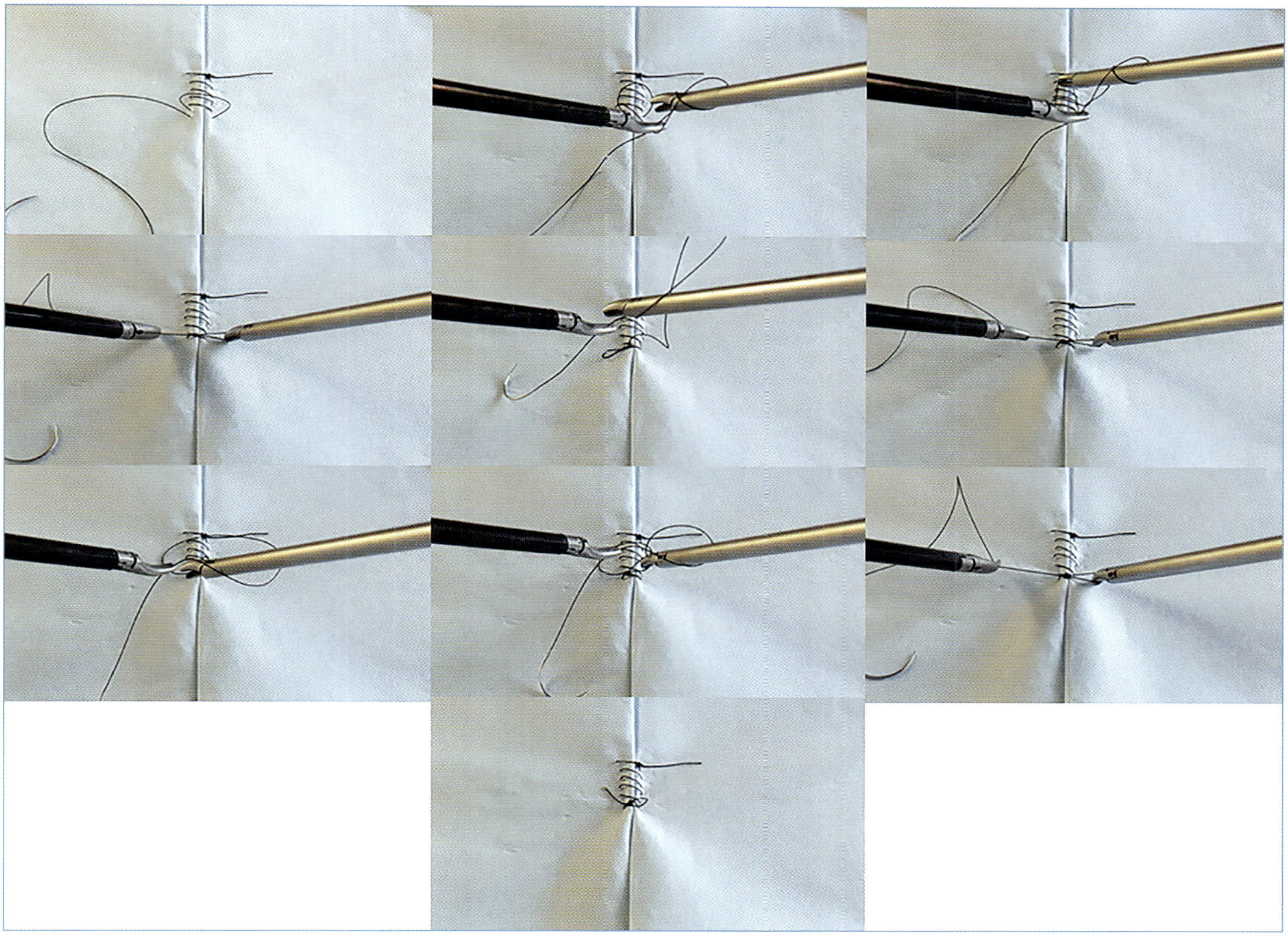

FIGURE 21. Termination of a running continuous suture with the three-legged tie method.

loop after the last throw that will act as the short tail. Another effective option is to use the Aberdeen/Cuschieri termination knot (**Fig. 22**).

LIS using a running continuous pattern requires even more attention than when an interrupted suture pattern is used. Failure is more likely to occur due to cluttering or chaotic crossed throws, initial and final knot slippage, or incorrect tension of the suture line. An ergonomic position of the ports and a perpendicular angle of the needle with respect to the tissue plane are mandatory. Therefore, the easiest way to accomplish an intracorporeal running suture pattern is to start from the upper part of a vertical incision and advance down. If the incision is horizontal, a right-handed surgeon will progress better from the left to the right side.

Key points

In LIS, a continuous suture pattern may be preferred if the suture line exceeds 3 cm.

- A general rule is that the length of thread needed is three times the length of the intended suture line.
- The length of the thread should not exceed 20 cm.
- The distance between suture bites should be equal to the depth of the bites.

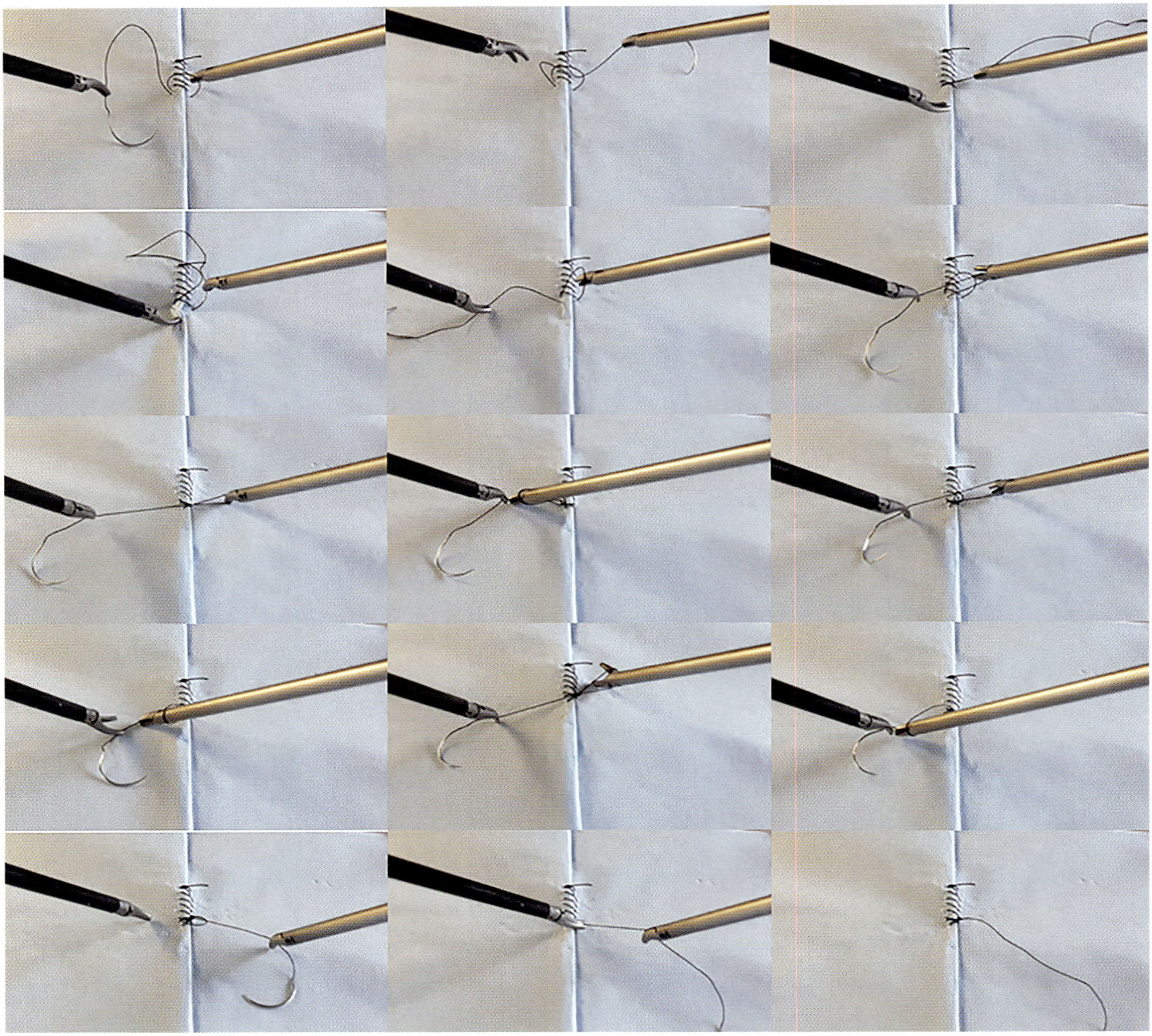

FIGURE 22. Aberdeen/Cuschieri termination knot.

TISSUE APPROXIMATION

Correct knot tying is not only a matter of tying the knot; equally important is the tissue approximation maneuver. In LS, since tactile feedback is diminished, the force applied to the tissues can be different from that used in conventional surgery. On the one hand, the surgeon can tear or necrotize the tissue if too much force is applied; on the other, there may be leaks or lack of healing due to poor tissue approximation. For this reason, the authors recommend that after each turn, the surgeon applies a steady tightening force, parallel to the tissue plane, equidistant between the long and short tails, and performed within the home base, without crossing the instruments.

The three basic patterns of LIS are: single stitch, stitch in figure of 8, X or Z, and continuous suture, and each of them can be knotted in different ways to approximate the tissue. With respect to single stitches, whatever the type of knot used (square knot, surgeon's knot, etc.), tissue approximation has the same features as in conventional surgery. The execution time is shorter, and neither repositioning of the needle nor control of the tension in the suture line are required. However, if the surgical situation warrants the restoration of widely separated edges, or if intraoperative hemostasis is needed due to profuse bleeding or bleeding hidden in the tissue, the so-called stitch in figure of 8, X, or Z may be more suitable (**Fig. 17**). This stitch requires two needle passages through the tissue before knotting, and the needle must be repositioned between each step. When this knot is made in LS, both passages should be parallel to facilitate maneuvering. Although this is an effective and time-saving knot, in case of medium to long incisions continuous suturing may be more suitable and time-effective.

NEEDLE WITHDRAWAL

Once the stitch or the suture line is finished, the needle is removed by pulling with the NH from the remaining thread, near the swage. For greater safety, the removal maneuver can be performed under laparoscopic guidance. Although this is the last step in LS, the needle should not be handled carelessly; otherwise, it can get lost inside the abdomen (especially amid the bowel). If not found there, the surgeon should not move or insert any instruments. A usual location where needles get stuck is inside the trocar sleeve. After looking inside of the optical trocar, the scope can be moved to the working trocar. If the needle is not there either, the abdominal cavity should be checked next. Manipulating tissues should be avoided, because the needle may be located right down intra-abdominally, on the viscera nearest to the tip of the trocar sleeve. If the needle cannot be found, a simple distraction in the last step of the laparoscopic procedure will make it necessary to convert to an open procedure.

LAPAROSCOPIC EXTRACORPOREAL SUTURING

LES is a very useful and versatile suturing modality in veterinary medicine because it can equal, or even exceed, the safety and efficiency of advanced devices such as bipolar energy, clips or specific clamps in biopsies, hemostasis of large pedicles, or resection of pedicled structures (e.g., cecum, gallbladder). It may be more useful in areas of limited access, where performing LIS is not comfortable. It is indicated when considerable force is needed to approximate the edges of the defect. LES has traditionally been associated with fewer training requirements than LIS, but it also has a learning curve and the need for intrinsic skills that must be practiced and refined outside the operating room. The are numerous different types of extracorporeal knots, each with its particular way of tying, and each may behave differently if made using braided or monofilament material.

While knotting in LS, either LIS or LES, important factors play different roles: biomechanical properties, tensile strength and coating of the suture material, friction between suture limbs, internal interference of the knot, tension applied until the knot is tightened, steps of knot configuration, slack between throws of the knot, tying instruments (including knot pusher design), and surgeon's skill.

LES is strongly influenced by the suture material, particularly by the biomechanical properties of the material with respect to the "quality" of the tissue. Thus, many surgeons consider that nonabsorbable braided sutures are the best choice regarding knot security and loop security in LES. All these factors make it necessary that, before applying LES in a clinical situation, the surgeon has perfect knowledge of how to perform it and the most suitable suture materials for each knot. This is particularly important in locking knots because they may self-block before reaching the target, thus having to make a new one. Therefore, it is mandatory to master how to tie the knots in a dry lab setting before using them in surgical cases, especially because some configurations with braided sutures are particularly difficult to slide.

There are many different types of extracorporeal knots, which, in general have been adapted from seafaring or fishing knots. Each has its own particular way of tying and may behave differently depending on whether monofilament or multifilament material is used. A good extracorporeal knot must fulfill some basic requisites. It must be well formed, so that the suture does not loosen later on, does not cut into itself when tightening, and does not lock prematurely. It must be easy to tighten and ensure maximum strength, but without tearing or cutting the tissue, as it should only bring the edges of the incision closer together. For a knot to be both effective and strong without loosening, it must have the attributes of knot security and loop security. Knot security is the effectiveness of the knot to resist slippage when load is applied and is dependent on three factors: friction, internal interference, and slack between each of the throws. Loop security is the ability to keep a suture loop tight while tying a knot. Any tied knot may have good knot security but poor loop security (a loose suture loop) and will therefore be ineffective in approximating the edges of the defect to be repaired.

In general, laparoscopic extracorporeal knots can be classified into two main categories: noncompound (static) sliding slip knots and compound sliding slip knots (**Table 5**).

Noncompound sliding slip knots (**Fig. 23**): it should be noted that in the existing literature noncompound knots are sometimes cited as nonsliding knots, as opposed to compound sliding knots. For this reason, so as not to confuse readers, the authors have avoided referring to noncompound knots as nonsliding, since, obviously, noncompound knots also have sliding maneuvers in each of the consecutive throws.

Noncompound knots are formed by making consecutive stacked simple knots (half stitches or half hitches) or by performing a square/surgeon's knot, always advanced on the tissue with a knot pusher. Noncompound knots have better biomechanical properties than compound knots, but the latter may be preferred in LES because they are easier to perform, in one single action, before complete knot progress. However, although compound knots can potentially damage the soft tissue during advancement, tying noncompound knots requires maneuvers of crossing the suture limbs (posts) and switching traction of both posts (hand crossing), which can release the tension on the suture limbs and lead to slippage of the first throws. The major disadvantage of noncompound knots is the propensity of the loop to loosen before the second half hitch is seated to the point at which it provisionally locks the knot. However, noncompound knots can be used in all situations, whereas compound knots can be only used if the suture slides freely through the tissue and knot pusher.

Compound sliding slip knots (**Fig. 24**) involve more than simple knots or half hitches over the thread that comes out of the trocar. An important consideration is to avoid performing compound slip knots when the quality of the tissue is poor. Another limitation of these knots is that they may slip back after being pushed into position, compromising loop security. Knots must be tight and must not slide back; a loosening greater than or equal to 3 mm could be considered a failure of suture function.

TABLE 5. Knots used in laparoscopic extracorporeal suturing
Noncompound (static) sliding knots
■ Stacked half hitches: reversed or nonreversed, on the same post or on alternating posts (i.e., the loops of flat knots—like the granny, square, or surgeon's knot—can be capsized to a sliding configuration)
■ Revo knot and modified Revo knot
Compound sliding slip knots
■ Roeder knot
■ Melzer–Buess knot (modified Roeder knot)
■ Equine knot (modified Roeder–Melzer–Buess knot)
■ Tayside knot
■ Weston knot
■ Mishra's knot
■ Pretzel knot
■ Pretied endoloop (commercial device or handmade knot plus knot pusher)
■ SMC knot
■ Tennessee slider knot
■ Nicky's knot
■ Giant knot
■ Trivedi's knot
■ Duncan's loop (fisherman's knot)

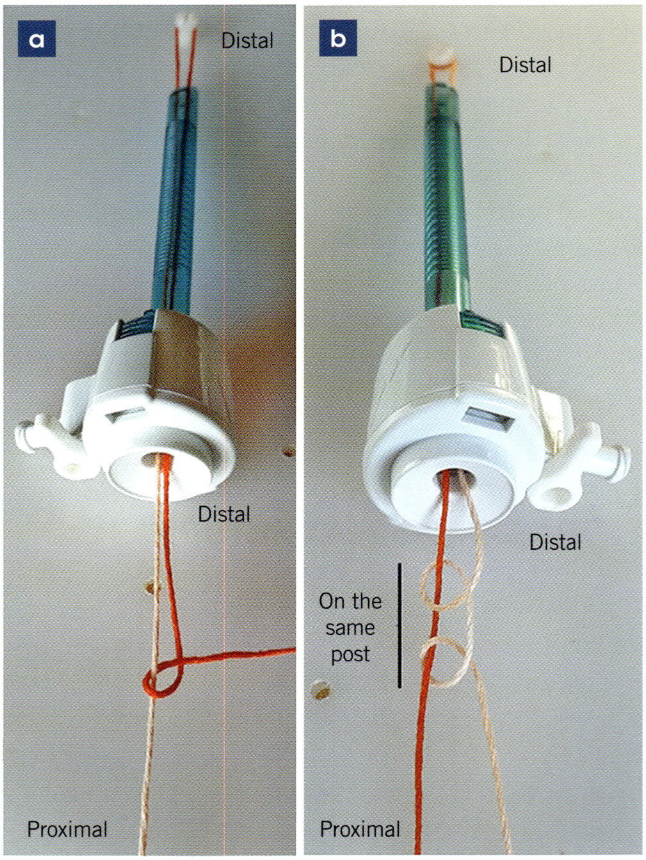

FIGURE 23. Noncompound sliding (static) slip knots. a) Simple overhand turn. b) Double turn, overhand and underhand, on the same post.

In view of this, two methods have been developed to prevent knot loosening: throwing additional loops over the sliding knot after it is seated (nonlocking slip knots) and changing the sliding knot into a nonsliding knot after it is seated (locking slip knots).

Although LES is the simplest for of LS, it has disadvantages with respect to LIS: possible loss of pneumoperitoneum through the trocar valve, dependence on auxiliary instruments such as the knot pusher, or temporary loss of the home base each time knotting is performed outside the patient. The time of performance is usually shorter than in LIS, but once LIS is mastered the average time of both methods are comparable. LES is less cost-effective than LIS because one suture is used after each completion of the knot. Indeed, LES knots are restricted to interrupted patterns like simple stitches or stitches in figure of 8, X or Z. Additionally, LES reproduces better the force exerted by the fingers in conventional surgery, so it is estimated that LES is suitable for vessels above 4 mm in thickness.

The underlying principles of LES consist of using a sufficiently long suture thread (70–90 cm, or even up to 1.5 m), with the needle-free tail remaining outside the patient at all times. As a general rule, the ideal suture size is 2-0 or greater. For slicing knots, a larger diameter correlates with a greater holding strength (knot and loop security). The optimal material depends on the type of knot, as certain sliding knots may have different holding strengths depending on the material used. In general, stiff hydrophobic monofilament has poor holding strength and may not be recommended in LES because it is more prone to fail than braided. During the tissue-piercing maneuvers, the thread may be introduced into the cavity by accident. To prevent this, the thread can be secured with a mosquito clamp. The needle is introduced through the trocar in the same way as for LIS. Once the needle is placed in the appropriate position in the NH, the tissue is pierced, and the needle is externalized by pulling the thread about 2–4 cm from the needle. A good length for the exteriorized working tail of thread is 20–30 cm. At this point, two ends (limbs) are ready to tie the knot (**Fig. 25**): the post limb (PL)—the straight end (fixed tail) of the thread that is under the most tension (stress) and around which the loops are thrown—and the nonpost limb (NPL)—the free end (wrapping tail) of the thread that wraps the loops around the PL. The authors emphasize that needle action is not always necessary (e.g., when occluding the cystic duct, renal vessels, or the thoracic duct).

There are multiple knots and modalities of performing LES, each with pros and cons among different extracorporeal knots and also compared to intracorporeal knotting. In all of them,

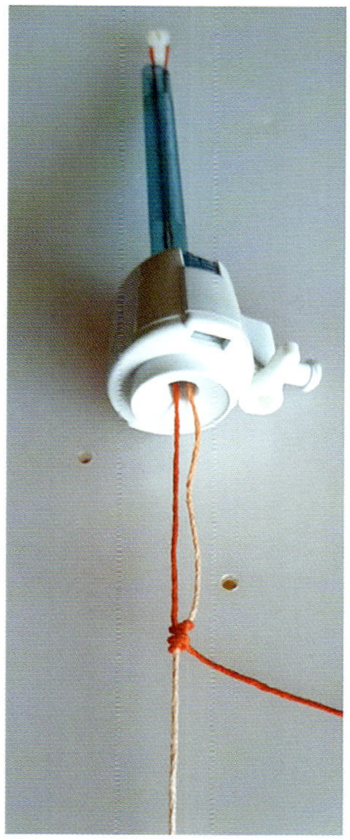

FIGURE 24. A Roeder knot (compound sliding slip knot) before being pushed on the tissue.

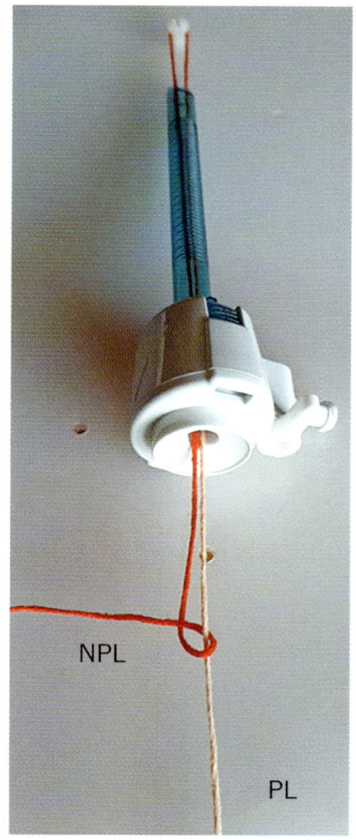

FIGURE 25. Post limb (PL), the straight and fixed tail of the thread. Nonpost limb (NPL), the wrapping tail that wraps around the PL to create compound or noncompound extracorporeal knots.

the knot is tied extracorporeally and, whether it is a noncompound static knot or a compound knot, it is tightened with some type of knot pusher. Before the suture is cut, any knot may be reinforced by adding three simple square turns, also known as Loutzenheiser's recommendations of three reversed half hitches on alternating posts (3-RHAP) (**Fig. 26**), extracorporeally with the knot pusher or intracorporeally with the laparoscopic NH. As discussed below, any secure knot in LES may be composed of the base knot for tissue reduction: two half hitches in noncompound sliding static slip knots or the formed compound sliding slip knot. After the base knot has been placed, its security is determined by the so-called surgical knot, that is, any blocking sequence of half knots, being the most recommendable the 3-RHAP (**Fig. 26**).

There are various shapes and diameters of knot pusher tips to lead the knots inside the cavity. They should be small enough to avoid snagging of the knot but big enough to allow the threads to freely pass. Usually, in compound knots, the PL is used by the knot pusher while the sliding knot is pushed and

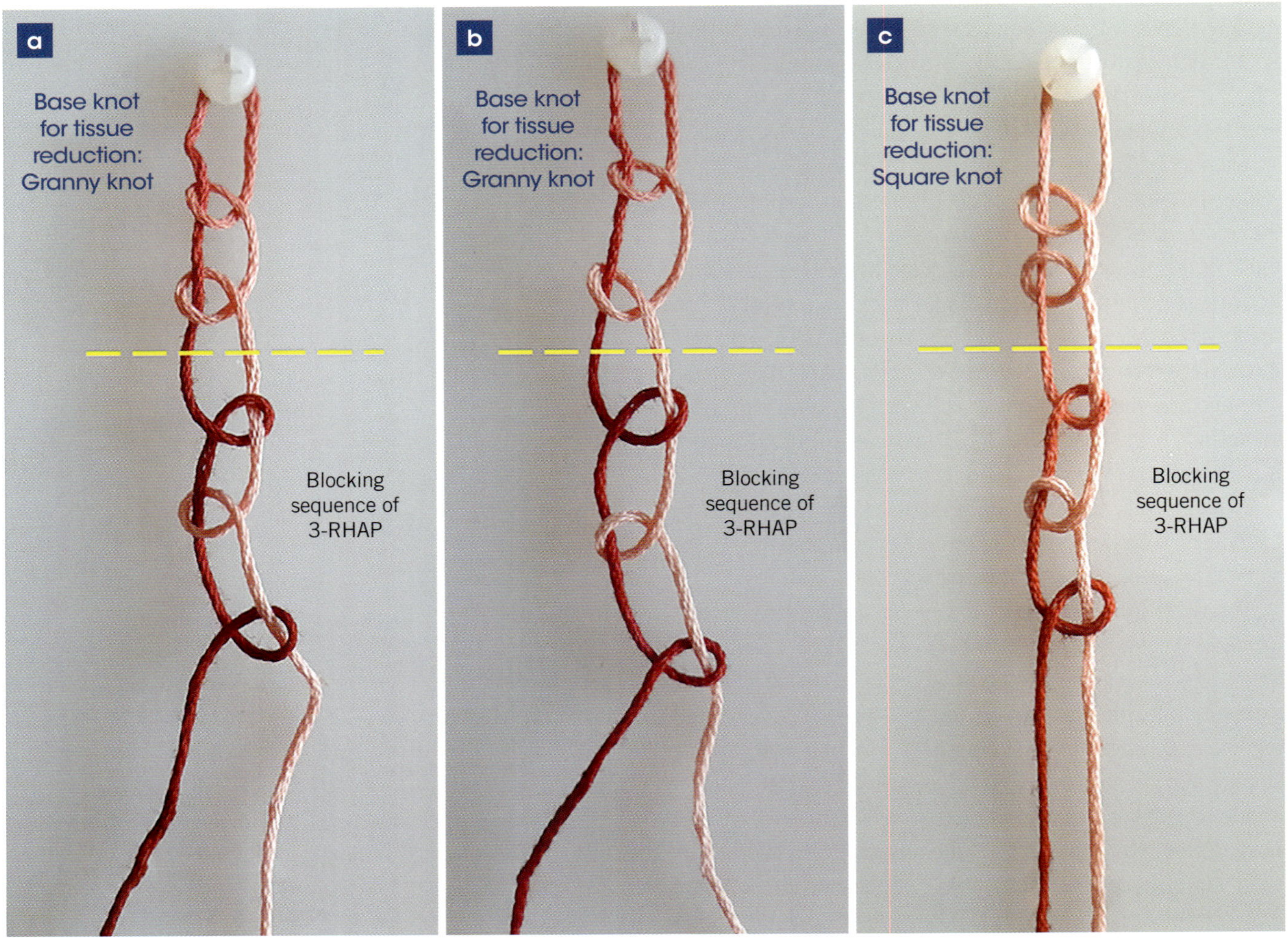

FIGURE 26. Examples of the three reversed half hitches on alternating posts (3-RHAP) recommended for securing any knot. a) Underhand, overhand post switch, overhand post switch. b) Overhand, underhand post switch, overhand post switch. c) Overhand, underhand post switch, overhand post switch.

firmly placed and seated on the target tissue (**Fig. 27**). This final action must be gentle, a "knot kissing" (**Fig. 36**), in order not to tear the tissue due to the extreme forces of the knot pusher and sliding knot over the tissue.

NONCOMPOUND (STATIC) SLIDING SLIP KNOTS

Half hitch, half knot, or simple knot (Fig. 23)

Clarke HC described simple extracorporeal knot tying in 1972 and developed a knot pusher for LES. According to this technique, one or several knots are tied outside the abdomen, and each of them is introduced with the knot pusher, thus forming a knot similar to those of open surgery. Especially for extracorporeal noncompound knots, to ensure that the half knot advances and remains tight on the tissue, one hand (the left one for a right-handed surgeon) must always keep gentle tension on both ends of the suture (PL and NPL) outside the patient. The other hand (the right one for a right-handed surgeon) is used to apply reverse traction (forward pressure) on the knot pusher. The knot pusher captures and pushes the knot into place slowly and steadily. The second and third throws can be used to lock and secure the first one. With this technique, consecutive surgical knots can be tied (wrapped) extracorporeally and introduced into the abdominal cavity, making this technique quite simple and reliable (**Fig. 27**).

Despite being used for open surgery, the half hitch is the most fundamental way of suturing in LES or LIS. It is a simple knot, in which the active tail of the thread (NPL) is tied over and/or under the straight passive tail (PL). Although essentially described as "insecure" on its own, it is a valuable component

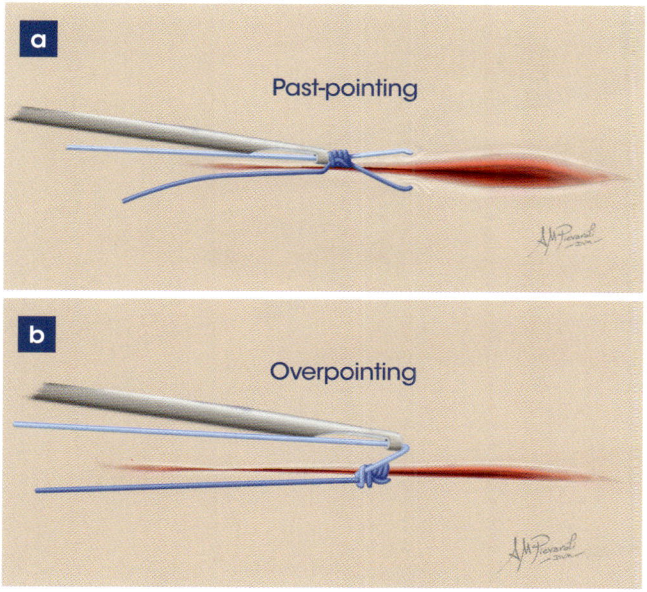

FIGURE 27. Techniques for securing laparoscopic extracorporeal sliding knots. a) Past-pointing for noncompound (static) half hitches. Keeping tension on the PL, the half hitch on the NPL is advanced past the knot base with the knot pusher. b) Overpointing for compound sliding knots. Keeping tension on the PL, the knot is pushed down on the tissue with the knot pusher ("knot kissing").

in a wide variety of useful and reliable snags, kinks, and knots. Half hitches may be stacked on each other to create a sequence of simple knots or may also be used with 3-RHAP to secure extracorporeal noncompound or compound knots. Half hitches can be formed in two different configurations: a loop limb tied over the PL (overhand limb) or a loop limb tied under the PL (underhand half hitch) (**Fig. 23**).

The different combinations of using half hitches in LES according to each work and author can be unmanageable. Human gynecologic laparoscopy frequently uses a sequence of simple knots with final locking 1:1:1 or 2:1, without alternating posts. It may be started, for example, with a first throw of an overhand turn of the NPL over the PL. It should be borne in mind that the knot pusher exerts a past-pointing tightening force (slightly laterally) beyond the place where the knot is left. At the same time, a gentle counterforce is exerted outward on the PL. The second throw is identical to the first one, also overhand, since the blocking sequence corresponds to the underhand third throw, also on the same post (**Fig. 28**). Regarding this sequence of knots, the authors remark that, unlike LIS recommendations, the first two turns of the base knot for tissue reduction are wrapped in the same direction and on the same PL and may form a granny knot on purpose, as in **Figure 26**. It is important to consider that the first two half hitches can also be joined in a first double turn, without separate throws, before the blocking sequence, and the last blocking half hitch also on the same post would be wrapped underhand in this case (**Fig. 28**).

A standard knot pusher is not always available. As an alternative, a laparoscopic Babcock or Duvall forceps can be used to push the knot, but the surgeon must consider the trocar size because these types of forceps only fit through a 10 mm trocar. In this technique consecutive half hitches are knotted extracorporeally, and each knot is advanced as follows: both suture tails are passed, from the outside to the inside, through the fenestrations at the tip of the Babcock forceps. Both suture tails are pulled taut together in one hand, and the grasper is passed through the trocar valve and cannula into the cavity, driving the knot into place. As the knot approaches the tissue, the tips of the Babcock forceps are opened to apply a lateral, balanced tension that secures the knot.

COMPOUND SLIDING SLIP KNOTS

Roeder knot (1:3–5:1) (Fig. 29)

The Roeder knot, or external fisherman's knot, is the first extracorporeal sliding knot described, by Hans Albert Roeder in 1918 for tonsillectomy and patented in 1931. It has undergone several modifications and improvements over time for application in LS. The safety of the Roeder loop depends mainly on the number of initial turns around the PL, and its safety as a compound knot depends on the additional half hitches. Although the original Roeder knot consisted of four or five turns around both the PL and NPL, the prevailing and more practical configuration of the Roeder knot for LES, described by Dr. Semm, has three turns around both strands. Mishra et al. demonstrated that the Roeder knot can be safe even with as few as two turns around both strands if it is followed by 3-RHAP. Therefore, in general, four or five turns (monofilament) or three turns (braided) may be sufficient for a Roeder knot. Other authors argue that once this knot has been tightened on the tissue, it can be reinforced intracorporeally with a single or double laparoscopic intracorporeal knot.

The Roeder knot, like the rest of compound (sliding) knots, is formed outside the patient and passed into the peritoneal cavity with the aid of a knot pusher made of hollow plastic (commercial) or fenestrated metal (reusable). The advantage of the Roeder knot is that only one knot is sufficient to secure the vascular pedicle, the biopsied material, or to approximate the edges of the incision.

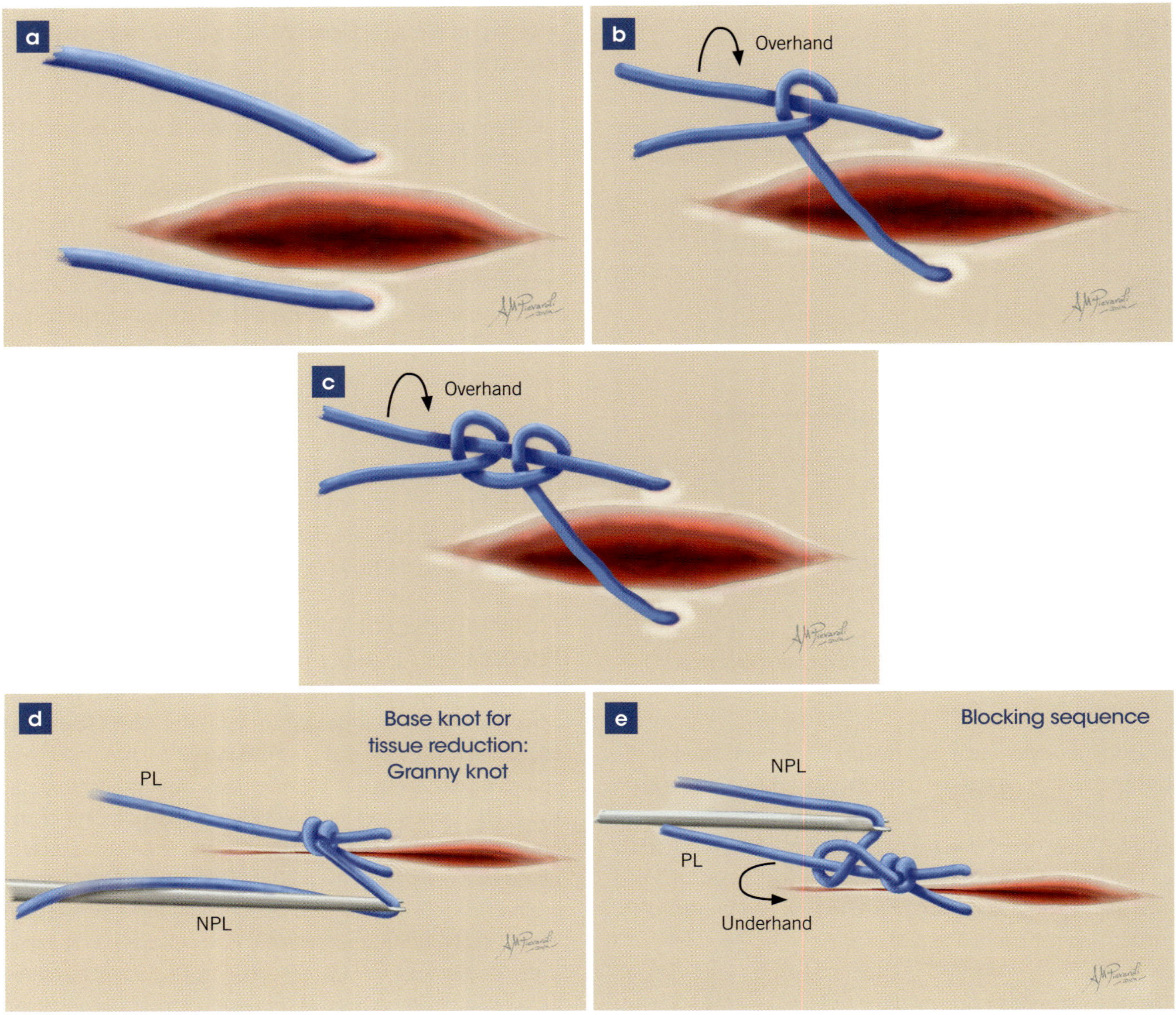

FIGURE 28. Sequence of simple knots with final locking (1 overhand:1 overhand:1 underhand), with past-pointing but without alternating posts.

The technique for making a Roeder knot is as follows:

- Two parts are differentiated before knotting, a longer fixed tail (PL) that remains on the right side of the trocar valve and a shorter loop tail (NPL) that remains on the left side of the trocar valve. The ideal length of the PL is approximately twice the length of the NPL. For security reasons while looping, the needle of the NPL may be cut.
- A simple turn of the NPL is wrapped around the PL. This first knot must remain slightly loose, without overtightening it. At the same time, an assistant usually keeps their index finger in the trocar valve hole to help maintain the tension of the two limbs and keep them with some degree of separation as well as to prevent loss of pneumoperitoneum.
- The NPL is thrown three to five times around both suture limbs distally (toward the trocar hole and patient). It should be kept in mind that up to eight turns may be performed, depending on the source.
- A final locking simple turn is made. The NPL only is looped around the PL, between the space closest to the holding finger (i.e., between the space of the fourth and fifth throw if five throws have been made). It is important that this final turn takes place on the same side of the PL, in this case, the

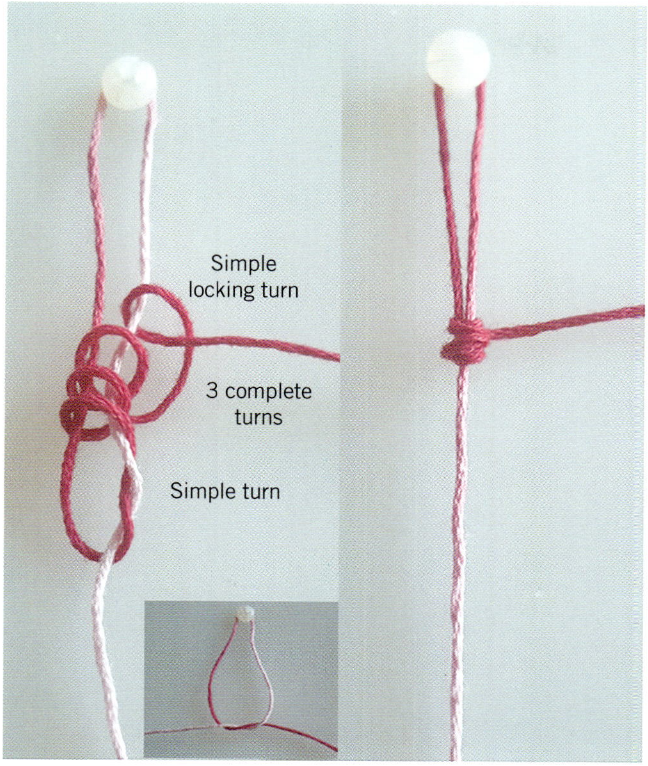

FIGURE 29. Roeder knot.

long tail on the right side of the valve, and not on the opposite side.

- The index finger is removed, and the Roeder knot is tightened and shaped (fully compound). The excess thread is trimmed before advancing the knot. The knot pusher captures the PL while it is pulled taut, and the knot is introduced into the cavity. The PL must remain as longitudinal (axial) on the trocar as possible. The procedure is identical if a closed plastic introducer is used.
- A series of additional turns in opposing directions are optional, especially the Loutzenheiser's recommendations of 3-RHAP.
- The excess long thread on which the knot was advanced is cut with laparoscopic scissors.

Melzer–Buess knot (2:3:2) (Fig. 30)

A modification of the Roeder knot, and frequently called the Meltzer or Melzer knot, the original Melzer–Buess knot was described in 1991 by the general surgeons Melzer and Buess for extracorporeal ligation during laparoscopic colectomy. Nowadays, the Melzer–Buess knot is preferred over the Roeder knot and is maybe the gold standard extracorporeal compound knot for securing tubular structures like blood vessels or the cystic duct during cholecystectomy, since catgut is no longer available.

Polydioxanone (PDS) is a good suture material choice for the Melzer–Buess knot. The technique for making this knot is as follows:

- A double half knot is made by wrapping the NPL around the PL.
- Three complete throws are made with the tail of the NPL over both the PL and NPL distally (toward the trocar and patient).
- The knot is locked by two (opposing) half hitches of the NPL. They must always be wrapped around the same side, over the PL.
- The knot is configured and advanced into place with the knot pusher while maintaining gentle tension on the PL.

Equine (modified Roeder–Melzer–Buess) knot (2:2:1) (Fig. 31)

An interesting variant, whose initial design did not include 3-RHAP, is the one described in 1999 by Rijkenhuizen and Grinwis for equine laparoscopic castration. A mixture of the Melzer–Buess and Roeder knots, the equine knot combines safety and simplicity. Safety because it starts like the Melzer–Buess knot, with a double half knot of the NPL around the PL, to provide extra friction and minimum backsliding. Simplicity because it is followed by only two turns of the Roeder knot around both strands and a final half hitch around the standing limb. However, this is no obstacle to potentially adding the recommended 3-RHAP after any completed knot for optimum knot security.

Tayside knot (1:4:1) (Fig. 32)

The Tayside knot is more secure than the Roeder knot. The technique for making this knot is as follows:

- As for the Roeder knot, a first overhand simple knot is made over the PL. This will create the first loop between this first knot (proximal) and both tails that come from the trocar valve (distal).
- With the assistant surgeon pulling to keep the PL straight, the surgeon uses the index and thumb fingers of the left hand to fix the first knot of the first loop, and with the right hand the NPL is passed four times over the PL, creating a second loop.
- The locking knot is made when the NPL is passed through the second loop, forming a third loop, through which the NPL is passed. This tail is finally pulled with the right hand,

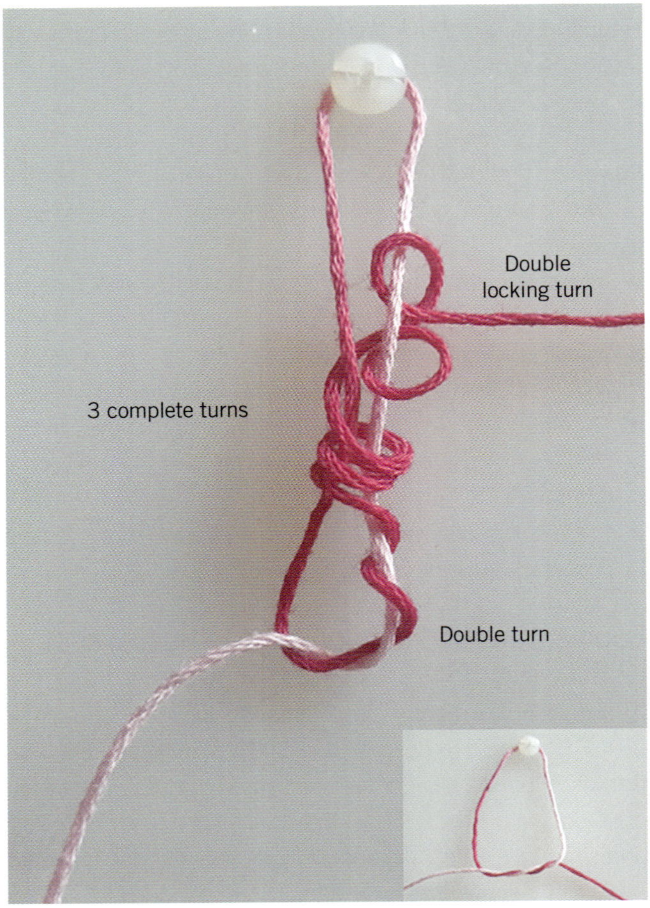

FIGURE 30. Melzer–Buess knot.

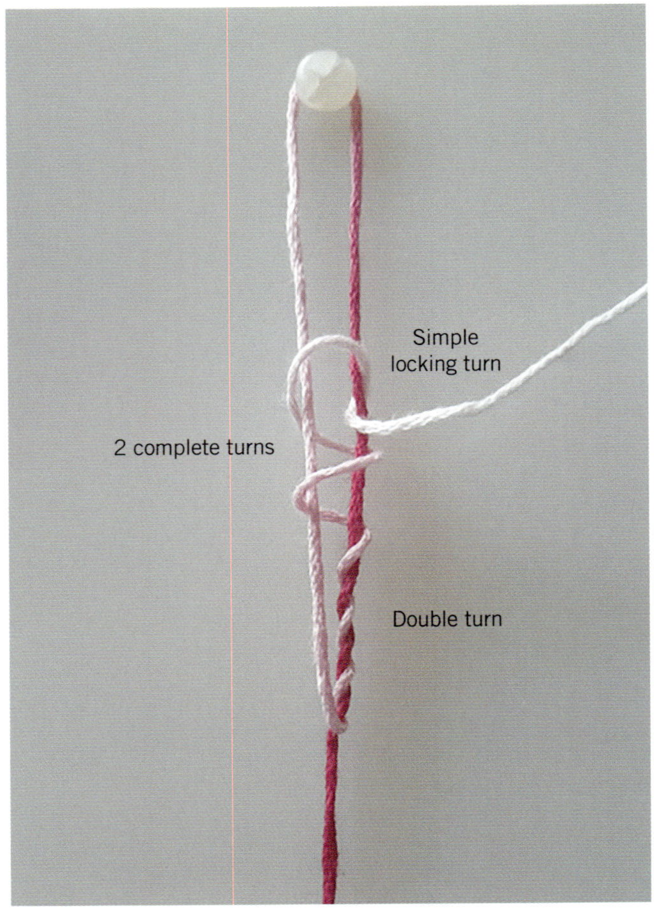

FIGURE 31. Equine knot (modified Roeder–Melzer–Buess knot).

maintaining the tension of the left index on the first loop and the countertraction of the assistant in the PL. With this, the final knot is formed and locked and is ready to be advanced.

Unlike other knots, the Tayside knot has the particularity that it does not slide on its own if the surgeon pulls on the PL. In fact, this action can tear the tissue. Therefore, the surgeon must first make sure that the knot is well formed and locked by laterally pulling on the NPL. Once this is done, the knot pusher is mandatory to advance the Tayside knot forward.

Weston knot (1:1:1:1) (Fig. 33)

Described first by Dr. Peter Weston in 1991, the Weston slip knot is mainly used in human laparoscopic gynecology and arthroscopic surgery. It is relatively easy to tie extracorporeally and to slip into the body cavity, it can be tightly secured (self-locking), and it is not bulky. Overall, it is a comfortable knot because the PL does not move when wrapping the NPL.

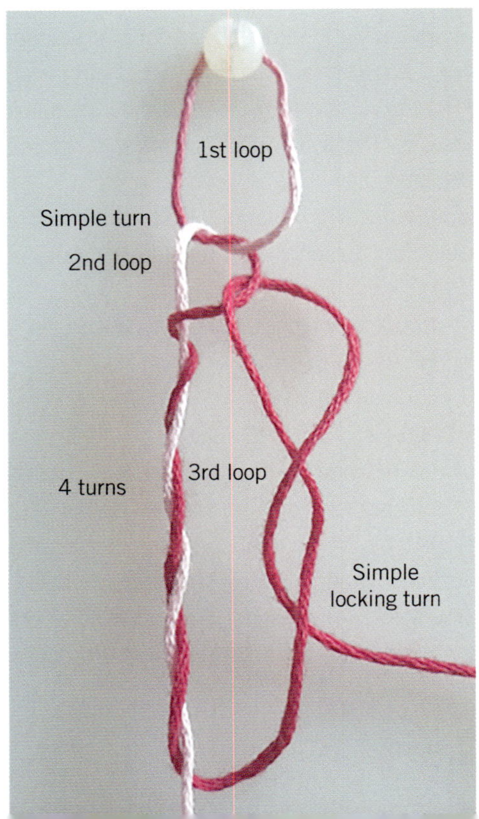

FIGURE 32. Tayside knot.

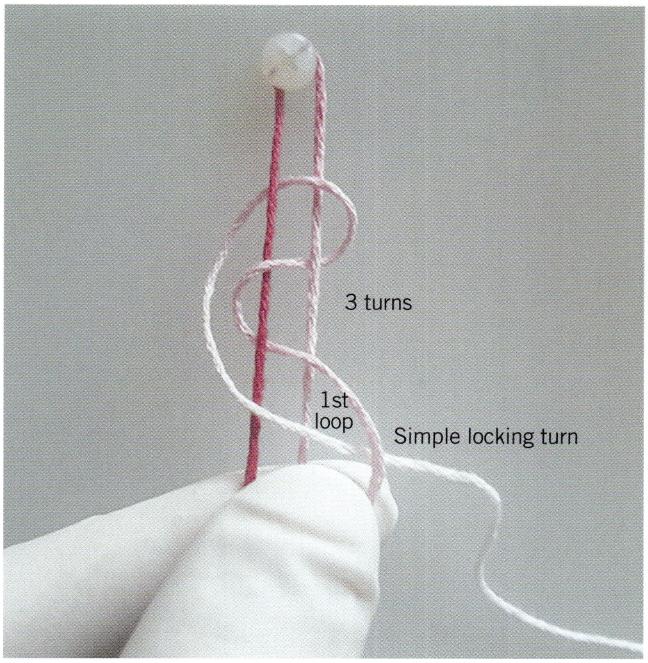

FIGURE 33. Weston knot.

The technique for making a Weston knot is as follows:

- Two parts are differentiated before knotting, a longer loop tail (NPL) that remains on the right side of the trocar valve and a shorter fixed tail (PL) that remains on the left side of the trocar valve (contrary to the Roeder and Melzer–Buess knots). The ideal length of the NPL is approximately twice the length of the PL. For security reasons while looping, the needle of the PL may be cut.
- Before starting any of the loops, both tails are kept parallel between the left thumb and index finger, because the NPL will be passed three times between the PL and NPL.
- The NPL on the right is passed between both posts to the left side, to create a first single turn (underwrap) around the left PL. This makes a first loop on the right NPL, between the surgeon's thumb and index finger (proximal) and the first underwrap turn (distal). This first loop will be used as the locking loop.
- The NPL on the left side is passed between both posts, this time from left to right, to create a second single turn (underwrap) around the right NPL.
- A third single turn (underwrap) is thrown around the left PL.
- The NPL is passed through the first loop created on the right NPL.
- The knot is then stacked and may be advanced only by pulling on the PL. Once blocked on the target tissue, the Weston knot is locked by pulling on the NPL.

Mishra knot (1:1:1:1:1:1:1) (Fig. 34)

Recently, Dr. R. K. Mishra developed a simple, reproducible, safe knot that works well with any suture material. It can be used to occlude tubular structures of up to a maximum diameter of 22 mm. The Mishra knot is essentially a modification of the Roeder–Melzer–Buess knot. Therefore, its tying technique is very similar: a mixture of simple turns and complete loops alternating each other that aims to achieve better knot security by application of a lock after every wind. The Mishra knot has been compared to other extracorporeal knots and it has been concluded that, overall, it combines the loop and knot security of other standardized laparoscopic extracorporeal knots. In particular, the Mishra knot and the Tayside knot have higher knot quality scores than the Roeder knot.

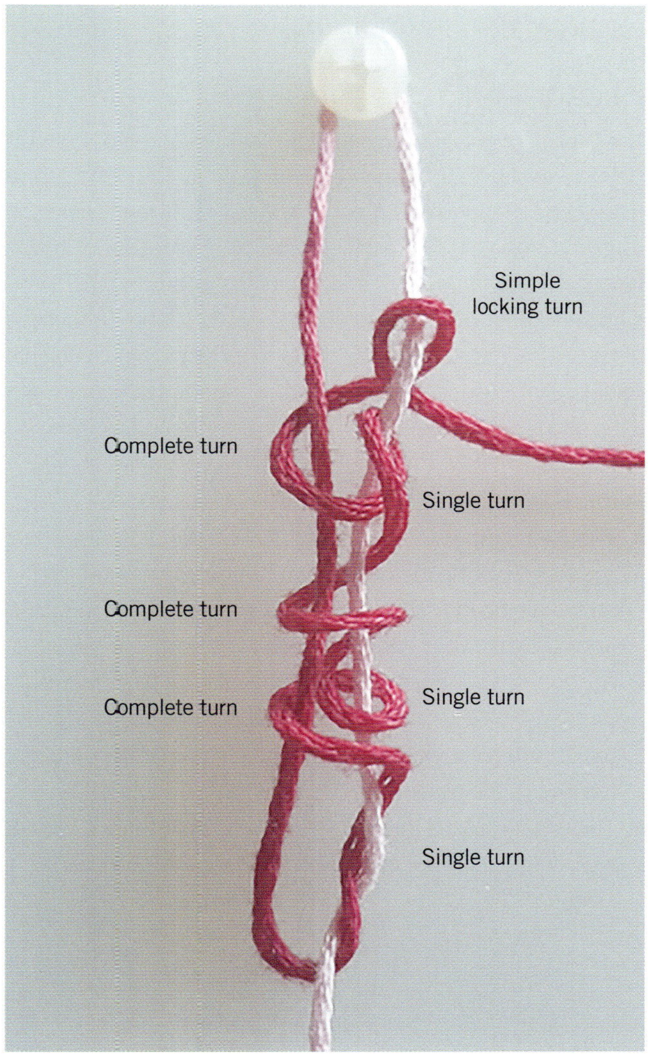

FIGURE 34. Mishra knot.

The technique for making a Mishra knot is as follows:

- A simple (overwrap) turn of the NPL is wrapped around the PL.
- The tail of the NPL takes the first complete loop by wrapping both the PL and NPL.
- For the second simple turn, the NPL is wrapped around the PL only.
- The NPL takes the second complete loop by wrapping both the PL and NPL.
- For the third simple turn, the NPL is wrapped around the PL only.
- The NPL takes the third complete loop by wrapping both the PL and NPL.
- A fourth simple turn of the NPL is finally wrapped around the PL only.
- The Mishra knot is configured and ready to slip while keeping the PL straight. Backing it up with the 3-RHAP reinforces knot security.

Pretzel knot (1:1) (Fig. 35)

The Pretzel knot is a simple to learn, easy to prepare, low profile locking slip knot. It only requires two half hitches that are advanced from the patient and trocar valve (distal) toward the surgeon (proximal). Overall, the pretzel knot slides easily, maintains good locking tension, and, in comparison with other standardized knots (SMC, giant, Dines, Nicky's, and Tennessee slider knots), has significantly better loop security in its original configuration. As for any other knot, it may be backed up with three additional RHAP.

The technique for making the pretzel knot is as follows:

- The fixed limb (PL) remains on the left hand, and a single overhand half hitch is made with the wrapping limb (NPL) on the right hand. This will create a first loop between the PL and NPL that will be used as the locking loop.
- An opposing (underhand) second half hitch is made by passing the NPL under the PL. It should be borne in mind that this turn should be made proximal (toward the surgeon, not toward the patient).
- The NPL is passed through the first loop between the PL and NPL of the first overhand half hitch. The knot will look like a pretzel.

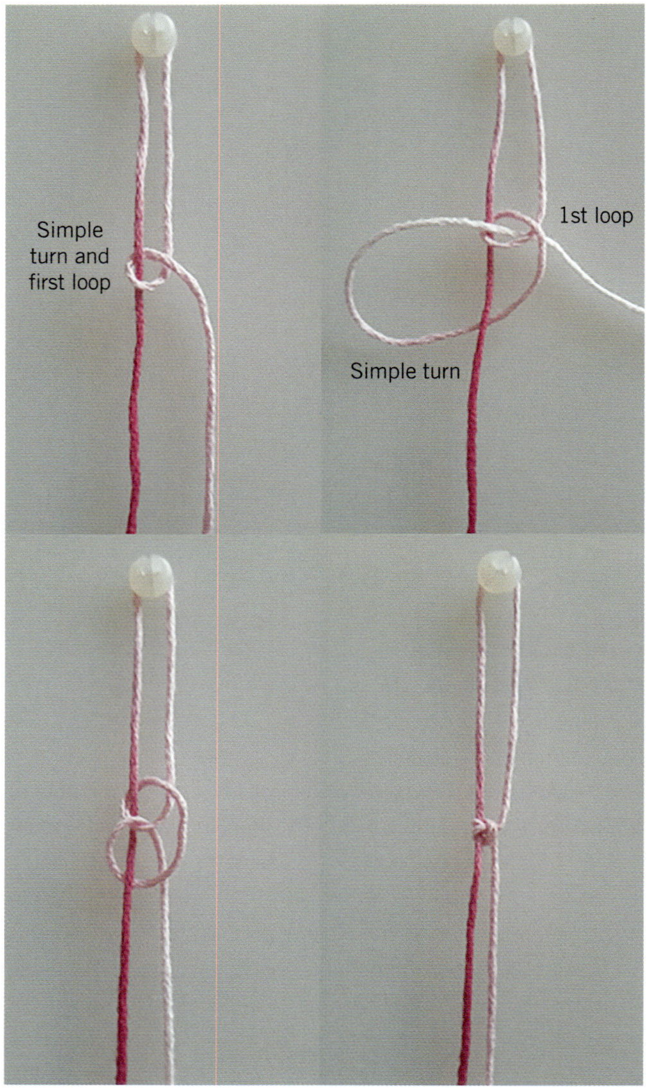

FIGURE 35. Pretzel knot.

- The knot is configured by gentle traction on the NPL in line with the PL. At this point, the knot is slid inside the body cavity by pulling on the PL or using a knot pusher.
- The knot must be flipped for security after it has been advanced to the desired position. The NPL is pulled to strangle and lock the PL. This will flip and lock the knot, similar in effect to post switching. Additional reversed half hitches may be added as well.

Key points

- In LES, the surgeon must bear in mind the arthroscopic Loutzenheiser's recommendations from the Arthroscopic and Orthopedic surgery. As these repairs suffer from high loads on the knots, emphasis is placed on the following rule: at least three nonidentical (reversed) half hitches on alternating posts (3-RHAP) should be thrown after the initial base knot.
- The base knot reduces the tissues before the 3-RHAP. The base knot for noncompound sliding (static) slip knots consists of two half hitches. For compound sliding slip knots, the base knot is fully formed extracorporeally.
- In LES, the surgeon should be familiar with at least one noncompound sliding (static) knot and one compound sliding slip knot to adapt knot configuration according to the intraoperative findings.
- Simplified knot formulas:
  - Roeder knot: 1:3–5:1.
  - Melzer–Buess knot: 2:3:2.
  - Equine knot (modified Roeder–Melzer–Buess knot): 2:2:1.
  - Tayside knot: 1:4:1.
  - Weston knot: 1:1:1:1.
  - Mishra knot: 1:1:1:1:1:1:1.
  - Pretzel knot: 1:1.

ENDOLOOP (FIG. 36)

Commercial pretied loops are available for hemostasis of vascular pedicles, biopsy, or pedunculated tissues. Pretied knots may be more convenient in terms of security, but they are more expensive than handmade knots. The free end of commercial knots will remain outside the patient, inside the plastic guide tube (knot pusher), and is detachable from the guide tube. To prevent gas leakage, these knots have an adapter or overtube that fits over the trocar valve.

Placement is very simple. The knot is passed through the trocar using the introducer (otherwise, the loop bends and is difficult to handle inside). After placing the loop around the tissue

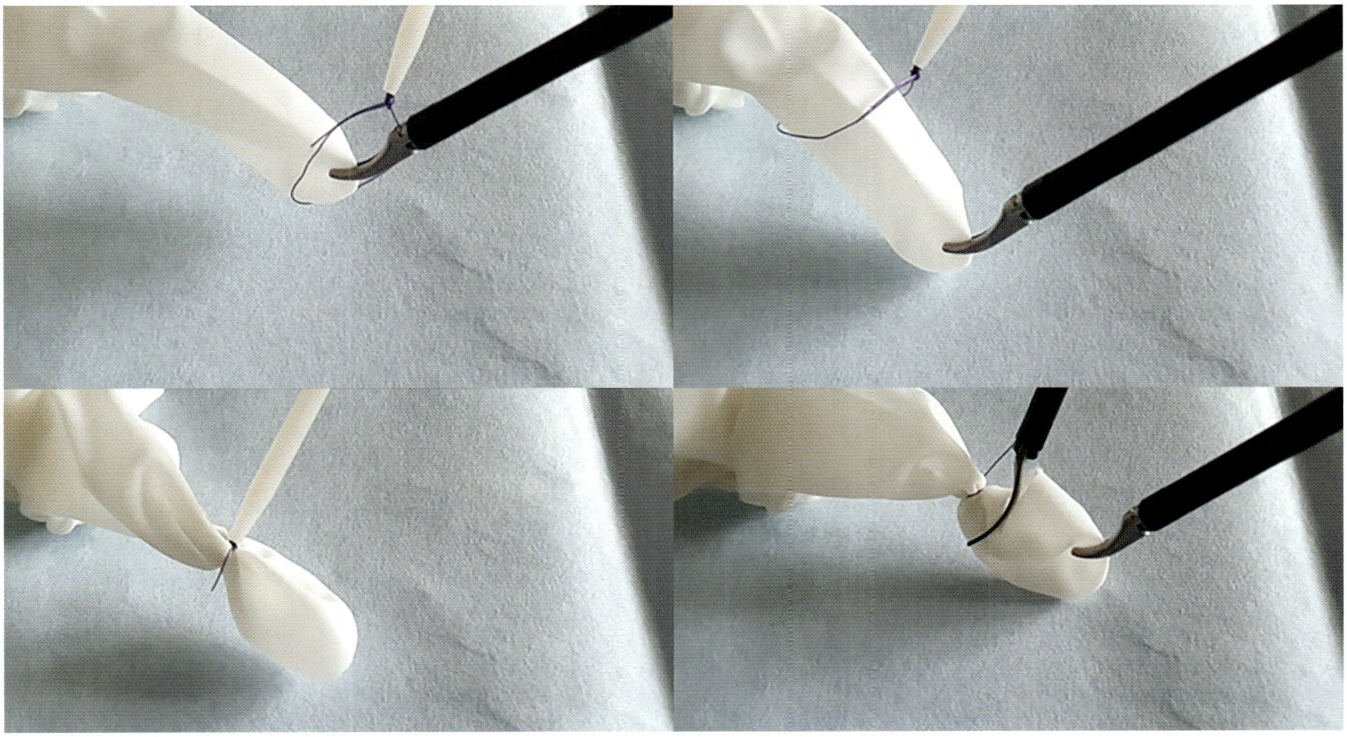

FIGURE 36. Endoloop and technique for biopsy with ipsilateral trocar setting.

to be ligated, the proximal end of the knot pusher (outside the patient) is broken off and used to exert traction on the free end of the thread, while the distal part of the tube (tip inside the patient) is used to push the knot over the tissue.

Commercial pretied knots are available in absorbable monofilament and braided and nonabsorbable braided materials. They usually employ the Roeder knot and have their own pushing guiding aid. However, endoloops can be handmade by making an extracorporeal knot and reusing the guide from other commercially available pretied knots or advancing the knot with any standard reusable knot pusher.

BARBED SUTURES (FIG. 37)

Self-anchoring sutures were first described in the early 1950s and then reported in in vitro (human cadavers) and in vivo (canine model) clinical reports for the repair of long flexor tendons. In recent times, the use of self-anchoring sutures seems unstoppable in many MIS fields, especially in laparoscopy. They are very effective in reducing operative times and improving surgical efficiency. An example in veterinary medicine is the clinical application in total laparoscopic incisional gastropexy or colopexy. Two types of barbed sutures were compared with intracorporeally tied knots using absorbable monofilament suture. Both types of barbed sutures significantly decreased the mean time required for intracorporeal gastropexy suture (V-Loc = 19 minutes, Quill = 20 minutes) when compared to monofilament suture (PDS = 39 minutes). In addition, it was demonstrated with ultrasound/laparoscopy that both barbed sutures correctly maintained the gastropexy at least 6 months postoperatively.

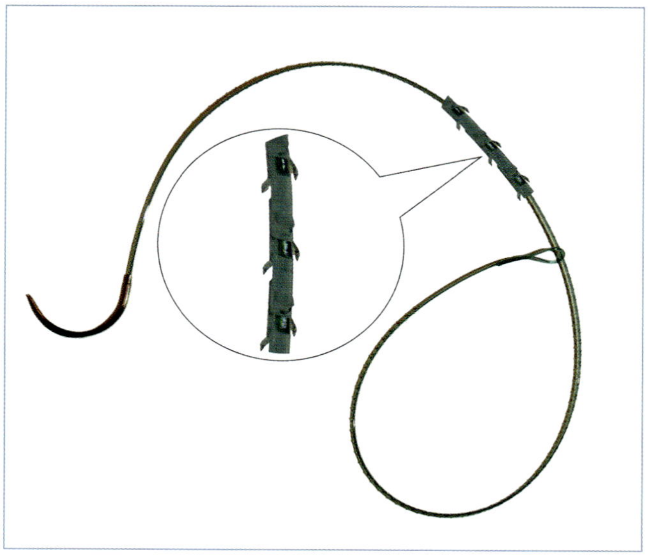

FIGURE 37. Example of a unidirectional barbed suture (V-Loc) with a loop as the anchoring system (stopper) for the first stitch.

The main characteristic of barbed sutures is that their anchoring barbs or spicules avoid the need for a conventional surgical knot for tissue approximation. This is especially beneficial in MIS procedures to overcome space and movement limitations. Currently, the most widely used self-anchoring sutures are V-Loc, Quill, Filbloc, and Stratafix. They can be classified according to absorbability (absorbable or nonabsorbable) and barb direction (unidirectional or bidirectional), and they can also be coated with antimicrobial agents. However, barbed sutures mainly differ in the type of spicule (shape, thickness, number, angulation, etc.) and in the method of anchoring the first point (loop, button lock system, fixation tab).

The potential adverse effects of barbed sutures must be taken into consideration. The method of handling and anchoring of each commercial brand must be known before clinical application. Once the barbed suture passes through the tissue, there is no going back due to the anchoring of the barbs, which can lead to surgery failure. Cases of postoperative digestive obstruction, similar to foreign body adhesions, have also been described. This complication is thought to be related to the barbs of the suture thread. If excessive intracavitary thread is left, the suture can react nonspecifically with the surrounding tissues, especially the intestine and mesentery. This is why it is recommended to leave a short end thread. Though rare, barbed suture entanglement should be considered a potentially serious differential diagnosis in these cases.

ADDITIONAL SUTURING AND KNOT TYING TECHNIQUES

SUTURING IN LAPAROENDOSCOPIC SINGLE-SITE SURGERY (LESS)

Laparoendoscopic single-site surgery (LESS), or single-incision laparoscopic surgery (SILS), is a laparoscopic approach with one single trocar, through which all the instruments and optics enter, resulting in minimal triangulation. This configuration makes it difficult to undertake LIS with the methods explained above. In addition, LIS during the LESS approach is quite dependent on the type of port trocar and on the instruments and optics available (angled or straight). To overcome these constraints, barbed sutures are used to avoid knotting, although techniques such as the so-called side winding suturing have been developed in an attempt to simplify LIS during LESS. This suturing method requires a roticulating dissector/grasper (Roticulator) or any laparoscopic forceps with prebent angulation. Roticulating or prebent laparoscopic instruments adapt to restricted space and limited ranges of motion. They are used for tissue traction and assist the NH in passing the needle through the incision, as in standard LS. If the Roticulator is used for the knotting maneuver, its curvature is deployed close to the incision (home base). The long tail is grasped with the NH and the suture is wrapped twice over the tip of the Roticulator, which then approaches and grabs the short tail. As usual, the NH pulls on the long tail at the same distance but in the opposite direction of the short tail to form a square (reef) knot or a surgeon's knot. The procedure is then repeated until the desired number of knots is reached.

Another modality, used by the authors, allows replication of the traditional laparoscopic knot tying technique with standard straight material. The angle of movements may increase and parallel working may be reduced if the needle is taken with one of the instruments and the loops are made with the other hand over the swage, taking advantage of the rigidity of the needle base. This maneuver is also facilitated if the NH jaws are kept open (gladiator rule).

Ingenious alternatives with straight instruments only have been described in human medicine, such as intracorporeal knotting on a D-loop in pediatric laparoscopy or a specific successive pattern of turns and rotations of the instruments on the thread for intracorporeal cinch knots in gynecologic laparoscopy.

SLING SUTURE

The sling suture technique was described by Nathanson and Cuschieri. A straight percutaneous needle with thread is passed through the abdominal or thoracic wall from outside to inside and vice versa. This needle is used for two purposes: to control any active bleeding from the abdominal or thoracic wall and to lift or retract any organ or tissue in order to facilitate operative view (falciform ligament, liver, stomach, intestine, ureter, bladder, uterus, etc.). It should be noted, however, that handling a straight needle with a long thread inside a small space may involve difficult maneuvers.

HEAVING LINE KNOT

The heaving line knot is a type of stopper knot that works as a starting knot in continuous sutures. The stopper knot is formed extracorporeally and is only recommended when the consistency of the tissue and serosa is good. A clip (standard titanium, Hem-o-lok, Lapra-Ty, Ti-Knot, Cor-Knot fasteners) or a piece of hemostatic sponge may be used proximal to the knot (toward the needle, between the tissue and the knot) to enhance the safety of a heaving line knot. They may be used in partial nephrectomy, mucosal apposition in reduced spaces like transanal laparoscopic surgery, or to approximate intestinal loops before anastomosis. About 5 cm extra thread length is required for extracorporeal knot creation. Also, the abovementioned ancillary stoppers may be used to fasten the end of running and interrupted sutures.

PURSE STRING SUTURE LINE

When required, circular tightening of the tissue can be achieved with a purse string suture by continuous entrance and exit stitches in 5 mm points.

ROBOTIC, ARTICULATED, AND MECHANICAL DEVICES

Beyond the use of NHs vs. knot pushers in LS, new robotic or mechanical devices are becoming more popular to reduce time and improve surgical results. The clinical application of the da Vinci robot (Intuitive) was demonstrated in the first report of robotic-assisted radical prostatectomy in a dog, particularly while completing the urethra–bladder anastomosis with barbed suture. There are pioneering experiences with more affordable robotic NHs (Flexdex) in total laparoscopic gastropexy in dogs. Other nonrobotic, mechanized, articulated systems that allow a wide degree of mobility inside the patient are available. Their needle and thread are usually incorporated in the tip, the loop itself is already configured, or interchangeable cartridges of barbed and nonbarbed sutures are available (ProxiSure, Endo360°, SILS Stitch, Endo Stitch, Suture Assistant, Quick-Stitch). There are also technology-based laparoscopic mechanical staplers (powered staplers) whose robotization has enabled a smart clamp effect that provides feedback to the surgeon, resulting in improved outcomes for the patient (EndoWrist, Signia, Echelon, Lunar). They have a precise and stable handheld robotic articulation at the distal tip to minimize tremor. The system detects if the stapler jaws are adequately closed on the target tissue while the staples and blade automatically run smoothly through the tissues.

HOW MANY TURNS AND THROWS DO I NEED?—KNOT SECURITY IN LAPAROSCOPIC SURGERY

The knot quality score (KQS) is an objective formula to assess knot security and deduce the degree of knot tightening and slipping. It is considered that knot security fails when the knot slips more than 3 mm or ruptures. Knot security also considers the loop- and knot-holding capacity without failing. Research on knotting provides extensive background information in this respect, but the existing studies are variable in terms of the number of surgeons performing the knots, whether they consider the KQS or not, the type of knot and suture material used, etc. Some studies affirm that the most important factor in knot security may be the type of suture material, being monofilament more likely to fail, although they also found differences regarding the type of knot. Thus, it can be concluded that, for LIS, intracorporeal flat square knots (four throws) and surgeon's knots tolerate distraction forces better and have a higher median KQS compared to intracorporeal square slip knots. For LES (static knots with a knot pusher), alternating flat square throws or a surgeon's knot pushed to the target tissue tolerate distraction forces better and have a higher median KQS compared to compound sliding knots.

The question of how many turns and throws are needed cannot be answered conclusively because knots can be influenced by knot type, number of turns/throws, final knot volume, technique used, surgeon's skill, suture size and material, structure, absorbability, etc. Some studies state that a near zero knot failure rate may be achieved according to the number of throws (layers): some authors advocate using a minimum of three throws, others recommend four to six throws, six to eight throws, and others specify six full square knots (twelve layers) (see knot nomenclature in **Table 3**). To summarize, LIS and conventional surgical knotting are both secure, and a knot may be considered safe with three or four throws. Although, ideally, the security is maximized with six throws, the safety of the knot will not be further enhanced if this number is exceeded. In the case of LES, static square knots and static surgeon's knots provide the best loop and knot security, but the majority of compound knots offer acceptable to good loop security as well. However, differences have been reported depending on whether three additional reversed (opposing) half hitches were placed on top of the knot.

WHAT IS THE BEST KNOTTING CONFIGURATION?

Intracorporeal flat knot configuration: An interesting 2019 study measured the drag forces of knot sliding/failing for different braided (nonabsorbable silk and absorbable Vicryl) and monofilament (nonabsorbable polypropylene and polyester) suture materials in several sizes (3-0, 2-0, 0, and 2) using four knot configurations. The authors of the study used the nomenclature by Loutzenheiser et al.: square knots with two throws (1=1) and three throws (1=1=1) and surgeon's knots with two throws (2=1) and three throws (2=1=1), the symbol = meaning that the next throw wraps in the opposite direction from the previous one. Interestingly, the results showed that, in all suture materials studied, the drag forces of knot sliding/failing using a same material were as follows: (2=1=1) > (1=1=1) > (2=1) > (1=1). This conclusion can be considered a general rule for the most representative flat knots, but the main limitation of the study was that absorbable monofilament materials were not included.

Extracorporeal slip knot configuration: The optimal formula after any noncompound knot that includes the base knot or the first two half hitches for tissue reduction should be followed by three reverse half hitches (Loutzenheiser's 3-RHAP) (**Fig. 26a**), but other formulas are accepted (**Figs. 26b,c**). For any of the configurations, the first two half hitches (base knot) on the same post just reduce the tissue (reduction maneuver), while the final 3-RHAP locks the knot (locking maneuver). For compound knots, the optimal and most recommended formula after the knot has been advanced on the tissue is the Loutzenheiser's 3-RHAP (**Fig. 26a,c**), but others may also be considered (**Fig. 26b**). In summary, any final locking tool of three hitches that does not involve alternating posts is considered as not secure.

Key points

- For LIS flat knot configuration, the literature claims that, in general, the degree of knot security is as follows: (2=1=1) > (1=1=1) > (2=1) > (1=1). The symbol = means that the next throw wraps in the opposite direction from the previous one.
- Three or four throws may be sufficient for good knot security. Ideally, optimal knot security is achieved with six throws, but exceeding this number will not further enhance knot security.
- For LES slip knot configuration, the literature claims that, in general, the optimal formula after any noncompound knot that includes the first two half hitches for tissue reduction should be followed by three reverse half hitches (Loutzenheiser's 3-RHAP). Likewise, the optimal formula after any compound knot should include the Loutzenheiser's 3-RHAP.

SUGGESTED READINGS

9 LEARNING AND ADVANCING MINIMALLY INVASIVE SURGERY SKILLS

Boel A. Fransson

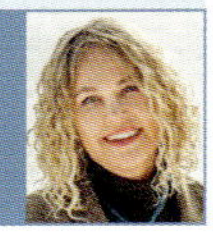

Veterinary training in small animal minimally invasive surgery (MIS) was first made a requirement in 2009 when the American College of Veterinary Surgeons (ACVS) added 20 MIS cases for completing residency training. At that time, 86% of small animal ACVS diplomates were already performing MIS procedures in clinical practice. Most diplomates reported they had been trained by faculty during their residency programs, but many had not received formal training themselves, and there was, and remains to be, a considerable variation in focus, instrumentation, and caseload among programs. More than a decade later, surgical trainees are still expressing the need for additional training options. This chapter describes a stepwise approach to training of novices (**Box 1**), either in training programs or self-educated, until they have developed into competent MIS surgeons (**Fig. 1**).

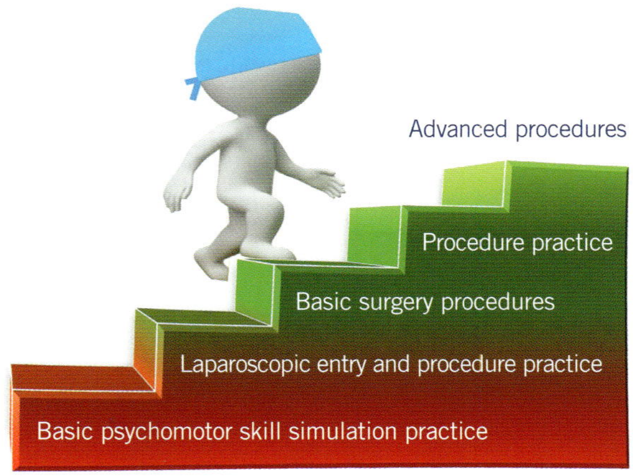

FIGURE 1. Training steps for a novice surgeon striving to become competent in MIS surgery.

Box 1. Steps for a novice surgeon toward becoming competent in advanced MIS while maintaining patient safety

1. Basic psychomotor skills simulation practice
2. Basic laparoscopic training course in live animal models
3. Simulation (cadaver) training in laparoscopic entry and basic surgical procedures, if needed as evidenced by outcome in basic training course
4. Performance of basic laparoscopy in live animals until competent
5. Simulation training of advanced psychomotor skills and procedures
6. Advanced MIS training course in live animal models
7. Simulation (cadaver) training until comfortable for live animal surgery, if needed as evidenced by outcome in advanced training course

BASIC PSYCHOMOTOR SKILLS

General instrument handling in MIS needs specific training, as open surgery does not prepare the surgeon for the lack of both depth perception and sensory feedback. In addition, the surgeon needs to adapt to the reduced field of view and gain the ambidexterity required. The skills difference between MIS and open surgery has often been compared to the difference between eating with chopsticks instead of knife and fork. Therefore, how can we get really good at using our "chopsticks" quickly?

It appears generally accepted that the most effective way of gaining these skills, while maintaining patient safety, is by simulation-based training. Unfortunately for educators, merely providing unlimited voluntary access to simulator equipment results in poor attendance. Lack of time and extensive clinical responsibilities are the biggest barriers to voluntary simulation training. Effective training requires clear performance goals, tasks with solid relevance to clinical practice, and mandatory training during protected time. Educator feedback during training and obligatory assessments after training are also important for motivation.

Simulation can be done in simple box trainers (**Fig. 2**), which mainly provide access to basic skills training in low-fidelity (not lifelike) models. For MD training, there are more lifelike models commercially available that can be used in box trainers and thus provide simulation of surgical procedures. Some of these may in the future prove to be valuable also for veterinary training. Virtual reality trainers (**Fig. 3**) can provide both basic skills training and actual surgical procedures, including bleeding, clip slippage, and other simulated complications. They can also provide video tutorials and organized curricula with didactic information. Some advantages and disadvantages with either simulation method are provided in **Table 1**. Unfortunately, neither lifelike physical models nor virtual reality simulation has been developed for veterinary use; therefore, the benefits of such models are currently unknown. However, some seem appropriate for veterinary use due to anatomical and procedural similarities (e.g., cholecystectomy).

For the novice without access to virtual reality trainers, box training remains a great option for gaining psychomotor skills. A multitude of tasks have been described for practicing and have been proven to increase operating room performance. The best validated tasks are the ones used in the only presented training curricula for veterinarians to date, the VALS program (valsprogram.org), which is based on the Fundamentals of Laparoscopic Surgery program for MD surgeons. These tasks (**Fig. 4**) have been described in detail elsewhere. With a box trainer there are however endless variety and opportunities for practice, as evidenced by Dr. Hiroo Kanai's recommended origami exercises (**Fig. 5**).

A range of psychomotor skills are in need of training, including ambidexterity, precision, and cues for depth perception. The ability to tie surgical knots may seem to be too advanced for the laparoscopic novice, but it is not until the surgeon is able to do such advanced skills that the level of skills has truly dramatically improved. Simpler tasks such as peg transfer merely serve to build a foundation for the more advanced tasks of knot tying or origami.

LAPAROSCOPIC ENTRY AND BASIC PROCEDURE PRACTICE

A major limitation to all currently available simulators is the lack of laparoscopic entry training. Initial entry of cannulas and instruments into the body cavity is the most common source for MIS-related complications. In addition, laparoscopic entry techniques are widely variable among veterinary surgeons, and training for the specific entry method of choice needs specific practice. In clinical training programs, residents receive entry training by the traditional apprentice approach. However, for the practicing surgeon wanting to start MIS, apprentice training may not be an option. Under those circumstances, cadaver practice is a good high-fidelity simulation model and can be a great practice tool. Cadaver practice is also a reasonable approach for practicing

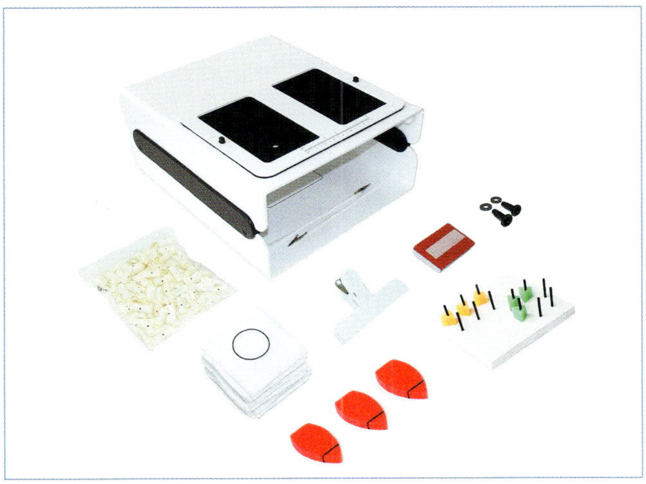

FIGURE 2. A commercially available box trainer (VALS box, Limbs & Things, Savannah, GA, USA).

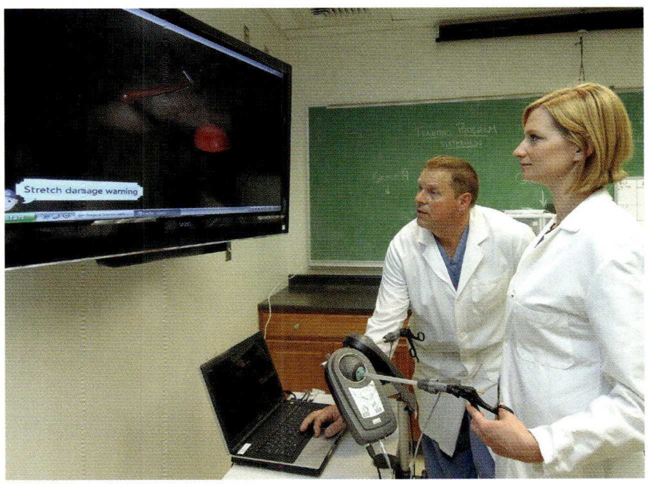

FIGURE 3 Virtual reality training allows for basic and advanced training. A great advantage is the possibility for simulated complications, such as the one depicted in the image. The trainee is inappropriately stretching the "blood vessel" too much, leading to a stretch damage warning.

TABLE 1. Advantages and disadvantages of different types of simulation training devices

Simulation type	Uses	Advantages	Disadvantages
Box trainer	■ Gaining psychomotor skills	■ Low cost ■ Versatile ■ Tactile (haptic feedback) ■ Uses real instruments	■ No feedback on performance ■ Disposable materials needed ■ In itself does not provide surgery procedure training ■ No laparoscopic entry training
Virtual reality	■ Gaining psychomotor skills ■ Practicing surgical procedures (if validated) ■ Gaining advanced skills	■ Allows basic skills and surgery procedure practice ■ Simulates bleeding/complications ■ Immediate feedback ■ Measurable metrics on performance ■ No disposable materials needed (unlimited use)	■ High cost to purchase and for software update ■ Haptic feedback only available at considerable extra cost ■ No laparoscopic entry training
Physical models	■ Practicing surgical procedures (if validated)	■ Lifelike ■ Simulates surgery with actual instruments ■ Can be used in any box trainer	■ Human anatomy ■ One time use only ■ Cost
Augmented reality	■ Gaining psychomotor skills ■ Practicing surgical procedures (if validated) ■ Gaining advanced skills (if validated)	■ Virtual overlay over physical model combines advantages	■ Accessibility ■ Cost

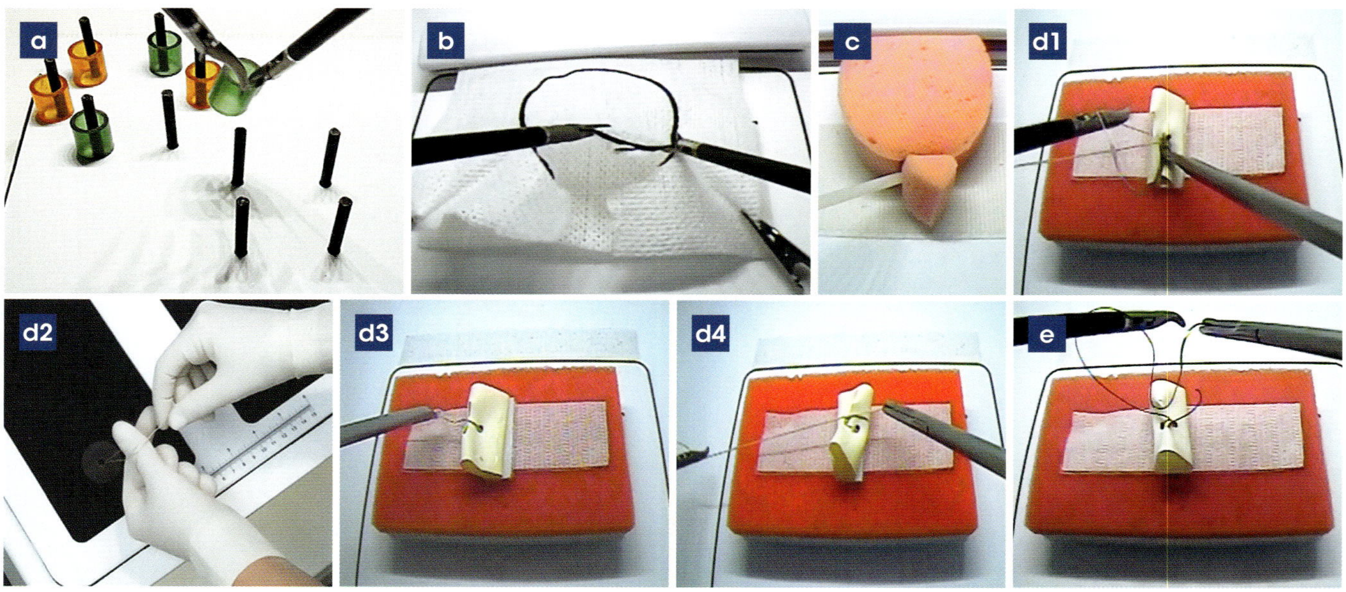

FIGURE 4. The five tasks in the VALS program are as follows. a) Peg transfer. b) Pattern cutting. c) Ligature loop application. d) Extracorporeal knot tying: d1) a suture bite is completed intracorporeally; d2) the suture is exteriorized through the cannula and a slip knot is tied; d3) a knot pusher is used to cinch the knot; d4) single throws are applied on top of the slip knot. e) Intracorporeal suture and knot tying.

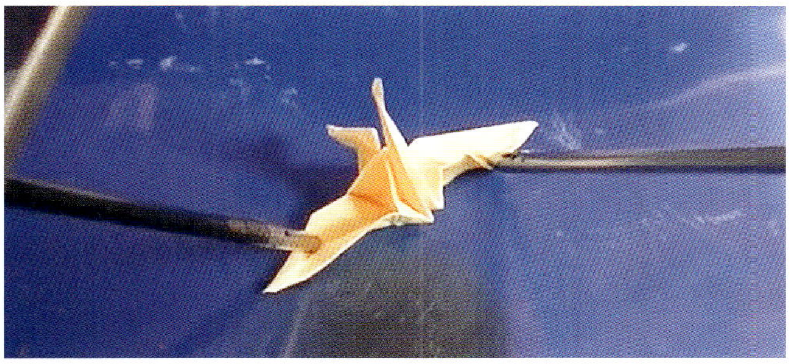

FIGURE 5. A multitude of practice exercises can be used in a box trainer. Here, Dr. Hiroo Kanai (Hospital Director, Kanai Veterinary Surgery, Himeji, Japan) is folding one of his more than 3000 origami cranes in order to keep his advanced surgical skills sharp.

basic surgical procedures, such as laparoscopic ovariectomy, and a variety of laparoscopic-assisted procedures, prior to performance in live animals. The author's research group has described a low-cost physical model simulating laparoscopic entry and ovariectomy. Hopefully, there will be commercially available simulation models for laparoscopic entry practice in the future.

PERFORMING BASIC PROCEDURES IN LIVE ANIMALS

After obtaining basic skills and practicing laparoscopic entry, the trainee ideally participates in a training course utilizing a live animal model. Such courses are often organized in cooperation with industry selling the MIS equipment. One company in particular, Storz, has been supportive of veterinary MIS and has sponsored a multitude of courses providing hands-on practice. Currently, Storz is working both through individual workshops and in conjunction with a number of institutions in the USA, Australia, and Thailand as training centers. In the USA, courses are held at educational centers such as the Translational Medicine Institute (TMI) at Colorado State University, or at the University of Georgia. In Europe, the European School for Advanced Veterinary Studies (ESAVS), among other centers, provides hands-on training for veterinarians starting in laparoscopic surgery.

If the trainee has progressed smoothly through these initial steps of training, performing basic surgical procedures such as ovariectomy, diagnostic procedures, and a variety of laparoscopic-assisted surgeries in live animals is the next logical step. The learning curve is individual for each person, but as a general rule of thumb approximately 100 procedures were considered a number for MD surgeons to strive for to be considered competent. This rule of thumb has been supported in veterinary medicine, as the first 80 surgeries have been associated with a learning curve.

ADVANCED PROCEDURE TRAINING

A veterinarian with ample experience in basic laparoscopy may desire to progress to advanced MIS, such as adrenalectomy, cholecystectomy, lung lobectomy, vascular ring anomaly correction, hiatal hernia repair, or nephrectomy. All these procedures have in common a need for extreme instrument precision and control. This is the rational for requiring ACVS Fellows in small animal MIS (laparoscopy/thoracoscopy) to pass the certifying VALS test with a minimum score of 348 instead of the regular 270 used for other surgeons and residents.

Therefore, laparoscopic suturing or similar exercises to develop, master and maintain excellent psychomotor skills are highly encouraged at this level. Importantly, advanced laparoscopic psychomotor skills tend to decay unless practiced with a minimum of 6-month intervals after gaining competence.

Ideally, advanced procedures are also simulation-trained prior to live animal model practice. Currently, there are no validated curricula or models, but recent developments in commercially available physical models and virtual reality simulation for laparoscopic cholecystectomy holds some promise. Both physical and virtual reality models are simulated for human anatomy, but fortunately the anatomy for cholecystectomy is similar to that of dogs. There is ongoing work to determine if these models can be validated for use in veterinary surgeons' training.

Live animal model practice and a high level of didactic knowledge are required prior to attempting any advanced MIS surgical procedures. In general, a surgeon should not consider performing any surgery in MIS that they are not experienced in by open surgery. A few of the previously mentioned training centers offer advanced MIS surgery courses for veterinarians. Only if the training has been smooth in the live animal model should the surgeon attempt surgery on animal patients. If needed, cadaver practice should be performed until the surgeon is certain about their skills prior to proceeding with surgery on live animals.

SUGGESTED READINGS

10 INDOCYANINE GREEN—INITIAL APPLICATIONS OF FLUORESCENCE-GUIDED SURGERY

Fausto Brandão, Constantin Vasile Ifteme

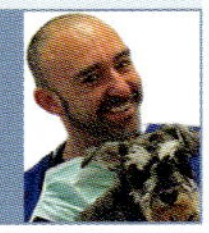

The fluorescence behavior of various natural-occurring particles and substances was reported in the early 16th century, and it was also documented later in the 19th century in some mineral compounds, chlorophyll, and quinine. In the mid-1800s, this physical phenomenon was observed when certain substances were exposed to prism-refracted light, generating an ultraviolet wavelength and fluorescence emission. In the 1950s, the fluorescence effect was used after staining to detect malignant cells in vaginal smears. When analyzed under microscopy, neoplastic cells with increased nucleic and ribonucleic acids were detected with this method. The use of hematoporphyrin fluorescence in biliary and cancer surgery was first published in 1955. This method was further developed and is still used as an endobronchial tumor indicator to facilitate the bronchoscopic localization of early squamous cell carcinoma. Other researchers investigated ultraviolet cystoscopy following tetracycline administration, which lead to visual guidance for biopsies and early detection of tumor recurrence after treatment of bladder carcinoma (with persistent tumor cells in the urinary sediment, but no visible neoplasia under white light urethrocystoscopy). The evaluation of cardiac ischemia and reperfusion was another vast area of research. Finally, a large number of investigations in fluorescence-guided technology led to a Nobel Prize in chemistry in 2008 for the discovery and development of green fluorescent protein.

> Fluorescence has been studied over several decades, but investigations still continue and will greatly contribute to further advances in modern medicine, including biochemistry, biomolecular medicine, and anatomical localization in surgery.

The basic study of indocyanine green (ICG) fluorescence imaging began in the 1970s. It was then applied to ophthalmology, and in the 2000s it started being used in breast cancer surgery to detect sentinel lymph nodes. Its application in the digestive system began in 2006, demonstrating the detection of sentinel lymph nodes in stomach and colon cancers.

In recent years, ICG has come to be widely utilized in various clinical fields. It can be used as a contrast agent not only for cerebral and coronary angiography but also for lymphangiography and cholangiography. The usefulness of this method has also been recognized in hepatobiliary surgery, such as the staining of hepatic segments and the detection of liver tumors. The assessment of the vascular perfusion of skin grafts under ICG fluorescence is one of most notable applications in reconstructive surgery. ICG has been used as a vital dye to measure circulating blood volume and as a diagnostic test reagent to evaluate liver function tests.

Several decades have passed since it was discovered that ICG possessed the characteristic property of generating fluorescence following conjugation with plasma proteins, but the mechanism of the fluorescence-quenching phenomenon and the creation of ICG fluorescence in response to other substances such as methanol and ethanol has not been fully clarified.

In recent years, ICG fluorescence endoscopy has been developed for thoracoscopic and laparoscopic surgery, enabling sentinel node navigation surgery in gastrointestinal tract cancer. It has been clearly demonstrated to date that, when combined with ICG fluorescence imaging, endoscopic surgery provides a more accurate approach for minimally invasive surgery.

FUNDAMENTALS OF NIR/ICG

ICG ($C_{43}H_{47}N_2NaO_6S_2$) is a water-soluble compound with a molecular weight of 755 g/mol (**Fig. 1**). It has been clinically approved in many countries for over 50 years for use in medical diagnostics, including determining cardiac output, hepatic function, and liver blood flow.

When ICG is injected into a tissue, it immediately binds tightly to blood plasma. The majority of ICG is accumulated in hepatic parenchymal cells and is then excreted in the bile without being metabolized.

The typical medical applications of ICG include hepatic function and liver blood flow diagnostics, which are determined via its optical absorption functions. ICG also exhibits well-established fluorescence properties and is commonly employed in ophthalmology for retina or choroid diagnostic imaging.

The peak optical absorption wavelength of ICG is approximately 800 nm, with peak fluorescence wavelengths of approximately 840 nm in the blood. These near-infrared (NIR) wavelengths can penetrate more deeply into the tissue compared with visible wavelength fluorescence compounds, such as fluorescein. These wavelengths fall behind the visible spectrum, therefore requiring an endoscopic imaging system with customized filters, with high sensitivity to the NIR wavelength, critical for detecting and measuring ICG fluorescence.

The use of optical technology in the NIR wavelength for tissue measurement of ICG is advantageous, as it can avoid the influence of autofluorescence and allows assessment in relatively deep tissues. However, the main limitations for detection and measurement relate to wavelength and main tissue absorbent molecules, namely water and hemoglobin. The peak excitation and emission wavelengths of ICG are, respectively, 800 nm and 840 nm in the blood. Since hemoglobin strongly absorbs light at wavelengths shorter than 650 nm, and water absorbs light at wavelengths longer than 900 nm, the ICG optical window is optimized. That said, ICG fluorescence can also provide angiographic assessment of blood and lymphatic vessels located relatively deep within the tissues (up to 10 mm).

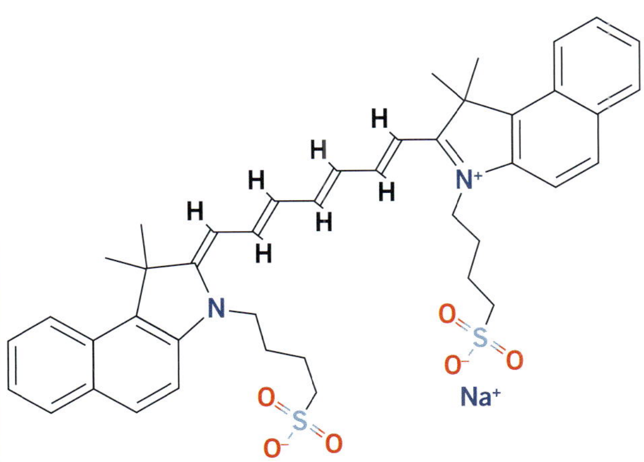

FIGURE 1. Structural formula of indocyanine green.

Human reports document very low ICG toxicity, with rarely occurring side effects, specifically shock symptoms, nausea, angialgia, and fever.

The fluorescence intensity of ICG is almost linearly increased with concentration when using a low concentration. However, at higher concentrations, the fluorescence intensity peaks and subsequently decreases, a phenomenon termed the quenching effect. This is because ICG acts as a fluorescent substance as well as an optical absorber. Therefore, when ICG concentrations are too high, it absorbs fluorescent light itself, which is the main cause of quenching.

The typical concentration and dose of ICG injection for a diagnostic liver function test using the light absorption properties of ICG are 5 mg/mL and 0.5 mg/kg, respectively. However, to avoid the quenching effect and improve fluorescence efficiency, 2.5 mg/mL is typically suggested for breast cancer, and even lower concentrations, of 0.5 mg/mL, for enhanced sentinel lymph node detection.

Thus, a very-high-concentration ICG solution shows lower fluorescence intensity, while a low-concentration ICG solution yields higher fluorescence intensity. Clinically, a very dark ICG color-stained lymph node with very low fluorescence intensity due to quenching is rarely observed.

IMAGING TECHNOLOGY

As fluorescence-guided surgery became a routine practice, manufacturers invested in developing dedicated ICG technology systems that eliminate the prior need for system customization that employed built-in or snap-on filters.

Currently, NIR/ICG systems are available with dedicated light sources and imaging modules and cameras. Modern laparoscopic fluorescence imaging systems include a dedicated light cable and an assortment of different scopes ranging from 0° or 30° 5 to 10 mm diameter rigid laparoscopes, ICG exoscopes, which contain an optical filter system for white light, and ICG imaging. In current clinical practice, the Karl Storz Rubina 4K ICG system is preferred by the authors due to its imaging quality under white light. The system can be activated with the aid of a foot pedal switch, cycling through different modes and through intraoperative conventional imaging under white light (WL-mode), and NIR fluorescence imaging (ICG/NIR-mode).

In the new generation 4K NIR/ICG cameras (Rubina, Karl Storz), these features are also available with customized buttons located in the camera head (**Fig. 2**).

When the system is used in NIR/ICG fluorescence mode, it can offer images in either blue or green, which enhances the image in highly perfused and fluorescent areas (blue mode), to more intense fluorescence and detailed delineation against surrounding tissue (green mode). Rubina cameras also present other NIR/ICG advanced modes, such as monochromatic fluorescence, which enables a black and white imaging mode for better operating contrast, sharpness, brightness, and signal detection (**Fig. 3a**).

Because of the continuous changing of images and the stable position of the laparoscope, anatomical orientation can be maintained. However, a direct fluorescence signal overlay on the conventional anatomical image is now possible. The overlay mode allows for operation while superimposing green fluorescence on the displayed white light image. This offers operating comfort for the surgeons, since switching from a dark background fluorescent image to a white light image is more time-consuming and requires keeping the laparoscope positioned at an exact point on the operating field (**Fig. 3b**).

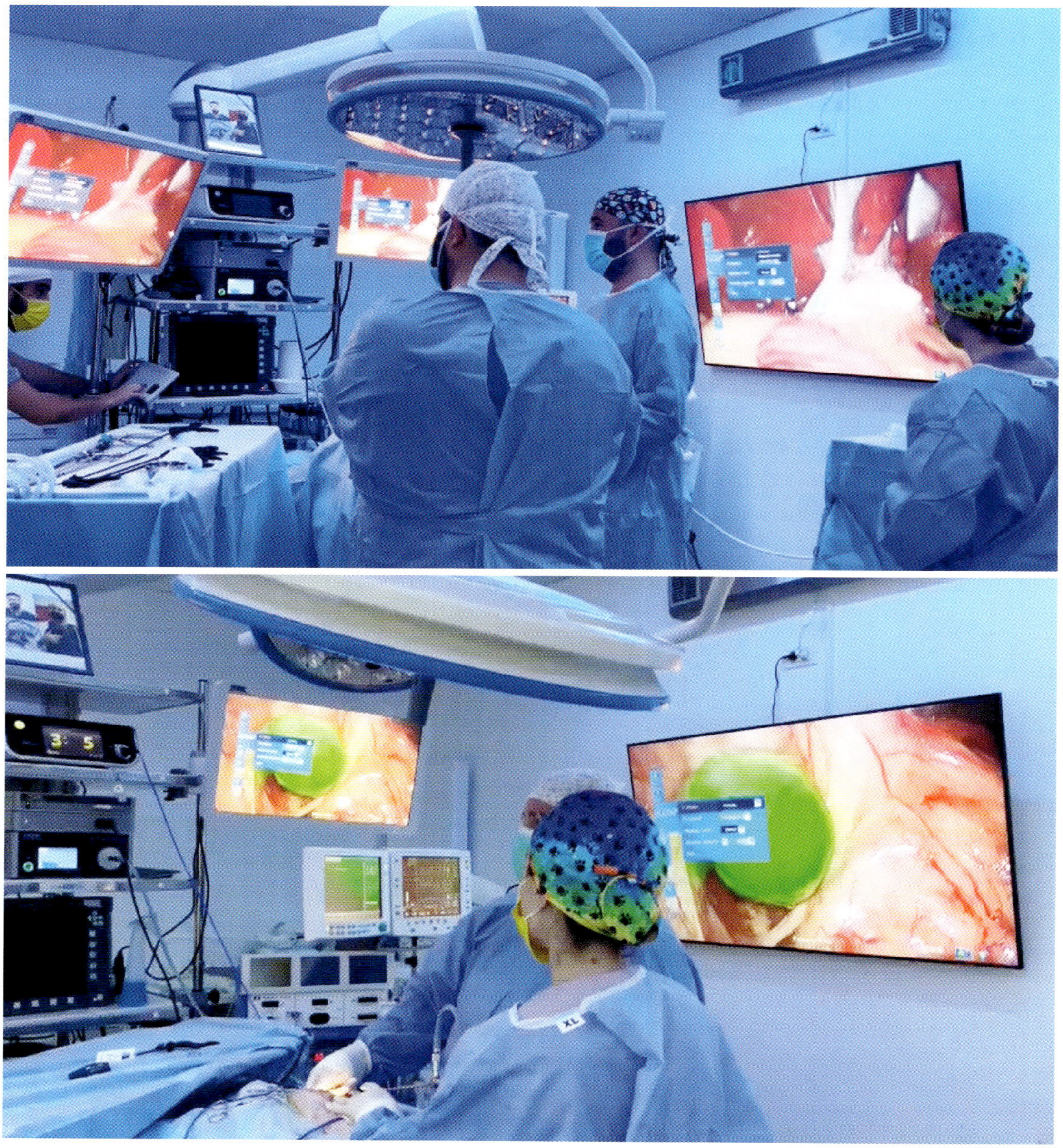

FIGURE 2. Operating room setup with a Rubina 4K ICG system (Karl Storz).

The recent introduction of intensity mapping enables the surgeon to interpret the grade of fluorescence displayed on the screen and correlate it with an intensity fluorescence scale throughout the procedure. This results in improved perception of tissue marking over surgical time. Overlaid images of white light and NIR/ICG are combined and processed with intelligent analysis software. With a specialized camera control unit, minuscule tonal differences in fluorescence, not visible to the human eye, are detected and highlighted by a color scale mapping system (**Fig. 3c**).

Ranging from blue (the weakest fluorescence signal) to yellow-orange (the strongest fluorescence signal) tones, color mapping maximizes early detection of lymphatic circulation and sentinel lymph nodes. The color grading system also greatly influences the distinction of sentinel lymph nodes from subsequent lymph nodes, which can be very helpful in surgical decision-making.

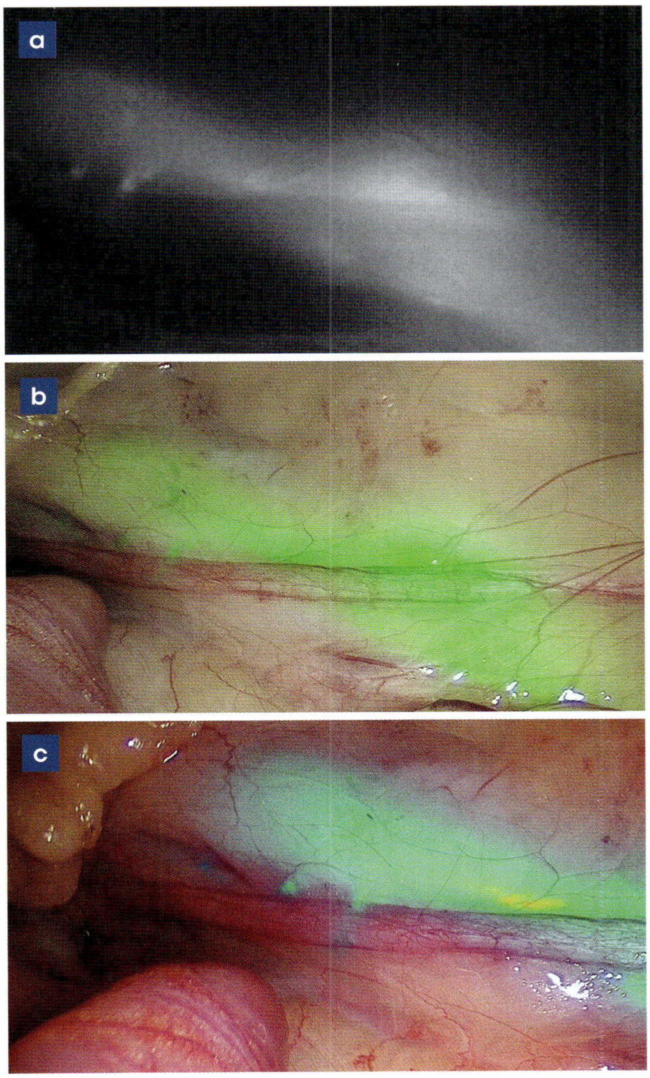

FIGURE 3. Images of a medial iliac lymph node at a) monochromatic, b) overlay, and c) intensity mapping modes.

Videoendoscopic oncological surgery can benefit from NIR technology, since ICG is used to map neoplastic tissues and their lymphatic drainage. Consequently, mapped lymph nodes can be surgically removed, allowing for subsequent histopathological analysis. Sentinel lymph node mapping is now enhanced with fluorescence intensity mapping, since it achieves an improved distinction between lymph nodes and surrounding lymphatic pathways.

However, the different light source technology leads to a diversity of benefits depending on the system used. Laser light sources (Synergy, Arthrex) have a higher contrast of the green signal in overlay mode but less satisfactory anatomical color visualization (yellowish tones). LED laser-free light sources (Rubina, Karl Storz) offer a pristine white light anatomical image second to none, but with a relatively diminished contrast signal of green intensity color in overlay mode, compared to laser light sources. Nevertheless, LED laser-free systems offer the previously described intensity mapping mode.

PROCEDURE PRINCIPLES

ICG fluorescence navigation surgery has been widely used in different clinical fields. Variable dosages of ICG concentrations for perilesional or intravenous injections have been widely attempted. An ICG solution made of 25 mg of ICG dissolved in 5, 10, 20 or 40 mL of distilled water has been conventionally used for intravenous or subcutaneous injections. However, the optimal parameters for the use of ICG have not been fully established in the human field, and they have only been anecdotally reported in veterinary medicine. As a result, more studies are required in human and veterinary medicine to establish and validate documented protocols for each procedure (**Fig. 4**).

In veterinary medicine, optimal concentrations and protocols have not been documented and published, and in the authors' experience the general guidelines of the International Society of Fluorescence Guided Surgery (ISFGS) are followed and adapted as caseloads are built. Up to now, several types of procedures have been performed, including cholecystectomy, sentinel lymph node mapping in several types of tumors (mammary carcinoma, melanoma, anal sac carcinoma), and vascular

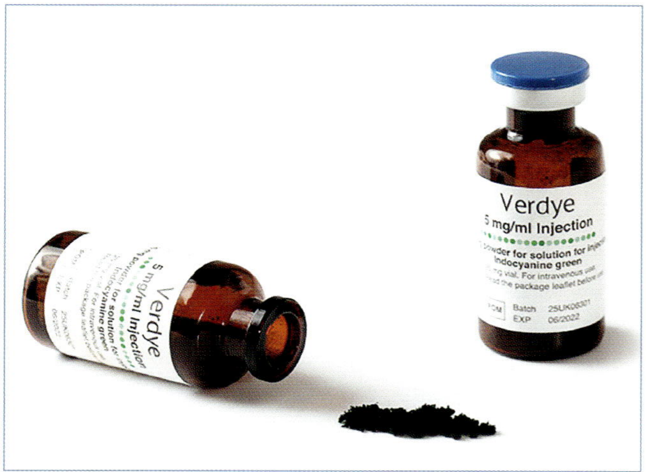

FIGURE 4. Commercial presentation of ICG: 25 mg per vial, 5 mg/mL when diluted with 5 mL of sterile water (Verdye, Diagnostic Green).

assessment in surgical anastomoses and surgical traumatized tissue resection. Therefore, further research and clinical applications need to be compiled in order to provide a veterinary guide for surgical applications.

It is known that ICG by itself does not possess the property of emitting fluorescence without coupling with albumin or α- or β-lipoprotein. It is also documented that temperature and pH might influence fluorescence intensity, but these factors have not yet been established in veterinary patients. Moreover, regarding data extrapolated from human applications, it was found that the use of dark and cold conditions was optimal for traumatized tissue resection, as the ICG fluorescence brightness was maintained for a longer period, especially with the monochromatic mode. That said, diluted concentrations still need to be further investigated for procedure optimization.

CLINICAL APPLICATIONS

Over the last decade, many clinical applications using an ICG approach have been introduced. Some of the more commonly performed surgeries include liver mass resection, thoracoscopic thoracic duct ligation, and exoscopic fluorescence-guided neoplasia and sentinel lymph node resection. In human subspecialties, NIR/ICG is commonly used for procedures such as breast cancer sentinel lymph node navigation surgery, coronary artery bypass grafting, brain surgery, plastic surgery, and gastrointestinal surgery.

Common clinical applications of ICG

- Reconstructive surgery
- Sentinel lymph node resection
- Skin cancer surgery
- Lymphatic surgery
- Hepatobiliary surgery
- Gastrointestinal surgery
- Gynecologic surgery
- Endocrine surgery
- Neurological surgery

CASE EXAMPLES

Below, several clinical examples of veterinary ICG-guided surgeries are illustrated. The authors believe this technique will become the standard of practice in the field. Note that doses and protocols for ICG have not yet been standardized, and the references below result from the authors' experience and adaptation from human protocols suggested by the ISFGS (https://isfgs.org).

LAPAROSCOPIC CHOLECYSTECTOMY

ICG fluorescence cholangiography is an intraoperative technique to allow visualization of the extrahepatic biliary structures during laparoscopic cholecystectomy. This significantly increases the identification rates of the extrahepatic biliary structures both before and after laparoscopic dissection at the liver hilum, compared to standard white light technology.

It is currently considered one of the most important intraoperative imaging techniques to reduce the incidence of biliary duct injury. The main limitation of ICG cholangiography is its reduced depth penetration (<10 mm). Therefore, in case of obese patients or acute cholecystitis, a reduced ratio of identification is observed.

In order to get the maximum benefit from this technology, the fluorescence signal should be identified only within the extrahepatic biliary structures. Due to the hepatic pharmacokinetic clearance profile, it is quite common to have an intense green fluorescence liver background during laparoscopic cholecystectomy after intravenous administration (**Fig. 5**). It has been proven that this kind of intraoperative visualization effect can impair the correct identification of the anatomy. That said,

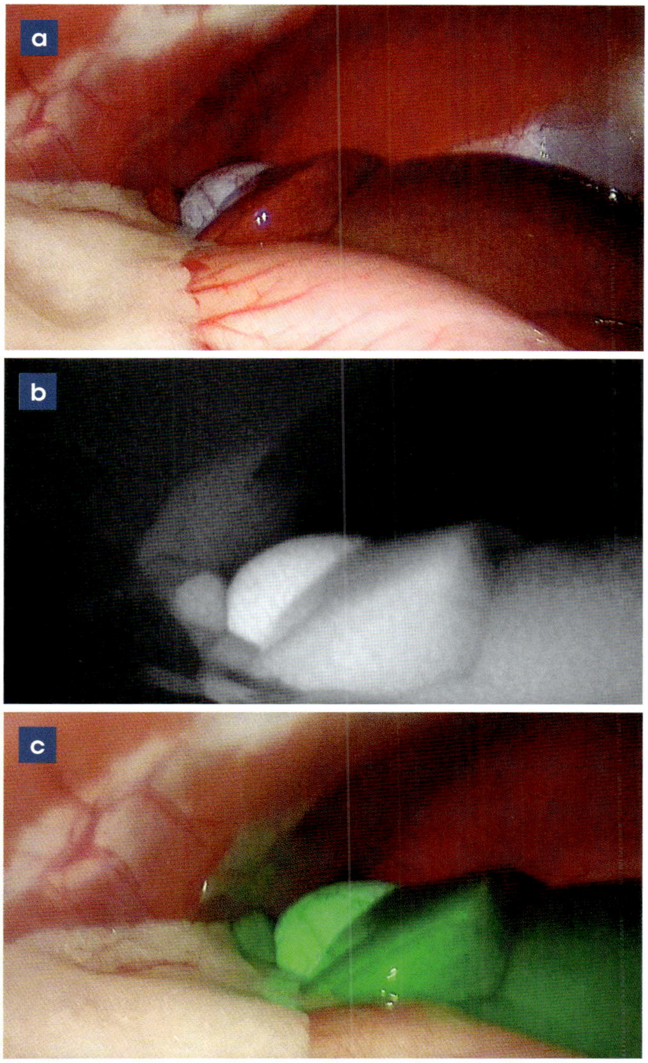

FIGURE 5. Laparoscopic images of the liver with a high dose of ICG before clearance. a) White light imaging, b) overlay, and c) monochromatic modes. Note the intense green background and the lack of contrast between parenchyma and extrahepatic biliary pathways.

the ideal fluorescence visualization profile should be characterized by an intense ICG signal localized to the extrahepatic structures, with an absence or very low signal in the liver background ratio. This result is dependent on dose and timing of ICG administration as well as on the patient's liver function.

Considering the previous concepts, with ICG fixed-dose protocols, the time until surgery would have to be increased to reduce the liver background signal ratio, which is extremely impractical, especially in veterinary patients.

In the case illustrated below, a fixed-dose ICG protocol was administered 18 hours prior to surgery at a dose of 0.25 mg/kg. The ICG via containing 25 mg of powder is diluted in 20 mL of sterile water and administered slowly through an intravenous catheter in a peripheral vein. In the authors' limited experience, when ICG was administered less than 10 hours prior to surgery, the liver parenchyma also demonstrated a high fluorescence signal and generated quenching, thus resulting in less contrast between the biliary ducts and the hepatic tissue. Therefore, it is important to understand the clinical condition present and the liver parenchyma tissue clearance time for ICG. It is now understood that the gallbladder, cystic ducts, and extrahepatic pathways might be enhanced with earlier administration times or with administration of extremely reduced dosages in a shorter time before surgery.

In some cases, employing the monochromatic mode allows for more detail of the hepatic ducts compared to overlay and intensity mapping modes. This results in enhanced dissection precision and avoids clipping in a lower area of the cystic duct, especially in patients with a short duct (**Fig. 6**).

The current experience with low doses and reduced perioperative administration time (60 minutes) seems to be optimal. This generates a very low or almost absent liver background signal, with optimized contrast in the biliary tree.

The authors postulate that doses lower than 0.012 mg/kg administered intravenously 60 minutes prior to surgery generate a very low liver background signal with an LED light system. Even with such low dosages, it was still possible to identify some liver ducts running on the liver parenchyma during dissection. This can be very helpful in cases of cholecystitis with more adhesions, as the risk of liver duct injury is minimized.

Further studies and clinical case reports are required to provide continued evidence for the systematic use of microdoses with current technology systems.

Substance	Concentration	Time of administration	Dose
ICG (high fixed-dose protocol)	1.25 mg/mL	18 h prior to surgery	0.25 mg/kg IV
ICG (low dose protocol)	1.25 mg/mL	180 min prior to surgery	0.05 mg/kg IV
ICG (microdose current trend)	0.625 mg/mL	60 min prior to surgery	0.012 mg/kg IV

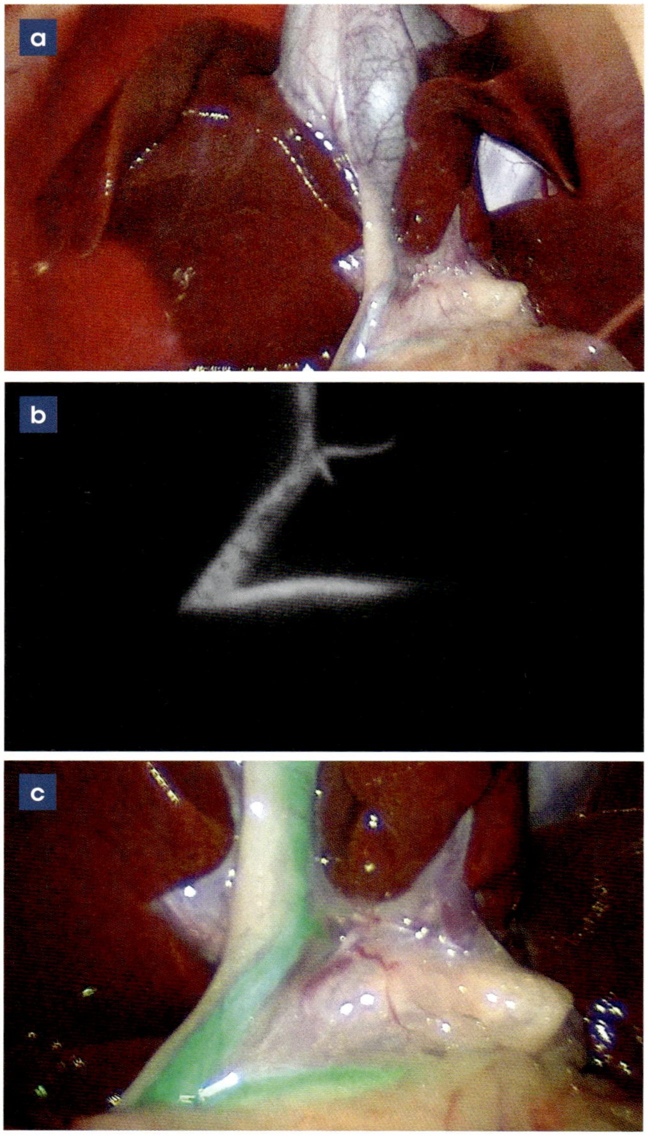

FIGURE 6. Laparoscopic cholecystectomy with a standard fixed dose injected 18 hours before surgery. Images under a) white light, b) monochromatic, and c) intensity mapping modes.

FELINE MAMMARY CARCINOMA

Regional lymph node assessment in invasive mammary neoplasia can be challenging, as tissues get invaded and adhesions and neovascularization develop. Contrast radiography for axillary lymph node identification can also be initially performed with the local injection of lipiodol (480 mg/mL), in a dose of 0.2 to 0.3 mL per injection site, in various quadrants around the neoplastic lesions (**Fig. 7**). Radiographs or fluoroscopic imaging can be obtained several hours after injection, denoting regional lymphatic drainage. ICG diluted at 0.25 mg/mL is injected 1 hour to 30 minutes prior to surgery to enhance the local lymph nodes at the surgical site. Monochromatic, overlay, and intensity mapping are then used throughout the procedure to guide a more accurate tissue resection and lymph node removal. Tissue margins from samples removed should be stained with histological dye and sent for histopathologic evaluation.

Iliac lymph node identification and resection might be challenging, especially in overweight and obese patients. Perilesional injection of ICG is extremely helpful for detailed open surgical or laparoscopic assessment and dissection (**Fig. 8**).

Substance	Concentration	Time of administration	Dose
Lipiodol	480 mg/mL	24 h prior to surgery	0.2–0.3 mL per site (quadrant)
ICG	0.25 mg/mL	30 min prior to surgery	0.5 mL per site (quadrant) intradermal/SQ

SENTINEL LYMPH NODE IN CUTANEOUS MELANOMA

In this case of cutaneous melanoma, ICG was used in a dilution of 0.25 mg/mL at a dose of 0.3 to 0.5 mL per site, in all four quadrants around the macroscopic lesions. Tissue assessment with NIR/ICG throughout the resection facilitates detection of possible lymph drainage, thus resulting in a more thorough excision of small affected areas that could otherwise be missed under white light illumination (**Fig. 9**).

Substance	Concentration	Time of administration	Dose
ICG	0.25 mg/mL	30 min prior to surgery	0.5 mL per site (quadrant) intradermal/SQ

CANINE MAMMARY CARCINOMA

In this case of suspected mammary carcinoma metastasis to the iliac lymph nodes, ICG was administered 30 minutes prior to surgery as previously described. Lymphatic drainage and medial iliac lymph nodes were then enhanced to facilitate dissection and lymphadenectomy (**Fig. 10**).

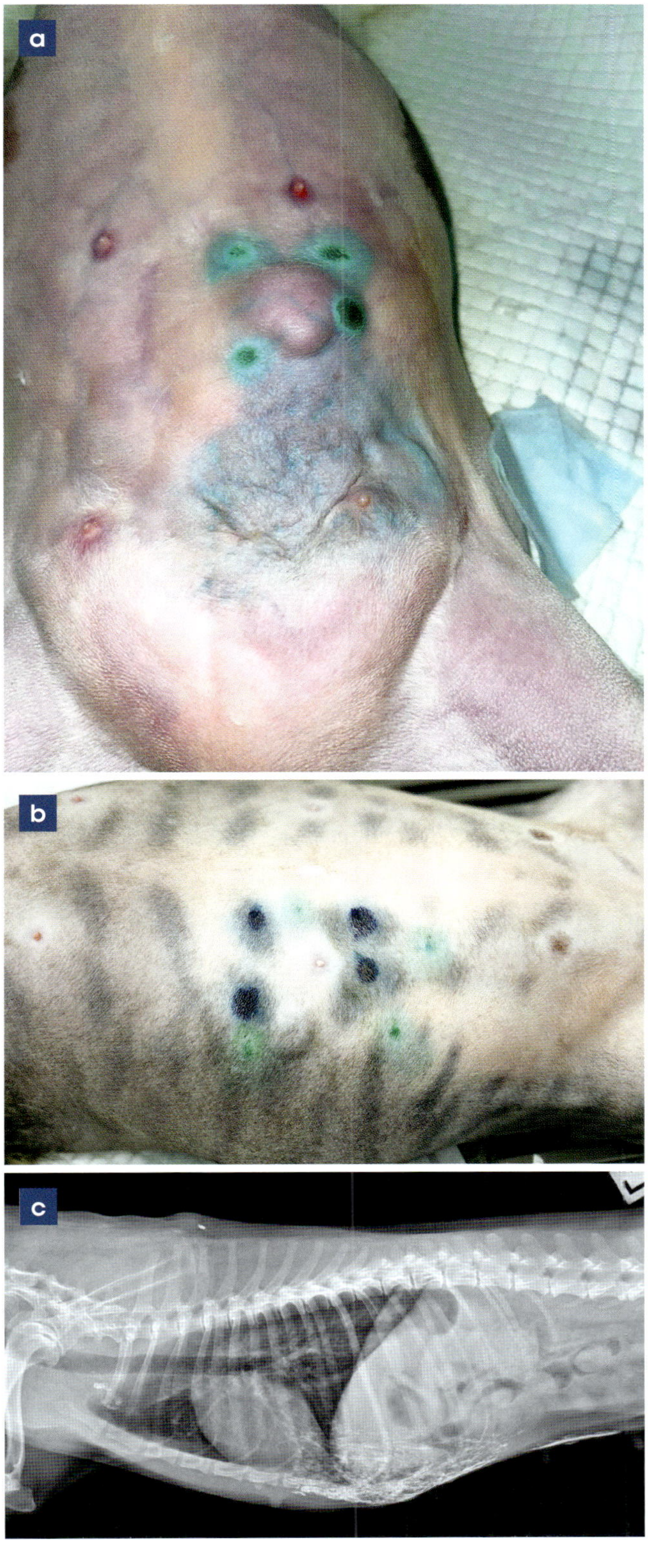

FIGURE 7. a,b) Four-quadrant injection of ICG and c) radiograph obtained after lipiodol injection for a lymphangiogram and axillary lymph node detection.

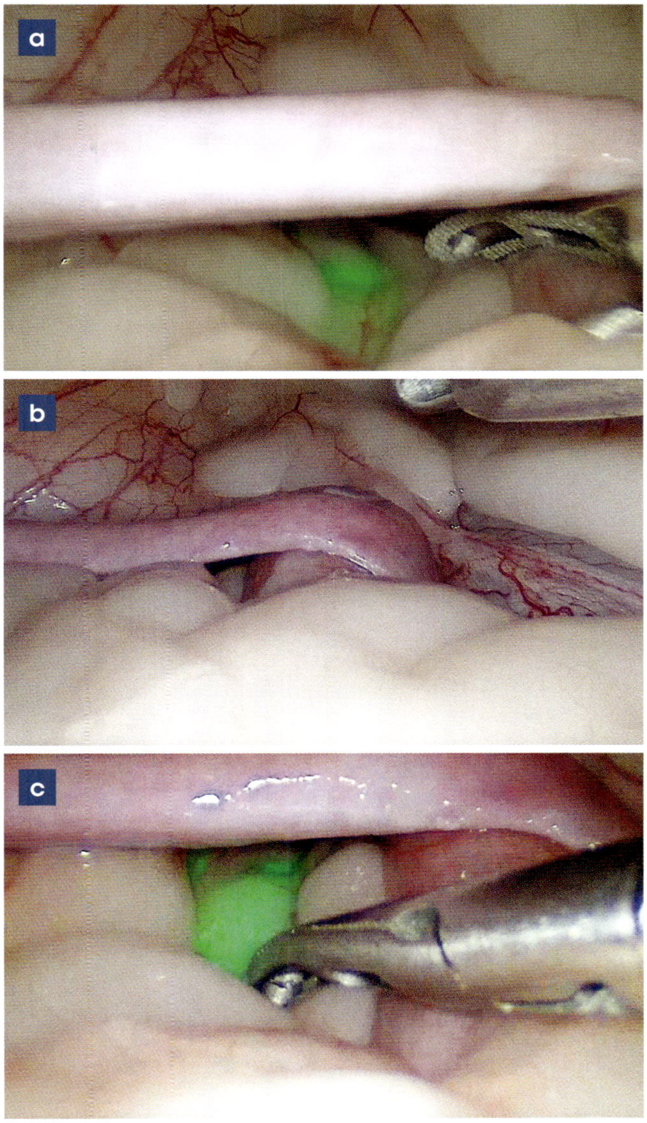

FIGURE 8. Identification and dissection of a medial iliac lymph node in a feline patient with mammary carcinoma.

Substance	Concentration	Time of administration	Dose
ICG	0.25 mg/mL	30 min prior to surgery	0.5 mL per site (quadrant) intradermal/SQ

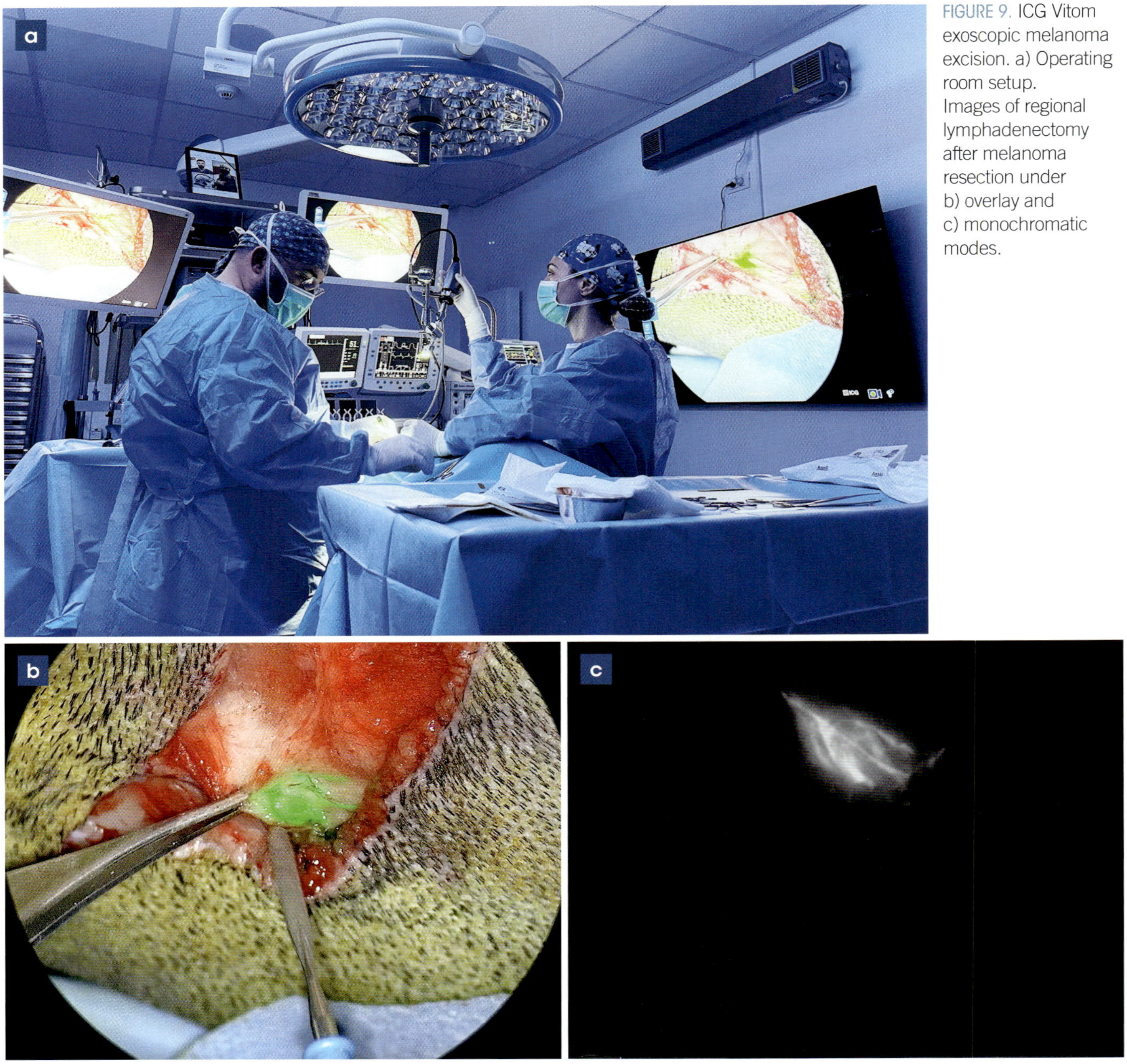

FIGURE 9. ICG Vitom exoscopic melanoma excision. a) Operating room setup. Images of regional lymphadenectomy after melanoma resection under b) overlay and c) monochromatic modes.

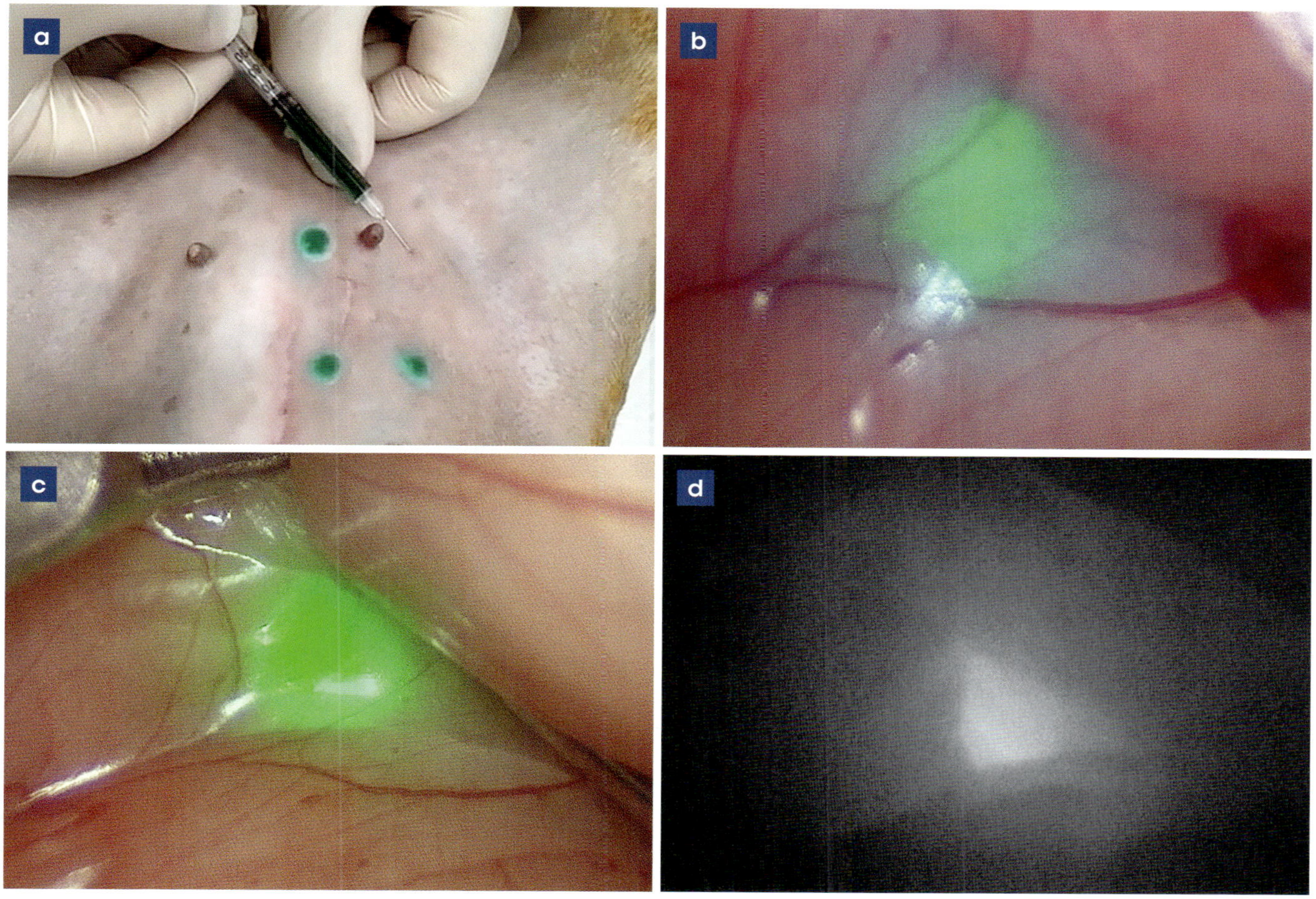

FIGURE 10. a) Four-quadrant injection in a case of canine mammary carcinoma. Medial iliac lymph node lymphadenectomy, with images in b) intensity mapping, c) overlay, and d) monochromatic modes.

VASCULAR ASSESSMENT OF TRAUMATIZED TISSUE

As outlined earlier in this chapter, ICG has demonstrated effectiveness for vascular and tissue perfusion assessment in plastic and reconstructive surgery. In the case presented here, ICG was used to assess vascular bowel perfusion to select for tissue debridement and resection after a bite wound to the abdominal wall with massive perforations and intestinal trauma. Mesenteric perfusion is better assessed with the monochromatic fluorescence mode, which details viable vascularity after intraoperative injection of ICG (**Fig. 11**).

Substance	Concentration	Time of administration	Dose
ICG	0.25 mg/mL	Intraoperatively	0.05–0.25 mg/kg IV

THORACOSCOPIC THORACIC DUCT LIGATION

Chylothorax is considered a challenging surgical condition, since individual variations of the duct and its ramifications might occur. Presurgical lymphography is required to maximize diagnostic accuracy. Ideally, intraoperative lymphography would be performed immediately after closure to ensure correct complete ligation. However, integrated multimodal imaging is rarely available in veterinary operating rooms. Moving the patient to a CT room and back into the operating room at the end of a procedure requires a multidisciplinary team to diminish the already prolonged surgical times. Moreover, the additional costs make this scenario impractical in most facilities.

ICG-guided thoracic duct ligation demonstrates superior advantages over other modalities, such as methylene blue, since ICG provides longer and better contrast of the lymphatics.

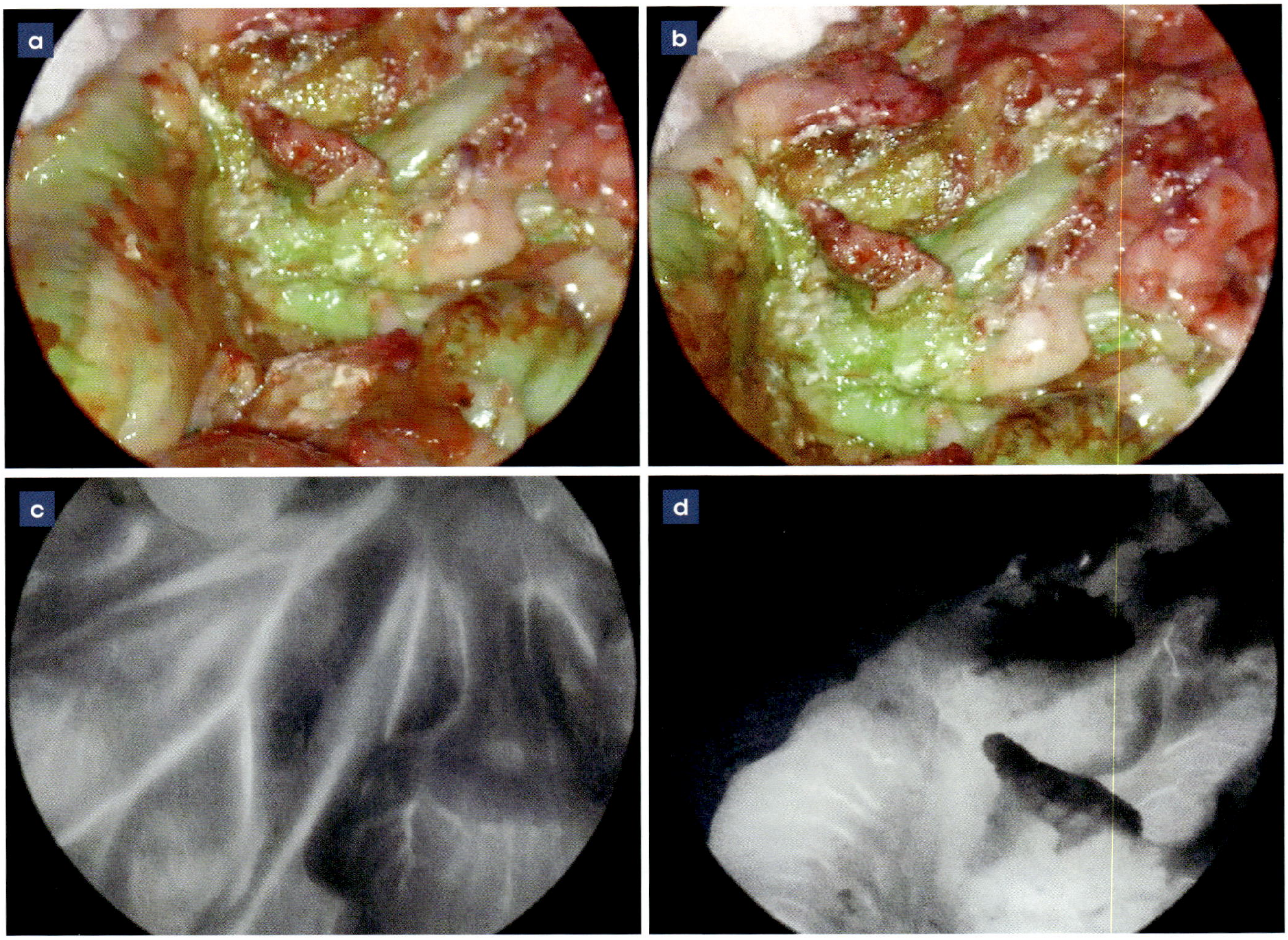

FIGURE 11. Open laparotomy vascular perfusion assessment in a case of bite wound trauma. Intestinal perfusion and tissue vascularization are assessed with a,b) overlay and c,d) monochromatic modes.

However, low-dose protocols for veterinary application have not yet been established, and current dosages follow the ISFGS guidelines.

In the case illustrated here, a vial of 25 mg of ICG powder is diluted in 40 mL of sterile saline (0.625 mg/mL). A flank approach is performed in the lateral abdominal wall and an atraumatic wound retraction device is used to expose the viscera. Identification of ileocolic or mesenteric lymph nodes is suitable for this technique, depending on surgeon preference and patient size. For a 55 kg dog, a loading dose of 2 mL is injected, and fluorescence is observed after a few minutes with overlay mode.

Thoracoscopic dissection is then carefully continued and completed, maximizing the exposure of branches for optimal clipping. Procedure success is confirmed by the absence of fluorescence in the clipped branches, using overlay and monochromatic modes for better accuracy.

Smaller branches located to the left of the aorta are less easily missed with an ICG-guided procedure than with methylene blue, since contrast intensity of the latter soon diminishes, and repeated doses might result in negative consequences for the patient.

Second-generation ICG imaging systems offer better visualization compared to those of the first generation, in which a blueish image was displayed over a black background. With overlay, intensity mapping, and monochromatic modes, modern systems allow for an accurate dissection in white light imaging while superimposing the ICG green (or other defined color) overlay (**Figs. 12–16**).

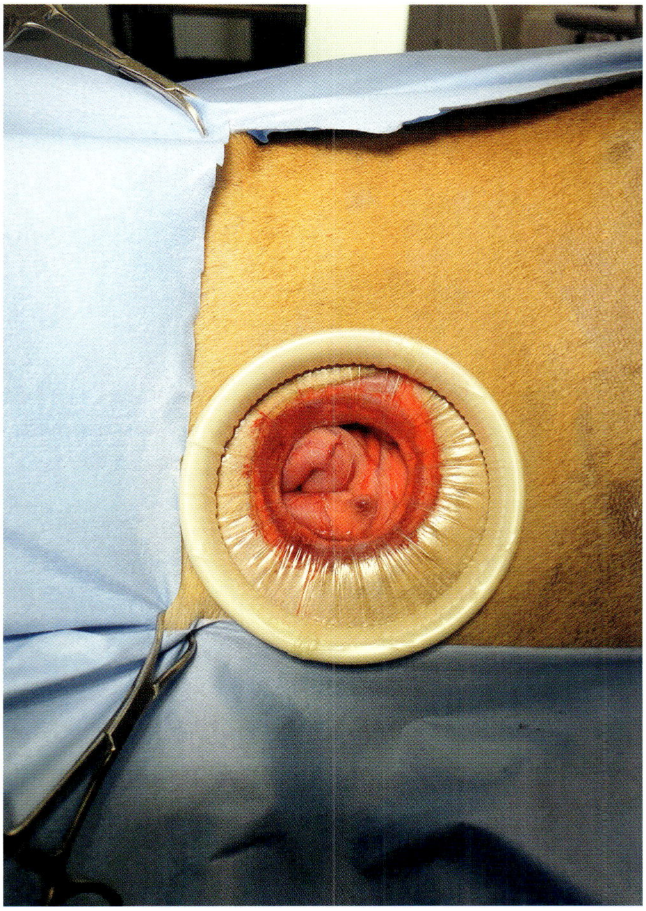

FIGURE 12. Wound retraction device placed on the flank for identification and ICG injection in the mesenteric lymph node.

Substance	Concentration	Time of administration	Dose
ICG	0.625 mg/mL (25 mg ICG+40 mL saline)	Intraoperatively	2 mL injected into mesenteric lymph node

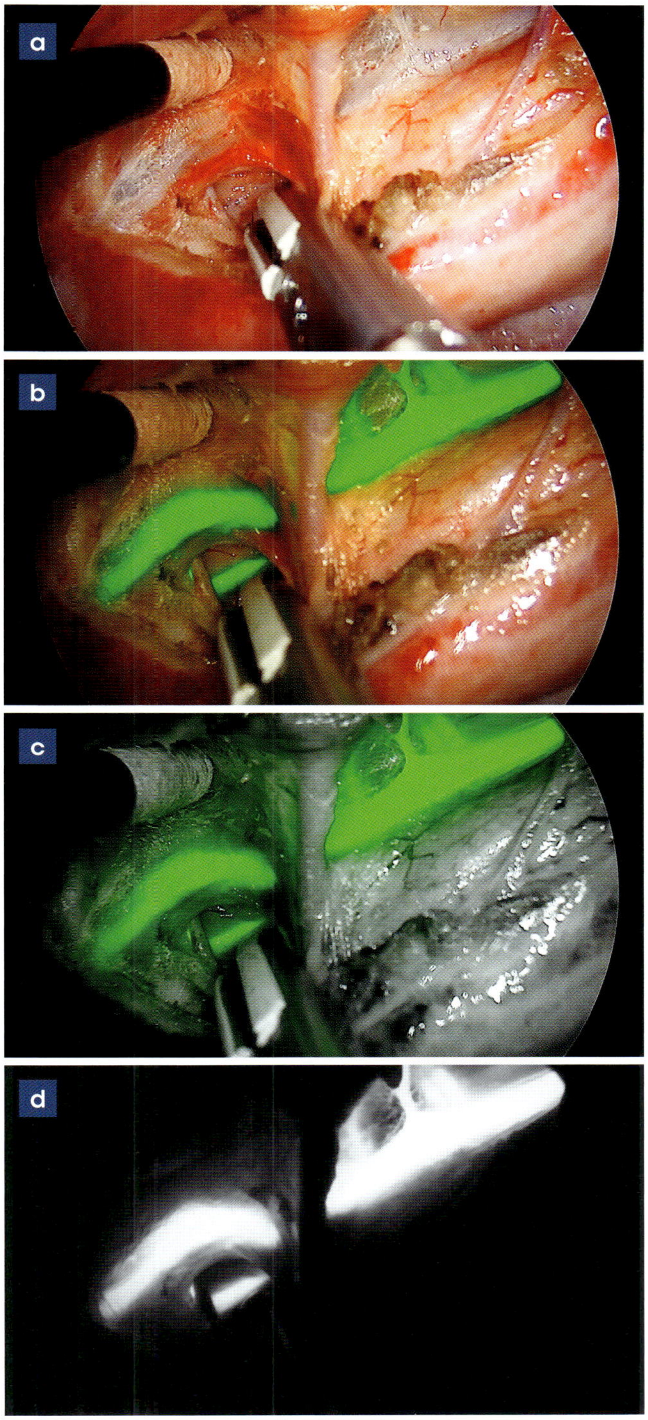

FIGURE 13. a) Initial white light dissection for thoracic duct ligation approach. b) Green overlay enhancement of the thoracic duct and its branches. c) Overlay in black and white image background. d) Monochromatic mode for maximum contrast.

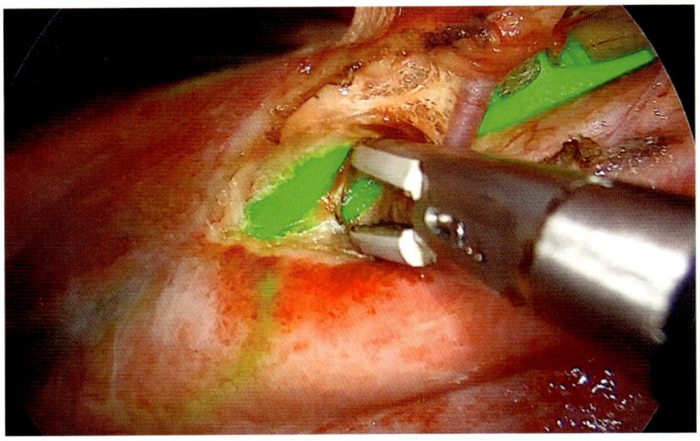

FIGURE 14. Finalization of dissection for clipping.

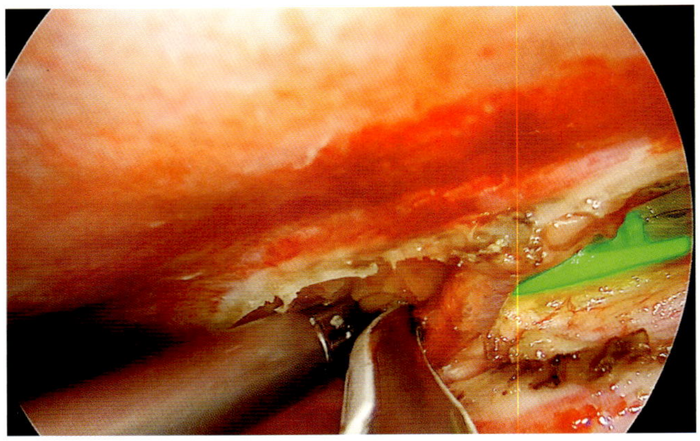

FIGURE 15. Titanium clipping of the thoracic duct and its branches.

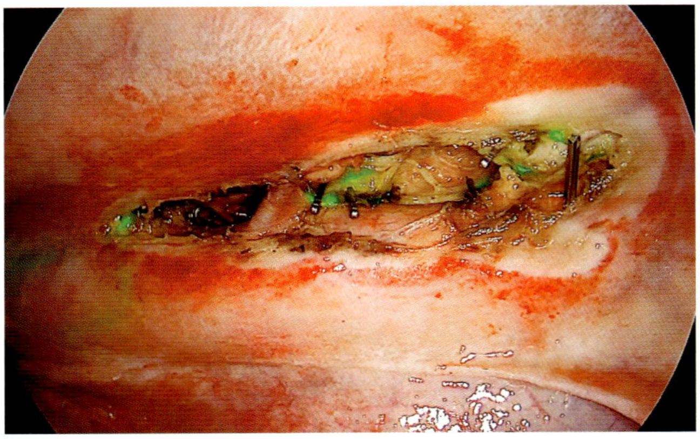

FIGURE 16. Confirmation of ICG signal absence in the surgical site after clipping, indicating complete ligation and no leakage.

SUGGESTED READINGS

Section II

LAPAROSCOPY

LEARNING FROM THE PAST

In terra caecorum beati monoculi.

Prof. A. Properzi (1923–2012)

11 ANESTHESIA IN LAPAROSCOPIC SURGERY

Alessandra Malavasi

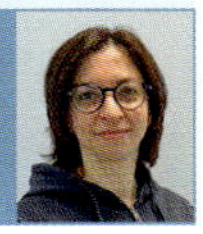

Indications

- Laparoscopic surgery

Contraindications

- Intracranial disease
- Pulmonary disease
- Cardiovascular disease
- Coagulopathy
- Hypovolemia, dehydration, and shock

Laparoscopic and laparoscopic-assisted surgery are gaining more and more popularity in veterinary medicine as diagnostic and therapeutic tools due to their undoubtable benefits compared to open surgery. Laparoscopic approaches, when performed by trained surgeons, are associated with faster surgery times, limited trauma, decreased inflammatory mediators and metabolic response suggestive of stress, reduced pain, lower infection rates, fewer postoperative complications, reduced hospitalization times, and decreased analgesic drug requirements, compared with traditional surgical approaches.

Laparoscopy requires the formation of a working area within the peritoneal cavity, which is commonly achieved by producing a pneumoperitoneum via carbon dioxide (CO_2) insufflation. In most cases, laparoscopic procedures also require specific patient positioning (Trendelenburg, reverse Trendelenburg, or lateral recumbency). Pneumoperitoneum, CO_2 insufflation, and patient positioning influence the patient's physiological functions (**Table 1**). Anesthetists should be aware of this to provide appropriate and safe anesthesia.

Abdominal gas inflation necessary to create a pneumoperitoneum determines an increase in intra-abdominal pressure (IAP), which has a hemodynamic and ventilatory impact dependent on the degree of IAP and on the volemic status of the patient.

TABLE 1. Physiological effects of pneumoperitoneum and patient positioning

	Cardiovascular	Respiratory	CNS	Other
Pneumoperitoneum	↑ MAP, SVR, CVP ↓ CO	↑ $PaCO_2$, airway pressure ↓ FRC, PaO_2, lung compliance	↑ ICP	↓ Renal, portal, and splanchnic circulation
Trendelenburg	↑ PVR, SVR ↓ CO	↑ V/Q mismatch, airway pressure ↓ FRC	↑ ICP, IOP	↓ Renal, portal, and splanchnic circulation
Reverse Trendelenburg	↓ Venous return	—	↓ ICP	—
Lateral recumbency	—	↑ V/Q mismatch	—	—

CO, cardiac output; CNS, central nervous system; CVP, central venous pressure; FRC, functional residual capacity; ICP, intracranial pressure; IOP, intraocular pressure; MAP, mean arterial pressure; $PaCO_2$, carbon dioxide arterial pressure; PaO_2, oxygen arterial pressure; PVR, pulmonary vascular resistance; SVR, systemic vascular resistance; V/Q, ventilation:perfusion ratio.

Cardiac output is a function of venous return and cardiac function, determined by the inotropic and chronotropic properties of the heart and by the afterload. Venous return depends on the mean systemic pressure, the pressure within the small veins and venules (i.e., the capacitance vessels of the systemic vasculature), venous resistance, and the hydraulic resistance of the veins between the site of mean systemic pressure and the right atrium (i.e., mostly the caudal vena cava).

Increases in IAP can raise both mean systemic pressure and venous resistance. Since the difference between mean systemic pressure and right atrial pressure is the pressure gradient for venous return, increasing mean systemic pressure (at constant right atrial pressure) augments venous return.

Increasing venous resistance obviously decreases venous return. The caudal vena cava is a major component of venous resistance, draining blood from abdomen and caudal part of body. Increases in IAP able to compress this large vein cause an increase in venous resistance, which in turn decreases venous return and thus cardiac output, decreasing stroke volume.

Volemia plays a pivotal role in caval opposition to compression by increased IAP. In fact, in hypovolemic conditions, caval pressure is low and the vena cava is easily compressed, resulting in high venous resistance.

Increases in IAP also increase afterload, raising total peripheral resistance.

With an IAP of 15 mmHg, an increase in heart rate, arterial blood pressure, caudal legs venous pressure, central venous pressure, right atrial pressure, and pulmonary vessels pressure, and a decrease in cardiac output were observed in healthy cats and dogs. With pressures of 8–10 mmHg in dogs and 4–8 mmHg in cats, hemodynamic parameters appear to be stable in healthy animals compared to baseline.

IAP increase can lead to hypoperfusion of splanchnic organs; the greater the insufflation pressure, the worse the hypoperfusion. In dogs an IAP of 16 mmHg was related with a decrease in superior mesenteric artery and portal vein blood flow, while an IAP of 15 mmHg showed a trend toward higher serum concentrations of hepatic and renal function indicators compared to insufflation pressures of 7 and 12 mmHg. In fact, low-pressure capnoperitoneum (8 mmHg) has been associated with improved perfusion of the parietal peritoneum in humans.

A systematic review and meta-analysis of animal studies showed an overall increase in serum creatinine and a decrease in urine output and renal blood flow during pneumoperitoneum.

Histopathology of splanchnic organs after pneumoperitoneum revealed pathological changes in the kidneys and pancreas of dogs with an insufflation pressure of 20 mmHg, and findings of hypoxic cell injury in rabbits with IAPs of 10, 15, and 20 mmHg.

The increase in IAP induced by pneumoperitoneum has also an impact on ventilatory dynamics due to the cranial shift of the diaphragm, which reduces functional residual capacity, promotes the formation of pulmonary atelectasis because of compression of the pulmonary parenchyma, increases intrathoracic pressure, and induces a 30%–50% decrease in thoracopulmonary compliance.

CO_2 is the first choice to create a pneumoperitoneum for laparoscopic surgery because it allows for electrocautery techniques, reduces the risk of fatal gas embolism, and is cost-effective. CO_2 is absorbed by abdominal vasculature, mainly at an IAP less than 10 mmHg, raising the blood CO_2 content.

A mild increase in blood CO_2 induces changes both in ventilatory parameters, with a rise in minute ventilation and tidal volume, and in hemodynamic parameters, with an increase in cardiac output, in an attempt to restore arterial CO_2 to normal.

If systemic CO_2 accumulation is severe enough, a decrease in stroke volume and a sympathetic discharge, with acceleration in heart rate and increase of afterload due to vascular resistance changes, are observed. If the lungs are not able to excrete the excess CO_2 from the blood, it is stored in skeletal muscle and in bone (two-compartment model).

In healthy animals, $PaCO_2$ and end-tidal CO_2 ($EtCO_2$) correlate, so capnography is useful for monitoring CO_2 blood concentrations. However, this is not the case in patients with impaired pulmonary excretion of CO_2, and arterial blood gas analysis is needed.

Head-down (Trendelenburg), head-up (reverse Trendelenburg or Fowler), or lateral recumbency may be needed for some laparoscopic surgeries, all of which have a cardiocirculatory and ventilatory impact on patients, added to that of the pneumoperitoneum itself (**Table 1**). In dogs with pneumoperitoneum, the Trendelenburg position increases the risk of gastroesophageal reflux but ameliorates cardiac output, whereas the reverse Trendelenburg position significantly aggravates the depression of cardiac output.

The very first articles related to veterinary anesthesia during laparoscopic surgery are physiological studies written in the 80s and 90s, carried on dogs and pigs as a model to unveil the hemodynamic and acid–base effects of pneumoperitoneum and capnoperitoneum in human medicine.

ANESTHETIC MANAGEMENT

Careful preoperative evaluation is key for successful anesthesia. The aim of preoperative evaluation is to assess the ASA status of the patient and if they are able to tolerate the hemodynamic and ventilatory effects of the laparoscopic procedure, evaluating the overall risk of the patient.

Due to the hemodynamic effects of the pneumoperitoneum, laparoscopy is contraindicated in hypovolemic and dehydrated patients, in those with shock syndrome or whose heart is not able to cope with a change in venous return or an increase in afterload, and in those in which an increase in intracranial pressure is a concern.

Capnoperitoneum is contraindicated in patients with pulmonary disease associated with impaired CO_2 excretory ability.

A thorough anamnesis and clinical assessment must always be done, paying particular attention to the circulatory and respiratory systems and to hydration status of the patient.

Besides the routine preanesthetic panel, in patients undergoing laparoscopic surgery a chest X-ray should be done to assess the integrity of the diaphragm and evaluate the radiological appearance of the lungs, thoracic vessels, and cardiac shadow. Any abnormality detected must be investigated with further exams.

There are no particular recommendations about the choice of anesthetic drugs for ASA 1 and ASA 2 patients, which are usually young and healthy animals undergoing elective procedures, such as ovariectomy and gastropexy. In the author's experience, in dogs, premedication with methadone (0.2 mg/kg) and dexmedetomidine (2 µg/kg IM or 0.5–1 µg/kg IV, depending on the patient's temperament) provides good analgesia, some sedation, and a sparing effect on propofol, used for anesthesia induction, as intubation is normally performed with 1–3 mg/kg IV of this drug, avoiding an undesirable spleen enlargement.

The choice of anesthetic drugs for patients classified as ASA 3 or greater is made according to the underlying disease.

Anesthesia maintenance is normally carried out with inhaled anesthetics (isoflurane or sevoflurane).

Further analgesia may be required during access to the abdomen and trocar positioning. A 0.5–1 µg/kg bolus of fentanyl is usually adequate to manage the noxious stimulus.

Due to ventilation impairment associated with the pneumoperitoneum, mechanical ventilation is recommended. A ventilatory strategy providing a tidal volume of 12 mL/kg , an inspiratory:expiratory ratio of 1:2, an inspiratory pause of 25% of inspiratory time, and a positive end-expiratory pressure (PEEP) of 5 cmH_2O after a vital capacity alveolar recruiting maneuver (40 cmH_2O for 20 seconds), with a respiratory rate adjusted on the basis of the $EtCO_2$ tension, has been demonstrated to improve lung function during and after capnoperitoneum in healthy dogs undergoing laparoscopy (**Fig. 1**).

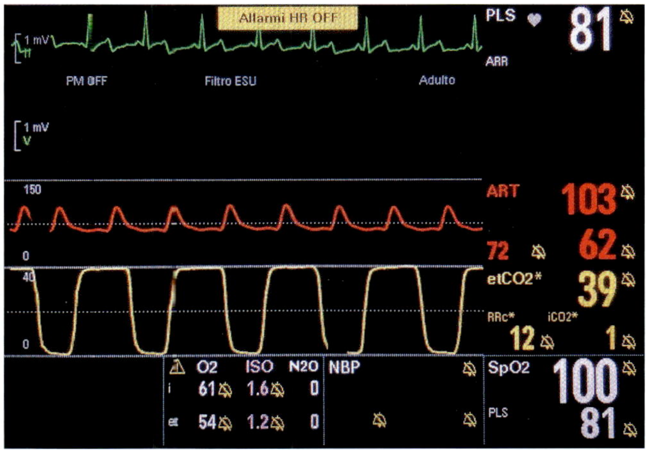

FIGURE 1. Invasive blood pressure monitoring is a useful tool to investigate volemia and perfusion of the anesthetized patient before the abdomen is insufflated. It is especially recommended in patients classified as ASA 3 or greater.

Capnography is an essential monitoring tool in laparoscopy, as $EtCO_2$ strongly correlates with $PaCO_2$ in healthy lungs with effective ventilation. Hemodynamics monitoring and cardiovascular stabilization before pneumoperitoneum induction and during laparoscopic surgery are crucial in every patient undergoing laparoscopy, but especially in those with concurrent diseases (most notably renal or pancreatic disease).

Perfusion pressure of splanchnic organs is defined by the difference between mean arterial pressure and IAP.

Usually monitored parameters include electrocardiography and arterial pressure measurement (**Box 1**). The latter can be performed in young, healthy animals with oscillometric or Doppler devices, whereas invasive blood pressure monitoring is recommended in elderly patients or in those with underlying diseases (**Fig. 2**).

Hypothermia in anesthetized patients must be managed routinely.

POSTOPERATIVE MANAGEMENT

- Make sure that abdomen is completely desufflated.
- Manage postoperative pain, choosing the drugs according to the underlying condition of the patient.
- When postoperative bleeding can occur, for example after taking biopsies, monitor the patient for 12–24 hours.

BOX 1. Recommended parameters to monitor

- Capnography
- Pulse oximetry
- Electrocardiography
- Blood pressure (noninvasive or invasive)
- Temperature
- Spirometry

COMPLICATIONS

Complications of laparoscopic surgery

- Bronchial intubation
- Gastroesophageal reflux
- Vagovagal reflex
- Pneumothorax, pneumomediastinum, pneumoderma
- Embolism

BRONCHIAL INTUBATION

When a pneumoperitoneum is created, the diaphragm is shifted cranially and the endotracheal tube can be displaced, causing bronchial intubation. When this occurs, only one lung is ventilated.

How to recognize it:

- At pneumoperitoneum induction, peak pressure rises more than expected, $EtCO_2$ rises, SpO_2 may decrease, and blood gas analysis reveals some grade of hypoxemia and hypercapnia.

What to do:

- Displace the endotracheal tube cranially.

GASTROESOPHAGEAL REFLUX

Gastroesophageal reflux may lead to regurgitation and aspiration of stomach contents. An increased IAP, as with pneumoperitoneum, associated with a Trendelenburg position is a predisposing factor. Regurgitation can be silent, not being detected by the anesthetist.

Preventive measures include appropriate preanesthetic fasting and, in patients with a history of vomiting or regurgitation, prokinetic drugs and H_2 blockers or proton pump inhibitors.

How to recognize it:

- Yellowish or brown fluid present in the patient's mouth or nares.

What to do:

- Check airway security (endotracheal cuff insufflation).
- Remove material from the mouth, nose, pharynx, and esophagus.
- Flush the esophagus with saline and protect it with sucralfate.
- Extubate with the cuff slightly inflated.

VAGOVAGAL REFLEX

At pneumoperitoneum induction, hypotension and bradycardia can seldom develop as a vagovagal reflex. Bradycardia and hypertension may appear during ovarian pedicle traction.

How to recognize it:

- Sudden drop in heart rate and mean arterial pressure, visible with invasive blood pressure monitoring, or loss of

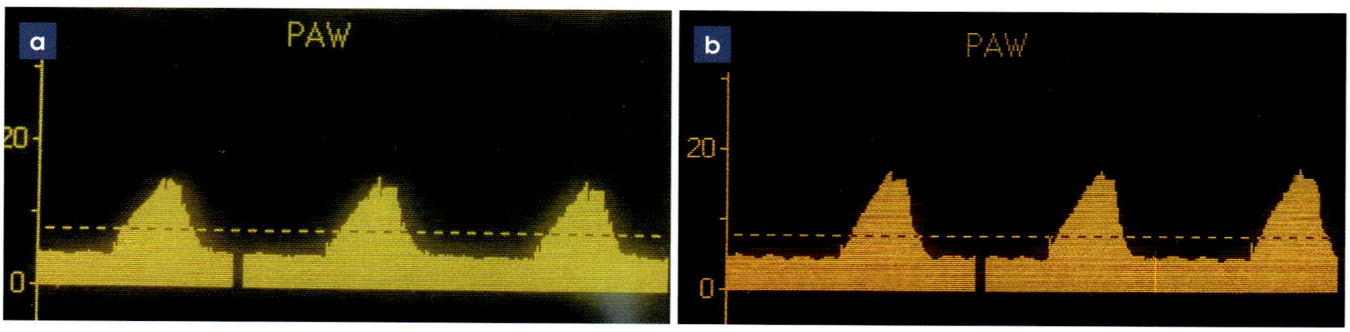

FIGURE 2. Airways pressure a) before and b) after pneumoperitoneum induction, with the patient under intermittent positive pressure ventilation (tidal volume 12 mL/kg, inspiratory:expiratory ratio 1:2, inspiratory pause 25% of inspiratory time, positive end-expiratory pressure 5 cmH_2O). The peak pressure increase in figure b reflects the decrease in thoracopulmonary compliance induced by the pneumoperitoneum.

noninvasive blood pressure signal, in case of hypotension and bradycardia.

- Drop in heart rate and rise of mean arterial pressure in case of bradycardia and hypertension.

What to do:

- In case of hypotension and bradycardia at pneumoperitoneum induction, deflate the abdomen and administer atropine (20–40 µg/kg IV).
- In case of bradycardia and hypertension, just monitor. If necessary, administer atropine (10 µg/kg).

PNEUMOTHORAX, PNEUMOMEDIASTINUM, AND PNEUMODERMA

In the veterinary literature, few case reports describe the presence of pneumothorax and pneumopericardium in canine patients after pneumoperitoneum induction. The cases reported are thought to be a result of gas passage through embryonic remnants or alternatively through potential diaphragmatic defects or weak points. Pneumoderma is due to gas insufflation out of the peritoneal cavity.

How to recognize them:

- Pneumothorax can be suspected in a ventilated patient when peak pressure increases, breath sounds decrease on thoracic auscultation, $EtCO_2$ decreases, and hypoxemia develops.
- Pneumopericardium causes acute cardiac tamponade.

What to do:

- Prompt drainage of fluid collection by thoracocentesis or pericardiocentesis is mandatory.
- Pneumoderma and retroperitoneal emphysema are not dangerous and generally reabsorb in a few hours.

EMBOLISM

Clinically significant CO_2 embolism is a rare but potentially fatal complication of anesthesia administered during laparoscopic surgery. It is caused by entrapment of CO_2 after inadvertent injection in an injured vein, artery, or solid organ, resulting in blockage of the right ventricle or pulmonary artery.

How to recognize it:

- CO_2 embolism should be suspected if bradycardia, tachycardia, or arrhythmias with hypotension, a sudden drop of $EtCO_2$, and possibly desaturation (decrease in SpO_2) occur, mainly at the beginning of the procedure.

What to do:

- Discontinue abdominal insufflation and give 100% O_2.
- Administer vasopressors and inotropic agents to maintain cardiac output as needed.
- Place the patient in the Trendelenburg position to decrease the risk of gas traveling to the head.

Key points

- Understanding the physiological consequences of capnoperitoneum is a cornerstone of anesthesia management.
- Close hemodynamics monitoring and adequate ventilation are required because of the physiological effects related to laparoscopy.

SUGGESTED READINGS

CLINICAL CASES

11.1 HYPOTENSION AND BRADYCARDIA AT PNEUMOPERITONEUM INDUCTION IN A FEMALE DOG

Samuele Venuta

A 2-year-old female mixed-breed dog weighing 25 kg was presented for laparoscopic ovariectomy. Based on preanesthetic examination and routine blood work, the patient was classified as ASA 1.

Premedication consisted of methadone (0.2 mg/kg IM) and dexmedetomidine (0.002 mg/kg IM) administered in the same syringe. After 10 minutes, the cephalic vein was cannulated and induction was performed with propofol (2.5 mg/kg IV). Orotracheal intubation anesthesia was maintained with isoflurane delivered in 60% O_2, providing an end-tidal isoflurane concentration of around 1%.

Mechanical ventilation using a ventilator in volume control mode was performed to maintain $EtCO_2$ below 55 mmHg (tidal volume 270 mL, respiratory rate 12 breaths per minute, PEEP 3 cmH_2O, inspiratory:expiratory ratio 1:2.5). Heart rate, electrocardiography, SpO_2, $EtCO_2$, invasive blood pressure, and temperature were monitored.

The surgical field was clipped and scrubbed, and the first port was placed. Pneumoperitoneum was induced with 5 L/min flow until 9 mmHg pressure was reached.

Suddenly, hemodynamic parameters dropped down: heart rate passed from 50 to 23 bpm and mean arterial pressure from 70 to 30 mmHg. $EtCO_2$ decreased to 28 mmHg. Pneumoperitoneum was discontinued and an IV bolus of atropine at 0.02 mg/kg was immediately given.

After a few minutes, heart rate, mean arterial pressure, and $EtCO_2$ raised to 98 bpm, 85 mmHg, and 50 mmHg, respectively. Pneumoperitoneum was induced again, and surgery was continued and completed uneventfully. Patient recovery was good, and the outcome satisfactory.

The presumptive diagnosis is vagovagal reflex due to pneumoperitoneum induction. Diagnosis is confirmed by the effectiveness of IV atropine treatment.

In case of vagovagal reflex during laparoscopic surgery, management consists of cessation of gas insufflation, deflation of the abdomen, and administration of an IV atropine bolus.

Key points

- Patient monitoring is key to promptly detecting any change in vital signs that could potentially lead to a critical condition and death.
- It is not possible to know in advance if a patient will have bradycardia and hypotension at pneumoperitoneum induction.

Tips and tricks

- ✓ Invasive blood pressure measurement allows continuous arterial blood pressure monitoring, thus providing beat-to-beat information.
- ✓ Calculating emergency drugs doses before anesthesia leads to faster interventions if needed.

12 PATIENT POSITIONING, ACCESS, PORT PLACEMENT, AND PNEUMOPERITONEUM IN LAPAROSCOPY

Roberto Properzi

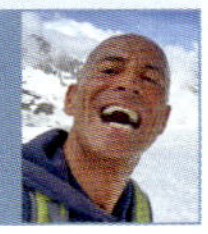

Both in human and veterinary medicine, the first surgical steps are of fundamental importance for the success of the procedure, although they are associated with a higher risk of iatrogenic complications.

Several studies about correct patient positioning, laparoscopic access, and port placement are available in the veterinary literature. Although this chapter provides guidelines, surgeons develop their own laparoscopic entry technique through experience.

> Peritoneal access remains the gravest concern for the laparoscopic surgeon and continues to be a leading cause of complication during laparoscopic surgery (F. Rossi).

PATIENT POSITIONING

For first port access, the animal is positioned in dorsal recumbency slightly inclined to the left so as to avoid the falciform ligament (**Fig. 1**). The penetration of this ligament during first port access can cause problems, especially in large-sized patients with a large falciform ligament.

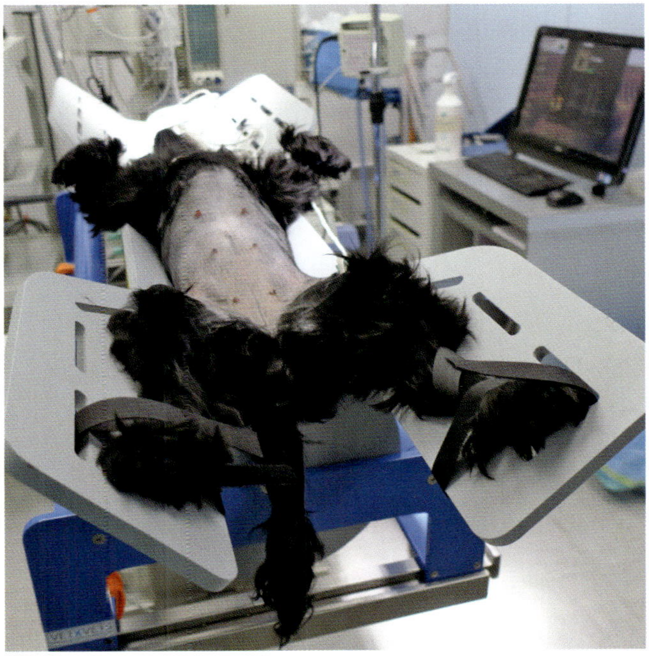

FIGURE 1. Patient positioned on the surgical table.

LAPAROSCOPIC ACCESS AND PORT PLACEMENT

The most commonly used techniques for first port insertion are the closed technique and the open technique. The closed technique is performed by the insertion of a Veress needle through which a pneumoperitoneum can be established. Once the abdominal cavity is filled with carbon dioxide (CO_2), the first port is created. Regarding the open techniques, the most frequently used is the Hasson technique, by which abdominal entry is essentially accomplished via minilaparotomy (**Video 1**). Once the port is inserted into the abdominal cavity, a pneumoperitoneum is created by insufflating CO_2.

VIDEO 1. Laparoscopic access using an open technique (Hasson technique). The first port is generally inserted midway between the xiphoid process of the sternum and the umbilicus, in a slightly right paramedian position to avoid the falciform ligament along the longitudinal fibers of the abdominal rectus muscle.

The author used to perform the closed technique with an 18-gauge needle instead of a Veress needle, inserting it midway between the xiphoid process of the sternum and the umbilicus, in a slightly right paramedian position to avoid the falciform ligament, after making a skin incision and lifting the fascia with a curved Crile hemostatic forceps. However, the author now uses an open technique (Hasson technique).

In the author's opinion, two tools make the difference when performing the Hasson technique: the modified Senn–Miller retractor (**Fig. 2**) and the curved Crile hemostatic forceps with a rat tooth tip (**Fig. 3**).

The first port is generally inserted midway between the xiphoid process of the sternum and the umbilicus, in a slightly right paramedian position to avoid the falciform ligament along the longitudinal fibers of the abdominal rectus muscle (**Fig. 4**).

The correct length of the skin incision is established by making an impression on the skin with the end of the cannula (**Fig. 5**). A number 15 scalpel blade is normally used to cut the skin and the abdominal rectus muscle fascia with one-eighth of a turn in a counterclockwise direction. A curved Klemmer forceps is then utilized to expand the incision down to the fascia. The peritoneum is grasped and lifted with a curved Crile hemostatic forceps with a rat tooth tip, and then it is cut with the scalpel blade.

In the abdomen, the Senn–Miller retractor works like a hook, lifting the tissues (from the parietal peritoneum to the skin) and further detaching the underlying bowel loops from the muscular fascia. This retractor also counterbalances the pressure that is necessary for the insertion of the cannula through its trocar inside the abdomen (**Fig. 6**).

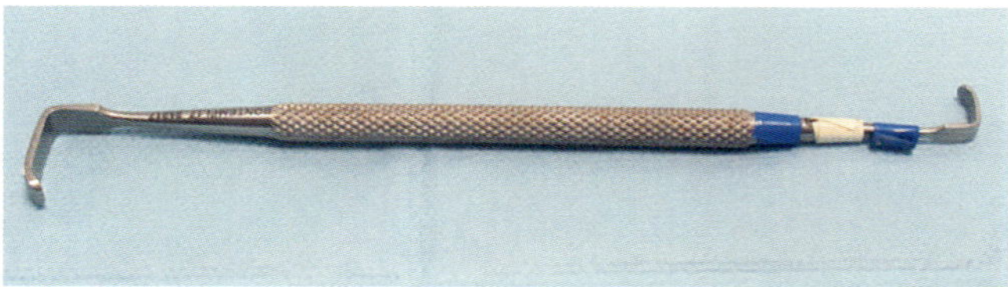

FIGURE 2. Modified Senn–Miller retractor. The blunt side has been made thinner to facilitate insertion in the small surgical incision.

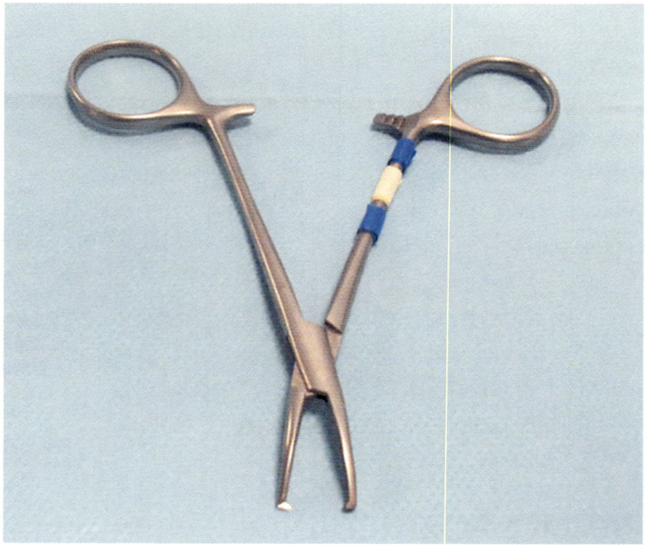

FIGURE 3. Mosquito forceps with a rat tooth tip.

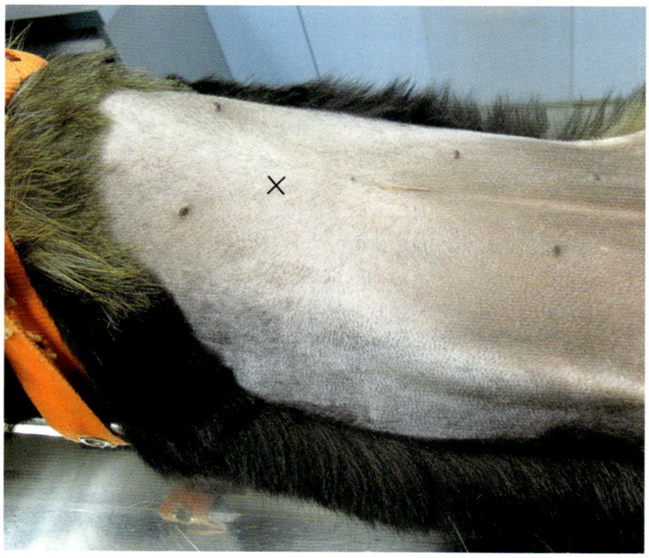

FIGURE 4. Insertion point of the first laparoscopic port (cross).

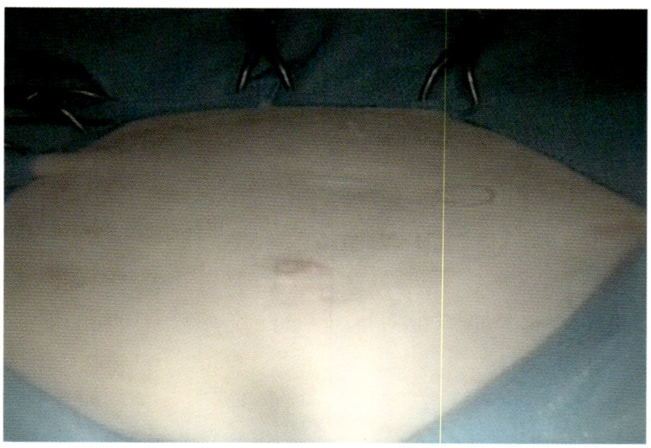

FIGURE 5. Cannula impression on the skin to establish the correct length of the incision.

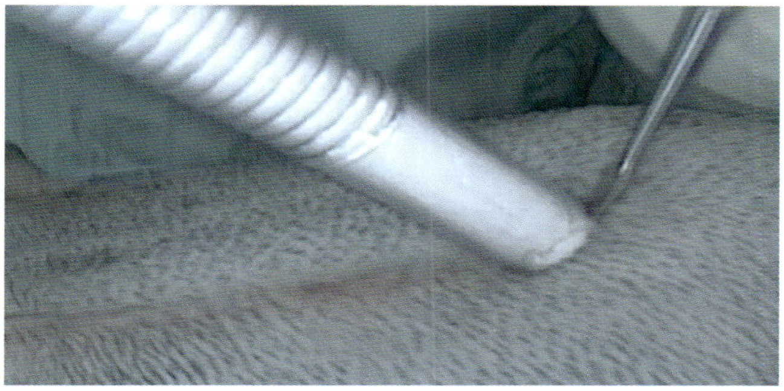

FIGURE 6. Insertion of the first cannula.

The trocar should be aimed laterally, in an oblique position, toward the right side of the patient (away from the spleen, which is on the left) in order not to damage the spleen or other internal organs. Once the cannula is inside the abdomen, the trocar is removed and the CO_2 gas tube is connected to the tap on the cannula to create the pneumoperitoneum.

The second and third (or more) ports are placed under laparoscopic visualization, in a position based on the surgical procedure being performed (**Fig. 7**) (**Video 1**).

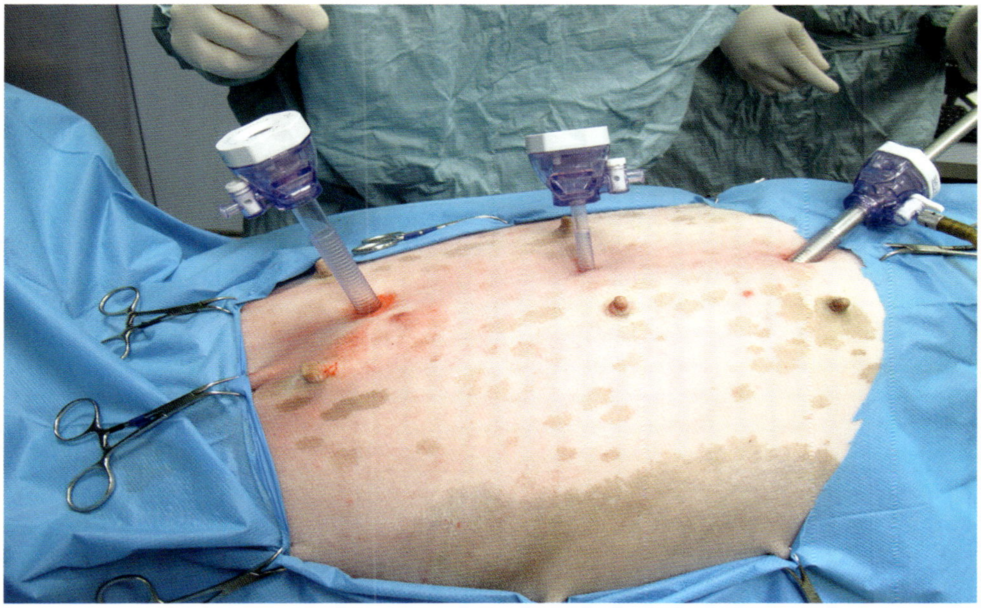

FIGURE 7. Final position of the ports.

Tips and tricks

- ✓ The patient should be positioned with a slight inclination to the left to avoid the falciform ligament.
- ✓ The use of a modified Senn–Miller retractor and a curved Crile hemostatic forceps with a rat tooth tip is strongly recommended.
- ✓ The first port is generally inserted in a slightly right paramedian position to avoid the falciform ligament.
- ✓ The trocar should be aimed laterally, in an oblique position, toward the right side of the patient in order not to damage the spleen or other internal organs.

PNEUMOPERITONEUM

Laparoscopic procedures need a surgical field provided by the establishment of a pneumoperitoneum. The pneumoperitoneum can be hyperbaric or isobaric depending on whether or not gas is insufflated into the abdominal cavity.

Different types of gases can be used to create a pneumoperitoneum in laparoscopic procedures, including CO_2, helium, argon, nitrogen, or nitrous oxide. Although helium and argon are inert gases, they can increase the risk of venous gas embolism due to their relative insolubility. Nitrous oxide reduces postoperative pain but is flammable and cannot be used in association with electrical devices, which makes this gas useful for diagnostic procedures but not for therapeutic ones.

CO_2 is the most frequently utilized gas in small animal laparoscopy because it is safe and inexpensive. However, this gas has some collateral effects, such as peritoneal irritation, and it is therefore necessary to remove any residual CO_2 after the procedure to decrease postoperative pain.

Gas insufflation of the abdomen to create a pneumoperitoneum produces an increase in intra-abdominal pressure, which has hemodynamic and ventilatory impacts that depend on the degree of intra-abdominal pressure and on the patient's volemic status. This increase in intra-abdominal pressure has also an impact on ventilatory dynamics due to the cranial shift of the diaphragm, which reduces functional residual capacity, promotes the formation of pulmonary atelectasis because of pulmonary parenchyma compression, increases intrathoracic pressure, and induces a 30%–50% decrease in thoracopulmonary compliance.

Since the elevation of intra-abdominal pressure, the Trendelenburg position, and hypercapnia increase intracranial pressure, laparoscopy must be avoided in patients with head injury or neurological disorders.

Finally, the lowest pressure possible should be used for abdominal insufflation. According to the literature, increasing the abdominal pressure above 7 mmHg does not contribute to a substantial increase in the working space in cats or dogs.

Despite the availability of devices for gasless procedures, it seems that in healthy animals the risks associated with gasless techniques are higher than those associated with pneumoperitoneum.

SUGGESTED READINGS

13 COMPLICATIONS IN LAPAROSCOPY

Francesco Collivignarelli

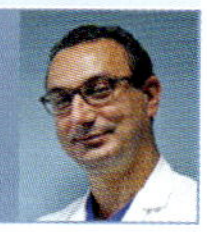

The first objective when performing laparoscopic surgery is to obtain an adequate pneumoperitoneum, which requires proper access in order to insufflate carbon dioxide. This is a critical step because of the potential for iatrogenic trauma to abdominal organs or vasculature during port placement. Laparoscopic access can be gained with several techniques:

- Open:
  - Minilaparotomy (Hasson technique)
- Closed:
  - Veress needle
- Blind:
  - Veress needle
  - Trocar insertion
  - Trocar insertion after establishment of pneumoperitoneum
- Visual

Two main techniques have been described to achieve pneumoperitoneum: the closed entry method with a Veress needle technique and the open Hasson technique. The Veress needle is a laparoscopic instrument with a spring-loaded blunt stylet that is introduced blindly into the peritoneal space and then connected to the insufflation tube. Once the pneumoperitoneum is established, the first port is created. The Hasson technique provides access to the peritoneal cavity by performing a minilaparotomy of the same diameter as the cannula, allowing the insertion of a cannula into the peritoneal cavity under direct visualization.

Complications related to the pneumoperitoneum include:

- spleen (**Fig. 1**), bowel, or bladder injuries
- pneumothorax
- subcutaneous emphysema.

Fatal embolism has also been reported. In the veterinary literature, guidelines for establishing a safe and rapid pneumoperitoneum are lacking, and few surgical studies have been conducted.

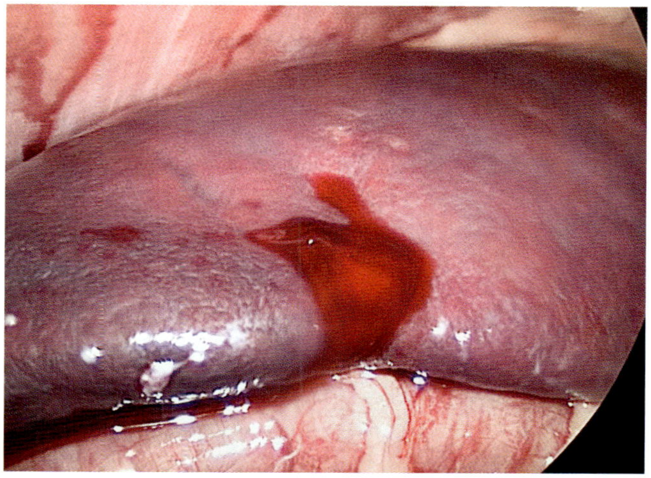

FIGURE 1. Splenic injury.

ANATOMICAL KNOWLEDGE

Although port placement for various instruments is considered essential, no consensus has been reached on trocar placement, even for the same procedures. This lack of consistency in criteria for port placement may leave substantial room for error, especially in the hands of novice surgeons. A sound knowledge of the anatomy of the abdominal wall helps to prevent any hemorrhages that could compromise visualization of the abdominal organs (**Fig. 2**).

CLOSED ENTRY WITH THE VERESS NEEDLE TECHNIQUE

The Veress needle technique was developed by János Veress in 1938. A 1 mm skin incision is made with a number 11 scalpel blade 1 cm to the right of the umbilicus, and then a 150 mm long reusable Veress needle is introduced. Successful placement is validated by introducing 5 mL of sterile saline solution

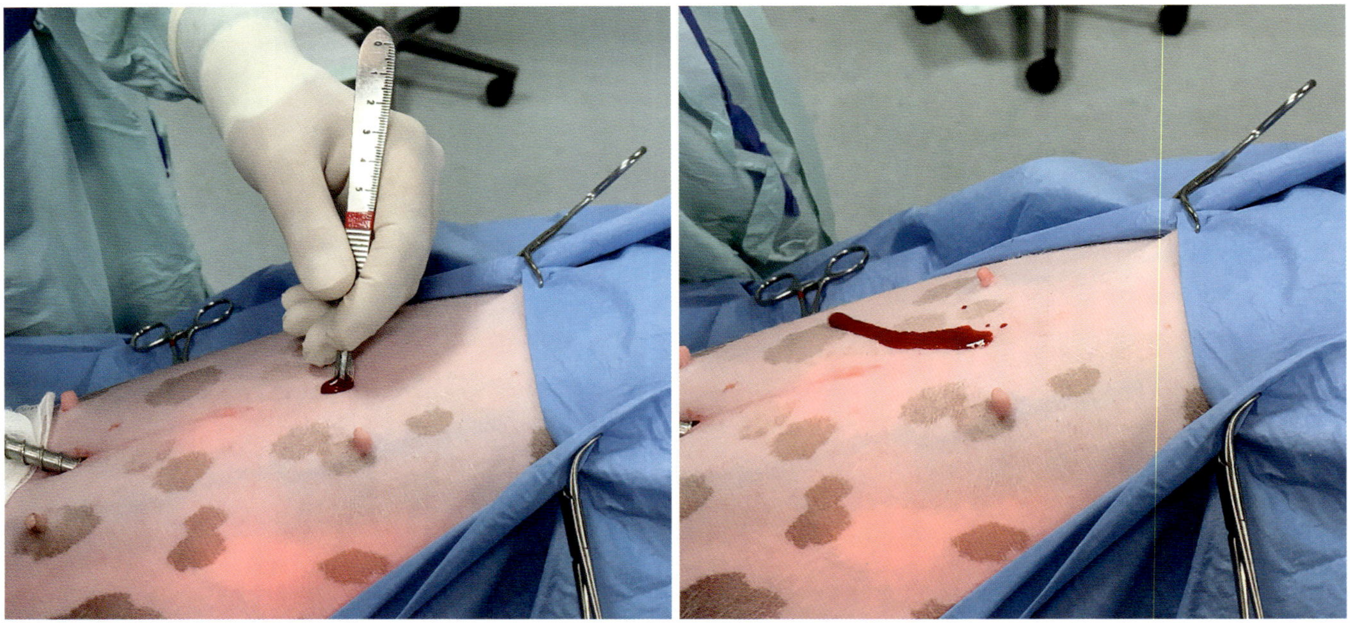

FIGURE 2. The surgeon should have a sound knowledge of the anatomy of the abdominal wall to avoid damaging vessels during port placement.

through the needle (injection test). The Veress needle is then connected to the insufflation tube and a pneumoperitoneum is established. Carbon dioxide insufflation is started and continued until a pressure of 4–8 mmHg is reached.

Once the pneumoperitoneum is achieved, a port is created blindly a few centimeters caudal to the umbilicus using a 6 mm trocar cannula. A laparoscope is inserted through the port, and visual exploration of the abdominal cavity is conducted. Any injury inflicted during the blind insertion of the needle and trocar is noted.

OPEN ENTRY TECHNIQUES

The open technique to establish the pneumoperitoneum was first described by Hasson in 1971. Over the next few years, several changes were made which saw several publications flourish. Currently the most used technique consists in making a 5 mm incision in the skin and subcutaneous tissue 5 mm caudal to the umbilicus with a number 11 scalpel blade, followed by a minilaparotomy for cannula insertion (**Fig. 3**). For this, the subcutaneous fat is exposed and resected to visualize the linea alba. The abdominal wall is lifted using a Klemmer forceps and incised with a number 11 scalpel blade. Surgical margins are grasped with two Klemmer forceps, or two sutures are placed in the fascia on either side of the cannula to lift the abdominal wall (**Fig. 4**), and then a blunt cannula is inserted (**Fig. 5**). After checking correct positioning of the instrument and exploring the abdominal cavity through the laparoscope, an insufflation tube is connected to the trocar. Carbon dioxide insufflation is started and continued until a pressure of 4–8 mmHg is reached.

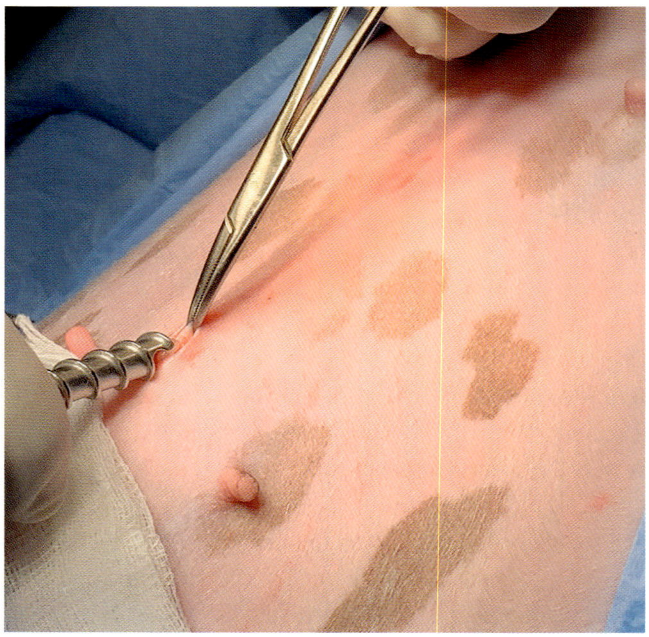

FIGURE 3. Abdominal entry is essentially accomplished by performing a minilaparotomy.

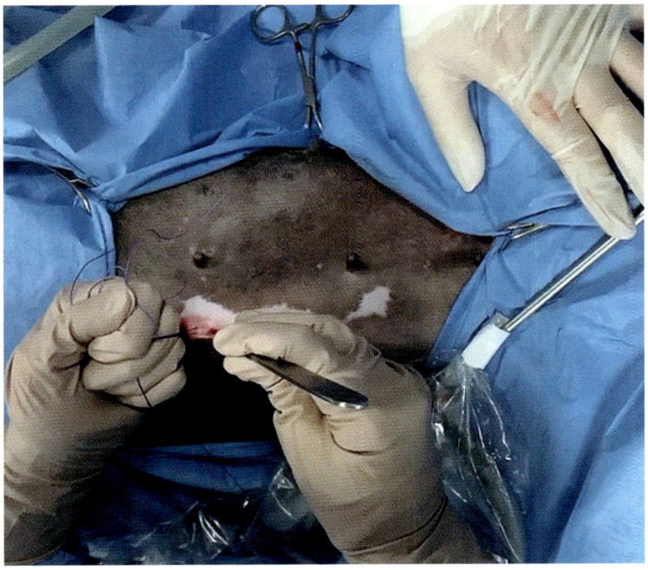

FIGURE 4. Sutures are placed in the fascia on either side of the cannula and attached to the cannula to seal the abdominal wall incision to the cone-shaped sleeve.

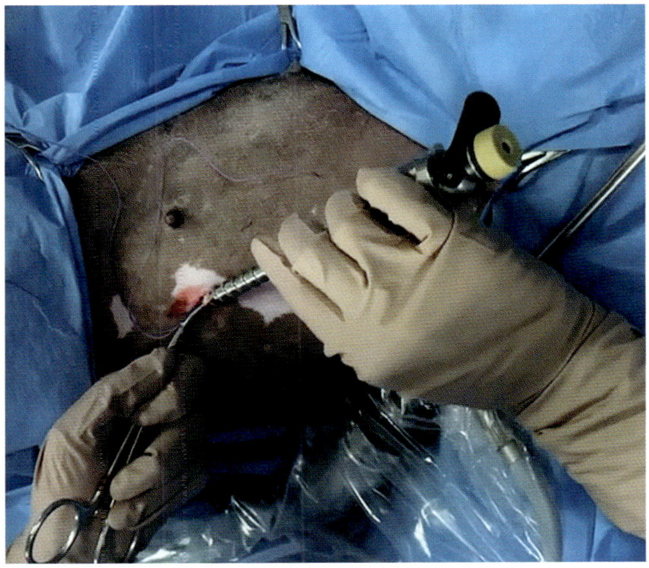

FIGURE 5. The cannula is inserted into the peritoneal cavity.

LAPAROSCOPIC ACCESS COMPLICATIONS

Several complications related to the initial access have been described in the literature. Anderson and Fransson described complications in a variety of laparoscopic procedures performed in cats and dogs; the Hasson technique was associated with only minor complications, whereas the Veress needle technique resulted in splenic injury in 2% of patients. Gas leakage is a disadvantage associated with the modified Hasson technique and is related to wide surgical wounds compared with the cannula diameter. Gas leakage was quickly managed by placing Allis forceps around the abdominal wall to limit the leak and restore the peritoneal pressure. Bianchi et al. described a modified technique that is faster and safer than the Veress needle technique for the creation of the first port in laparoscopic surgery. In conclusion, there is no perfect technique; there are techniques with which the surgeon is more familiar.

INTRAOPERATIVE COMPLICATIONS AND CONVERSION TO OPEN TECHNIQUES

Most of the complications encountered in minimally invasive surgery are related to bleeding. Although hemorrhage rarely creates hemodynamic instability, it can be very annoying in delicate procedures in which visualization of the organs is very important (e.g., adrenalectomy, nephrectomy). Bleeding may warrant conversion to open surgery, especially if the surgeon has little experience in minimally invasive surgery. In any case, all of the traditional surgery tools are available to the minimally invasive surgeon, including the ability to ligate with suture, apply hemostatic clips, use vessel-sealing devices, and apply topical hemostatic agents, so as to avoid conversion to open surgery as much as possible. If suction is available, careful aspiration of blood followed by grasping and ligation of larger hemorrhaging vessels is often possible. However, decision-making in these cases should be rapid, and if hemostasis cannot be accomplished quickly, conversion to open surgery should be considered.

Conversion from a minimally invasive to an open approach may be necessary for a variety of different reasons, which can be grouped as follows

- **Emergent conversion.** An intraoperative complication occurs that cannot be resolved without open access.
- **Elective conversion.** A complication has not occurred, but the minimally invasive approach does not guarantee the continuation of the procedure. This type of conversion can be desirable, for example, in certain tumors with large adhesions, depending on the experience of the surgeon.

POSTOPERATIVE COMPLICATIONS

The most frequent complications in minimally invasive surgery are port-site complications, including:

- seroma formation
- surgical site infection
- rarely, herniation.

Suturing the fascial sheath of the body wall at the entry points is strongly recommended. However, these complications seem to resolve spontaneously within a few days.

Port-site metastasis is a potential complication when neoplastic lesions are resected and withdrawn through small port incisions. Other factors such as surgery, local immune response, and pneumoperitoneum may also play a decisive role in the etiopathogenesis of port-site metastasis.

SUGGESTED READINGS

14 EXPLORATORY AND DIAGNOSTIC LAPAROSCOPY

Christopher B. Thomson, Ameet Singh

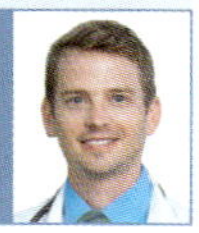

Indications

- Targeted sampling of various abdominal organs, for histopathology, cytology, culture, toxicopathological examination (e.g., copper quantification)
- Diagnostic staging for various types of neoplasia
- Treatment monitoring (e.g., copper storage disease, inflammatory bowel disease)

Contraindications

- Severe coagulopathy
- Decompensated cardiovascular disease
- Inability to handle anesthesia

Laparoscopy not only provides a minimally invasive opportunity to visualize the peritoneal cavity and abdominal organs but also improves the magnification and illumination from which the surgeon evaluates the various structures. Through adjustments of patient positioning and retraction instruments, nearly all abdominal organs can be visualized; this is particularly true when extracorporeal handling of the gastrointestinal tract is performed.

Minimally invasive surgery also offers a highly attractive option for targeted organ biopsies within the abdomen due to the ability to visualize lesions, manipulate the organs, control hemorrhage, and obtain large tissue samples. Laparoscopy has been utilized to collect samples from nearly all abdominal organs, particularly from the liver, kidneys, gallbladder, pancreas, spleen, adrenal glands, peritoneum, prostate, urinary bladder, lymph nodes, falciform fat, and used for gastrointestinal sampling through a laparoscopic-assisted approach.

Additionally, laparoscopic-assisted procedures expand the spectrum of organs that can be assessed and sampled to include those of the gastrointestinal tract and the peritoneum (**Fig. 1**). Recent evidence suggests that laparoscopic-assisted intestinal surgery is safe and feasible and does not have increased complications compared to open laparotomy while being less invasive. However, diagnostic/exploratory laparoscopy requires more time, and conversion to open laparotomy may be needed for select cases.

When compared to percutaneous image-guided biopsies, benefits from the use of laparoscopy include control of hemostasis, collection of larger samples, improved targeting of pathologic lesions, and an ability to manipulate the organs being sampled. For example, when performing liver biopsies, it is feasible to ensure that samples are being collected from each individual lobe and biopsy sites can be selected based on visual pathology. When compared to an open laparotomy, minimally invasive

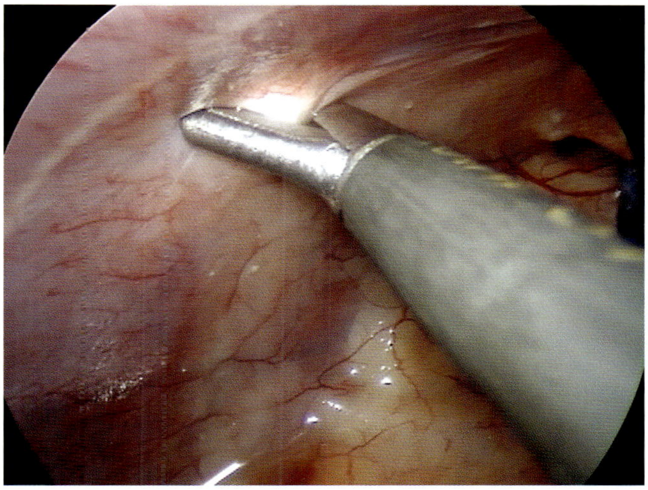

FIGURE 1. Laparoscopic targeted biopsy of the peritoneum. Image courtesy of Dr. Andrea Pievaroli.

surgery has been shown to result in less postoperative pain, shorter return to normal activity, and fewer postoperative wound complications.

Patient evaluation prior to laparoscopy should be tailored towards the individual patient but generally comprises a minimum database through physical examination, complete blood count, chemistry profile, and urinalysis. For patients with liver or renal disease, coagulation testing should be considered as well. However, for laparoscopic liver biopsies, patients with biochemical coagulopathies rarely have clinically significant bleeding, and bleeding is not correlated with coagulation. If neoplasia is suspected, appropriate staging is recommended, including lymph node sampling and thoracic radiographs. Abdominal diagnostic imaging prior to the procedure is often dictated by the underlying indication, including radiographs, ultrasound, and/or CT.

Laparoscopic liver and pancreatic biopsy were first described in the dog in 1972, using a human proctoscope (St. Mark's Major proctoscope set with infants sigmoidoscope) as a laparoscope by Drs. J. R. F. Dalton and F. W. G. Hill.

PATIENT PREPARATION AND POSITIONING

Preoperative patient preparation for minimally invasive surgery of the abdomen has many similarities to that of traditional open abdominal surgery. Preparation includes routine preoperative fasting and use of perioperative antibiotic prophylaxis depending on the planned procedure and patient status. Additional preparation steps include evacuating the urinary bladder and performing a wider hair clip than might be utilized for a traditional ventral midline laparotomy. Evacuation of the urinary bladder allows for increased physical space within the peritoneal cavity during the laparoscopic procedure and minimizes the risk of accidental trauma to the bladder during establishment of laparoscopic ports. A wider hair clip allows the laparoscopic ports to be placed in a more lateral position to facilitate appropriate instrument triangulation.

Patient position for minimally invasive surgery of the abdomen largely depends on the planned procedure. By varying a patient's position, the surgeon can use passive retraction of the abdominal viscera by gravity to facilitate exposure of the anatomic structures of interest for a particular procedure. This position may need to be changed during the procedure, requiring an operating table that can be adjusted to the desired angles. For procedures involving the retroperitoneal space, it is often advantageous to position patients in sternal recumbency, with the pelvis supported, allowing abdominal viscera to passively fall away from retroperitoneal structures of interest. An ideal operating table for use with minimally invasive surgery allows tilting the table side to side (e.g., to provide sequential access to each side of the reproductive tract) as well as the front and back ends of the table (e.g., Trendelenburg position to maximize exposure of the caudal abdomen). It is important to carefully secure patients to the table to prevent inadvertent slipping or falling during the procedure. Commercially available tabletop add-on patient positioning platforms are becoming more common through veterinary laparoscopic supply companies. These devices offer the ability to retrofit an existing nontilting surgical table for laparoscopic use.

OPERATING ROOM LAYOUT

For abdominal exploration, the patient is placed in dorsal recumbency. The possibility to rotate the patient into an oblique lateral recumbency is required for visualizing dorsally and retroperitoneally located structures. Some surgeons prefer the use of a 10°–30° reverse Trendelenburg position (elevation of the head) to evaluate cranially located structures (liver, gallbladder, stomach) by allowing other abdominal organs to fall caudally.

It is recommended that instrument tables be unattached from the patient table and freely mobile; this provides the surgeon full access to the patient's abdomen and an ability to perform surgery from both sides. The video monitor is often positioned cranially for most procedures but can be moved to the side based on the expected location of surgery (e.g., liver vs. kidney vs. pancreas) (**Fig. 2**).

PORT PLACEMENT (FIG. 3)

- T1, on the midline, 1–2 cm caudal to the umbilicus
- T2, on the midline, 1–2 cm caudal to T1
- T3 (optional), 4–6 cm cranial to T1
- Optional single-port device, in the region of the umbilicus

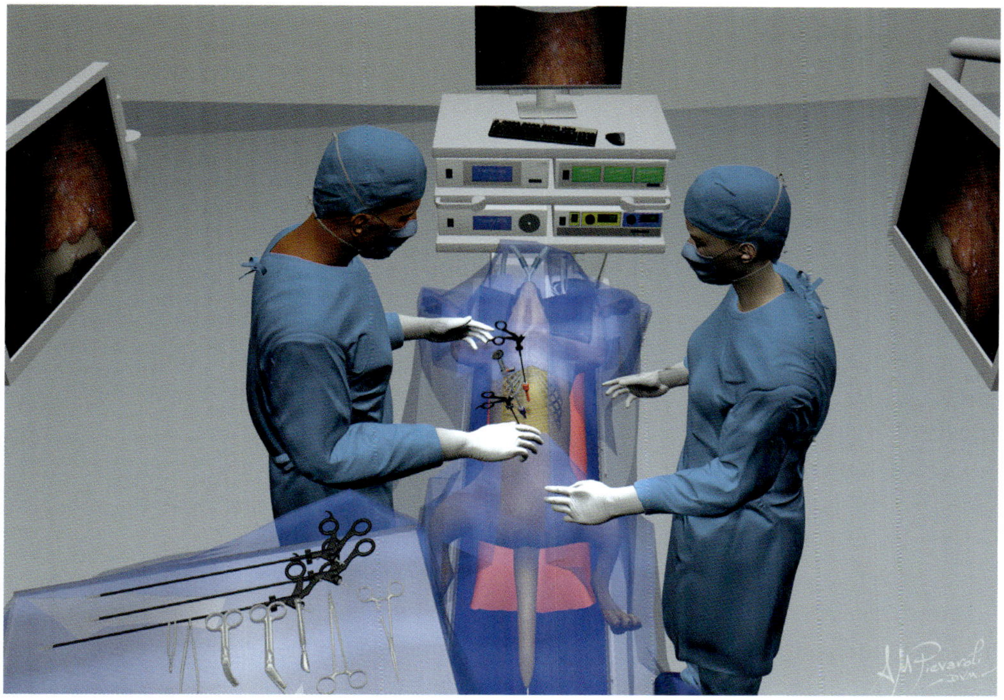

FIGURE 2. Operating room layout for laparoscopic abdominal exploration. Initially, the patient is positioned in dorsal recumbency. Depending on the organ to be viewed, it may be useful to tilt the table for oblique lateral recumbency. Some surgeons prefer the use of Trendelenburg or reverse Trendelenburg positioning to allow abdominal organs to fall cranially or caudally.

Instruments

On the table:

- Standard surgical set
- Telescope 5 mm – 30°, camera, light source
- Two or three 5 mm cannulas
- Grasping forceps, blunt probe, cup biopsy forceps
- Laparoscopic fan retractor

Ready to use:

- Needle core biopsy device
- 20–22-gauge, 3–6-inch spinal needle
- 12 cc syringe
- Endoscopic cannula for aspiration/irrigation
- Single-port platform (e.g., SILS Port)
- Vessel-sealing device
- Pretied or extracorporeally tied loop ligature
- Gelatin sponge (e.g., Gelfoam)

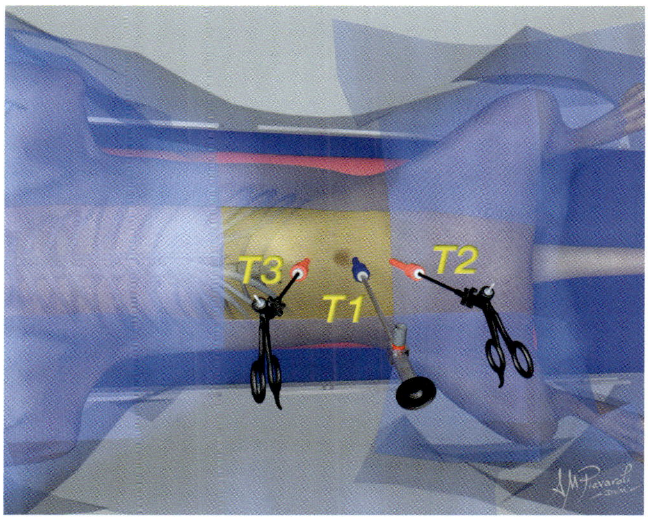

FIGURE 3. Port placement for general laparoscopic abdominal exploration.

The following procedures are described below:

A. Abdominal exploration
B. Liver and gallbladder evaluation and biopsy
C. Kidney and adrenal gland evaluation and biopsy
D. Pancreas evaluation and biopsy
E. Spleen evaluation and biopsy
F. Lymph node evaluation and biopsy
G. Gastrointestinal tract evaluation and biopsy

A ABDOMINAL EXPLORATION

Full abdominal exploration is often recommended in any patient undergoing abdominal surgery. Similar to conventional laparotomy, in minimally invasive surgery the surgeon should plan on performing a consistent, methodical exploration to ensure completeness of evaluation. A complete exploration may not always be necessary if comprehensive diagnostic imaging was performed preoperatively. Full laparoscopic exploration to evaluate all intra-abdominal organs has been shown to add on average 36 minutes when performed by an experienced surgeon, compared to just 12 minutes for exploration via conventional open laparotomy.

Port placement can be modified based on the organs of interest but typically consist of 1–3 ports that are placed on the ventral midline. The use of a rotating tray or tilting the operating table can help to facilitate patient rotation into a partial right or left lateral recumbency when necessary. When attempting to view the kidneys, adrenal glands, and portions of the gastrointestinal tract, patients may need to be repositioned intraoperatively for optimization of visibility. It can be useful to do an initial tilting of the patient to the right to avoid interference of the spleen when evaluating the left-sided structures.

When utilizing a multiport setup, full intestinal visualization and palpation requires intracorporeal manipulation. This can be tedious and risk serositis if not performed appropriately. Because of this, if a full intestinal exploration is expected, the use of a wound retractor and single-port platform is recommended. This allows for extracorporeal digital palpation of the entire length of the intestines.

PROCEDURE

- After port placement and pneumoperitoneum have been achieved, the 5 mm telescope is inserted in T1 and a first exploration of the abdomen is performed.
- Organs that are often visible on entry without any manipulation include the spleen, falciform fat, liver, gallbladder, stomach, omentum, jejunum, urinary bladder, and tumors (**Figs. 4–6**).
- Under endoscopic vision, the other two cannulas for the operative instruments are inserted in T2 and T3.
- To facilitate visualization of the left or right kidney, adrenal gland, and ovary, patients should be positioned in the opposite oblique lateral recumbency, up to 45° or greater (**Fig. 7**).
- A blunt probe, laparoscopic fan retractor, and laparoscopic grasping forceps can be used to manipulate abdominal organs such as the spleen and intestines and aid visibility.
- A blunt probe is useful for manipulation of the liver lobes (**Fig. 8**) and examination of the lateral extent and parietal and visceral surfaces.
- Using a blunt probe and grasping forceps, the gallbladder and biliary tree can be manipulated to view the cystic and common bile ducts (**Fig. 9**).
- The stomach can be fully examined, from fundus to pylorus, through the aid of a blunt probe and grasping forceps. To visualize the entirety of the gastroesophageal junction, it may be necessary to position the patient in oblique right lateral recumbency and dissect the hepatic triangular ligaments; however, this is rarely needed (e.g., if there is suspected pathology in this region).

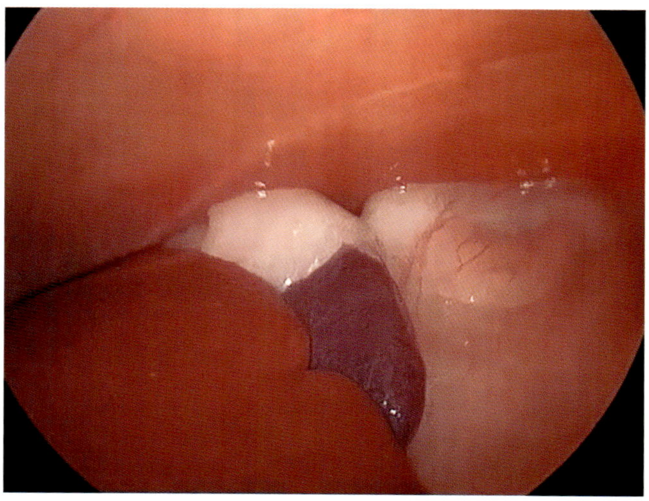

FIGURE 4. Endoscopic view of the left hepatic lobe, spleen, parietal peritoneum, and abdominal fat. Image courtesy of Dr. Roberto Properzi.

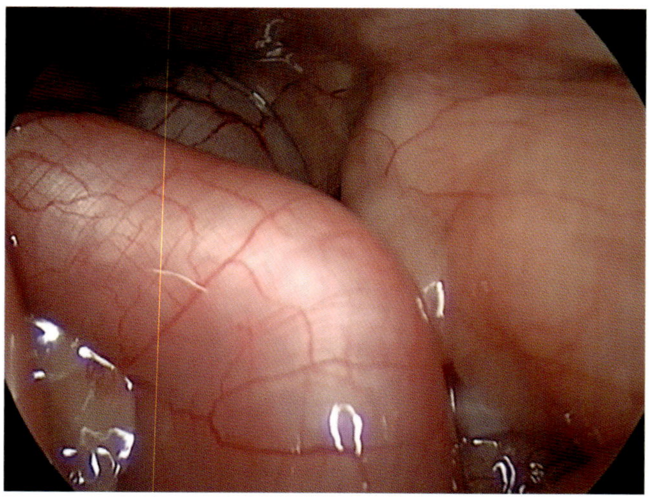

FIGURE 5. Endoscopic view of the urinary bladder and intestinal loops. Image courtesy of Dr. Roberto Properzi.

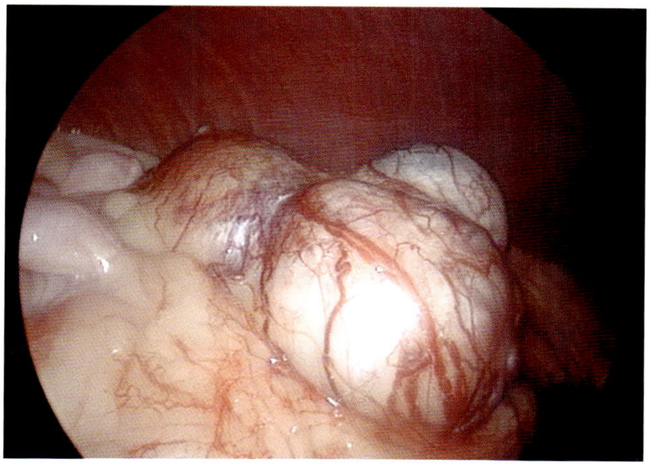

FIGURE 6. Endoscopic view of an abdominal tumor. Image courtesy of Dr. Andrea Pievaroli.

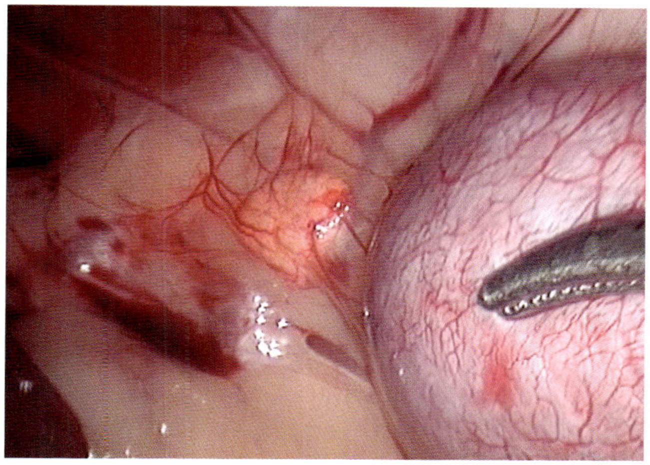

FIGURE 7. Endoscopic view of the left adrenal gland and kidney. Image courtesy of Dr. Andrea Pievaroli.

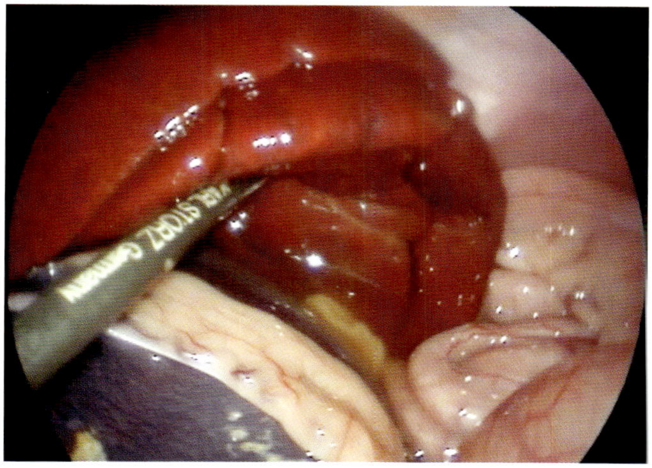

FIGURE 8. Laparoscopic examination of the liver. A blunt probe is used for delicate manipulation of the lobes. Image courtesy of Dr. Roberto Properzi.

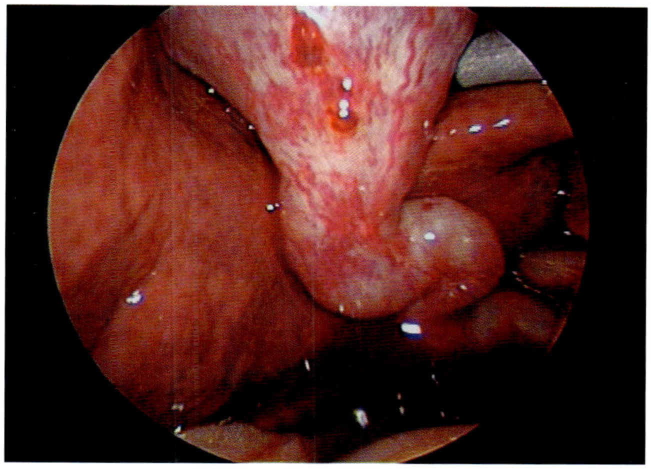

FIGURE 9. Enlarged and tortuous cystic duct. Image courtesy of Dr. Andrea Pievaroli.

- For intracorporeal examination of the intestines, the omentum must be first manipulated cranially. Then, using two Babcock grasping forceps, a section of the intestinal tract can be grasped and traced in a specific direction (**Fig. 10**). This requires careful attention to the tension exerted when grasping and pulling the intestines, often requiring multiple repositioning of the local intestines and manipulation with a blunt probe.
- After tilting the patient to a 45° oblique right lateral recumbency, the spleen can be retracted to allow better visualization of the left-sided structures. This includes evaluating a portion of the left limb of the pancreas, more of the gastric fundus, descending and transverse colon, kidney, adrenal gland, and ovary/uterine horn.

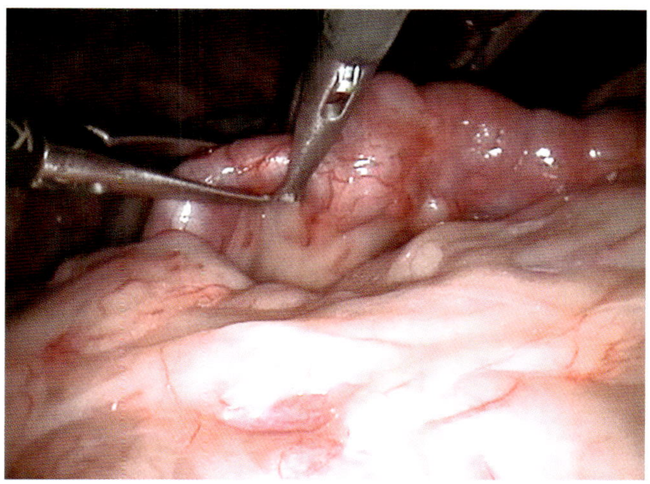

FIGURE 10. Examination of the intestines using two Babcock grasping forceps. Image courtesy of Dr. Andrea Pievaroli.

- Following a body tilting of 45° oblique to the left, the duodenum can be visualized and lifted to examine the body and right limb of the pancreas (**Fig. 11**). The right adrenal, kidney, ovary/uterine horn can then be examined.
- For extracorporeal examination of the intestines, a ≈2 cm incision, similar to the size of an extra small wound retractor and SILS Port, is made in the region of the subumbilical port site. A loop of jejunum is grasped from within the abdominal cavity and externalized. The jejunum can then be traced extracorporeally to the ileocolic junction and caudal duodenal flexure. Care must be taken to ensure that there is not excessive constriction of the intestines or vasculature while exteriorizing the intestines through the small incision; portions of the intestines may need to be replaced into the abdomen intermittently.

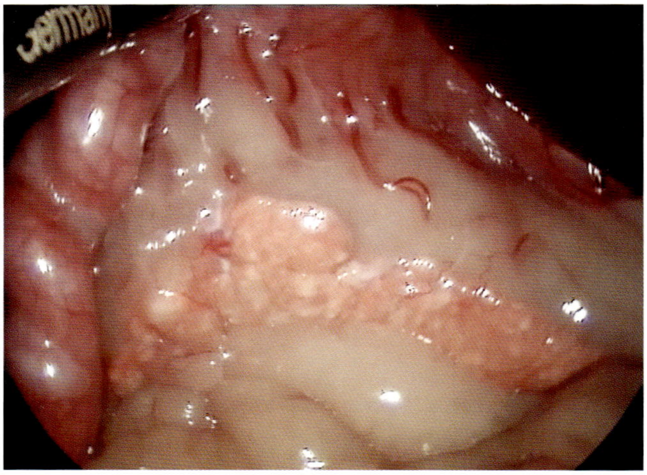

FIGURE 11. The duodenum is lifted to examine the pancreas. Image courtesy of Dr. Andrea Pievaroli.

B LIVER AND GALLBLADDER EVALUATION AND BIOPSY

Laparoscopic liver biopsy is one of the most commonly performed minimally invasive procedures. It allows for a large sampling of the liver with a targeted approach, collecting samples from any liver lobe and any visible pathologic changes of the liver. Indications for laparoscopic liver biopsy are numerous but typically include changes in serum enzymology. Increased serum ALT activity is one of the earliest indicators of chronic hepatitis. Biopsies can be used for making a diagnosis, aiding in prognosis, and monitoring for treatment response. An important factor in the utility of liver biopsies includes the number of portal triads obtained for analysis. At least 12–15 portal triads are recommended for full evaluation of liver biopsy specimens. This often requires obtaining between two and four samples with common laparoscopic cup biopsy forceps. Additionally, given the differences that can be observed within different liver lobes, it is recommended to perform biopsies in several locations and associated lobes. Risks associated with any hepatic sampling technique are primary hemorrhages. Despite common derangements of coagulation associated with the underlying liver disease, the overall incidence of bleeding is low, around 1.2%–3.3%

PROCEDURE

- The patient is positioned in dorsal recumbency, and the abdomen is aseptically prepared, taking into account the potential for conversion to open laparotomy if needed.
- After port placement and pneumoperitoneum have been achieved, the 5 mm telescope is inserted in T1 and a first exploration of the abdomen is performed.
- Under endoscopic vision, at least one other cannula is placed for instrumentation.
- The liver and gallbladder should be assessed with the blunt probe, evaluating both the diaphragmatic and visceral surfaces.
- Sampling is most commonly performed from the distal edges of various liver lobes, using cup or punch biopsy forceps. The forceps can be passed underneath the edge of the liver to be sampled, opened, and slowly elevated towards the liver edge until the margin has fallen into the biopsy forceps jaws. After the liver margin has been grasped, hemostasis can be aided through prolonged closure of the biopsy jaws or through twisting of the forceps. The sample is then pulled from the liver parenchyma (**Figs. 12 and 13**).
- A blunt probe can be placed at the biopsy site for direct compression to aid in hemostasis (**Fig. 14**). Additionally, using the forceps, gelatin sponge or other hemostatic agents can be used at the biopsy site to help in hemostasis.
- If the liver disease is not diffuse or if there are focal lesions that are not at the margins of the liver, the biopsy forceps can be directed towards the desired area and sampling can be performed from a central lesion. In large or cystic lesions, the risk of significant hemorrhage after biopsy may be higher.
- Alternatives to biopsy forceps include the use of a vessel-sealing device for a distal tip wedge resection, pretied or extracorporeally tied loop ligatures, or a stapled partial resection of the distal liver lobe.

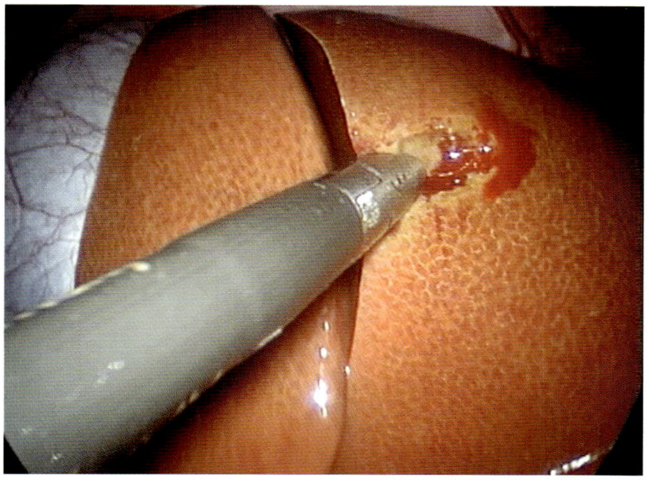

FIGURE 12. Liver biopsy with a cup biopsy forceps. Image courtesy of Dr. Andrea Pievaroli.

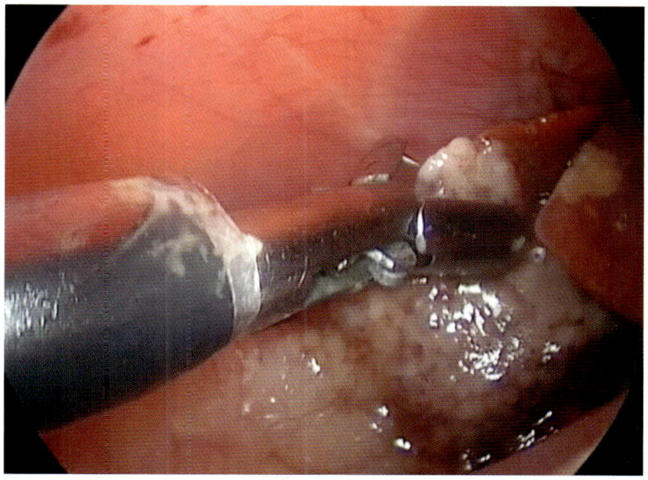

FIGURE 13. It is important to biopsy both normal and pathological liver tissue. Image courtesy of Dr. Roberto Properzi.

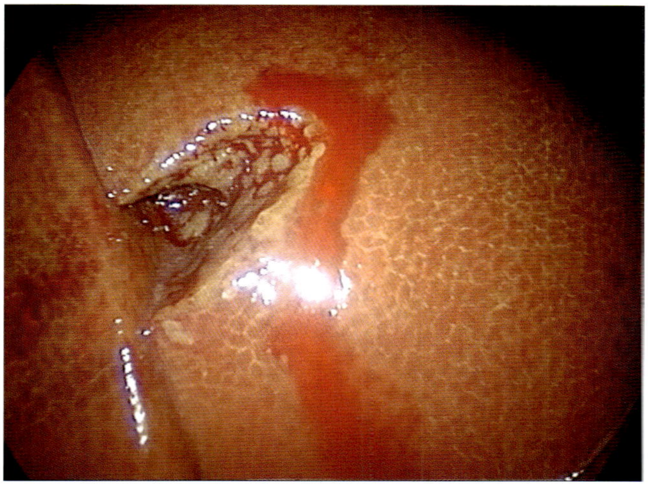

FIGURE 14. Hemostasis check after liver biopsy. If bleeding occurs, a blunt probe can be placed at the biopsy site for direct compression. Image courtesy of Dr. Andrea Pievaroli.

- For a laparoscopic cholecystocentesis, a long (2–4 inches) 20–22-gauge spinal needle is passed percutaneously, caudal to the diaphragm. The needle should be advanced at an angle that will enter the gallbladder through a section of liver (preferred) or directly into the gallbladder itself. A blunt probe or grasping forceps can be used to stabilize the gallbladder during puncture. Following puncture into the gallbladder, a bile sample is collected with a 12 cc syringe. It is generally recommended to maximally decompress the gallbladder during aspiration to minimize bile leakage due to decreased intracholecystic pressure.

C KIDNEY AND ADRENAL GLAND EVALUATION AND BIOPSY

Laparoscopic kidney biopsy is performed under general anesthesia and allows direct visualization of the kidney and selective sampling. When compared to percutaneous ultrasound-guided kidney biopsy samples, laparoscopic biopsy specimens were found to have double the number of glomeruli despite using the same core needle size (32 vs. 16, respectively).

Biopsy can be performed with either a 14- or 16-gauge core needle biopsy (**Fig. 15**) or a 5 mm cup biopsy forceps. Hemostasis is applied through direct compression with a blunt probe (**Fig. 16**). Histological scoring can be performed with either technique; however, the number of glomeruli obtained is significantly higher with cup biopsy forceps than with core needle biopsy (60 vs. 26, respectively). When using a core needle biopsy technique, both 14- and 16-gauge needle sizes were found to yield samples with a similar number of glomeruli, whereas the specimens obtained with 18-gauge needles were found to have significantly fewer glomeruli and greater crush artifact.

Adrenal gland biopsy is rarely performed before attempting to remove the diseased gland. Accuracy in differentiating cortical from medullary adrenal tumors with cytology alone ranges from 90% to 100%. Even fine needle aspirates of the adrenal gland are associated with bleeding, catecholamine release, ventricular tachycardia, and even fatalities. However, partial adrenalectomy has been previously reported, and laparoscopic adrenal biopsy can be performed with endoclips or a vessel-sealing device.

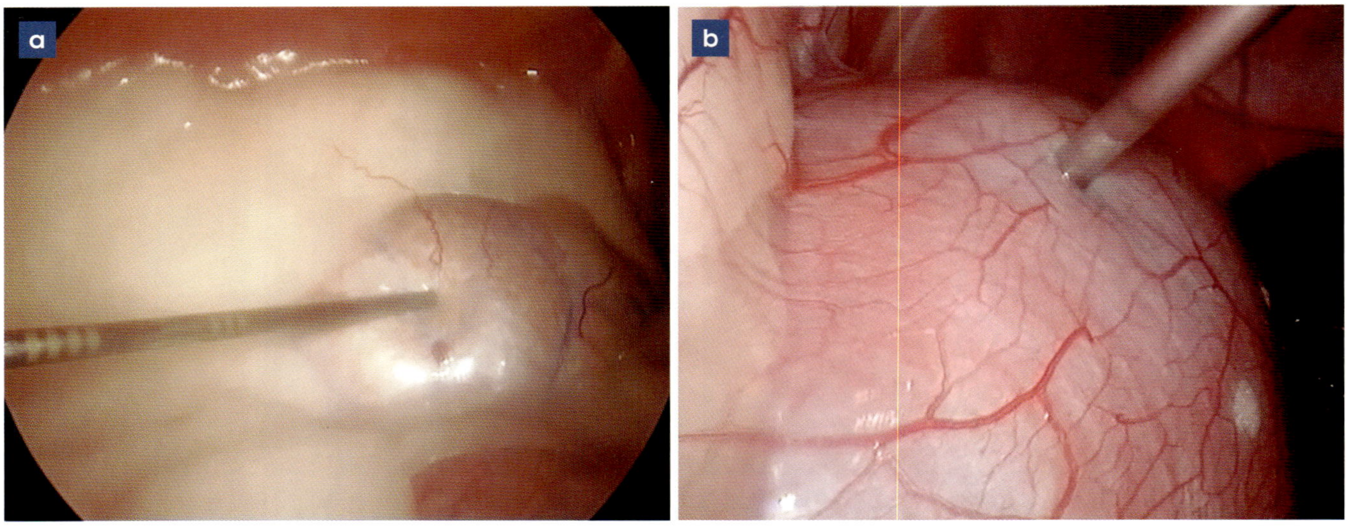

FIGURE 15. Examples of kidney biopsy using a Tru-Cut device. Image a courtesy of Dr. Roberto Properzi. Image b courtesy of Dr. Andrea Pievaroli.

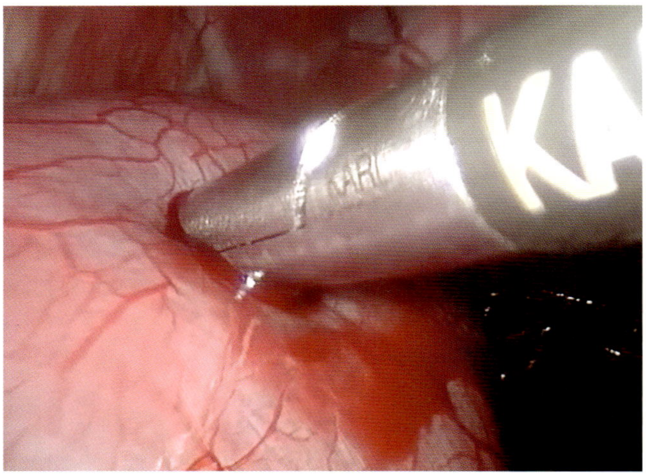

FIGURE 16. After kidney biopsy, hemostasis is controlled through direct compression with a blunt probe. Image courtesy of Dr. Andrea Pievaroli.

PROCEDURE

- The patient is positioned in dorsal recumbency, and the abdomen is aseptically prepared, taking into account the potential for conversion to open laparotomy if needed.
- After port placement and pneumoperitoneum have been achieved, the 5 mm telescope is inserted in T1 and a first exploration of the abdomen is performed.
- Under endoscopic vision, the other two cannulas for the operative instruments are inserted in T2 and T3.
- The patients is rotated into oblique lateral recumbency (30°–45°) to expose the kidney of interest.
- The kidney can be manipulated with a blunt probe or Babcock forceps.
- If cup biopsy forceps are used, either the cranial or caudal pole of the kidney is chosen and the blunt probe or forceps are used to stabilize the opposite pole. The cup biopsy forceps (5 mm) are inserted and used to sample the renal parenchyma. Following biopsy, direct compression is performed at the biopsy site for roughly 5 minutes. Additionally, gelatin sponge can be preloaded into the laparoscopic forceps and placed over the biopsy site to aid in hemostasis.
- If core needle biopsy is performed, a 14- or 16-gauge needle is inserted percutaneously through the body wall near the proposed site of the biopsy. The needle should be positioned tangentially to the surface of the kidney (i.e., parallel to the long axis of the kidney) before firing the automated spring mechanism. Following biopsy, compression should be held for roughly 5 minutes. Hemostasis can be confirmed following compression; if additional support is needed, gelatin sponge may be placed over the biopsy site.
- For adrenal biopsy, endoclips (10–12 mm) are placed at the site of the proposed biopsy and samples are harvested by transecting tissue distal to the clips with endoscopic Metzenbaum scissors. Similarly, a vessel-sealing device (e.g., harmonic scalpel) can be used to partition and transect the adrenal gland.

D PANCREAS EVALUATION AND BIOPSY

Both laparoscopic and laparoscopic-assisted techniques can be used for biopsy of the pancreas (**Fig. 17**). Experimentally, it has been shown that laparoscopy has less of an effect on bowel transit time and stress biomarkers when compared with an open distal pancreatectomy in dogs. Pancreatic sampling can be performed for histopathology and culture if necessary. The right limb of the pancreas is often easily accessible without excessive manipulation of other abdominal organs, whereas the left limb of the pancreas often requires dissection through the omentum. Various techniques have been used for sampling the pancreas, including a vessel-sealing device, pretied loop ligatures, and endoscopic clips. The use of a vessel-sealing device has been shown to be safe, potentially faster, and less likely to be associated with postoperative pancreatitis than conventional suture fracture techniques for pancreatic surgery.

PROCEDURE

- The patient is positioned in dorsal recumbency, and the abdomen is aseptically prepared, taking into account the potential for conversion to open laparotomy if needed. If the right limb of the pancreas is to be evaluated, partial oblique left lateral recumbency can aid in easy identification of the pancreas and duodenum.
- After port placement and pneumoperitoneum have been achieved, the 5 mm telescope is inserted in T1 and a first exploration of the abdomen is performed.
- Under endoscopic vision, at least one other cannula is placed for instrumentation.
- The pancreas can be assessed with the blunt probe and the duodenum manipulated with Babcock forceps.
- Sampling can be performed from the margin of the pancreas via cup or punch biopsy forceps. The forceps can be passed underneath the edge of the pancreas, opened, and slowly elevated towards the pancreas edge until the margin has fallen into the biopsy forceps jaws.
- After the biopsy has been performed, direct compression with a blunt probe aids in hemostasis. Additionally, gelatin sponge or other hemostatic agents can be passed to the biopsy site using the forceps to help in hemostasis.

E SPLEEN EVALUATION AND BIOPSY

Splenic biopsy is rarely performed but has been described via laparoscopy and percutaneously guided by ultrasound. Biopsy can be performed at the splenic margin for suspected diffuse splenic disease, or targeted biopsy can be used if lesions have been identified on diagnostic imaging or intraoperative evaluation (**Fig. 18**). The main risk associated with biopsy is hemorrhage.

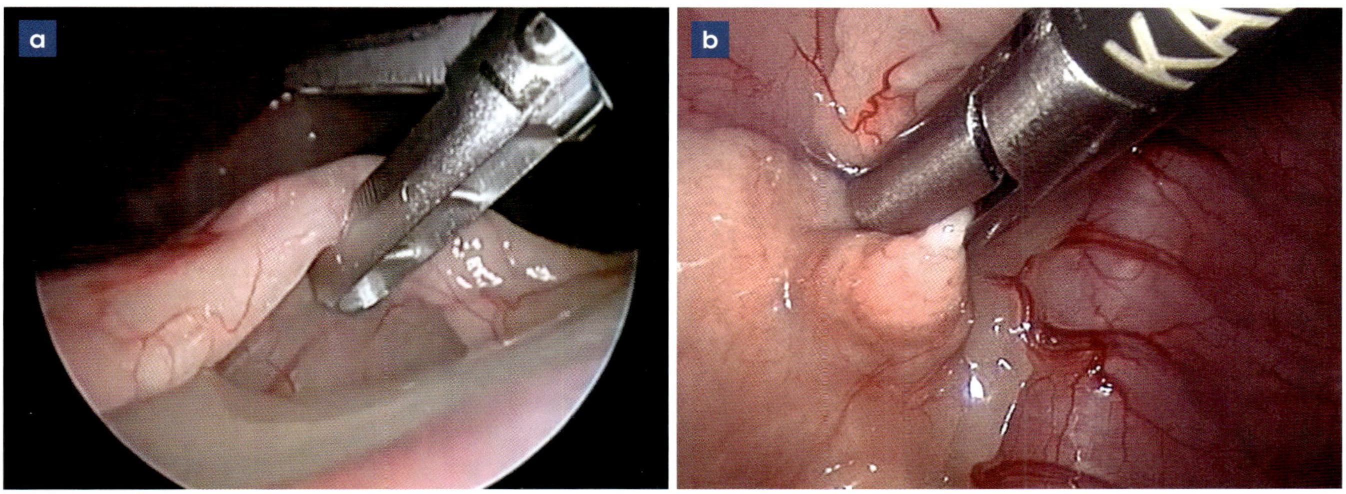

FIGURE 17. Pancreatic biopsy using a dedicated biopsy cup forceps with a central fenestration. Image a courtesy of Dr. Roberto Properzi. Image b courtesy of Dr. Andrea Pievaroli.

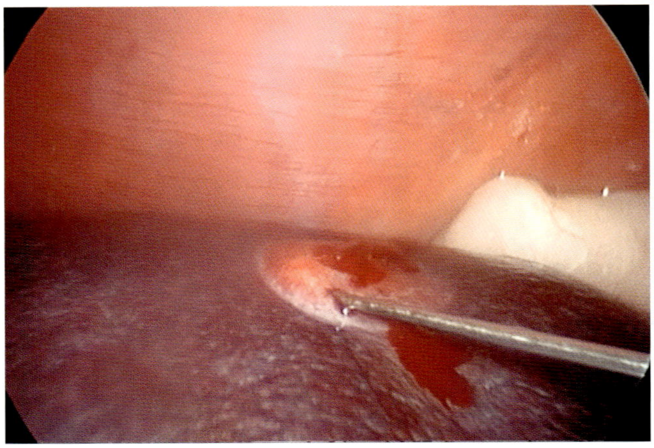

FIGURE 18. Needle aspiration of splenic lesions is performed with more precision via laparoscopy. Image courtesy of Dr. Andrea Pievaroli.

PROCEDURE

- The patient is positioned in dorsal recumbency, and the abdomen is aseptically prepared, taking into account the potential for conversion to open laparotomy if needed.
- After port placement and pneumoperitoneum have been achieved, the 5 mm telescope is inserted in T1 and a first exploration of the abdomen is performed.
- Under endoscopic vision, at least one other cannula is placed for instrumentation.
- The spleen should be assessed with the blunt probe, evaluating both the dorsal and ventral aspects.
- Sampling can be performed from the margin of the spleen via cup or punch biopsy forceps. The forceps can be passed underneath the edge of the spleen, opened, and slowly elevated towards the spleen edge until the margin has fallen into the biopsy forceps jaws (**Fig. 19**).
- After the biopsy has been performed, hemostasis can be aided through direct compression with a blunt probe. Additionally, gelatin sponge or other hemostatic agents can be passed to the biopsy site using the forceps to help in hemostasis.
- If the splenic disease is not diffuse or if there are focal lesions, the biopsy forceps can be directed towards the desired area and sampling can be performed from a central lesion. In large or cystic lesions, the risk of significant hemorrhage after biopsy may be higher.
- Alternatives to biopsy forceps include the use of pretied or extracorporeally tied loop ligatures or a stapled partial resection of the spleen.

F LYMPH NODE EVALUATION AND BIOPSY

Detection of an enlarged lymph node during laparoscopy or by imaging is an indication for biopsy, along with nondiagnostic cytology aspirates and during staging of canine oncologic patients (**Fig. 20**). 3 mm or 5 mm oval cup biopsy forceps are used, and patient positioning depends on other laparoscopic procedures performed concurrently or on which lymph node is sampled.

Laparoscopic extirpation of sublumbar lymph nodes, including the medial iliac, internal iliac (hypogastric), and sacral lymph nodes, can be performed. This technique provides a large

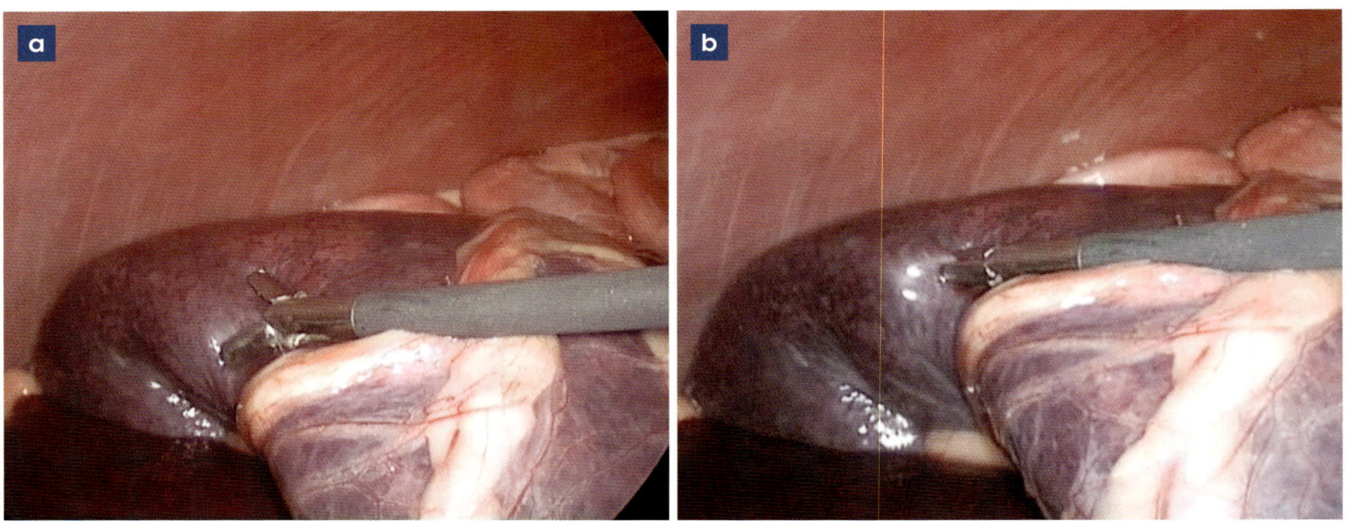

FIGURE 19. Spleen biopsy with dedicated forceps a) before and b) after grasping the tissue. Image courtesy of Dr. Roberto Properzi.

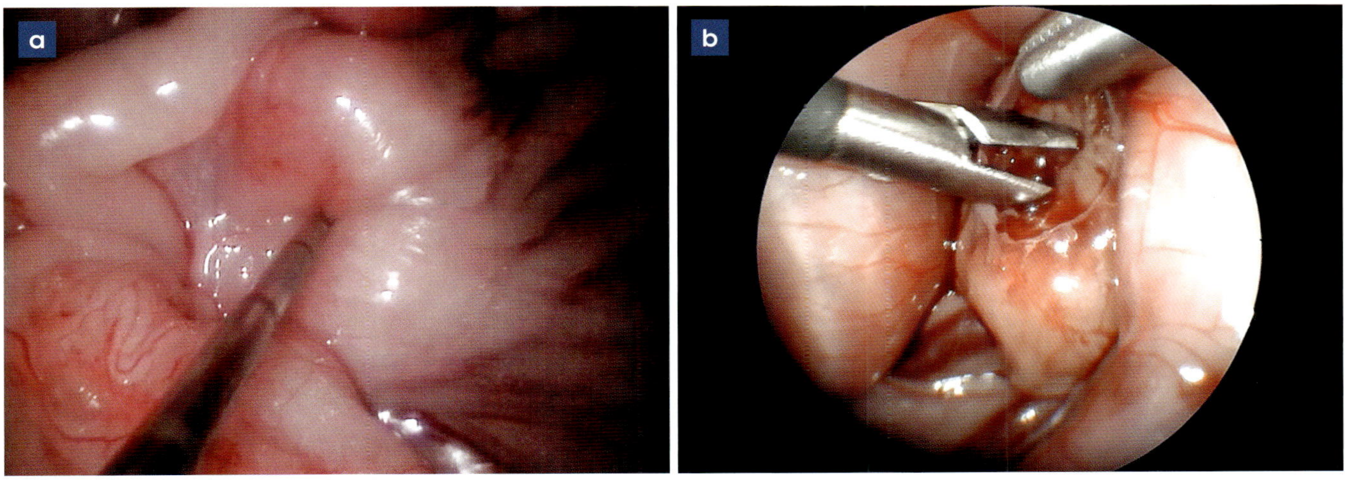

FIGURE 20. Examples of mesenteric lymph node biopsy using a Tru-Cut device. Image a courtesy of Dr. Roberto Properzi. Image b courtesy of Dr. Andrea Pievaroli.

advantage over conventional surgery due to the morbidity that is observed for lymph node dissection from a celiotomy approach. This is particularly true for patients diagnosed with metastatic neoplasia, such as anal sac adenocarcinoma. Data is being accrued regarding the safety and efficacy for sublumbar lymph node extirpation.

PROCEDURE

- A lateral three-port caudal abdominal approach can be used for the ipsilateral lymph nodes.
- The medial iliac lymph nodes are identified by incising the retroperitoneum caudal to the deep circumflex iliac artery and vein and dorsal to the external artery or vein using a vessel-sealing device.

G GASTROINTESTINAL TRACT EVALUATION AND BIOPSY

Laparoscopic-assisted techniques are commonly used for extracorporeal biopsy of the gastrointestinal tract in dogs and cats. Following laparoscopic exploration and any intracorporeal procedure (e.g., hepatic or pancreatic biopsy), the single-port device (e.g., SILS) is removed and a wound retraction device is inserted. The gastrointestinal tract is exteriorized and extracorporeal biopsy is performed (**Fig. 21**). Depending on the location of the wound retractor, the majority of the duodenum (mid and distal portions), jejunum, and proximal colon can be exteriorized.

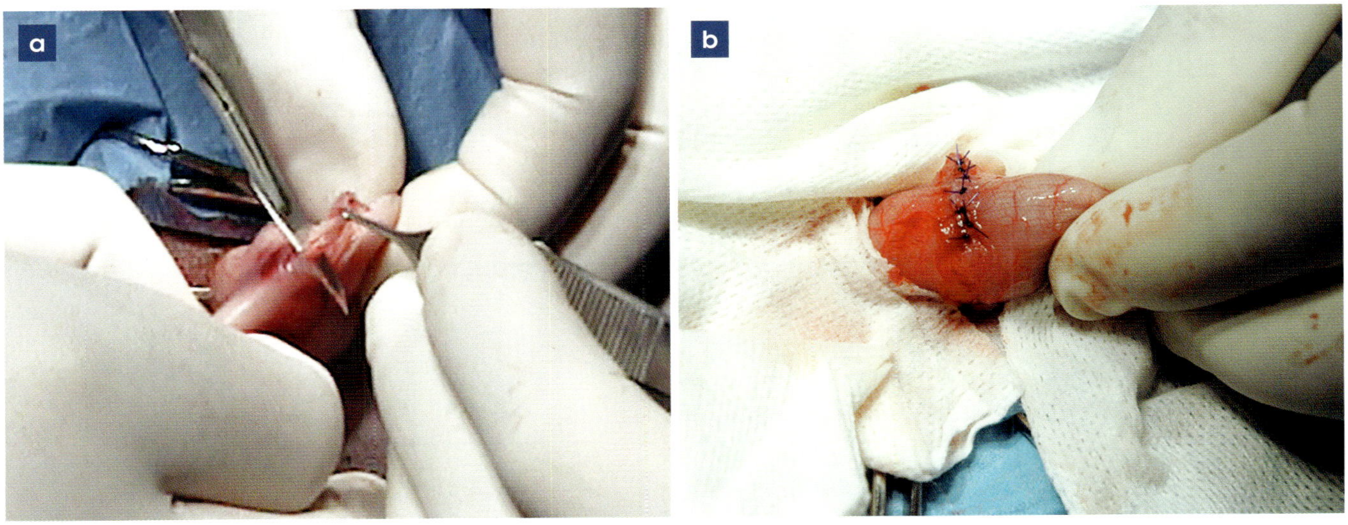

FIGURE 21. Laparoscopic-assisted intestinal incisional biopsy. Images courtesy of Dr. Andrea Pievaroli.

PROCEDURE

- The patient is positioned in dorsal recumbency, and the abdomen is aseptically prepared, taking into account the potential for conversion to open laparotomy if needed.
- Following laparoscopic exploration and any intracorporeal procedures, the single-port device is removed and a wound retraction device is inserted.
- Available bowel is digitally grasped and exteriorized through the wound retraction device. Desired areas of intestine are biopsied extracorporeally.
- Once biopsy has been performed, the bowel is returned to the abdomen and covered with omentum. The minilaparotomy incision is closed routinely.

POSTOPERATIVE MANAGEMENT

Abdominal exploration and multiorgan biopsy is generally well tolerated. Patient requirements are more often dictated by the underlying disease than by postprocedural care. Pain control can be aided by port-site local analgesia, appropriate pre- and perioperative analgesia, and postoperative pain management via oral or injectable pain medications for 3–7 days. If performed on elective basis, most patients are discharged from hospital on the same day of the procedure. Additional supportive care for patients with liver, kidney, pancreatic, or gastrointestinal disease is often associated with their preprocedural status. Owners should be cautioned to monitor the port-site incisions, and activity restriction is often warranted for 10–14 days following surgery.

Complications of exploratory and diagnostic laparotomy

- Conversion to open laparotomy
- Hemorrhage necessitating red blood cell transfusion
- Port-site complications (splenic puncture, incision site infection, seroma)
- Nondiagnostic sampling
- Anesthetic complications

Key points

- Laparoscopic and laparoscopic-assisted procedures are well established in veterinary surgery, with novel minimally invasive approaches and procedures described regularly in the peer-reviewed literature.
- Advances in preoperative workup (e.g., abdominal CT and/or MRI) have facilitated more appropriate patient selection for minimally invasive surgical procedures, allowing more focused dissections and less surgical trauma.
- As the field advances, advantages related to magnification, visualization, and accessibility are expected to establish laparoscopic and laparoscopic-assisted procedures as superior to traditional open surgery for certain procedures.
- Developing advances, such as single-incision laparoscopic surgery (SILS) and/or natural orifice transluminal endoscopic surgery (NOTES), are actively pursued in veterinary patients.

SUGGESTED READINGS

CLINICAL CASES

14.1 CISTERNA CHYLI ABLATION

David García Rubio

CASE DESCRIPTION

Cat aged 14 years affected by severe pleural effusion. After analyzing the drained fluid, it was concluded that this was a case of chylothorax, and a CT scan and echocardiogram were performed. Since the tests came back normal, cardiac conditions, neoplasia, and lung lobe torsion were ruled out, and the disease was classed as idiopathic. Therefore, a combined approach to treatment was proposed, through thoracic duct ligation in addition to cisterna chyli ablation.

Key points

- Performing a CT scan after contrast dye injection in the lymph nodes (0.6 mL/kg of nonionic contrast dye) helps to identify the anatomy and locate the cisterna chyli, which may vary between patients. The use of the pads, rectal submucosa, popliteal lymph nodes, and mesentery as injection pathways has been described.
- The injection of methylene blue into the lymph nodes at a dose of 0.5 mg/kg from a 1% solution is recommended to facilitate visualization of the cisterna chyli.

PORT PLACEMENT

The patient is placed in sternal recumbency for a left paracostal approach. In this case, as the abdomen had been previously opened to perform a lymphangiogram with methylene blue in the cecocolic junction lymph node, the same incision was used for single-incision laparoscopic surgery with three 5 mm ports (T1, T2, and T3). A pneumoperitoneum with CO_2 at 6 mmHg was used throughout the procedure.

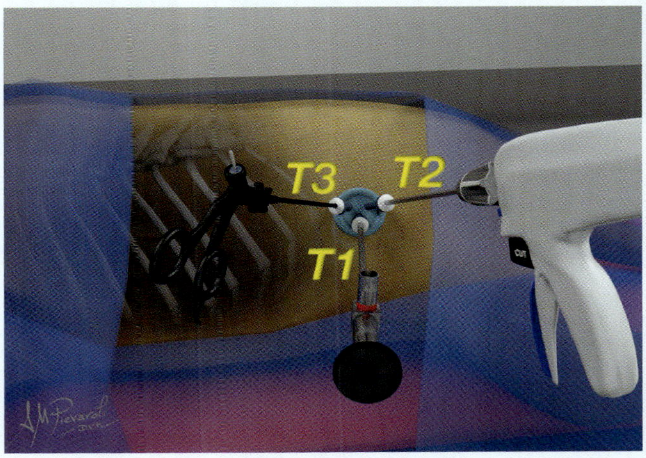

PROCEDURE

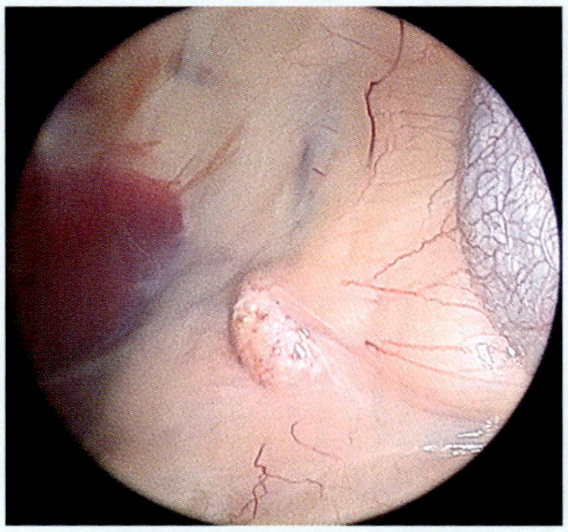

FIGURE 1. Endoscopic view of the anatomical region where dissection is to be performed, between the cranial pole of the left kidney and the caudal pole of the left adrenal gland.

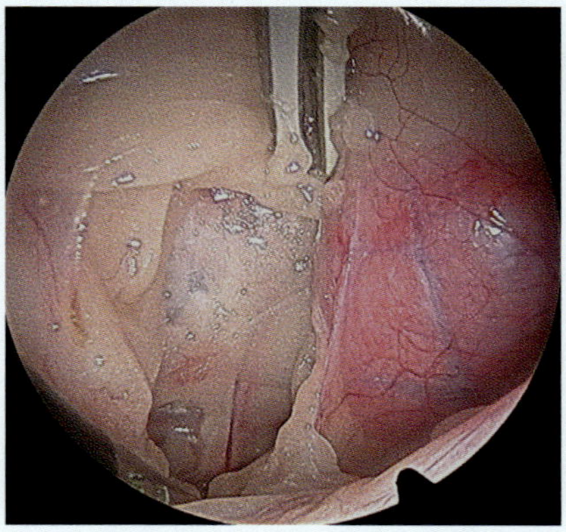

FIGURE 2. Deep tissue dissection of paracostal muscles.

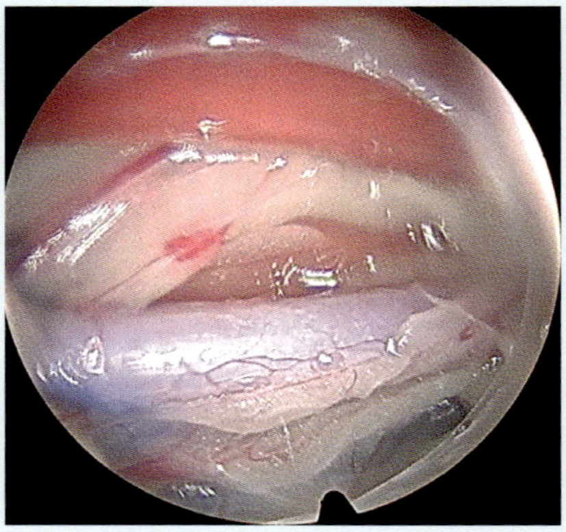

FIGURE 3. The heartbeat is then used to locate the abdominal aorta. Dissection around it is carefully performed.

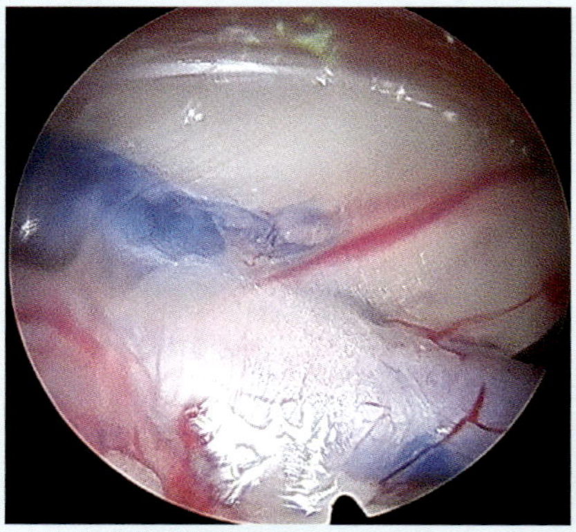

FIGURE 4. The cisterna chyli is usually located dorsally to the aorta (although this varies between patients) and consists of a dilation of the lymphatic system. In the image, the cisterna chyli has been dyed with methylene blue.

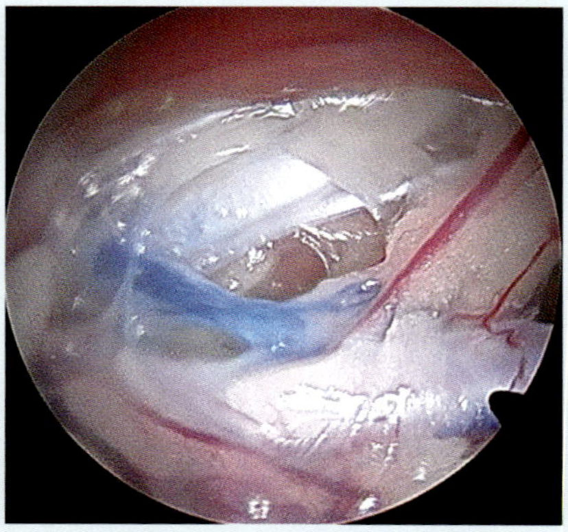

FIGURE 5. Detailed view of the cisterna chyli following its full dissection.

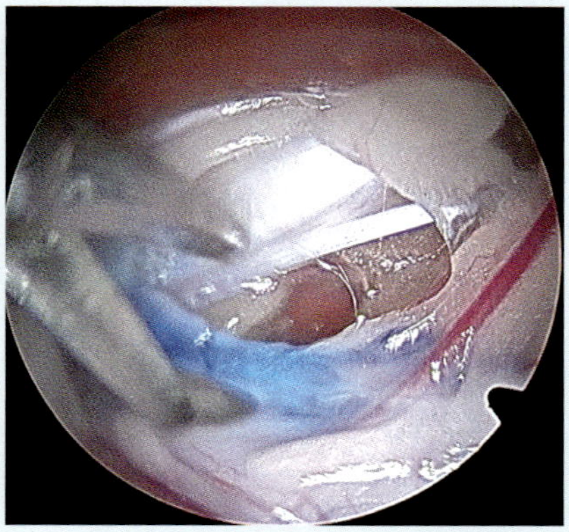

FIGURE 6. The cisterna chyli should then be torn or cut.

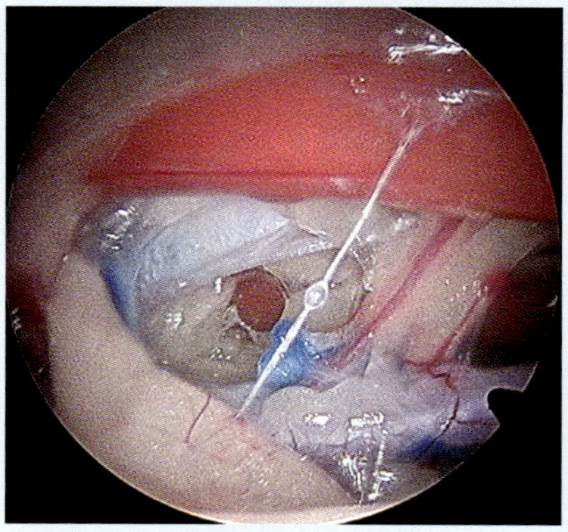

FIGURE 7. Final appearance after completing ablation.

Tips and tricks

- ✓ It may be difficult to locate the abdominal aorta as it travels through the body. It is helpful to use the heartbeat as a guide.
- ✓ If the lymphangiogram is carried out via the mesenteric lymph nodes, the same incision may be used, whether via Alexis retractors (Applied Medical, Rancho Santa Margarita, CA) or single-port SILS systems (Medtronic, Minneapolis, MN). Otherwise, it is generally more convenient to use three individual 5 mm trocars.

14.2 LAPAROSCOPIC INTRAPERITONEAL FOREIGN BODY RETRIEVAL (TWO-PORT TECHNIQUE)

Erin A. Gibson, William T. N. Culp

CASE DESCRIPTION

A 10-month-old spayed female Labrador Retriever presented with a 3-day history of forelimb pain and lameness. She was known to have ingested a grill brush containing metallic bristles approximately 1 week prior to presentation. After diagnostic evaluation, metallic bristles were noted in the axillary region (explaining the lameness) and in the peritoneal space, in the upper right quadrant. The bristle in her axillary region was removed, and laparoscopic retrieval of the intraperitoneal foreign body was elected.

Key points

- Image guidance (e.g., radiographs and ultrasound) is useful to localize foreign bodies prior to surgery, particularly when they are radiopaque. This will also allow the surgeon to evaluate the suitability of attempting minimally invasive retrieval or open retrieval of retained foreign bodies.
- Easy retrieval was achieved in this case due to the foreign body being located ventrally in the peritoneal cavity as well as being of a size amenable to removal through the established ports.

PORT PLACEMENT

A 1 cm ventral midline incision was made approximately 3 cm caudal to the umbilicus. A modified Hasson technique was used to initiate a subumbilical camera port (T1), and the tip of a 6 mm Endotip trocarless cannula (Ternamian Endotip Cannula, Karl Storz, El Segundo, CA) was introduced into the peritoneal cavity. A 5 mm 30° telescope (Hopkins Forward-Oblique Telescope, Karl Storz, Tuttlingen, Germany) was introduced and aimed to the site of the second port placement (cranial and right of the midline). A second port was established under direct visualization utilizing a second 6 mm Endotip cannula 2 cm caudal to the costal arch and 6 cm lateral (right) to the midline under direct visualization of the telescope (T3). Once peritoneal access was established, foreign body retrieval from the abdomen was performed through the second port with laparoscopic grasping forceps (Clickline Dissecting and Grasping forceps, Karl Storz, El Segundo, CA). The foreign body was pulled into the cannula and removed.

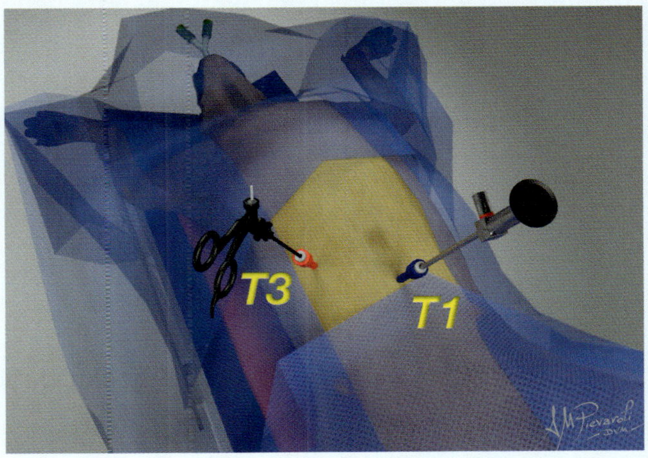

PROCEDURE

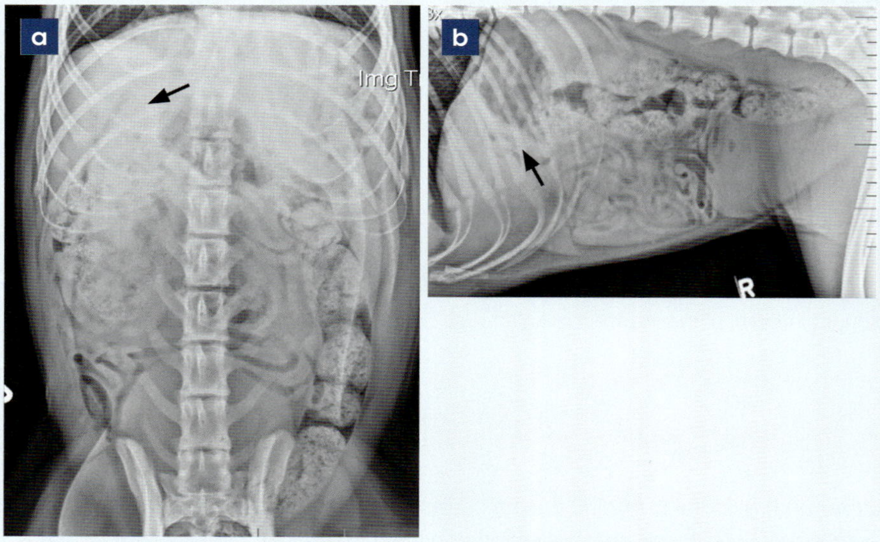

FIGURE 1. a) Ventrodorsal and b) lateral projection radiographs of a 10-month-old Labrador Retriever who had ingested a grill brush with metallic bristles. In both images, a metallic foreign body (arrow) can be identified in the upper right quadrant of the peritoneal cavity.

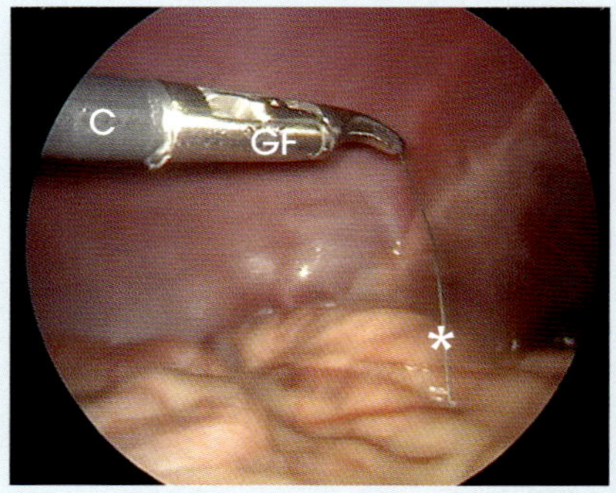

FIGURE 2. Laparoscopic image of metallic foreign body removal from the peritoneal cavity obtained from a 5 mm telescope in a cannula on the ventral midline. A 6 mm cannula (C) can be seen to the right of the midline in the cranial abdomen, through which a grasping forceps (GF) has been introduced to grasp the foreign body (*), which will be removed through the cannula.

Tips and tricks

- ✓ When possible, utilize a cannula that is large enough to allow for removal of a foreign body through the cannula itself. This will avoid having to remove the cannula during foreign body extraction, preventing the foreign body from contacting the wall and falling back into the peritoneal cavity.
- ✓ If possible, consider having fluoroscopy available in the operating room during removal of intraperitoneal foreign bodies that are radiopaque, as this can help with localization.

14.3 LAPAROSCOPIC EXPLORATION IN A CAT

Antoine Adam

CASE DESCRIPTION

A cat presented with the usual clinical signs of chronic digestive disease. Laparoscopic exploration of the abdomen was performed as part of the workup (clinical suspicion of inflammatory disease or tumoral process, ultrasound, blood tests). This minimally invasive procedure allows access and biopsy of the liver, pancreas, spleen, kidneys, major lymph nodes, stomach, duodenum, jejunum, and ileum, with a 1.5–2 cm opening and a very short hospitalization time.

Key points

- Place the cannulas in the correct location, usually just cranial to the umbilicus. This is key to accessing all abdominal structures.
- Always use a ring-shaped retraction device.
- For liver biopsy, advance the cannula and use it as a bayonet.
- Avoid performing a biopsy in the pancreatic duct region.

PORT PLACEMENT

A small towel was placed under the back of the patient to elevate the abdomen. A heating mat and a ground plate for electrosurgery, if needed, should also be placed. The pneumoperitoneum is created and the ports placed without lateral tilting of the patient; sometimes right tilting can be used.

The first cannula (T1) was placed on the midline, approximately 1 cm caudal to the umbilicus, and a 3 mm telescope was introduced. The second cannula (T2), for 3 or 5 mm instruments, was placed on the midline, approximately 2 cm cranial to the umbilicus. If needed, a third port (for 3 mm instruments) can be placed between T1 and T2.

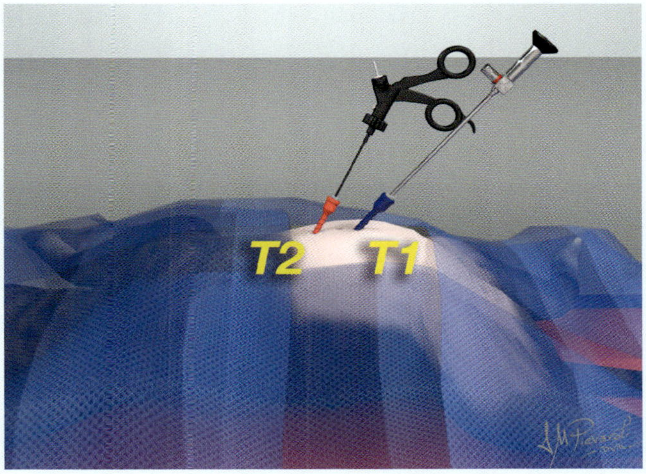

PROCEDURE

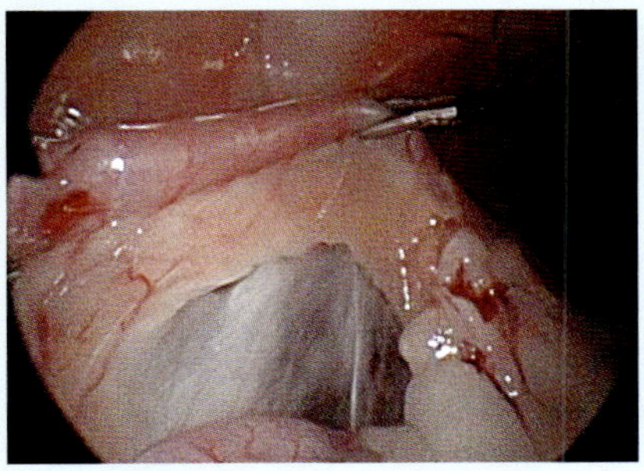

FIGURE 1. Pancreatic body. The biopsy instrument is used to gently manipulate the duodenum and visualize all the pancreas before biopsy.

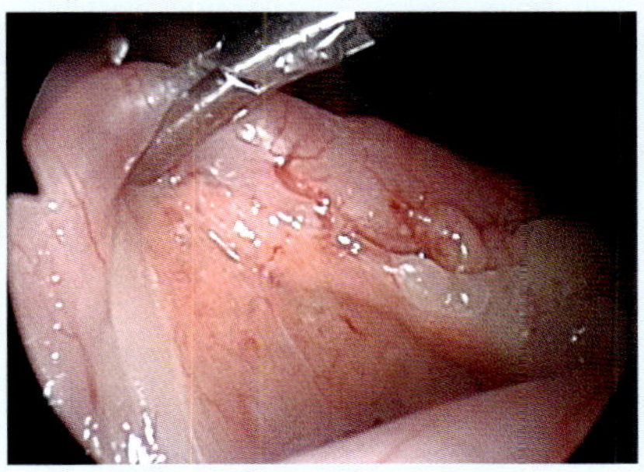

FIGURE 2. Closer view of the pancreas. If there is an adhesion or a mass, a third port can be placed and 3 mm atraumatic forceps can be used for manipulation. Biopsy samples are taken at the edge of the pancreas or inside the mass. The pancreatic duct region should be avoided.

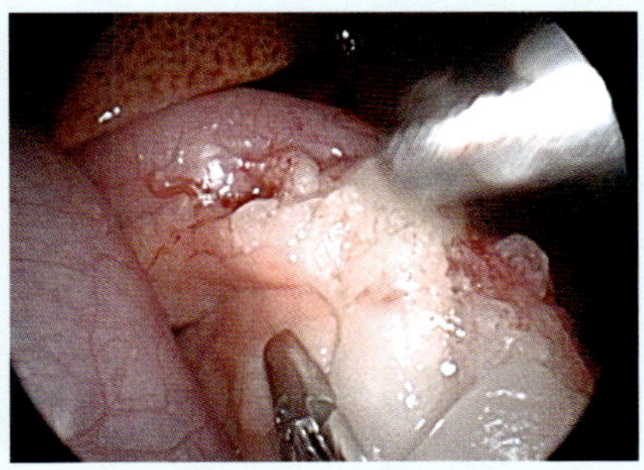

FIGURE 3. Pancreatic biopsy. If there is bleeding, the biopsy cup (closed) can be used to put direct compression over the biopsy site for a few minutes. This usually helps to stop bleeding.

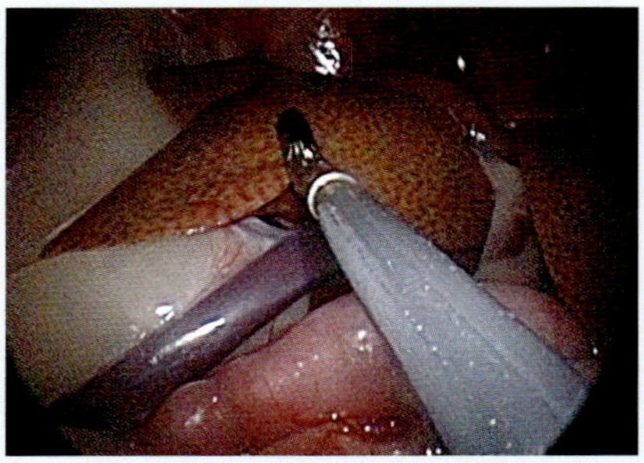

FIGURE 4. Liver biopsy. At least 4–5 samples should be collected; one specimen is used for culture. Samples can be taken from the middle of a lobe.

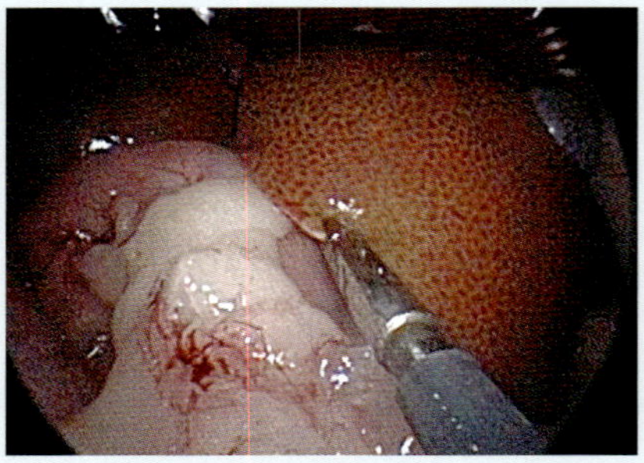

FIGURE 5. Liver biopsy. The instrument cannula is advanced near the liver (deep in the abdomen) and used as a bayonet to obtain the liver sample.

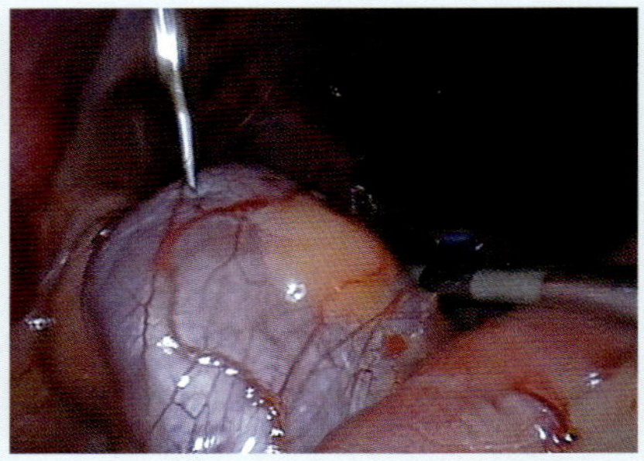

FIGURE 6. Kidney biopsy. Holding the kidney with a probe or an atraumatic instrument, a biopsy gun is used percutaneously in a tangential plane near the kidney pole. If there is bleeding, apply direct pressure with the palpation probe for a few minutes.

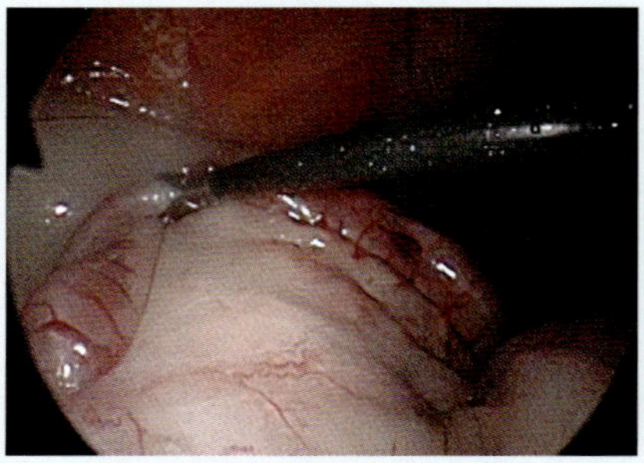

FIGURE 7. Part of the intestinal tract can be explored. The third port and two atraumatic instruments (3 mm) are necessary to manipulate the bowels. The mesenteric lymph nodes can be visualized if they are enlarged, and a biopsy can be performed.

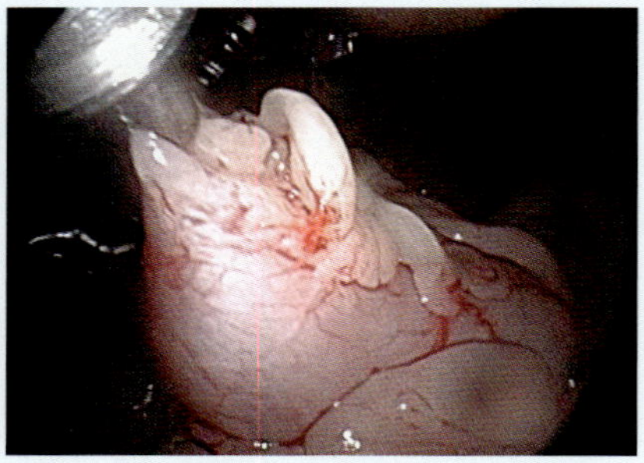

FIGURE 8. The stomach is being grabbed with atraumatic forceps. Stay sutures are placed to help with full-thickness biopsy. Samples from the intestinal tract are taken as in open surgery, with the ring distractor in place.

Tips and tricks

- ✓ Tilt the operating table to the right (halfway) to have a better visualization of the pancreas.
- ✓ Advance the instrument cannula near the liver (deep in the abdomen) to help obtain the liver biopsy specimen.
- ✓ If bleeding occurs, use the biopsy cup (closed) to apply compression at the biopsy site.
- ✓ Always have a 3 mm suction device available.

14.4 LAPAROSCOPIC TREATMENT OF HEMOABDOMEN

Michael Brückner

CASE DESCRIPTION

A 2-year-old Bearded Collie was referred for suspected hemoabdomen after prescrotal castration. On presentation, the dog was in stable condition and the hematocrit was within the reference range. Abdominal ultrasound revealed a moderate amount of free corpuscular fluid; therefore, the dog was prepared for laparoscopic surgery. Approximately 1 L of blood was removed from the abdominal cavity with a suction/irrigation tube to allow inspection of the inguinal rings. The laparoscopic approach allowed excellent visualization of the spermatic cord and testicular vessels, which were sealed using a vessel-sealing device.

Key points

- The origin of bleeding must be known.
- The patient should be in stable condition.
- Be ready for conversion to open surgery.

PORT PLACEMENT

Single-port access was made with two 6 mm Ternamian Endotip trocars in the umbilicus: a cranial telescope port (T1), and a caudal instrument port (T2). The patient was tilted to each side to allow inspection of both inguinal canals.

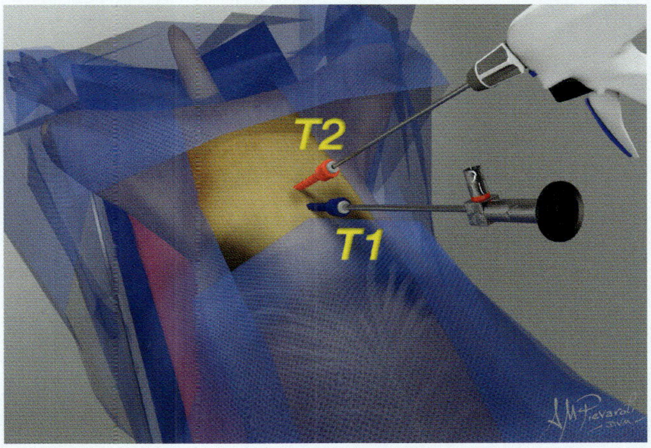

PROCEDURE

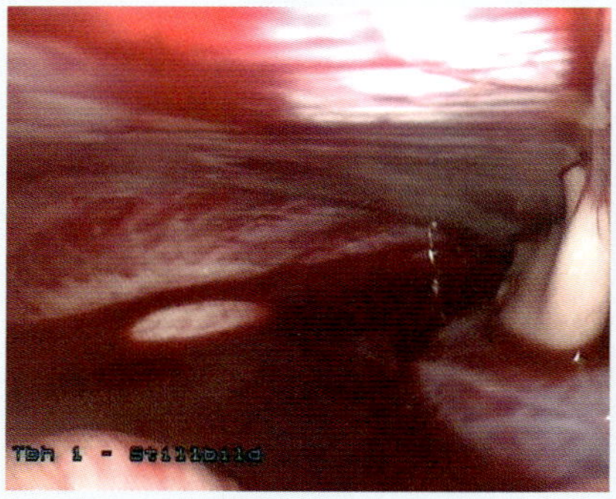

FIGURE 1. Initial laparoscopic view of the left caudal abdomen before removal of the blood. The ventral bladder ligament and urinary bladder are to the right of the image.

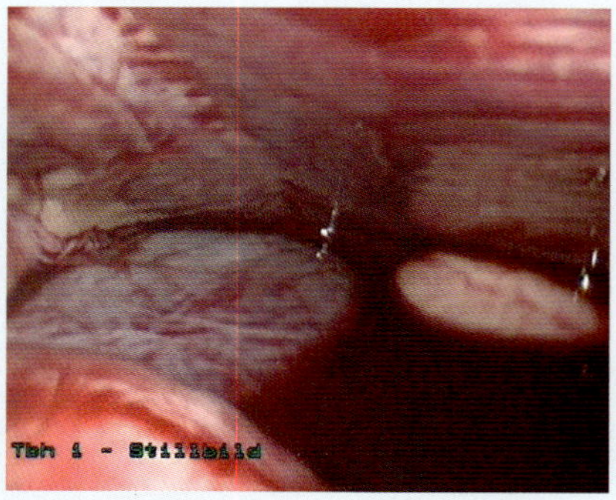

FIGURE 2. Initial laparoscopic view of the right caudal abdomen before removal of the blood. The ventral bladder ligament and urinary bladder are to the left of the image.

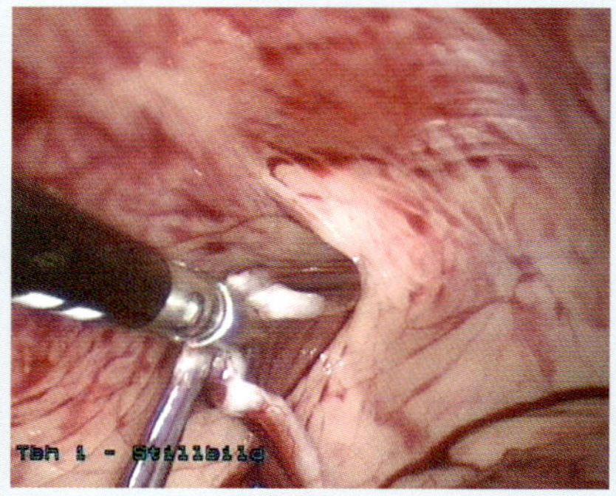

FIGURE 3. Left inguinal ring after partial removal of the blood. The left ductus deferens and testicular vessels are sealed using a vessel-sealing device.

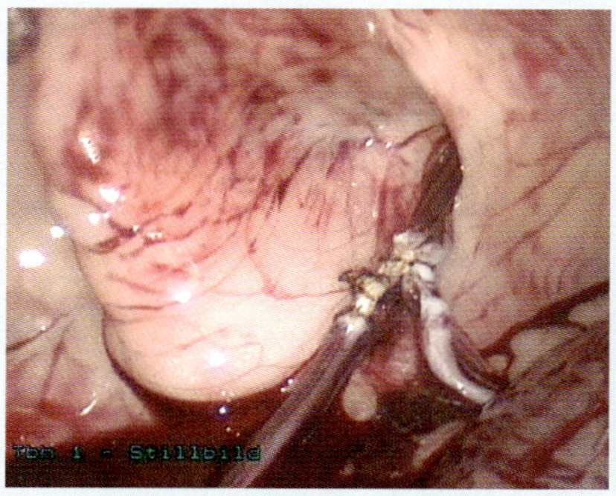

FIGURE 4. Left ductus deferens and testicular vessels after using the vessel-sealing device twice.

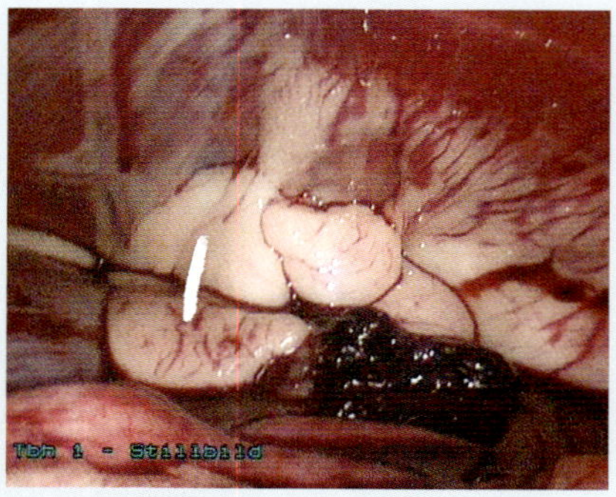

FIGURE 5. A blood clot is lying in front of the right inguinal ring. The urinary bladder is to the left of the image.

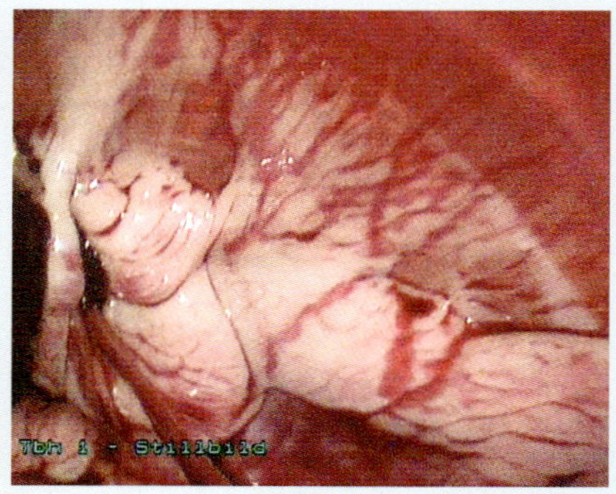

FIGURE 6. After pushing the blood clot away, the right ductus deferens and testicular vessels become visible. Some blood can be seen oozing out from the right inguinal ring.

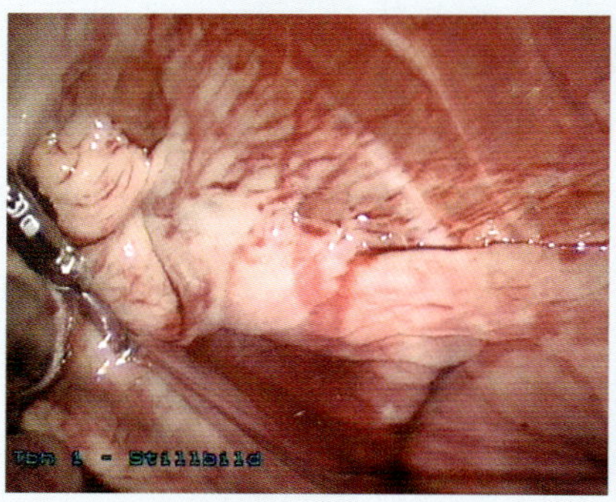

FIGURE 7. The right ductus deferens and testicular vessels are sealed using the vessel-sealing device.

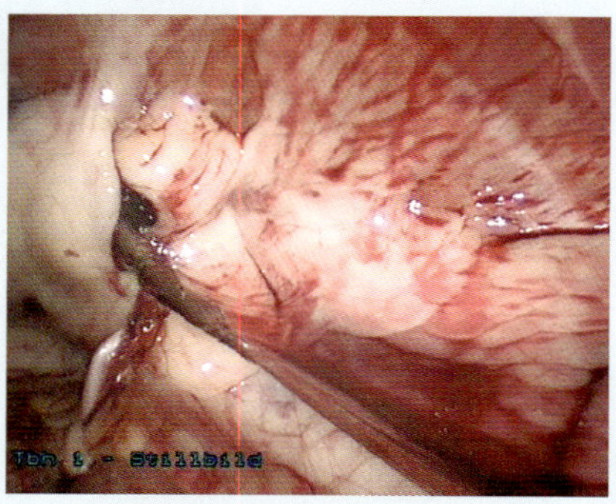

FIGURE 8. Right ductus deferens and testicular vessels after the first application of the vessel-sealing device.

Tips and tricks

- ✓ Partially remove the blood.
- ✓ Use a vessel-sealing device.
- ✓ Use gravity to your advantage.

14.5 MINIMALLY INVASIVE ABDOMINAL APPROACH TO SUBCOSTAL FOREIGN BODY REMOVAL

Matteo Balestrieri, Boris Dalpozzo

CASE DESCRIPTION

A 9-year-old male Cocker Spaniel was referred for investigation of a suspected foreign body after 1 week of hyperthermia and lethargy. The CT highlighted a thoracic wall abscess with two foreign bodies at the 9th–10th left intercostal space associated with bronchopathy in the left caudal pulmonary lobe bronchus. Considering the localization, a standard ultrasound-guided approach was not viable due to the costal artifacts and interference that made it difficult to reach the foreign body from the outside; therefore, a minimally invasive abdominal approach was chosen. After creating a pneumoperitoneum with a Veress needle, three 5 mm ports were placed. Under ultrasound guidance, a needle was placed from the outside into the abscess as guidance to locate the exact position. After the procedure, the dog was discharged the same day and made a good recovery without complications.

Key points

- Subcostal localization of the foreign body.
- Ultrasound-guided needle placement.
- Short surgery time.
- Good visualization.
- Rapid discharge.

PORT PLACEMENT

The patient was placed in dorsal recumbency. The first 5 mm port (T1) was placed 1 cm caudal to the umbilicus, the second port (T2) was placed 3 cm caudal to T1, and the third port (T3) was placed 2–3 cm cranial to T1.

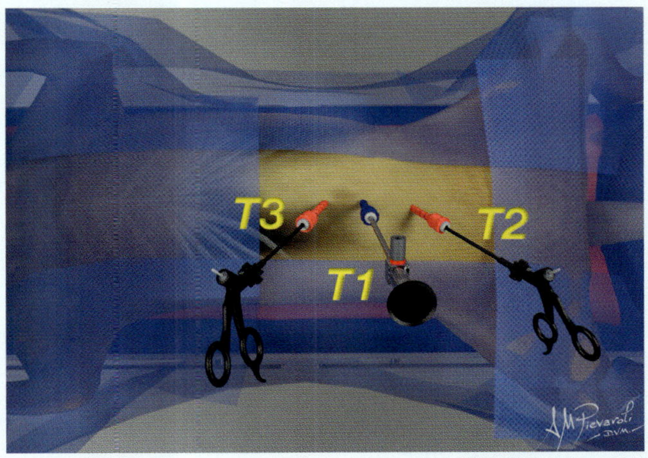

PROCEDURE

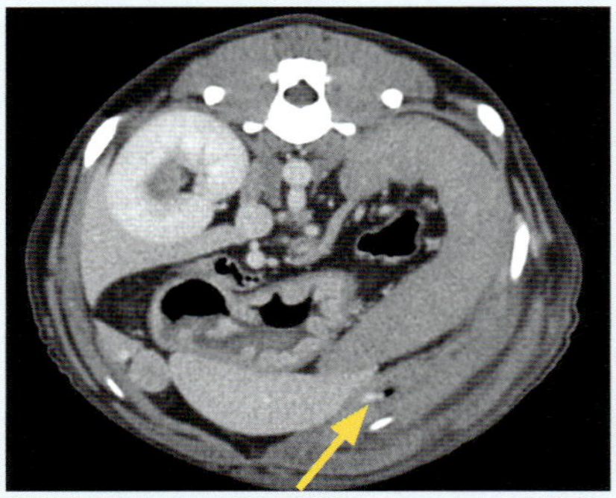

FIGURE 1. CT image of the abscess with a foreign body in the left thoracic wall on the 10th intercostal space (arrow). Image courtesy of Dr. F. Rossi.

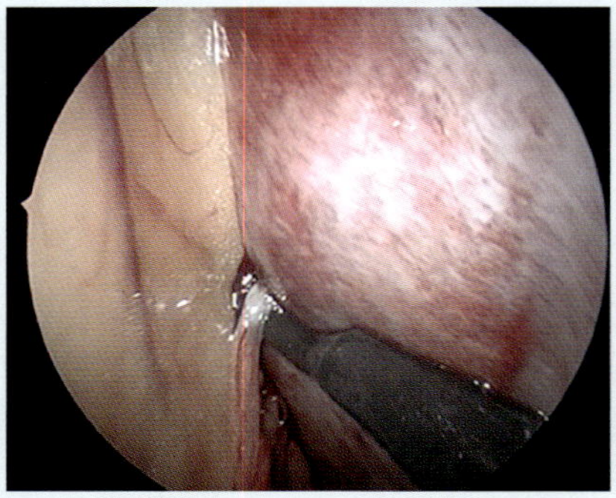

FIGURE 2. Upon entering the abdominal cavity, an omental adherence in the left cranial abdominal wall is noted and resected with a monopolar hook.

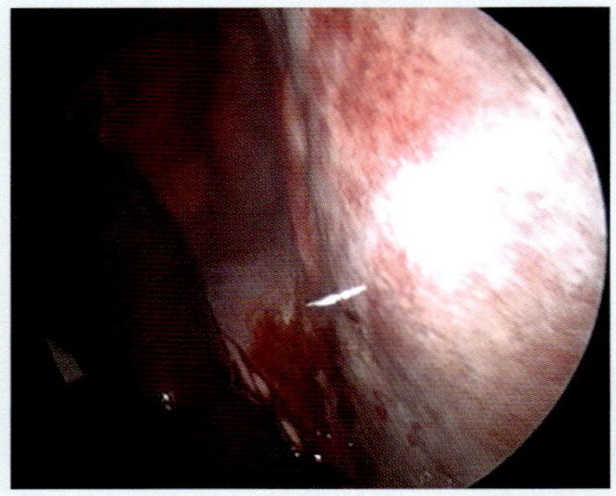

FIGURE 3. The previously placed needle is pushed inside the abdominal cavity to locate the dissection area.

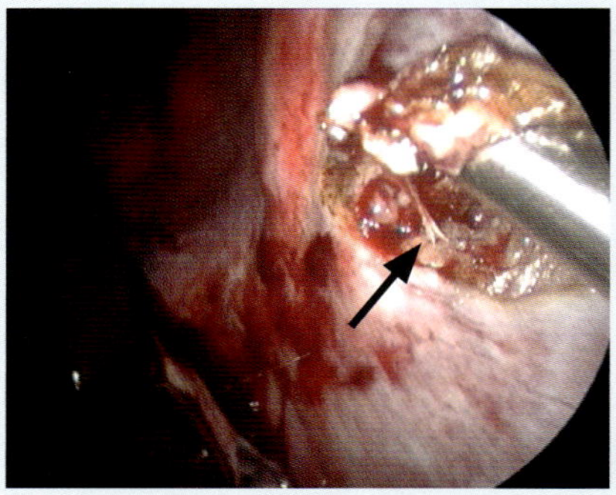

FIGURE 4. While dissecting the muscles with the monopolar hook, a 5 mm suction cannula is used to prevent abdominal contamination with the content of the abscess and blood. Keeping the area clean allows visualization of the foreign body (arrow).

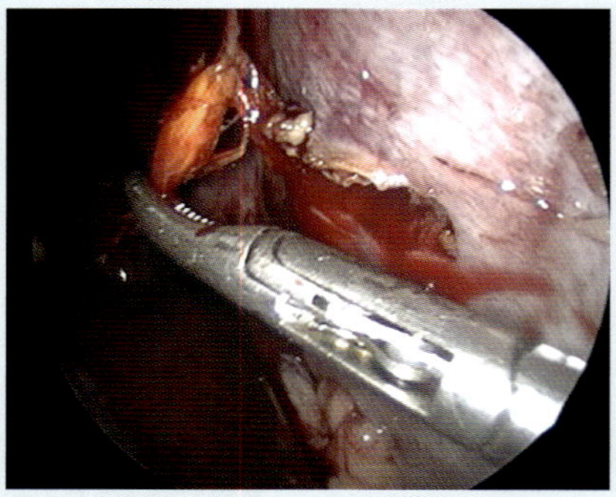

FIGURE 5. The foreign body is grasped with a 5 mm tissue grasper and carefully rotated, with the longitudinal axis parallel to the instrument. Every movement should be followed with the camera until complete extraction to avoid losing the foreign body in the peritoneal cavity.

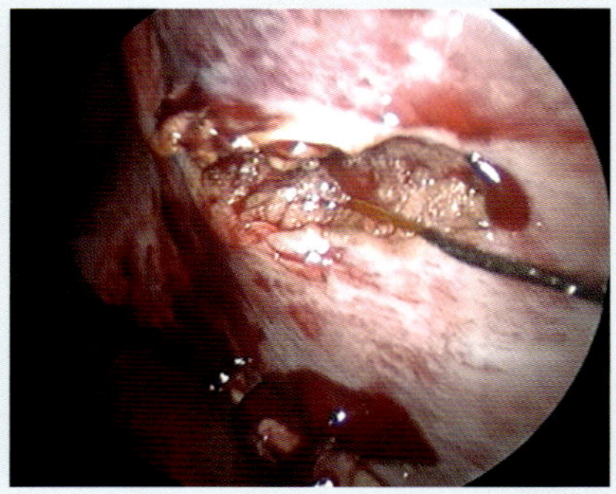

FIGURE 6. After aspiration, the second foreign body is visualized, probably another part of the same grass awn.

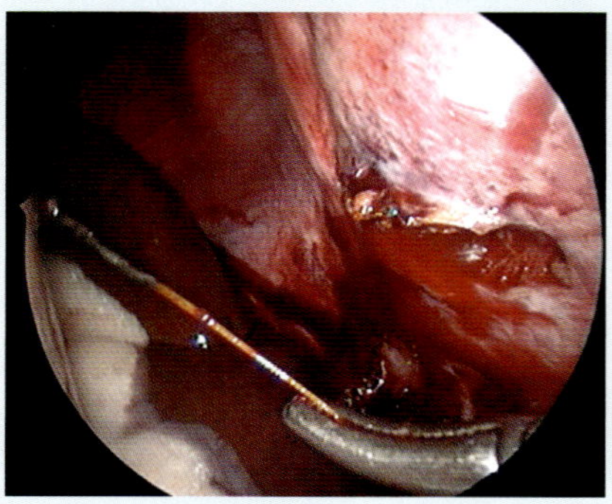

FIGURE 7. The same steps are followed for removal of the second foreign body: grasping, rotation, and extraction. Rotation is essential to achieve the correct position for extraction of the foreign body without the risk of breaking it or losing it at the surgical port.

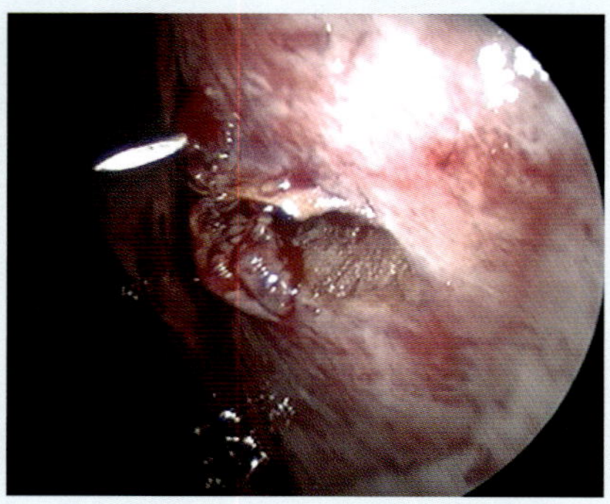

FIGURE 8. Final view of the dissected area after complete aspiration of the content. The wound will heal by second intention, with none or little discomfort for the patient. Surgical site omentalization can help in the healing and drainage of larger wounds while reducing the risk of adherence to abdominal viscera.

Tips and tricks

- ✓ A higher CO_2 insufflation rate helps prevent abdominal wall collapse while using the aspiration cannula.
- ✓ Keep good visualization while manipulating a foreign body inside the abdominal cavity.

14.6 LAPAROSCOPIC REPOSITIONING OF A VENTRICULOPERITONEAL SHUNT CATHETER

Michael Brückner

CASE DESCRIPTION

An 11-month-old male Cairn Terrier was presented due to a poorly functioning ventriculoperitoneal shunt system. During a radiographic contrast study of the system, there was evidence of a distal shunt obstruction. Laparoscopy was used to free the abdominal catheter of the shunt system and perform a partial omentectomy and omentopexy of the remaining omentum. Concurrently, the dog was sterilized. Results of a new radiographic contrast study 1 year after the procedure provided evidence that the ventriculoperitoneal shunt system was functional.

Key points

- Single-port access.
- Blunt dissection.

PORT PLACEMENT

Single-port access was made with two 6 mm Ternamian Endotip trocars in the umbilicus: a cranial telescope port (T1), and a caudal instrument port (T2). The patient was tilted to the right and left sides to reach the contralateral inguinal canals for the sterilization procedure.

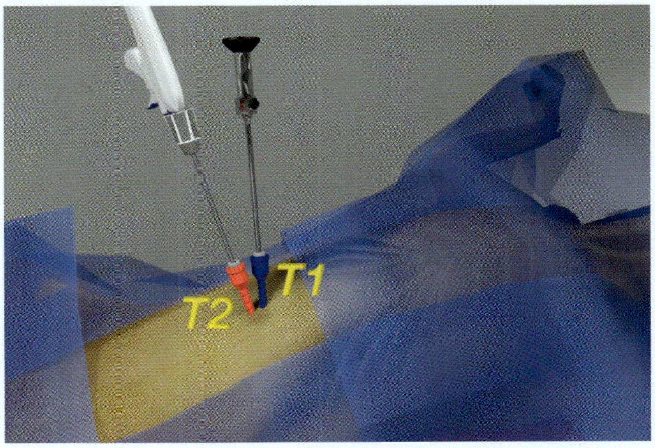

PROCEDURE

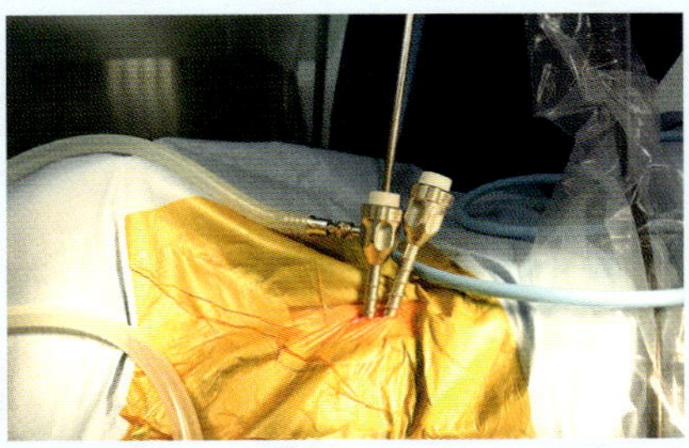

FIGURE 1. Single-port access in the umbilicus with two 6 mm Endotip trocars and the camera in the caudal port.

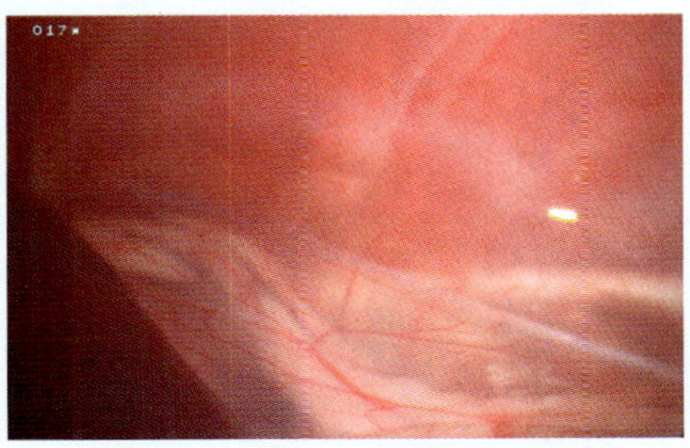

FIGURE 2. Abdominal catheter of the shunt system running in a gelatinous fluid pocket. The spleen is to the left of the image.

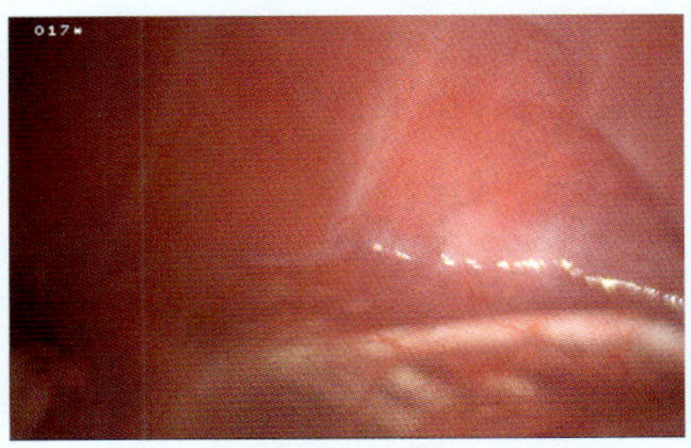

FIGURE 3. Caudal aspect of the shunt system, where it is entering into the abdominal cavity (to the right of the image).

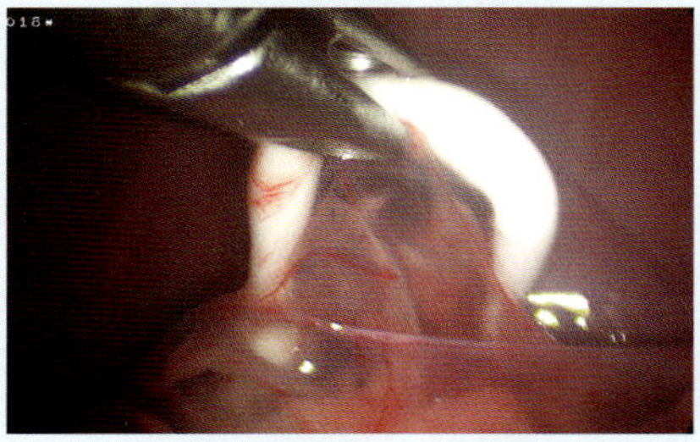

FIGURE 4. After blunt dissection, the catheter is grasped and pulled out of the gelatinous fluid pocket.

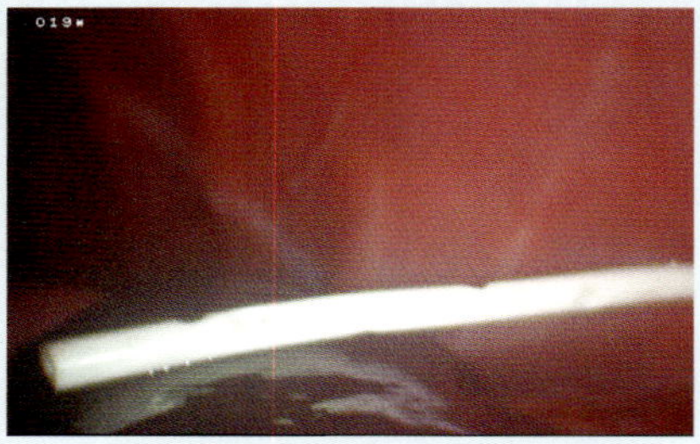

FIGURE 5. The catheter is placed in a more cranial direction, lying on the ventral surface of the spleen.

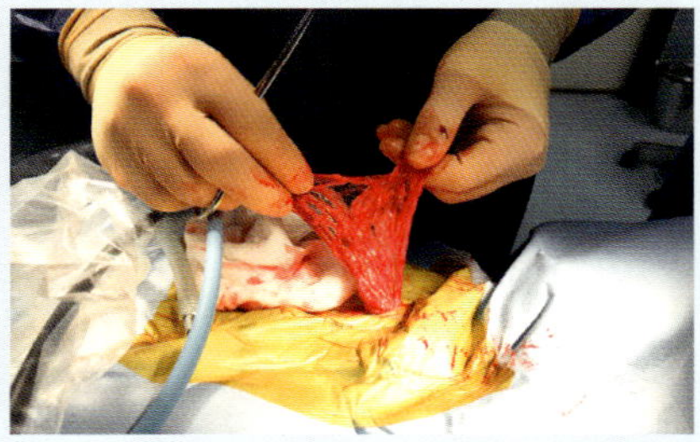

FIGURE 6. After grasping the omentum, removing both trocars, and connecting the two ports, the omentum is exteriorized. Omentectomy is then performed, and the remaining omentum is included in the closure of the abdominal fascia.

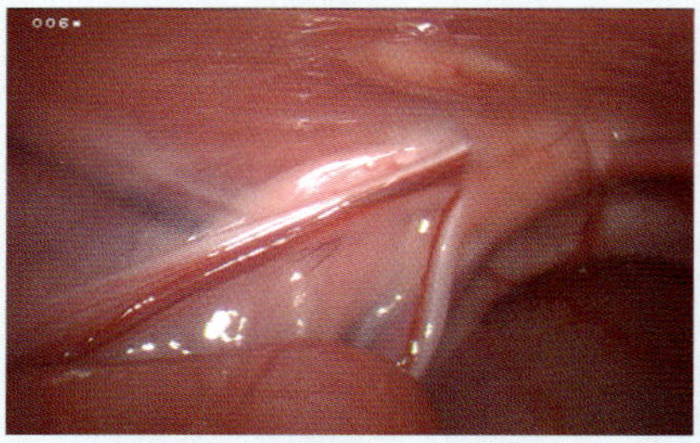

FIGURE 7. Visualization of the left inguinal canal, showing the testicular vessels to the left of the image and the ductus deferens to the right.

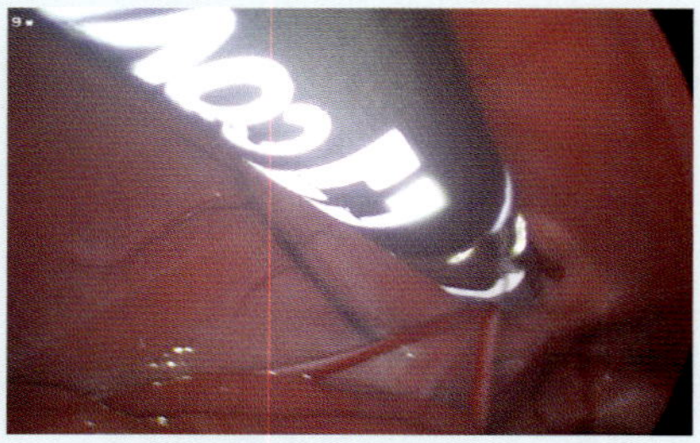

FIGURE 8. A vessel-sealing device is used to seal the testicular vessels and ductus deferens twice before transection.

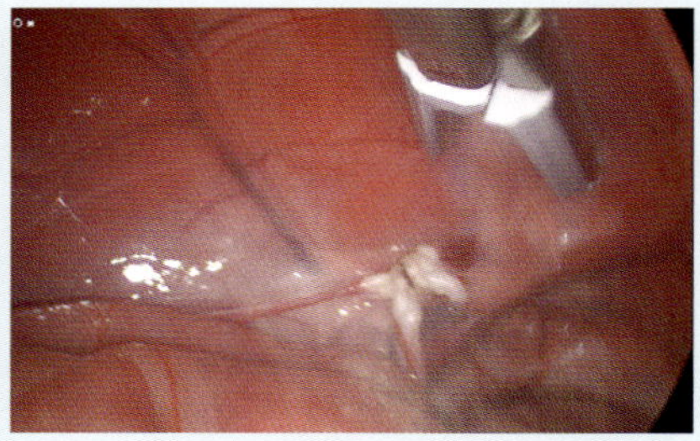

FIGURE 9. Image after sealing of the testicular vessels and ductus deferens before transection.

Tips and tricks

✓ Use gravity to your advantage.
✓ Connect both ports.
✓ Enlarge the incision as needed.

14.7 LAPAROSCOPIC LIVER BIOPSY

Enrico Sponza, Francesca Molinari

CASE DESCRIPTION

Advantages of laparoscopic liver biopsy include owner compliance, fast execution, better patient recovery, no need for postoperative monitoring, and high sensitivity in the cases reported by the authors. Among the disadvantages are the high cost of the equipment, a long learning curve, and the difficulty of performing core biopsies.

Key points

- The technique involves placement of 2–3 ports.
- The patient can be placed in lateral or dorsal recumbency.
- Multiple biopsy samples should be collected.
- No with intrahepatic lesions.

PORT PLACEMENT

The patient is placed in lateral or dorsal recumbency, based on the lesion location. The first port (T1, telescope port) is placed on the epigastric linea alba. The second port (T2, right-hand port, or T3, left-hand port) is placed in the left or right paramedian position, cranial to T1. After setting the endoscopic devices and locating the spot to be sampled, forceps are placed in position, the branches are closed, and pressure is maintained for about 20 seconds before traction to reduce bleeding. Sampling should be repeated to increase the diagnostic potential of the investigation.

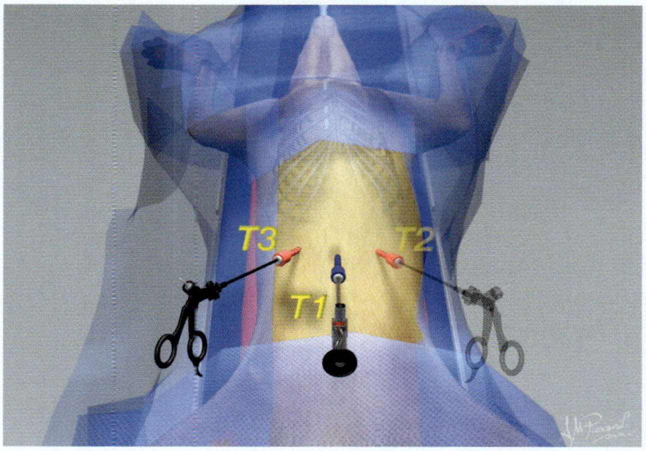

PROCEDURE

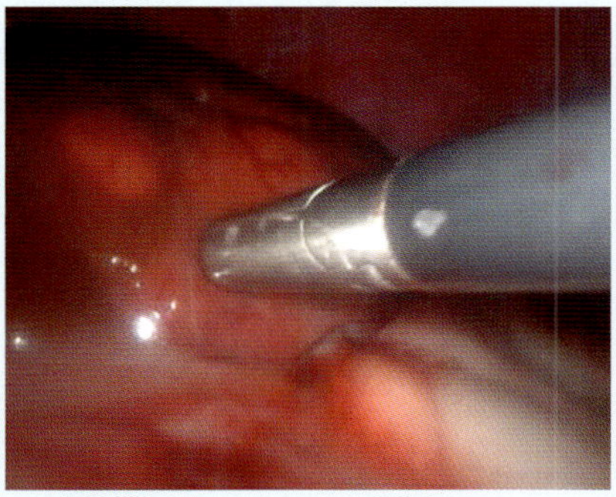

FIGURE 1. The biopsy forceps is introduced through the port..

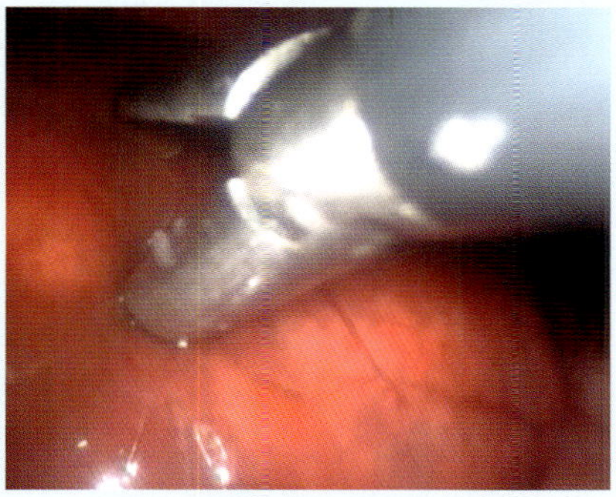

FIGURE 2. The liver surface is examined and palpated with the forceps. The forceps are then opened to grasp liver tissue.

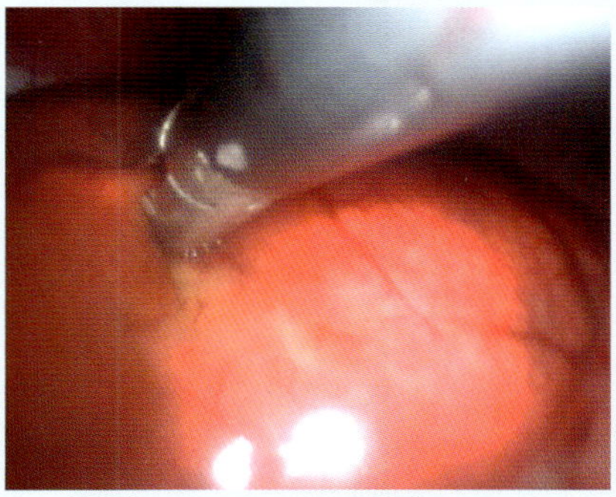

FIGURE 3. Biopsy performed in the central portion of a liver lobe.

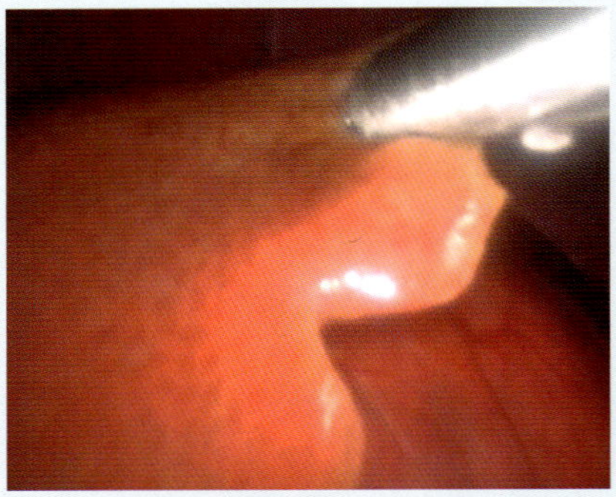

FIGURE 4. Biopsy performed at the edge of a liver lobe.

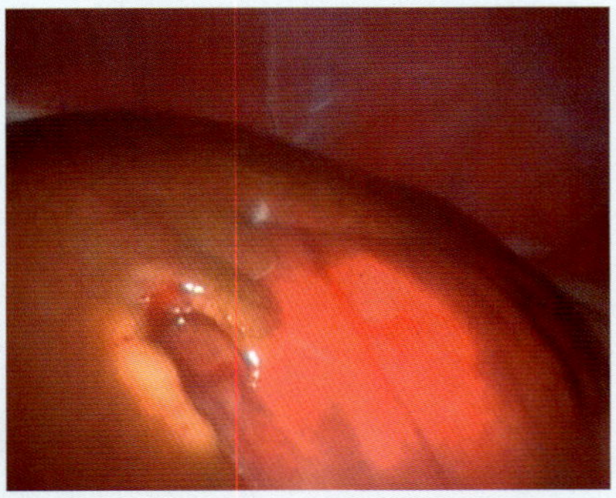

FIGURE 5. Minimal bleeding after taking the biopsy. Bleeding must always be assessed. To reduce bleeding, forceps pressure should be maintained for a few second before taking the biopsy.

Tips and tricks

✓ Use a Trendelenburg or reverse Trendelenburg position.
✓ Keep the forceps closed for about 20 seconds before traction.

15 LAPAROSCOPIC OVARIECTOMY

Andrea M. Pievaroli

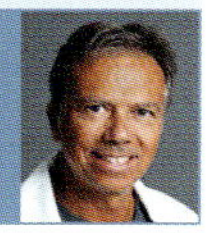

Indications

- Removal of both ovaries for suppression of the estrous cycle
- Prevention of diseases of the reproductive system
- Treatment of ovarian pathologies
- Treatment of ovarian remnant syndrome

Contraindications

- Cardiovascular and pulmonary diseases
- Congenital diaphragmatic defects
- Uterine pathologies (cases requiring ovariehysterectomy/ laparoscopic ovariohysterectomy)

Laparoscopic ovariectomy is the endoscopic surgical procedure most frequently performed in dogs. Even in cats, it has become an alternative to traditional ovariectomy and is increasingly offered to cat owners. Laparoscopic sterilization is becoming widely accepted by pet owners, who often request a minimally invasive approach with less postoperative pain and a faster recovery for other surgeries on their pets. The advantages of laparoscopic ovariectomy have been widely demonstrated through various scientific studies and have led to an ever-increasing number of veterinary clinicians being able to perform this procedure. It can be said that this technique is now considered the gold standard for female dog sterilization. Less pain, less discomfort, and fewer complications are indisputable advantages. Dogs undergoing laparoscopic ovariectomy have a significantly lower pain score and increased postoperative activity levels compared to dogs spayed with the traditional technique.

The first laparoscopic procedure for the sterilization of dogs and cats reported in the literature dates back to 1985. The authors chose a minimally invasive laparoscopic approach to perform occlusion of the uterine horns by electrocoagulation, without removing the ovaries. The first laparoscopic procedures for ovary removal in the dog were described by European veterinary schools in the 1990s. In the 2000s, the technique was progressively perfected as the instruments and equipment for minimally invasive surgery—until then used exclusively in human medicine—became less expensive and more easily accessible.

While ovariectomy is mainly indicated to suppress the estrous cycle, avoid reproduction, and prevent diseases of the reproductive system, it can also be performed for the treatment of ovarian pathologies.

Since the introduction of the laparoscopic technique for dog and cat sterilization, the advisability of performing an ovariectomy (OVE) over removing the ovaries and the uterus (ovariohysterectomy, OVH) has been called into question. This topic has often been contentious in the veterinary literature. European veterinary surgeons have been performing OVE for years without any complications affecting the uterine tract left in situ. Veterinary surgeons in the United States, on the other hand, have historically been taught to perform OVH to reduce the risk of pyometra or neoplasia affecting the uterus. However, studies with long-term follow-up periods have shown no evidence of pyometra or of a higher incidence of uterine neoplasia (approximately 0.003%) in ovariectomized patients. For this reason, and considering the ease of the procedure, if there are no indications for the removal of the uterus, laparoscopic sterilization of dogs is usually done everywhere by removing only the ovaries (lapOVE).

The risk of acquired urinary incontinence (AUI) following lapOVE does not differ from that when OVE is performed by laparotomy. A study published in 2019 compared the prevalence rates and severity of AUI between dogs spayed with laparoscopic and open laparotomy approaches and concluded that the minimally invasive approach does not reduce the likelihood of this complication.

LapOVE can be performed in patients of all breeds, ages and sizes, with some limitations in too small or excessively obese patients. Each patient can be considered a potential candidate for laparoscopic sterilization. Technical difficulties and surgical times can be influenced by the body conformation, the state of nutrition (body condition score, BCS), and by the amount of adipose tissue located in correspondence with the ovary. It is essential to acquire experience and skills in lapOVE to be able to perform, when necessary, the removal of the uterus (lapOVH), a topic that will be discussed in Chapter 17.

The first laparoscopic ovariectomy of dogs was reported in 1993 by S. Thiele, G. Kelch, et al.

DESCRIBED SURGICAL PROCEDURES

Various techniques have been described for the laparoscopic removal of the ovaries in dogs and cats, involving the use of one, two or three ports. The choice depends on the surgeon's personal preferences and the surgical difficulty in the patient. In the early years, when lapOVE procedures began, the operative ports were placed transversely to the midline, on a left and right paramedian line. This arrangement was soon replaced by positioning ports only on the midline, for greater advantages in performing the procedure.

In the veterinary literature, scientific studies published since 2009 have compared the various techniques to evaluate the advantages and disadvantages in their execution and the benefits for the patient in the postoperative period. The first reported one-port technique was performed using a particular 10 mm telescope with an operating channel (operating laparoscope) placed 1–2 cm caudal to the umbilicus. Endoscopic forceps and sealing devices were inserted parallel to the scope to perform the OVE. Although this technique has been shown to be safe and feasible even in small size patients, there is no triangulation for the graspers and more experience and skills are required to deal with any possible intraoperative complications. A paper published in 2011 compared the one-, two-, and three-port techniques to evaluate surgical time and severity of postoperative pain (using a modified Melbourne Pain Scale and palpation of surgical sites) in dogs undergoing lapOVE. The conclusion was that there were no significant differences in complication rates between the groups, but there were significantly lower pain score levels with the two-port technique than with the three-port technique. In addition, there was a similar median pain score between dogs in which two instrument cannulas were used and those in which a single cannula was used. In recent years, another single-access technique has taken hold and is commonly used today, which consists in the use of single-incision multiport devices to introduce more operative instruments in the same port (single-incision laparoscopic surgery [SILS] and similar single-port devices).

PATIENT PREPARATION AND POSITIONING

The patient should be fasted for 10–12 hours before surgery; water is allowed. The bladder should be emptied before the procedure to allow better visualization into the pelvic area. The abdomen is widely clipped; the surgical clip should extend cranially to the xiphoid process and include the entire vulva caudally. Even if the access is limited to the midline, wide clipping of the hair must also be performed laterally. This is preferable in case of conversion (as a rule for each laparoscopic procedure) and in case of percutaneous needle insertion for the two-port technique.

The patient is placed in dorsal recumbency and the skin is aseptically prepared before draping (**Fig. 1**). It is preferable to use a tilting table (better if motorized and remotely controlled) to easily reposition the patient during the different steps of the procedure (**Fig. 2**). Alternatively, positioners supplied by some companies can be used. They are placed on the operating table and allow the patient to be tilted laterally (**Fig. 3**).

In addition to lateral inclinations to better visualize the ovaries, it can be useful to tilt the table in a Trendelenburg position to displace the spleen cranially.

Some fundamental structures that should be identified during lapOVE are indicated in **Figure 4**. Attention must be paid to effective coagulation of vascular structures (ovarian artery and vein, uterine branch of ovarian artery and vein), which may be responsible for bleeding following ovary removal. In some obese patients, or if the lateral tilt of the table is not adequate, it may be useful to follow the round ligament to locate the ovary.

OPERATING ROOM LAYOUT

The endoscopy tower with all devices can be placed at the patient's foot or head, depending on the size of the operating room. The important thing is to leave enough space for the

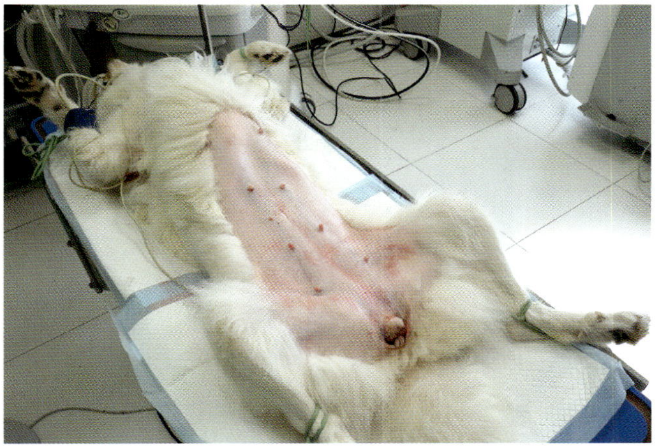

FIGURE 1. Dog in dorsal recumbency. The abdomen is widely clipped.

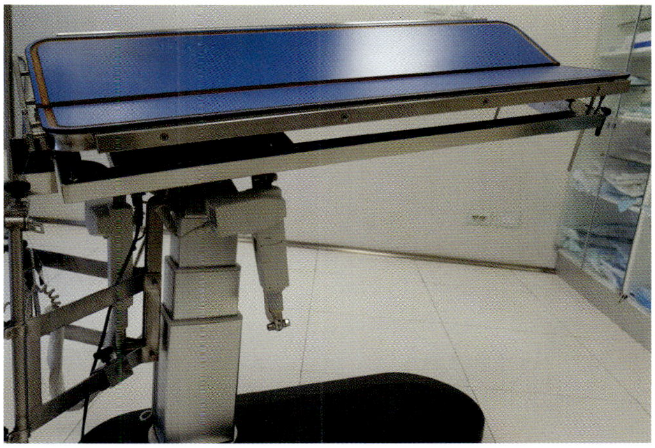

FIGURE 2. For laparoscopic ovariectomy, it is preferable to use a motorized tilting surgical table with a remote control.

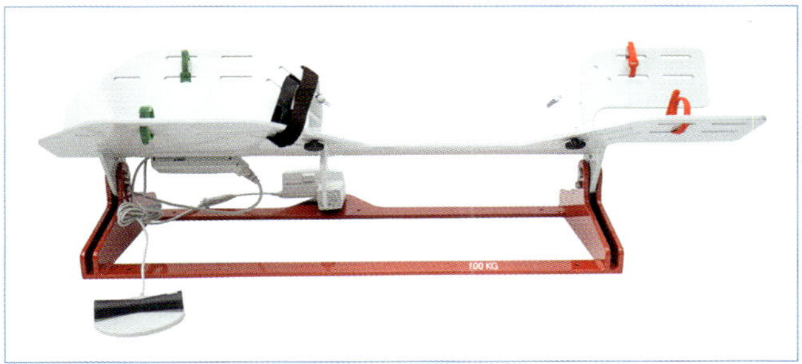

FIGURE 3. Example of an electrical tilt device positioner. Design by Dr. Berardino Izzo (Italy).

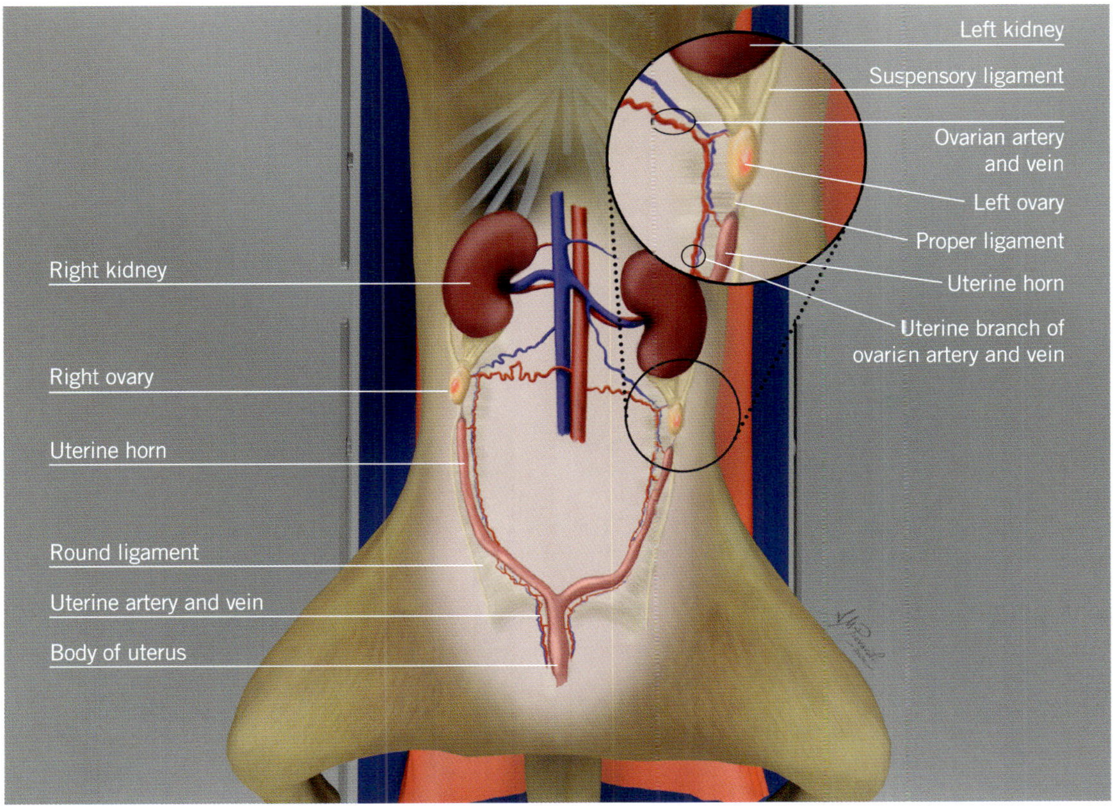

FIGURE 4. Female dog reproductive system.

surgeon and the assistant to move from one side of the table to the other. If the monitor is fixed on the tower, it is usually placed at the caudal end of the table (**Fig. 5**).

However, it is preferable to be able to move the monitor during the procedure to follow the surgeon's change of position and comply with the ergonomic principles of minimally invasive endoscopic surgery. This may be possible using a ceiling or boom-mounted monitor, a monitor installed on a mobile tower, or two monitors arranged on each side of the patient. The anesthesia machine is placed near the patient's head. The instrument table is placed caudolateral to the table, on the same side as the surgeon. To perform the OVE, the surgeon and their assistant position themselves on the opposite side in relation to the ovary to be removed (**Fig. 6**).

The following procedures are described below:

A. Two-port ovariectomy technique
B. Three-port ovariectomy technique
C. Single-port laparoscopic ovariectomy technique (J. Runge and J. Becker)

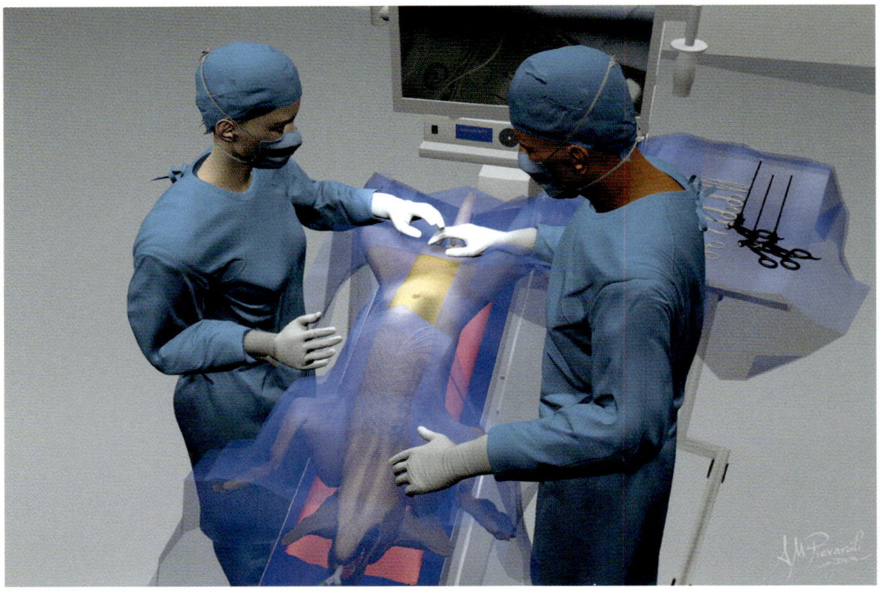

FIGURE 5. Operating room layout for laparoscopic ovariectomy. Initial setup for port placement.

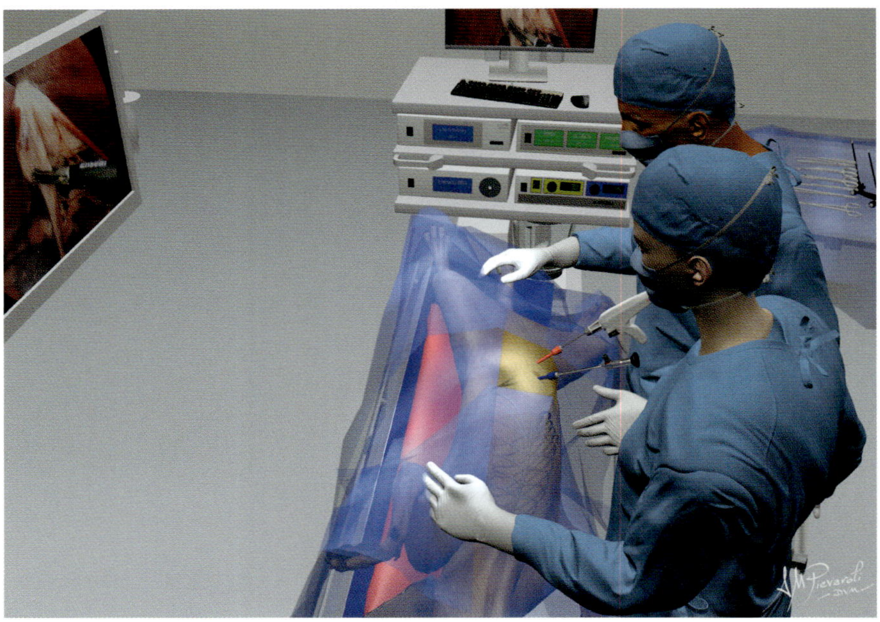

FIGURE 6. Layout during the ovariectomy: the table is tilted laterally; the surgeon and the assistant are positioned on the opposite side in relation to the ovary to be removed.

A TWO-PORT OVARIECTOMY

Two-port ovariectomy is currently the most commonly used technique and has the advantage of being very minimally invasive, as reported in the literature. Ports are placed in the midline, 1–2 cm cranial and 2–4 cm caudal to the umbilicus, depending on the size of the patient. The cranial cannula is used for the telescope, while the caudal cannula is used for the operative instruments. The distance between the trocars must be adequate for correct triangulation around the ovary. The ovary to be removed is kept suspended in the abdomen using a suture inserted percutaneously with a needle. This solution avoids using the third cannula, thereby reducing the invasiveness of the surgery. Some surgeons use a specific OVE hook instrument (Karl Storz Endoscopy) instead of the suture. After suspending the ovary to be removed, coagulation and cutting are performed (**Video 1**).

VIDEO 1. Two-port laparoscopic ovariectomy.

Instruments

On the table:

- Standard abdominal surgical pack
- Telescope 5 mm – 30°
- Two 5 mm cannulas (or one 5 mm cannula + one 10 mm cannula)
- Grasping forceps
- Large-gauge (usually 1 or 0) suture swaged on a needle
- Vessel-sealing device

Ready to use:

- Endoscopic cannula for aspiration/irrigation
- Third cannula to switch to the three-port technique

Minilaparoscopy 3 mm set (Fig. 7) for dogs and cats weighing less than 3–4 kg:

- Standard abdominal surgical pack
- Telescope 2.7 mm – 30°
- Two 3 mm cannulas
- Grasping forceps
- Endoscopic scissors
- A suture swaged on a needle
- Bipolar coagulation forceps

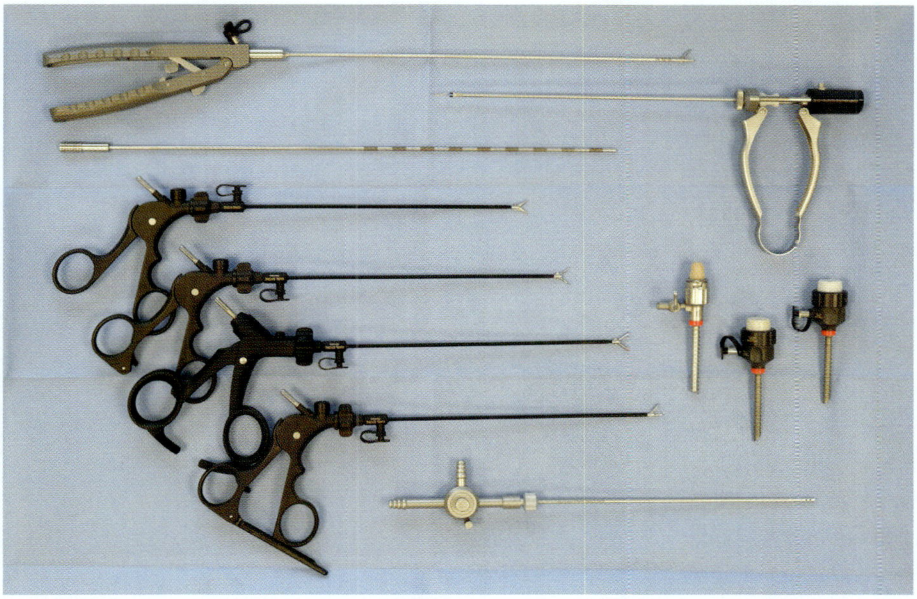

FIGURE 7. Minilaparoscopy set for patients weighing less than 3–4 kg.

PORT PLACEMENT (Fig. 8)

- T1, on the midline, 1–2 cm cranial to the umbilicus
- T2, on the midline, 3–6 cm caudal to the umbilicus

PROCEDURE

- Placement of the first trocar (cranial [T1] or caudal [T2]) is based on the surgeon's preferences. It is advisable to tilt the table into a Trendelenburg position to perform this step of the procedure. The author prefers to use threaded cannulas (Storz Endotip) to prevent slippage from within the peritoneum.
- A pneumoperitoneum is established using the surgeon's preferred technique; the author uses the Ternamian or a modified Hasson technique. After the first port has been placed and the pneumoperitoneum achieved, the 5 mm telescope is inserted and a first exploration of the abdomen is performed to check for any evidence of iatrogenic trauma caused by placement of the first cannula.
- The falciform ligament, which could prevent correct vision and cloud the lens of the telescope, can often be found in this area of the peritoneum (**Fig. 9**). It is necessary to screw the port deeper to find the right inclination to overcome the ligament.

Tips

To avoid crossing the falciform ligament, the port can be inserted slightly lateral (1–2 cm) to the midline.

- Under endoscopic vision, the second cannula is inserted for a correct triangulation around the ovary to be removed. It is preferable to use the cranial port for the telescope and the caudal port for the instruments (**Fig. 10**). Some authors prefer to reverse the tools (telescope in the caudal port and forceps in the cranial port).
- The surgeon performs the surgery on the contralateral ovary with respect to their position.
- For better visualization of the ovary, especially in obese patients, in the presence of meteoric intestinal loops or splenomegaly, the patient should be tilted to an oblique position (at least 45°) to displace the organs by gravity and facilitate manual surgical procedures **(Fig. 11)**. Some authors prefer to place the patient in lateral recumbency instead of in an oblique position.

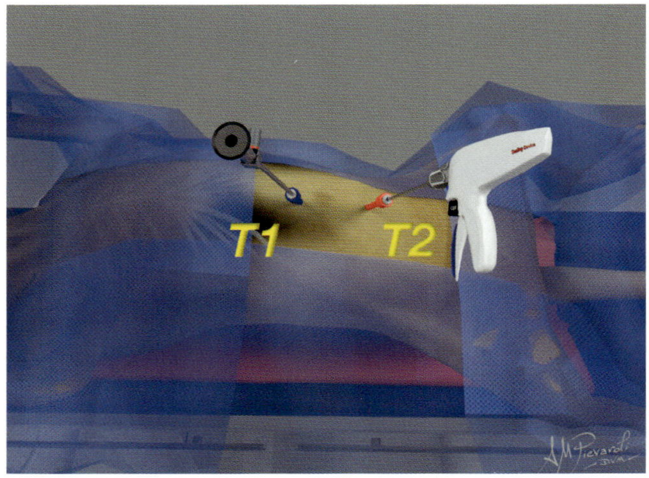

FIGURE 8. Port placement for two-port ovariectomy.

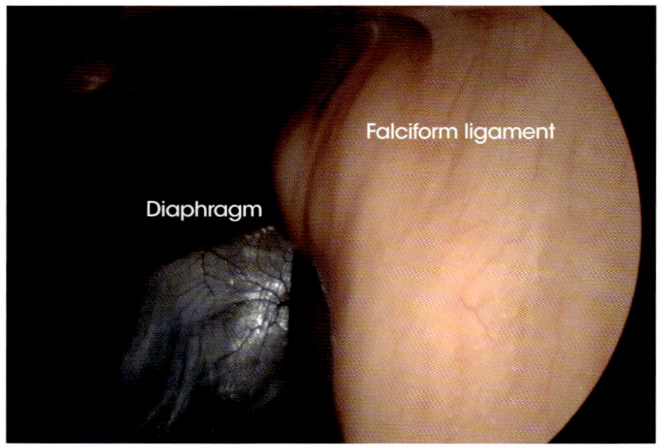

FIGURE 9. The falciform ligament can often be found in umbilical area. This could prevent correct vision and cloud the lens of the telescope.

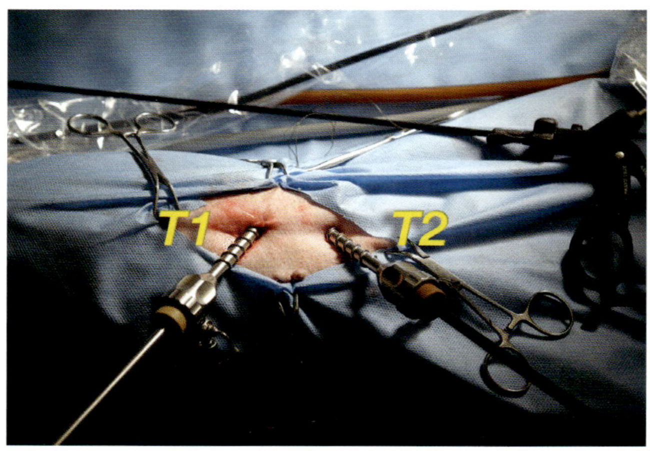

FIGURE 10. Image of the operating field for two-port laparoscopic ovariectomy.

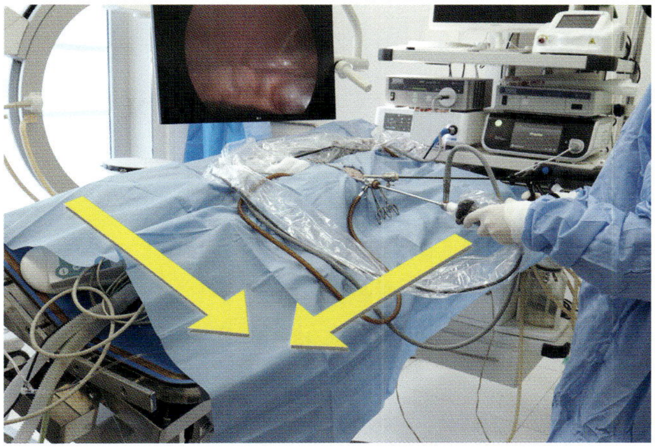

FIGURE 11. The table should be tilted laterally, at least 45°. Use a Trendelenburg and oblique position to displace the organs by gravity.

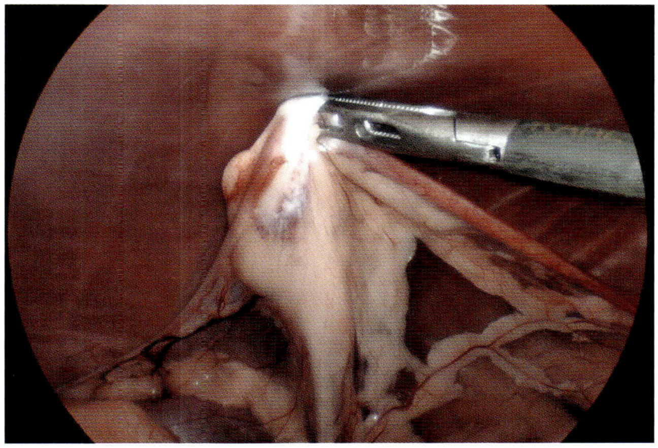

FIGURE 12. The proper ligament is grasped to elevate the ovary (the left ovary is shown in the figure).

- Atraumatic forceps or a blunt probe are used to move the organs and locate the ovary and uterine horn, which are located caudal to the kidney. Forceps are then used to grasp the proper ligament and elevate the ovary to visualize the kidney, the suspensory ligament of the ovary and the ovarian vasculature (**Fig. 12**).
- Palpating the abdomen from the outside, a point on the wall is identified in correspondence with the ovary. Then, under direct endoscopic vision, a suture is inserted percutaneously with a large size half-circle needle (**Fig. 13a**). The needle is passed through the proper ligament or the cranial uterine horn, avoiding the ovarian artery and vein, and then outside of the body wall again (**Fig. 13b**).
- After anchoring the ovary with suture thread, the forceps are removed from the port.
- The two ends of the suture outside the body wall are pulled to elevate the ovary and placed under tension with Klemmer forceps or a hemostat (**Fig 14**).
- A vessel-sealing device (VSD) is introduced in the caudal port. The suspensory ligament is usually sealed and transected first. Then, the kidney is identified and the omentum or other organs that may interfere are moved. The jaws of the forceps are used to seal and dissect the mesovarium (including the ovarian artery and vein) and suspensory ligament, taking care to remain at a sufficient distance from the ovary (**Fig. 15**).

Two-port minilaparoscopy with 3 mm cannulas: In small dogs and cats, 3 mm bipolar forceps should be used to coagulate vessels and tissues. The small endoscopic scissors are then introduced to dissect the ovaries free (**Fig. 16**) (**Video 2**).

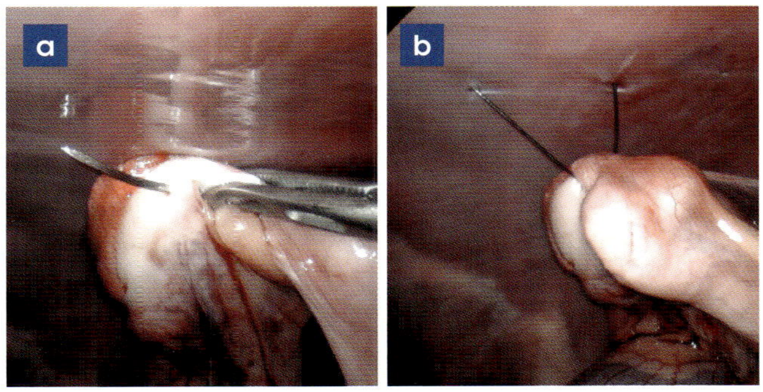

FIGURE 13. A suture is inserted percutaneously with a large size half-circle needle and passed through the proper ligament.

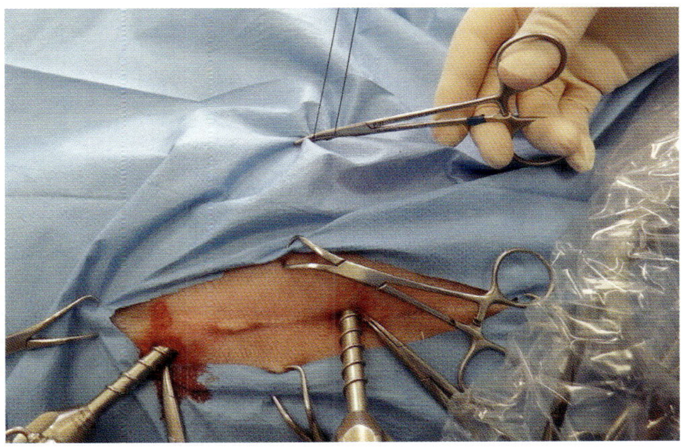

FIGURE 14. The two ends of the suture are clamped outside using a hemostat.

VIDEO 2. Two-port minilaparoscopic ovariectomy in a cat.

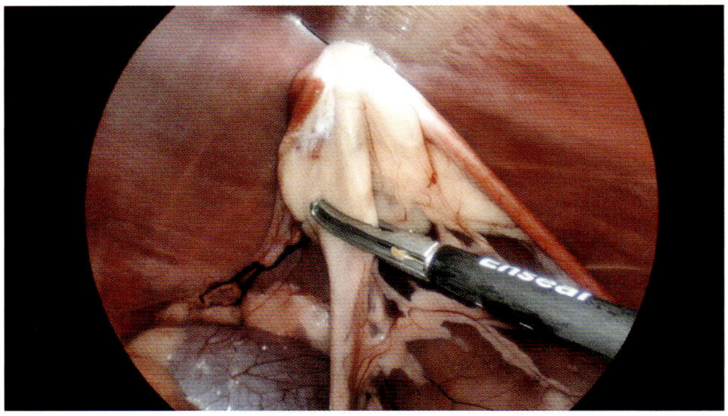

FIGURE 15. Use of a vessel-sealing device to grasp the suspensory ligament between the kidney and ovary to perform the resection.

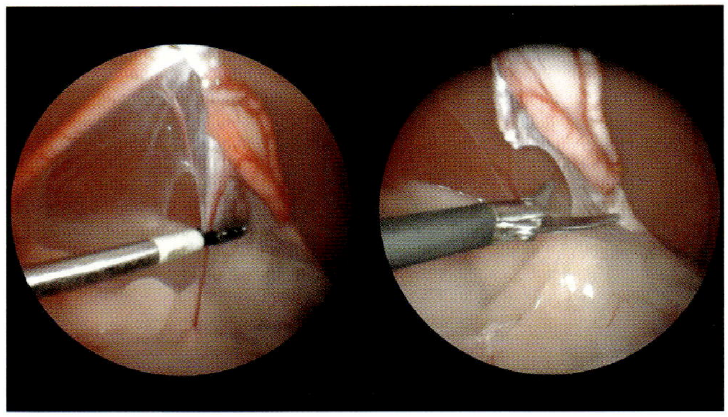

FIGURE 16. Two-port minilaparoscopy. a) Use of 3 mm bipolar forceps to coagulate the suspensory ligament. b) The ovaries are then dissected free with scissors.

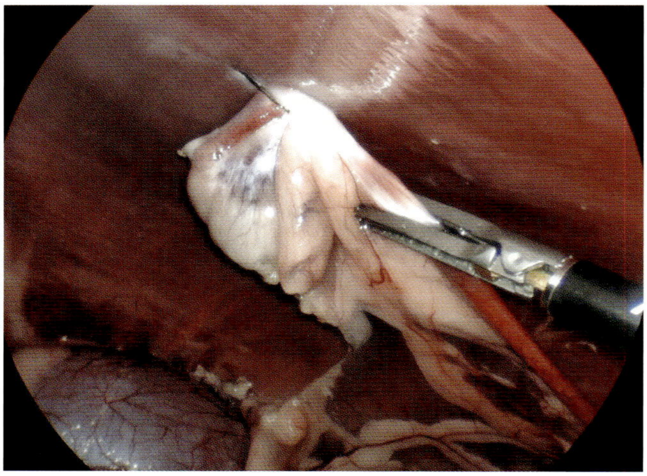

FIGURE 17. The jaws are closed and the vessel-sealing device operated to perform resection of the uterine horn.

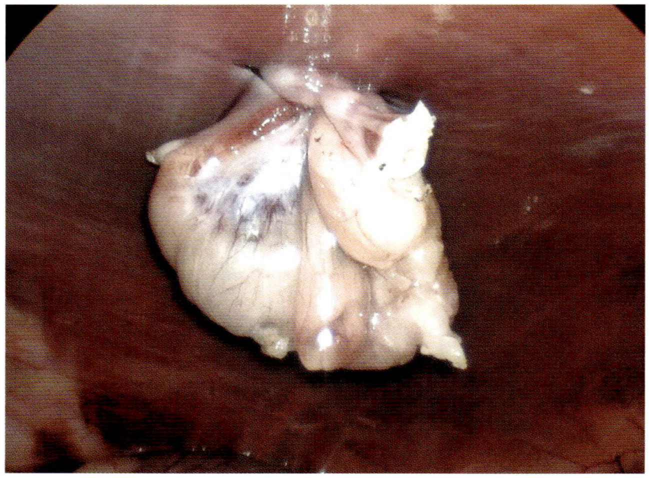

FIGURE 18. The dissected ovary is still anchored by the suture to the body wall.

- Then, using the VSD, the first part of the uterine horn is grasped and the resection is performed including the mesometrium, until the ovary is completely isolated (**Fig. 17**). The ovary must remain anchored to the body wall by the suture (**Fig. 18**).
- The surgeon should carefully check for any evidence of bleeding from the dissected vessels before tilting the table in the opposite position to remove the contralateral ovary.
- At this point, the surgeon and the assistant should move to the opposite side and the table should be tilted laterally towards them.
- The surgeon then performs the same procedure to remove the second ovary (**Fig. 19**).
- After the procedure has been completed on both sides, the table is tilted back to the initial neutral position. It is preferable for the surgeon and the assistant to be placed on each side of the table.

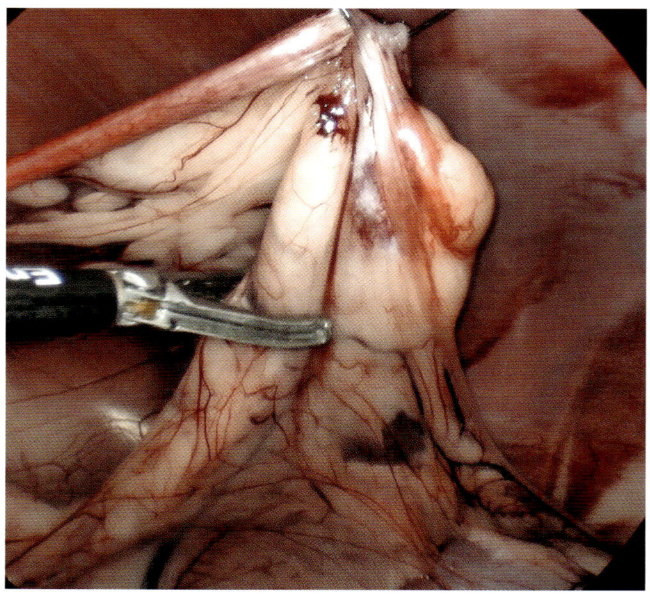

FIGURE 19. Endoscopic view of the second ovary (right ovary).

PROCEDURE

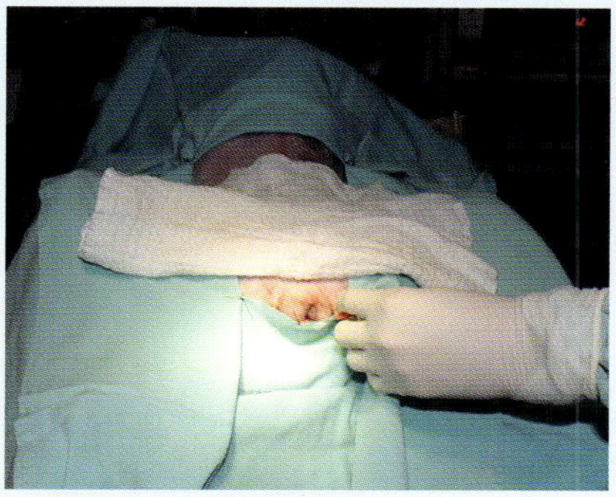

FIGURE 1. The patient is placed in dorsal recumbency, with the head directed towards the video system, with wide exposure of the abdomen and vagina. A wide area of abdominal and perineal hair is clipped, including the paralumbar fossa and caudal third of the rib cage up to the transverse processes, in addition to the inner aspect of the hindlimbs.

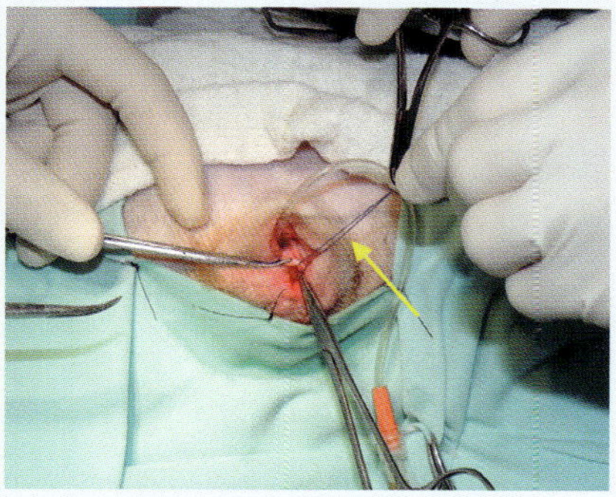

FIGURE 2. A tacking suture is placed in the mucosa of the fornix in a ventral position (arrow); it will be critical for vaginal wound closure at the end of the procedure. Using fine-tipped curved hemostats, the fornix area is grasped and exteriorized for placement of the tacking suture, which is further used to expose the vaginal wound.

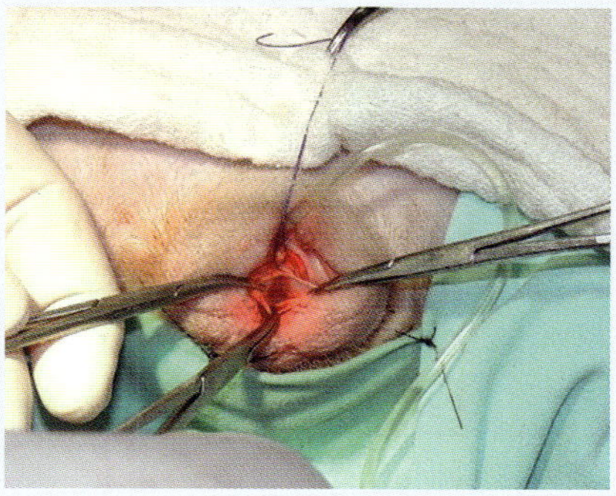

FIGURE 3. An incision is made in the vaginal mucosa and submucosa. The remaining layers of the vagina will be bluntly dissected using the rounded trocar tip until the abdominal cavity is reached. Hemostatic forceps are used to grasp the edges of the vaginal wound to guide trocar insertion.

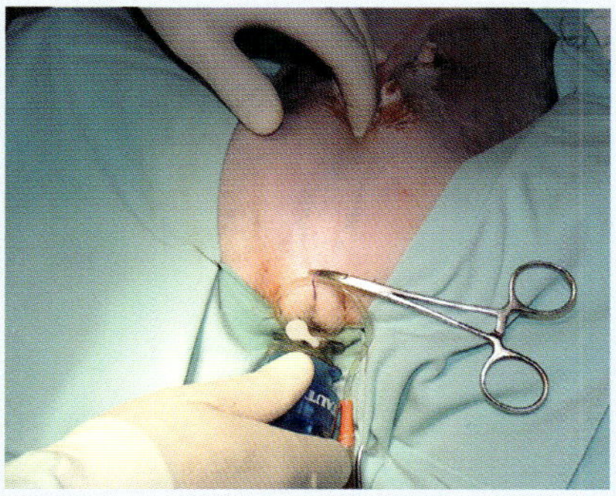

FIGURE 4. A disposable translucent 10–12 mm smooth trocar cannula with a blunt obturator is inserted through the vaginal wound in order to perforate the remaining layers by blunt dissection, thus providing access to the peritoneal cavity.

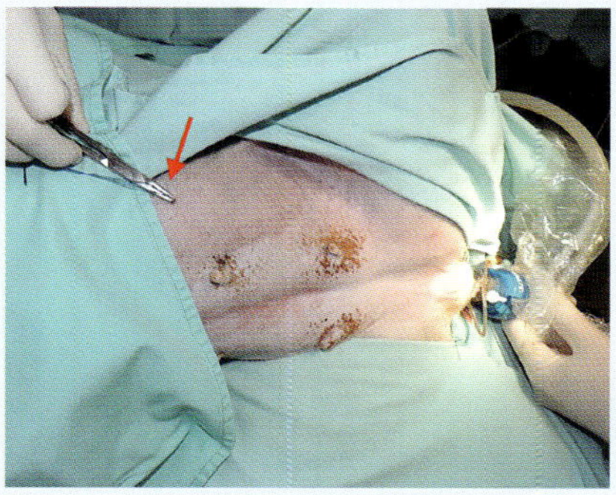

FIGURE 5. A 10 mm straight-angled operative laparoscope is inserted through the cannula to confirm complete access to the abdominal cavity. Long (≥38 cm of working length) 5 mm laparoscopic Kelly forceps are used to grasp the uterine horn at the level of the proper ovarian ligament. With the patient slightly rotated, the ovary is raised and attached to the abdominal wall using a transparietal suture (arrow) for exposure of the mesovarium.

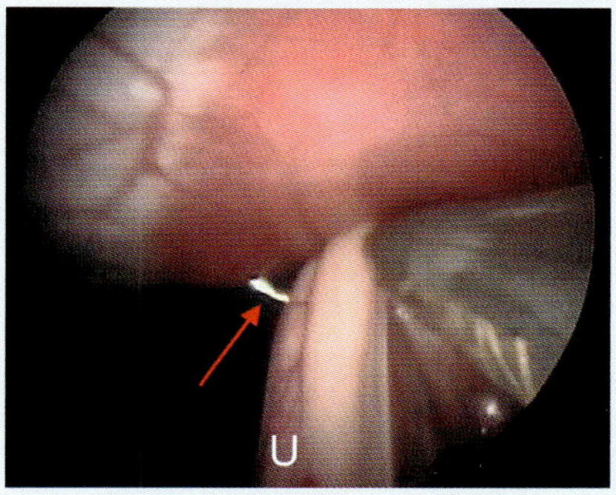

FIGURE 6. The uterine horn (U) is raised to the abdominal wall and a transparietal suture is placed using a long thread. Laparoscopic view of the transparietal suture (arrow) used to expose the ovary and its ligaments and vessels.

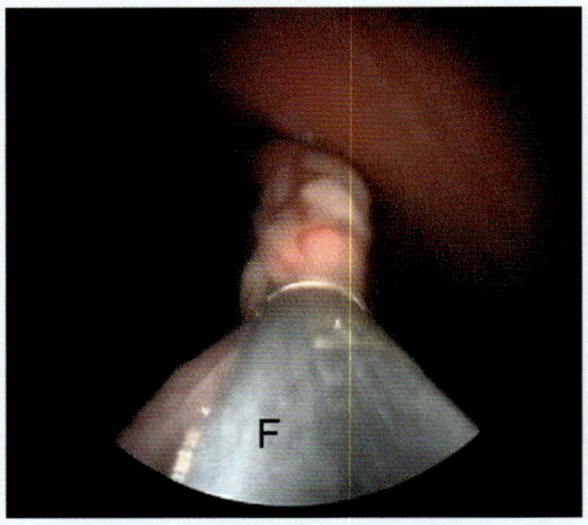

FIGURE 7. Bipolar forceps (F) with a cutting blade and a vessel-sealing device or ultrasonic scalpel should be used to coagulate and transect the uterine horn and vessels as close as possible to the proper ligament. Transection of the uterine horn is performed close to the proper ligament.

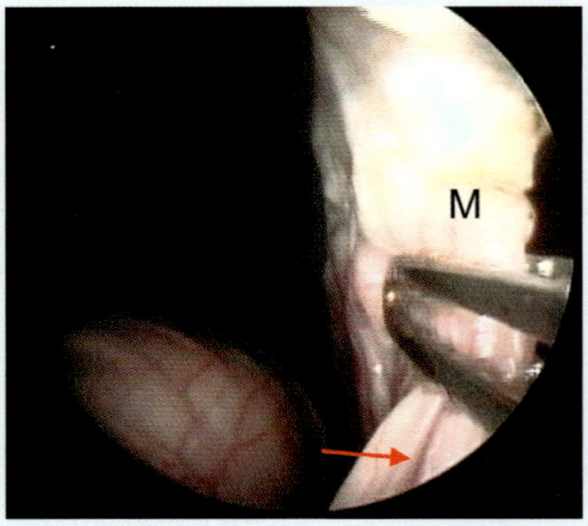

FIGURE 8. The ovarian pedicle, mesovarium and suspensory ligament are subsequently coagulated and severed, until the ovary is completely released. Coagulation of the vessels of the ovary and mesometrium (M). The arrow highlights the left ovarian vein.

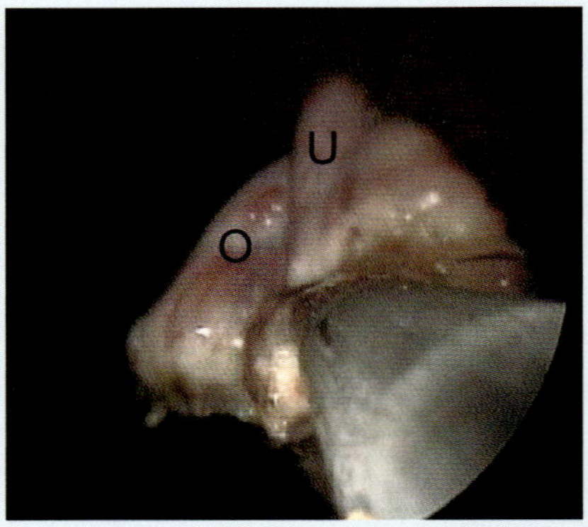

FIGURE 9. The ovary is removed from the cavity while keeping the transparietal suture anchored to it. If the cannula is removed along with the ovary, it should be replaced to approach the opposite ovary. The isolated ovary (O) will be inserted through the vaginal cannula. The ovary should be grasped at the level of the remaining uterine horn (U) or suspensory ligament.

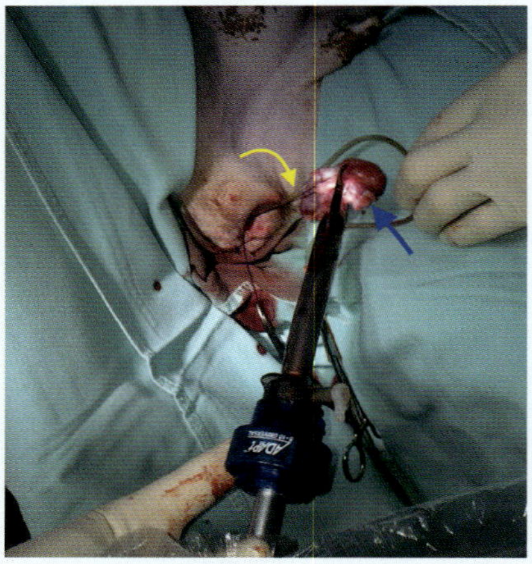

FIGURE 10. Removal of the ovary (blue arrow) along with the cannula and Kelly forceps from the abdominal cavity. The transparietal suture (yellow arrow) is still attached to the ovary.

Tips and tricks

- ✓ Transvaginal access is performed in the fornix, preferably at the midpoint of the vagina. The incision will extend to the submucosa and the vaginal tunica muscularis by blunt dissection. This provides better cannula fixation, reducing CO_2 leak.
- ✓ "Blind" insertion of the port must be cautiously performed. The colon should be pulled laterally using the surgeon's nondominant hand while directing the cannula parallel to the ventral midline, into the peritoneal cavity.
- ✓ The use of a translucent cannula is useful for checking proper positioning of the port within the peritoneal cavity prior to insufflation.
- ✓ The authors prefer approaching the left ovary first, which is less exposed due its proximity to the spleen and colon. Tilting of the patient to the side opposite to that of the approached ovary will displace the bowel away from the ovary in cases of difficult exposure.

▶

- ✓ The transparietal suture can include the proper ovarian ligament, the area below it (in this perspective) or even the uterine horn (taking care to avoid the uterine vessels). Thus, the final aspect of the horn will be adequately exposed.
- ✓ Coagulation and transection of a short segment of the uterine horn, followed by coagulation and transection of the uterine vessels and mesometrium will simplify the approach to the mesovarium, ovarian vessels and suspensory ligament. Those structures will be exposed almost in a "straight line" ahead of the forceps.
- ✓ After transection from all attachments, the ovary is grasped at the remaining uterine stump or suspensory ligament, without releasing the transparietal suture.
- ✓ The ovary should be brought to the cannula and preferably retrieved through it (if the size of the ovary allows it), without removing the transparietal suture (which remains grasped outside the cavity with a hemostat).
- ✓ The transparietal suture should be removed only when the ovary is completely outside the vagina. This way, if the ovary drops during removal, it will be repositioned in the flank by the external traction of the suture thread.
- ✓ The traction of the vaginal repair suture will allow adequate exposure of the wound, which will be sutured in its mucous and submucosal layers.

15.2 TWO-PORT LAPAROSCOPIC OVARIECTOMY IN THE CAT

Antoine Adam

CASE DESCRIPTION

LapOVE is a minimally invasive procedure that is commonly performed not only in dogs but also in cats. In fact, cats often recover surprisingly quickly from lapOVE. It should be noted that special surgical equipment for small-sized patients is necessary.

Key points

- Pneumoperitoneum is established with an 18-gauge needle at the tip of the CO_2 line.
- A 5 mm cannula is used for the cranial port, to introduce the VSD and remove the ovary.
- A 3 mm cannula is used for the caudal port, to introduce a small (3 mm) telescope.
- Light cannulas should be used.
- The telescope is placed near the region of interest to achieve good visualization (3 mm telescopes have less light).
- The fat is dissected before placing the 3 mm cannula to help with closure and avoid future herniation.

PORT PLACEMENT

A small towel is placed under the back of the cat to elevate the abdomen. A heating mat and, if needed, a ground plate for electrosurgery should also be placed.

The first cannula (T1) is placed on the midline, approximately 1–2 cm caudal to the umbilicus, and a 3 mm camera is introduced. The second cannula (T2), for the 5 mm VSD, is placed on the midline, approximately 2 cm cranial to the umbilicus.

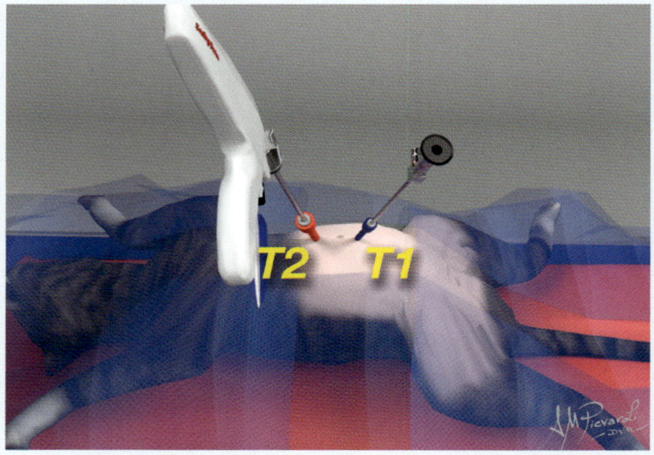

PROCEDURE

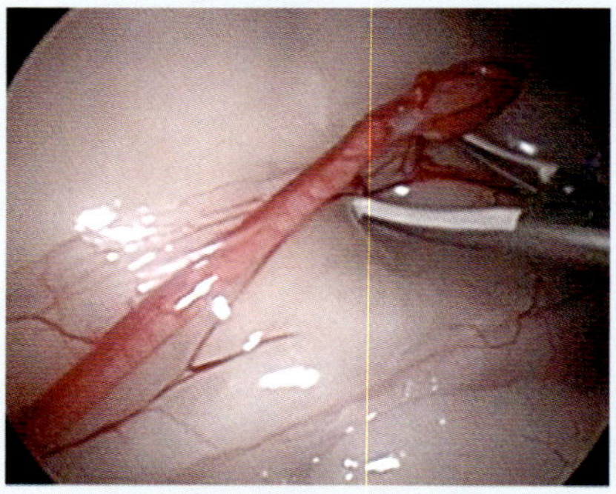

FIGURE 1. Dissection of the ovarian vessels. The ovary is located at the caudal pole of the kidney. No traction device is needed. The goal is to place the tip of the vessel-sealing device underneath the ovarian vessels.

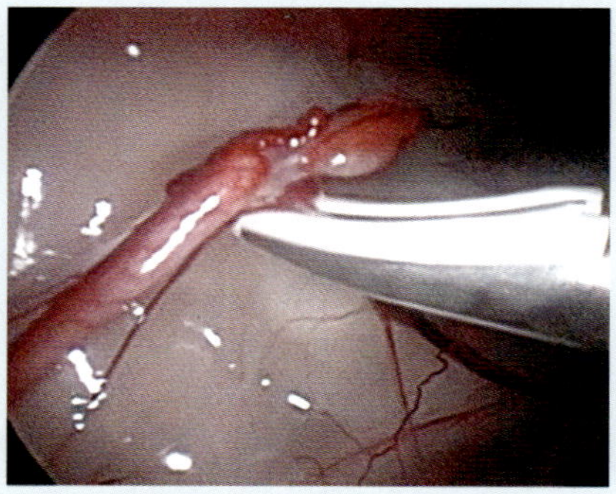

FIGURE 2. Under good visual control, the ovary is suspended with the tip of the vessel-sealing device, and the ovarian vessels are cut.

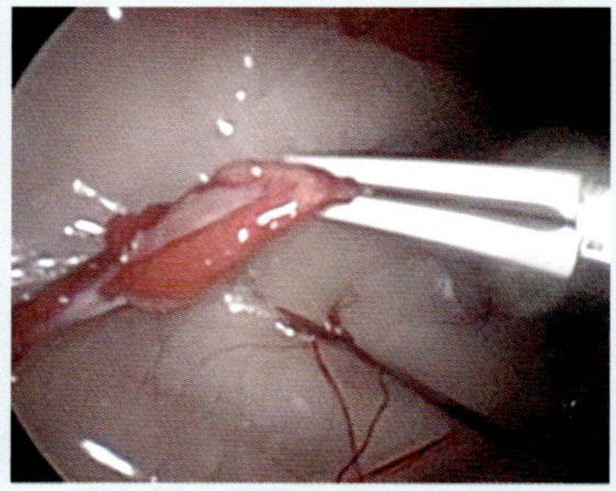

FIGURE 3. The suspensory ligament is cut in the same manner. Care should be taken to ensure that all the ovary is removed.

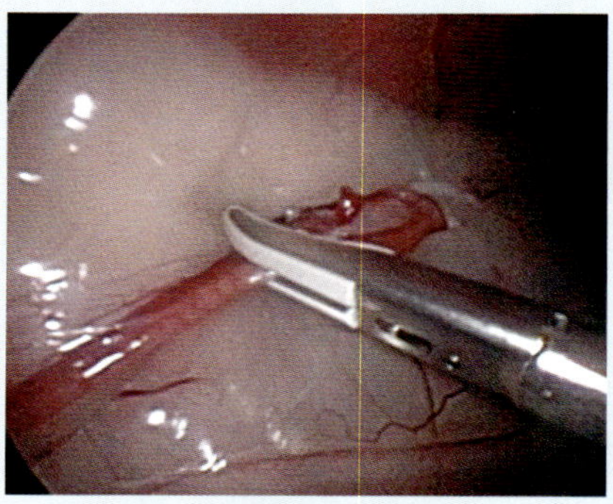

FIGURE 4. After cutting the uterine horn, the ovary is left in place. The vessel-sealing device is replaced with a 5 mm Babcock forceps, which is used to grab the ovary. If there is any tissue still holding the ovary, gentle traction is applied to tear it.

Tips and tricks

- ✓ Use an 18-gauge needle, not a Veress needle, to create the pneumoperitoneum.
- ✓ Do not use three portals. Use the VSD to seal and dissect the ovaries.
- ✓ An abdominal insufflation pressure of 6–8 mmHg is enough.
- ✓ Use the tip of the VSD to retract the spleen (if it obscures the view of the left ovary) by grabbing the fat and the vessel at the hilus.
- ✓ Dissect the fat before placing the 3 mm cannula to help with closure.

15.3 LAPAROSCOPIC OVARIECTOMY IN A DOG WITH TYPE III SCLEROSING ENCAPSULATING PERITONITIS

Michael Brückner

CASE DESCRIPTION

A 14-month-old intact female mixed-breed dog was diagnosed with type III sclerosing encapsulating peritonitis (SEP) at the age of 5 months after a routine workup including biopsy performed during exploratory laparotomy. About 1 year later the owner wanted to spay her dog and an OVE was recommended, especially due to the presence of extensive adhesions. A laparoscopic approach was chosen to reduce the amount of intraoperative tissue manipulation and inflammation as well as to minimize the size of the incision, as the dog was on prednisolone treatment. A standard two-port approach was chosen and dissection of the adhesions reduced to a minimum. Both ovaries were temporarily fixated with a percutaneous needle–suture combination and transected using a VSD.

Key points

- Minimal tissue manipulation keeps inflammation low.
- Blunt dissection avoids further inflammation.
- The use of percutaneous suspension reduces the number of ports.

PORT PLACEMENT

A 6 mm Ternamian Endotip trocar was placed in the umbilicus (camera port), and an 11 mm cannula with multifunction valve was placed half-way between the umbilicus and the pubic rim. The patient was tilted to the right and left sides to reach the respective contralateral ovaries.

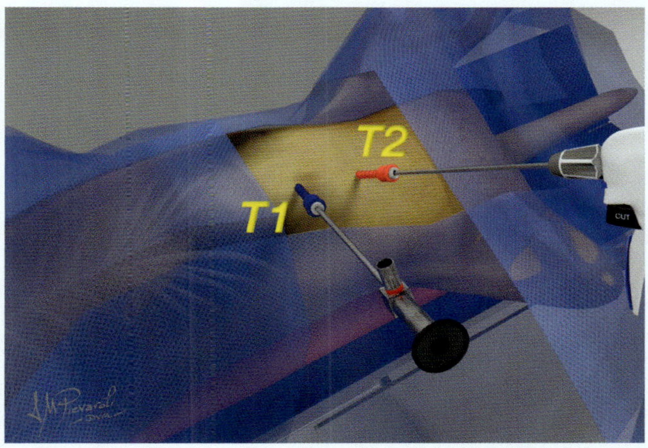

PROCEDURE

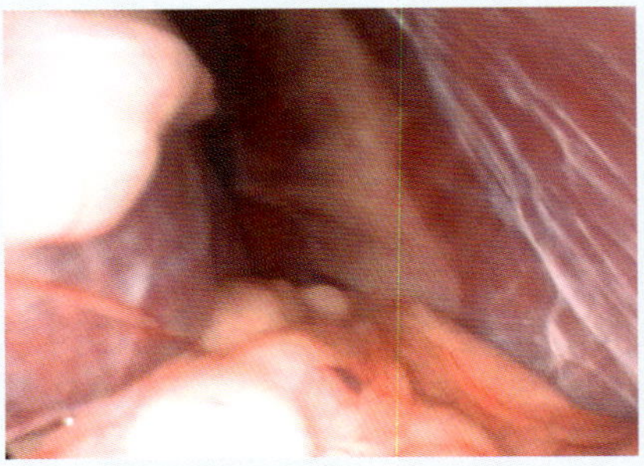

FIGURE 1. Transition between the abdominal wall and diaphragm. Multiple fibrin strands are visible over the peritoneum. The stomach and spleen are enclosed in a sac of fibrous tissue.

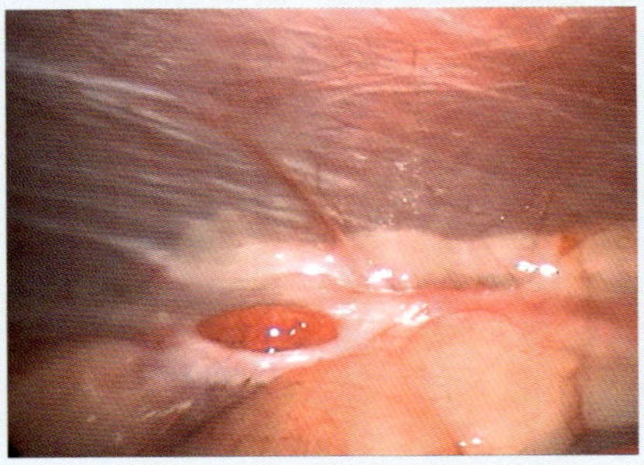

FIGURE 2. The left bursa ovarica is visible as well as the fibrin strands on the peritoneal lining of the abdominal wall.

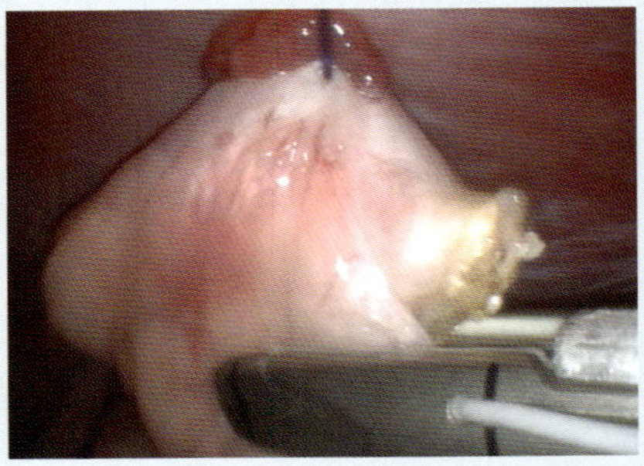

FIGURE 3. The left ovary is temporarily suspended from the abdominal wall with a needle–suture combination, and the uterine horn is transected with a vessel-sealing device.

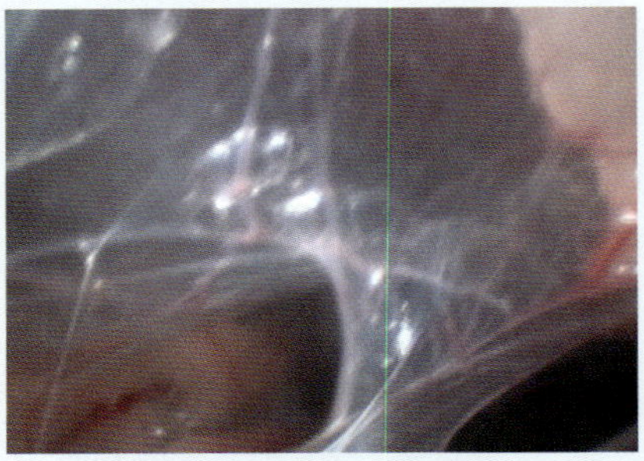

FIGURE 4. Multiple adhesions between the organs prevent the visualization of the right ovary.

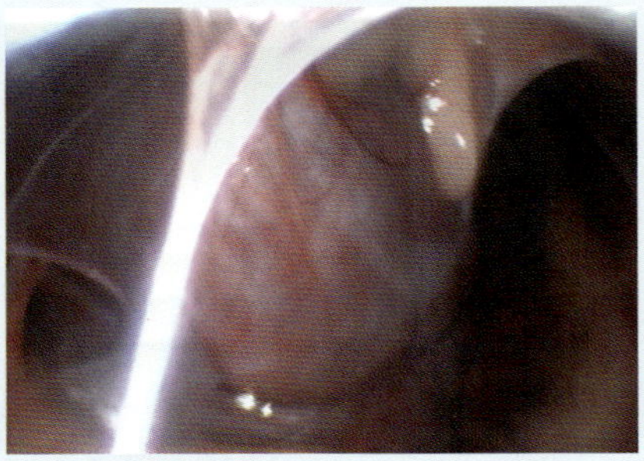

FIGURE 5. The urinary bladder is attached to the ventral abdominal wall and has multiple adhesions around.

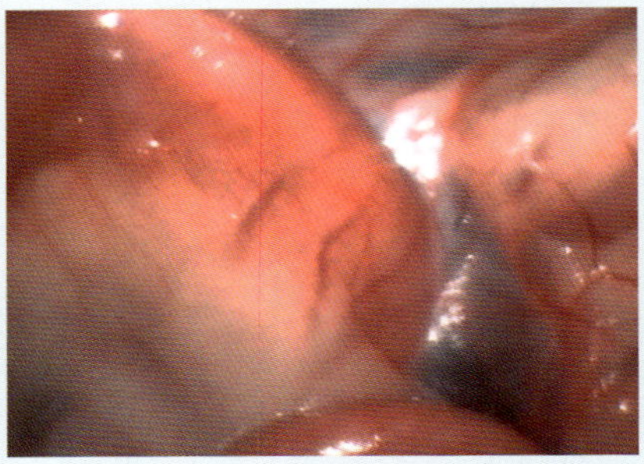

FIGURE 6. The camera is switched to the caudal port, and the adhesions between the small intestinal loops are partially dissected with the grasping forceps.

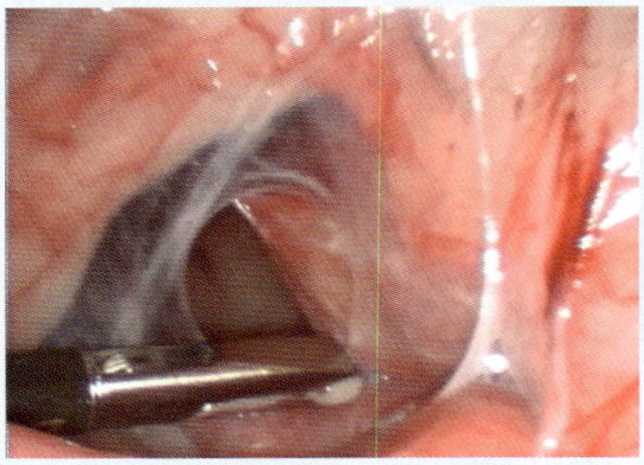

FIGURE 7. The camera is switched back to the cranial port. The small intestinal loops are further dissected to allow visualization of the right ovary.

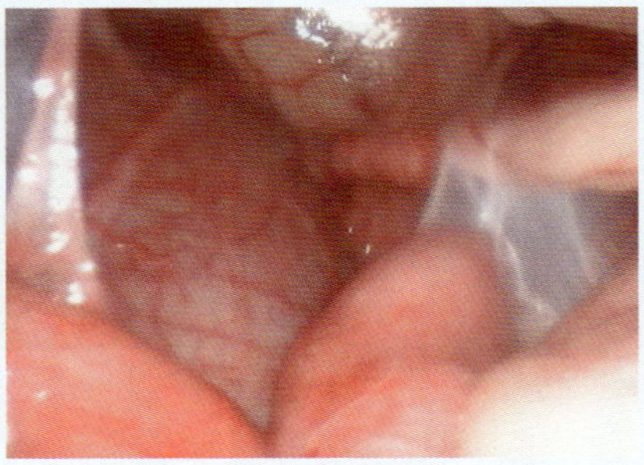

FIGURE 8. Further adhesions between the urinary bladder, uterus, and small intestinal loops, allowing classification as type III sclerosing encapsulating peritonitis.

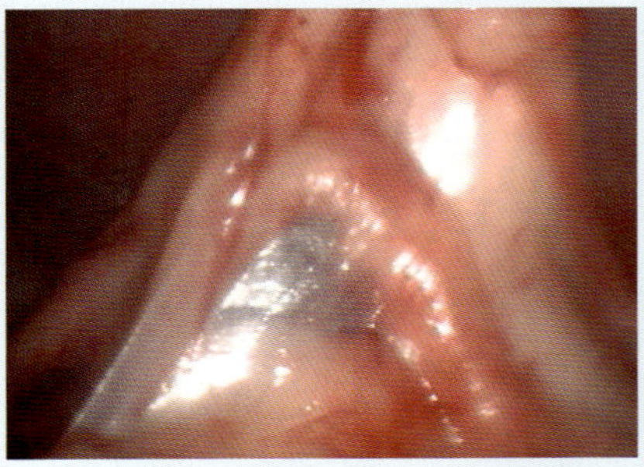

FIGURE 9. The right ovary is percutaneously attached to the abdominal wall. A small intestinal loop is adhered to the mesometrium. The suspensory ligament is to the right of the image.

Tips and tricks

- ✓ Use gravity to your advantage.
- ✓ Switch between ports.
- ✓ Use a VSD.

15.4 LAPAROSCOPIC OVARIECTOMY IN LARGE- AND GIANT-BREED DOGS

Paolo Boschi, Roberto Properzi

CASE DESCRIPTION

One of the complications associated with lapOVE in large- and giant-breed dogs is the difficulty of removing the ovary through the operating cannula due to its large size. This complication increases surgical time and the risk of ovarian tissue rupture. To facilitate ovary removal, it is recommended to transect the ovarian bursa with a bipolar VSD and remove the ovarian tissue without the ovarian bursa through the operating portal.

Key points

- One of the complications of lapOVE in large- and giant-breed dogs is the difficulty of removing the ovary through the operating cannula.
- In large- and giant-breed dogs, the ovarian tissue should be separated from the ovarian bursa and removed through the operating cannula.

PORT PLACEMENT

A standard three-midline-ports laparoscopic approach was used. The first cannula (T1) was placed 1–2 cm cranial to the umbilicus and a 10 mm 30° telescope was introduced. A 5 mm cannula (T2) was placed 4 cm caudal to T1. A 10 mm cannula (T3) was placed 4 cm caudal to T2.

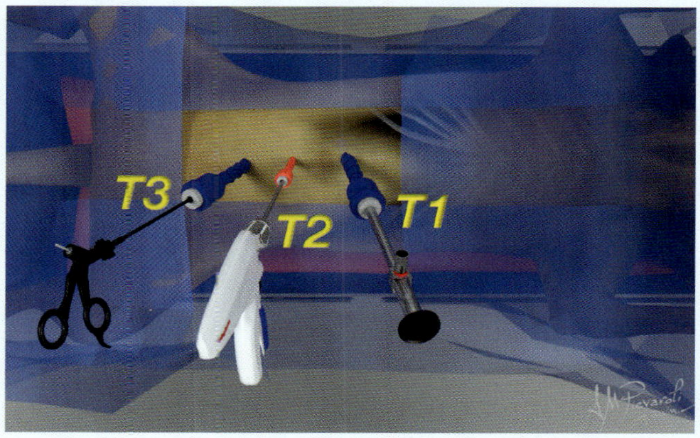

PROCEDURE

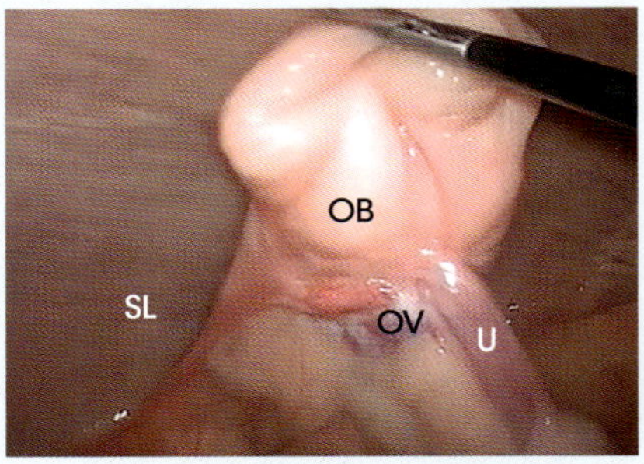

FIGURE 1. The ovarian bursa (OB) is grasped and pulled using laparoscopic Babcock forceps. Note the ovarian vessels (OV), uterus (U), and suspensory ligament (SL).

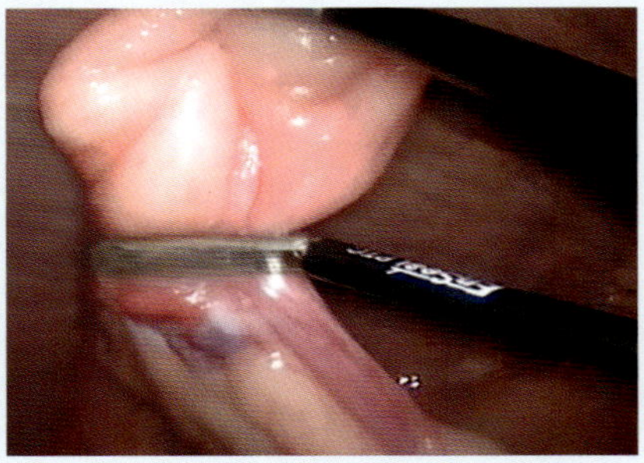

FIGURE 2. The ovarian bursa is transected using a bipolar vessel-sealing device. It can be partially or completely transected.

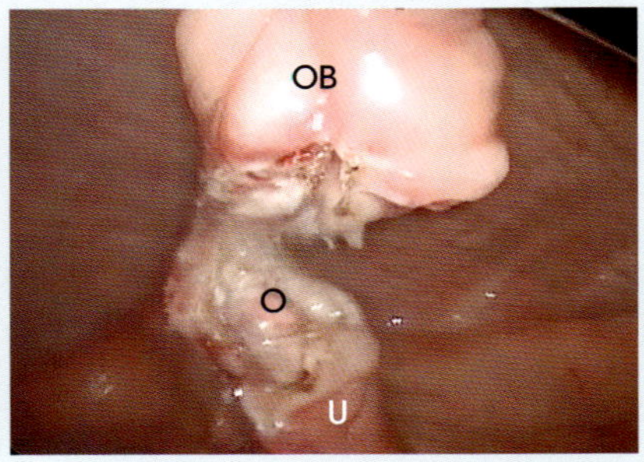

FIGURE 3. Ovarian bursa (OB) partially transected. O, ovary; U, uterus.

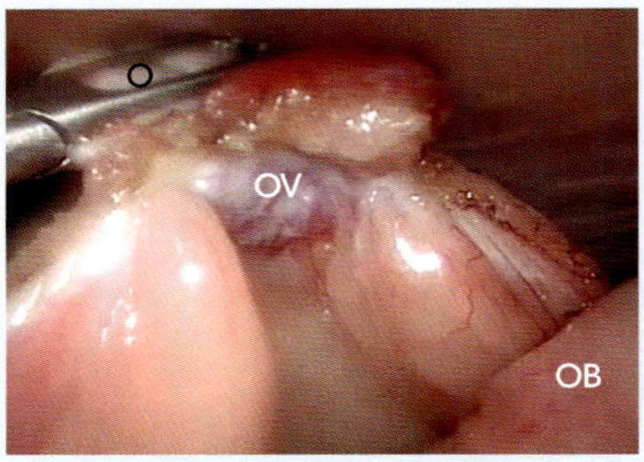

FIGURE 4. The ovary (O) is grasped with the laparoscopic Babcock forceps. Note the transected ovarian vessels (OV) and ovarian bursa (OB).

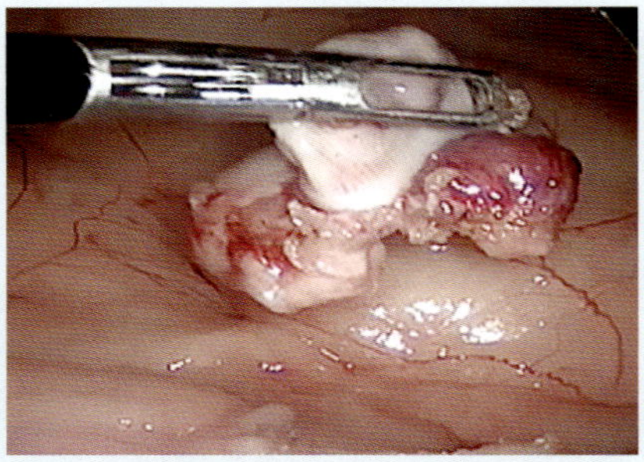

FIGURE 5. The ovary is freed from the ovarian bursa with a gentle rocking motion and is easily extracted from the abdomen through the 10 mm operating cannula.

Tips and tricks

- ✓ Transect the ovarian bursa to make ovary removal easier in large- and giant-breed dogs.
- ✓ Gently pull the freed ovary, without the ovarian bursa, through the operating cannula and out of the abdomen.

15.5 TWO-PORT LAPAROSCOPIC OVARIECTOMY WITHOUT OVARY SUSPENSION SUTURE IN A FEMALE DOG

Giovanni Allevi

CASE DESCRIPTION

A new lapOVE technique has been evaluated in 50 female dogs. This technique is performed using only two ports, with no suspension of the ovaries.

Key points

- This technique does not involve suspension of the ovary using a transabdominal suspension suture with a round needle or forceps.
- It is important to check for any uterine condition to evaluate the need for an OVH.

PORT PLACEMENT

The patient was placed in dorsal recumbency for setting up the operating field: a two-port technique with two 5 mm trocars was performed (VersaPort, Covidien). The first cannula (T1) was placed 1 cm caudal to the umbilicus with a modified Hasson technique and a 5 mm 30° telescope (Karl Storz Veterinary Endoscopy) was introduced; the abdomen was inflated with carbon dioxide (CO_2) with a pressure of 10 mmHg. The second cannula (T2) was placed on the midline, a few centimeters caudal to T1.

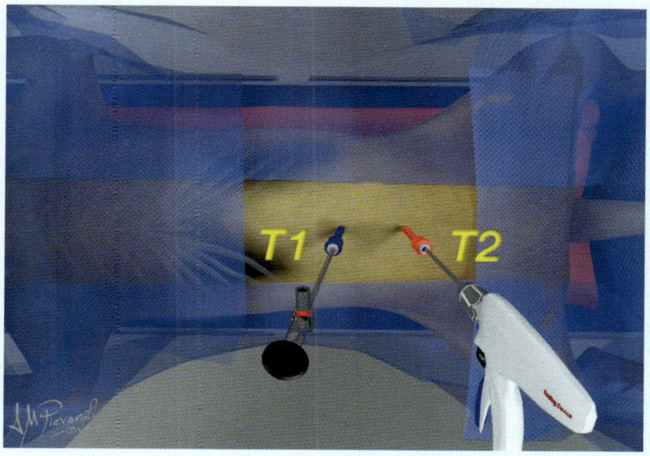

PROCEDURE

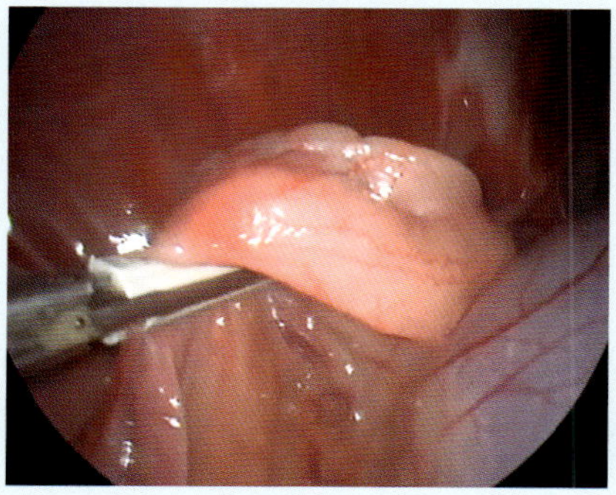

FIGURE 1. The ligation device suspends the ovary and moves it away from the abdominal wall and the other organs in a safe position.

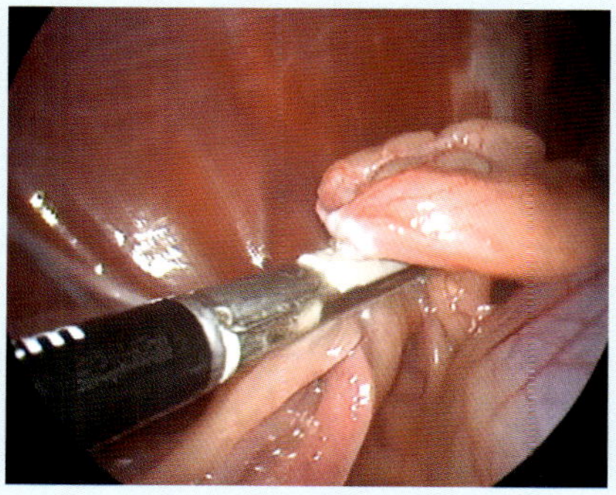

FIGURE 2. Continuous cranial sliding of the laparoscopic ligation device – ovarian ligament.

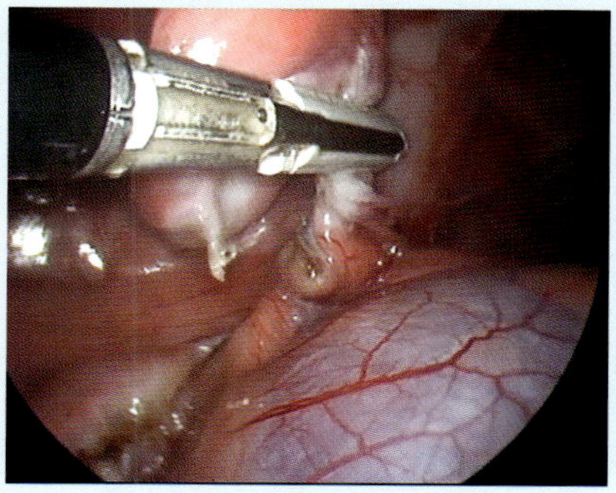

FIGURE 3. Continuous cranial sliding of the laparoscopic ligation device – suspensory ligament.

Tips and tricks

- ✓ During the use of the ligation device, a proper distance from the abdominal wall is essential in order to avoid causing injuries or pain to the patient.
- ✓ The procedure consists in a constant progression of the laparoscopic ligation device along the tissue and a continuous switching between cauterization and cutting.

15.6 LAPAROSCOPIC OVARIECTOMY IN AN AFRICAN LIONESS (*PANTHERA LEO*) USING A SINGLE-PORT MULTIPLE-ACCESS DEVICE

Mathieu Manassero

CASE DESCRIPTION

A 22-month-old lioness weighing 100 kg was presented for elective OVE for breeding control. After suitable immobilization, a catheter was placed in the cephalic vein and intravenous propofol (titrated to effect) was given to facilitate intubation. Anesthesia was maintained by sevoflurane in 100% oxygen delivered via the orotracheal tube. Electrocardiography, capnography, pulse oximetry, esophageal temperature, noninvasive blood pressure, and respiratory rate were monitored during anesthesia. The lioness was placed on a mechanical ventilator throughout the surgical procedure with an end-tidal CO_2 between 35 and 40 mmHg and a maximal airway pressure of 20 cmH_2O.

Key points

- Because of the depth of subcutaneous fat, extensive subcutaneous dissection was necessary to insert the single-port multiple-access device.
- The single-port multiple-access device was placed cautiously under visual control to avoid causing lesions and damage to abdominal organs.
- Traction on the muscular margins was maintained during insertion of the cannula to provide counter pressure and avoid iatrogenic lesions.
- After single-port device introduction, the lioness was put in a 10° Trendelenburg position and the operating table tilted at a 15° angle approximately on the right side for the left ovary and the left side for the right one to enhance exposure.
- Specific bent or articulated instruments are not necessary to perform an OVE.
- The single-port device and the first transected ovary should be removed before performing the contralateral OVE to prevent any loss of the ovary in the abdomen.
- The skin was closed with an intradermal continuous suture pattern.

PORT PLACEMENT

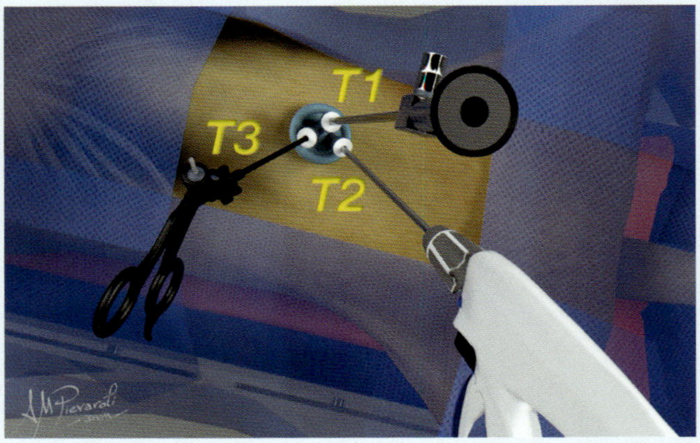

A single-port multiple-access technique was used with the SILS Port (Covidien, Norwalk, CT, USA). The lioness was positioned in dorsal recumbency and the abdominal area was aseptically prepared. A 2 to 3 cm skin incision was made just caudal to the umbilicus and carried down to the peritoneum.

After introduction of the single-port device, a pneumoperitoneum (12 mmHg) was induced using CO_2 through the specific cannula of the device.

PROCEDURE

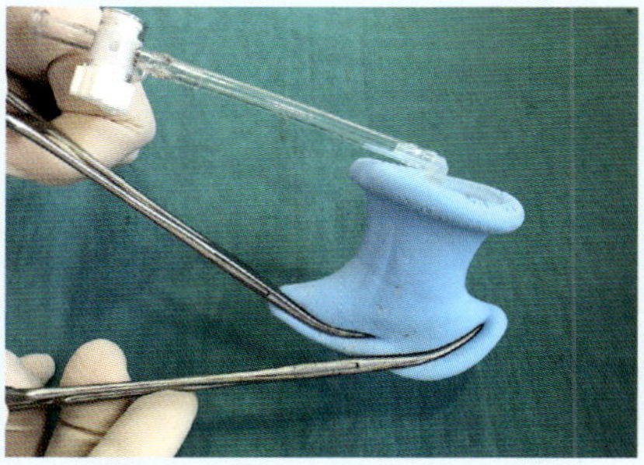

FIGURE 1. The single-port device is folded at the level of the lower ridge with the use of two curved forceps, which clamp the device in a staggered fashion.

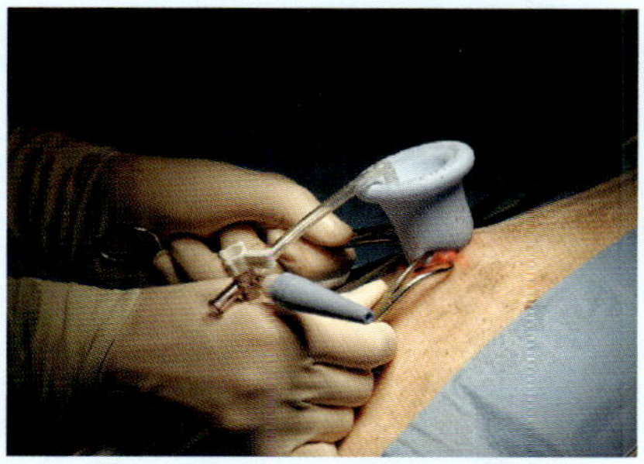

FIGURE 2. The muscular margins of the incised linea alba are grasped and everted with Babcock forceps. The lower ridge of the single-port device is subsequently introduced into the abdomen and then released from the forceps.

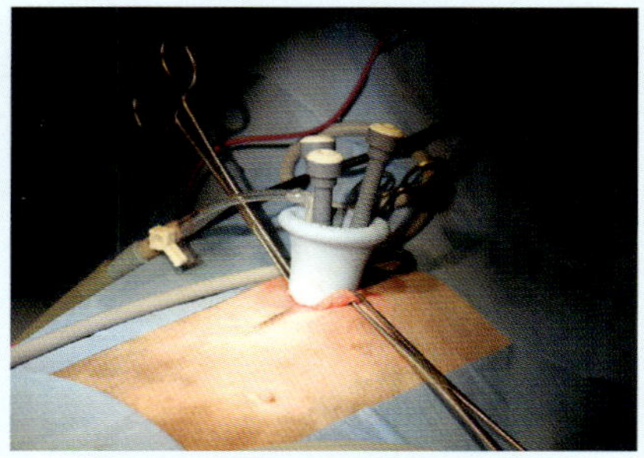

FIGURE 3. Three 5 mm cannulas are introduced through the access channels with a blunt trocar, which is subsequently withdrawn, and the pneumoperitoneum (12 mmHg) is induced.

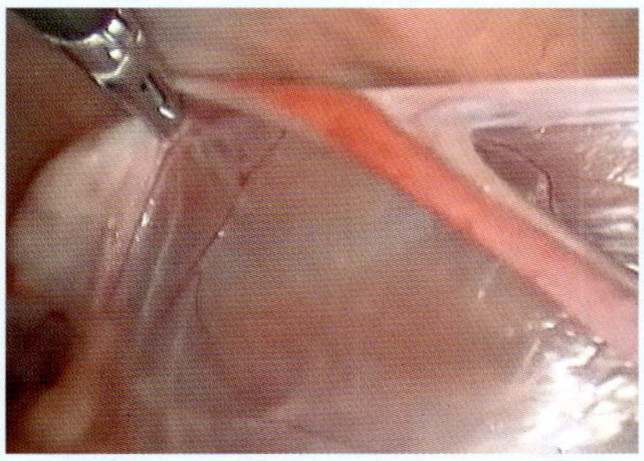

FIGURE 4. The table is tilted to the right side to expose the left ovary. The proper ligament is then grasped and suspended using a standard 5 mm laparoscopic grasper.

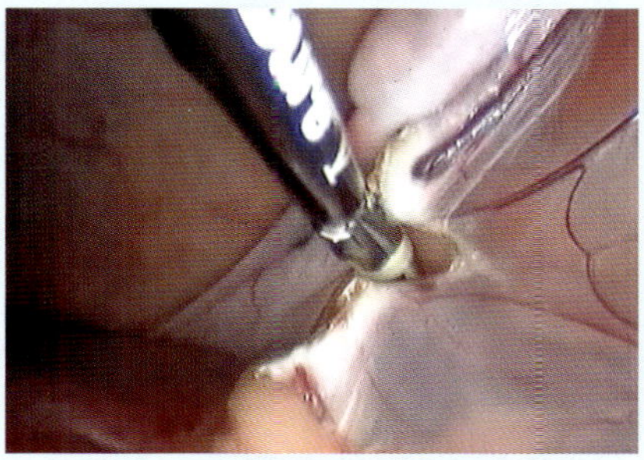

FIGURE 5. The proper ligament is pulled caudally and the ovarian pedicle is sealed and transected first with a 5 mm laparoscopic vessel sealer/divider device.

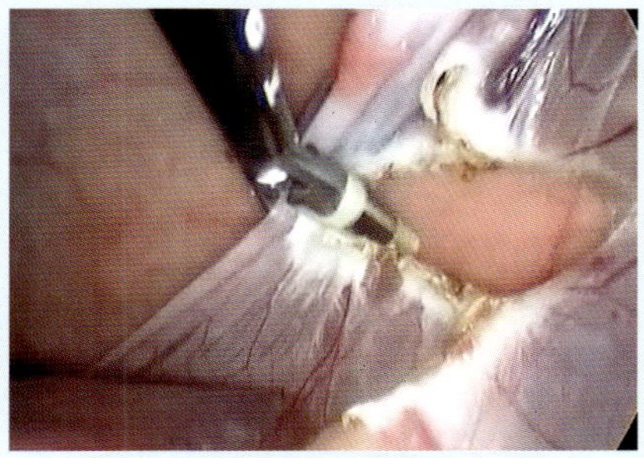

FIGURE 6. The cranial part of the mesovarium is subsequently sealed and transected to the suspensory ligament with the vessel sealer/divider device while moving the ovary caudally.

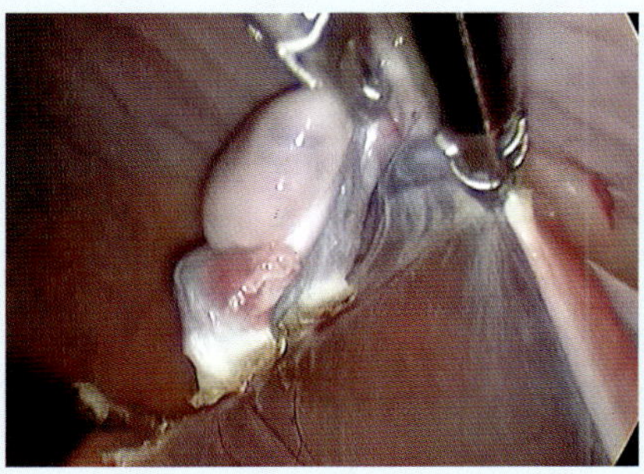

FIGURE 7. Finally, the proper ligament is pulled cranially and the proximal part of the uterine horn and caudal part of the mesovarium are sealed and transected with the vessel sealer/divider device while moving the ovary cranially.

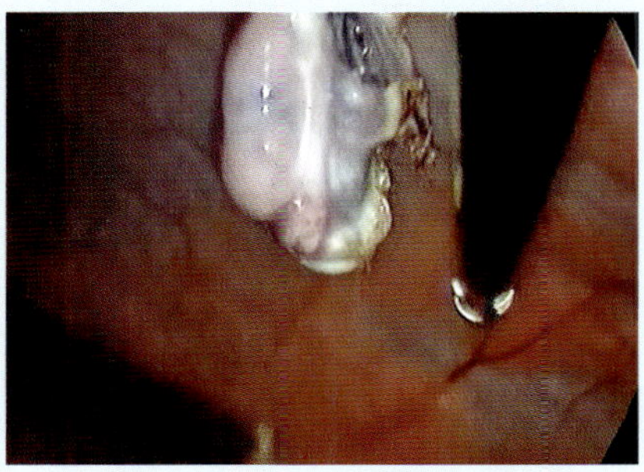

FIGURE 8. While the transected left ovary is firmly grasped with the laparoscopic grasper, the vessel sealer/divider device, the telescope, single-port device, and associated cannulas are removed and the grasper and ovary are subsequently retrieved from the abdomen. The single-port device is reintroduced as previously described and the right ovariectomy is performed in the same way.

Tips and tricks

- ✓ The muscular margins of the incised linea alba can be grasped with stay sutures (0 polyglactin 910) instead of Babcock forceps to provide more working space for single-port device insertion.
- ✓ To increase maneuverability and decrease potential conflict between the instruments and telescope, the use of a 30° telescope and a right-angle adaptor placed onto the connection between the light cable and telescope is advised.
- ✓ Place the telescope port in the most lateral and upper access of the single-port device. To accommodate this position the single-port device can easily be rotated after its insertion.
- ✓ Do not hesitate to switch the position in the single-port device of the laparoscopic grasper and the vessel sealer/divider device to increase safe use of the vessel sealer/divider device.
- ✓ Use of 43 to 45 cm long laparoscopic instruments is advised in lionesses.
- ✓ Apply the vessel sealer/divider device as close as possible to the ovary and uterine body to avoid causing damage to a large mesometrial vessel or ureter.
- ✓ For device removal, remove first the cannula, which allows the abdomen to deflate, relieves pressure on the muscular edges of the laparotomy incision, and thus facilitates removal of the device.
- ✓ Even if this is possible, the use of a 10 mm vessel sealer/divider device into a 10 mm cannula is not advised because it reduces triangulation if specific bent or articulated instruments are not used.

15.7 LESS OVARIECTOMY USING A SIMPLE HANDMADE ACCESS DEVICE

Marco Augusto Machado Silva, Maurício Veloso Brun

CASE DESCRIPTION

There is a growing interest towards laparoendoscopic single-site surgery (LESS) approaches in the small animal setting. Several autoclavable and single-use LESS access devices are available. Almost all of them were developed for use in human patients and require a 2–4 cm long incision (usually at the umbilicus, for cosmetic purposes). While cosmetic appeal is not a frequent (if any) concern in small animals, decreased pain and wounds are the most important benefits reported. Limitations of LESS devices and instruments in the veterinary practice include lack of triangulation, need for expensive long curved instruments to compensate the lack of triangulation, and absence of LESS devices designed for use in small animals, especially small dogs and cats. To fill these gaps, a simple and relatively inexpensive handmade LESS access device was developed for both OVE and OVH in small dogs and cats. The main advantages of this device are use of two channels, no need for expensive operative laparoscopes, no need for curved LESS instruments, short (about 6–10 mm) incision length, works as a specimen retrieval device, quick and easy to assemble and to adjust to the abdominal wall, and provides optimal seal, avoiding CO_2 leak.

Key points

- Components of the handmade LESS device: two trocar cannulas (3–5 mm), a funnel obtained from a plastic (polyethylene terephthalate, PET) bottle, a latex balloon, two urinary catheters (8 and 12 Fr), and a 2-0 nylon thread.
- Preparation: the catheters are sterile, the latex balloon is steam sterilized, and the plastic cone should be sterilized using “cold” methods (soaking, peroxide plasma, ethylene oxide).
- Assembly of the device:
  1. Assembly a ring of 1.5–2.0 cm diameter using the 8 Fr and 12 Fr urinary catheters.
  2. Cover the funnel with the balloon.
  3. Pass the sheath of the balloon through the ring.
  4. Fold the balloon sheath backwards, covering the ring and the small hole of the funnel (a short latex sheath of about 5–10 mm must remain between the ring and the small hole of the funnel).
  5. Make two holes in the balloon, at the large hole of the funnel.
  6. Insert the two trocar cannulas through the two holes in the balloon.
  7. Attach the cannulas to the balloon with two encircling sutures. The device is ready for use.

PORT PLACEMENT

The patient and the surgical field were aseptically prepared as for two-port lapOVE, including clipping of the paralumbar area. A 6–10 mm midline celiotomy was performed 1–3 cm caudal to the umbilicus. The ring of the handmade device was inserted through the abdominal incision, leaving the funnel outside the abdominal cavity. At this point, the device will seem locked inside the abdominal cavity, as the ring reexpands when released within the cavity and the sheath of the device is short enough to keep the abdominal wall trapped between the ring and the small hole of the funnel. The CO_2 cable was connected to the valve of one of the cannulas for abdominal insufflation. The telescope and an instrument were inserted through the cannulas.

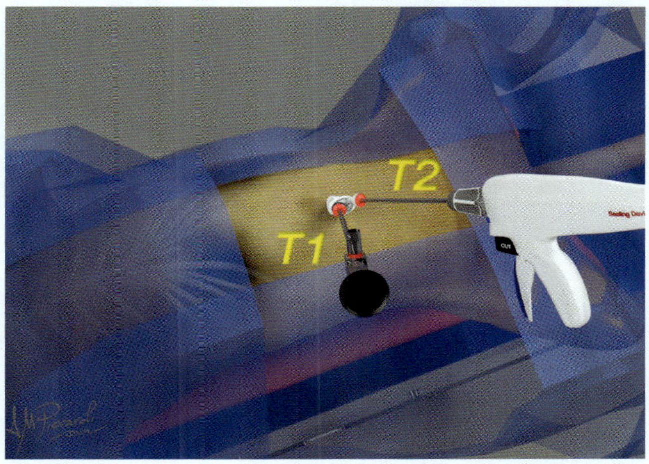

PROCEDURE

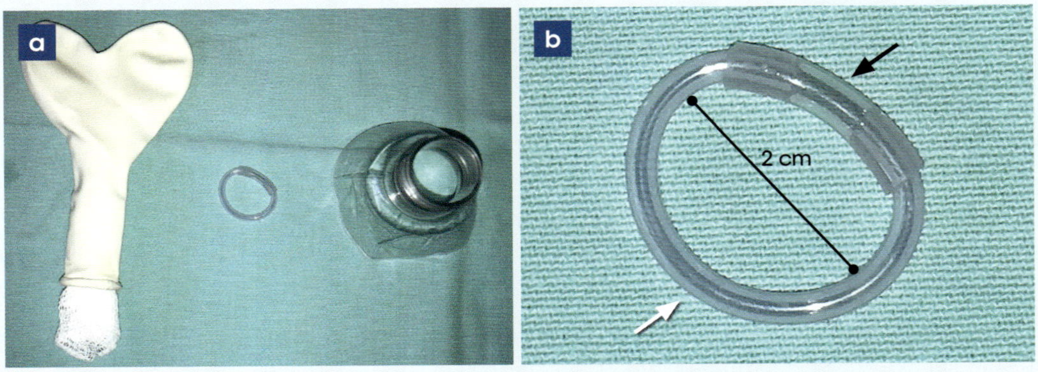

FIGURE 1. Components of the handmade LESS access device. a) Left: a heart-shaped latex balloon. Middle: a ring made from 8 Fr and 12 Fr urinary catheters. Right: a funnel obtained from a plastic (PET) bottle. b) Detail of the catheter ring. A piece of a 12 Fr catheter (black arrow) is coupled to a piece of an 8 Fr catheter (white arrow). Inner diameter of 2 cm.

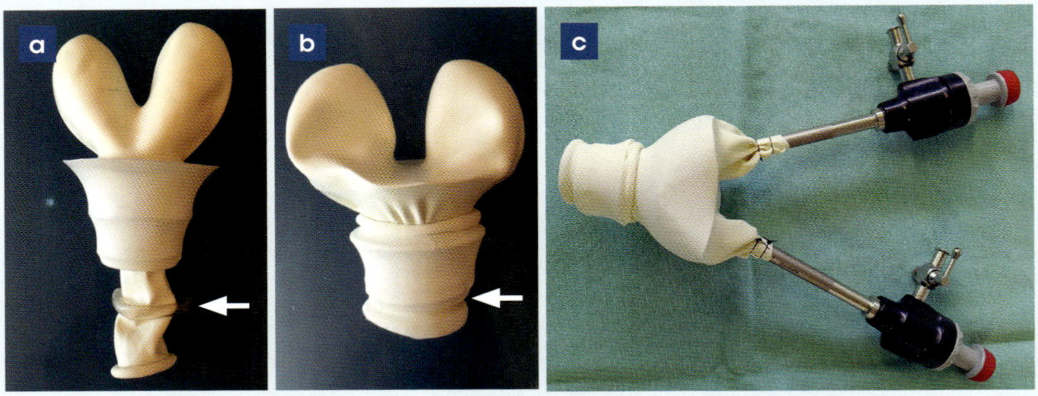

FIGURE 2. Assembly of the handmade LESS access device. a) The plastic funnel is covered by the latex balloon. The sheath of the balloon is passed through the catheter ring (arrow). b) The sheath of the balloon is folded backwards to cover the ring and the small hole of the funnel. A short sheath (arrow) remains between the ring and the small hole of the funnel. c) Device ready for use.

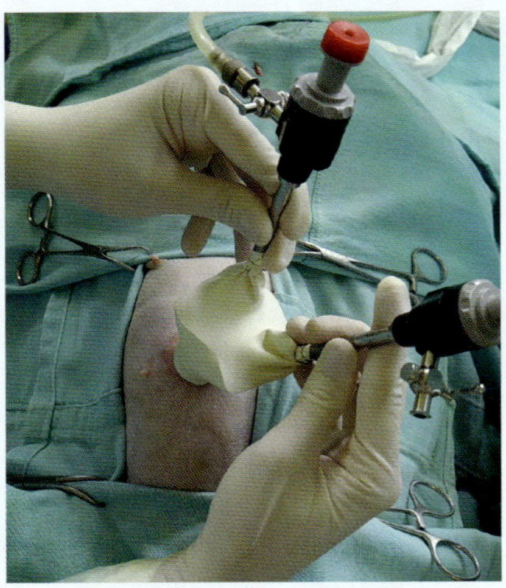

FIGURE 3. The handmade LESS access device in the abdominal cavity of a cat (bottom of image, caudal; top of image, cranial). Note the CO_2 cable attached to the valve of the most cranial cannula.

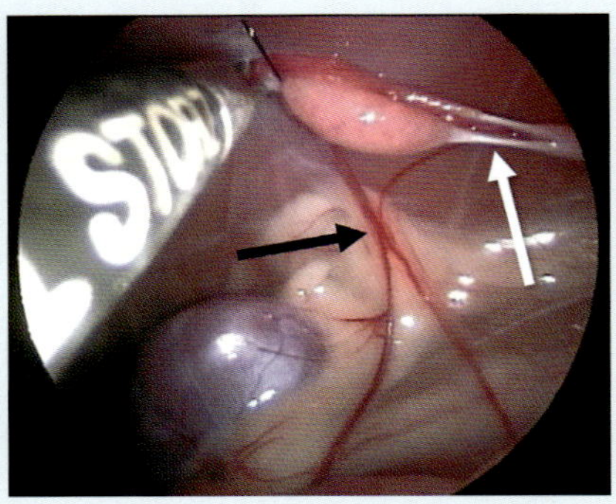

FIGURE 4. The operating table is tilted laterally to the right side to expose the left ovarian pedicle, as traditionally performed in the two-port lapOVE approach. The ovary is lifted against the abdominal wall using grasping forceps and a tacking suture is applied to the suspensory ligament. Note the wide exposition of the ovarian pedicle (black arrow) and proper ligament (white arrow).

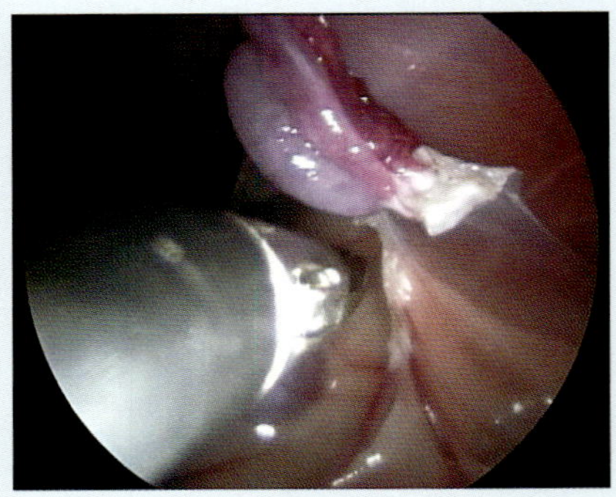

FIGURE 5. Bipolar forceps with a cutting blade (or vessel-sealing device or ultrasonic scalpel) are used to coagulate and transect the uterine horn and vessels as close as possible to the proper ligament. Then, the ovarian pedicle and suspensory ligament are coagulated and transected.

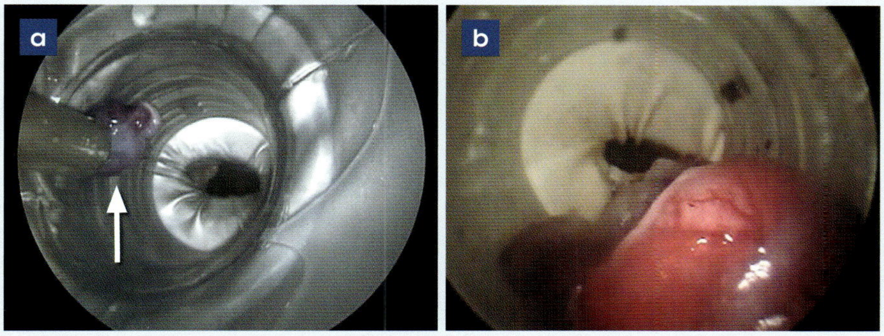

FIGURE 6. The ovary is grasped by the suspensory ligament, uterine horn stump, or proper ligament, and the tacking suture is released. a) The ovary (arrow) is retrieved through the cannula of the device. The contralateral ovary is removed in the same manner. The device is retrieved by gentle traction and the wound is closed routinely. b) Large ovaries, like the one shown in the image (from a dog), can be stored inside the device for further retrieval after resection of both ovaries.

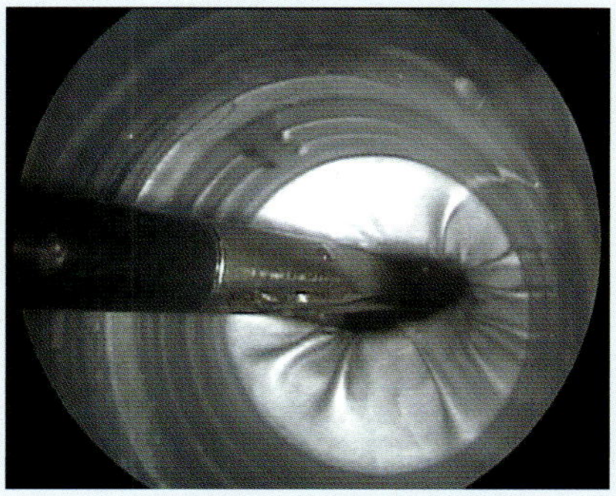

FIGURE 7. Instrument switching, if required, is performed under endoscopic guidance. In the image, Metzenbaum scissors are inserted into the abdominal cavity after pulling the endoscope back into the access device.

Tips and tricks

- ✓ The funnel can be of different materials (e.g., steel, polypropylene, etc.).
- ✓ If small-diameter (≈3 mm) instruments, telescope, and trocars are used, the celiotomy should be shorter (≈6 mm).
- ✓ In cases of small umbilical hernias, access can be performed through the defect.
- ✓ Ensure that the ring of the device is correctly and completely placed through the linea alba incision, not in the subcutaneous or retroperitoneal space.
- ✓ The authors prefer to place the device so that the trocars are aligned with the patient's long axis; that is, one cannula is cranial and the other caudal.
- ✓ Preferably insert the telescope through the cranial cannula. Although some sword fighting may occur, this will make instrument motion easier, resembling the two-port lapOVE technique.
- ✓ If instrument change is necessary, pull the telescope back within the device to assist instrument entry.
- ✓ The authors prefer to grasp the suspensory ligament rather than the proper ligament or the uterine horn to lift the ovary against the abdominal wall. Thus, the transparietal suture is passed through the suspensory ligament. This provides better exposition of the proper ligament and ovarian pedicle.
- ✓ If the ovary is too large to be withdrawn through a 3–5 mm cannula, it should be released within the device. The same maneuver is then performed for resection of the contralateral ovary, and the device with both ovaries inside is finally removed.

16 LAPAROSCOPY FOR OVARIAN REMNANT SYNDROME

J. Brad Case

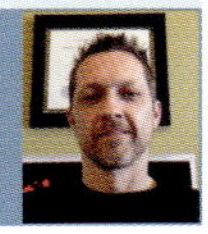

Indications

- Removal of the ovarian remnant tissue for obviation of estrous-related behaviors
- Prevention of ovarian-related diseases (e.g., pyometra, mammary neoplasia)

Contraindications

- No explicit contraindications for laparoscopic ovarian remnant surgery have been determined
- Stable dogs and cats with an intact diaphragm and no cardiopulmonary disease are ideal

Ovarian remnant syndrome (ORS) is a regularly reported condition that results from incomplete removal of all ovarian tissue at the time of gonadectomy. It most commonly affects the right ovarian pedicle due to the more cranial nature of the right ovary versus the left. Increased body weight has been associated with an increased risk of ORS. Although clinical signs consistent with estrous cycling and a history of gonadectomy without confirmation of complete ovary removal are enough to justify laparoscopic exploration, hormone panels including luteinizing hormone assay and diagnostic ultrasonography are useful in confirming a diagnosis of ORS (**Fig. 1**). Laparoscopic exploration to identify and excise the remnant ovarian tissue is desirable due to the excellent magnification and illumination provided as well as the ability to access the deep abdominal gutters via a minimally invasive approach (**Fig. 2**). Furthermore, laparoscopy is the preferred approach over laparotomy due to the associated reduction in tissue injury and postoperative pain.

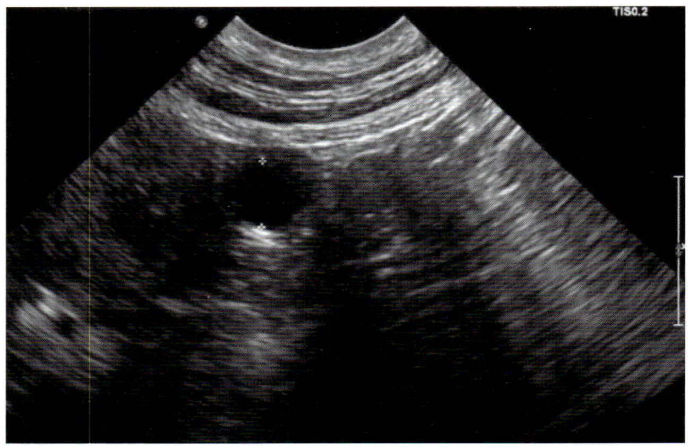

FIGURE 1. Transabdominal ultrasonographic image of an ovarian remnant in a dog. Note the round to ovoid anechoic appearance of the remnant ovary.

> The first report of laparoscopic ovarian remnant removal in dogs was published in 2014 by J. Naiman et al.

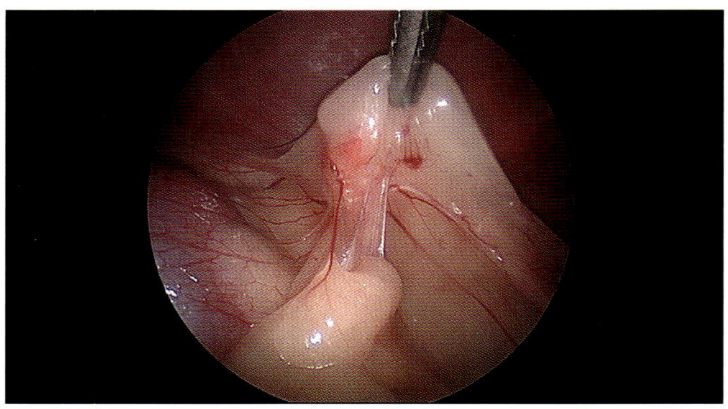

FIGURE 2. Laparoscopic view of an ovarian remnant. The left kidney is to the left of the image, an articulating grasper is seen retracting the remnant ventrally, the suspensory ligament is attached cranial to the kidney, the vascular pedicle is diving dorsally, and the uterus and mesometrium are coursing caudally to the right of the image.

DESCRIBED SURGICAL PROCEDURES

Both multiport (two or three) and single-port techniques have been described. However, no direct comparisons between techniques have been reported to date. Theoretical advantages of the single-port approach are improved safety during peritoneal access, lack of need for port-site enlargement, and ease of tissue removal versus multiport approaches. Potential disadvantages include cost of disposable single-port devices and loss of triangulation. The latter is overcome by the use of articulating instrumentation and angled telescopes.

PATIENT PREPARATION AND POSITIONING

A physical examination and basic blood work (packed red blood cell volume, total solids, blood glucose, and blood urea nitrogen) should be performed prior to elective laparoscopic ovarian remnantectomy. In general, dogs should be fasted at least 8 hours prior to anesthesia and have an IV catheter placed for fluid and medication therapy during the procedure. The urinary bladder should be expressed or drained with a urinary catheter at the time of anesthesia induction. Premedications that result in splenic enlargement (e.g., acepromazine) should be avoided. Perioperative analgesia may include opioid and/or nonsteroidal medications. Local anesthesia with bupivacaine is recommended at individual port sites prior to incision. The vast majority of dogs treated with perioperative nonsteroidal medication and oral tramadol return to baseline pain indices by 48 hours after laparoscopic ovariectomy. The patient is positioned in dorsal recumbency and clipped from the xiphoid process to the pubis and dorsally past the level of the 13th rib. If a hydraulic float table is available, the patient may be positioned directly on the operating table. In contrast, a rotating tray may be used for lateral rotation of the patient if a standard operating table is being used. The abdomen is aseptically prepared as for traditional laparotomy. This ensures that adequate preparation and quick conversion to laparotomy can be performed if needed.

OPERATING ROOM LAYOUT

Perhaps the most important factor when considering operating room layout is that the operating surgeon and surgeon assistant must be able to easily move from one side of the operating table to the other. This is necessary because for laparoscopic surgery of the right ovary the surgeon and assistant must operate from the left side of the patient. Similarly, when operating the left ovary, the surgeon and assistant must operate from the right side of the patient. Although bilateral ORS is exceedingly rare, it may occur, and exploration of both abdominal gutters may be necessary to find the remnant ovarian tissue if preoperative localization is unknown.

Although many layout options likely exist, the author's preference is to have the dog positioned at the foot of the operating table and the anesthesia circuit and staff positioned at the head of the operating table. The instrument back table is positioned at the foot of the operating table, with enough room for the surgeon and assistant to walk around the back table from side to side of the patient (**Fig. 3**). Either one or two viewing monitors can be used. If only the monitor on the tower is available, the tower and monitor must be easily moveable from one side to the other to

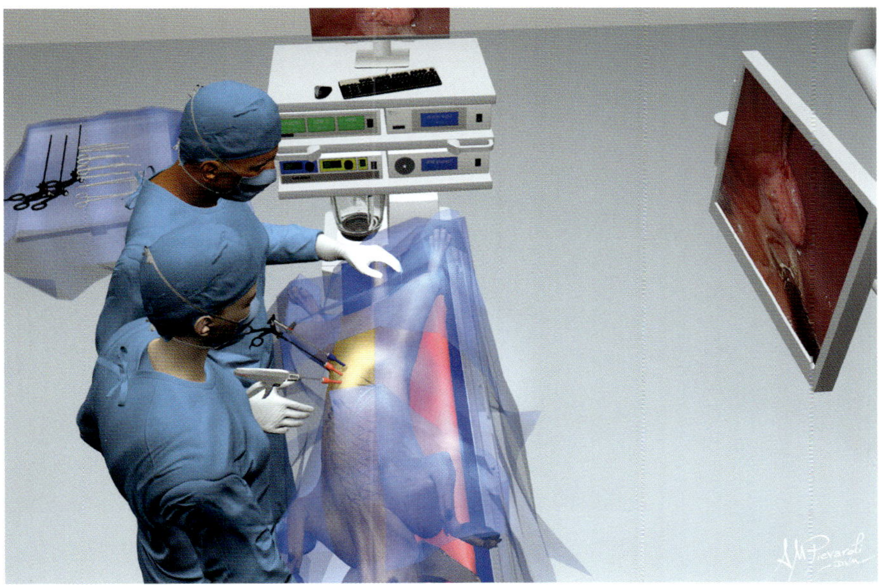

FIGURE 3. Operating room layout for laparoscopic ovarian remnant surgery.

facilitate ergonomic exploration of both the right and left abdominal gutters.

A three-port approach to ovarian remnantectomy is most commonly reported and is similar to that described for laparoscopic ovariectomy. Recently, a single-port approach in 13 dogs has been described. Both port placements are described herein.

Instruments

On the table:

- Standard abdominal surgical pack
- High-definition video camera
- Telescope 5 mm – 30°
- Three 5 mm cannulas
- Laparoscopic Babcock or DeBakey forceps, straight 5 mm
- Vessel-sealing device

Additional instrumentation for single-port approach:

- Single-incision surgery port (SILS, Medtronic) (**Fig. 4**)
- Laparoscopic endograsper (EndoClinch, Medtronic), articulating 5 mm (**Fig. 5**)

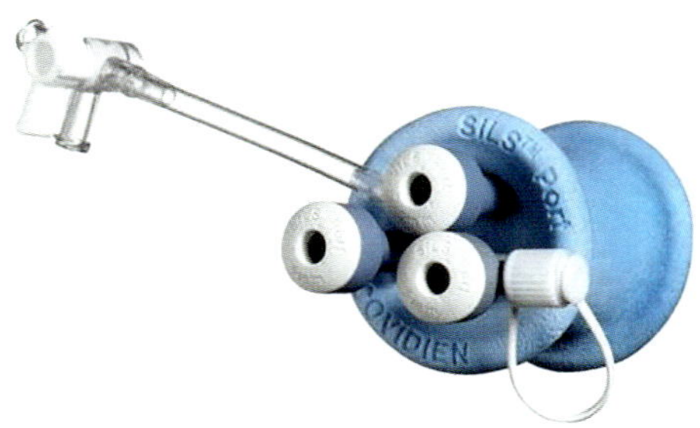

FIGURE 4. SILS port device.

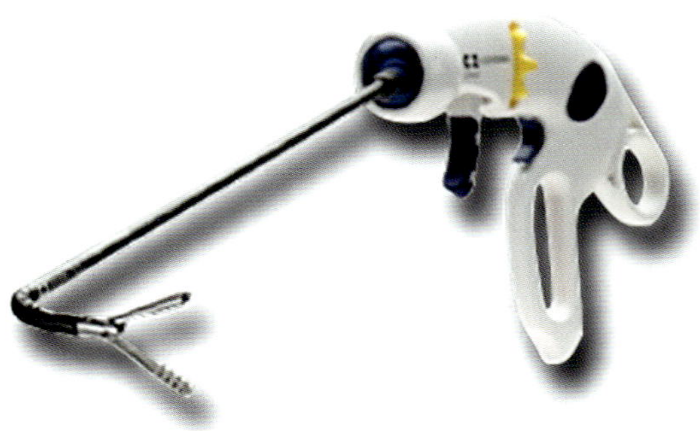

FIGURE 5. EndoClinch instrument.

PORT PLACEMENT

Three-port approach (**Fig. 6**):

- T1, on the midline, 2 cm caudad to the umbilicus
- T2, on the midline, 8 cm cranial to T1
- T3, on the midline, 4 cm cranial to T1

Triangulation between the laparoscope, instruments, and lesion is important, especially for the beginning laparoscopist. Ignorance of this principle makes for a more difficult and complicated surgery. A popular concept is the baseball field analogy, where the telescope (T1) may be thought of as third base, while T3 and T2 are the pitcher's mound and first base, respectively, for operations of the right ovary. For operations involving the left ovary, the analogy is reversed. Thus, the telescope (T1) is first base, T3 is the pitcher's mound, and T2 is third base.

Single-port approach (**Fig. 7**):

- T1, T2, T3, on the midline, 1–2 cm caudad to the umbilicus

Triangulation between the laparoscope, instruments, and lesion is lost with single-port laparoscopy. This makes for a more complicated surgery. To reconcile the loss of triangulation, articulating instruments and angled telescopes are needed when performing single-port procedures. The angled telescope allows for the camera and light post to be moved away from the midline while viewing the target tissue. An articulating grasper allows for the handle of the grasper to be moved towards the floor and thus frees up space for the vessel-sealing device to move freely during dissection of the mesovarium and pedicle (**Fig. 8**).

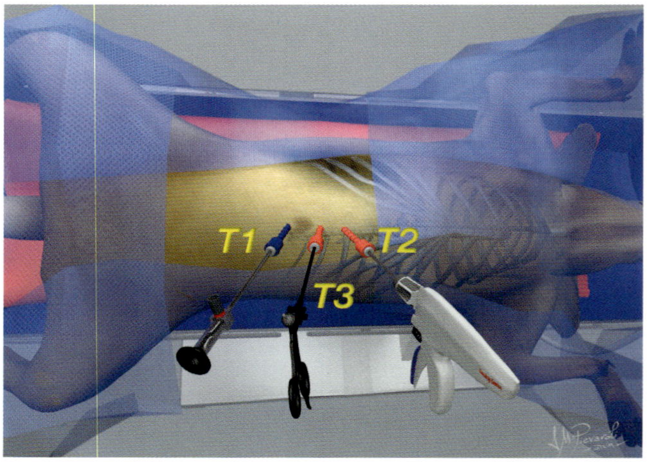

FIGURE 6. Three-port placement for ovarian remnant surgery.

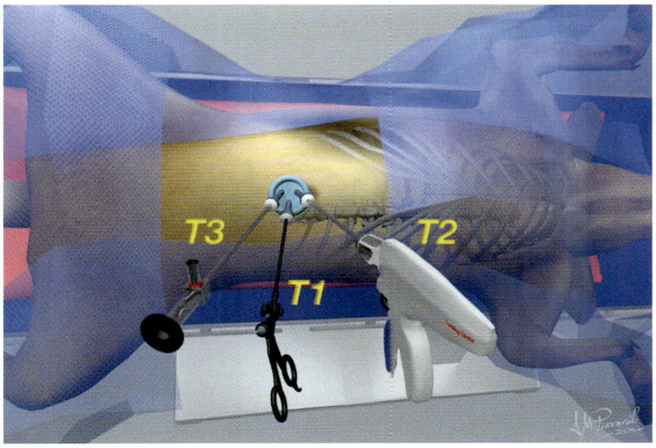

FIGURE 7. Single-port placement for ovarian remnant surgery.

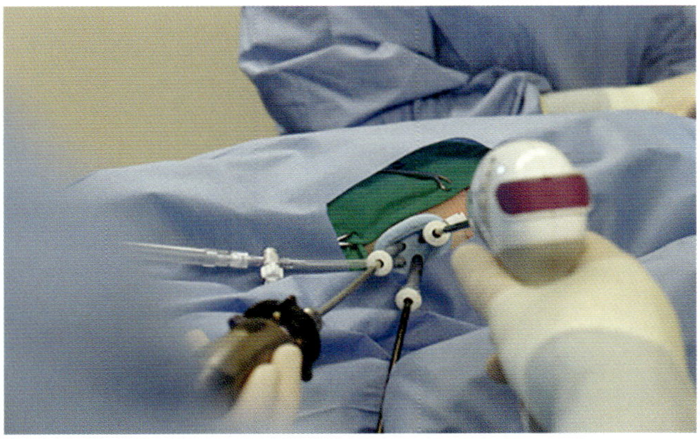

FIGURE 8. Intraoperative image of port and instrument position for right ovarian remnant removal. The camera is in the caudal port, the grasper in the central port, and the bipolar sealing device in the cranial port.

PROCEDURE

- After all ports are placed and pneumoperitoneum has been achieved, the patient is rotated approximately 45° to the left and right for initial exploration of the abdominal gutters.
- Remnant ovarian tissue is typically fleshy and pink in color but is often obscured by peritoneal adipose tissue (**Fig. 9**).
- Once suspect remnant tissue has been identified, the surgeon uses a grasping forceps in their nondominant hand to grasp and elevate the tissue ventrally away from the region of the ureters and retroperitoneum.
- A vessel-sealing device is used to bluntly and sharply dissect the mesovarium and ovarian pedicle subjacent to the remnant ovarian tissue (**Fig. 10**).

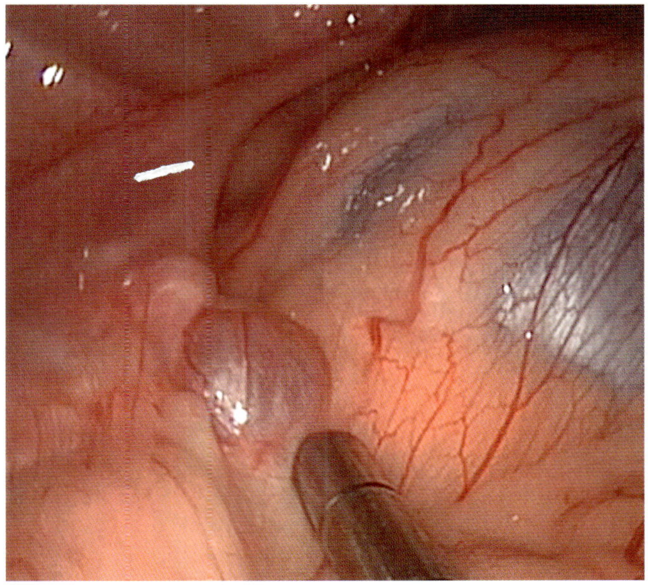

FIGURE 9. Laparoscopic view of a right ovarian remnant (at the tip of the blunt probe). The right kidney is to the right of the image.

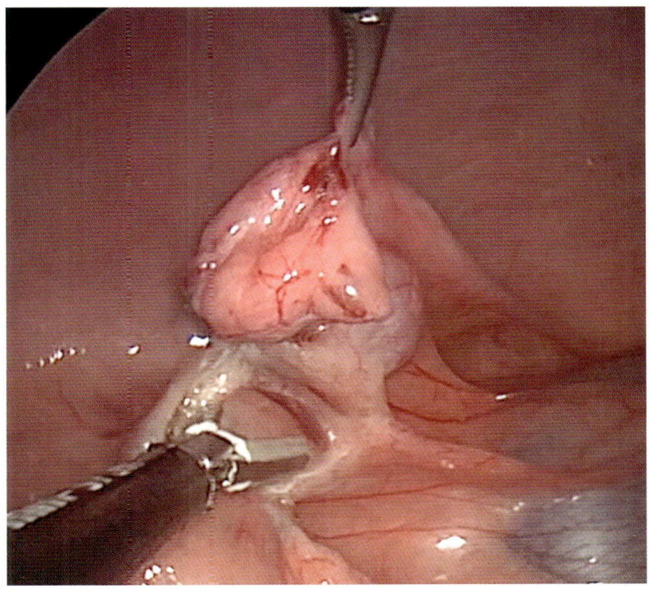

FIGURE 10. The right ovarian remnant is grasped and elevated away from the kidney and dorsal structures to facilitate safe dissection. A bipolar device is visible at the level of the dissection plane.

- The remnant ovarian tissue can be extracted after dilation of the grasping instrument port site (**Fig. 11**).
- Remnant ovarian tissue is typically fleshy and firm and a margin of mesovarium should be present around the suspected tissue.

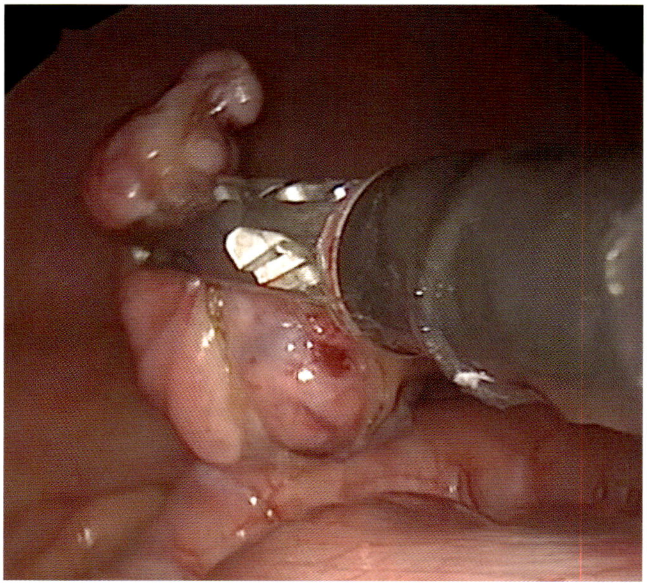

FIGURE 11. The completely dissected ovarian remnant is grasped with an articulating grasper just prior to removal.

POSTOPERATIVE MANAGEMENT

- Analgesic requirements for dogs undergoing laparoscopic ovarian remnant surgery appear to be minimal.
- Intraoperative infiltration of all port sites with local anesthetic affords 4–6 hours of analgesia postoperatively and, when coupled with nonsteroidal anti-inflammatory medication (2–3 days), is generally effective for uncomplicated laparoscopic ovarian remnant removal.
- If further analgesia is indicated, opioid medications can be included postoperatively. However, it is rare to require opioids beyond 48–72 hours following uncomplicated laparoscopic ovarian surgery.

Complications of laparoscopic ovarian remnant surgery

- Ovarian pedicle hemorrhage is a possible complication during dissection of an ovarian remnant, but this complication appears to be rare when a vessel-sealing device is used for transection of the ovarian vasculature.
- Incomplete removal or failure to remove the offending remnant is also a possibility due to poor exposure of the ovarian pedicles and/or failure to obtain diagnostic preoperative imaging.

Key points

- Laparoscopic ovarian remnant removal is minimally invasive and associated with excellent outcomes.
- The single-port technique facilitates tissue extraction and appears to be faster than the multiport approach.

SUGGESTED READINGS

CLINICAL CASES

16.1 OVARIAN REMNANT SYNDROME AFTER LAPAROSCOPIC OVARIECTOMY IN A CAT

Paolo Boschi, Roberto Properzi

CASE DESCRIPTION

The first case of accidental implantation of ovarian tissue at the port site after laparoscopic ovariectomy in a cat is described. A 2-year-old spayed female domestic cat showed recurrent behavioral signs of estrus 4 months after laparoscopic ovariectomy. ORS was presumed. Diagnostic laparoscopy confirmed the presence of a mass, macroscopically similar to ovarian tissue, attached to the peritoneal area caudal to the umbilicus where the laparoscopic port had been inserted to perform previous laparoscopic ovariectomy. Laparoscopy was converted to laparotomy to remove the abnormal tissue and the uterus. Histopathological findings showed ovarian follicles of various maturation stages in the mass and confirmed endometrial hyperplasia. Histology underscored that ovarian remnant tissue had resumed function. No clinical signs consistent with ORS were reported 6 months after excision of the abnormal tissue. In conclusion, removal of the ovaries through a laparoscopic port site may cause fortuitous ovarian tissue implantation at the abdominal wall in the cat.

Key points

- First case of accidental implantation at the port site after laparoscopic ovariectomy in a cat. The diagnostic laparoscopy revealed the presence of a mass, visually similar to ovarian tissue, that was removed.
- Histology of the excised mass revealed large ovarian follicles of various maturations stages. It is mandatory to take preventive measures to avoid ovarian remnants that resume function and must be excised.

PORT PLACEMENT

The first 5 mm cannula (T1) was placed on the midline, 1 cm cranial to the umbilicus, and a 30° telescope was introduced. The second 5 mm cannula (T2) was placed on the midline, 2 cm caudal to T1.

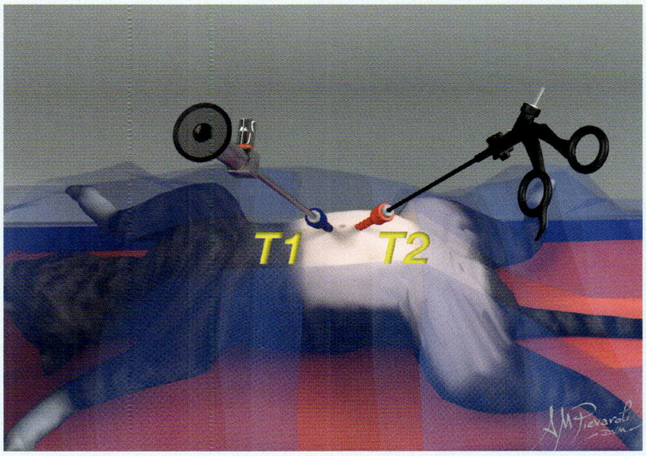

PROCEDURE

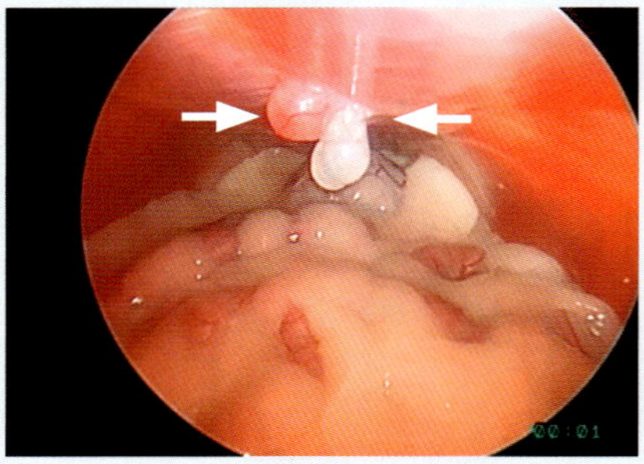

FIGURE 1. Laparoscopic image showing the presence of a mass (arrows) attached to the peritoneum.

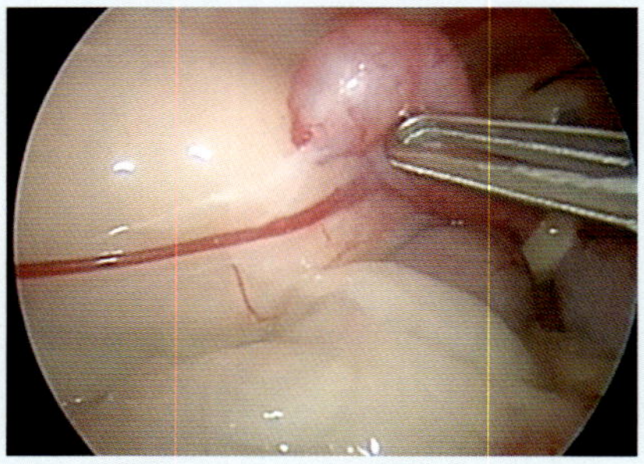

FIGURE 2. Laparoscopic image showing hyperplasia of the uterine horn without presence of ovarian tissue.

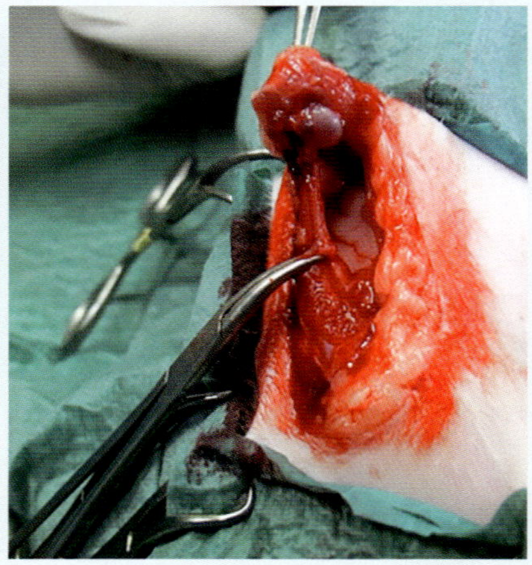

FIGURE 3. Intraoperative image showing the macroscopic features of the mass.

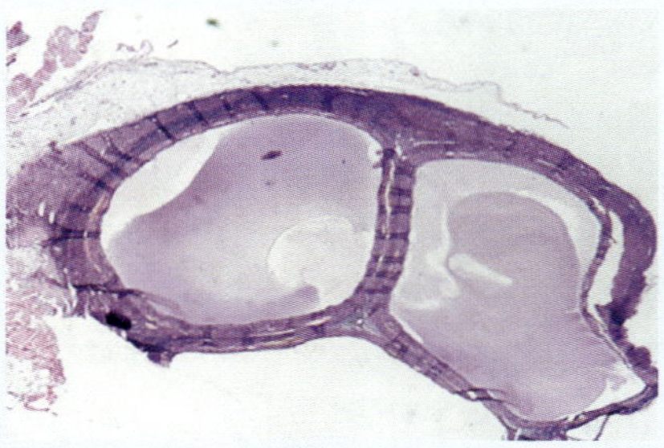

FIGURE 5. Histological image of the excised mass. There are large ovarian follicles of various maturation stages.

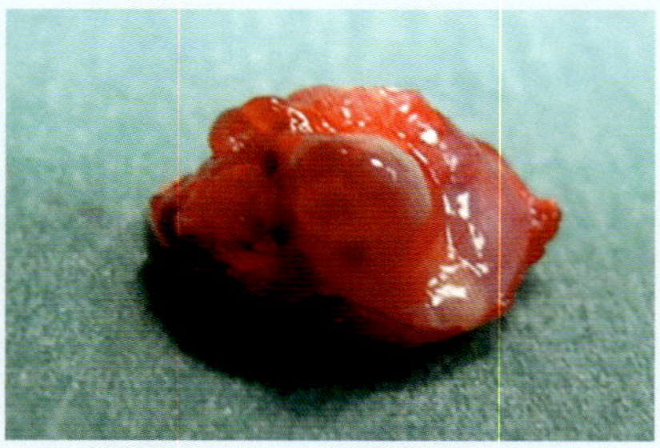

FIGURE 4. Excised mass.

Tips and tricks

- ✓ Check for ovarian remnants after laparoscopic extraction.
- ✓ Use large-diameter trocars, retrieval bags, or morcellators to remove ovarian tissue.

16.2 OVARIAN REMNANT SYNDROME IN A DOG

Ivan Jevtic

CASE DESCRIPTION

A 5.5-year-old female Pit Bull weighing 29 kg showed estrus signs again 3 months after ovariohysterectomy. Estrus occurred every 6 months, with presence of milk in the mammary glands, swelling of the vagina with mucopurulent discharge, and attraction of males. These signs had been present for 2.5 years. A presumptive diagnosis of ORS was made, and laparoscopic removal of the remaining ovary was performed. After the procedure, the patient no longer manifested any clinical signs of ORS.

Key points

- In a spayed female dog, clinical signs suspicious of ORS include swelling of the vulva, presence of milk in the mammary glands, attraction of males, and blood-tinged vaginal discharge.

PORT PLACEMENT

For this surgery, a two-port technique was performed. A 12 mm cannula (T1) was placed 2 cm caudal to the umbilicus and a telescope with a working channel (Karl Storz) was introduced. Port T2 was placed 5 mm caudally from the first 5 mm port for grasper. The operating table was tilted to the left to allow better visualization of the right ovary.

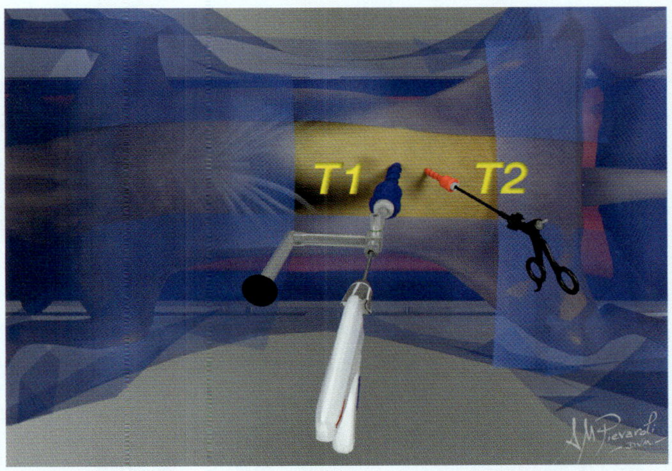

PROCEDURE

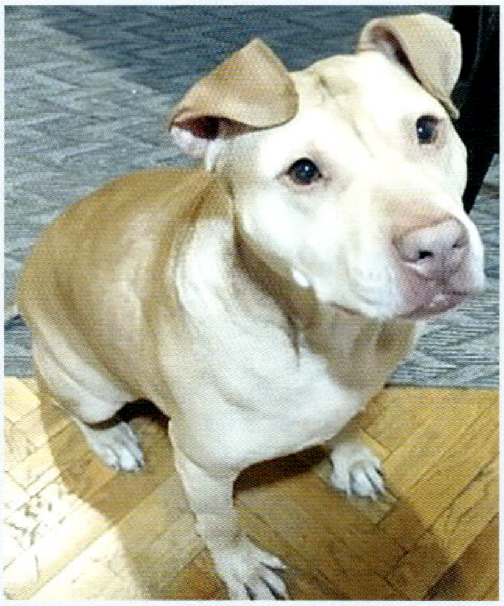

FIGURE 1. The patient is a 5.5-year-old spayed female Pit Bull dog.

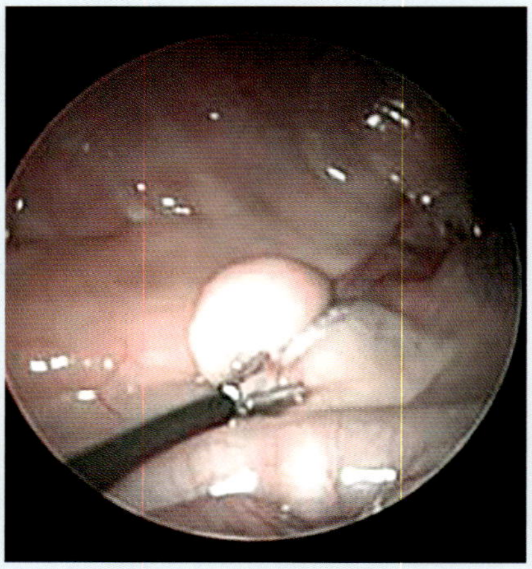

FIGURE 2. Laparoscopic exploration reveals the presence of part of the right ovary.

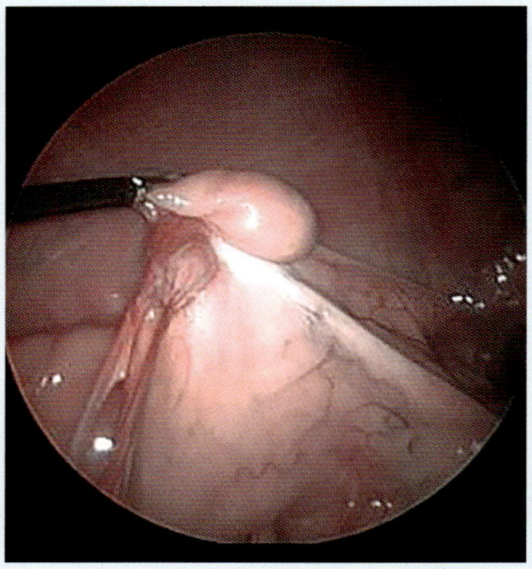

FIGURE 3. The ovary is grasped with a laparoscopic grasper introduced through T2.

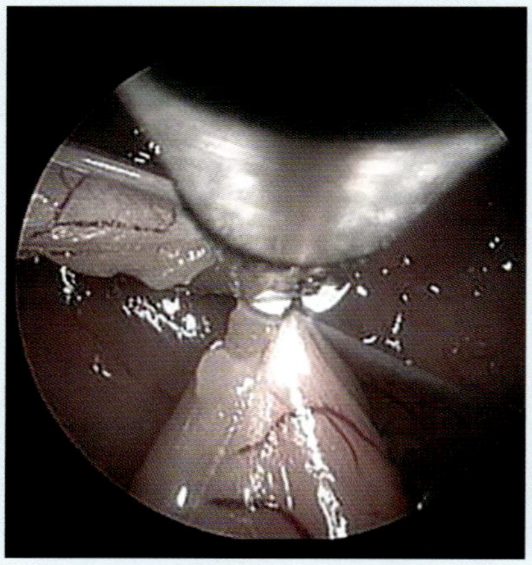

FIGURE 4. The ovary is separated from the surrounding tissue using LigaSure introduced through the working channel of the telescope.

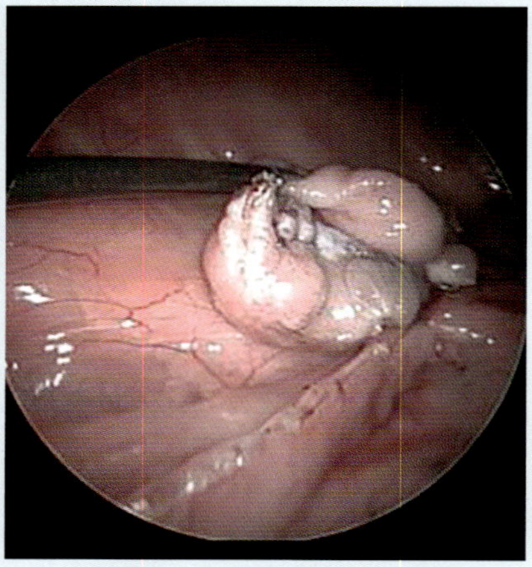

FIGURE 5. The ovary and surrounding adipose tissue are separated from the blood vessels and ligaments.

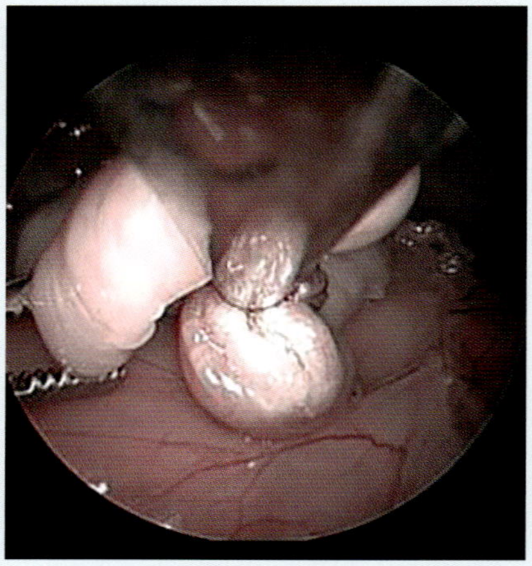

FIGURE 6. The ovary is removed using a grasper introduced through the working channel of the telescope

Tips and tricks

✓ If a telescope with a working channel is used, it is possible to perform the procedure with two ports.

17 LAPAROSCOPIC OVARIOHYSTERECTOMY

Andrea M. Pievaroli

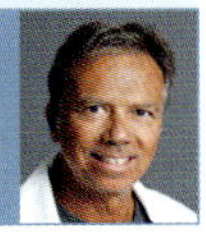

Indications

- Removal of the ovaries and uterus for suppression of the estrous cycle
- Prevention of diseases of the reproductive system
- Treatment of ovarian and uterine pathologies

Contraindications

- Cardiovascular and pulmonary diseases
- Congenital diaphragmatic defects
- Severe ovarian and uterine pathologies

Laparoscopic ovariohysterectomy (lapOVH) is indicated to suppress the estrus cycle and to prevent and treat diseases of reproductive system. Even if, in normal conditions, lapOVH could be performed with a totally laparoscopic technique, in common practice the laparoscopic-assisted technique is the most frequently used by almost all surgeons. Some studies published in the veterinary literature have confirmed that this laparoscopic-assisted technique is very effective for the removal of the uterus, even in certain pathological conditions, without giving up the advantages of the reduced invasiveness of laparoscopy (less postoperative pain and quicker recovery).

It can be said that lapOVH has even greater advantages than laparoscopic ovariectomy (lapOVE) when both are compared to their respective traditional techniques. In fact, a larger incision in the abdominal wall is required to perform an ovariohysterectomy, whereas the incision for an ovariectomy is only a few centimeters long.

As described for lapOVE, lapOVH can be performed in dogs of all breeds, ages, and sizes, with some limitations in too small or excessively obese patients. It can also be safely performed in cats. In cases of ovarian or uterine pathologies (e.g., ovarian tumors or cysts, uterine fluid collections, pyometra), patients should be considered candidates for lapOVH. Many factors can affect the feasibility of this procedure. In the absence of ovarian or uterine pathologies, the same considerations for lapOVE apply to lapOVH. Technical difficulties and surgical times can be influenced by the body conformation, the state of nutrition (body condition score), and by the amount of adipose tissue located in correspondence with the ovary.

The procedure is more challenging in the presence of ovarian or uterine pathologies. In this case, as described below, it is necessary to perform some preoperative evaluations to decide the surgical approach.

> The first laparoscopic ovariohysterectomy for pyometra in dogs was reported in 1995 by S. Minami, Y Okamoto, et al.

DESCRIBED SURGICAL PROCEDURES

The laparoscopic technique for performing ovariohysterectomy is very similar to that described for performing ovariectomy. Depending on the surgeon's personal preferences and the surgical difficulty, one, two, or three ports can be used. In the veterinary literature, various techniques have been described and the results regarding the pros and cons are comparable to those of ovariectomy.

The main difference between lapOVH and lapOVE is that the former procedure is divided into two steps. First, the ovarian suspensory ligament is laparoscopically resected, and then the uterus and ovaries are removed under laparoscopic assistance. Therefore, for the extraction of the uterus from the abdomen, a small incision is made on the midline of the pubis using the traditional technique.

In cases of ovarian pathologies and uterine infections or fluid collections (e.g., mucometra, pyometra), it is important to carry out a preliminary investigation to decide whether to adopt the laparoscopic technique. Usually, a complete ultrasound examination is sufficient to diagnose ovarian or uterine pathologies and to determine the size of the organs to be removed. The size of large ovarian cysts can be reduced by aspirating the fluid content with a needle introduced percutaneously into the abdomen. Uterine horns increased in size, due to the presence of endouterine fluid collections, are a relative contraindication to lapOVH. The size of the uterus (measured by ultrasound) must always be related to the size and breed of the patient. In fact, in large dogs, if enough working space is available, it is possible to laparoscopically remove a uterus even as large as 4–6 cm in diameter. The incision in the abdominal wall, necessary for the extraction of the uterus, will therefore depend on the size of the uterine horns.

PATIENT PREPARATION AND POSITIONING

Patient preparation is the same as described for lapOVE. The patient should be fasted for 10–12 hours before surgery; water is allowed. The bladder should be emptied before the procedure to allow a better visualization near the cervix. The abdomen is widely clipped; the surgical clip should extend cranially to the xiphoid process and include the entire vulva caudally. Even if the access is limited to the midline, wide surgical shaving of the hair must also be performed laterally. This is preferable in case of conversion (as a rule for any laparoscopic procedure) and in case of percutaneous needle insertion for the two-port technique. In fact, the conversion rate to open surgery of lapOVH is higher than that of lapOVE, especially in case of disease of the reproductive system.

The patient is placed in dorsal recumbency and the skin is aseptically prepared before draping. It is preferable to use a tilting table (better if motorized and remotely controlled) to easily reposition the patient during the different steps of the procedure. Alternatively, positioners supplied by some companies can be used. They are placed on the operating table and allow the patient to be tilted laterally.

In addition to lateral inclinations to better visualize the ovaries, it can be useful to tilt the table in a Trendelenburg position to displace the spleen cranially.

Some fundamental structures that should be identified during lapOVH are indicated in **Figure 1**. Attention must be paid to effective coagulation of vascular structures (ovarian artery and vein), which may be responsible for bleeding following ovary

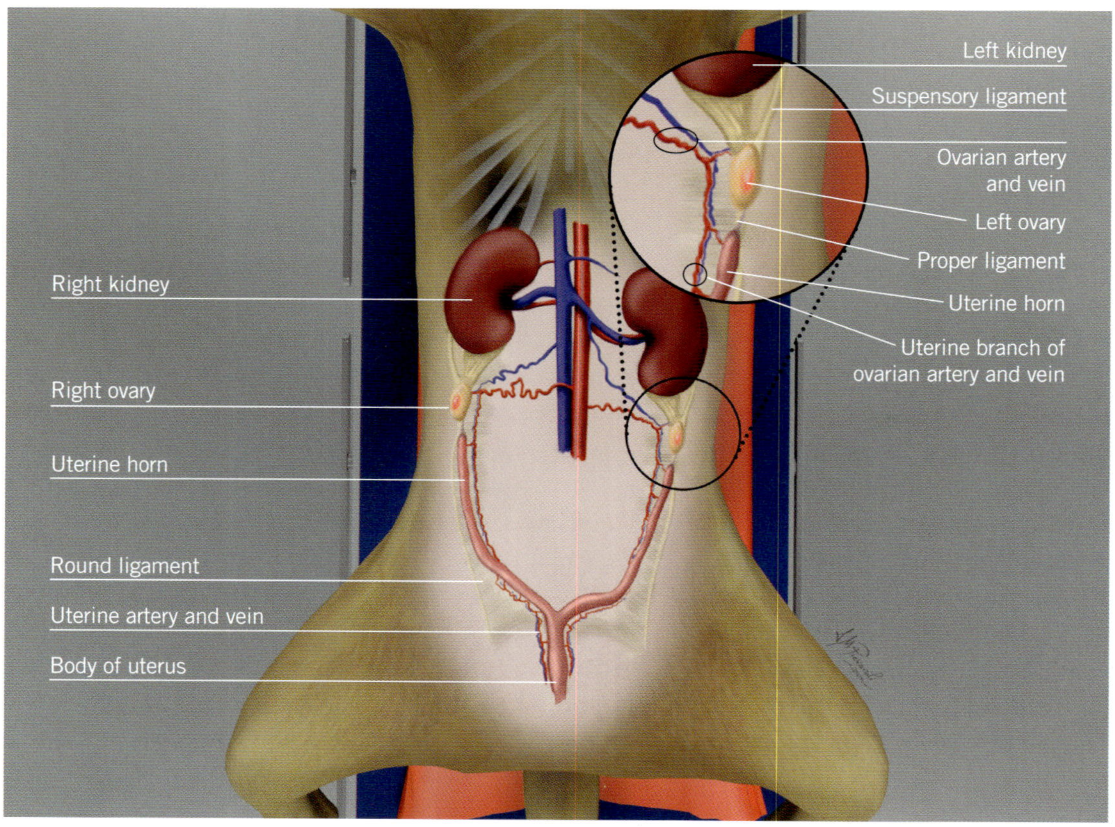

FIGURE 1. Female dog reproductive system.

resection. The uterine arteries and veins near the cervix must also be properly ligated before repositioning the stump in the abdomen. In some obese patients, or if the lateral tilt of the table is not adequate, it may be useful to follow the round ligament to locate the ovary.

OPERATING ROOM LAYOUT

The endoscopy tower with all devices can be placed at the patient's foot or head, depending on the size of the operating room. The important thing is to leave enough space for the surgeon and the assistant to move from one side of the table to the other. If the monitor is fixed on the tower, it is usually placed at the caudal end of the table (**Fig. 2**).

However, it is preferable to be able to move the monitor during the procedure to follow the surgeon's change of position and comply with the ergonomic principles of minimally invasive endoscopic surgery. This may be possible using a ceiling or boom-mounted monitor, a monitor installed on a mobile tower, or two monitors arranged on each side of the patient. The anesthesia machine is placed near the patient's head. The instrument table is placed caudolateral to the table, on the same side as the surgeon. To perform the lapOVH, the surgeon and the assistant position themselves on the opposite side in relation to the ovary to be removed (**Fig. 3**).

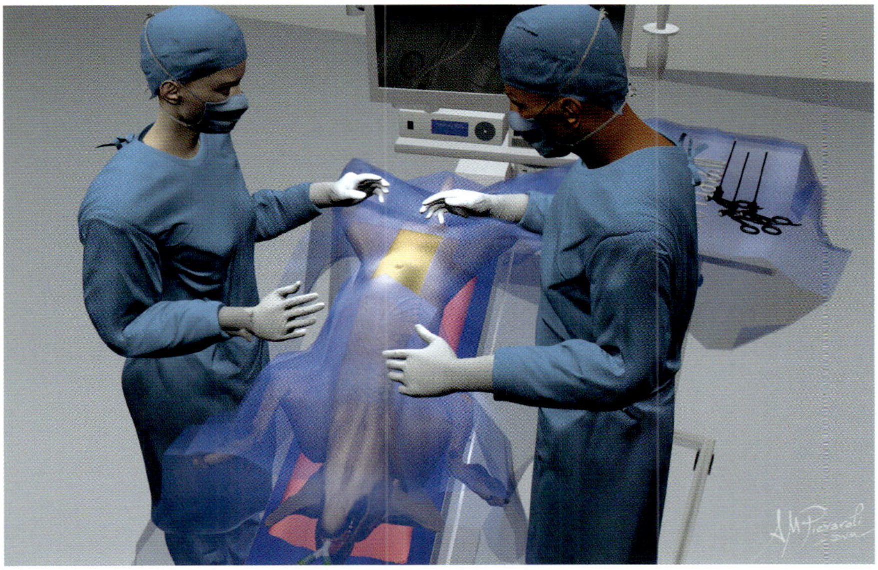

FIGURE 2. Operating room layout for laparoscopic ovariohysterectomy. Initial setup for port placement.

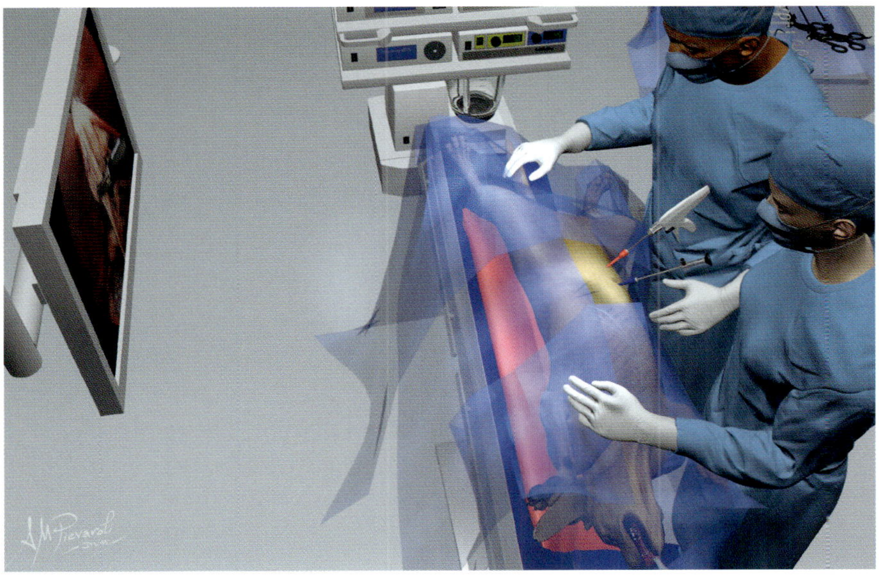

FIGURE 3. Layout during laparoscopic ovariohysterectomy: the table is tilted laterally; the surgeon and the assistant are positioned on the opposite side in relation to the ovary to be removed.

The following procedures are described below:

A. Two-port ovariohysterectomy technique

B. Three-port ovariohysterectomy technique

A TWO-PORT OVARIOHYSTERECTOMY

Two-port ovariohysterectomy is currently the most used technique by the author for lapOVH in normal conditions and in cases of nonserious pathologies of the reproductive system. As lapOVE, it has the advantage of being very minimally invasive, as reported in the literature. Ports are placed in the midline, 1–2 cm caudal to the umbilicus and 1–2 cm cranial to the edge of the pubic bone. The cranial cannula is used for the telescope, while the caudal cannula is used for the operative instruments. For resection of the suspensory ligament, the ovary is kept suspended in the abdomen using a suture inserted percutaneously with a needle. This solution avoids using the third cannula, thereby reducing the invasiveness of the surgery. Some surgeons use a specific ovariectomy hook instrument (Karl Storz Endoscopy) instead of the suture. After suspending the ovary to be removed, coagulation and cutting of the suspensory ligament, including part of the mesometrium, are performed. The caudal incision is then enlarged to extract the reproductive system from the abdomen, and the procedure continues in the traditional way by ligating the uterus near the cervix (**Video 1**).

PORT PLACEMENT (FIG. 4)

- T1, on the midline, 1–2 cm caudal to the umbilicus
- T2, on the midline, 1–2 cm cranial to the pubic bone

PROCEDURE

- The cranial trocar is placed first (T1). The author prefers to use threaded cannulas (Storz Endotip) to prevent slippage from within the peritoneum. It is advisable to tilt the table into a Trendelenburg position to perform this step of the procedure.
- A pneumoperitoneum is established using the surgeon's preferred technique; the author uses the Ternamian or a modified Hasson technique. After the first port has been placed and the pneumoperitoneum achieved, the 5 mm telescope is inserted and a first exploration of the abdomen is performed to check for any evidence of iatrogenic trauma caused by placement of the first cannula.

Instruments

On the table:

- Standard abdominal surgical pack
- Telescope 5 mm – 30°
- Two 5 mm cannulas (or one 5 mm cannula + one 10 mm cannula)
- Grasping forceps
- Large-gauge suture swaged on a needle
- Vessel-sealing device

Ready to use:

- Endoscopic cannula for aspiration/irrigation
- Third cannula to switch to the three-port technique

Minilaparoscopy 3 mm set (see Fig. 7 in Chapter 15) for dogs and cats weighing less than 3–4 kg:

- Standard abdominal surgical pack
- Telescope 2.7 mm – 30°
- Two 3 mm cannulas (or one 3 mm cannula + one 5 mm cannula)
- Grasping forceps
- Endoscopic scissors
- A suture swaged on a needle
- Bipolar coagulation forceps (3 mm)/vessel-sealing device (5 mm)

VIDEO 1. Two-port ovariohysterectomy.

- The falciform ligament, which could prevent correct vision and cloud the lens of the telescope, can often be found in this area of the peritoneum (**Fig. 5**). It is necessary to screw the port deeper to find the right inclination to overcome the ligament.

Tips

To avoid crossing the falciform ligament, the port can be inserted slightly lateral (1–2 cm) to the midline.

- Under endoscopic vision, the second cannula is inserted. After locating the cranial edge of the pubic bone by palpation, the incision for the trocar is made 1–2 cm cranial to the bone. It is preferable to use the cranial port for the telescope and the caudal port for the instruments (**Fig. 6**).
- The surgeon performs the surgery on the contralateral ovary with respect to their position.
- For better visualization of the ovary, especially in obese patients or in the presence of meteoric intestinal loops or splenomegaly, the patient should be tilted to an oblique position (at least 45°) to displace the organs by gravity and facilitate manual surgical procedures.
- Atraumatic forceps or a blunt probe are used to move the organs and locate the ovary and uterine horn, which are located caudal to the kidney. Forceps are then used to grasp the proper ligament and elevate the ovary to visualize the kidney, the suspensory ligament of the ovary, and the ovarian vasculature (**Fig. 7**).

Tips

If the surgeon has more difficulties than expected when manipulating the uterus with a single forceps, it is recommended to convert the procedure into a three-port technique.

- Palpating the abdomen from the outside, a point on the wall is identified in correspondence with the ovary. Then, under direct endoscopic vision, a suture is inserted percutaneously with a large size half-circle needle. The needle is passed through the proper ligament, avoiding the ovarian artery and vein, and then outside of the body wall again (**Fig. 8**).

Tips

If an endouterine fluid collection is present (e.g., mucometra, pyometra), care must be taken not to perforate the uterine horn with the needle.

- After anchoring the ovary with suture thread, the forceps are removed from the port.
- The two ends of the suture outside the body wall are pulled to elevate the ovary and placed under tension with Klemmer forceps or a hemostat.

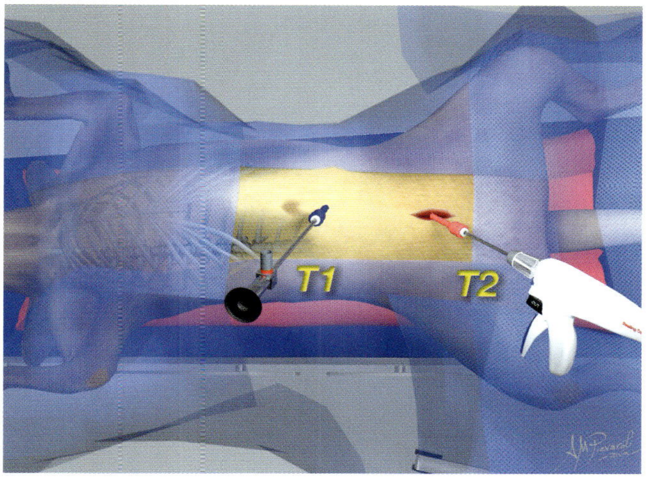

FIGURE 4. Port placement for two-port ovariohysterectomy.

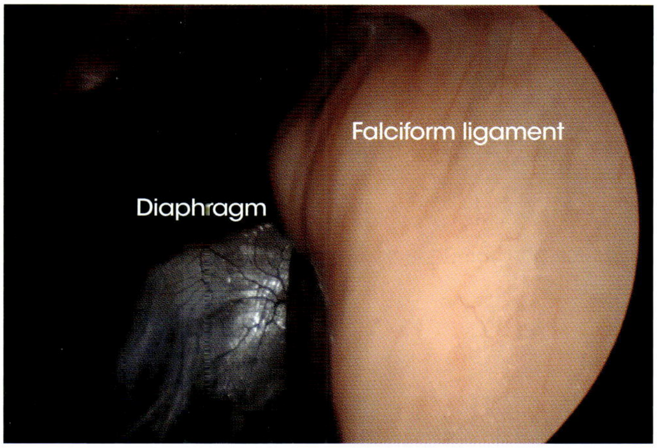

FIGURE 5. The falciform ligament can often be found in the umbilical area. This could prevent correct vision and cloud the lens of the telescope.

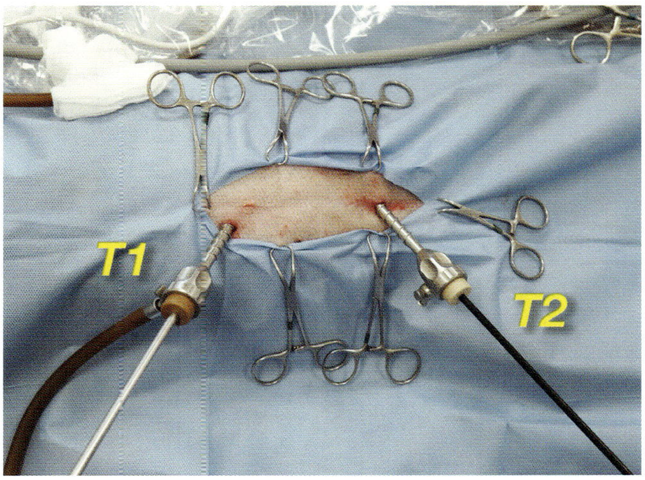

FIGURE 6. Image of the operating field for two-port laparoscopic ovariohysterectomy.

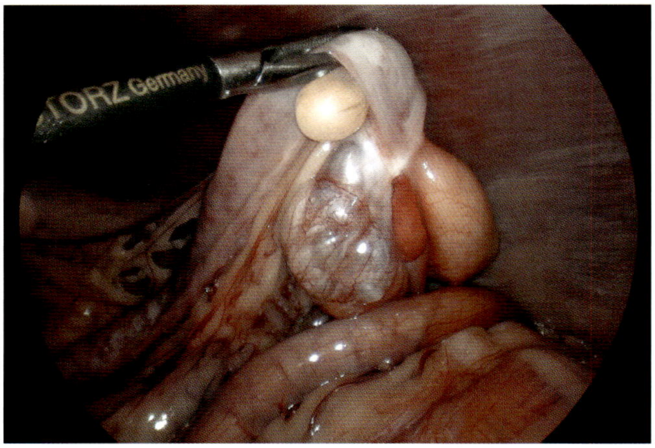

FIGURE 7. The proper ligament is grasped to elevate the ovary (the right ovary is shown in the figure).

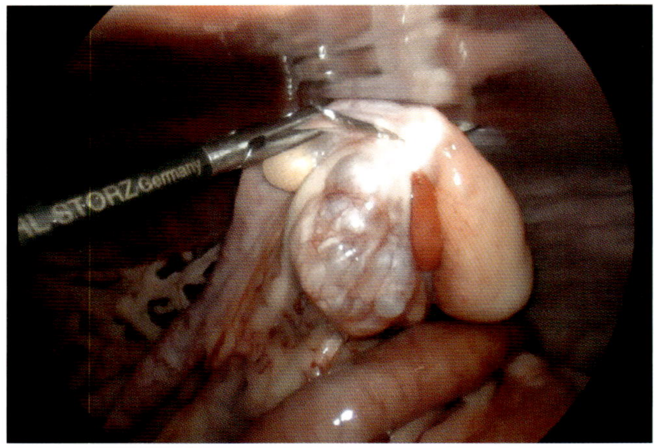

FIGURE 8. A suture is inserted percutaneously with a large size half-circle needle and passed through the proper ligament.

- A vessel-sealing device (VSD) is introduced in the caudal port. The kidney is identified and the omentum or other organs that may interfere are moved. The jaws of the forceps are used to seal and dissect the mesovarium (including the ovarian artery and vein) and suspensory ligament, taking care to remain at a sufficient distance from the ovary (**Fig. 9**).

  Two-port minilaparoscopy with 3 mm cannulas: In small dogs and cats, 3 mm bipolar forceps should be used to coagulate vessels and tissues. The small endoscopic scissors are then introduced to dissect the ovaries free (**Fig. 10**). Alternatively, if the working space allows it, even in small patients a VSD may be used through a caudal 5 mm cannula. In fact, the caudal incision will have to be subsequently enlarged to extract the uterus.
- Then, resection is continued, including part of the mesometrium. The ovary must remain anchored to the body wall by the suture.
- The surgeon should carefully check for any evidence of bleeding from the dissected vessels before tilting the table to the opposite position to resect the contralateral ovary.
- At this point, the surgeon and the assistant should move to the opposite side and the table should be tilted laterally towards them.
- The surgeon then performs the same procedure to resect the second ovary.
- After the procedure has been completed on both sides, the table is tilted back to the initial neutral position. It is preferable for the surgeon and the assistant to be placed on each side of the table.
- The forceps are inserted in the caudal cannula to grasp an ovary and bring it to the port. The suture is released and the cannula is removed while pulling the ovary towards the abdominal wall (**Fig. 11**).
- For the second step of the procedure, the extraction of the ovaries and uterus, the port incision must be widened.
- While holding the forceps that are grasping the ovary, a small incision is made on the midline where the caudal port is inserted. Rapid deflation of the peritoneal cavity occurs. The incision must allow for extraction of the uterus even if it is increased in volume (**Fig. 12**).
- Avoiding injury to the uterine wall and vessels, both uterine horns (and ovaries) are gently pulled and brought out of the abdomen (**Fig. 13**).

Tips

A Gelpi retractor can be used to keep the midline incision open.

- At this point, the telescope is removed (not yet the cranial cannula) and the procedure is continued in the traditional manner. The uterus is ligated near the cervix (**Fig. 14**) and removed, and the uterine stump is repositioned into the abdomen.
- The caudal incision in the abdominal fascia is closed routinely. Then, a pneumoperitoneum is established again using the cranial cannula and an exploration of the abdomen is performed to exclude active bleeding and to check the uterine stump (**Fig. 15**). The abdomen is then deflated and the ports removed.
- Finally, the small cranial incision in the abdominal fascia and the skin at the port sites are closed routinely.

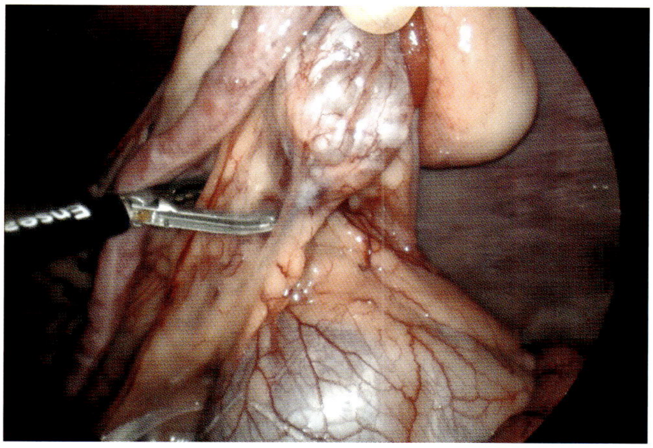

FIGURE 9. Use of a vessel-sealing device to grasp the suspensory ligament between the kidney and ovary to perform the resection.

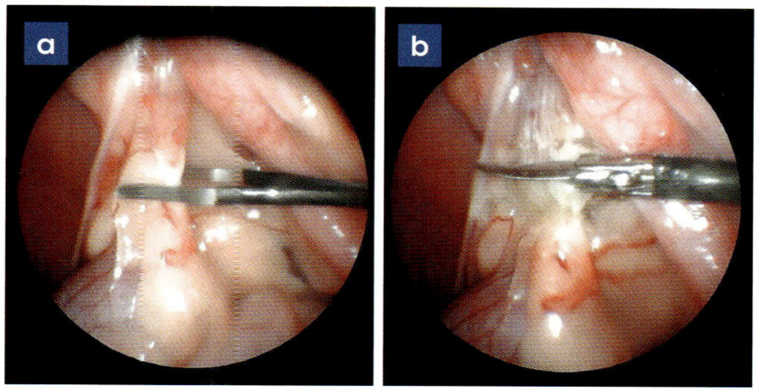

FIGURE 10. Two-port minilaparoscopy. a) Use of 3 mm bipolar forceps to coagulate the suspensory ligament. b) The ovaries are then dissected free with scissors.

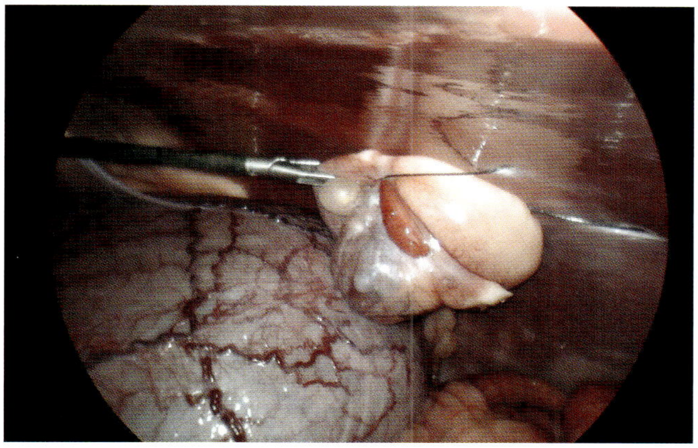

FIGURE 11. The ovary is grasped and, after releasing the suture, brought to the caudal port. The caudal cannula is removed while pulling the ovary towards the abdominal wall.

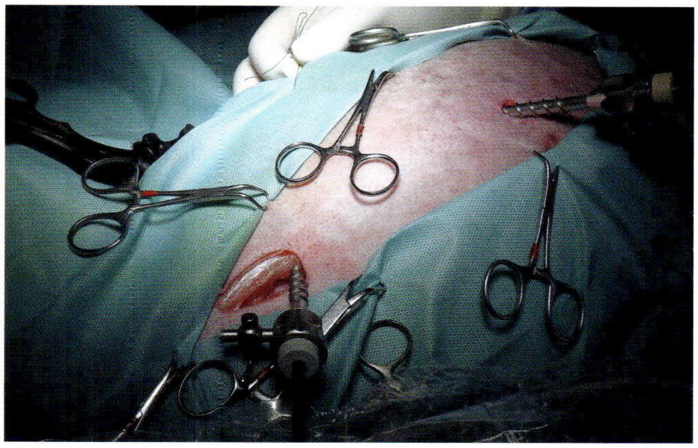

FIGURE 12. To extract the uterus, a small incision is made on the midline where the caudal port is inserted. The length of the incision depends on the size of the uterus.

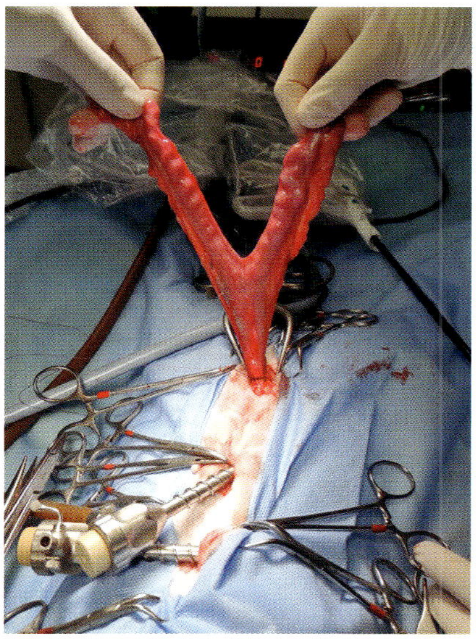

FIGURE 13. After continuing the resection of the broad ligament, and taking care not to injure the uterine arteries and veins, the uterine horns (and ovaries) are brought out of the abdomen.

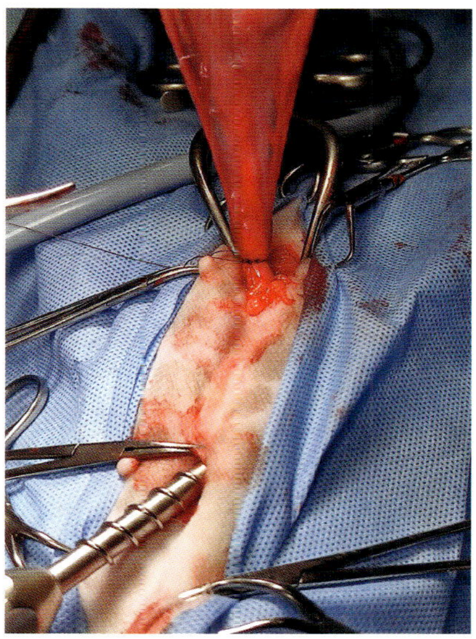

FIGURE 14. As in open surgery, the uterus is ligated near the cervix and removed.

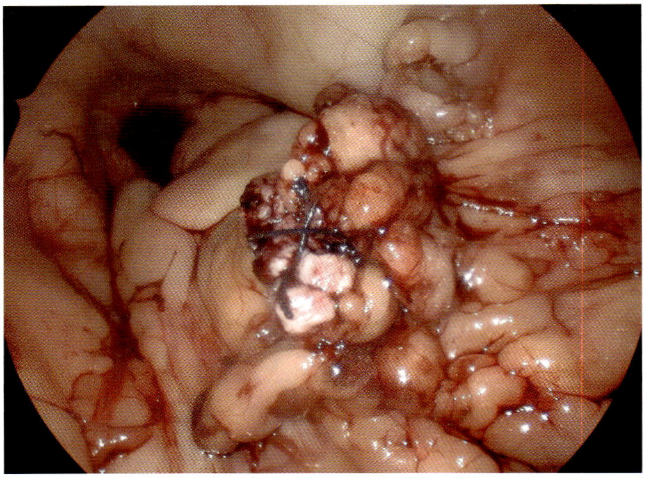

FIGURE 15. Before removing the cranial cannula, an abdominal exploration should be performed to exclude active bleeding and to check the uterine stump.

B THREE-PORT OVARIOHYSTERECTOMY

The use of three ports to perform lapOVH is considered the standard technique by many surgeons. This is because lapOVH is more challenging than lapOVE, especially in cases of ovarian and uterine pathologies or very obese patients. The use of a third port for the grasping forceps replaces the suture passed percutaneously to suspend the ovary. The use of two "hands" can facilitate the laparoscopic procedure, as manipulating the uterine horns is easier. With this technique, if there is enough working space, it is possible to remove a significantly enlarged uterus.

Ports are placed in the midline, cranial and caudal to the umbilicus and slightly cranial to the pubis. The central cannula is used for the telescope, while the cranial and caudal cannulas are used for the operative instruments. The grasping forceps are used to locate and suspend the ovary, while the ovary is resected using the VSD in the other port. The caudal incision is then enlarged to extract the reproductive system from the abdomen, and the procedure continues in the traditional way by ligating the uterus near the cervix (**Video 2**).

VIDEO 2. Three-port ovariohysterectomy.

Instruments

On the table:

- Standard abdominal surgical pack
- Telescope 5 mm – 30°
- Three 5 mm cannulas (or two 5 mm cannulas + one 10 mm cannula)
- Grasping forceps
- Vessel-sealing device

Ready to use:

- Endoscopic cannula for aspiration/irrigation

Minilaparoscopy 3 mm set for dogs and cats weighing less than 3–4 kg:

- Standard abdominal surgical pack
- Telescope 2.7 mm – 30°
- Three 3 mm cannulas (or two 3 mm cannulas + one 5 mm cannula)
- Grasping forceps
- Endoscopic scissors
- Bipolar coagulation forceps/vessel-sealing device (5 mm)

PORT PLACEMENT (FIG. 16)

- T1, on the midline, 1–2 cm caudal to the umbilicus
- T2, on the midline, 1–2 cm cranial to the pubic bone
- T3, on the midline, 3–5 cm cranial to T1

PROCEDURE

- Placement of the first port (cranial or central) is based on the surgeon's preferences. It is advisable to tilt the table into a Trendelenburg position to perform this step of the procedure. The author prefers the use of threaded cannulas (Storz Endotip) to prevent slippage from within the peritoneum.
- A pneumoperitoneum is established using the surgeon's preferred technique; the author uses the Ternamian or a modified Hasson technique. After the first port has been placed and the pneumoperitoneum achieved, the 5 mm telescope is inserted and a first exploration of the abdomen is performed to check for any evidence of iatrogenic trauma caused by placement of the first cannula.
- Under endoscopic vision, the second and the third cannulas are inserted. To get a more natural view, it is preferable to use the central port for the telescope and the cranial and caudal ports for the instruments (**Fig. 17**).

- The falciform ligament, which could prevent correct vision and cloud the lens of the telescope, can often be found when introducing the cranial port. It is necessary to screw the port deeper to find the right inclination to overcome the ligament.

Tips

To avoid crossing the falciform ligament, the port can be inserted slightly lateral (1–2 cm) to the midline.

- The surgeon performs the procedure on the contralateral ovary with respect to their position.
- For better visualization of the ovary, especially in obese patients or in the presence of meteoric intestinal loops or splenomegaly, the patient should be tilted to an oblique position (at least 45°) to displace the organs by gravity and facilitate manual surgical procedures.
- Atraumatic forceps or a blunt probe are used with both hands to better move the organs and locate the ovary and uterine horn, which are located caudal to the kidney. Using the forceps in the cranial port, the proper ligament is grasped and the ovary is elevated to visualize the kidney, the suspensory ligament of the ovary, and the ovarian vasculature (**Fig. 18**).
- A VSD is introduced in the caudal port. The kidney is identified and the omentum or other organs that may interfere are moved. The jaws of the forceps are used to seal and dissect the mesovarium (including the ovarian artery and vein) and the suspensory ligament, taking care to remain at a sufficient distance from the ovary (**Fig. 19**). Part of the mesometrium is also sealed and transected.

  Minilaparoscopy with 3 mm cannulas: In small dogs and cats, the surgeon should use 3 mm bipolar forceps to coagulate vessels and tissues. The small endoscopic scissors are then introduced to dissect the ovaries free. Alternatively, if the working space allows it, even in small patients a VSD may be used through a caudal 5 mm cannula. In fact, the caudal incision will have to be subsequently enlarged to extract the uterus.
- The surgeon should carefully check for any evidence of bleeding from the dissected vessels before tilting the table to the opposite position to resect the contralateral ovary.
- At this point, the surgeon and the assistant should move to the opposite side. The table is then tilted laterally towards them.

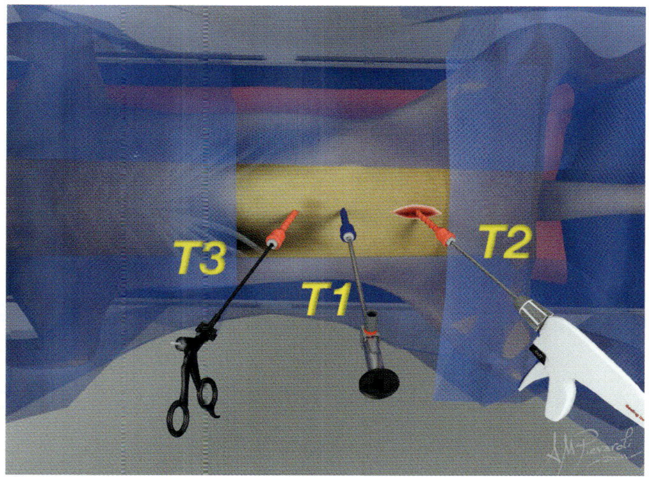

FIGURE 16. Port placement for three-port ovariohysterectomy.

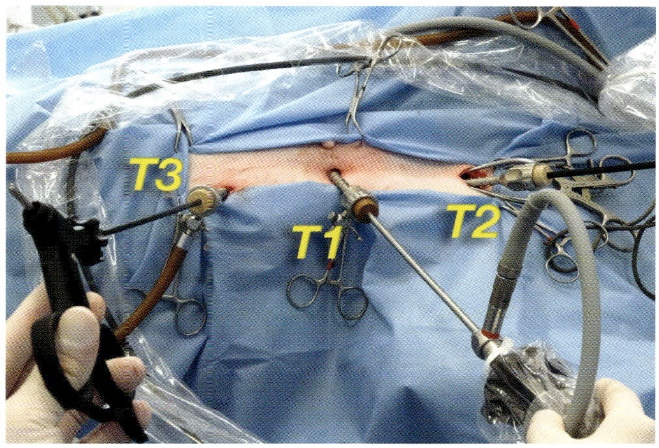

FIGURE 17. Image of the operating field for three-port laparoscopic ovariohysterectomy.

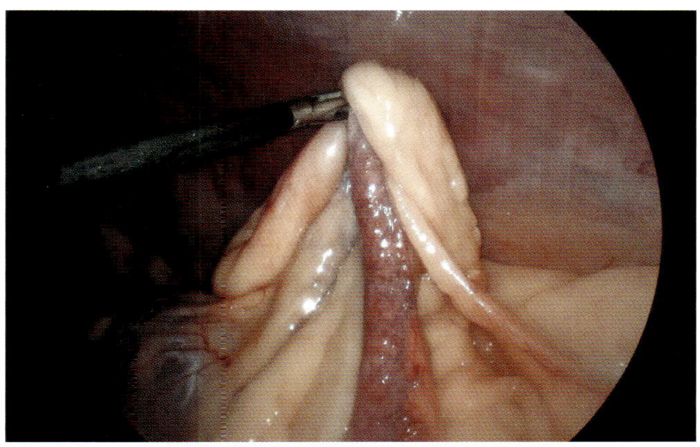

FIGURE 18. The ovary is elevated using the forceps in the cranial port to visualize the suspensory ligament and mesovarium (the left ovary is shown in the figure).

- The surgeon then performs the same procedure to resect the second suspensory ligament.
- After the procedure has been completed on both sides, the table is tilted back to the initial neutral position. It is preferable for the surgeon and the assistant to be placed on each side of the table.
- The forceps are inserted in the caudal cannula to grasp an ovary. The cannula is removed while pulling the ovary towards the abdominal wall.
- For the second step of the procedure, the extraction of the ovaries and uterus, the port incision must be widened.
- While holding the forceps that are grasping the ovary, a small incision is made on the midline where the caudal port is inserted. Rapid deflation of the peritoneal cavity occurs. The incision must allow for extraction of the uterus even if it is increased in volume (**Fig. 20**).
- Avoiding injury to the uterine wall and vessels, both uterine horns (and ovaries) are gently pulled and brought out of the abdomen.

Tips

A Gelpi retractor can be used to keep the midline incision open.

- At this point, the telescope and the other forceps are removed (not yet the cranial and central cannulas) and the procedure is continued in the traditional manner. The uterus is ligated near the cervix and removed, and the uterine stump is repositioned into the abdomen.
- The caudal incisions in the abdominal fascia are closed routinely. Then, a pneumoperitoneum is established again using one of the cranial cannulas and an exploration of the abdomen is performed to exclude active bleeding and to check the uterine stump (see **Fig. 15**). The abdomen is then deflated and the ports removed.
- Finally, the small incisions in the abdominal fascia and the skin at the port sites are closed routinely.

LAPAROSCOPIC OVARIOHYSTERECTOMY FOR OVARIAN OR UTERINE PATHOLOGIES

LapOVH can be successfully performed in many patients with disorders affecting the ovaries or uterus. In these cases, the degree of difficulty of the procedure is higher, and the choice of using two or three ports depends on the severity of the disease and on the surgeon's experience. In most patients, the uterus can be removed by a two-port technique (**Fig. 21**). In more challenging cases, a three-port technique is recommended (**Fig. 22**).

It is always necessary to perform some preoperative evaluations to decide if the patient is a candidate for a minimally invasive approach. In the author's experience, there are some factors that influence the feasibility of the procedure. In addition to the patient's size and body condition score, the patient's morphological conformation (breed) should also be considered. It is more difficult to perform laparoscopy in some breeds due to the anatomical features of their abdomen, which do not always allow the

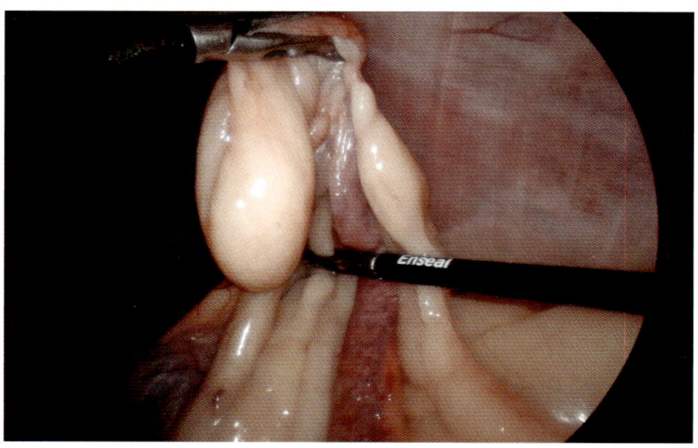

FIGURE 19. The vessel-sealing device is used to seal and dissect the mesovarium (including the ovarian artery and vein) and the suspensory ligament.

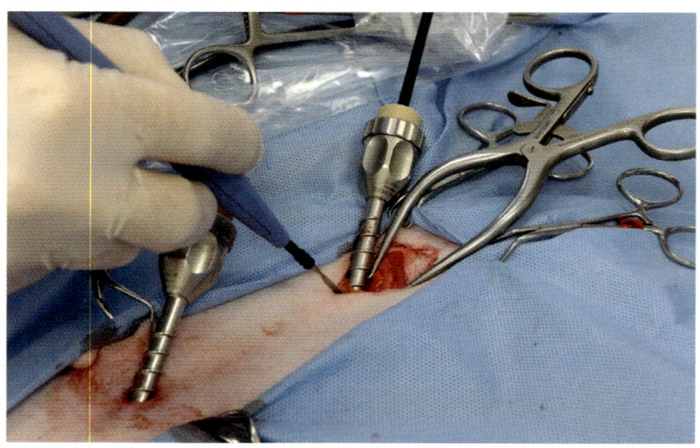

FIGURE 20. To extract the uterus, a small incision is made on the midline where the caudal port is inserted. The length of the incision depends on the size of the uterus.

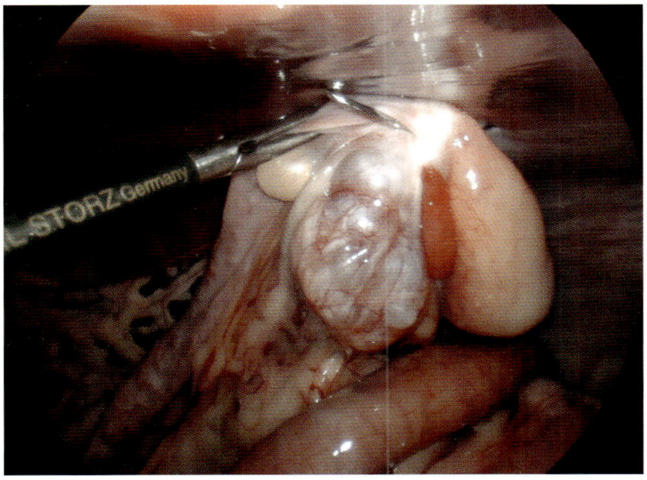

FIGURE 21. Ovarian cyst associated with endometritis. Two-port laparoscopic ovariohysterectomy was performed.

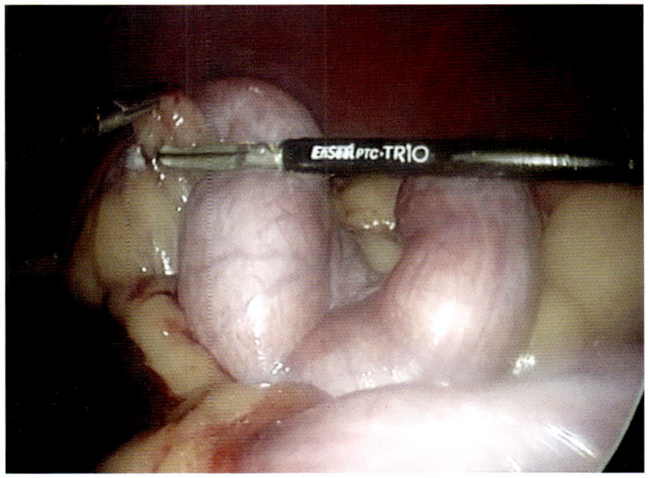

FIGURE 22. Pyometra in a dog. Three-port laparoscopic ovariohysterectomy was elected in this case.

creation of an adequate working space after CO_2 insufflation. The size of the uterus (or of the ovary), measured preoperatively by ultrasound, must always be evaluated in relation to the conformation and size of the abdomen in order to determine if a specific patient is an appropriate candidate for lapOVH. A uterus increased in volume due to an endouterine fluid collection (e.g., a uterine horn of 2 cm in diameter) can be considered small in a large-sized dog but large in a small-sized dog. Therefore, the decision whether to perform lapOVH should never be based on the size of the uterus alone; the patient's size and morphological conformation should be considered as well (**Fig. 23**).

The morphological parameters to be considered are the height of the abdomen (measured from the xiphoid process to the corresponding spinous process of the thoracic vertebra) and the length of the abdomen (measured from the xiphoid process to the pubis) (**Fig. 24**). The height of the abdomen must be sufficient to allow good lifting and hooking of the ovary in order to locate the suspensory ligament to be cauterized and resected. Abdominal height, in relation to the diameter of the uterine horns, is determinant in the choice of technique (laparoscopic or traditional). Larger uterine horns in relation to the height of the abdomen result in an exponential increase in surgical difficulty. The same principle can be applied in cases of ovarian cysts or tumors, taking as a reference the diameter of the affected ovary. If an ovarian cyst is present, it can be aspirated percutaneously using a needle during the procedure to reduce the size of the ovary (**Fig. 25**).

The patient's state of nutrition (body condition score) and, in particular, the amount of adipose tissue at the ovary (a parameter that cannot be evaluated before surgery) are additional factors that determine the degree of difficulty of the procedure. The patient's size and weight are therefore relative factors if considered alone.

Care must be taken when manipulating the uterine horns, especially in case of purulent collection (pyometra). The risk of uterine rupture resulting in dissemination of the material in the abdomen can be reduced by using atraumatic forceps (**Fig. 26**).

The availability of instruments for minilaparoscopy allows surgeons to perform lapOVH even in toy-sized patients if the criteria described above are met (**Fig. 27**).

POSTOPERATIVE MANAGEMENT

- Patients that are considered stable and healthy preoperatively can typically be discharged on the same day, and antibiotic therapy is not necessary.
- In cases of ovarian and uterine pathologies, the patient should be hospitalized to continue supportive care, antibiotics, and other therapies.
- Analgesia is continued for few days after surgery.
- Exercise is restricted for 3–4 days after surgery.

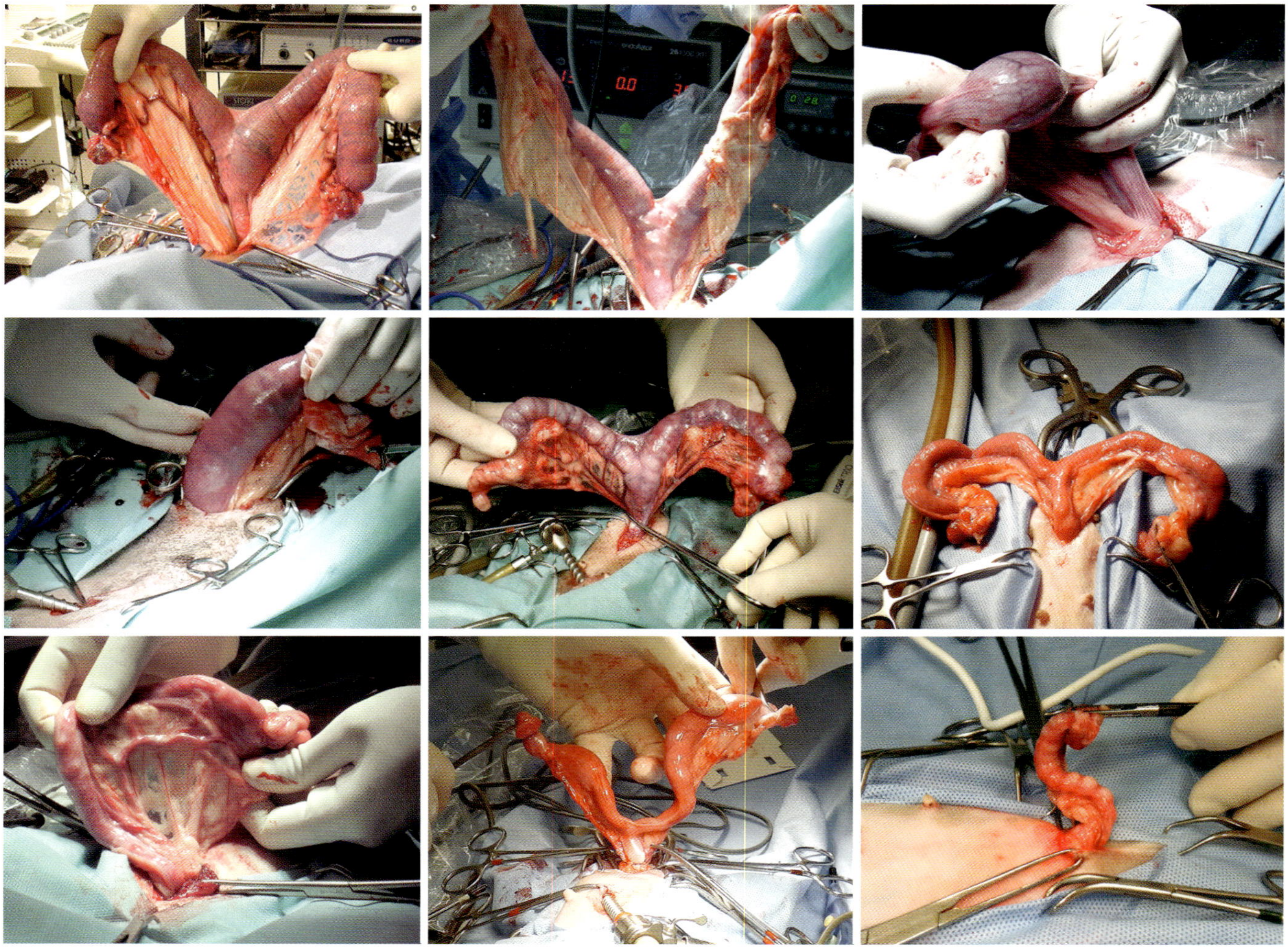

FIGURE 23. Comparison of uteri in dogs of different sizes. It is evident that an enlarged uterus can be considered relatively small in a large-sized dog but large in a small-sized dog.

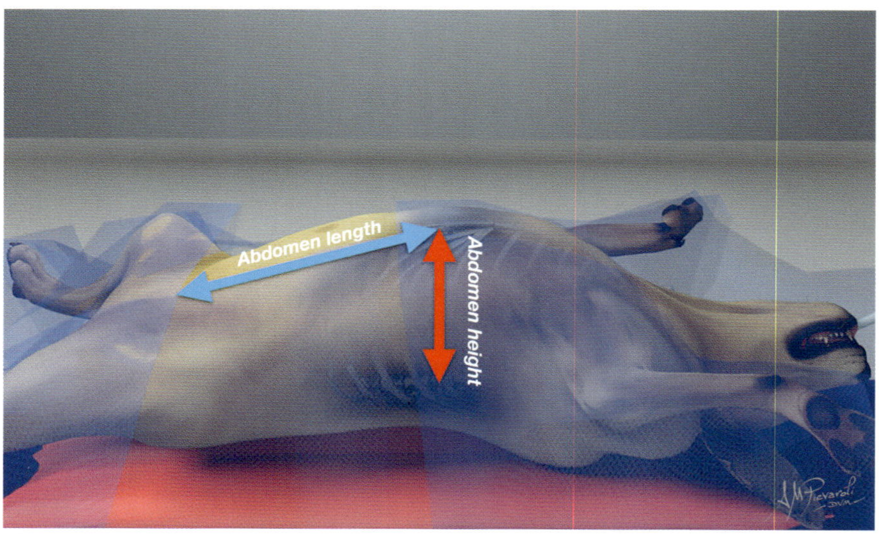

FIGURE 24. An adequate working space after CO_2 insufflation is essential to perform laparoscopic ovariohysterectomy in patients with disorders affecting the ovaries or uterus. The morphological parameters to be considered are the height of the abdomen (measured from the xiphoid process to the corresponding thoracic vertebra) and the length of the abdomen (measured from the xiphoid process to the pubis).

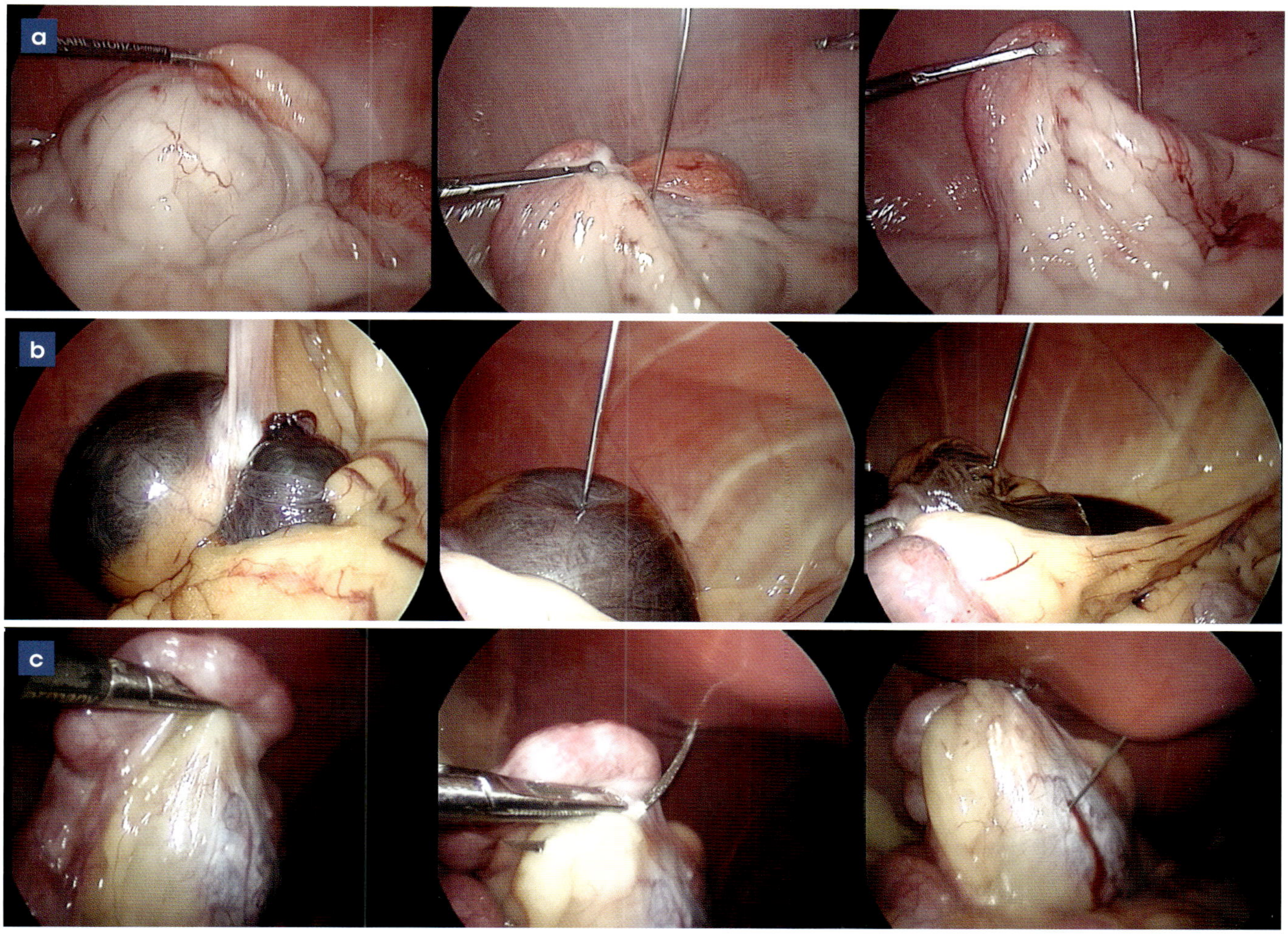

FIGURE 25. Ovarian cysts can be aspirated using a percutaneous needle to reduce the size of the ovary. Different techniques (two- and three-port laparoscopic ovariohysterectomy) to grasp the ovary and aspirate the cyst with a needle are shown.

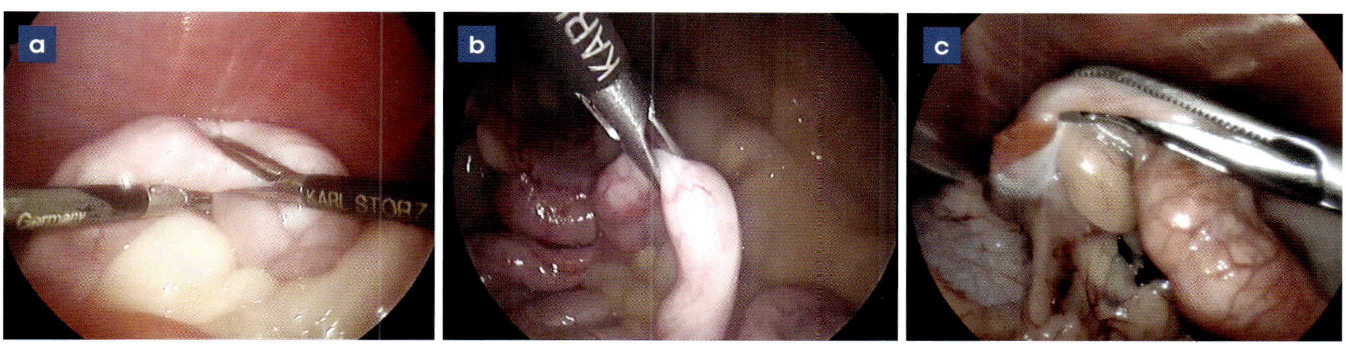

FIGURE 26. Three cases of pyometra treated laparoscopically. The patient's size and morphological conformation were considered adequate in relation to the size of the uterus. Atraumatic forceps should be used to manipulate the uterine horns, especially in cases of purulent collection (pyometra), in order to reduce the risk of uterine rupture and dissemination of the material in the abdomen.

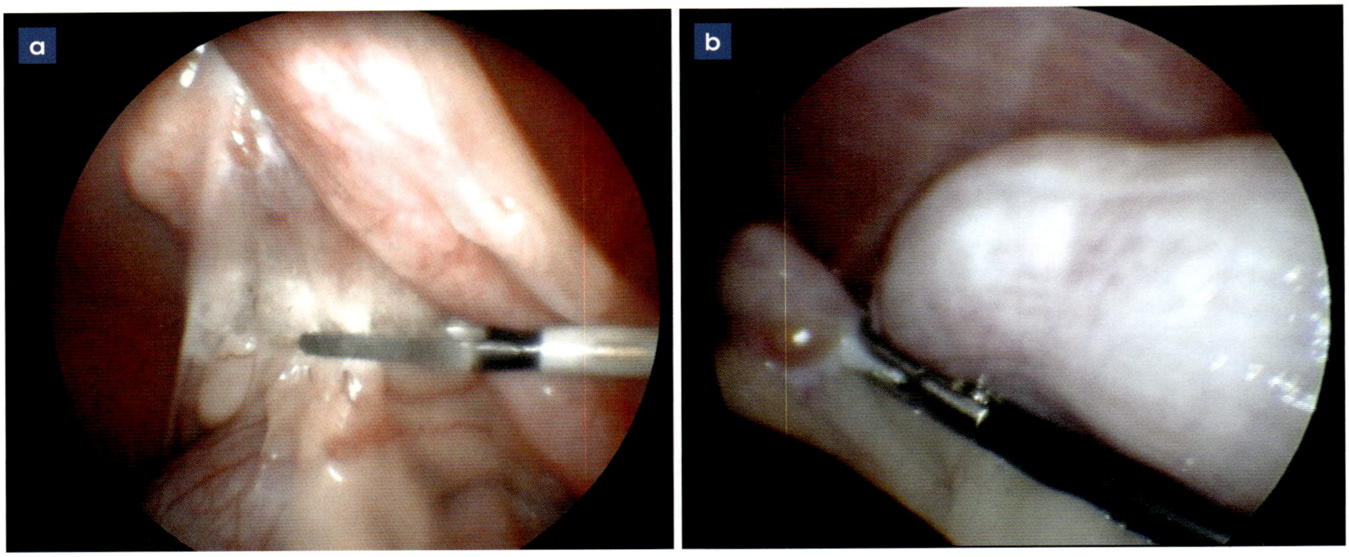

FIGURE 27. Two-port laparoscopic ovariohysterectomy performed in two very small patients (Chihuahua <3 kg). Instruments for minilaparoscopy are used.

Complications of lapOVH

- Low complication rates, mostly related to laparoscopic procedures.
- Bleeding from the pedicle due to incomplete closure of the vascular structures.
- Conversion to laparotomy rates are higher if uterine pathologies, iatrogenic lesions to the uterine horns (pyometra), or hemorrhage are present.
- Acquired urinary incontinence, as a benign condition, has been reported to occur in 9% to 15% of cases.

Key points

- Tilt the patient 45° for better visualization of the ovaries.
- Use a vessel-sealing device to close the vascular structures.
- In case of uterine pathologies, handle the uterine horns gently and be careful not to perforate them during percutaneous needle insertion.

SUGGESTED READINGS

18 LAPAROSCOPIC CRYPTORCHIDECTOMY

Andrea M. Pievaroli

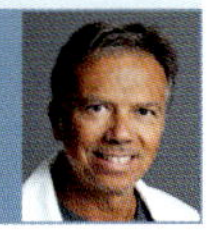

Indications

- Removal of retained testicles in the abdomen or inguinal canal
- Removal of twisted or neoplastic retained testicles

Contraindications

- Large neoplastic testicles with adhesions or effusion
- Cardiovascular and pulmonary diseases

Cryptorchidism, or undescended testes, is a common congenital defect in dogs (7%) and less frequent in cats (1.3%). It can be unilateral (86%), with a higher incidence in the right testicle, or bilateral (14%). Since retained testicles in the abdomen have an increased incidence of neoplasia and a higher risk of torsion, removal of undescended testicles or castration is the treatment of choice for affected animals.

To determine the exact location of the retained testicle, palpation of the inguinal region is performed in conjunction with ultrasound examination. Laparoscopy is a simple and safe method to remove the retained testicles, with many advantages for the patient due to the reduced morbidity of the procedure. It is also indicated in doubtful cases, in which the presence of fat and lymph nodes in the inguinal region can mimic the presence of the testicle. If it is not possible to locate the testicle using ultrasound, laparoscopic exploration of the abdomen may be considered.

> The first laparoscopic cryptorchidectomy in a dog was described in 1993 by A. Gimbo, G. Catone, et al.

PATIENT PREPARATION AND POSITIONING

The patient should be fasted for 10–12 hours before surgery. The bladder should be emptied before the procedure to allow better visualization. The ventral abdomen is widely clipped, including the entire scrotum caudally. The patient is placed in dorsal recumbency and the skin is aseptically prepared, including an aseptic wash of the prepuce.

It can be useful to tilt the table in a Trendelenburg position (10°–15°) to displace the abdominal organs away from the pelvic region, thereby improving visualization.

OPERATING ROOM LAYOUT

Because the procedure is performed in the caudal abdomen, the monitor (or the scope tower) is placed at the caudal end of the table to leave enough space for the surgeons to move during the procedure. The anesthesia machine is placed near the patient's head. The instrument table is placed caudolateral to the table, on the same side as the surgeon. The surgeon positions themselves on the opposite side in relation to the retained testicle, with the assistant facing the surgeon (**Fig. 1**).

The following procedures are described below:

A. Two-port laparoscopic cryptorchidectomy technique
B. Single-port laparoscopic cryptorchidectomy technique

A TWO-PORT LAPAROSCOPIC CRYPTORCHIDECTOMY

Laparoscopic cryptorchidectomy is typically performed by placing two ports in the caudal region of the abdomen. The use of a third port is not necessary unless the testicle is located in the

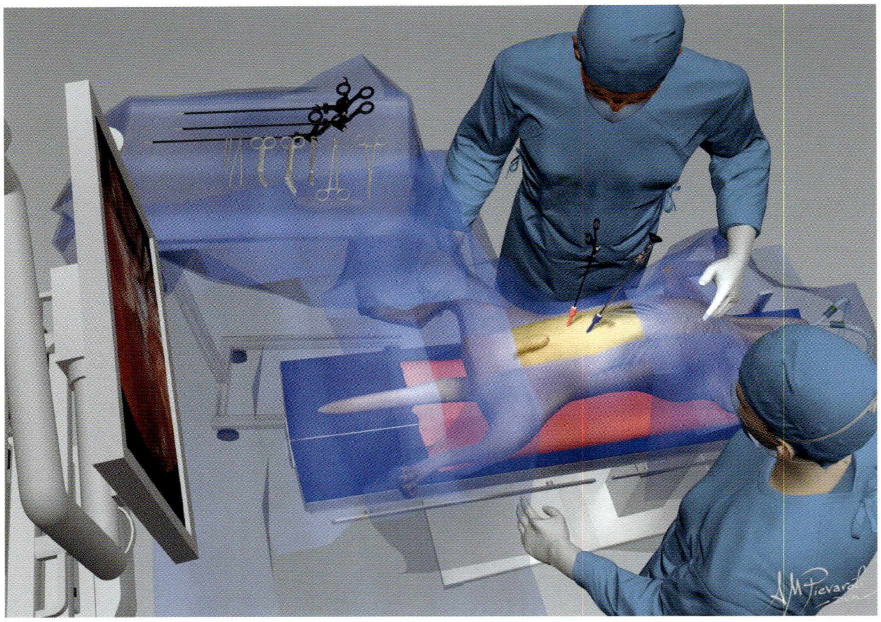

FIGURE 1. Operating room layout for laparoscopic cryptorchidectomy.

inguinal canal and needs to be searched for and isolated. Some authors prefer a single-port multiple-access technique, considered feasible and safe.

In the two-port technique, after introducing the telescope in the first port, the testicle is searched for lateral to the bladder, where it is also possible to follow the vas deferens. The second port is then placed, and the testicle is grasped and lifted using forceps and secured to the body wall using a percutaneous suture. The vascular plexus and vas deferens are closed with a sealing device or endoclips before being transected. The testicle is then removed through one of the ports (**Video 1**).

A laparoscopic-assisted technique has also been described. After having identified and grasped the retained testicle, it is brought out through the second port (enlarged enough to exteriorize the testicle) to perform ligation and resection as in the traditional open technique.

PORT PLACEMENT (FIG. 3)

- T1, on the midline, 1–2 cm caudal to the umbilicus.

VIDEO 1. Two-port laparoscopic cryptorchidectomy.

- T2, in a paramedian position (3–5 cm) on the opposite side of the retained testicle, at the same level or caudal to T1. In case of bilateral cryptorchidism, T2 may also be placed on the midline, caudally to T1.

PROCEDURE

- A pneumoperitoneum is established using the surgeon's preferred technique; the author uses the Ternamian or a modified Hasson technique with threaded cannulas (Storz Endotip) as ports because they are more stable once placed in the patient. After the first port has been placed and the pneumoperitoneum achieved, the 5 mm telescope is inserted and a first exploration of the abdomen is performed to check for any evidence of iatrogenic trauma caused by placement of the first cannula.
- Under endoscopic vision, the second cannula is inserted in a paramedian position on the opposite side of the retained testicle, at the same level or caudal to T1 (**Fig. 4**).
- The region is explored for initial evaluation and identification of the retained testicle, which is usually located lateral to the bladder. The vas deferent can be followed to locate the testicle within the abdomen (**Fig. 5**).
- Babcock forceps or other atraumatic forceps can be used for manipulation of the organs.

Instruments

On the table:

- Standard surgery set
- Telescope 5 mm – 30°
- Two 5 mm threaded cannulas/trocars (or one 5 mm + one 10 mm)
- Grasping forceps (e.g., Babcock, Maryland)
- Large-gauge suture (usually 1 or 0) swaged on a needle
- Vessel-sealing device

Ready to use:

- Third cannula to switch to the three-port technique
- Endoscopic clip applier
- Endoscopic scissors
- Monopolar/bipolar electrosurgery unit

Minilaparoscopy 3 mm set (Fig. 2) for dogs and cats weighing less than 3–4 kg:

- Standard abdominal surgical pack
- Telescope 2.7 mm – 30°
- Two 3 mm cannulas
- Grasping forceps
- Endoscopic scissors
- A suture swaged on a needle
- Bipolar coagulation forceps

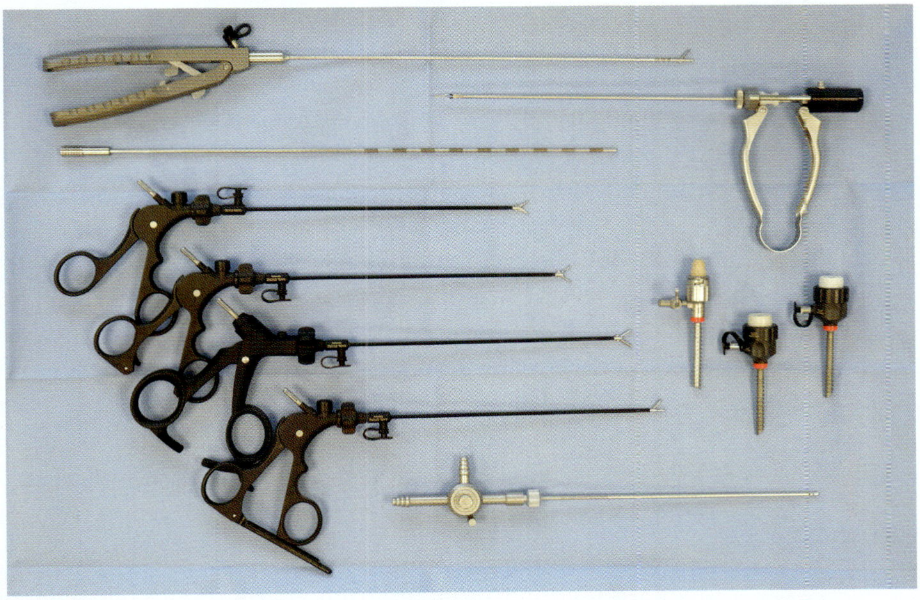

FIGURE 2. Minilaparoscopy set for patients weighing less than 3–4 kg.

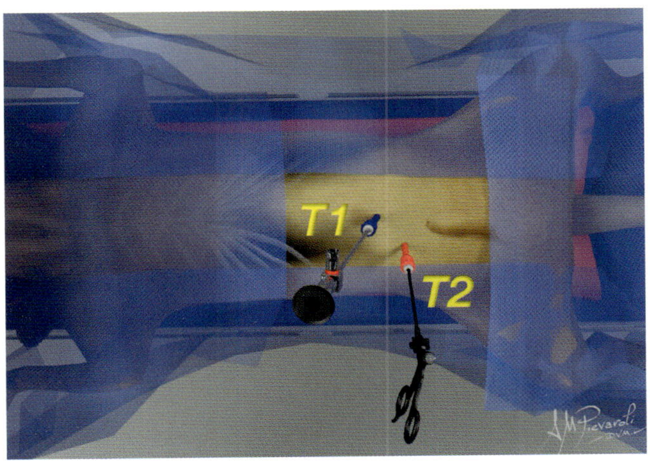

FIGURE 3. Port placement for two-port laparoscopic cryptorchidectomy.

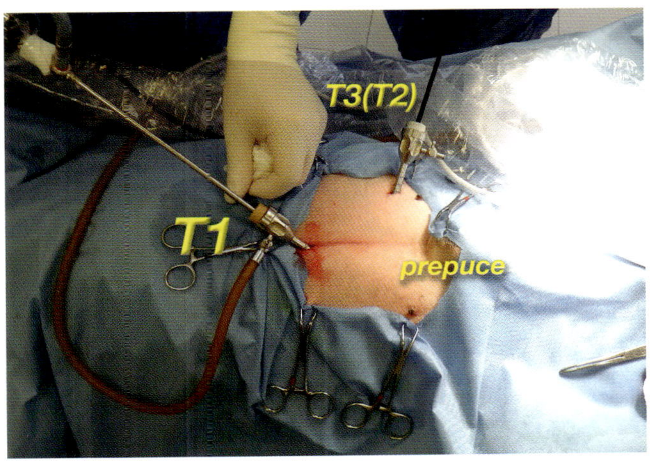

FIGURE 4. Image of the operating field for two-port laparoscopic cryptorchidectomy.

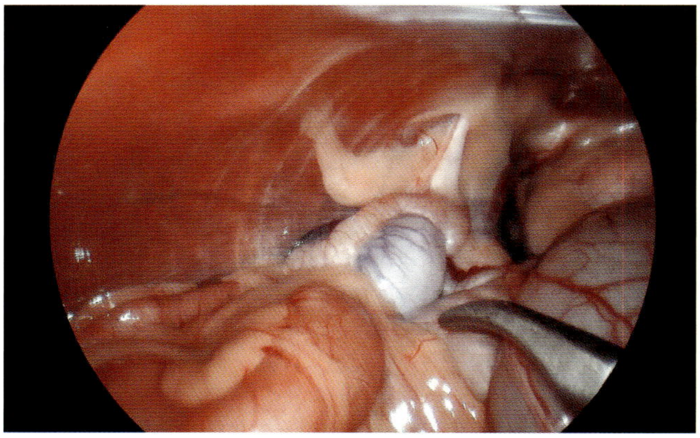

FIGURE 5. The retained testicle is usually located lateral to the bladder (the left testicle is shown in the image).

Tips

If the vas deferens along with the testicular artery and vein enter the inguinal canal, the testicle has partially completed its transabdominal descent. In this case, the testicle may be brought back into the abdomen by performing gentle traction on the vas deferens (Fig. 6).
If this is not possible, it is necessary to perform a surgical exploration using the traditional open technique to search for the testicle in the inguinal region.

- The testicle is grasped and brought to the ipsilateral abdominal wall using forceps (**Fig. 7**). A suture inserted percutaneously with a needle can be used to suspend and stabilize the testicle (in the same way as in two-port laparoscopic ovariectomy) (**Fig. 8**).

Tips

In neoplastic testicles, avoid passing the needle through the neoplastic tissue to reduce the risk of spreading cancer cells.

- After removing the grasping forceps, a vessel-sealing device is inserted and used to coagulate and resect the vas deferens, pampiniform plexus, and gubernaculum testis (**Fig. 9**). Alternatively, endoscopic clips and endoscopic scissors can be used to resect these structures (**Fig. 10**). In small-breed dogs and cats, in which minilaparoscopy can be performed (**Fig. 11**), 3 mm bipolar forceps and scissors can be used (**Fig. 12**).
- If the testicle is partially or completely twisted, adhesions to adjacent structures may need to be removed. If necessary, a third port can be placed for two-handed manipulation.
- After resection, adequate hemostasis should be ensured. In large dogs, particular care must be paid in closing the large pampiniform plexus.
- The forceps are inserted in the port to grasp the testicle (**Fig. 13**). The suture is released and the cannula is removed while pulling the testicle out of the abdomen; the port incision may need to be enlarged depending on the size of the testicle.
- When neoplastic testicles are removed, the abdominal cavity and organs must be inspected to evaluate for metastasis.
- The abdomen is deflated and the small incisions are closed routinely.
- To complete the surgery, prescrotal castration is performed to remove the other testicle.

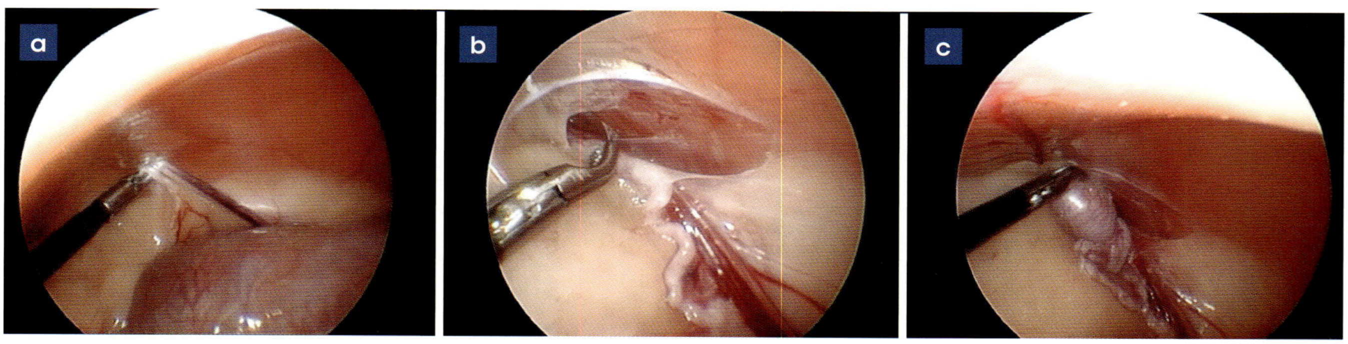

FIGURE 6. Minilaparoscopy in a cat. a) The cryptorchid testicle is located in the inguinal canal. b) Gentle traction is performed on the vas deferens and tissues are dissected. c) The testicle is brought back into the abdomen.

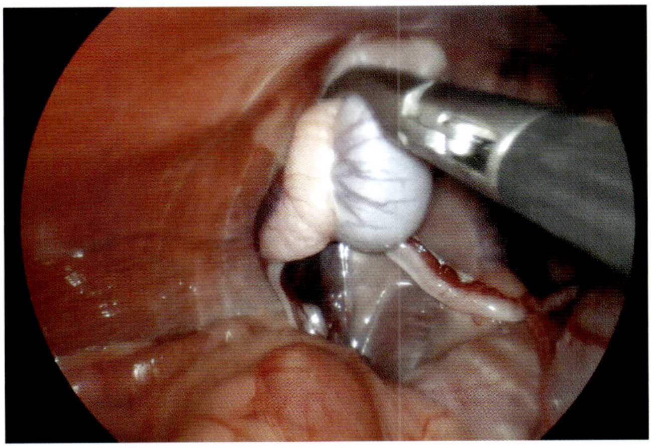

FIGURE 7. The testicle is grasped and brought to the ipsilateral abdominal wall.

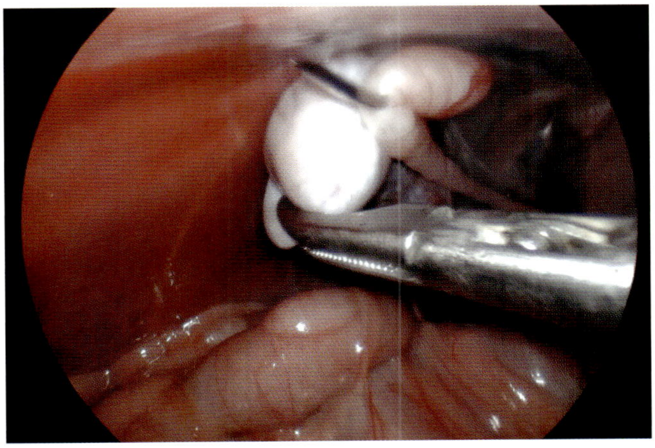

FIGURE 8. A suture is inserted percutaneously with a needle to suspend and stabilize the testicle.

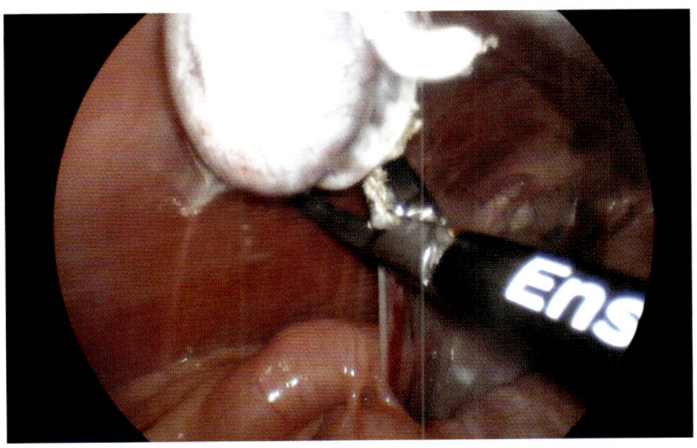

FIGURE 9. A vessel-sealing device is used to coagulate and resect the vas deferens, pampiniform plexus, and gubernaculum testis.

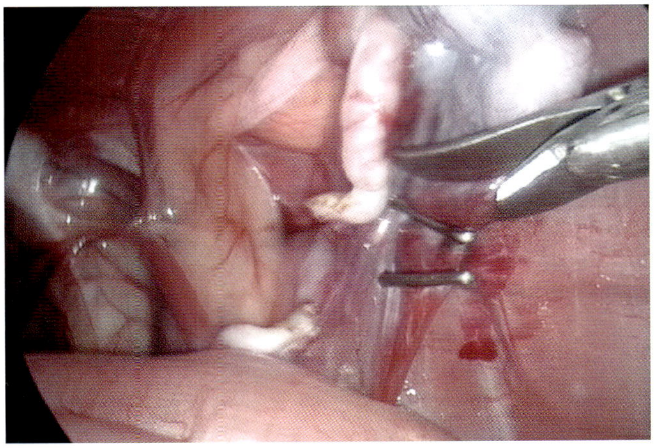

FIGURE 10. As an alternative to electrical devices, laparoscopic clips can be used to interrupt vascular structures, which are then resected using scissors.

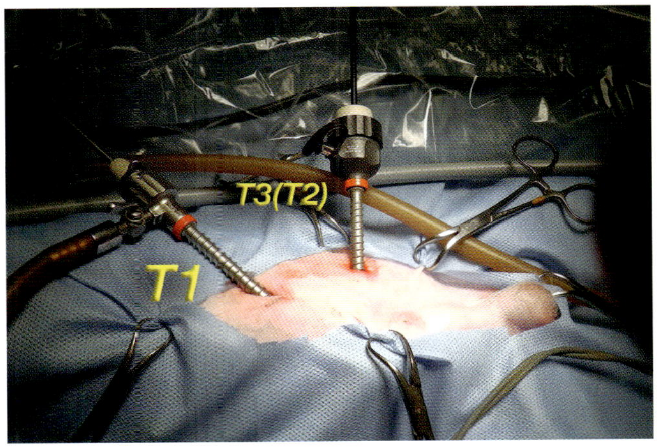

FIGURE 11. Image of the operating field for minilaparoscopic cryptorchidectomy in a small-size patient.

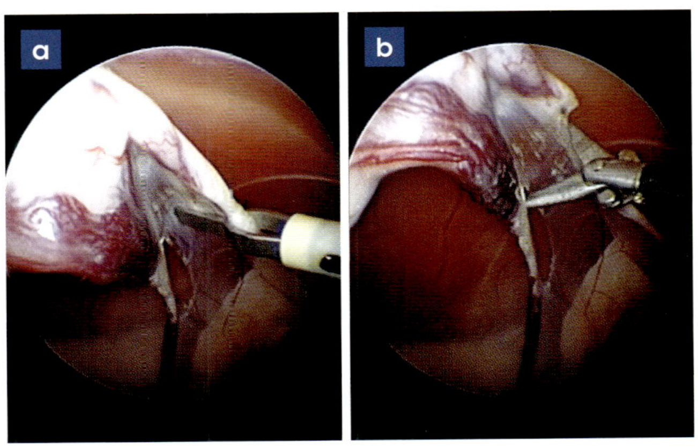

FIGURE 12. Two-port minilaparoscopy. a) Use of 3 mm bipolar forceps to coagulate the vas deferens, pampiniform plexus, and gubernaculum testis. b) The structures are then resected with scissors.

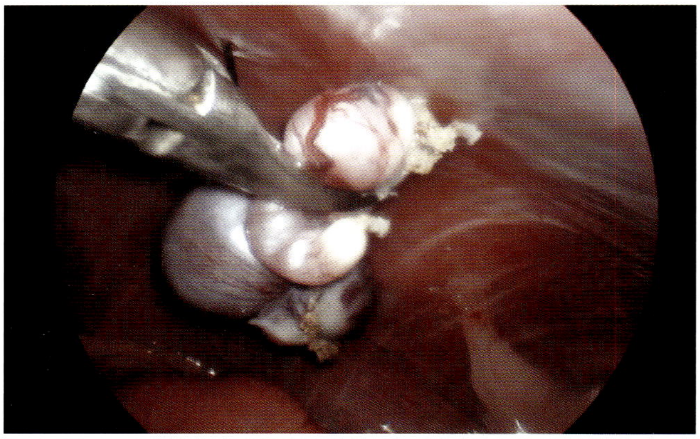

FIGURE 13. The resected testicle is grasped using forceps.

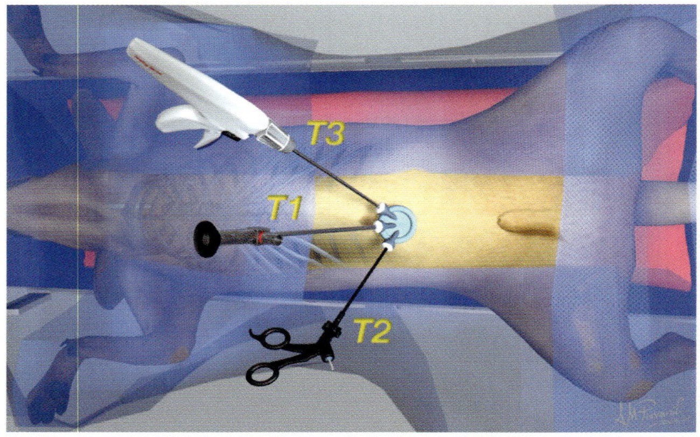

FIGURE 14. Single-port placement for laparoscopic cryptorchidectomy.

B SINGLE-PORT LAPAROSCOPIC CRYPTORCHIDECTOMY

Jeffrey J. Runge, Joshua G. Becker

Instruments

- Standard surgery set
- Telescope 5 mm – 30°
- Single-incision port device
- A bipolar vessel-sealing device appropriate for the patient size
- Articulating laparoscopic grasping forceps (e.g., SILS Clinch Graspers)
- A specimen retrieval bag should be considered if testicular neoplasia is suspected

PORT PLACEMENT (FIG. 14)

- T1, T2, T3. The port is placed in standard fashion at the level of the umbilicus.

PROCEDURE

- After the port has been placed and a pneumoperitoneum established, the telescope is inserted and the abdomen is surveyed in standard fashion, checking for anatomical landmarks and identifying the visible anatomy. Care must be taken to avoid and check for evidence of iatrogenic trauma secondary to port placement (**Fig. 15**).
- The testicle and relevant anatomy are identified. In some cases, the intra-abdominal testicle can be readily identified in the mid-caudal abdomen (**Fig. 16**). To locate the testicle, either the testicular artery and vein can be followed from their craniodorsal origin near the kidney or the vas deferens can be followed from its insertion into the prostatic urethra. The gubernaculum testis can also be followed cranially from the inguinal canal to locate the testicle within the abdomen.
- The patient's position on the operating table can be manually adjusted into a modified dorsal-lateral recumbency to better visualize the contralateral testicle (e.g., if first removing the left testicle, the patient would be adjusted into a modified right lateral recumbency). If the surgeon has a surgical table with a lateral tilt function, this can be utilized on its own or concurrently to help facilitate this process (**Fig. 17**).
- The patient's abdomen can also be gently shaken after positioning to adjust the omentum and other potentially obstructive viscera, thus improving visualization of the testicles.
- The articulating forceps or other blunt probing instruments can be used to manipulate and position tissue for better visualization.
- With the articulating grasper, a 90° positional bend at the distal third of the instrument can be created with the tip deflecting toward the testicle.
- The spermatic cord is then grasped using the forceps, which can be locked in a closed position, and the spermatic cord is elevated to visualize and isolate the tissue. The tissue is suspended with the bent portion of the articulating instrument still deflected (**Fig. 18**).

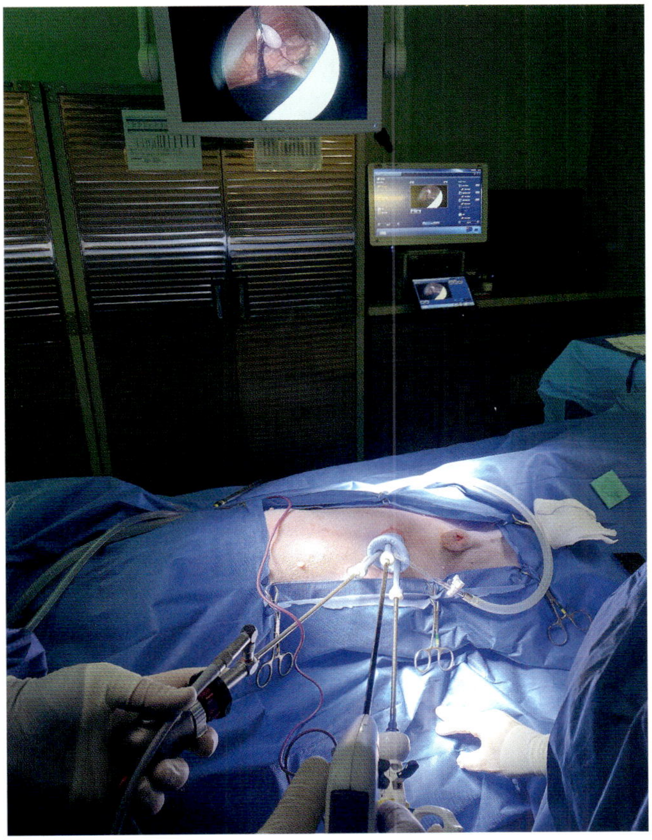

FIGURE 15. Placement of the SILS port for a laparoscopic cryptorchidectomy of a left abdominal testicle. This instrument arrangement utilizes a telescope, an articulating grasper, and a bipolar vessel-sealing device.

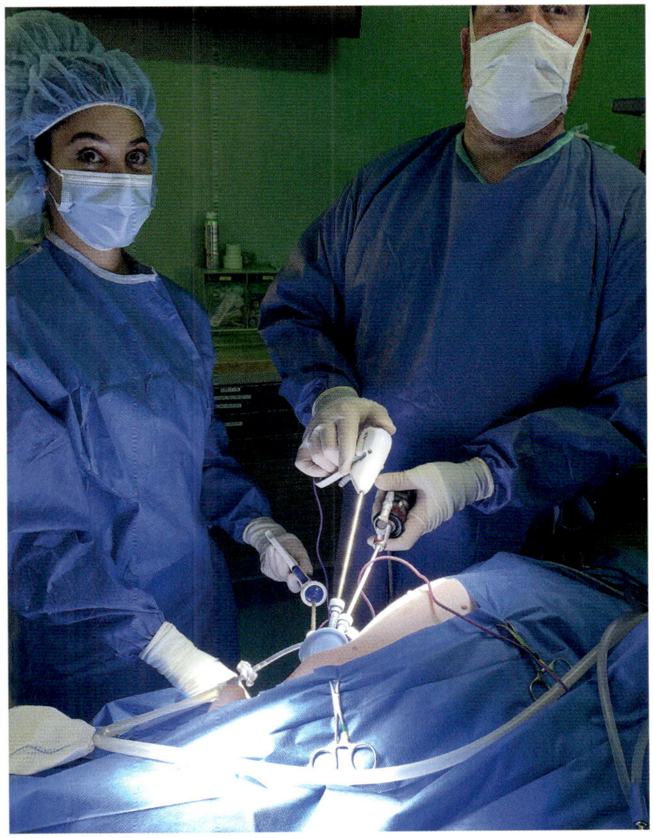

FIGURE 17. Position of surgeon and assistant surgeon for single-port laparoscopic cryptorchidectomy of a left abdominal testicle.

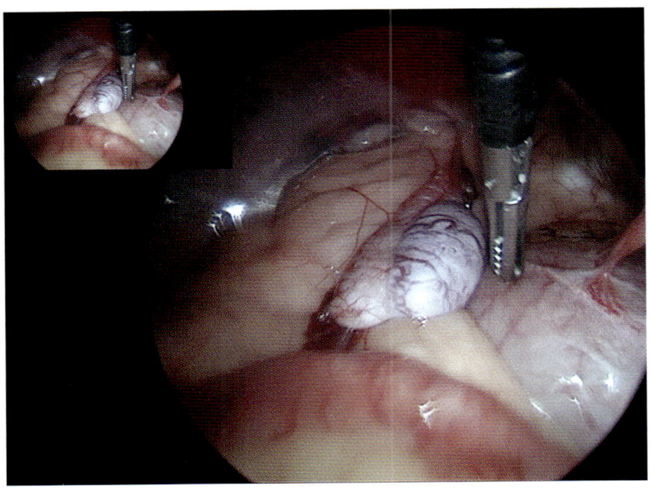

FIGURE 16. Laparoscopic view of a left testicle retained in the caudal abdomen, adjacent to the bladder.

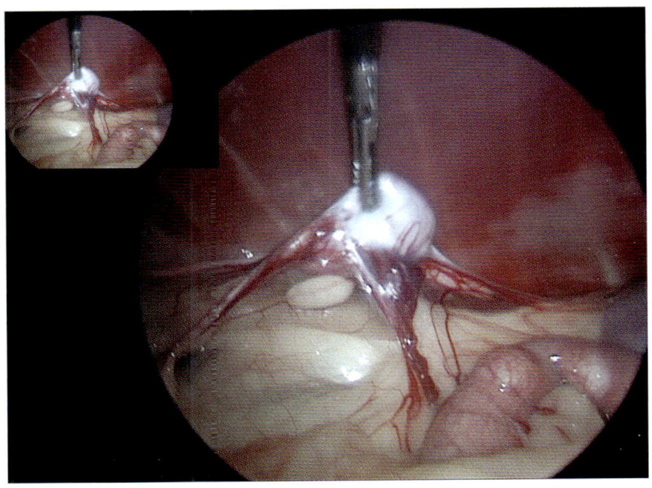

FIGURE 18. An articulating grasper is used to suspend a retained abdominal testicle.

- With the testicle and relevant anatomy isolated, the vessel-sealing device is then used to carefully seal and cut the vas deferens/vascular bundle, epididymal ligament/gubernaculum, and any other residual ligamentous attachments.
- Once the testicle and associated tissue have been dissected from their attachments, the testicle can be partially retracted from the laparoscopic field to better visualize the dissection site and monitor for any delayed bleeding. Care should be taken to ensure that the testicle is properly grasped prior to dissection and retraction from the visual field to minimize the risk of inadvertent dropping in the abdominal cavity
- If the SILS port is used, the port should be removed from the incision along with the forceps grasping the testicle in order to remove the testicle.
- If testicular neoplasia is suspected, the testicle should be placed into a specimen retrieval bag prior to removal.
- It is recommended to inspect the testicle to check for completeness of dissection.
- In case of bilateral cryptorchidism, the contralateral testicle can be removed in the same manner. If the contralateral side is unaffected, a routine castration can then be performed.

POSTOPERATIVE MANAGEMENT

- Most patients have short general anesthesia times and recover rapidly after surgery.
- Patients that are considered stable and healthy preoperatively can typically be discharged on the same day.
- Patients that are undergoing surgery for suspected neoplasia should be evaluated for stability to determine recommendations for overnight hospitalization and monitoring.
- Local analgesics at the time of incision site closure and injectable analgesics in the immediate postoperative phase are recommended.
- The patient can be discharged with a short course of additional medications for pain control.
- For laparoscopic cryptorchidectomy without concomitant pathologies antibiotic therapy is not necessary.

Complications of laparoscopic cryptorchidectomy

- Low complication rates, mostly related to laparoscopic procedures.
- Hemorrhage in the first hours following surgery due to incomplete closure of the vascular structures.
- Iatrogenic trauma to peripheral organs.

Key points

- Perform preoperative imaging to ensure that the testicle is located intra-abdominally.
- In large-sized dogs, be very mindful of the sealing or clipping of the pampiniform plexus to avoid intra-abdominal bleeding after the procedure.

SUGGESTED READINGS

CLINICAL CASES

18.1 TESTICULAR TORSION IN A CRYPTORCHID DOG

Andrea M. Pievaroli

CASE DESCRIPTION

A 6-year-old German Shepherd Dog was presented for elective castration and laparoscopic removal of the undescended right testicle. A previously performed ultrasound examination had identified the right testicle in the intra-abdominal region. During the laparoscopic procedure, reactive adhesions were observed in the pelvic region, with the involvement of the omentum. This anomaly was found to be caused by the torsion of the testicle retained in the abdomen, occurred at an unknown time and without the dog showing evident clinical signs. After identifying the testicle, the adhesions and testicular structures were resected using a vessel-sealing device. The testicle was then removed through one of the ports by the laparoscopic technique.

Key points

- Preoperative imaging is critical to identify the intra-abdominal testicle.
- When not clearly visible, particular care should be taken to seal or clip the pampiniform plexus to avoid the risk of intra-abdominal bleeding in the postoperative period.

PORT PLACEMENT

The patient was placed in dorsal recumbency. The first cannula (T1) was placed on the midline, 1–2 cm caudal to the umbilicus. The second cannula (T2) was placed in a right paramedian position, 2–3 cm caudal to T1. The third cannula (T3) was placed in a left paramedian position, 2–3 cm caudal to T1.

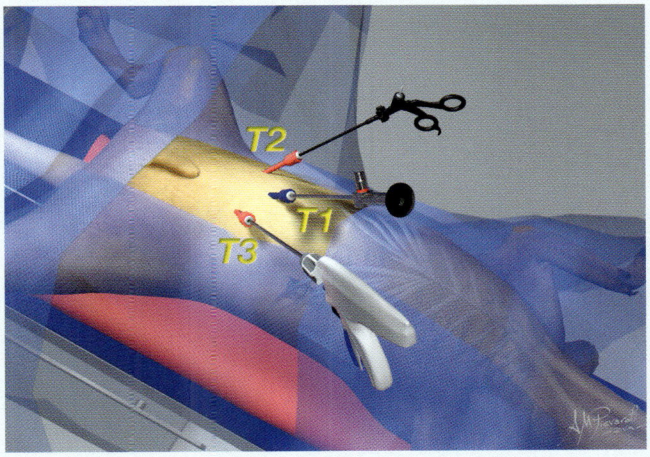

PROCEDURE

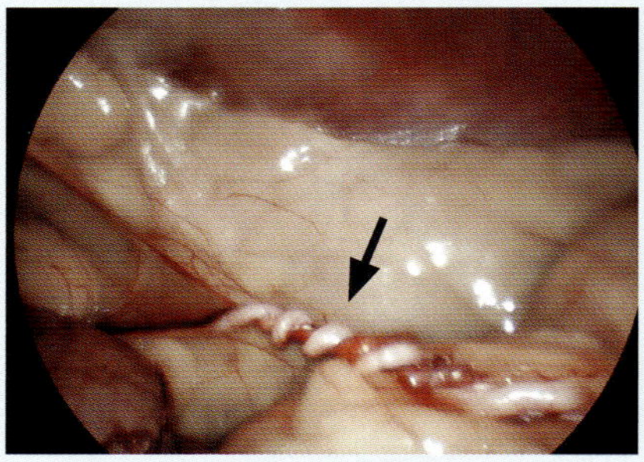

FIGURE 1. The twisted aspect of the vas deferens and vascular structures is clearly visible (arrow).

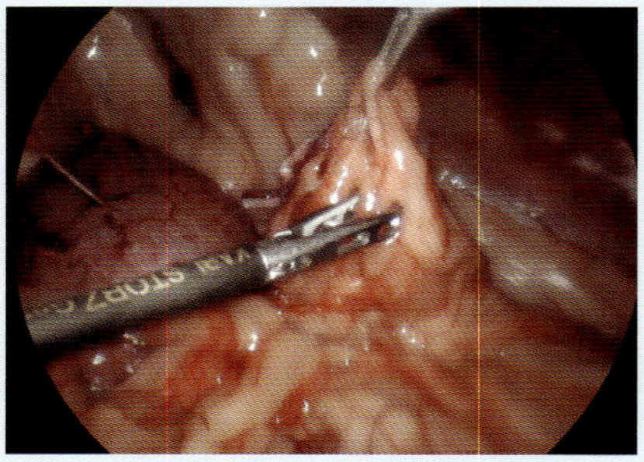

FIGURE 2. The testicle (not visible) is incorporated within the adhesions of the omentum.

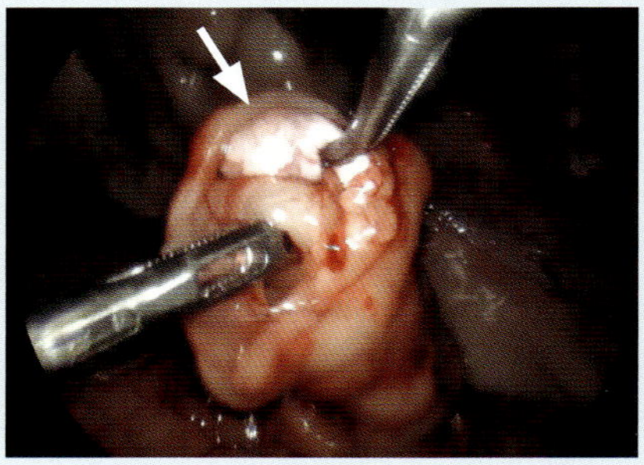

FIGURE 3. With the help of the second forceps, a dissection is performed to locate and free the testicle (arrow).

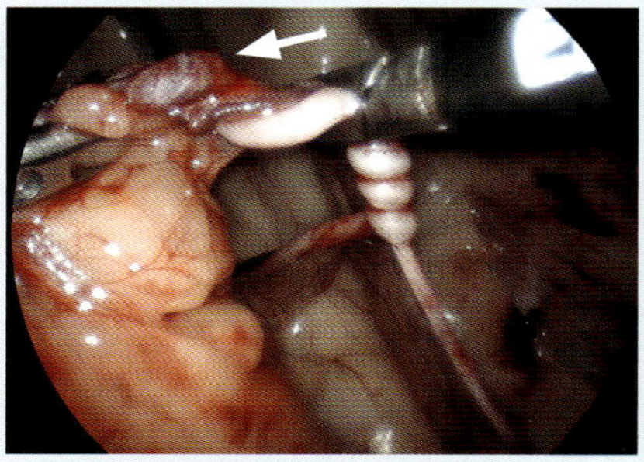

FIGURE 4. Continuing the dissection, the pampiniform plexus is also visible (arrow).

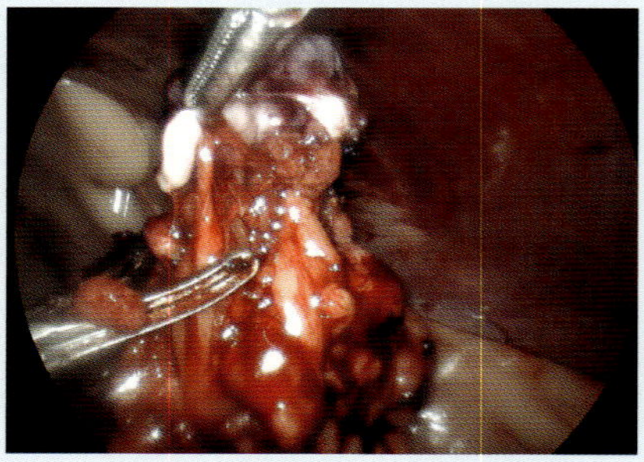

FIGURE 5. The adhesions, vas deferens, and vascular structures are resected with the vessel-sealing device. It may be helpful to secure the testicle to the abdominal wall using a percutaneous suture.

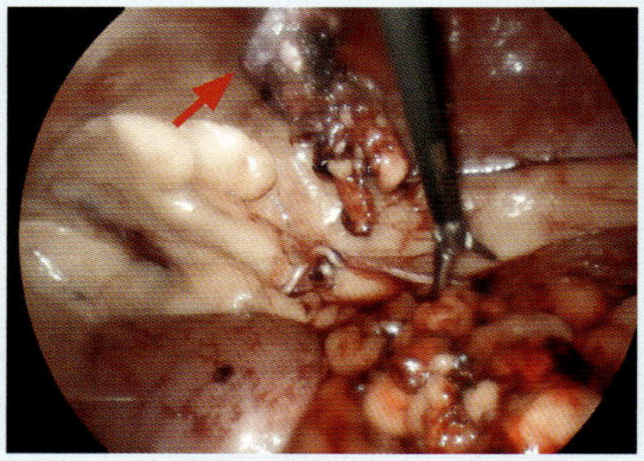

FIGURE 6. After the testicle has been resected, the area should be inspected to make sure there is no bleeding. The testicle (arrow) is removed through one of the ports.

Tips and tricks

- ✓ Start with a two-port technique. Then, after performing a first laparoscopic exploration, and only if necessary, add the third port.
- ✓ Secure the testicle to the abdominal wall using a percutaneous suture.
- ✓ Use a vessel-sealing device.

18.2 LAPAROSCOPIC CRYPTORCHIDECTOMY

D. L. Casas García

CASE DESCRIPTION

A 7-month-old male Teckel presented without testicles in the scrotum on physical examination. During ultrasound examination, both testicles were visualized in the abdomen, confirming a bilateral cryptorchidism. No other anomalies were detected in the ultrasound evaluation. Bilateral laparoscopic cryptorchidectomy was scheduled.

Key points

- In cases of testicular neoplasia or testicular torsion, adhesions to adjacent structures can impair visualization or the access for dissection.
- It is important to remember that a complete abdominal exploration must be done to evaluate for metastasis, especially in the regional lymph nodes, kidneys, spleen, pancreas, and liver.
- When cryptorchidism is unilateral, the last step is to remove the scrotal testicle by the conventional surgical technique.

PORT PLACEMENT

From a minimally invasive point of view, cryptorchidism in small animals can be managed by multiport or single-port laparoscopic surgery. In this case, the multiport technique was chosen, with the use of minilaparoscopic percutaneous forceps for the suspension of both testicles. Three ports were used for the procedure: a telescope port (T1), a 3 mm right-handed instrument port (T2), and a 5 mm left-handed instrument port (T3).

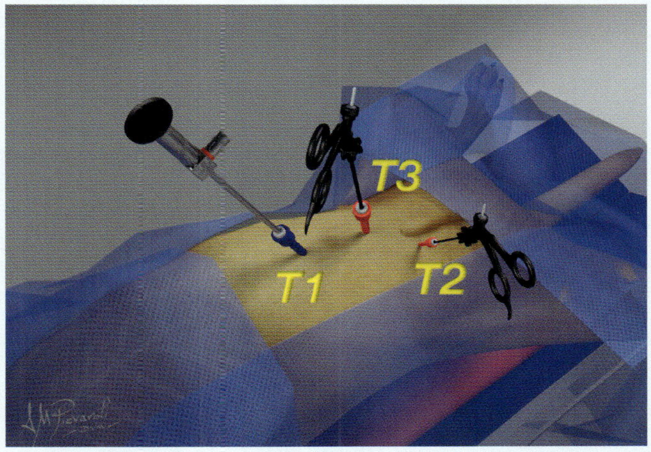

PROCEDURE

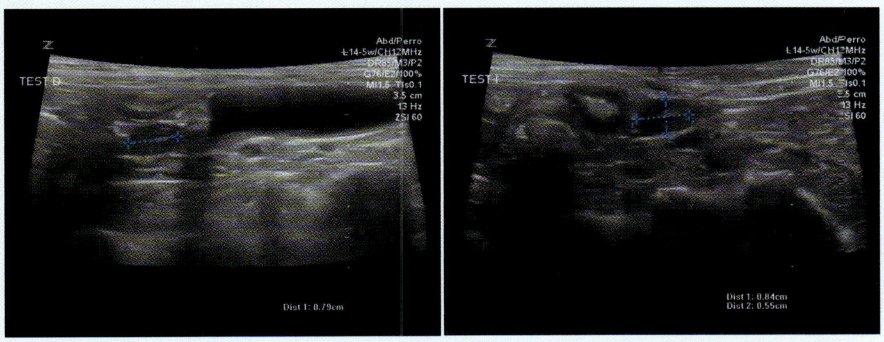

FIGURE 1. Ultrasound is the main tool for diagnosis of cryptorchidism because it allows identification and localization of undescended testicles in the inguinal and intra-abdominal regions with a sensitivity of 100% and 96%, respectively.

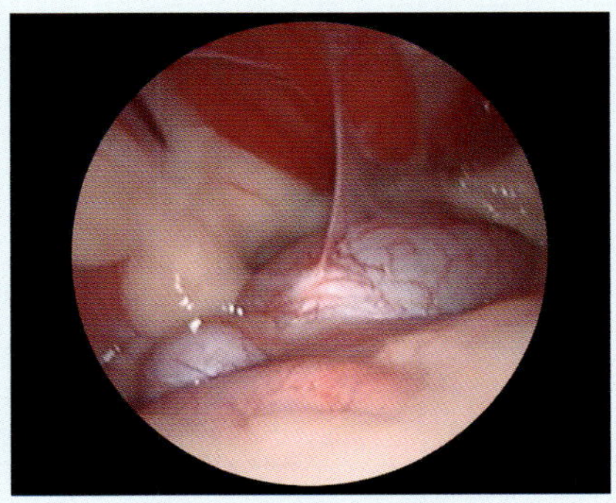

FIGURE 2. With the patient in dorsal recumbency, it can be difficult to visualize undescended testicles during laparoscopic exploration of the caudal region of the abdomen.

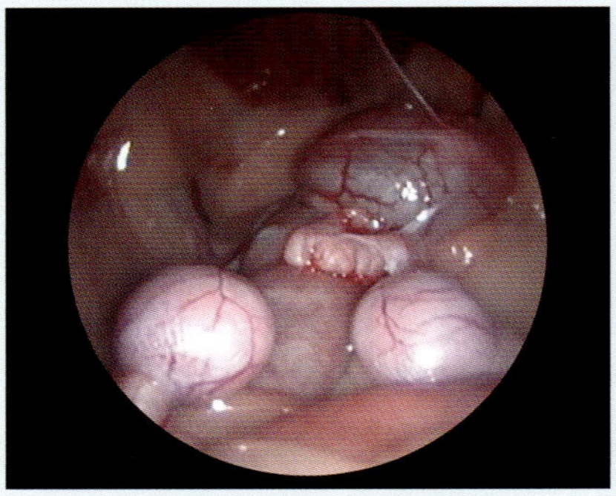

FIGURE 3. Using a Trendelenburg position, intra-abdominal testicles are easily visualized because the intestines move cranially by gravity.

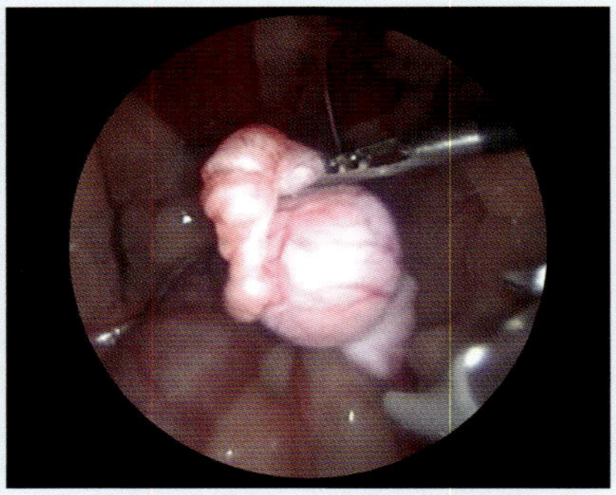

FIGURE 4. The testicles are suspended using minilaparoscopic forceps inserted percutaneously paramedial to the linea alba.

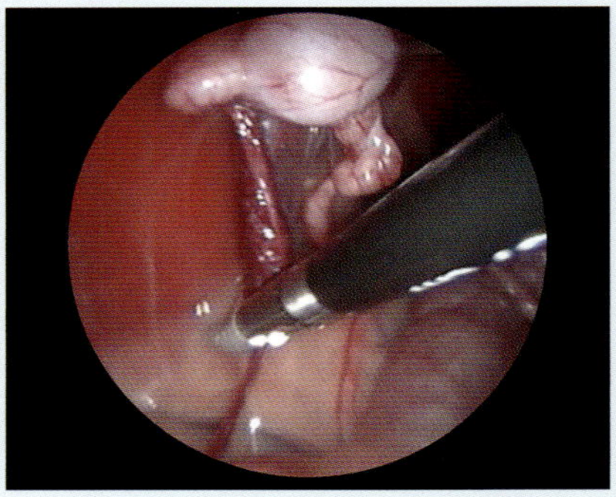

FIGURE 5. With the testicles suspended, the different structures, including the testicular arteries and veins, are coagulated and cut.

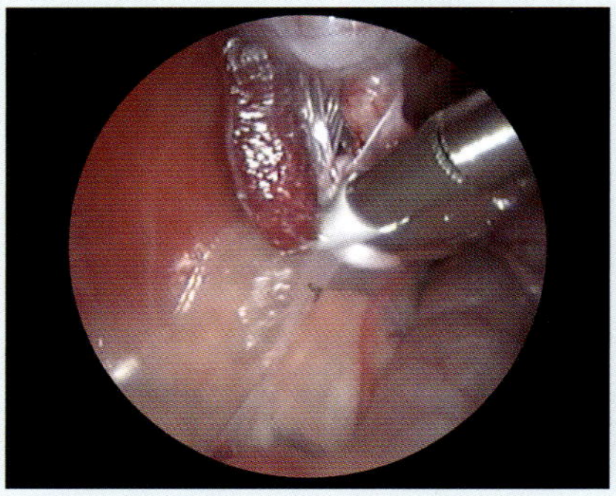

FIGURE 6. The vasa deferentia and their corresponding arteries as well as the epididymal ligaments are then sealed and sectioned.

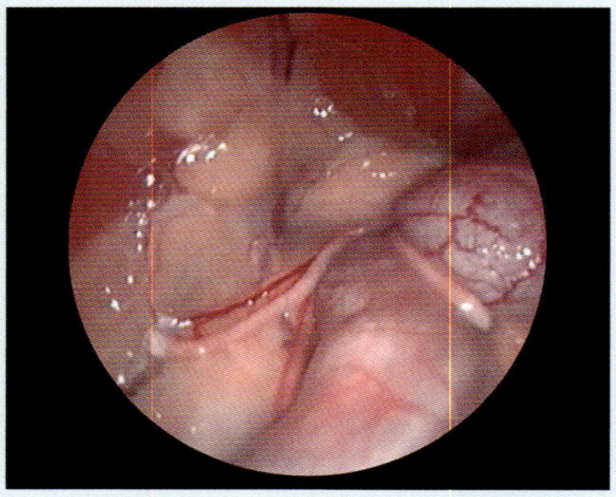

FIGURE 7. Hemostasis of the sectioned structures and the absence of iatrogenic trauma, especially to the ureters, must always be checked.

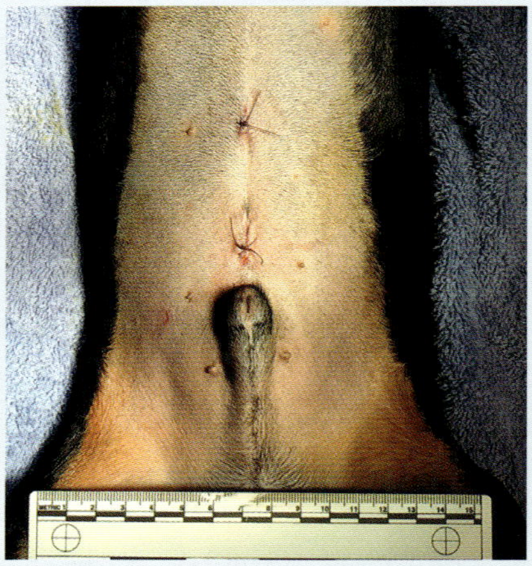

FIGURE 8. The use of a laparoscopic technique for cryptorchidism management in small animals allows an early postoperative recovery of the patients with satisfactory esthetic results.

Tips and tricks

- ✓ Put the patient in a Trendelenburg position to displace the intestines cranially. This helps in localizing the testicles and increases the working field.
- ✓ To minimize the number of implanted trocars, the testicles can be suspended using minilaparoscopic forceps or a transabdominal suture.
- ✓ In cases of partial or complete testicular torsion, the testicle must be sectioned in that twisted position to limit reperfusion injury.

19 LAPAROSCOPIC-ASSISTED CYSTOSCOPY AND PERCUTANEOUS SUPRAPUBIC CYSTOSCOPY

Andrea M. Pievaroli

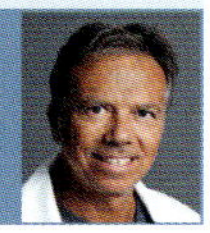

Indications	Contraindications
■ Removal of calculi	■ Complex abdominal diseases
■ Resection of polyps	■ Active urinary tract infections
■ Biopsy of the bladder and masses	■ Not indicated for resection of bladder masses

Laparoscopic-assisted cystoscopy is a minimally invasive surgical procedure that allows access to the bladder from the prepubic (suprapubic) region. It has been proven to be a valid alternative to traditional laparotomic cystotomy, especially in small male patients in which the size and course of the urethra do not allow the use of adequate flexible endoscopic instruments to perform retrograde cystoscopy.

While laparoscopic-assisted cystoscopy is mainly indicated to remove urinary stones, it can also be performed for the treatment of some bladder pathologies or for the collection of biopsy samples. It offers all the benefits of minimally invasive surgery, including minimal postoperative pain and rapid recovery. It has been reported that traditional surgical techniques do not allow complete removal of bladder stones in 10%–20% of cases. This is also due to poor visualization, especially at the level of the bladder neck and the first tract of the urethra. Higher complication rates associated with traditional surgical cystotomy and higher recurrence rates of suture-induced uroliths have led to the perfection of less invasive surgical techniques to access the bladder lumen, especially for the removal of calculi. The original technique, laparoscopic-assisted cystotomy, was first described in 2003 and involves the use of CO_2 to establish a pneumoperitoneum. This laparoscopic access also allows exploration of the abdominal cavity and can be associated with other procedures before identifying and lifting the cranial portion of the bladder. In the following years, when the purpose of the procedure was only to access the bladder lumen, a new technique without the use of CO_2, called percutaneous suprapubic cystoscopy or percutaneous cystolithotomy (PCCL), was developed and proved to be faster and just as effective. In this chapter, both techniques are described: laparoscopic-assisted cystotomy and PCCL.

> The first laparoscopic-assisted cystoscopy in dogs was reported in 2003 by C. A. Rawlings et al.

PATIENT PREPARATION AND POSITIONING

The patient should be fasted for 10-12 hours before surgery. If intraoperative cystocentesis for urine culture is not planned, it is preferable to start antibiotic therapy a few days before surgery to minimize the risk of intraoperative infections due to incision of the bladder and urine leakage into the abdomen. The ventral abdomen is widely clipped, including the entire prepuce or vulva caudally. The patient is placed in dorsal recumbency and the skin is aseptically prepared, including an aseptic wash of the prepuce or vulva. Prior to surgery, the bladder should be catheterized to drain the urine, and at least two or three lavages with warm saline mixed with 1%–2% povidone-iodine, followed by flushing with saline, should be performed. After flushing, the bladder should be filled with saline solution, avoiding overdistension.

It can be useful to tilt the table in a Trendelenburg position (10°–15°) to displace the abdominal organs away from the pelvic region, thereby improving visualization of the bladder.

OPERATING ROOM LAYOUT

Since both procedures are performed in the caudal abdomen, the monitor (or the scope tower) is placed at the caudal end of the table. The anesthesia machine is placed near the patient's head. The instrument table is placed caudolateral to the table, on the same side as the surgeon. The surgeon positions themselves on the right or left side of the patient, depending on personal preference (right- or left-handed person). The assistant positions themselves on the opposite side. It is advisable to tilt the table into a Trendelenburg position (**Fig. 1**).

The following procedures are described below:

A. Laparoscopic-assisted cystoscopy technique

B. Percutaneous suprapubic cystoscopy or percutaneous cystolithotomy technique (PCCL)

C. Single-port percutaneous cystolithotomy technique (J. Runge and J. Becker)

A LAPAROSCOPIC-ASSISTED CYSTOSCOPY

The first step of this technique involves a laparoscopic approach with the use of CO_2 to establish a pneumoperitoneum. This insufflation allows the surgeon to explore the abdominal cavity and organs, perform other procedures (e.g., biopsy), and accurately choose the portion of the bladder to be exteriorized. With the aid of stay sutures, a small cystotomy is performed and a cystoscope is introduced. Through the incision, the bladder and urethra can be examined, lavages can be performed, and uroliths can be removed (**Video 1**).

VIDEO 1. Laparoscopic-assisted cystoscopy.

PORT PLACEMENT (FIG. 3)

- T1, on the midline, 2–3 cm caudal to the umbilicus.
- T2, on the midline, a few centimeters caudal to T1, at the level of the bladder apex. In some male dogs, T2 can be placed slightly lateral to the prepuce, depending also on the location of the cranial portion of the bladder.

PROCEDURE

- A pneumoperitoneum is established using the surgeon's preferred technique; the author uses the Ternamian or a modified Hasson technique with threaded cannulas (Storz Endotip) as ports because they are more stable once placed

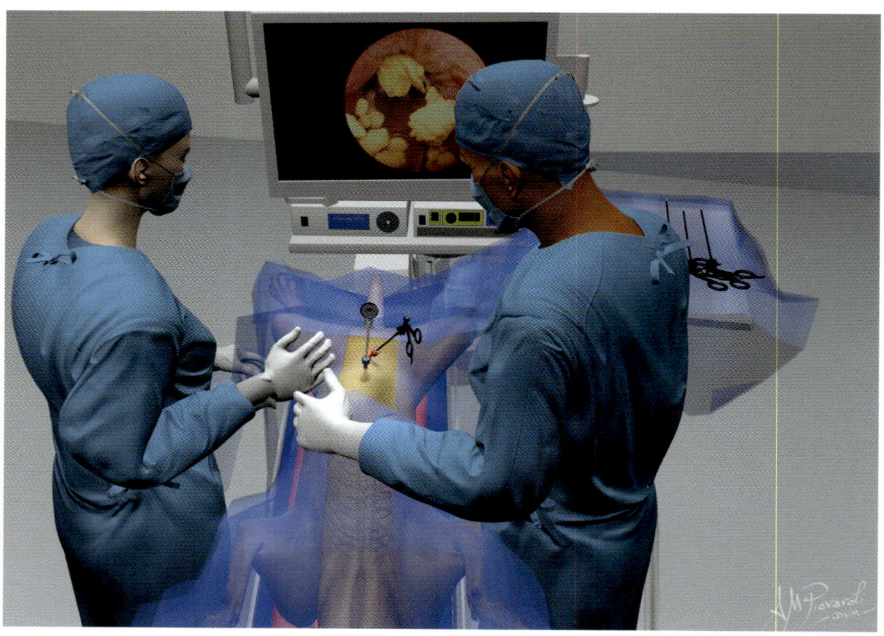

FIGURE 1. Operating room layout for laparoscopic-assisted cystoscopy and percutaneous suprapubic cystoscopy.

Instruments

On the table:

- Standard surgery set
- Cystoscope or telescope 2.7/5 mm – 0°/30°, with sheath
- 5 mm threaded cannulas/trocars
- Grasping forceps (e.g., Babcock, alligator)
- Basket catheter for uroliths
- Laser system device
- Suction/irrigation system

Ready to use:

- Flexible endoscope (video/optical) 2.5–3 mm (**Fig. 2**)

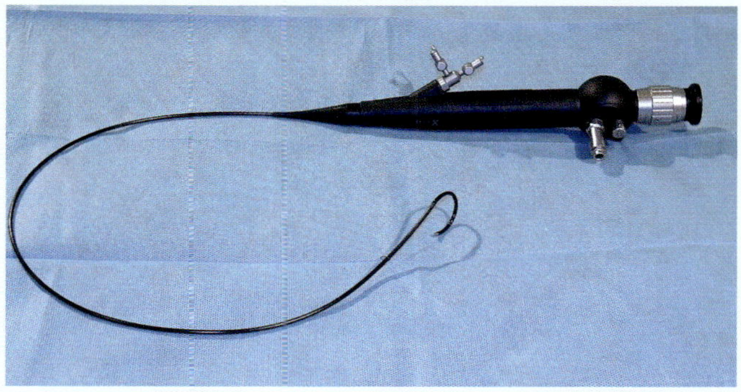

FIGURE 2. Flexible endoscope (2.5 mm ureteroscope, Karl Storz Flex-X2).

in the patient. After the first port has been placed and the pneumoperitoneum achieved, the 5 mm telescope is inserted and a first exploration of the abdomen is performed to check for any evidence of iatrogenic trauma caused by placement of the first cannula.

- Under endoscopic vision, the second cannula is inserted in a median position, caudal to the first cannula, at the level of the bladder apex.
- The region is explored for initial evaluation and identification of the bladder. Babcock forceps or other atraumatic forceps can be used to manipulate the bladder.
- The cranial portion of the bladder is grasped and brought to the port site, close to the abdominal wall, using forceps (**Fig. 4**).
- The caudal cannula is elevated along the forceps, still in place (**Fig. 5**), and the site of incision on the skin and abdominal wall is enlarged. The incision should be limited to 2–3 cm in length. If necessary, depending on the size of the urolith to be extracted, the incision can be enlarged at a later time (**Fig. 6**).
- To keep the bladder attached to the abdominal wall, two to four stay sutures can be placed in the four quadrants to

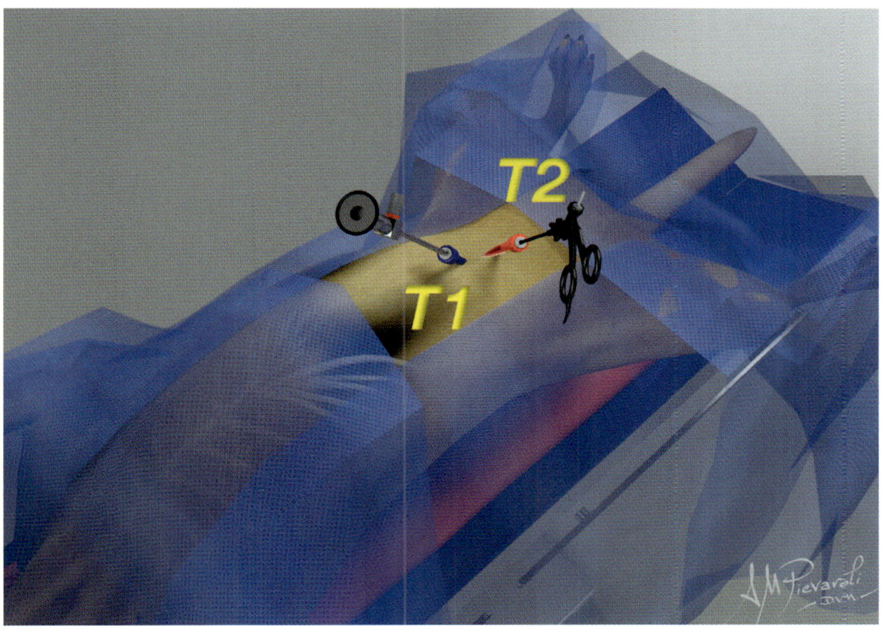

FIGURE 3. Port placement for laparoscopic-assisted cystoscopy.

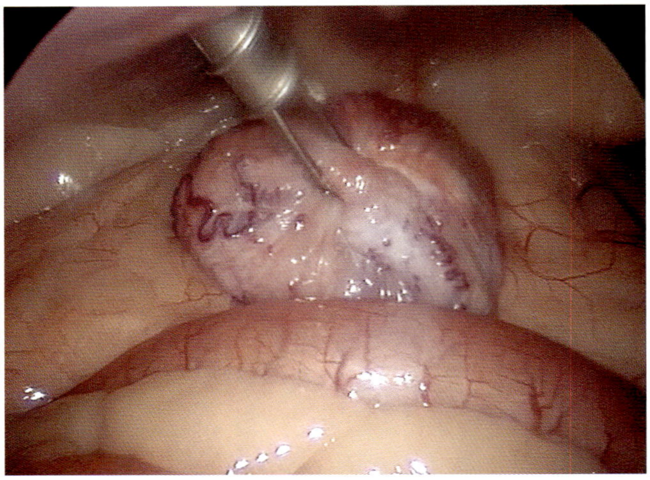

FIGURE 4. The apex of the bladder is grasped using forceps.

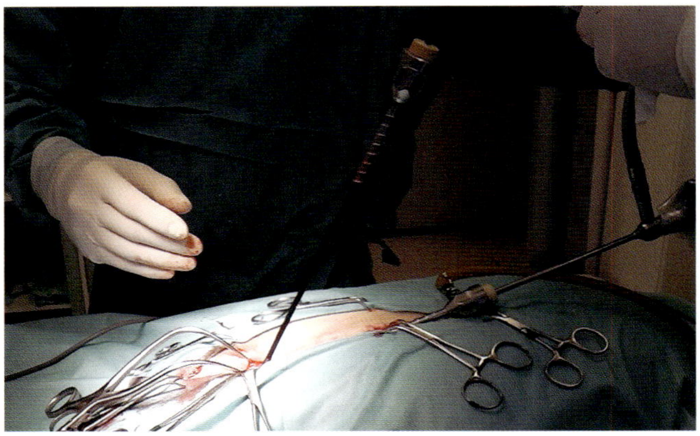

FIGURE 5. The caudal cannula is elevated along the forceps still grasping the bladder.

prevent urine contamination of subcutaneous tissues and peritoneal cavity, and the area can be packed with gauze to reduce urine contamination. Alternatively, the bladder can be fixed to the skin (cystopexy) using a temporary continuous suture (modified laparoscopic-assisted cystotomy).

- Once the bladder is secured, a small incision is made in the bladder using a number 11 scalpel blade (**Fig. 7**). A suction cannula should be promptly utilized to aspirate the leak of urine and the fluid contained in the bladder (**Fig. 8**).
- The cystoscope (or 2.7–5 mm endoscope with sheath) is then inserted into the bladder (**Fig. 9**). The endoscope may be inserted through a threaded trocar screwed to the bladder wall. This trocar acts as a port to access the bladder (**Fig. 10**).
- For better visualization of the bladder cavity, it is important to perform continuous infusion of saline solution. This can be achieved by connecting the infusion set to the Luer lock. Egress occurs through the urinary catheter introduced at the beginning of the procedure. The flow can be reversed during the procedure.

Tips

The flow of saline solution can be reversed to facilitate the movement of small nonvisible stones located along the urethra.

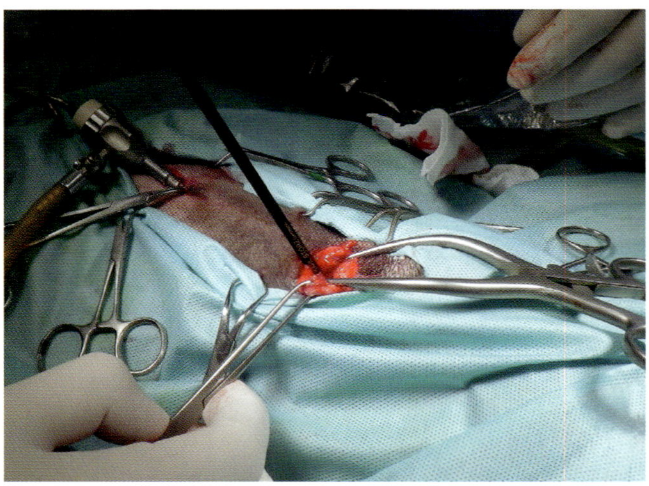

FIGURE 6. The incision on the skin and abdominal wall is enlarged. The wall of the bladder is lifted and exposed using the forceps.

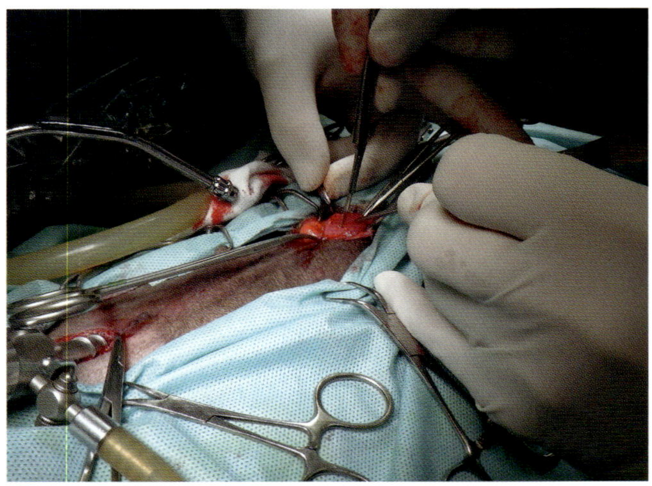

FIGURE 7. A number 11 scalpel blade is used to incise the bladder.

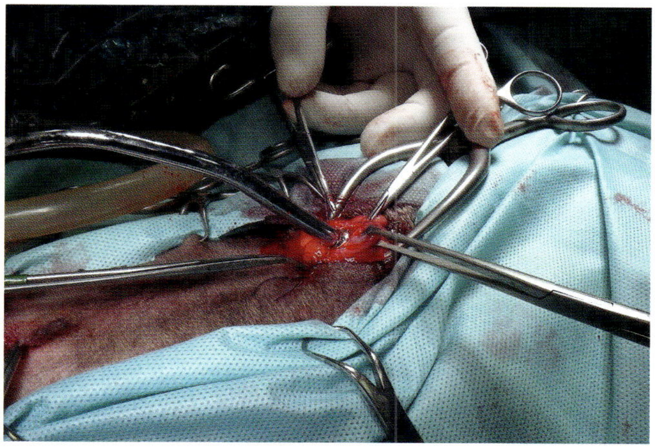

FIGURE 8. The leak of urine is aspirated with a suction cannula. The cannula is then introduced into the bladder to aspirate fluids.

- Using alternatively the 30° or 0° endoscope, the entire mucosal surface of the bladder and proximal urethra is examined for uroliths (**Fig. 11**) and lesions (polyps or masses).
- With the scope inside the bladder, a variety of instruments can be used to grasp and remove the uroliths (**Fig. 12**). The instrument can be inserted through the operating channel or parallel to the scope (**Fig. 13**). The incision may need to be enlarged.
- It may be necessary to remove the cystoscope for each calculus retrieval and then to reintroduce it into the bladder using forceps.

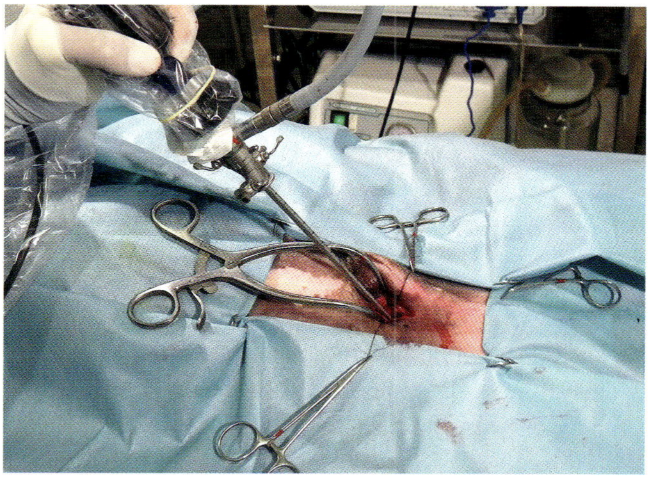

FIGURE 9. The cystoscope (in the image, a 2.7 mm endoscope with sheath) is inserted into the bladder.

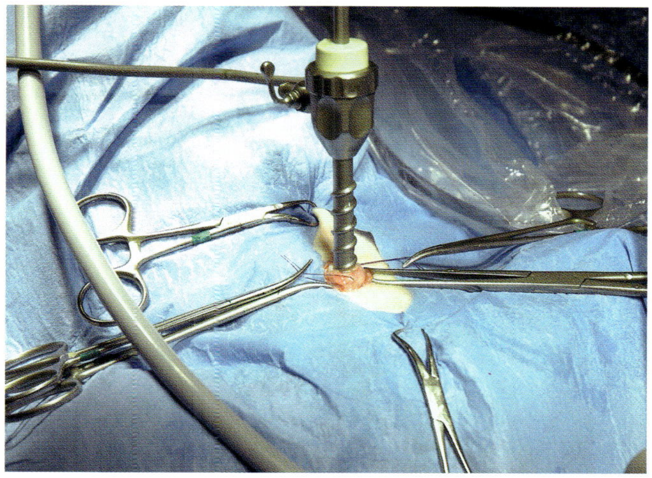

FIGURE 10. A threaded trocar screwed to the bladder wall may be used as a port to introduce the endoscope.

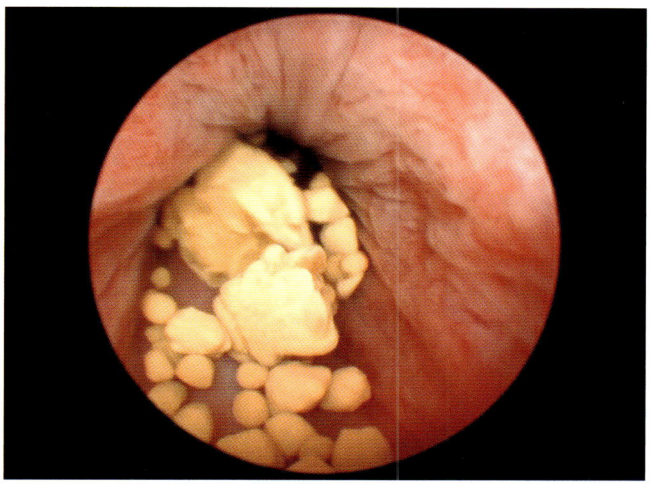

FIGURE 11. Small uroliths in the bladder, grouped in the trigonal region.

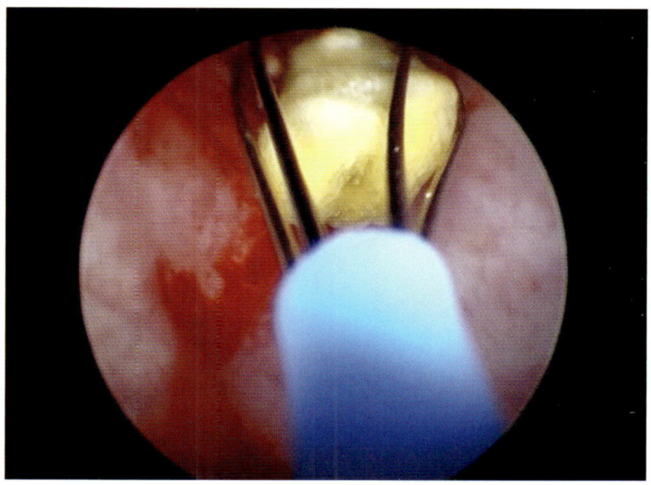

FIGURE 12. A variety of instruments can be used to grasp and remove the uroliths. The image shows a stone basket retrieval device.

- Endoscopic examination enables a thorough inspection of the bladder and urethra for localization of small uroliths, which may not be visible by traditional cystotomy. A sterile flexible endoscope (2.5–3 mm), introduced antegrade from the bladder, can be used to explore the entire urethra. This is especially useful in male patients.
- To help remove small stones located along the urethra, the catheter can be moved while irrigating to push the calculi into the bladder (retropulsion) (**Fig. 14**).
- Additionally, this procedure allows visualization of bladder and urethral lesions and changes in the mucosal folds, targeted biopsy of tumors (**Fig. 15**), and, in some cases, resection of polypoid masses (**Fig. 16**).
- After making sure that all the uroliths have been removed, the small incision in the bladder is closed using monofilament suture (**Fig. 17**).
- The incisions in the abdominal fascia and in the skin are closed routinely (**Fig. 18**).

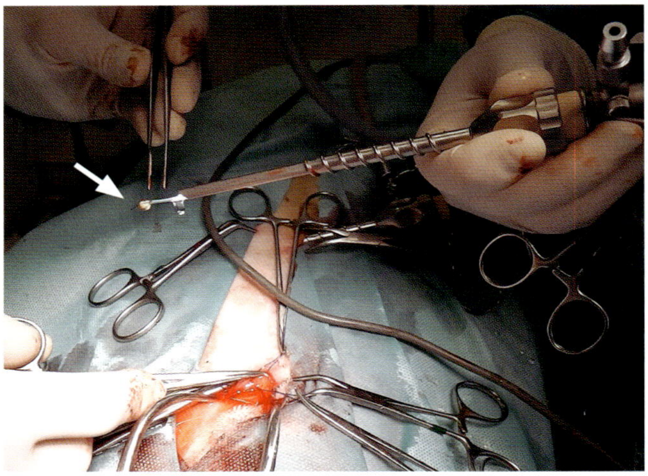

FIGURE 13. Flexible instruments can be inserted through the operating channel of the cystoscope or parallel to the scope to retrieve the urolith (arrow).

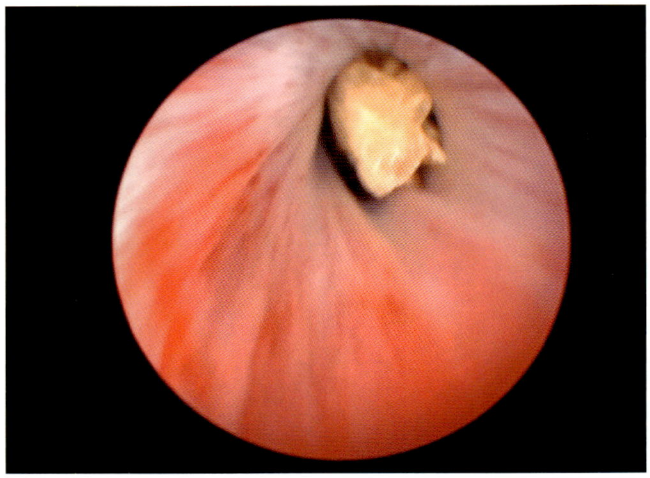

FIGURE 14. The urethral catheter can be used to push the calculi into the bladder (retropulsion).

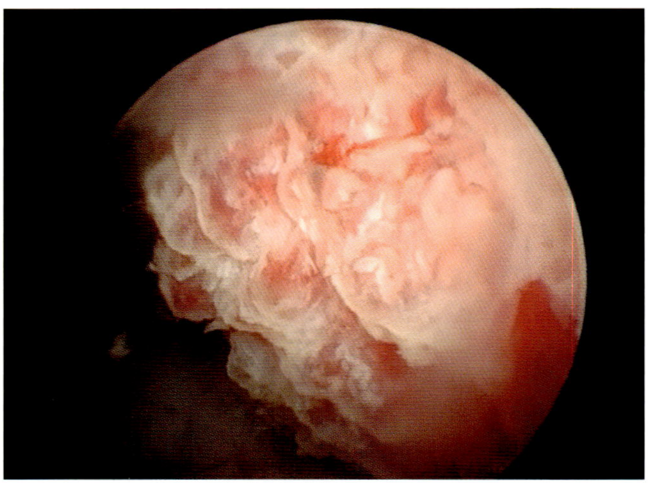

FIGURE 15. Neoplastic lesion in the bladder mucosa. Laparoscopic-assisted cystoscopy and percutaneous suprapubic cystoscopy allows for biopsy sampling as an alternative to transurethral endoscopy.

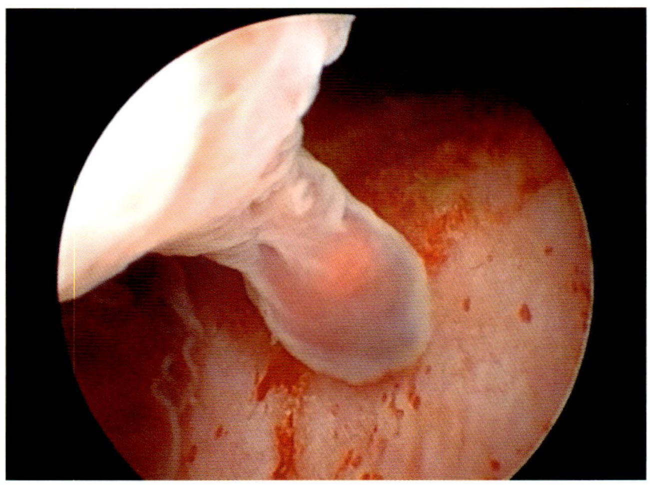

FIGURE 16. Polypoid mass.

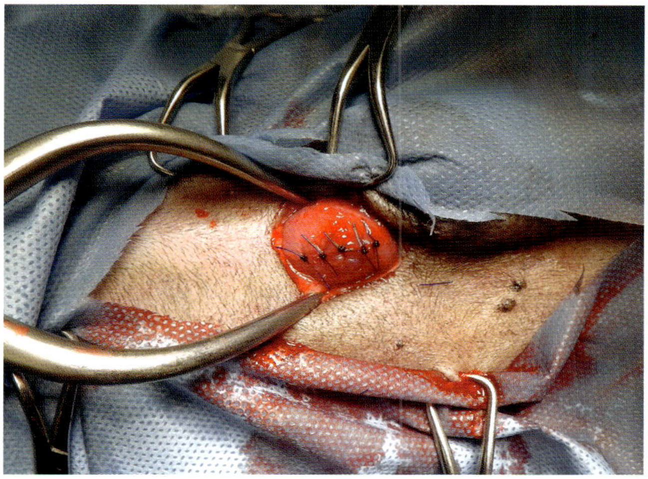

FIGURE 17. The small incision in the bladder is closed with monofilament suture.

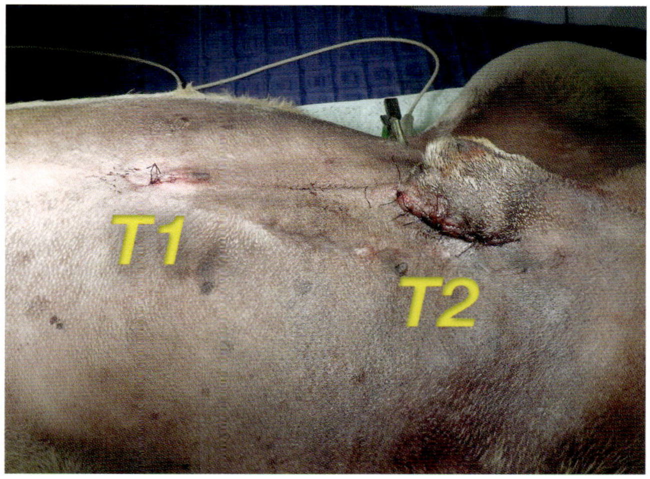

FIGURE 18. The abdominal fascia and the skin are closed routinely. In male dogs, access is typically made near the prepuce.

B PERCUTANEOUS SUPRAPUBIC CYSTOSCOPY OR PERCUTANEOUS CYSTOLITHOTOMY (PCCL)

This technique, faster than the previous one, does not include laparoscopic access through CO_2 insufflation. Using anatomical landmarks, manual palpation of the bladder, or ultrasound at the surgical site, a 1–2 cm minilaparotomy is performed over the bladder apex (**Fig. 19**). A small portion of the bladder is identified, grasped with atraumatic forceps, exteriorized, and anchored with the aid of stay sutures. A small cystotomy is performed and a cystoscope is introduced. Through the incision, the bladder and urethra can be examined, lavages can be performed, and uroliths can be removed (**Video 2**).

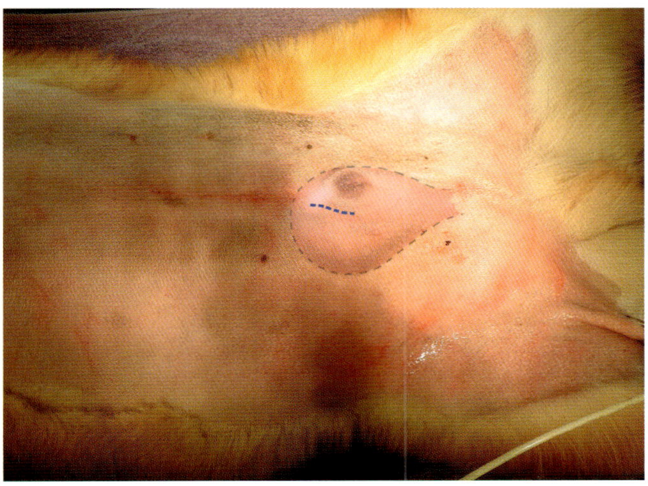

FIGURE 19. For percutaneous suprapubic cystoscopy, manual palpation of the bladder or ultrasound at the surgical site are useful to identify the bladder apex (gray dotted line). The small incision in male dogs is usually made craniolateral to the prepuce (blue dotted line).

Instruments

On the table:

- Standard surgery set
- Cystoscope or telescope 2.7/5 mm – 0°/30°, with sheath
- 5 mm threaded cannulas/trocars
- Grasping forceps (e.g., Babcock, alligator)
- Basket catheter for uroliths
- Laser system device
- Suction/irrigation system

Ready to use:

- Flexible endoscope (video/optical) 2.5–3 mm

VIDEO 2. Percutaneous suprapubic cystoscopy (PCCL).

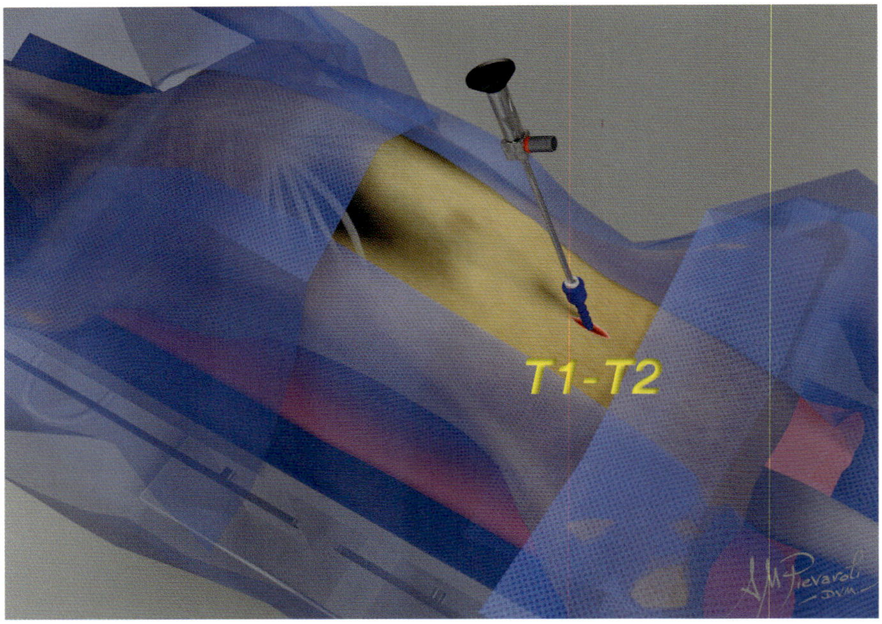

FIGURE 20. Port placement for percutaneous suprapubic cystoscopy.

PORT PLACEMENT (FIG. 20)

The cystoscope can be introduced directly into the bladder through the incision, without using a laparoscopic cannula. If a cannula is used, it must be inserted into the bladder through the incision in the apex and will act as the telescope port.

PROCEDURE

- The author prefers to use threaded cannulas (Storz Endotip) as ports because they are more stable once placed in the patient. Different cannula sizes can be used depending on the endoscope (2.7 or 5 mm).
- After emptying the bladder and performing at least two or three lavages with warm saline mixed with 1%–2% of povidone-iodine, the bladder is filled with sterile saline solution, avoiding excessive overdistension (approximately 10–15 mL/kg).
- The anatomical location of the bladder apex on the ventral midline is determined by anatomical landmarks, manual palpation of the bladder, or ultrasound.
- A small ventral midline skin incision of approximately 1–2 cm is made at the point identified as the bladder apex. In male dogs, this incision is made just cranial to the prepuce or slightly paraprepucial; in cats and female dogs, the incision is performed about 1–3 cm caudal to the umbilicus (**Fig. 21**).
- A Gelpi retractor is applied to the skin incision to better visualize the underlying abdominal wall. An incision is made in the abdominal cavity through the linea alba and the Gelpi retractor is then shifted to include the abdominal wall (**Fig. 22**).

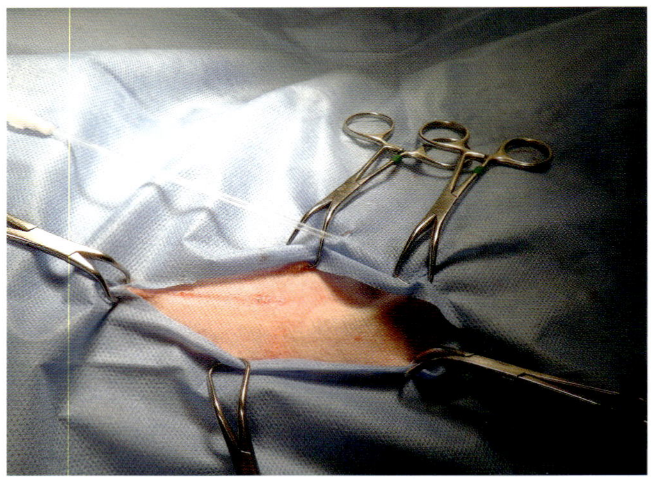

FIGURE 21. Draped operative field. Note the sterile urethral catheter already in place (male dog in the image), necessary to perform bladder irrigation during surgery.

- After identifying the bladder through the minilaparotomy incision, the bladder apex is grasped using atraumatic forceps and brought closer to the incision.
- To keep the bladder attached to the abdominal wall and reduce urine contamination, two to four stay sutures can be placed and the area can be packed with gauze (**Fig. 23**). Alternatively, the bladder can be fixed to the skin (cystopexy) using a temporary continuous suture.

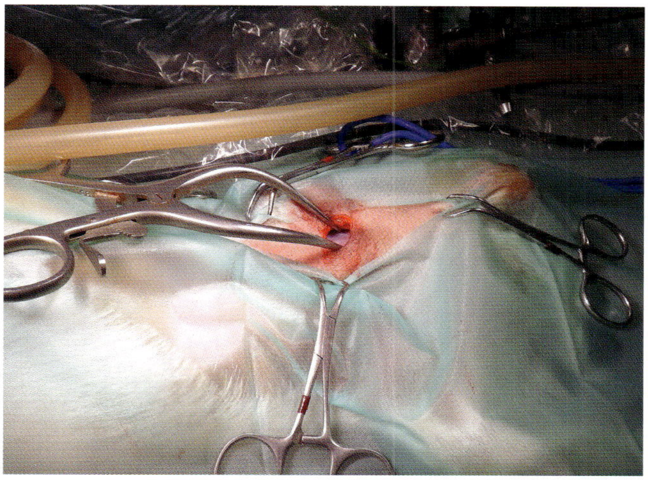

FIGURE 22. A Gelpi retractor is helpful after the incision of the skin and abdominal wall.

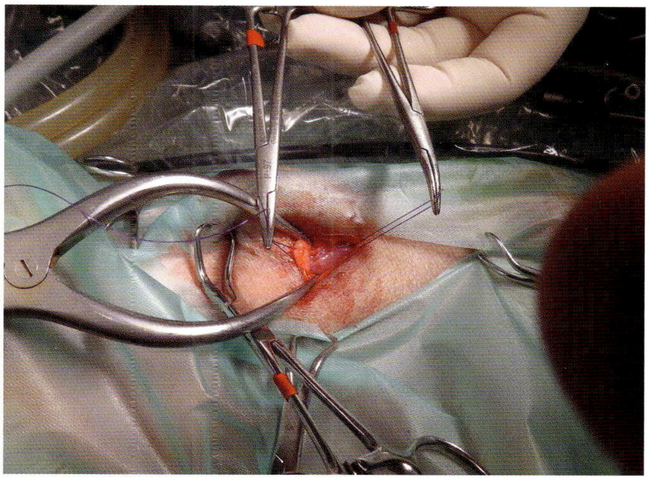

FIGURE 23. Urine contamination can be reduced by placing two to four stay sutures to secure the bladder.

- The procedure continues as described previously for laparoscopic-assisted cystoscopy.
- Once the bladder is secured, a small incision is made using a number 11 scalpel blade. A suction cannula should be promptly utilized to aspirate the leak of urine and the fluid contained in the bladder.
- The cystoscope (or 2.7–5 mm endoscope with sheath) is then inserted into the bladder (**Fig. 24**). The endoscope may be inserted through a threaded trocar screwed to the bladder wall. This trocar acts as a port to access the bladder.
- For better visualization of the bladder cavity, it is important to perform continuous infusion of saline solution. This can be achieved by connecting the infusion set to the Luer lock. Egress occurs through the urinary catheter introduced at the beginning of the procedure. The flow can be reversed during the procedure.

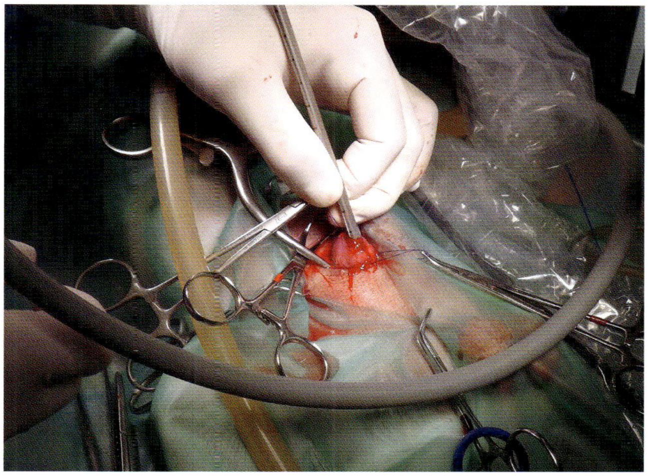

FIGURE 24. The cystoscope (in the image, a 2.7 mm endoscope with sheath) is inserted into the bladder.

Tips

The flow of saline solution can be reversed to facilitate the movement of small nonvisible stones located along the urethra.

- Using alternatively the 30° or 0° endoscope, the entire mucosal surface of the bladder and proximal urethra is examined for uroliths and lesions (polyps or masses).
- With the scope inside the bladder, a variety of instruments can be used to grasp and remove the uroliths. The instrument can be inserted through the operating channel or parallel to the scope. The incision may need to be enlarged.
- If numerous very small stones are present, it may be useful to aspirate them directly with a cannula (**Fig. 25**). However, an inflow of sterile saline solution must be ensured to prevent the bladder from emptying.
- It may be necessary to remove the cystoscope for each calculus retrieval and then to reintroduce it into the bladder using forceps.
- Endoscopic examination enables a thorough inspection of the bladder and urethra for localization of small uroliths, which may not be visible by traditional cystotomy. A sterile

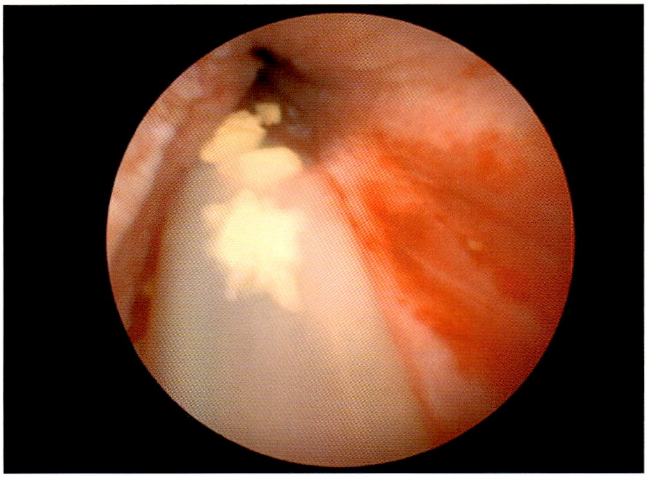

FIGURE 25. Use of a cannula to aspirate small stones disseminated in the bladder. An adequate inflow of sterile saline solution must be ensured to prevent the bladder from emptying.

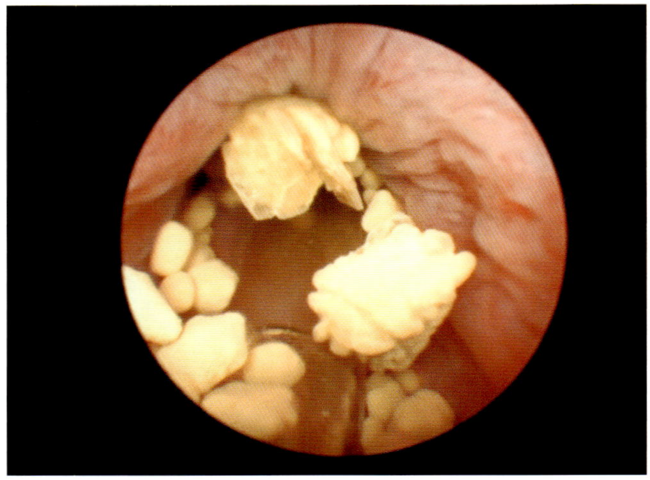

FIGURE 26. The urethral catheter can be used to push the calculi into the bladder (retropulsion).

flexible endoscope (2.5–3 mm), introduced antegrade from the bladder, can be used to explore the entire urethra. This is especially useful in male patients.

- To help remove small stones located along the urethra, the catheter can be moved while irrigating to push the calculi into the bladder (retropulsion) (**Fig. 26**).
- This procedure also allows visualization of bladder and urethral lesions and changes in the mucosal folds, targeted biopsy of tumors, and, in some cases, resection of polypoid masses.
- After making sure that all the uroliths have been removed, the small incision in the bladder is closed using monofilament suture.
- The incisions in the abdominal fascia and in the skin are closed routinely (**Fig. 27**).

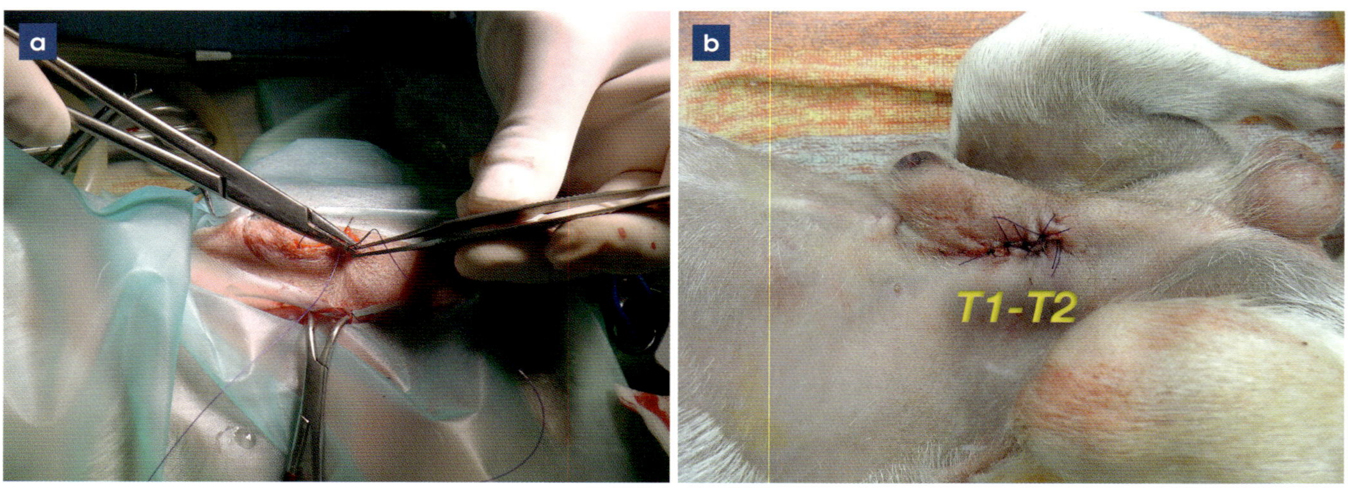

FIGURE 27. The incisions are closed routinely.

C SINGLE-PORT PERCUTANEOUS CYSTOLITHOTOMY

Jeffrey J. Runge, Joshua G. Becker

OPERATING ROOM LAYOUT

The surgeons position themselves on the patient's right side, and the endoscopy tower is placed directly across from them, on the left side.

PORT PLACEMENT (FIG. 28)

- 360° wound retractor, on the midline, at the level of the apex of the urinary bladder

PROCEDURE

- An approximately 1–2 cm ventral midline incision is made over the apex of the urinary bladder. A 360° wound retractor is then used to expose and isolate the urinary bladder.
- Three stay sutures are placed in a triangular arrangement on the ventral aspect of the bladder, near the apex. These sutures help maintain traction on the bladder for both cannula placement and intraoperative manipulation.
- A 2–3 mm stab incision is made using a number 11 scalpel blade, approximately centered and equidistant from each of the stay sutures. A laparoscopic threaded cannula is then immediately inserted into the bladder at the incision site, with the goal of preventing or minimizing urine leakage (**Fig. 29**).

Instruments

- Standard surgery set
- Rigid cystoscope 2.7 mm – 30°
- 2.5–2.8 mm flexible ureteroscope, often only needed in male patients (a 1.9 mm scope may be better suited for smaller patients)
- 360° wound retractor (the authors prefer the Alexis wound retractor)
- Laparoscopic 5 mm port with Luer lock attached to suction (optional)
- Laparoscopic 5 mm threaded cannula
- Stone basket (>70 cm length)
- Grasper
- Pressure bag for lavage
- Red rubber or Foley catheters
- Hydrophilic guide (Weasel) wire (0.018, 0.035, and 0.045 mm)

- The rigid cystoscope is inserted through the port and the bladder lumen and urethra are surveyed. Calculi are identified (**Fig. 30**) and removed using a stone retrieval basket through the working channel of the cystoscope (**Fig. 31**).
- Sterile saline can be used to distend the bladder and create working space for the procedure. The repeated distention

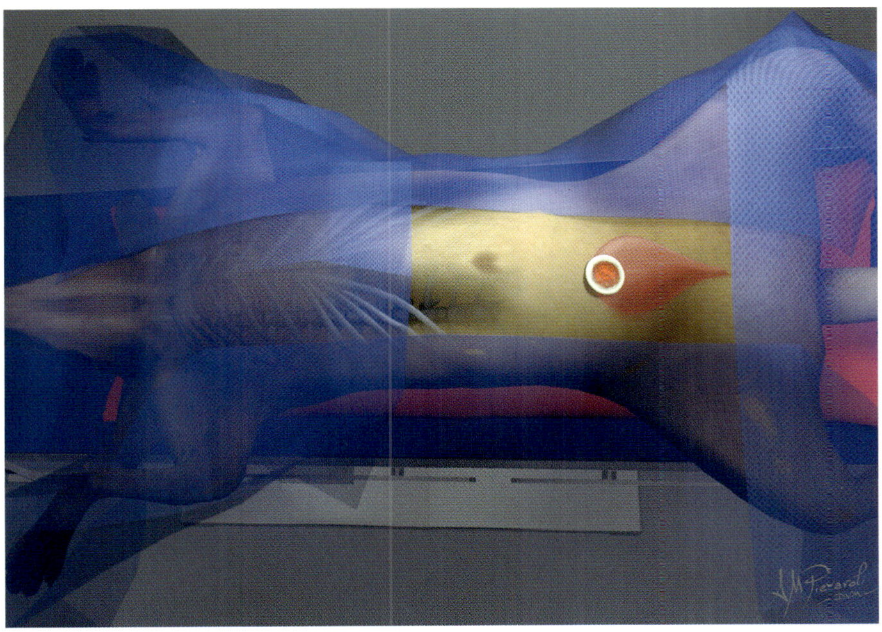

FIGURE 28. Port placement for single-port percutaneous cystolithotomy.

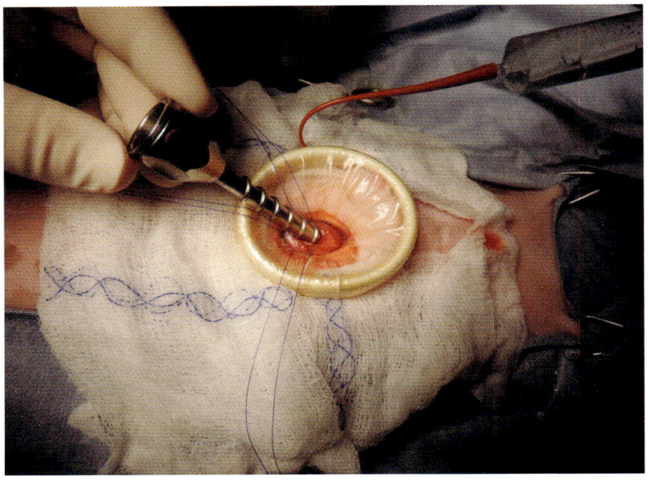

FIGURE 29. A wound retractor is placed in the caudal abdomen, just cranial to the preputial sheath of this patient. A 5 mm Endotip port is placed though the bladder.

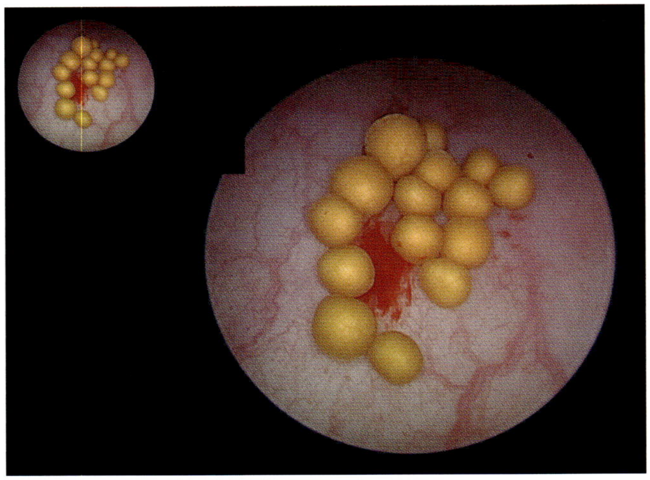

FIGURE 30. Normograde view inside the bladder showing cystic calculi at the trigone.

and draining allows for flushing of debris, blood, and potentially stones.

- Smaller calculi can often be suctioned out of the port using a urethral catheter to flush saline in a retrograde fashion.
- For removal of calculi that exceed the diameter of the 5 mm threaded cannula, the cannula can be replaced with a 10 mm cannula, the cannula can be removed and the calculi can be manipulated through the incision with the stone basket or graspers, or the calculi can be fragmented using lithotripsy (if available).
- After the bladder is cleared of calculi, the urethra is examined with either the rigid cystoscope (females) or the flexible ureteroscope (males or cats) to ensure complete removal of visible calculi. The basket retrieval device can be used to remove any remaining urethral calculi either via ureteroscopic guidance or through the working channel of the cystoscope.
- In feline patients with concern for inflammatory urethral obstruction, a urinary catheter can be placed under ureteroscopic guidance at this time.
- The bladder wall is closed in standard fashion using an interrupted appositional suture pattern and absorbable suture material.
- The caudal abdomen can be lavaged and inspected. Then, the abdomen is closed routinely. Local analgesics at the time of incision site closure are recommended.

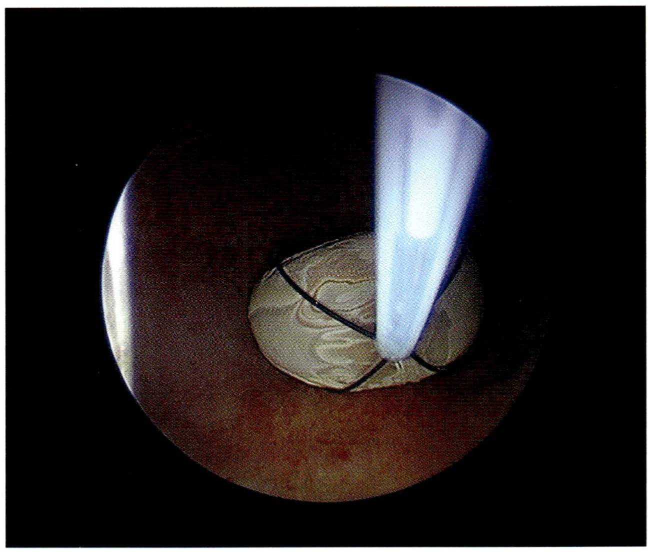

FIGURE 31. Basket retrieval of a cystic calculus using an operating cystoscope during percutaneous cystolithotomy.

- At least one lateral abdominal radiograph should be taken postoperatively and prior to waking the patient from anesthesia to confirm removal of all radiopaque calculi.
- In feline patients with preoperative concern for urethral obstruction or urethral trauma, an indwelling urethral catheter should be placed prior to closure and the patient hospitalized as clinically indicated.

POSTOPERATIVE MANAGEMENT

- Bupivacaine can be infused into the urethra for additional transient analgesia.
- Patients can typically be discharged from the hospital on the same day as the surgery.
- Patients that are considered stable preoperatively can be treated on an outpatient basis, although fluid therapy is recommended 12–24 hours postoperatively to maintain renal function and encourage voiding of residual blood and calculi fragments.
- Antibiotic therapy is indicated in the days following surgery.
- Supportive care is given if necessary. Multimodal analgesia is continued for the first few days postoperatively.
- Ultrasonographic evaluation of the bladder and urinary tract is recommended 12–14 days after surgery.

Complications of laparoscopic-assisted or percutaneous suprapubic cystoscopy

- Low complication rates (incorrect port placement, iatrogenic urethral trauma, hemorrhage, incisional complications).
- Urine leakage into the abdomen due to bladder suture dehiscence.
- Hematuria in the first days after surgery.

Key points

- Preoperative patient evaluation is important to determine which procedure to perform.
- Begin surgery knowing approximately the size and number of stones to be removed.
- Introduce the urethral catheter before surgery.
- Perform repeated bladder and urethral lavages before closing the bladder to remove small, even invisible, uroliths.

SUGGESTED READINGS

CLINICAL CASES

19.1 PERCUTANEOUS CYSTOSCOPIC CYSTOLITHOTOMY IN A YORKSHIRE TERRIER

Christopher B. Thomson

CASE DESCRIPTION

A 7-year-old neutered male Yorkshire Terrier dog was presented for cystolithiasis. The patient had been recently treated for straining to urinate, was found to have multiple urethral and bladder stones, and underwent retrograde flushing of obstructive urethroliths, but a single stone remained lodged in the urethra. On physical examination, moderate pain was detected on caudal abdominal palpation. Abdominal radiographs revealed multiple radiopaque stones, the largest measuring 4.5 mm in the urethra immediately proximal to the os penis. Percutaneous cystoscopic cystolithotomy was performed. Stone analysis was consistent with struvite uroliths.

Key points

- Small rigid and flexible endoscopes allow improved visualization of the urinary bladder wall and entire urethra, even in small dogs and male cats.
- The use of a cystoscopy sheath (versus the use of a rigid endoscope only) allows for easier bladder distension and fluid egress as well as passage of stone baskets and graspers.
- A PCCL approach can be utilized for antegrade laser lithotripsy.
- PCCL allows for stone removal without restrictions on stone number or size, patient's sex, species, or size, and can be performed quickly by experienced surgeons.

PORT PLACEMENT

A 5 or 10 mm threaded Ternamian Endotip can be used T1(T2), depending on availability and on urolith size. If multiple stones larger than 5 mm but smaller than 11 mm are present, the use of the 10 mm port can facilitate stone removal without the need for continuous replacement of the port.

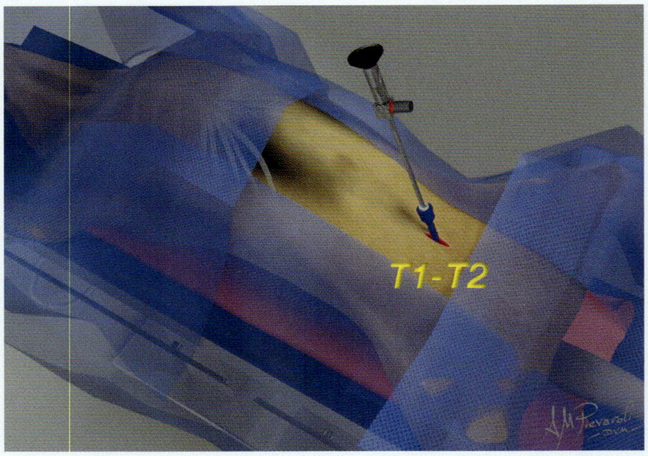

PROCEDURE

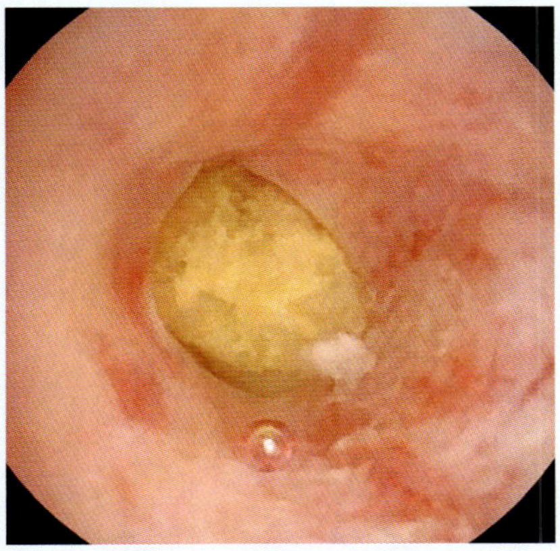

FIGURE 1. Following a 1 cm laparotomy incision and urinary bladder access, a 6 mm Ternamian Endotip is introduced into the urinary bladder, with retraction from three stay sutures. Urethrolith removal is attempted by flushing, basketing, and even retrograde probing with a meniscal probe, but the stone remains lodged in the urethra.

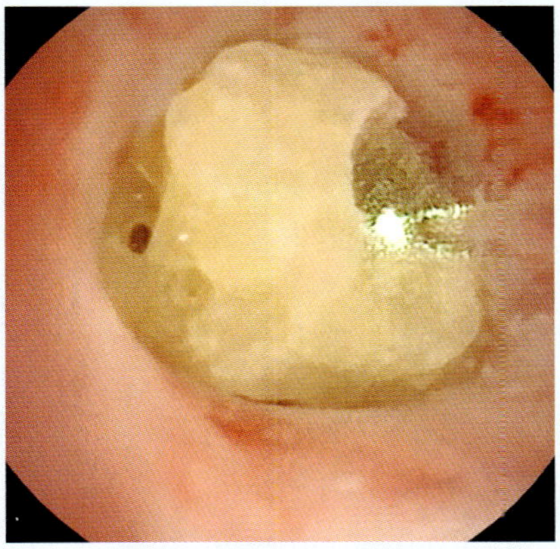

FIGURE 2. A Ho:YAG laser lithotripter is used to break up the stone into smaller pieces for retrieval.

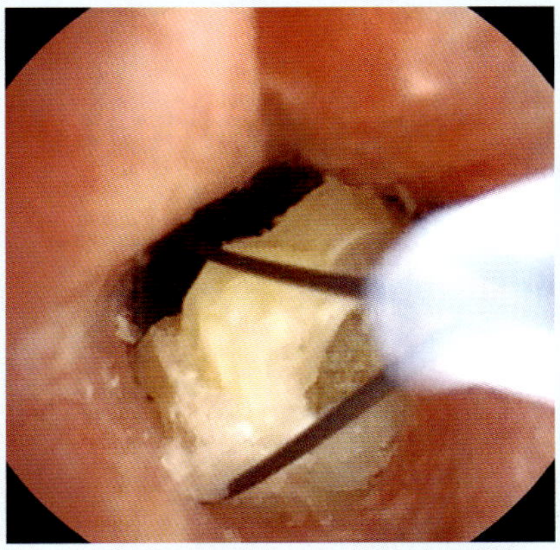

FIGURE 3. The small pieces are removed via basket retrieval and flushing.

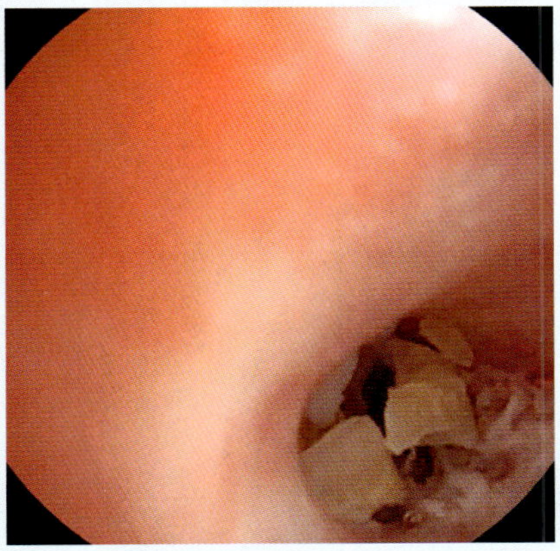

FIGURE 4. Smaller stone fragments are removed via antegrade and retrograde flushing.

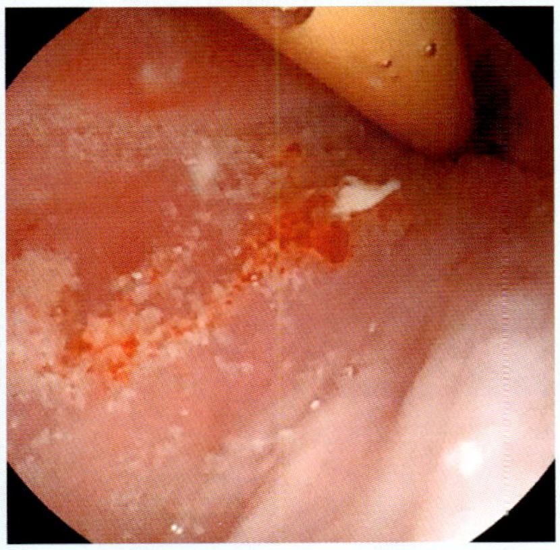

FIGURE 5. There is grit-like sand in the urinary bladder. It is flushed out with vigorous retrograde and antegrade flushing using a red rubber catheter through the cystotomy incision, after removing the trocar.

Tips and tricks

- ✓ Ensure that the bladder is full prior to surgery (either from urine retention or via a urinary catheter).
- ✓ Flushing (retrograde and antegrade) with and without the trocar allows for easier removal of small grit and sand-like cystoliths. Small stones can be suctioned up with suction applied to the trocar.
- ✓ Stay sutures within the bladder allow for ease of trocar placement and replacement without causing unnecessary trauma.

19.2 LAPAROSCOPIC-ASSISTED CYSTOSTOMY IN A CHIHUAHUA

D. L. Casas García

CASE DESCRIPTION

A 5-year-old male Chihuahua weighing 1.2 kg was presented for recurrent urolithiasis refractory to medical and dietary management. Abdominal radiographs revealed the presence of numerous uroliths in the urinary bladder (3–8 mm in diameter) and discarded the presence of uroliths in the urethra. Because of the reduced size of the patient's urethra (<2.8 mm), a laparoscopic-assisted cystostomy was scheduled due to the impossibility of performing a retrograde transurethral cystoscopy to surgically solve the urolithiasis.

Key points

- A laparoscopic-assisted approach for cystoscopy is the technique of choice for patients in which a transurethral retrograde cystoscopy cannot be performed, whether because the specific equipment is not available or because the retrograde approach is not possible.
- Besides, it is an alternative to PCCL for surgeons who are not familiarized with the technique.
- The exteriorization of the urinary bladder has several advantages over the pure laparoscopic approach, as it reduces the risk of urine contamination to the abdominal cavity and avoids the need for an intracorporeal suture, which takes more surgical time and requires a longer learning curve.
- The use of a trocar for cystoscopy allows for the bladder lumen to be distended without leakage of urine/saline through the cystostomy.

PORT PLACEMENT

For the laparoscopic-assisted cystostomy, a multiport technique was used with two 6 mm trocars placed on the midline: T1 (telescope) and T2 (operative instrument).

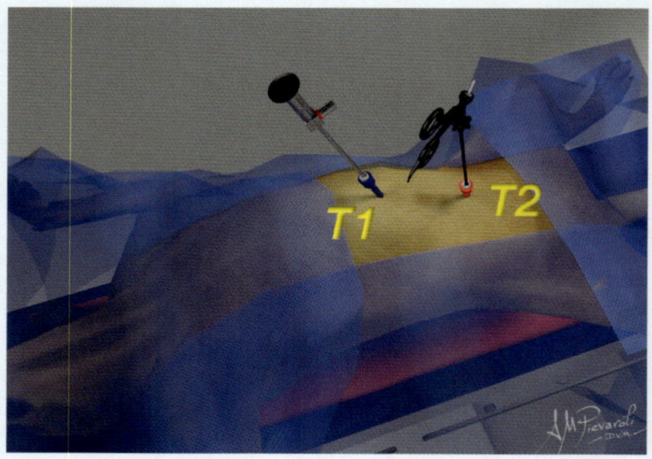

PROCEDURE

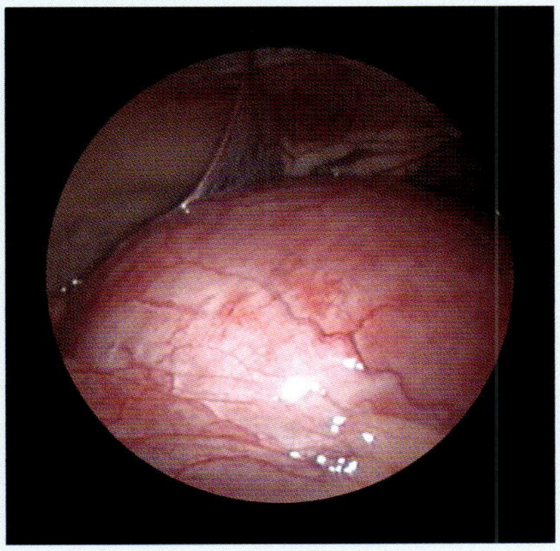

FIGURE 1. With the urinary bladder distended, the abdominal region for placement of the second trocar, at the bladder apex, is selected under laparoscopic visualization and digital palpation.

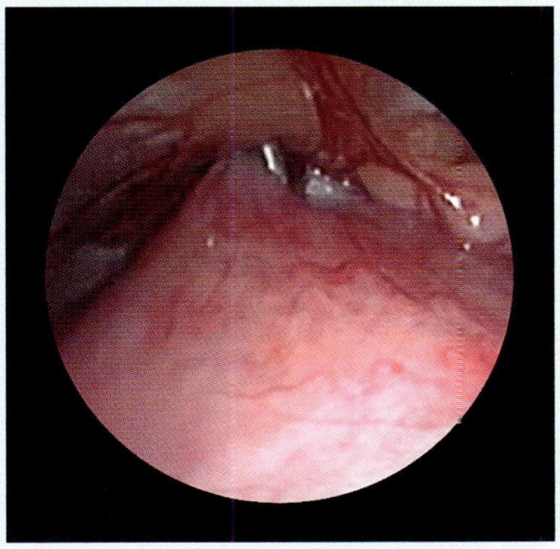

FIGURE 2. After positioning the patient, a 5 mm laparoscopic atraumatic grasper is used to hold the bladder wall for its exteriorization.

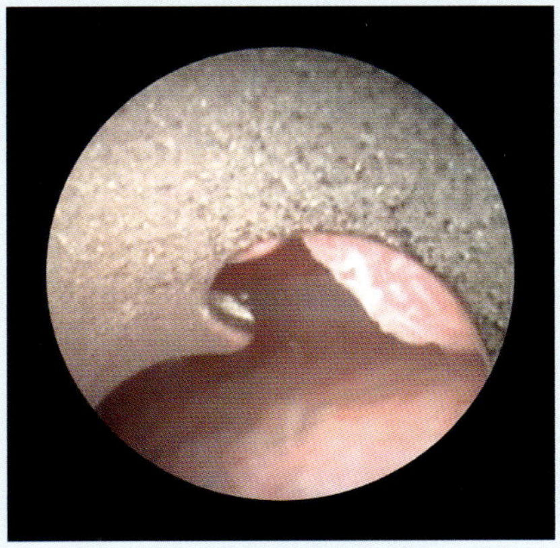

FIGURE 3. The bladder is fixed to the abdominal wall by one or two percutaneous sutures, creating a temporary cystopexy. A 6 mm Ternamian Endotip trocar without valve is then placed to ensure a hermetic cystostomy during the complete endoscopic procedure.

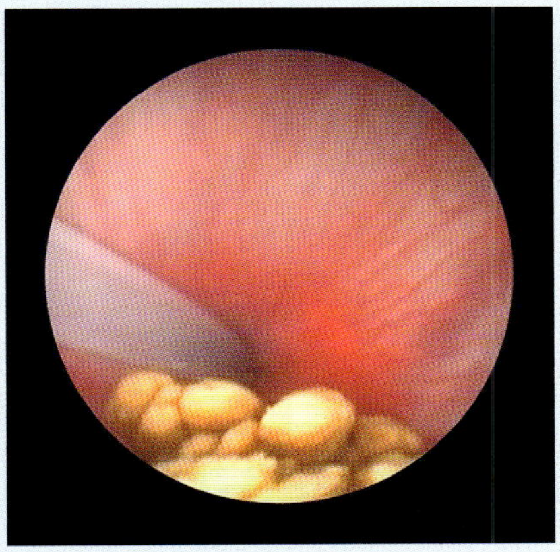

FIGURE 4. At the beginning of the procedure, retrograde urinary bladder catheterization was performed in order to control the filling/emptying of the bladder. This helps to avoid damage to the urinary bladder during trocar placement and reduces the risk of migration of lithiasic fragments to the urethra.

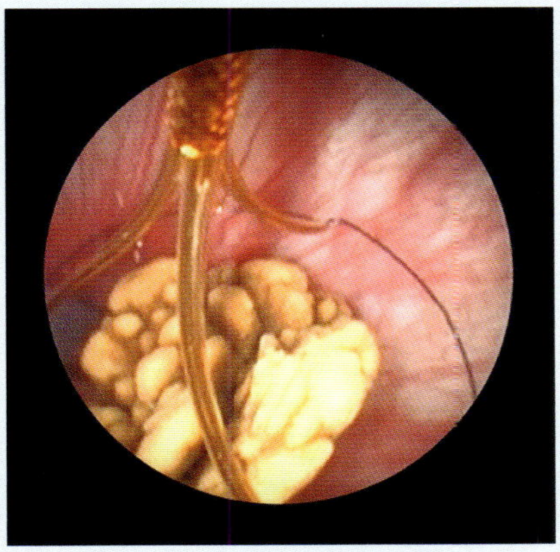

FIGURE 5. Using a 2.7 mm cystoscope with its sheath and corresponding working channel, the uroliths are removed through the trocar using an endourology retrieval basket.

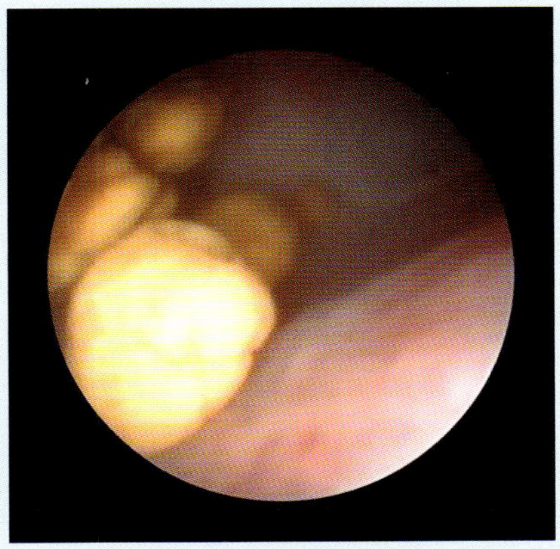

FIGURE 6. Smaller-diameter uroliths and the sediment are suctioned directly through the working channel of the sheath of the cystoscope.

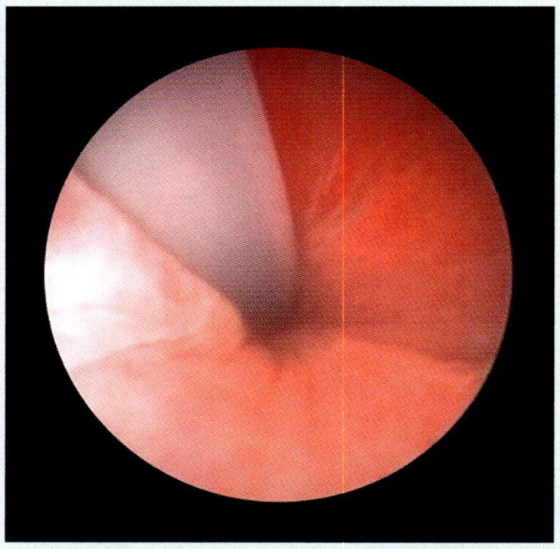

FIGURE 7. Once the procedure is completed, an anterograde technique is used to check for the absence of uroliths and iatrogenic trauma in both the urethra and urinary bladder.

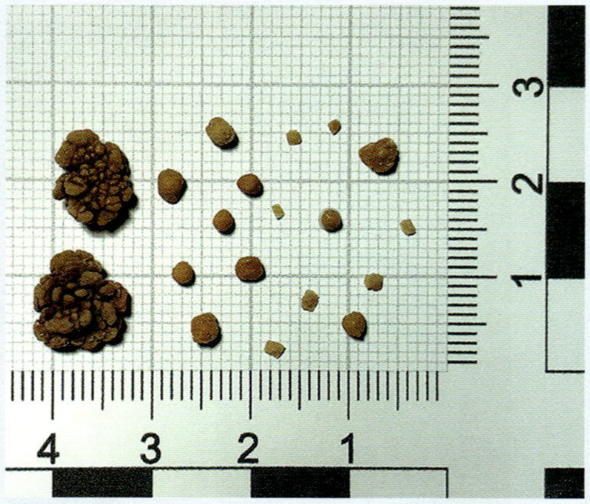

FIGURE 8. Retrieved uroliths should be sent to a laboratory to determine their composition.

Tips and tricks

✓ This procedure allows anterograde access to and complete exploration of the proximal urethra. This can be especially useful in cases of proliferative urethritis, as it avoids the management of uroliths in the penile urethra by a retrograde technique.

✓ Urinary catheterization avoids the risk of migration of sediment and small uroliths during cystoscopy.

20 LAPAROSCOPIC CYSTOTOMY

Andrea M. Pievaroli

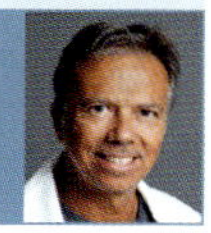

Indications	Contraindications
■ Removal of a single or limited number of large bladder stones	■ Uroliths that are too small or too numerous ■ Bladder infections with very inflamed and thickened bladder

Laparoscopic cystotomy has not been reported in the primary veterinary literature. Personal experiences have been described in a few publications and proceedings about minimally invasive surgery. Laparoscopic-assisted or video-assisted cystotomy, on the other hand, has been well described and is commonly used in dogs and cats (see Chapter 19).

The totally laparoscopic cystotomy technique has limited indications and requires greater experience and skill in intracorporeal laparoscopic suturing. Therefore, case selection is of critical importance. The main indication is removal of large stones, present as single uroliths or in a small number. If many small uroliths are present in the bladder, the video-assisted technique should be preferred due to its greater effectiveness and reduced surgical time.

The advantages of laparoscopic cystotomy conferred by minimal invasiveness include small port accesses and bladder incision.

> The first laparoscopic repair of a bladder rupture in a foal was published in 1995 by Ryland B. Edwards III et al.

PATIENT PREPARATION AND POSITIONING

The patient should be fasted for 10–12 hours before surgery. Antibiotic therapy should be started before the procedure to minimize the risk of intraoperative infections. The ventral abdomen is widely clipped, including the entire prepuce or vulva caudally. The patient is placed in dorsal recumbency and the skin is aseptically prepared, including an aseptic wash of the prepuce or vulva.

It can be useful to tilt the table in a Trendelenburg position (15°–20°) to displace the abdominal organs away from the pelvic region, thereby improving visualization of the bladder. Prior to surgery, the bladder should be catheterized to drain the urine, and at least two or three lavages with warm saline mixed with 1%–2% povidone-iodine, followed by flushing with saline, should be performed.

OPERATING ROOM LAYOUT

Since the procedure is performed in the caudal abdomen, the monitor (or the scope tower) is placed at the caudal end of the table, leaving enough space for the surgeons to move during the procedure. The anesthesia machine is placed near the patient's head. The instrument table is placed caudolateral to the table, on the same side as the surgeon. The surgeon positions themselves on the right or left side of the patient, depending on personal preference (right- or left-handed person). The assistant positions themselves on the opposite side. It is advisable to tilt the table into a Trendelenburg position (**Fig. 1**).

PORT PLACEMENT (FIG. 2)

- T1, on the midline, 1–2 cm caudal to the umbilicus
- T2, in a right paramedian position (3–5 cm), at the same level or caudal to T1

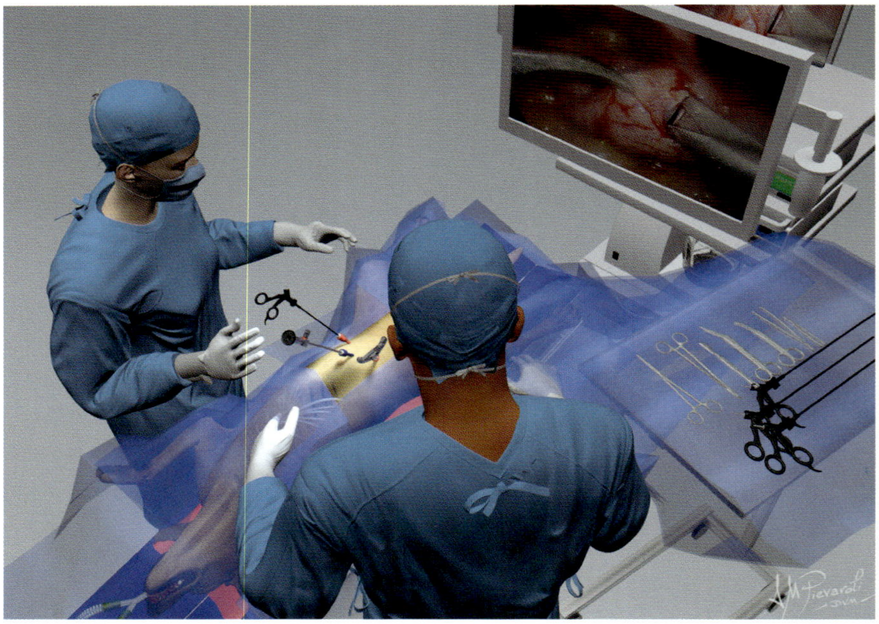

FIGURE 1. Operating room layout for laparoscopic cystotomy.

Instruments

On the table:

- Standard surgery set
- Telescope 5 mm – 30°
- Three 5 mm threaded cannulas/trocars (or one 10 mm cannula/trocar for larger instruments)
- Grasping forceps
- Endoscopic scissors
- Endoscopic cannula for aspiration/irrigation
- One or two needle holders for laparoscopic suturing

Ready to use:

- Endoscopic retrieval bag
- Monopolar/bipolar electrosurgery unit

- T3, in a left paramedian position (3–5 cm), at the same level or caudal to T1

PROCEDURE (VIDEO 1)

- The technique is performed with three ports oriented toward the caudal region of the abdomen for correct triangulation around the bladder. The author prefers to use threaded cannulas (Storz Endotip) to prevent slippage from within the peritoneum.
- A pneumoperitoneum is established using the surgeon's preferred technique; the author uses the Ternamian or a modified Hasson technique. After the first port has been placed and the pneumoperitoneum achieved, the 5 mm telescope is inserted and a first exploration of the abdomen is performed to check for any evidence of iatrogenic trauma caused by placement of the first cannula.
- The falciform ligament, which could prevent correct vision and cloud the lens of the telescope, can often be found in this area of the peritoneum. It is necessary to screw the

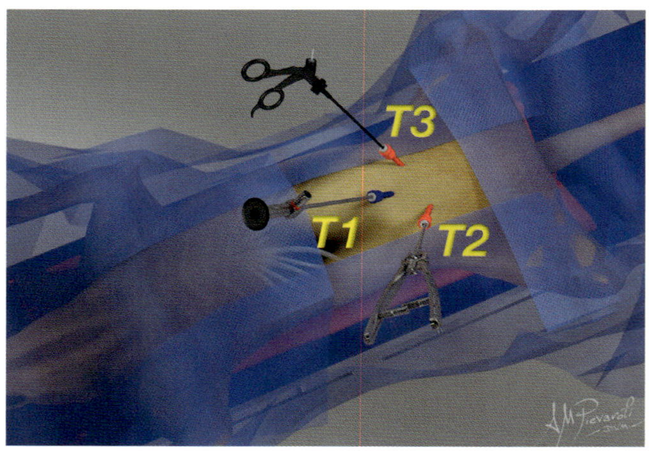

FIGURE 2. Port placement for laparoscopic cystotomy.

port deeper to find the right inclination to overcome the ligament.

Tips

To avoid crossing the falciform ligament, the port can be inserted slightly lateral (1–2 cm) to the midline.

VIDEO 1. Laparoscopic cystotomy.

- Under endoscopic vision, the second and third cannulas for the operative instruments are inserted in a paramedian position, on the right and left side.
- The region is explored for initial evaluation and identification of the bladder. The bladder should be emptied using the urethral catheter. Babcock forceps or other atraumatic forceps can be used for manipulation of the bladder (**Fig. 3**).
- A very small longitudinal incision is made near the bladder apex using endoscopic scissors (**Fig. 4**). Bleeding can be controlled with the monopolar/bipolar electrosurgical unit. A suction cannula is used to remove any residual bladder fluid content (**Fig. 5**).
- The bladder is grasped with forceps and the telescope is then introduced through the incision in the bladder to locate the urolith. Endoscopic forceps can also be used to keep the incision open while introducing the scope (**Fig. 6**).

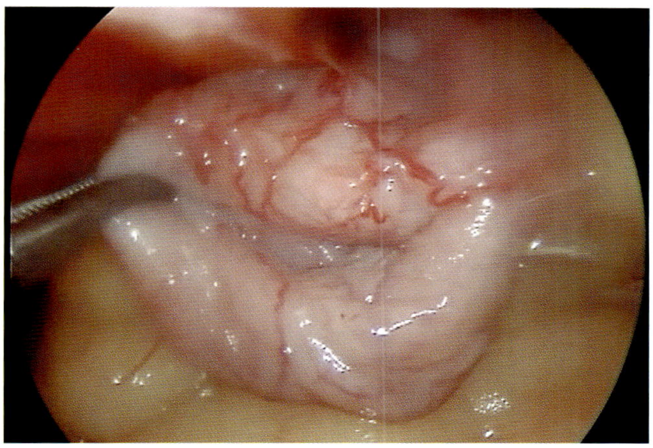

FIGURE 3. The apex of the previously emptied bladder is identified and grasped.

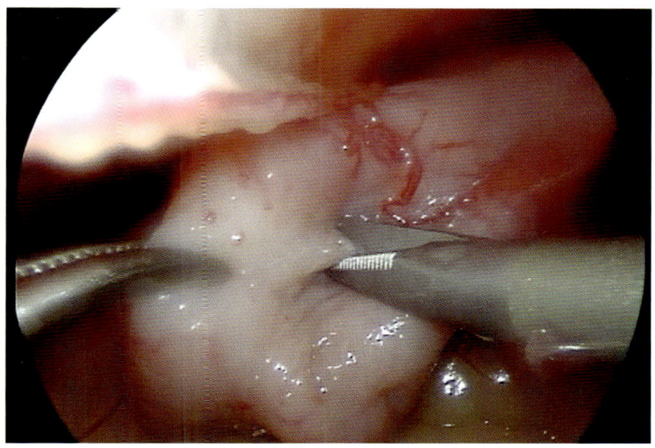

FIGURE 4. A small longitudinal incision is made in the proximity of the apex of the bladder using endoscopic scissors.

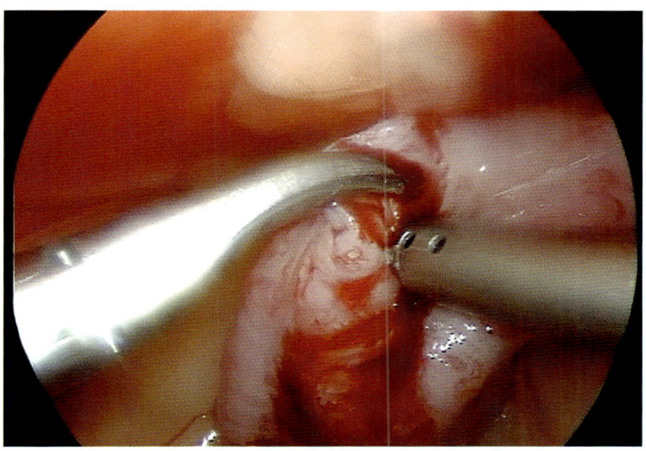

FIGURE 5. A laparoscopic suction cannula is used to remove residual bladder fluid.

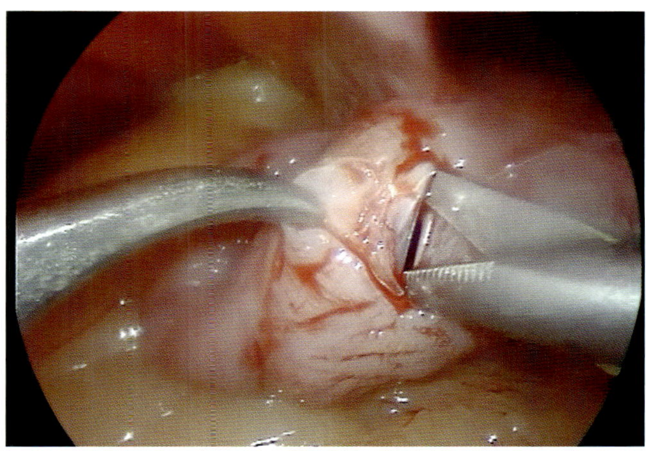

FIGURE 6. The incision in the bladder can be kept open with endoscopic scissors for introduction of the scope.

Tips

Alternatively, to hold the bladder in place, a temporary percutaneous suture can be passed through the ventral aspect of the bladder.

- With the scope inside the bladder, the forceps can be released and introduced through the incision in the bladder, parallel to the scope. The urolith is identified, grasped with the appropriate forceps, and removed (**Figs. 7 and 8**). The incision should only be enlarged if necessary. If more uroliths are present, the operation is repeated.
- Uroliths can be removed from the abdomen through one of the ports, which can be enlarged according to the size of the stone. Uroliths can also be removed with an endoscopic retrieval bag (e.g., Endobag) (**Fig. 9**).
- After making sure that all the uroliths have been removed, suturing can be performed.
- The bladder incision is closed using the endoscopic needle holder and monofilament suture. Depending on the length of the incision, a simple continuous pattern, in one or two layers, can be used (**Fig. 10**). For optimal results with simple continuous patterns, use of a barbed monofilament suture (V-Loc 90/180, Covidien; Biolong Barbed, Biomed) is recommended. Single knots can be tied in small incisions.
- Before removing the cannulas, a leak test is carried out by filling the bladder with saline. If a leak is present, the suture should be reinforced with additional knots. Then, the abdomen is aspirated and washed with warm saline solution.
- The skin is closed routinely.

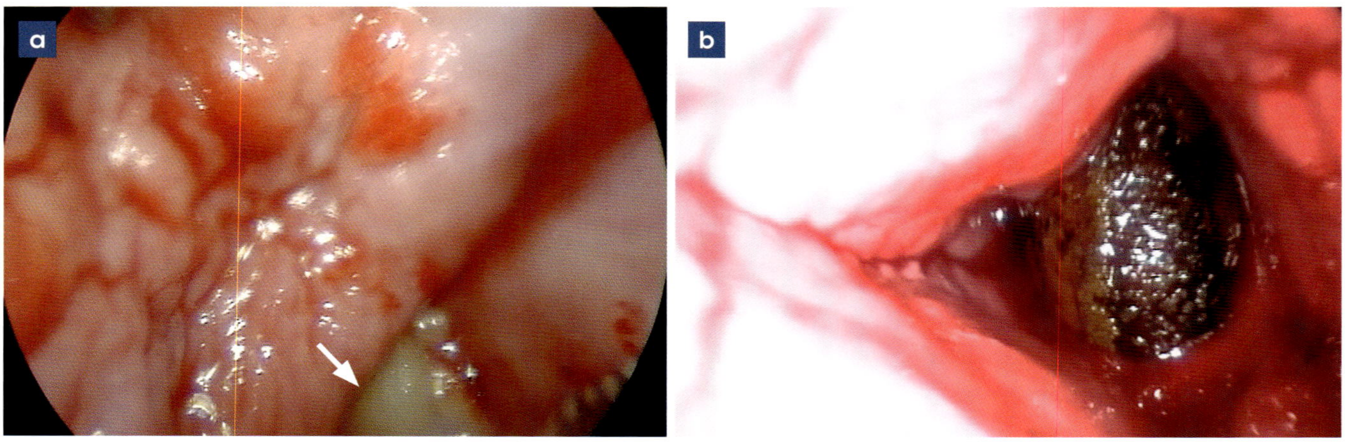

FIGURE 7. Endoscopic view inside the bladder. a) 10 mm urolith (arrow). b) A single large (3 cm) urolith.

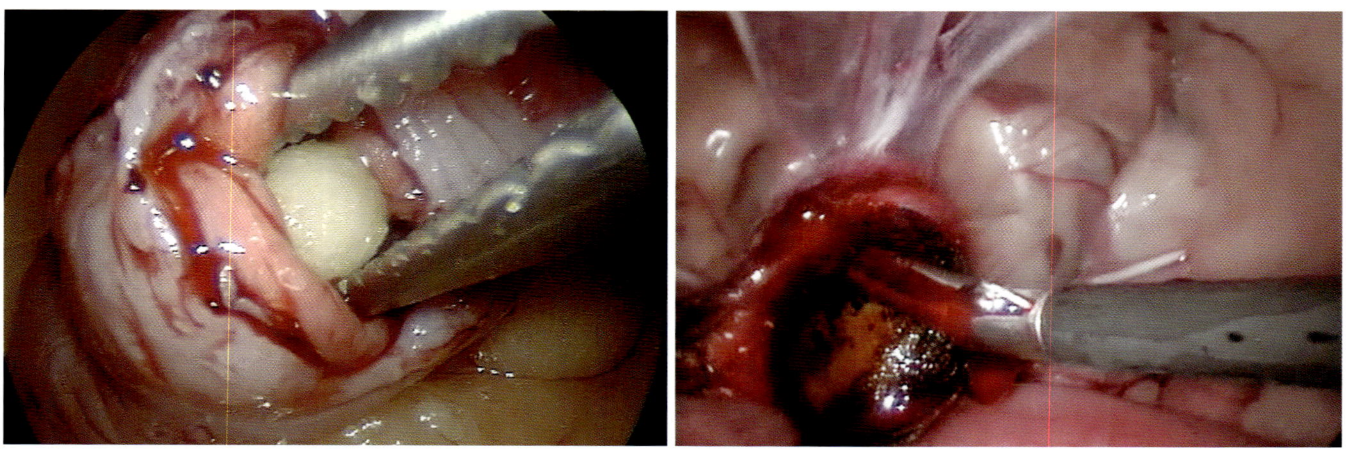

FIGURE 8. The appropriate grasping forceps should be chosen based on the stone to be removed.

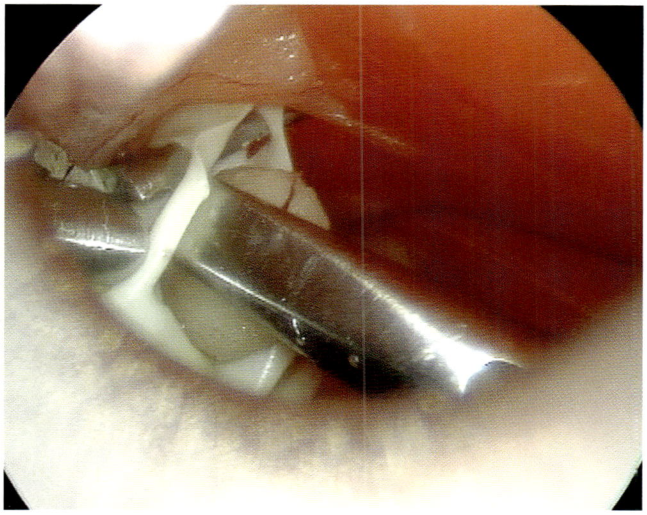

FIGURE 9. The urolith is removed using a homemade retrieval bag made from a finger of a powderless latex glove.

POSTOPERATIVE MANAGEMENT

- Patients can typically be discharged from the hospital 1–2 days after surgery.
- The urinary catheter is kept in place for the first 24–48 hours to drain the bladder.
- Antibiotic therapy is indicated in the days following surgery.
- Supportive care is given if necessary. Multimodal analgesia is continued for at least 1 week.
- Ultrasonographic evaluation of the bladder and urinary tract is recommended 12–14 days after surgery.

Complications of laparoscopic cystotomy

- Low complication rates.
- Urine leakage into the abdomen due to bladder suture dehiscence.
- Hematuria in the first days after surgery.

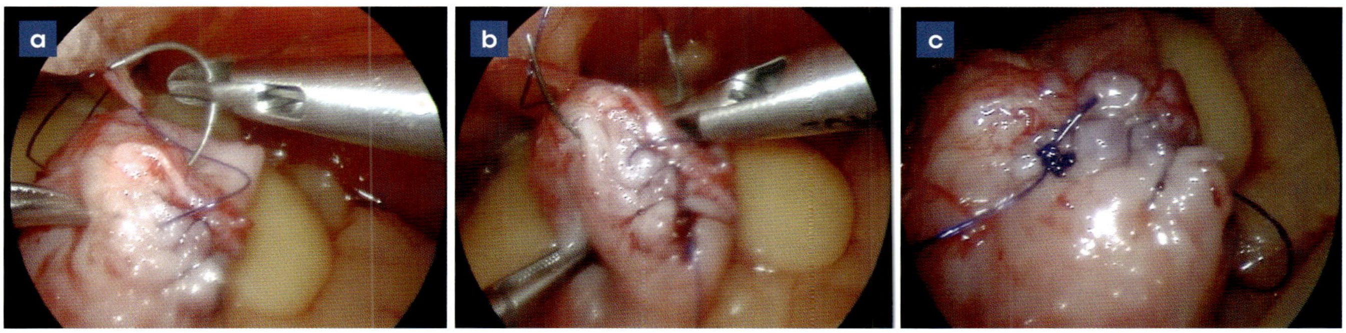

FIGURE 10. The bladder incision is closed intracorporeally with a continuous suture pattern using monofilament thread.

Key points

- Preoperative patient evaluation is important to determine which procedure should be performed.
- The procedure is indicated for the removal of large stones present as single uroliths or in a small number.
- Introduce the urethral catheter before surgery.
- Before removing the ports, perform a bladder leakage test with sterile saline.

SUGGESTED READINGS

21 LAPAROSCOPIC CYSTOPEXY

J. Brad Case

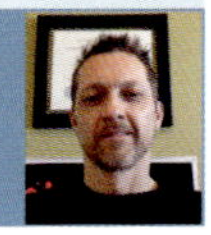

Indications	Contraindications
■ Treatment of pelvic bladder ■ Prevention and treatment of bladder retroflexion associated with perineal herniation	■ No explicit contraindications for laparoscopic cystopexy have been determined ■ Stable dogs and cats with an intact diaphragm and no cardiopulmonary disease are ideal

Cystopexy of the urinary bladder is indicated for conditions such as pelvic bladder and urinary bladder retroflexion associated with perineal herniation. Pelvic bladder in dogs appears to be congenital and rare. Urinary incontinence is the most common clinical sign observed and appears to be more prominent in spayed female dogs. In some cases, stranguria is observed due to invagination of the bladder trigone and kinking of the pelvic urethra causing urethral obstruction. Cystopexy via an open surgical approach has led to resolution of clinical signs in cases of urethral obstruction due to pelvic bladder.

Perineal herniation is more common in intact male dogs, and certain breed predilections exist. Bladder retroflexion with urethral obstruction occurs in up to 20% of cases. Cystopexy (and in some cases colopexy) has been recommended to prevent recurrence or future bladder retroflexion prior to perineal herniorrhaphy in dogs. In recent reports, a staged approach starting with urinary bladder cystopexy via laparotomy, with planned herniorrhaphy 4–6 weeks later, has been advocated.

Laparoscopic surgery is minimally invasive and results in less tissue trauma and pain, fewer complications, and shorter hospitalization time when compared to laparotomy for a variety of abdominal procedures. Recently, a laparoscopic-assisted (extracorporeal) approach for urinary bladder cystopexy has been described in seven healthy experimental dogs and three dogs with perineal herniation. Intracorporeal techniques further reduce tissue trauma by obviating the need for assist incisions and are associated with even less pain and more rapid return to function. To date, a single experimental report describing the technique for intracorporeal cystopexy and a case report of a dog with a pelvic bladder treated by intracorporeal cystopexy exists in the veterinary literature. In the former, intracorporeal cystopexy was found to be comparable to an open abdomen cystopexy; in the latter, intracorporeal cystopexy was associated with an excellent outcome.

> The first laparoscopic-assisted cystopexy of dogs was reported in 2002 by Clarence Rawlings et al.

DESCRIBED SURGICAL PROCEDURES

Both intracorporeal (three-port) and assisted techniques have been described. However, no comparisons between techniques or to traditional open cystopexy have been reported. Theoretical advantages of the intracorporeal approach are less tissue trauma, reduced pain, and lack of need for port-site enlargement. A potential disadvantage is the technical difficulty associated with intracorporeal suturing. The three-port approach to intracorporeal cystopexy has been described experimentally and is the author's preferred approach.

PATIENT PREPARATION AND POSITIONING

A physical examination and basic blood work (packed red blood cell volume, total solids, blood glucose, and blood urea nitrogen) should be performed prior to elective laparoscopic cystopexy. If urethral obstruction is present and/or the patient is clinically ill, a complete blood count and serum biochemistry profile should be evaluated. A contrast cystourethrogram is used to determine the diagnosis of pelvic bladder and, in some cases, bladder retroflexion. Medical procedures to mitigate urethral obstruction may be indicated prior to surgery if the patient is unhealthy or unstable.

In general, dogs should be fasted at least 8 hours prior to anesthesia and have an IV catheter placed for fluid and medication therapy during the procedure. The urinary bladder should be drained with a urinary catheter (if possible) at the time of anesthesia induction. Having the bladder slightly distended is useful in assessing the position of the bladder within the abdomen and for selecting the position for cystopexy. Premedications that result in splenic enlargement (e.g., acepromazine) should be avoided. Perioperative analgesia may include opioid and/or nonsteroidal medications as long as no contraindications for their use exist. Local anesthesia with bupivacaine is recommended at individual port sites prior to incision. The vast majority of dogs treated with perioperative nonsteroidal medication and oral tramadol return to baseline pain indices by 48 hours after laparoscopic cystopexy.

The patient is positioned in dorsal recumbency and clipped from the xiphoid process to the pubis and dorsally past the level of the 13th rib. A paramedian port is recommended for intracorporeal cystopexy; therefore, a wide clip is indicated to avoid contamination. If a hydraulic float table is available, the patient may be positioned directly on the operating table and the hydraulic function used to create about 30° of Trendelenburg and 30° of lateral positioning. Alternatively, a Trendelenburg position can be accomplished with a traditional operating table and the patient can be gently shifted on the table to acquire lateral oblique position. The abdomen is aseptically prepared as for traditional laparotomy. This ensures that adequate preparation and quick conversion to laparotomy can be performed if needed.

OPERATING ROOM LAYOUT

For laparoscopic cystopexy, the operating surgeon and surgeon assistant must be able to stand comfortably, one on each side of the operating table. For a left-sided cystopexy, the author prefers to stand on the right side of the patient to operate the needle holders. The assistant can operate the telescope from the patient's left side in either the T1 or T2 ports.

Although many layout options likely exist, the author's preference is to have the dog positioned with their hind end towards the foot of the operating table and the anesthesia circuit and staff positioned at the head of the operating table. The instrument back table is positioned at the foot of the operating table, with enough room for the surgeon and assistant to walk around the back table from side to side of the patient. Either one or two viewing monitors can be used, and they should be positioned at the foot of the table just above the instrument back table (**Fig. 1**).

Instruments

On the table:

- Standard surgical pack
- High-definition video camera
- Telescope 5 mm – 30°
- Three 5 mm threaded cannulas
- 5 mm laparoscopic Babcock or DeBakey forceps
- 5 mm laparoscopic cotton-tipped blunt dissection probes
- 5 mm L- or J-hook monopolar electrosurgical tip
- Two 5 mm laparoscopic needle holders
- 3-0 absorbable barbed suture swaged on a fine taper needle

PORT PLACEMENT (FIG. 2)

- T2, on the midline, 1 cm caudal to the umbilicus
- T1, on the midline, 4–6 cm cranial to T2
- T3, paramedian lateral to the rectus abdominus and to T2

PROCEDURE

- After the first port has been placed and the pneumoperitoneum achieved, the 5 mm telescope is inserted and an initial exploration of the abdomen is performed. Subsequent ports are then placed under optical guidance as described above.
- The position of the urinary bladder is assessed by grasping the bladder apex with a laparoscopic Babcock forceps and by placing cranial traction until the bladder is repositioned in an intra-abdominal location. In case of pelvic bladder,

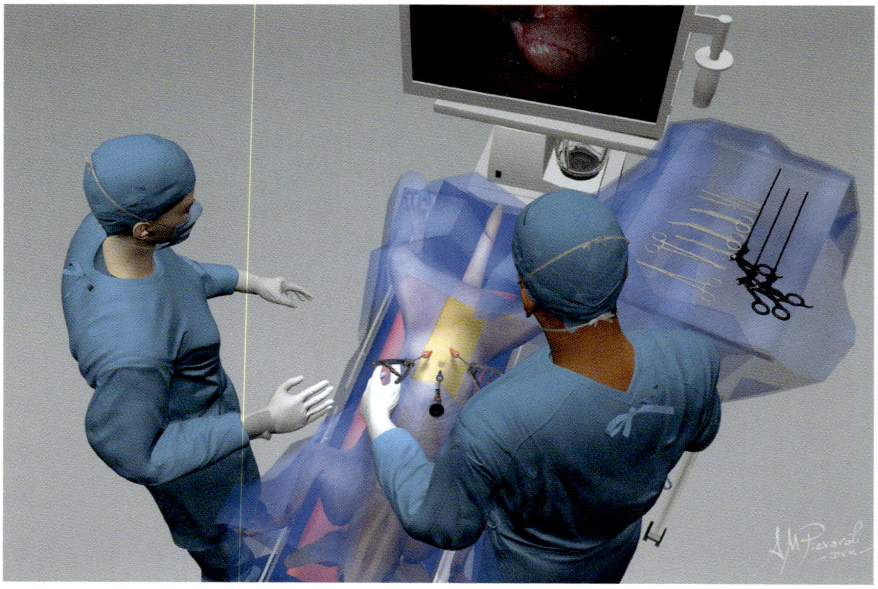

FIGURE 1. Operating room layout for laparoscopic intracorporeal cystopexy. The patient is placed in dorsal recumbency in a Trendelenburg position.

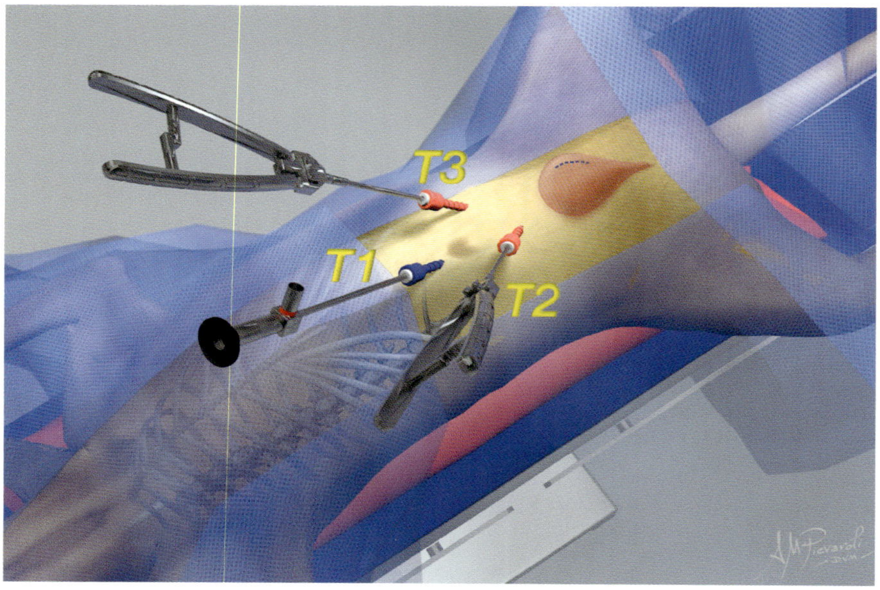

FIGURE 2. Port placement for three-port laparoscopic intracorporeal cystopexy. Note the two midline ports, one caudal and the other cranial to the umbilicus. A single paramedian port is placed on the lateral abdomen midway between T1 and T2.

most of the urinary bladder is located within the pelvic canal (**Fig. 3**). Thus, significant relocation into an intra-abdominal position is required prior to cystopexy (**Fig. 4**).

- Under endoscopic vision, a laparoscopic L-hook electrosurgical pencil is used to create a 3–4 cm long wound in the transversus muscle to the left of the urinary bladder (**Fig. 5**). A matching superficial wound can be made in the urinary bladder using the coagulation function of the L-hook device, although this may not be necessary to create a mature adhesion.
- A 3-0 barbed suture is passed from the caudal aspect of the transversus muscle incision to the caudal aspect of the matching bladder wound (**Fig. 6**). A simple continuous full-thickness pattern is used to completely suture the bladder to the transversus muscle (**Fig. 7**).
- The bladder is then gently instilled with sterile saline via the urinary catheter to examine the final position within the abdominal cavity (**Fig. 8**).
- Ports are removed and incisions closed routinely.

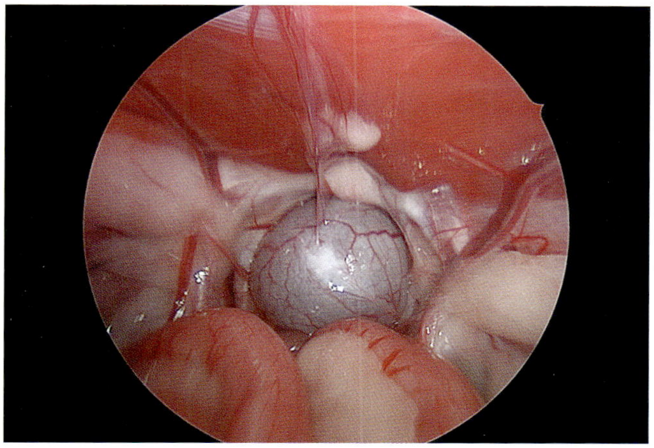

FIGURE 3. Laparoscopic image of an intrapelvic bladder in a young male dog. Note the pubic brim at the top of the image (ventral in the patient). Most (>90%) of the bladder is within the pelvic canal.

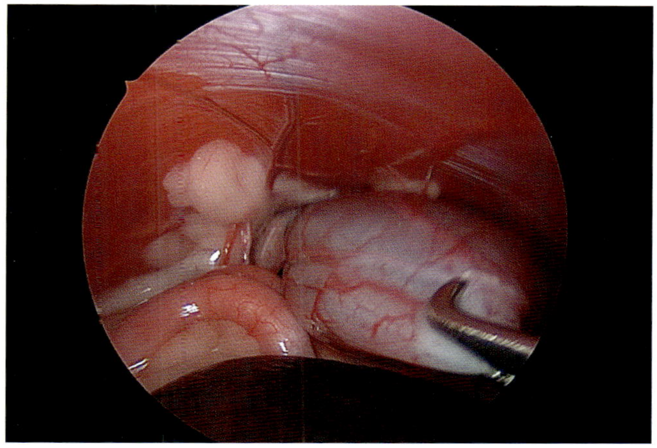

FIGURE 4. The pelvic bladder is reduced back to an intra-abdominal position.

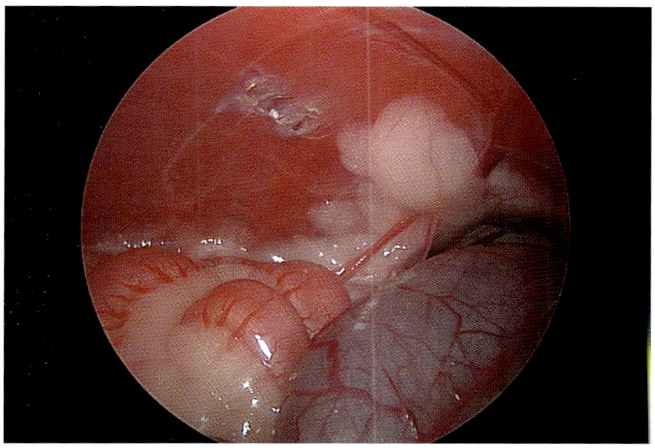

FIGURE 5. A 3–4 cm long wound is made in the transversus muscle to the left of the urinary bladder. This is the location where the urinary bladder will be fixed.

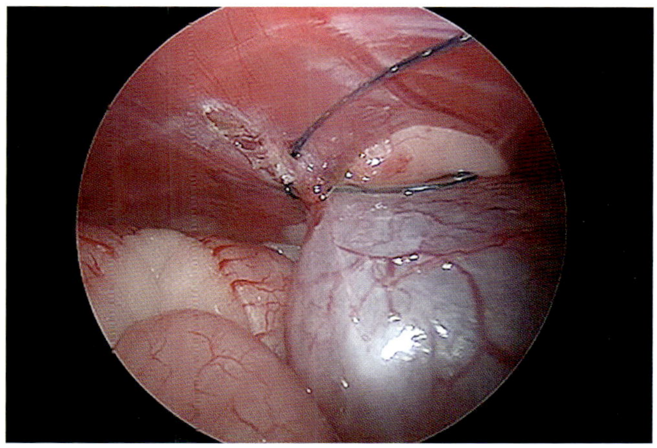

FIGURE 6. Beginning of the continuous suture pattern using barbed suture. The needle needs to be passed through the welded loop prior to further suturing. Generally, five or six passes are required to create a 4 cm cystopexy.

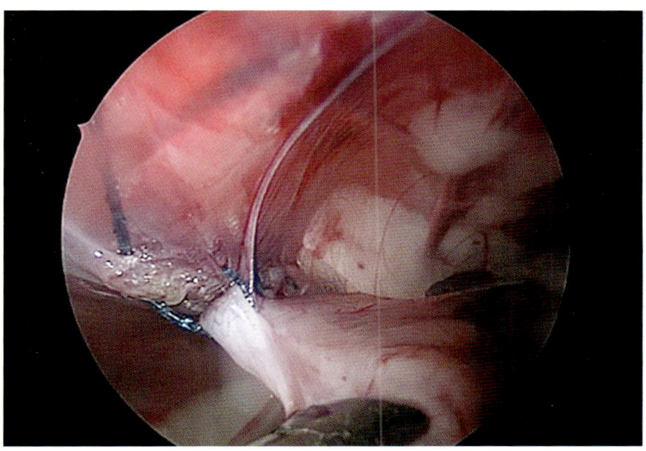

FIGURE 7. Completion of the intracorporeal cystopexy. A laparoscopic forceps is used to gently manipulate the bladder to ensure a strong adhesion.

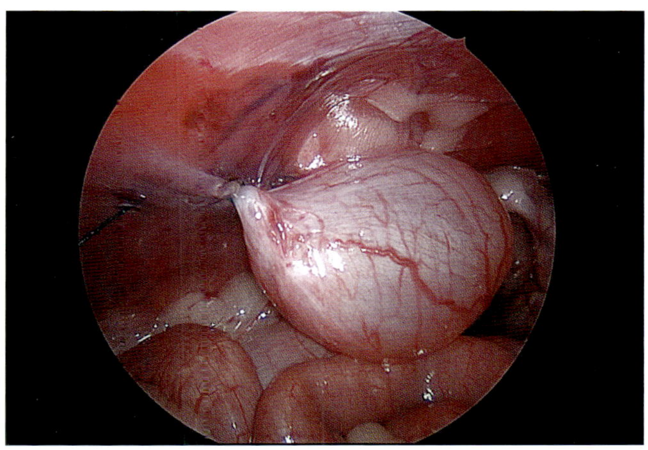

FIGURE 8. After cystopexy, the urinary bladder is infused with sterile saline to demonstrate proper positioning.

POSTOPERATIVE MANAGEMENT

- Analgesia following laparoscopic cystopexy is typically minimal and may include a nonsteroidal drug and an oral synthetic opioid (e.g., tramadol) for 2–3 days.
- Food and water can be offered ad libitum 8–12 hours after surgery as long as no contraindications exist.
- Dogs with pelvic bladder should be monitored for 24–48 hours to document normal micturition, although mild pollakiuria may be observed for 24–48 hours postoperatively.
- Normal residual urine volume is less than 0.3 mL/kg body weight and can be assessed by catheterizing and quantifying urine volume immediately following urination.
- Mild hematuria is expected for 24 hours after the procedure but should resolve within 48 hours.

Complications of laparoscopic cystopexy

- Complications are scarcely reported following laparoscopic cystopexy.
- Urine leakage from the cystopexy site has recently been reported in one dog.
- Surgical site infections have not been reported following laparoscopic cystopexy in dogs, but the risk is likely low.

Key points

- Cranial traction is required to position a pelvic bladder intra-abdominally during cystopexy.
- Cystopexy should be 3–4 cm in length, depending on the size of the dog.

SUGGESTED READINGS

22 LAPAROSCOPIC-ASSISTED VASOPEXY

Massimo Barilli

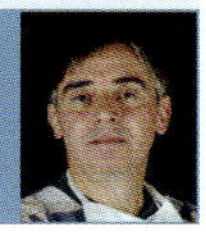

Indications	Contraindications
■ Relocation of an enlarged prostate and urinary bladder from the entrance of the pelvic canal to a more normal location in the abdominal cavity ■ Improvement of the subsequent fixation of the colon	■ Intracranial diseases ■ Cardiovascular and pulmonary diseases ■ Coagulopathy

Vasopexy is the surgical procedure by which an enlarged prostate and urinary bladder are relocated from the entrance of the pelvic canal to a more normal location in the abdominal cavity.

Colopexy, vasopexy, and cystopexy in conjunction with castration have been performed in some studies for the treatment of perineal hernia, and the recurrence rate reported is comparable to that of other studies using different methods. Recurrence of perineal hernia is rare following bilateral herniorrhaphy combined with colopexy and vas deferens pexy with or without cystopexy. Vasopexy and colopexy combined have been performed with a modified semitendinosus muscle transposition technique for the repair of ventral perineal hernia.

Before vasopexy, intact dogs are castrated with an open technique and the urinary bladder, if retroflexed, should be returned to its normal position.

Laparoscopic vasopexy has been described for the treatment of perineal hernia.

> Laparoscopic-guided deferentopexy was described in 2002 by J. F. Salomon et al. for the management of urethral sphincter mechanism incompetence in a male dog.

PATIENT PREPARATION AND POSITIONING

The dog's abdomen is clipped and aseptically prepared from the xiphoid process to the pubic brim. Prophylactic perioperative antibiotic therapy (cefazolin 22 mg/kg IV) is recommended.

For two-port colopexy, the dog is placed in dorsal recumbency, with the front and rear limbs secured, in a Trendelenburg position (head lower than the abdomen), and tilted to the right.

THREE-PORT LAPAROSCOPIC-ASSISTED VASOPEXY

A three-port laparoscopic approach is used for vasopexy alone or in combination with colopexy. Vasopexy is performed before colopexy.

Instruments

- Standard surgery set
- Telescope 5 mm – 30°
- Three 5 mm cannulas
- Grasping forceps

OPERATING ROOM LAYOUT

Cannulas are placed in a triangulation fashion, with the surgeon facing caudally (**Fig. 1**).

PORT PLACEMENT (FIG. 2)

- T1, on the midline, 1–2 cm caudal to the umbilicus
- T2, on the left lateral abdominal wall
- T3, on the right lateral abdominal wall

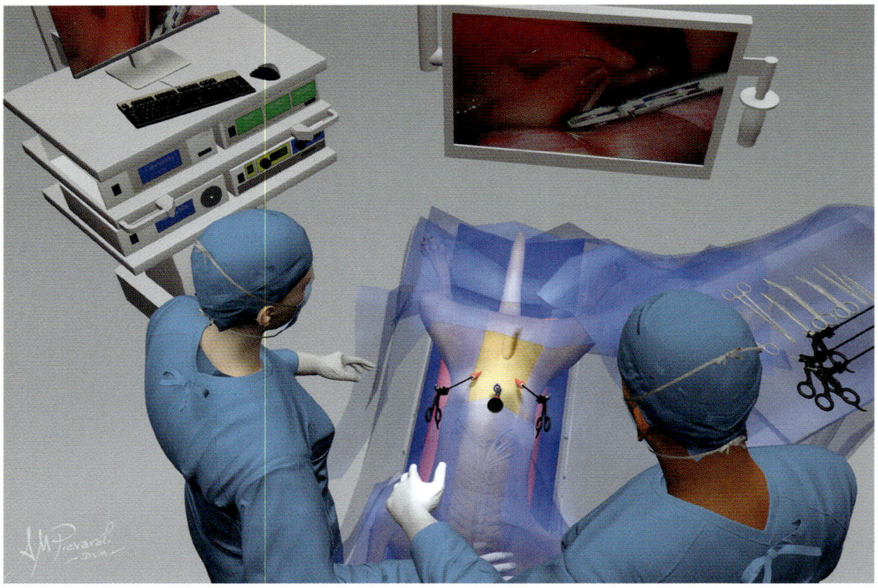

FIGURE 1. Operating room layout for laparoscopic-assisted vasopexy.

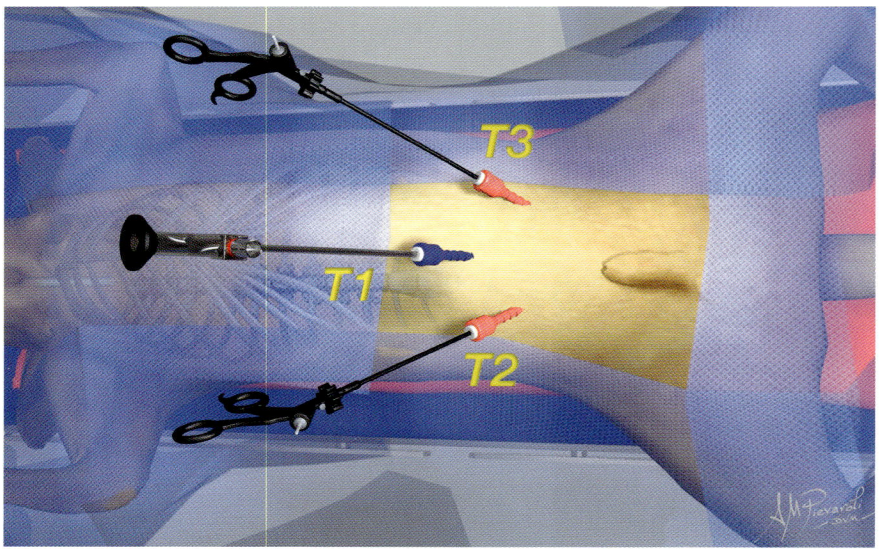

FIGURE 2. Port placement for three-port laparoscopic-assisted vasopexy.

PROCEDURE

- Before vasopexy, intact dogs are castrated using an open technique. The testicular artery and vein are ligated separately from the vas deferens.
- After the ports have been placed (**Fig. 3**) and the pneumoperitoneum achieved, the 5 mm telescope is inserted in T1 and a first exploration of the abdomen is performed to check for any evidence of iatrogenic trauma caused by placement of the cannulas.
- The vasa deferentia are identified in the inguinal canals on each side.
- Using a grasping forceps inserted in T2, the right vas deferens is grasped and retrieved from the right inguinal canal by applying gentle cranial traction (**Fig. 4**).
- The same maneuver is repeated on the left vas deferens using a grasping forceps inserted in T3.
- A small skin incision is made 3–4 cm caudal to T2 and a straight mosquito forceps is inserted through the abdominal wall into the abdominal cavity (**Fig. 5**). The mosquito forceps are used to grasp the left vas deferens and pull it out through the abdominal incision (**Fig. 6**).

- The same maneuver is repeated on the left vas deferens using a grasping forceps inserted in T3.
- A small skin incision is made 3–4 cm caudal to T3, and the same maneuver is repeated to pull the right vas deferens out of the abdominal cavity.
- At this point, laparoscopic-assisted colopexy can be performed if indicated.
- The pneumoperitoneum is evacuated and each vas deferens is sutured to the external muscle fascia of the abdominal wall using one or two monofilament sutures in an interrupted pattern.
- Before skin closure, the pneumoperitoneum is reestablished through T1 and the deferentopexies are examined laparoscopically to ensure that optimal positioning has been achieved and that excessive hemorrhage is not present (**Fig. 7**).
- After evacuating the remaining pneumoperitoneum, all the cannulas are removed and the port-site incisions closed in routine fashion.

POSTOPERATIVE MANAGEMENT

- Immediate postoperative management focuses on pain control.
- Hospitalization is recommended for 1 day after surgery to manage pain and monitor for signs of intestinal issues.
- The patient should be discharged with an E-collar and instructions for 14 days of activity restriction to allow proper healing of the skin and vasopexy sites.

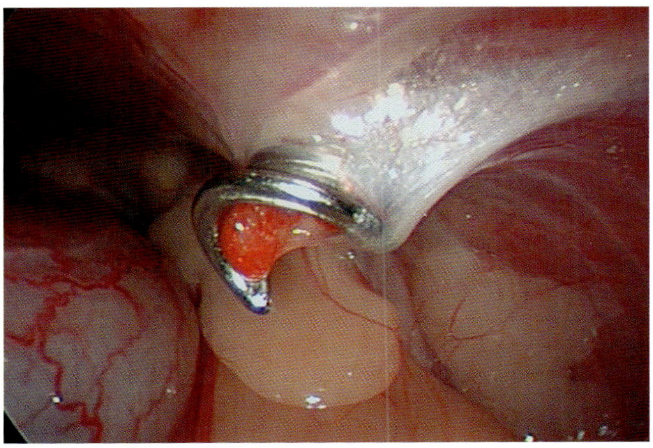

FIGURE 3. Placement of T3.

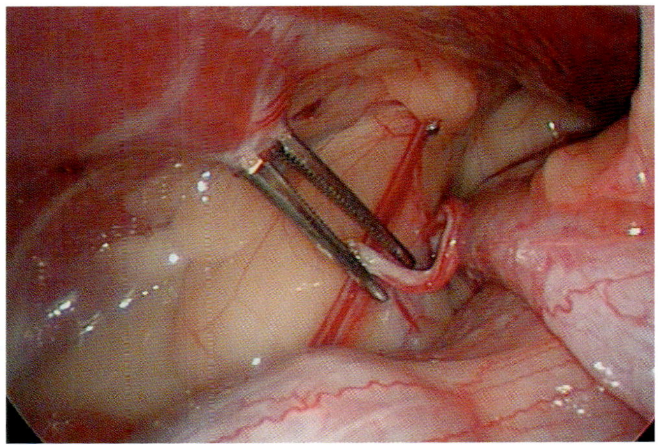

FIGURE 5. The left vas deferens is grasped with straight mosquito forceps inserted through the abdominal wall.

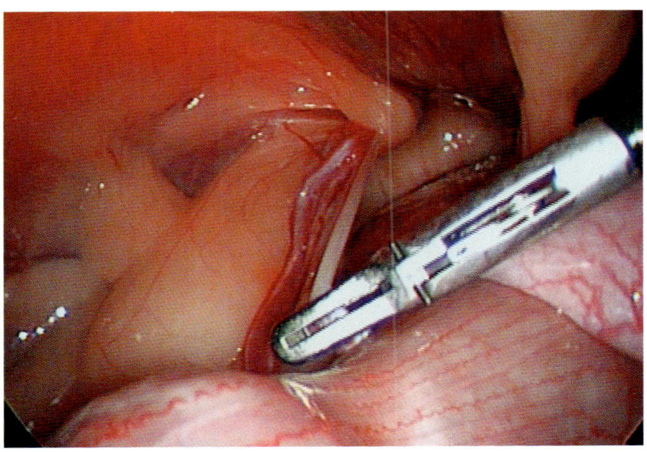

FIGURE 4. The right vas deferens is pulled out of the right inguinal canal.

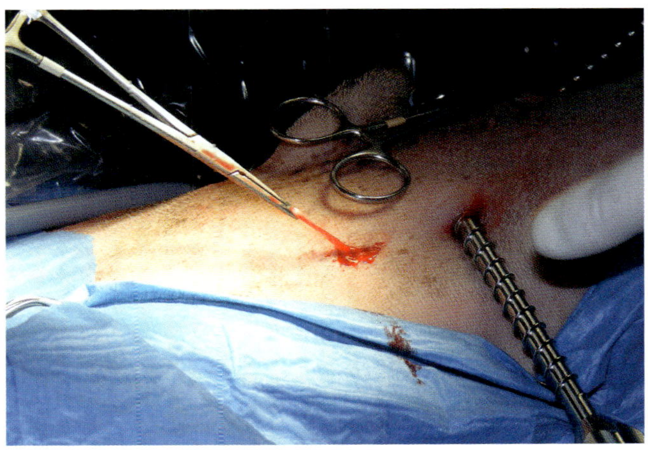

FIGURE 6. The vas deferens is pulled out through the abdominal wall.

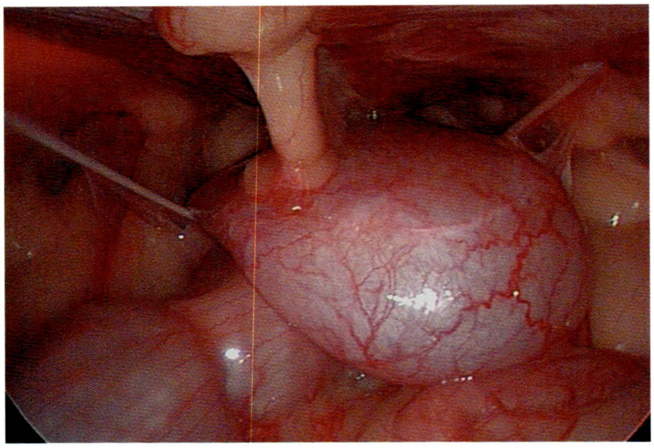

FIGURE 7. Laparoscopic visualization of vasopexy.

Complications of laparoscopic-assisted vasopexy

- In the hands of expert laparoscopic surgeons, intraoperative complications are rare; however, access-related issues are complications in any laparoscopic surgery.
- Complications include lesions during cannula introduction, incorrect port placement, residual subcutaneous emphysema, incisional fistula, and incisional infections.
- Postoperative complications include transient incontinence within 2–3 weeks of vasopexy.

Key points

- Consider vasopexy in addition to other procedures to treat recurrent perineal hernia or dislocated prostate.
- Do not exert excessive traction on the vas deferens to prevent it from tearing.

SUGGESTED READINGS

CLINICAL CASES

22.1 LAPAROSCOPIC REVERSIBLE NEUTERING IN A DOG

Roberto Giaconella, Emanuela Vitali, Veronica Giaconella

CASE DESCRIPTION

A 1-year-old male Maremmano-Abruzzese dog weighing 45 kg was operated on for reversible sterilization using a minimally invasive technique. Each vas deferens was blocked with an endoclip. A follow-up was carried out 1 month after the procedure by examining the ejaculate, and no spermatozoa were found. During the time that the endoclips were in place, the dog mated without reproducing. The endoclips were removed over a year after sterilization. At this point, testosterone levels (20 ng/mL) were within the normal range (0.8–25.6 ng/mL) and the dog was fertile again.

Key points

- Laparoscopic reversible neutering is a feasible method to prevent reproduction without interfering with hormonal levels.
- More case studies should be carried out to validate this method.
- The dog is fertile again and enjoys excellent health.

PORT PLACEMENT

The dog was placed in dorsal recumbency. The first port (T1) was placed 2 cm caudal to the umbilicus and a 5 mm 0° telescope was introduced. The second port (T2) was placed in a slightly right paramedian position, 10 cm caudal to T1, and a Babcock forceps was introduced. The third port (T3) was placed on the left side, at the same level as T2, and a 5 mm endoclip applier was inserted. Each vas deferens was blocked with an endoclip.

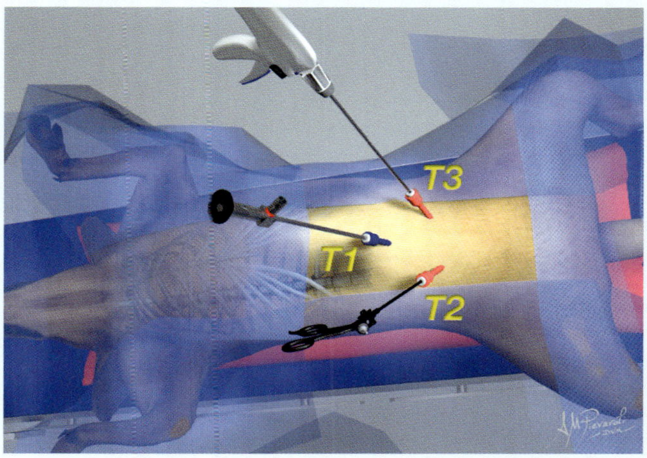

PROCEDURE

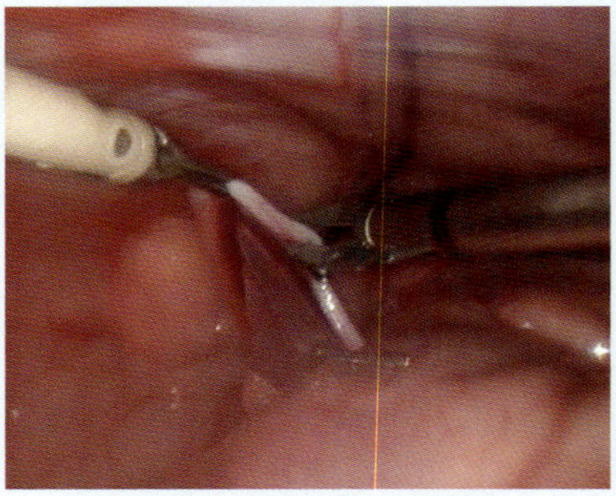

FIGURE 1. A 5 mm titanium clip is applied to the left vas deferens.

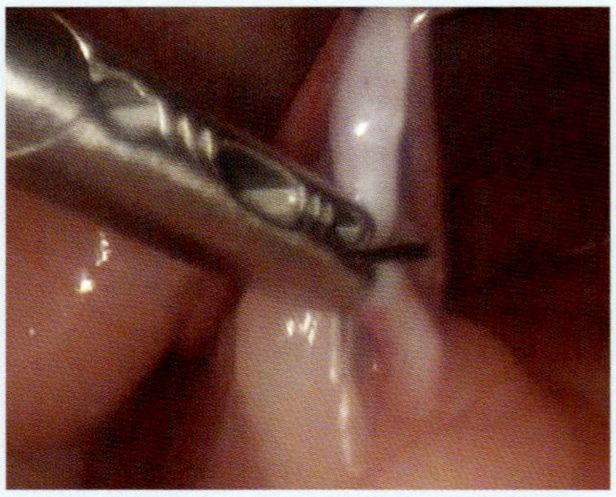

FIGURE 2. The clips are removed 1 year after application.

Tips and tricks

✓ When applying the clips, make sure to close the vas deferens.
✓ Use 5 mm clips, which are more delicate.
✓ Measure testosterone levels postoperatively to check if testicular vascularity was inadvertently impaired.

23 LAPAROSCOPIC URETERONEPHRECTOMY

Roberto Properzi

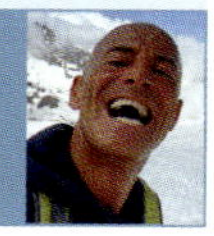

Indications	Contraindications
■ Hydronephrosis with or without pyelonephritis	■ Large renal masses (>5–7 cm)
■ Renal cysts and abscesses	■ Severe hydronephrosis
■ Modestly sized primary renal neoplasms	■ Complete hydroureter
■ Obstructive calculus disease	■ Multiple adhesions to adjacent structures (e.g., vena cava)
■ Idiopathic renal hematuria	■ Infection extending beyond the renal capsule
■ Traumatic renal injury with avulsion	■ Reduced function of the contralateral kidney

Transperitoneal laparoscopic ureteronephrectomy is gaining more and more popularity in veterinary medicine, like it did in human surgery, due to its significant advantages over traditional techniques. Adequate patient selection is essential, including assessment of the normal function of the contralateral kidney and careful evaluation of the anatomy of the operating field through advanced diagnostic imaging. It must be borne in mind that transperitoneal laparoscopic ureteronephrectomy represents one of the most challenging laparoscopic interventions; therefore, it should be performed by experienced surgeons.

> The first scientific work on laparoscopic ureteronephrectomy in humans was published in 1991 by Clyman et al.

DESCRIBED SURGICAL PROCEDURES

Laparoscopic ureteronephrectomy involving the use of three or four ports has been described. The advantages of this technique are the same as those of other minimally invasive surgical procedures, including reduced postoperative pain and a more rapid return to normal activity.

According to the surgical technique described in a 2013 study, the ureter was dissected as near as possible to the bladder and closed with three hemoclips. However, another technique in which this is not necessary has been reported, and no complications were noted after leaving a blind-ending ureteral stump behind.

PATIENT PREPARATION AND POSITIONING

The lateral abdomen on the side of the affected kidney is clipped; the surgical clip should extend from the transverse spinous processes of the vertebrae to the mid-abdominal area on the contralateral side and from the mid-thorax to the perineal area. The skin is aseptically prepared for surgery, including an aseptic wash of the prepuce in male dogs.

The patient is positioned in lateral recumbency, with the affected kidney up.

OPERATING ROOM LAYOUT

The surgeon and the assistant position themselves on one side of the operating table, facing the patient's abdomen. The endoscopic tower is placed on the opposite side of the operating table (**Fig. 1**).

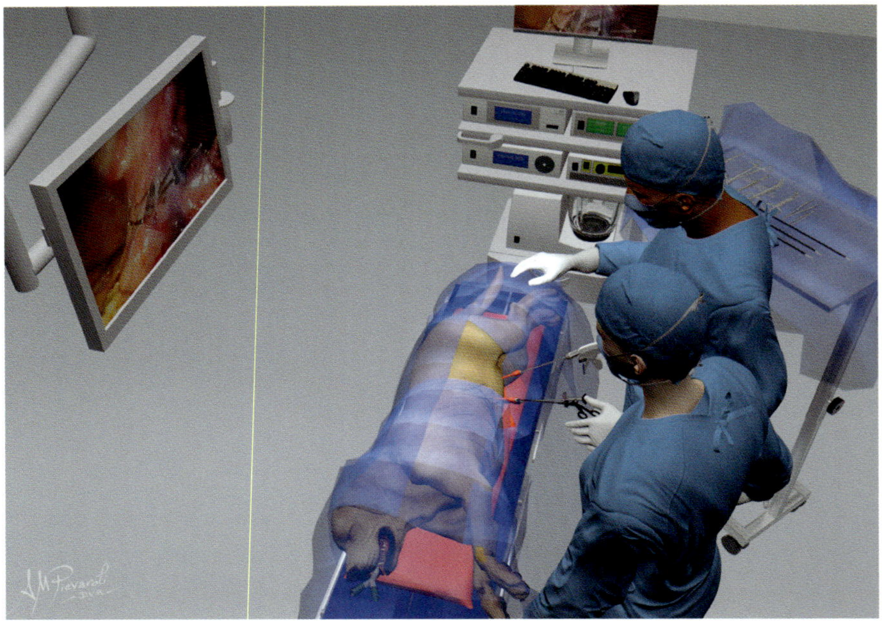

FIGURE 1. Operating room layout for laparoscopic ureteronephrectomy.

Instruments

On the table:

- Standard surgery set
- Telescope 5 mm – 30°
- Three 5 mm cannulas (or two 5 mm cannulas + one 10 mm cannula)
- Atraumatic grasping forceps
- Kelly forceps or right-angle dissecting forceps (**Fig. 2**)
- Vessel-sealing device
- Laparoscopic medium- to large-size metal or polymer hemoclips (**Fig. 3**)
- Monopolar electrosurgery unit
- Specimen retrieval bag (**Fig. 4**)

Ready to use:

- Endoscopic cannula for aspiration/irrigation
- Fourth cannula to switch to a four-port technique

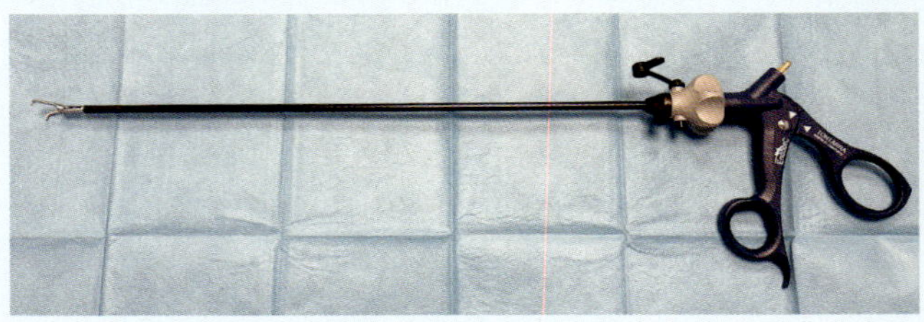

FIGURE 2. Right-angle dissecting forceps.

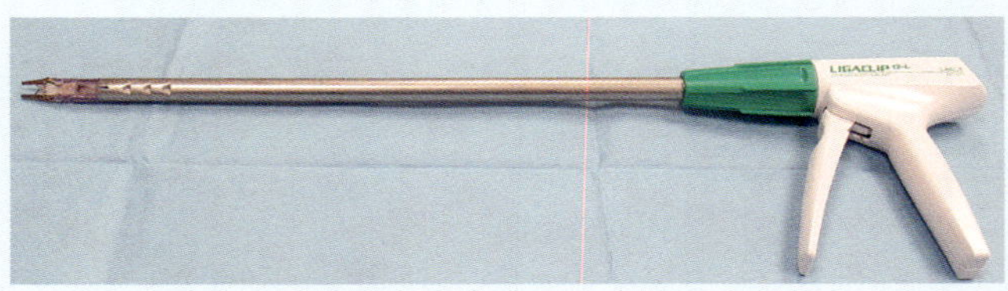

FIGURE 3. Laparoscopic hemoclips.

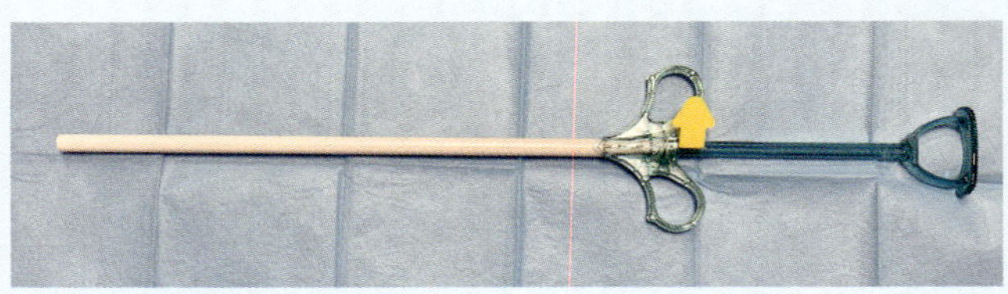

FIGURE 4. Specimen retrieval bag.

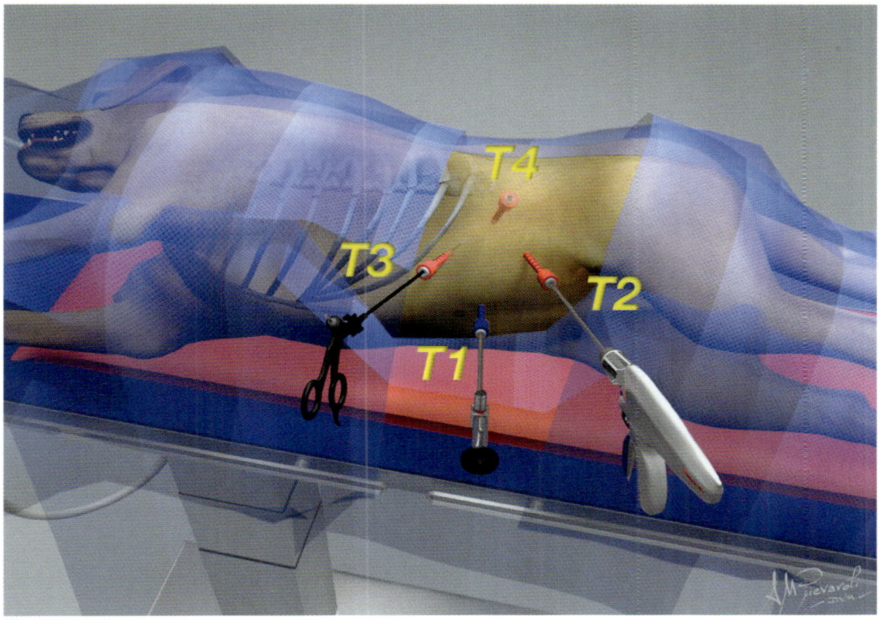

FIGURE 5. Port placement for laparoscopic ureteronephrectomy.

PORT PLACEMENT (FIG. 5)

- T1, on the midline, 1–2 cm caudal to the umbilicus (or more lateral if a 0° telescope is used)
- T2, in the caudal abdominal quadrant, just cranial to the pelvic limb
- T3, in the cranial abdominal quadrant, just caudal to the last rib
- T4 (optional, if tissue retraction is necessary), on the anticipated location of the affected kidney

PROCEDURE (VIDEO 1)

- After the first port has been placed and the pneumoperitoneum achieved, the 5 mm telescope is inserted and a first exploration of the abdomen is performed to inspect the kidney and the surrounding structures.
- Under endoscopic vision, the second and the third (and the fourth, if needed) cannulas for the operative instruments are inserted.
- If the kidney is hidden by the surrounding structures, the operating table can be tilted toward the surgeon or a foam wedge can be placed under the patient's back.
- Kidney dissection begins using the vessel-sealing device to separate the kidney from its retroperitoneal attachments (**Fig. 6**).
- The ureter is identified and its proximal end is dissected using the right-angle dissecting forceps and the vessel-sealing device (**Fig. 7**).
- Two or three clips are applied in the ureter to close it, and the ureter is then cut between the clips (**Fig. 8**).
- After identifying the renal hilus, the renal vessels are dissected.
- The renal artery and vein are closed with two or three laparoscopic hemoclips (**Fig. 9**) and sectioned using a vessel-sealing device (**Fig. 10**).
- The resected kidney is placed into a specimen retrieval bag (**Fig. 11**).
- Before closure, the entire surgical site is reexamined for any ongoing hemorrhage.
- After enlarging one of the instrument ports, the specimen retrieval bag is pulled out of the abdominal cavity.
- The port sites are closed routinely.

VIDEO 1. Laparoscopic ureteronephrectomy of an atrophic kidney.

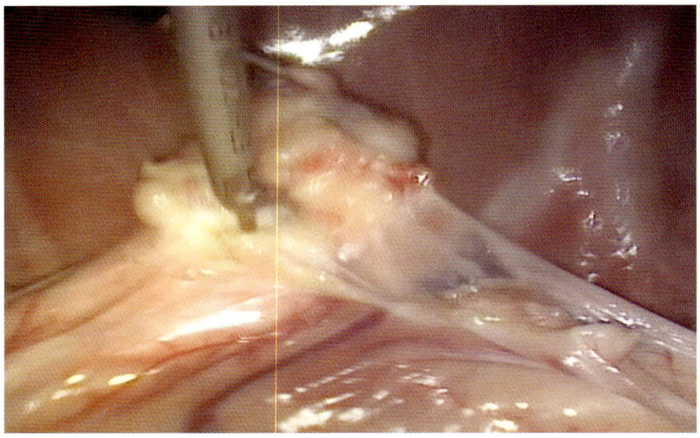

FIGURE 6. The kidney is dissected using a vessel-sealing device.

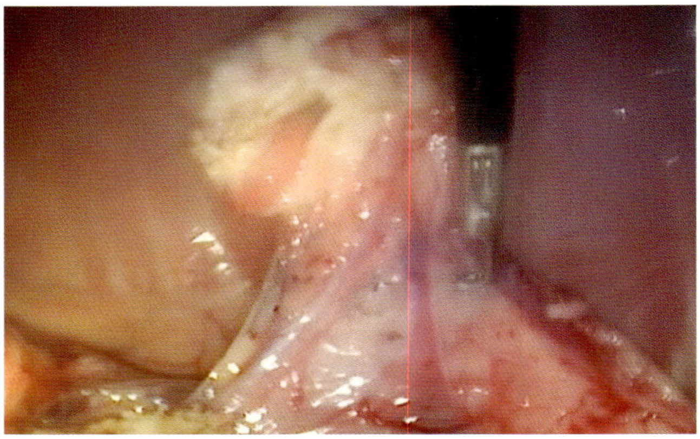

FIGURE 7. The ureter is dissected using a right-angle forceps.

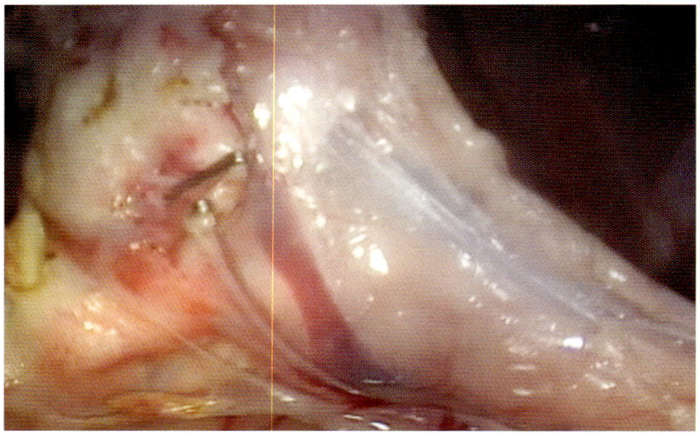

FIGURE 8. Two clips are applied to close the ectatic ureter.

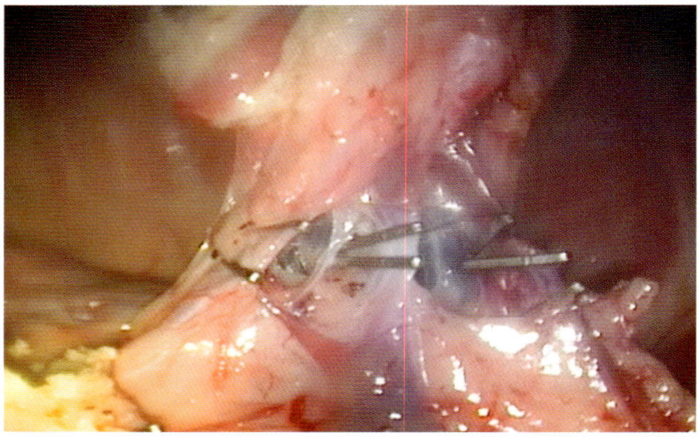

FIGURE 9. The renal artery and vein are closed with hemoclips.

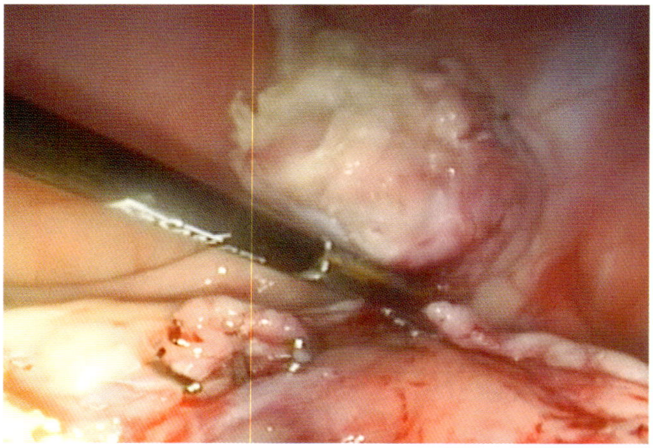

FIGURE 10. The renal artery and vein are sectioned with a vessel-sealing device.

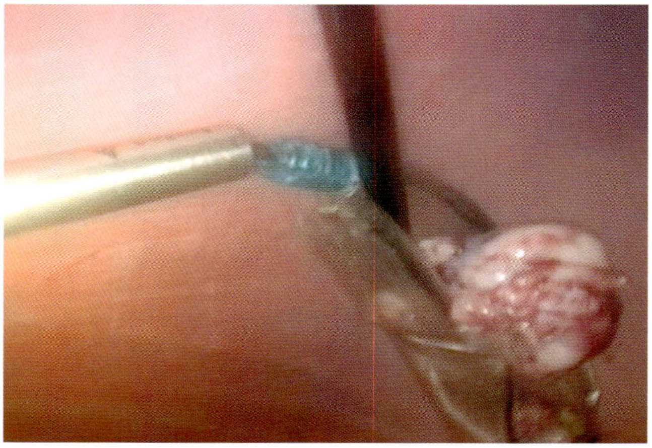

FIGURE 11. The kidney is placed into a specimen retrieval bag.

POSTOPERATIVE MANAGEMENT

- Postoperative analgesia is usually obtained with opioids, through a constant rate infusion of methadone or fentanyl, boluses of methadone, or an epidural injection of morphine.
- Nonsteroidal anti-inflammatory drugs are best avoided in kidney surgeries.
- Hospitalization time is usually 2–3 days.
- Long-term monitoring of renal function should be performed.

Complications of laparoscopic ureteronephrectomy

- Iatrogenic damage to surrounding structures.
- Hemorrhage from the renal capsule or the phrenicoabdominal vein during retroperitoneal dissection.
- Specimen retrieval bag tearing.

Key points

- Always check the function of the contralateral kidney preoperatively.
- It is not always important to close the ureter near the urinary bladder.
- If the kidney is hidden by the surrounding structures, the operating table can be tilted toward the surgeon or a foam wedge can be placed under the patient's back.

SUGGESTED READINGS

CLINICAL CASES

23.1 LAPAROSCOPIC OMENTALIZATION OF A RENAL CYST

Michael Brückner

CASE DESCRIPTION

A 7-year-old spayed female Norwegian Elkhound was presented because of a slowly growing cystic structure at the caudal pole of the left kidney. A small cyst had been initially detected at the time the dog was operated on for pyometra, but over the following 1.5 years, the cystic structure had reached a diameter of around 8 cm. Laparoscopic exploration revealed that the cyst was directly originating from the caudal pole of left kidney. Under laparoscopic guidance, percutaneous cyst drainage was performed followed by partial cystectomy and omentalization. According to the owner, the dog became much more active after the procedure. Follow-up ultrasound examinations did not reveal recurrence of the cyst about 6 months postoperatively.

Key points

- The cyst was drained percutaneously.
- The cystic wall was temporarily suspended from the abdominal wall with a percutaneous needle–suture combination.
- Intracorporeal suturing was performed.

PORT PLACEMENT

Two 6 mm Ternamian Endotip trocars were placed, one in the umbilicus (camera port) and the other half-way between the umbilicus and pubic rim. The patient was tilted towards the right side after port placement.

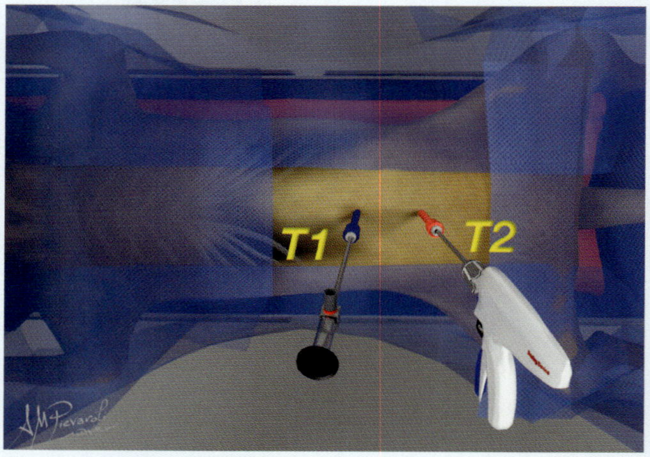

PROCEDURE

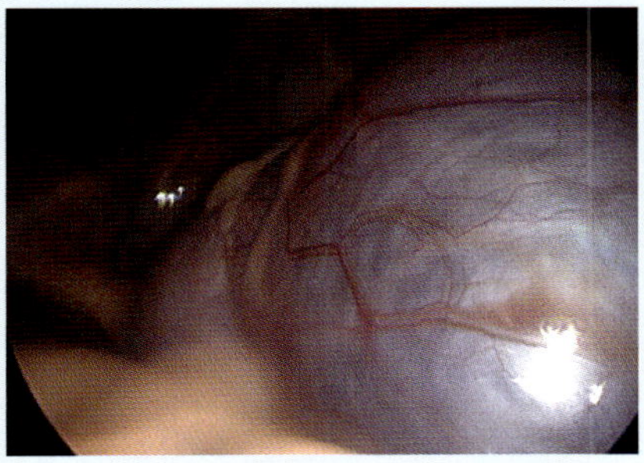

FIGURE 1. Cystic structure arising from the caudal pole of the left kidney. The normal left kidney is to the left of the image.

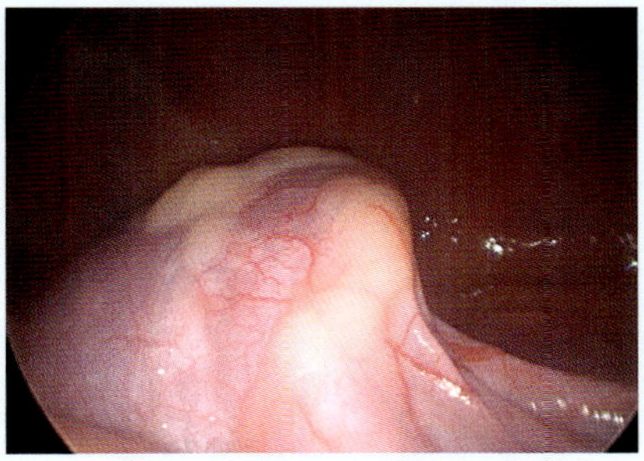

FIGURE 2. Appearance of the normal part of the left kidney after percutaneous drainage of the cyst.

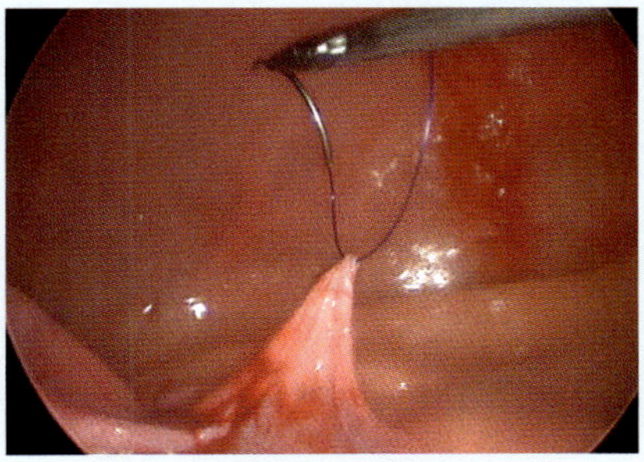

FIGURE 3. The cystic wall is suspended from the abdominal wall with a percutaneous needle–suture combination.

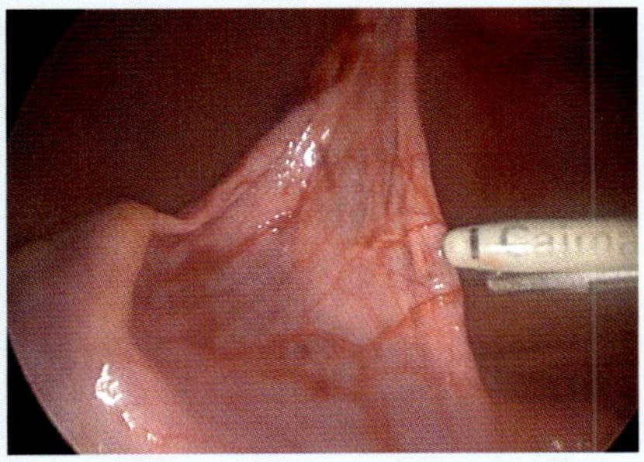

FIGURE 4. The cystic wall is opened using a vessel-sealing device.

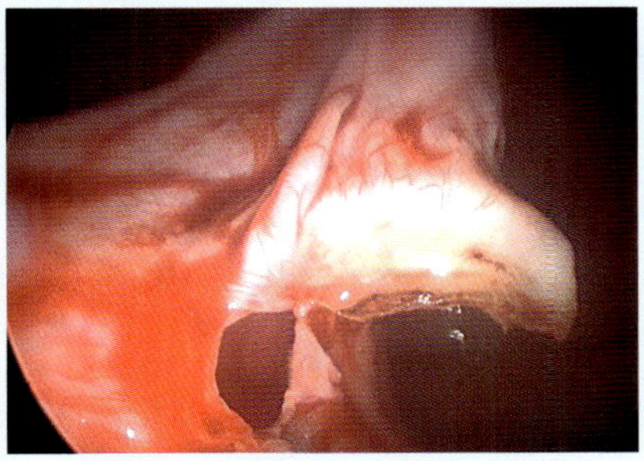

FIGURE 5. Opening in the cystic wall after one application of the vessel-sealing device.

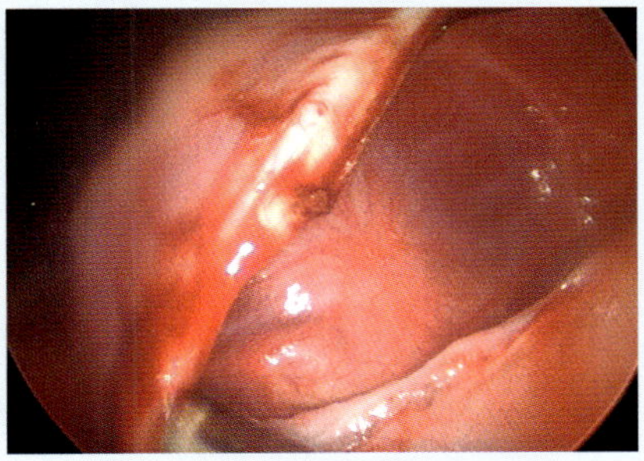

FIGURE 6. The interior of the cyst is inspected. A clear separation from the healthy part of the kidney is visible.

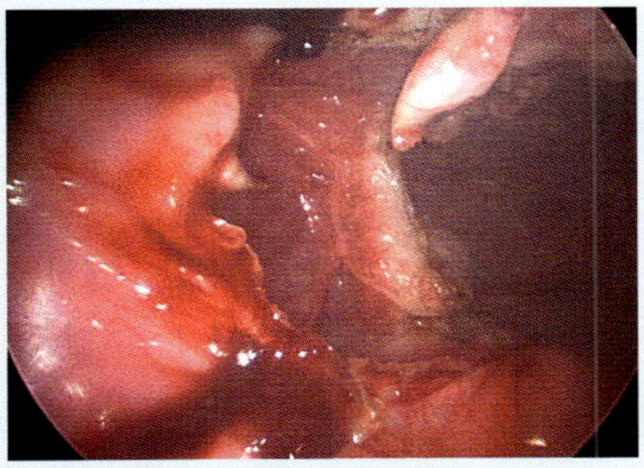

FIGURE 7. The cystic wall is further resected using the vessel-sealing device.

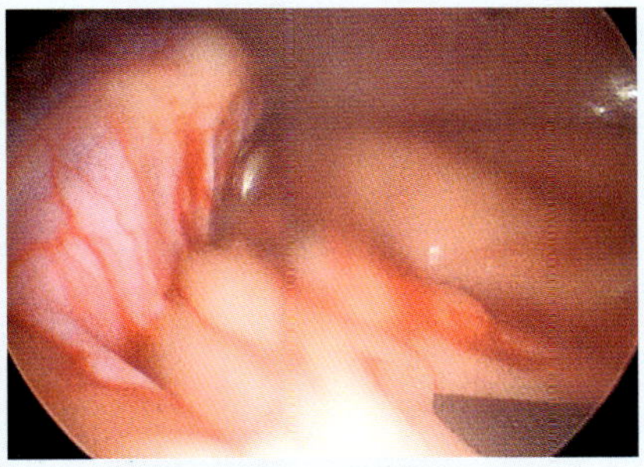

FIGURE 8. Omentum is placed into the remaining cystic wall.

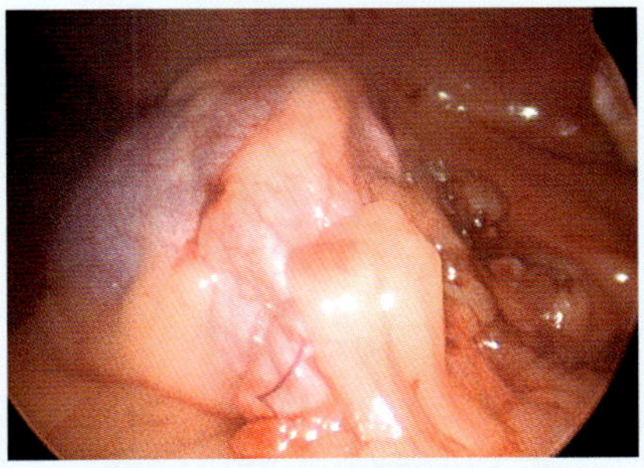

FIGURE 9. Final image after suturing the omentum to the ventral cyst wall with barbed suture.

Tips and tricks

- ✓ Drain the cyst with a spinal needle inserted percutaneously.
- ✓ Open and resect the cyst with a vessel-sealing device.
- ✓ Use a laparoscopic needle holder for intracorporeal suturing.
- ✓ Suture the omentalized defect with barbed suture.

23.2 LAPAROSCOPIC PERINEPHRIC PSEUDOCYST RESECTION

Justin B. Ganjei

CASE DESCRIPTION

A 14-year-old castrated male domestic shorthair cat was presented for surgical consultation of a right perinephric pseudocyst. The patient had been previously diagnosed with IRIS stage 2 chronic kidney disease that was managed with a low-protein diet. The owners had noticed progressive abdominal distension, perceived discomfort, and decreased appetite. A large right-sided perinephric pseudocyst was detected on abdominal ultrasound. Fluid analysis was consistent with a modified transudate, and bacterial culture was negative. Drainage had been performed on several occasions, with subsequent improvement of the clinical signs, but abdominal distension recurred within weeks. Perinephric pseudocyst resection was then recommended.

Before the procedure, due to the large size of the pseudocyst, percutaneous drainage was performed using an 18-gauge IV catheter to improve the working space, and about 400 mL of clear fluid was removed. Then, under direct visualization, the pseudocyst was drained completely (650 mL). The pseudocyst was laparoscopically resected using a 5 mm LigaSure device and retrieved through the caudal instrument port after removing the trocar.

Key points

- Preoperative drainage of the pseudocyst allows for markedly improved working space during the procedure.
- Only the ventral, cranial, caudal, and lateral aspects of the pseudocyst should be removed. The dorsal aspect can remain.
- Care should be taken to identify the ureter and the caudal vena cava, as these can be in very close proximity to the pseudocyst.

PORT PLACEMENT

A 0.5 cm incision was made 2 cm caudal to the umbilicus and a 5 mm balloon trocar (T1) was placed using a modified Hasson technique. The abdomen was insufflated to 8 mmHg with CO_2. A 5 mm 30° telescope was introduced. A second port (T2) was placed under direct visualization by inserting a 5 mm balloon trocar 2 cm cranial to T1. A third port (T3) was placed under direct visualization by inserting a 5 mm balloon trocar midway between T1 and the pubis. The patient was placed in slightly oblique left lateral recumbency.

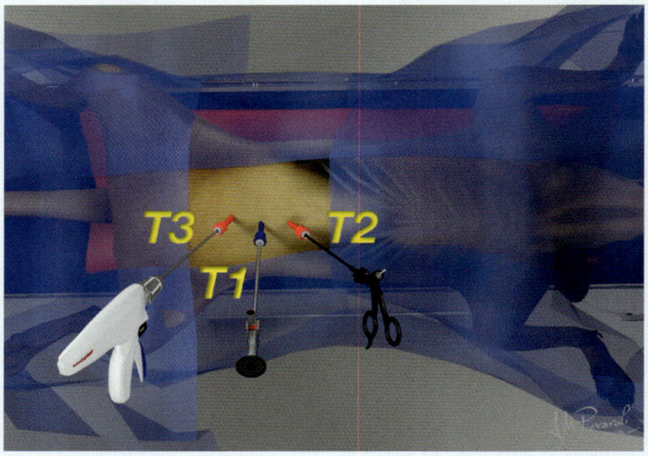

PROCEDURE

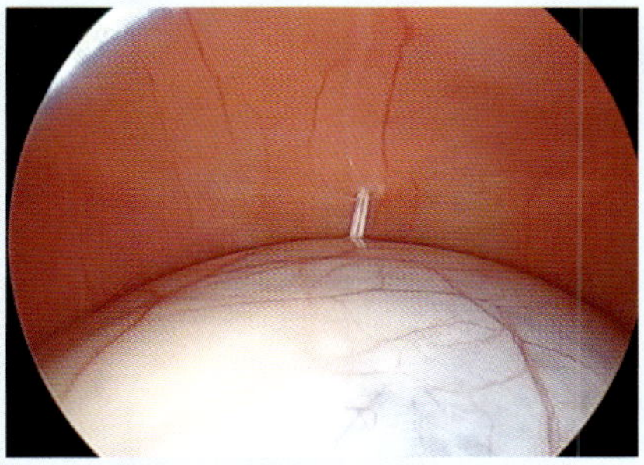

FIGURE 1. An IV catheter is inserted percutaneously to completely drain the perinephric pseudocyst.

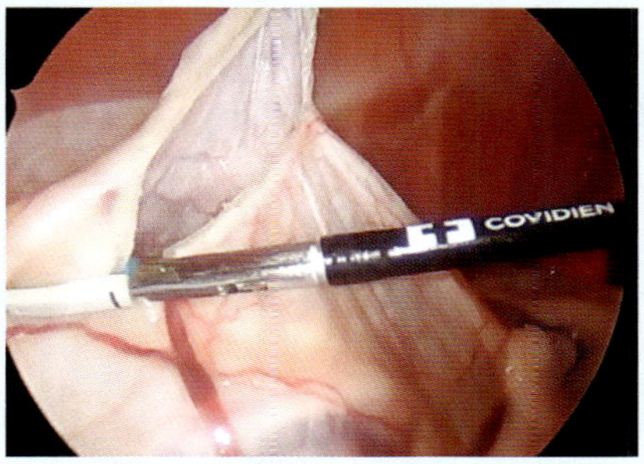

FIGURE 2. The pseudocyst is grasped with 5 mm Babcock forceps and resected using a 5 mm LigaSure device.

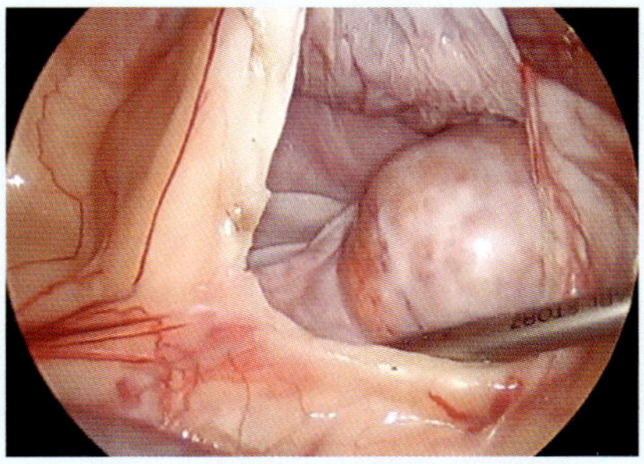

FIGURE 3. After incision of the pseudocyst capsule, pseudocystoscopy is performed. A small, irregular right kidney is seen within the pseudocyst, with fibrinous adhesions. A 5 mm laparoscopic suction device is used to remove residual fluid.

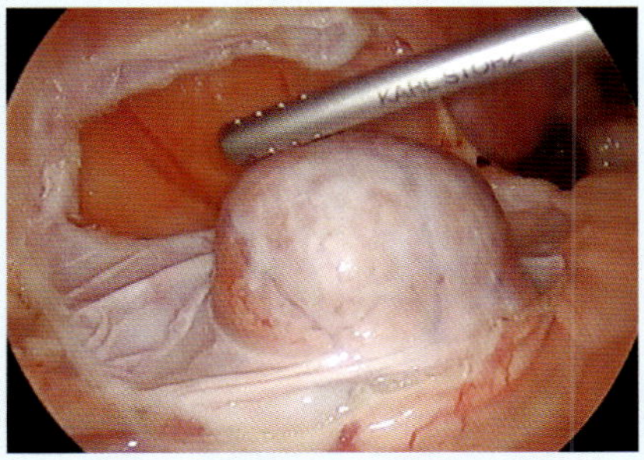

FIGURE 4. Laparoscopic image after completing perinephric pseudocyst resection with the LigaSure device. The ventral, cranial, caudal, and lateral aspects of the pseudocyst are resected, while the dorsal aspect is left intact. The resected pseudocyst is retrieved through the caudal port after trocar removal. The irregular kidney can be seen in the image.

Tips and tricks

- ✓ Tilting the patient into a slightly oblique lateral position facilitates exposure of the kidney and retroperitoneal region. The recumbency depends on the affected side (e.g., in case of a left perinephric pseudocyst, the patient should be placed in slightly oblique right lateral recumbency).
- ✓ Laparoscopic suction devices are very effective in removing large quantities of fluid quickly once the pseudocyst has been accessed.

23.3 LAPAROSCOPIC RENAL CYST DEROOFING, FULGURATION, AND OMENTALIZATION

Mathieu Manassero, Bastien Dekerle

CASE DESCRIPTION

A 10-month-old male crossbreed dog weighing 22 kg was presented with a 4-week history of emesis, flank pain, polyuria, and polydipsia. Diagnostic imaging showed a well-defined unilateral craniodorsal right renal mass containing anechoic fluid consistent with a simple renal cyst. Cytological examination of cystic fluid did not reveal tumoral cells and bacteriological culture was negative. Creatinine levels in the cyst fluid were not consistent with a communicating urinary cyst. The cyst was drained under ultrasonographic guidance but recurred 3 months later along with associated clinical signs. A laparoscopic approach for cyst deroofing, fulguration, and omentalization was performed.

Key points

- Place the dog in oblique lateral recumbency during the procedure to enhance exposure of the kidney.
- Drain the cyst percutaneously under laparoscopic guidance before cyst resection.
- Open the cyst dorsolaterally, at a distance from the renal hilus, using a vessel-sealing device.
- Inspect the interior of the cyst for the presence of neoplastic changes.
- Deroof the cyst circumferentially by resecting its wall as close to the renal parenchyma as possible using a vessel-sealing device.
- Fulgurate the remaining cystic wall on the kidney parenchyma with monopolar electrosurgery or argon beam coagulation to ablate the epithelial surface of the cystic wall.
- Perform a kidney biopsy and send the cystic wall for histopathological analysis to rule out neoplasia.
- Pack an omentum wrap on the remaining cystic wall and secure it to the renal capsule with two interrupted sutures.
- If extensive dissection of the retroperitoneum was carried out, perform a nephropexy by placing two interrupted sutures from the dorsal aspect of the kidney to the transversalis muscle.

PORT PLACEMENT

A three-port technique, with 5 mm cannulas, was used. The patient was placed in left lateral recumbency. The primary telescope port was placed using the Hasson technique 2 cm caudal and 5 cm lateral to the umbilicus, and a pneumoperitoneum (10 mmHg) was established. The second port was placed caudal to the last rib at the level of the chondrocostal junction. The third port was placed in the paralumbar fossa caudal to the kidney at the same level as the second port, cranial to the pelvic limb. The surgical team stood on the ventral/ventrolateral side of the patient, with the endoscopic tower placed opposite, on the dorsal side of the patient.

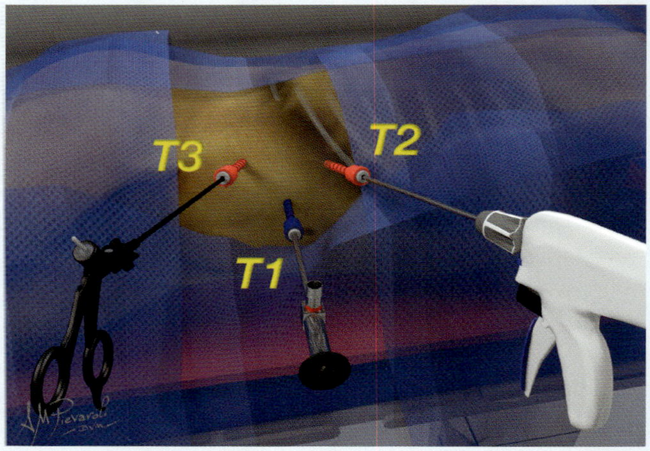

PROCEDURE

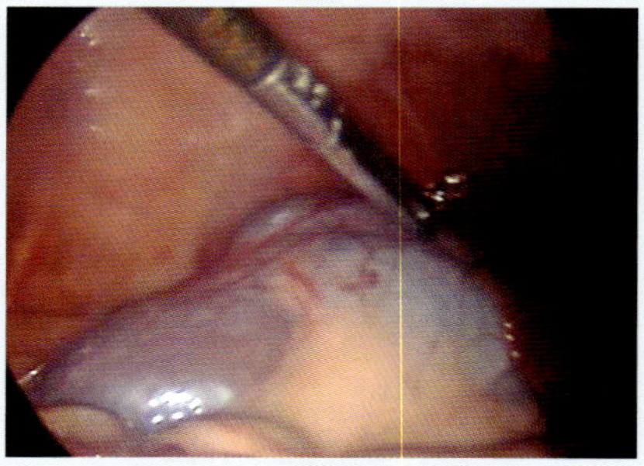

FIGURE 1. After medial retraction of the small intestine, the right kidney with the cystic lesion on its craniodorsal aspect (under the laparoscopic forceps) is identified.

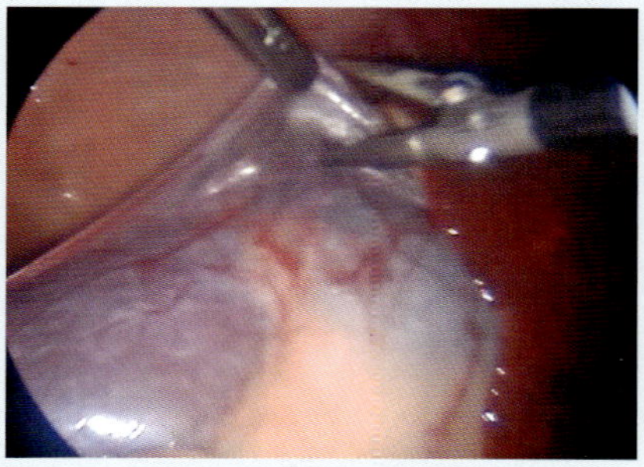

FIGURE 2. The hepatorenal ligament is transected with a vessel-sealing device to retract the caudate lobe of the liver cranially. The overlying perinephric fat and the peritoneum are subsequently bluntly dissected from the lateral aspect of the kidney.

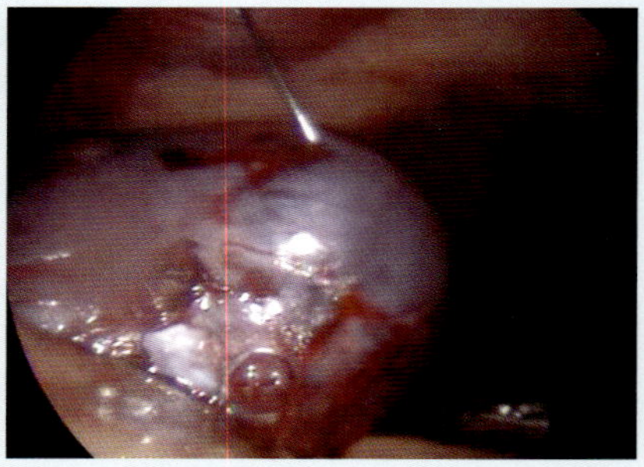

FIGURE 3. The cystic fluid is aspirated and the cyst almost fully emptied using a 22-gauge spinal needle inserted percutaneously under laparoscopic guidance.

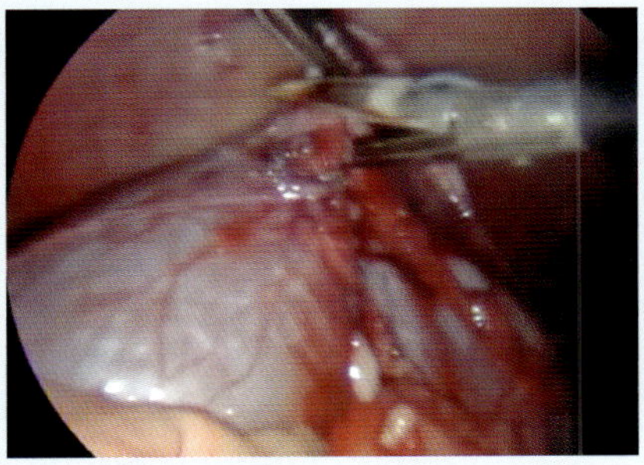

FIGURE 4. The cystic wall is grasped with fenestrated bowel grasper forceps and opened using the vessel-sealing device.

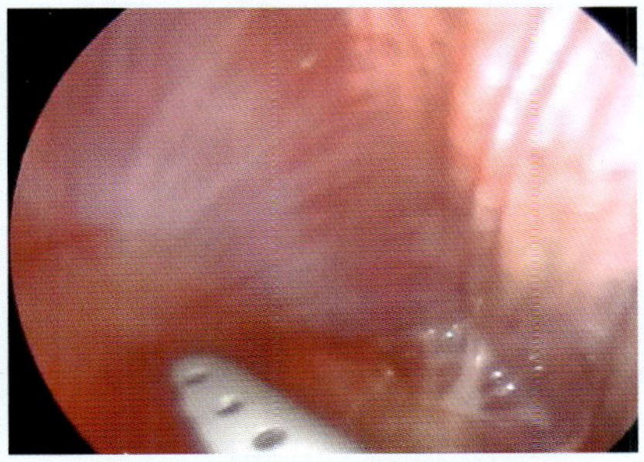

FIGURE 5. The inner part of the cyst is inspected and the remaining cystic fluid aspirated.

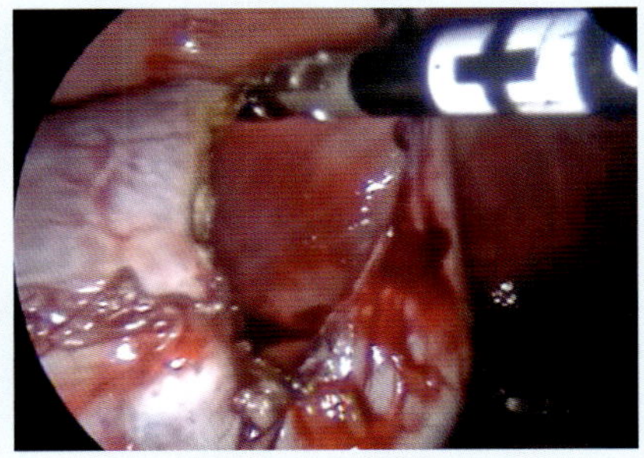

FIGURE 6. The cystic wall is excised circumferentially with the vessel-sealing device at the level of the renal capsule, taking care to maintain tenting of the cystic wall with the laparoscopic grasper.

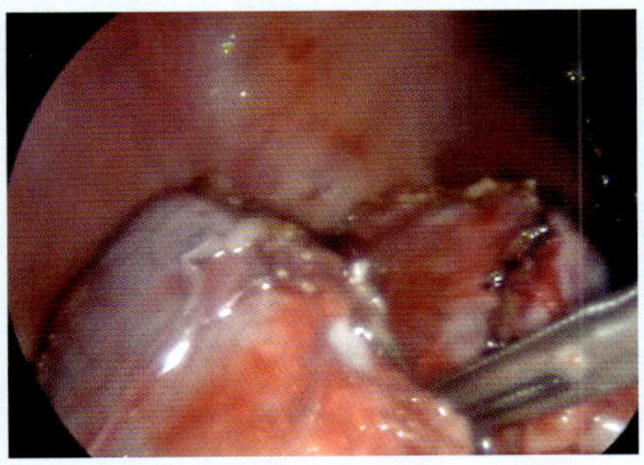

FIGURE 7. Final appearance of the right kidney after resection of the cystic wall in close contact with the renal capsule.

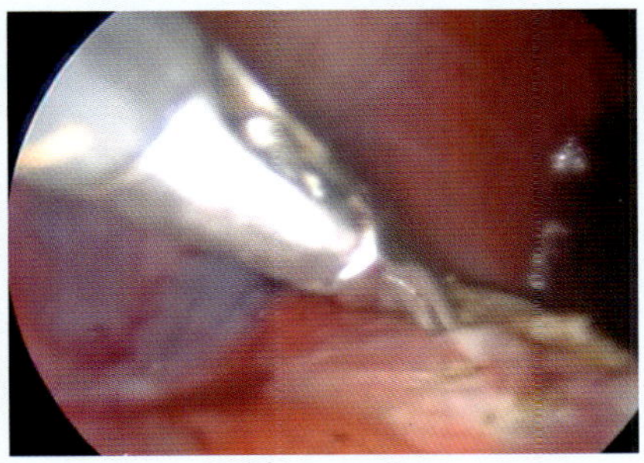

FIGURE 8. The cystic wall remaining in contact with the kidney parenchyma is fulgurated with monopolar electrocautery.

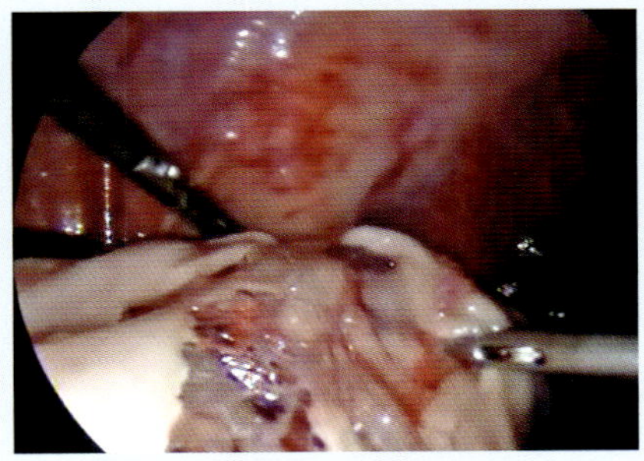

FIGURE 9. Omentum is placed on the kidney and sutured loosely to the renal capsule, and a nephropexy is performed.

Tips and tricks

- ✓ Using a 30° telescope can improve maneuverability and visualization. If a 0° telescope is used, the primary port should be placed 2–3 cm more laterally (7 cm lateral to the umbilicus).
- ✓ Do not place the primary port and the telescope too dorsal to prevent the surgeon's assistant from holding the telescope in a very elevated position.
- ✓ Take care to tent the cystic wall during resection.
- ✓ After fulguration, check for any urine leakage. In case of urine leakage, either pack the remaining cystic wall on the kidney parenchyma with hemostatic agents or a fibrin sealant, or suture the kidney. If the cyst is in the central part of the kidney, the cranial and caudal parts of the kidney can be sutured together with three interrupted horizontal mattress sutures to prevent further leakage.

24 CURRENT CONCEPTS IN MINIMALLY INVASIVE NEPHROLITHOTOMY

Fausto Brandão

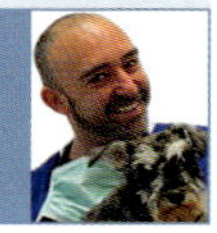

Indications

- Intermittent ureteropelvic junction obstruction due to freely movable nephroliths
- Infected nephroliths perpetuating pyelonephritis
- Large nephroliths causing pain
- Nephrolithiasis associated with progressive hydronephrosis and parenchymal loss
- Prevention of ureteral obstruction

Contraindications

- End-stage chronic kidney disease
- Patients too unstable to undergo complex surgery
- Surgeon's inexperience with renal-sparing interventional surgery

Nephrolithiasis has recently become a more common clinical presentation, although the factors for this increase have not yet been clearly identified (**Fig. 1**).

Complicated nephrolithiasis includes intermittent ureteropelvic junction (UPJ) obstruction due to freely movable nephroliths, infected nephroliths perpetuating pyelonephritis, large nephroliths causing pain, and nephrolithiasis associated with progressive hydronephrosis and parenchymal loss. These conditions comprise the most important clinical situations requiring surgical intervention, leaving the remaining presentations to medical assessment and management.

Classical open approach surgery involving nephrotomy and/or pyelotomy demonstrated high perioperative morbidity and tissue trauma with considerable nephron loss and a negative impact in functional integrity. Open surgical stone removal is rarely performed today and is mostly limited to extremely complex stones that are not eligible for minimally invasive approaches.

Although not clearly confirmed in the published literature, there is some clinical evidence of a relationship between nephrolithiasis and worsening of kidney injury. Published results suggest that biomarkers such as SDMA are typically higher in patients with nephrolithiasis, and patients with nephrolithiasis have a shorter life span. These preliminary results might suggest that even the presence of nonobstructive nephrolithiasis contributes to higher mortality rates and faster chronic kidney disease (CKD) progression.

Considering that nephrolithotomy might improve renal function in selected cases by eliminating pathway obstruction and infections, it is postulated that routine stone assessment with imaging modalities, and case selection for elective surgically assisted endoscopic nephrolithotomy (SENL), combined with CKD staging, might improve life span. Techniques for nephrolith management described in veterinary medicine include nephrotomy, pyelotomy, ureteronephrectomy, extracorporeal shock wave lithotripsy (ECSWL), percutaneous nephrolithotomy (PCNL), and SENL. Field experience and several studies have demonstrated that histological and functional changes occur after ECSWL. Shock wave lithotripsy has been reported to cause acute histological damage to the renal parenchyma, renal vasculature, and nephron structure. What is more, renal morphological changes after shock wave therapy included subcapsular hematomas and focal parenchymal damage. Vascular endothelial damage, nephron loss, and fibrosis within the cortex and medulla have also been demonstrated. Shock wave lithotripsy is likely to have better results with immobile nephroliths. The risk of shock wave–treated nephroliths becoming obstructive ureteroliths in addition to the cost and high complexity of

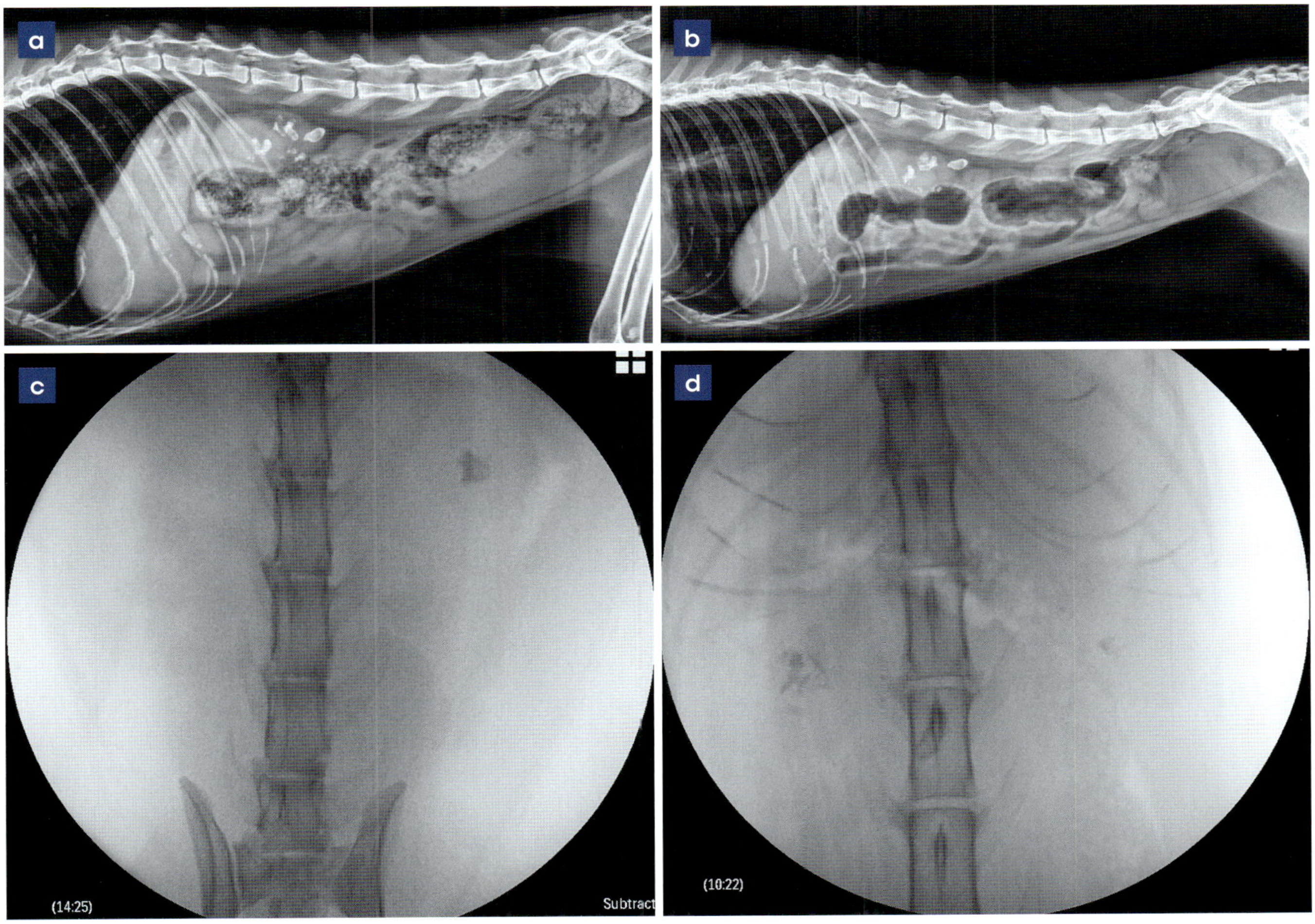

FIGURE 1. a,b) Laterolateral radiographs and c,d) intraoperative ventrodorsal still fluoroscopic images of feline patients with multiple nephroliths.

extracorporeal shock wave therapy units have almost excluded this technique from clinical use. Common sense has dictated that uncomplicated nephroliths should be left in place, monitored, and treated medically. However, when removal by open surgery was required, several complications have been reported such as hemorrhage, decrease in renal function, urine leakage, and nephrolith- or edema-induced ureteral obstruction.

In human urology, most conventional techniques for nephrolithotomy have been replaced by PCNL. Compared to other existing techniques for human patients, PCNL demonstrates the highest nephrolith free rate results. This is due to the lack of significant nephron transection, being highly renal sparing, and causing minimal puncture trauma.

The first experimental study on nephrolithotomy was published in 1987 by Gayle S. Donner et al.

DESCRIBED SURGICAL PROCEDURES

Recent veterinary publications refer to the use of PCNL and SENL for the removal of complicated nephroliths. PCNL was found to be laborious and difficult, with additional need for postoperative nephrostomy tubes, whereas SENL eliminated the need for nephrostomy tubes, stents, or any other devices postoperatively. Although requiring a laparotomy approach, SENL demonstrated results consistency and unmatched feasibility, thus opening an opportunity for refinement and routine approach to nephroliths in risk of obstruction, for preventative assessment of future obstruction, and for prevention of possible associated kidney disease progression.

PATIENT SELECTION

Patients undergoing modified SENL are recruited based on incidental findings on radiographic, ultrasound, and CT examinations, or when assessed with imaging for clinical features consistent with nephropathies. A thorough clinical examination and clinical history are essential for demographic results as well. Regular blood work including a complete blood count and a serum biochemistry panel should be obtained, followed by initial CKD staging. Urinalysis and urine culture are routinely performed to screen for lower urinary tract infections. When pyelonephritis is suspected, ultrasound-guided pyelocentesis should be performed and samples taken for immediate laboratory analysis. Total calcium and ionized calcium are used to rule out the presence of hypercalcemia. SDMA and UPC complete the assessment, since some publications correlate the presence of nephroliths with CKD progression.

EQUIPMENT

SENL is a high-skilled surgical procedure that requires advanced equipment and accessories that might only be available at referral clinics. A standard electrosurgery unit providing bipolar energy is ideal to perform hemostasis during laparotomy access, removing the falciform fat if needed for optimal surgical exposure, and preforming any additional hemostasis in the renal capsule throughout the procedure if bleeding persists from the renal puncture site. Equipment also includes an endoscopic imaging system, preferably full HD, since highly detailed images are required. Additionally, a C-arm is needed, with a software package enabling standard fluoroscopy mode and digital subtraction, which is essential for nephrolith localization, image-guided entry in the pelvis, and ureteral excretory pathway antegrade contrast study (**Fig. 2**).

Sterile sleeves are required for the endoscopic camera and light cable to ensure procedure sterility and to maintain optimal visualization quality by preventing moisture and fluid from falling between the camera lens and the scope eyepiece. Since fluid inflow and working channel instrumentation are required simultaneously, disposable sterile sealing valves are recommended to keep fluid from flowing out of the working channel stopcock while maintaining the sterility of the components.

For SENL, integrated rigid cystoscopes with a working channel are recommended due to their reduced diameter. In the author's experience a cystoscope with an external diameter of 9.5 Fr, a working length of 14 cm, and a working channel of 3 Fr is the optimal choice. For better maneuverability, a 3.5 mm diameter 300 cm long light cable is advised. For large-breed dogs, an integrated cystoscope with a diameter of 11.5 Fr,

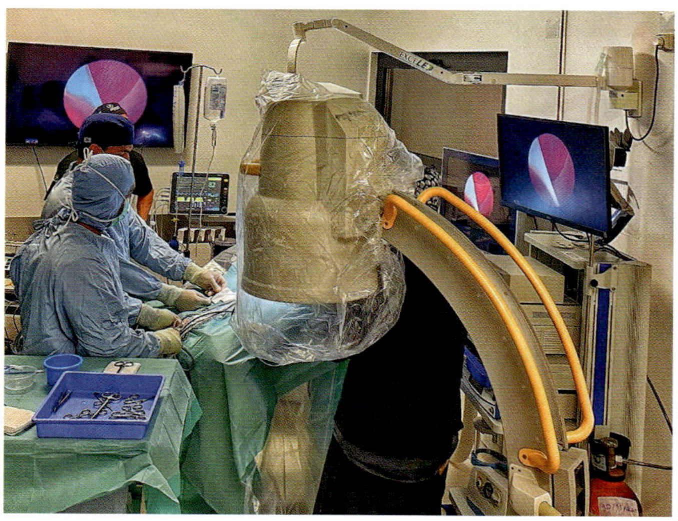

FIGURE 2. Operating room setup for surgically assisted endoscopic nephrolithotomy.

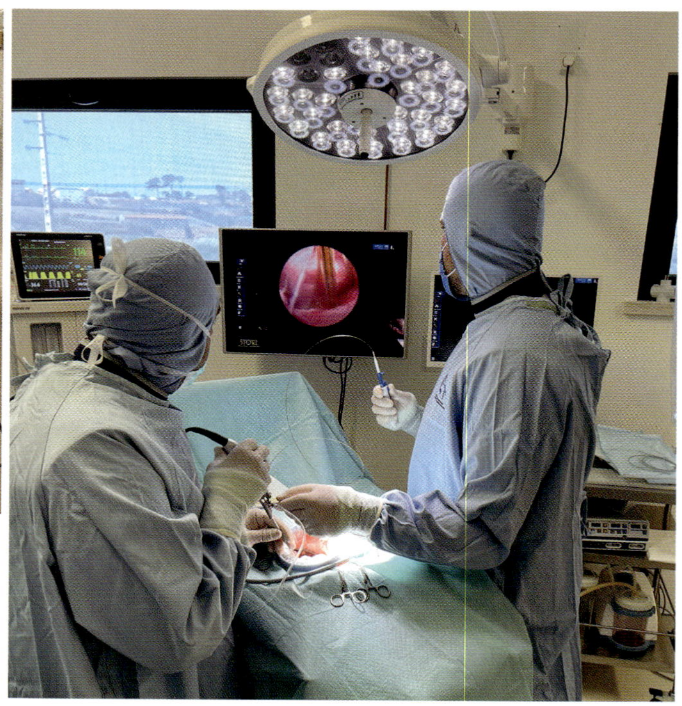

a working length of 15 cm, and a working channel of 5 Fr is the alternative choice. The most significant advantage of integrated working channels is that instruments always exit at the same angle and with minimal instrument motion. Rigid endoscopes requiring an operative sheath might have a more oval and spacious working channel that enables instruments to exit at different angles. While working in narrow cavities such as the UPJ or pelvis, this can present a serious challenge and increase the risk of wall capillary bleeding due to accidental instrument contact. For accessing the pelvis, interventional devices are required in order to promote a minimally invasive approach while keeping the procedure as tissue-sparing as possible. The pelvis approach is based on a Seldinger technique, requiring interventional accessories, such as an 18-gauge over-the-needle catheter and a 0.035" J tip guidewire. A set of 6–12 Fr polyethylene introducer dilators is recommended to bluntly enlarge the puncture site with minimal blood loss and less renal tissue trauma (**Fig. 3**).

Continuous aspiration of the abdominal cavity is required during the procedure, since the continuous droplet inflow through the working channel escapes from the puncture site. This allows for irrigating the renal pelvis for lavage, removing debris and sand nephroliths, and clearing the endoscopic viewing field. Saline or Ringer solution warmed to body temperature (38.5°C) is required to avoid hypothermia throughout the procedure. Forced-air patient warming systems are also essential, as abdominal surgical exposure significantly contributes to hypothermia.

Because the renal pelvis is a narrow space, grasping and retrieving the nephroliths requires front-opening nitinol baskets. The elliptic baskets with or without tip cannot operate properly inside the pelvis, as they require additional room to distend and open. These devices are used in human endourology, and no dedicated veterinary instruments are available. A 1.9 Fr diameter 120 cm long basket is used, and two versions are available: opening to 8 mm or 11 mm. For procedure ease, the 8 mm version is commonly used, reserving the 11 mm basket if larger stones need to be grasped. These baskets are very precise and enable head-on capture of stones of very small size (1 mm).

If fragmentation of larger stones is required, a holmium:YAG lithotripsy laser is required. The 2100 nm wavelength emission separates the water, generating small vapor bubbles, which are directed to the stone as the energy delivery source, resulting in stone fragmentation. A 20- or 35-watt unit is considered sufficient in small animal endourology for all clinical procedures. It is recommended to use smaller diameter multiple-use fibers of 230 microns, since they ensure higher flexibility and lesser working channel filling, thus leading to improved fluid flow for a better viewing field. The sealing valve also enables fixing the fiber in an optimal working length outside the tip of the working channel while avoiding fluid back flow from the working channel.

OPERATING ROOM LAYOUT

The patient is positioned in dorsal recumbency with a reverse Trendelenburg tilt. A C-arm is operating to-and-fro at the caudolateral aspect of the surgical table. Multiple minimally invasive surgery monitors are placed in front of the main surgeon and the assistant surgeon. The anesthesia circuit and staff are positioned at the head of the operating table, while the instrument table is placed caudolateral to the table on the opposite side and in front of the C-arm (**Fig. 4**).

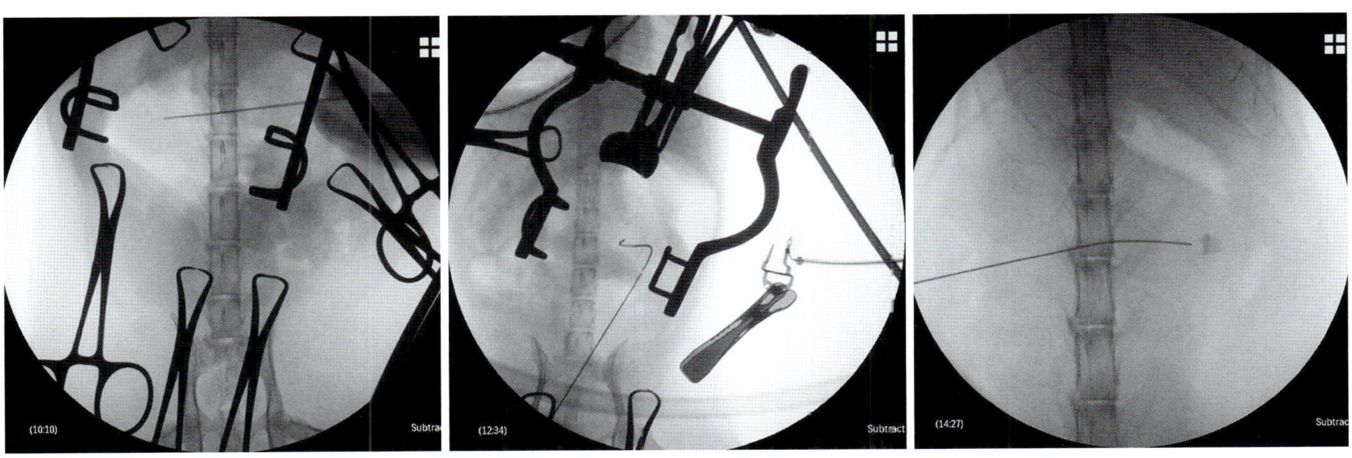

FIGURE 3. Intraoperative fluoroscopic puncture site estimated angle, and guidewire placed in pelvis for access.

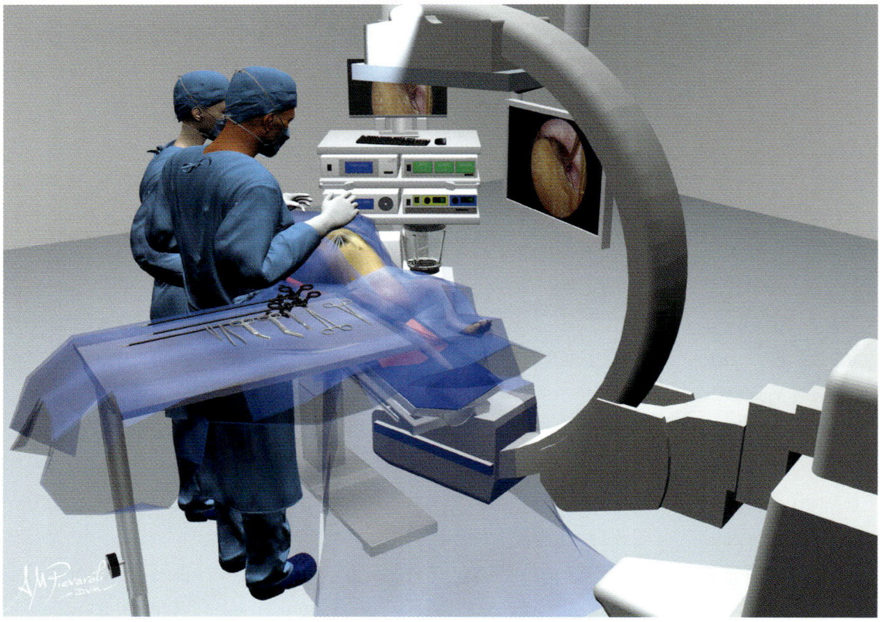

FIGURE 4. Operating room layout for minimally invasive nephrolithotomy.

Instruments

- Standard surgical set
- Balfour abdominal retractor
- Continuous surgical suction unit
- Endoscopic full HD system + sterile sleeves
- Forced-air warming system
- C-arm with standard and vascular software + C-arm sterile covers
- 9.5 Fr – 14 cm – 30° integrated cystoscope with 3 Fr working channel
- 18-gauge over-the-needle catheter
- 0.035″ J tip guidewire
- 6–12 Fr introducer dilators
- 1.9 Fr front-opening nitinol basket (8 mm)
- 3 Fr grasping forceps

MODIFIED SURGICAL-ASSISTED NEPHROLITHOTOMY TECHNIQUE

PROCEDURE

- A median laparotomy is performed using a number 15 scalpel blade, large enough to enable access to both kidneys. A Balfour abdominal retractor is used to expose the cranial abdomen and moistened gauze pads are placed for organ retraction and protection. The ventral surface of the kidney is exposed and a fluoroscopic image is obtained to locate the radiopaque nephroliths. Under fluoroscopic guidance, an 18-gauge over-the-needle catheter is used to estimate the optimal entrance point to maximize access to the stones and UPJ. Once the entrance angle is established, the pelvis is accessed with the 18-gauge catheter until urine is seen, and a sample is collected for culture and routine physical examination (**Fig. 5**).
- A 0.035″ J tip guidewire is inserted and the pelvis is accessed under fluoroscopic guidance. Then, the over-the-needle catheter is removed and a progressive sequence of interventional dilators are placed over the guidewire until a 10 Fr diameter is obtained. The last introducer is removed over the wire and replaced with the 3 Fr working channel of a 9.5 Fr integrated cystoscope. When larger stones are present, it might be helpful to use a 12 Fr dilator and choose an 11.5 Fr integrated cystoscope. In most cases, cats and small dogs are treated, meaning that a 9.5 Fr integrated cystoscope is the standard choice for the technique.
- A sterile fluid line is connected to the side stopcocks of the cystoscope and a drop fluid flow is achieved by gently opening the valve. High flow and pressure bags are not recommended since they might induce trauma to the tissue and overdistend the cavity, thus leading to some extent of organ damage.

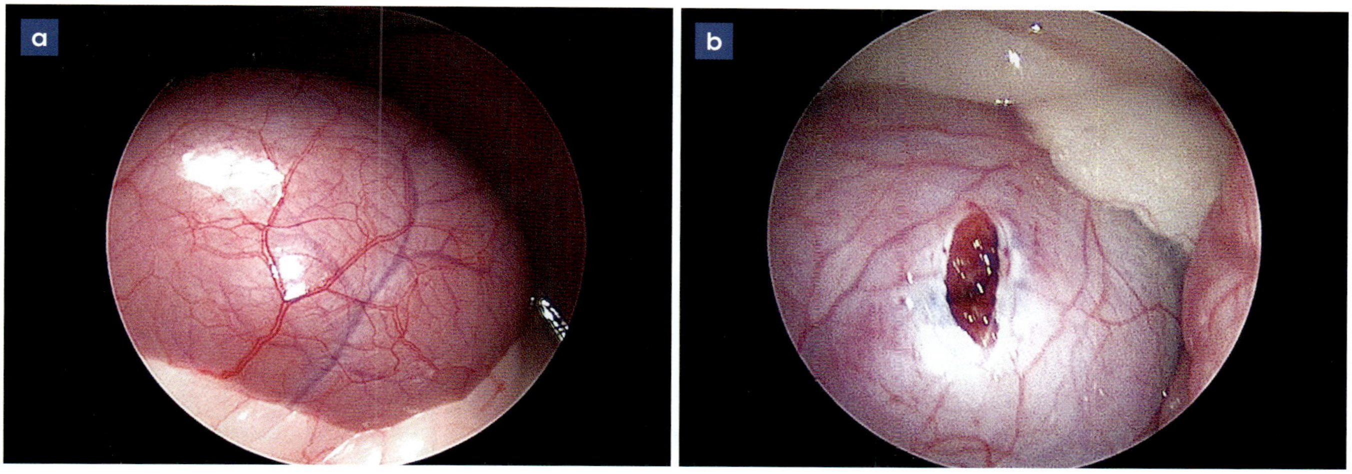

FIGURE 5. Intraoperative endoscopic view of a kidney and endoscopic puncture site after nephroscope removal. Note the absence of bleeding and the 3 mm puncture access.

- The scope is gently advanced over the guidewire until it reaches the pelvic cavity, and slow retraction of the guidewire is performed. Gentle maneuvering is mandatory to avoid pelvic trauma resulting in capillary hemorrhage that obscures the viewing field and generates clots that can later be associated with UPJ or ureteral obstruction. The retracted wire is gently advanced into the UPJ whenever this is visible and reachable (**Fig. 6**). This will prevent nephroliths from moving into the proximal ureter thus incurring proximal obstructions. The scope is retracted until the guidewire is freed and reintroduced alongside. In most cases, nephroliths are immediately identified and ideally grasped and removed with the aid of a front-opening nitinol basket. Individual nephrolith removal is performed until the cavity is left free of stones and sand. Droplet fluid infusion is usually enough to lavage the pelvic cavity and active surgical aspiration is ensured at the kidney scope entry, preventing the fluid from falling freely into the abdominal cavity (**Fig. 7**).

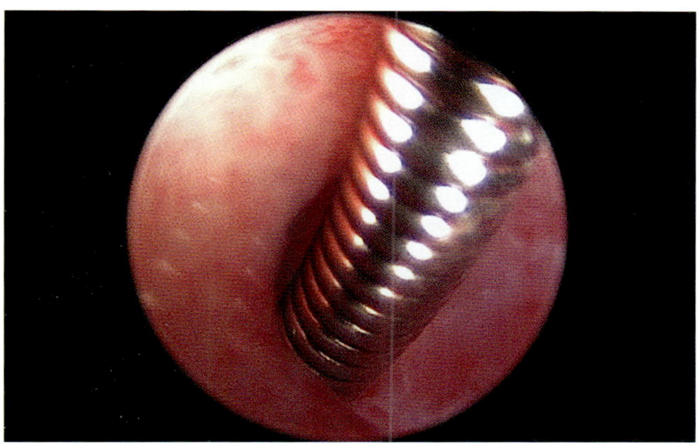

FIGURE 6. Endoscopic guidewire placement in the proximal ureter.

- In most cases, a 4 mm or less entry site puncture is sufficient for removing the nephroliths, but when larger stones are present intrarenal lithotripsy might be necessary to fragment the nephrolith into retrievable portions.
- Intrarenal lithotripsy results in pelvic epithelium edema due to contact vibration and contact of stones with the pelvic wall. Care must be observed when performing intrarenal lithotripsy and keep its use to a minimum. Capillary bleeding occurs when nephroliths hit the pelvis walls. The viewing field is kept clear with droplet fluid inflow of warm saline and by keeping the frequency (Hz) as low as possible. Depending on stone texture, laser lithotripsy settings are adjusted to the minimum necessary to promote single and effective fragmentation. Fragments are mechanically removed with the basket and lavage fluid instilled until no stone remains are present.
- When larger nephroliths exist, access to the UPJ might be difficult and the placement of the ureteral wire compromised; therefore, additional care should be observed to prevent small nephroliths or stone fragments from entering the proximal ureter. In that case, fluid inflow should be stopped or decreased substantially and the endoscope driven into the proximal ureter. At that level, some stones can still be retrieved if the ureteral diameter permits.
- Once the nephrolithotomy is concluded, a ureteral catheter is passed over the ureteral guidewire and an anterograde fluoroscopic ureterogram is performed under digital subtraction mode, so the excretory pathway is enhanced, and patency confirmed under real-time image guidance (**Fig. 8**).

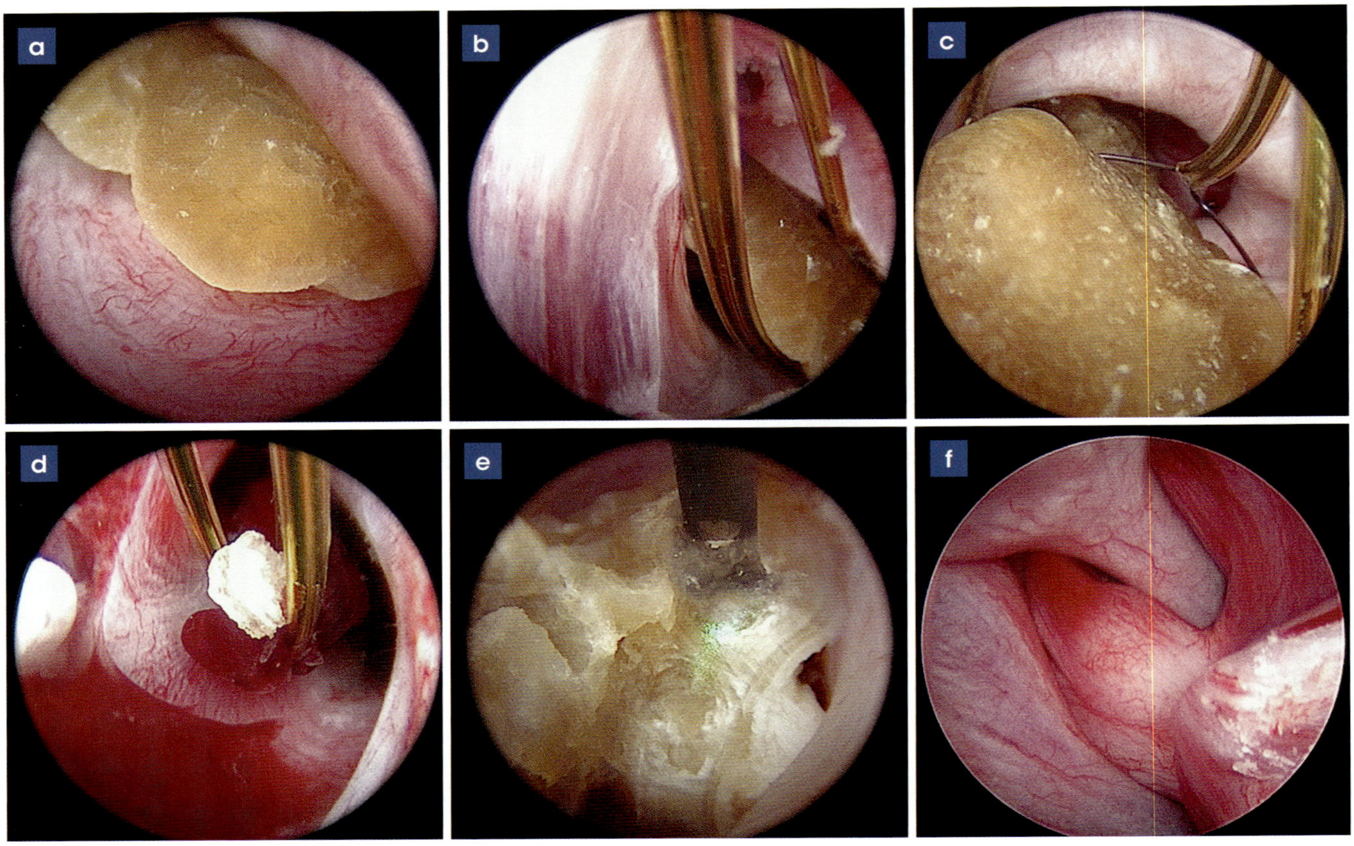

FIGURE 7. Intraoperative nephroscopic image series of identification of nephroliths, basket retrieval, intrarenal lithotripsy, and lavage of renal pelvis at the end of the procedure.

- Closure of the puncture sites is commonly performed with a 4-0 monofilament absorbable suture (polydioxanone) with one to three interrupted sutures. The suture should include a thin portion of renal parenchyma and the capsule and the apposition of sutures in a lateral aspect to the puncture site.
- The abdomen is checked for free fluid and lavage and aspiration are performed before removing the abdominal retractor. Abdomen, subcutis, and skin are closed routinely.

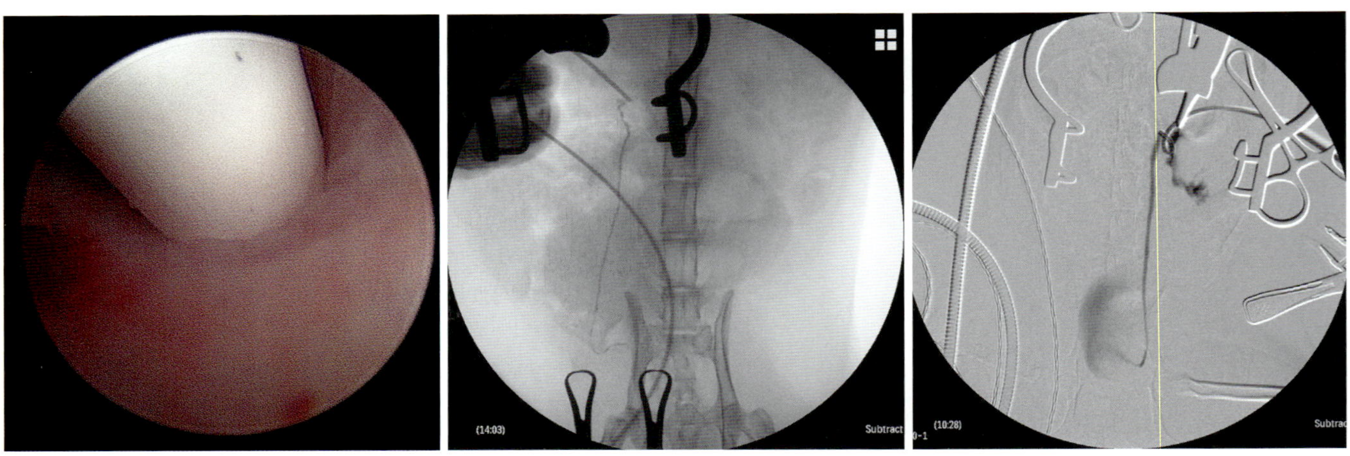

FIGURE 8. Ureteral catheter placed in the proximal ureter through the UPJ, and anterograde fluoroscopic ureterogram demonstrating the viable excretory pathway.

POSTOPERATIVE MANAGEMENT

- The puncture sites should be inspected intraoperatively for fluid drainage after their closure with sutures.
- Anti-inflammatory medication and perioperative fluid therapy should be carefully tapered and formulated according to the preexisting CKD.
- Postoperative abdominal ultrasound is recommended to inspect for free abdominal fluid.
- A complete blood count, serum biochemistry panel, and electrolytes should be checked regularly according to each patient.
- Perioperative antibiotic therapy should be adjusted based on the results from the sample collected intraoperatively by pyelocentesis.

Key points

- Routine X-rays and ultrasound imaging of the kidneys substantially contribute to early diagnosis and selecting the patients for medical and surgical assessment.
- Preexisting CKD should be monitored and continuously treated. CKD staging monitorization is mandatory to follow up with the progression of renal disease.
- When complicated nephrolithiasis with pyelonephritis is present, the clinical outcomes are very often encouraging since in most cases the infection rate diminishes dramatically.
- The results from nephroliths sent to composition analysis demonstrate a high incidence of calcium oxalate in both cats and dogs.
- In most cases, especially when lithotripsy is not performed, total emptying of the renal pelvis is likely achieved. However, the surgical time per renal unit is approximately 45–60 minutes. When both kidneys are addressed and surgical-assisted cystolithotomy is incorporated, complete surgical times can rise to 150–180 minutes.
- Residual sand stone might be particularly difficult to remove after intrarenal lithotripsy since minor capillary bleeding occurs, generating small clots and retaining fragmentation sand. Blood clots are retrieved with baskets to ensure minimum residual material after the procedure and to avoid complications due to secondary ureteral obstruction, since no ureteral stent is placed. Additional irrigation and aspiration are performed to ensure deep cleaning of the cavity and minimize recurrence.
- Due to its unique precision, not one case reported to date required an ureteral stent or a nephrostomy tube.
- In one case of parenchymal cyst with retained nephrolithiasis in the caudal pole, a minor subcapsular fluid leakage was observed in the subsequent 5 days postoperatively, with spontaneous resolution. It is believed that due to tissue elasticity the endoscope entry point might have leaked after suturing despite checking it intraoperatively.
- Nephrolithotomy for complicated cases is considered a lifesaving procedure. However, with the advent of this evolving technique, it is believed that safely addressing routine cases might avoid complications for ureteral obstructions and ureteral strictures, reserving the use of ureteral bypass systems and stenting to obstructive cases.
- With adequate case selection, it is believed that the modified surgical-assisted nephrolithotomy technique can help diminish the occurrence of life-threatening obstructive ureteral disease, which up to now has been considered a medical and surgical challenge.

SUGGESTED READINGS

CLINICAL CASES

24.1 NEPHRON-SPARING NEPHROTOMY TO REMOVE LARGE UROLITHS IN DOGS

Maurício Veloso Brun

CASE DESCRIPTION

This technique is indicated for patients with extensive nephrolithiasis (unresponsive to clinical treatment) whose renal pelvis is not dilated for urolith removal by pyelotomy and when the conditions of the disease or body conformation preclude laser vaporization and extraction by endourology. It can be applied to dogs of different dimensions and with unilateral or bilateral nephrolithiasis. In cases of bilateral disease, each kidney will be approached at a different time, since some loss of renal function is expected due to the access injury and temporary ischemia.

Key points

- The patient is positioned in lateral recumbency on the side contralateral to the affected kidney, with flank elevation.
- The renal parenchyma is sutured in a simple continuous pattern, preferably with an absorbable synthetic monofilament thread and a long cylindrical needle.
- The tourniquet, renal uroliths, and all hemostasis materials are removed from the cavity, using a retrieval bag if necessary.

PORT PLACEMENT

For left nephrotomy, three ports are used as follows. The first port (T1) (5 or 10 mm) is placed slightly lateral to the inguinal fold, at a midpoint between the iliac tuberosity and the costal margin. The second port (T2) (10 mm) is placed to the surgeon's dominant side in triangulation with the first and third (5 mm) ports.

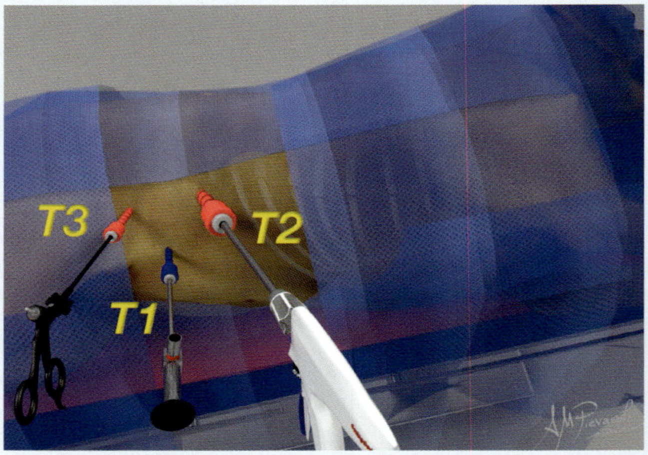

PROCEDURE

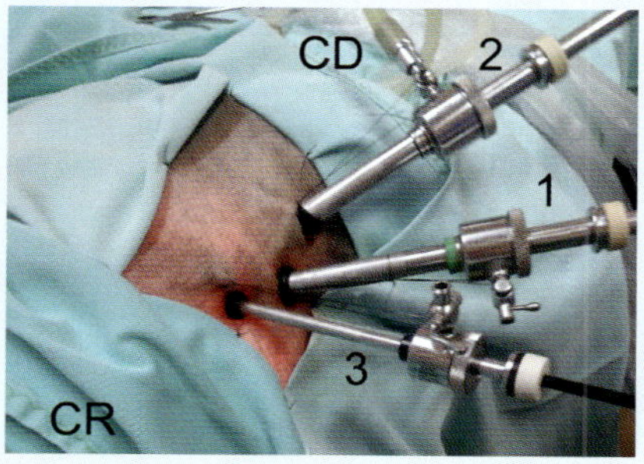

FIGURE 1. Placement of the three ports for left nephrotomy. CD, caudal; CR, cranial.

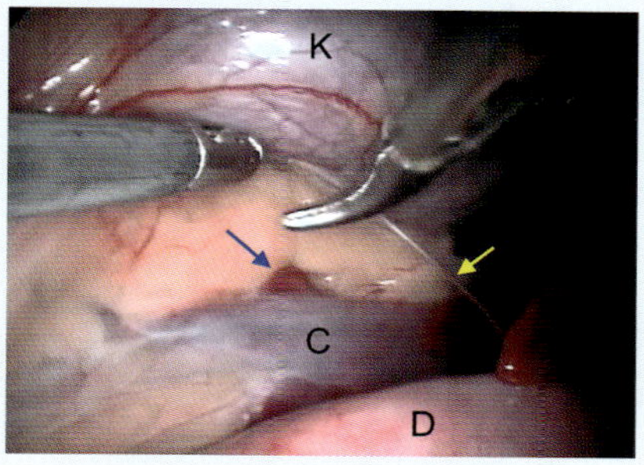

FIGURE 2. Exposure of the renal hilum for isolation and hemostasis of the renal vessels in a right nephrotomy. The blue arrow indicates the renal vein. The yellow arrow indicates the hepatorenal ligament. C, vena cava; D, duodenum; K, kidney.

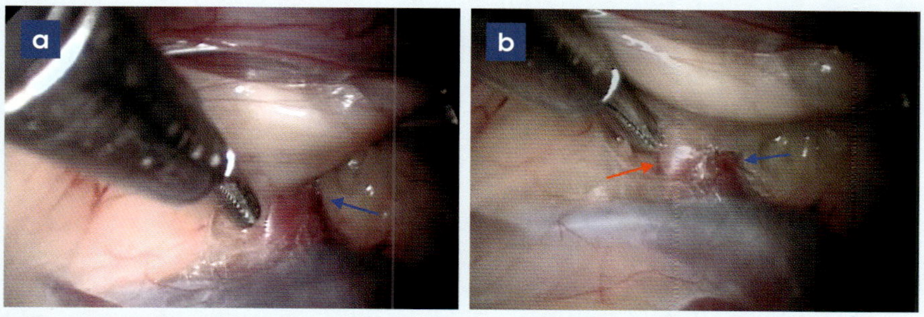

FIGURE 3. a) A brief dissection of the renal hilum is performed, starting with the renal vein (blue arrow). b) Behind the vein, in this perspective (laterally), the renal artery is visible (red arrow).

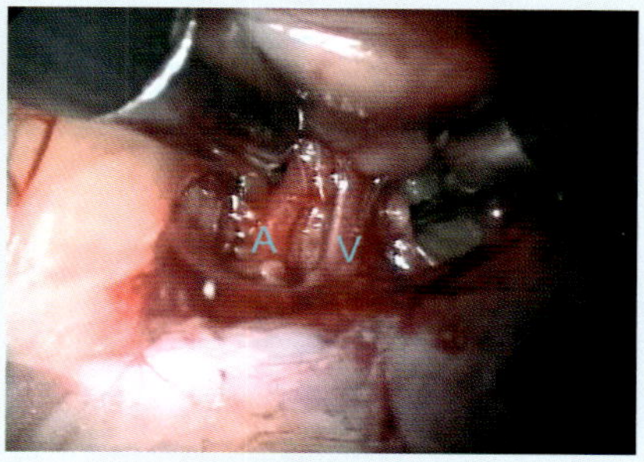

FIGURE 4. A Rummel tourniquet will be placed, including artery and vein together. Once the tourniquet is occluded, the warm ischemia time should be less than 30 minutes (preferably less than 20 minutes). The renal artery (A) and vein (V) are dissected for the passage of the umbilical tape.

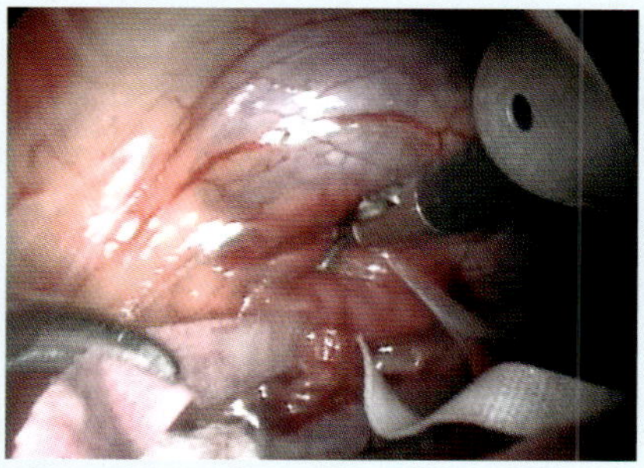

FIGURE 5. Passage of the umbilical tape behind the renal vessels for the Rummel tourniquet.

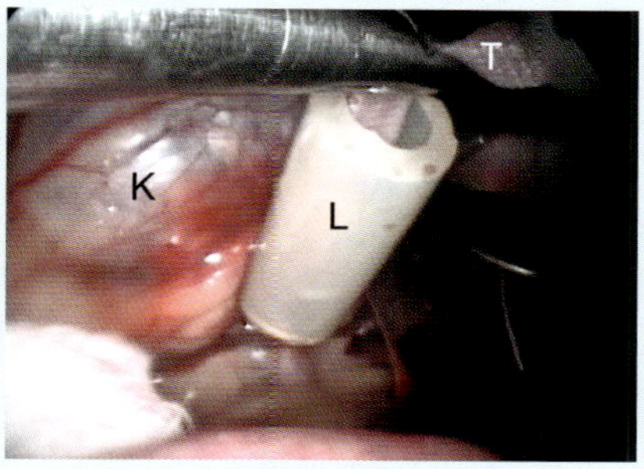

FIGURE 6. The two ends of the umbilical tape are passed through a latex tube (L) to form the Rummel tourniquet (T). K, kidney.

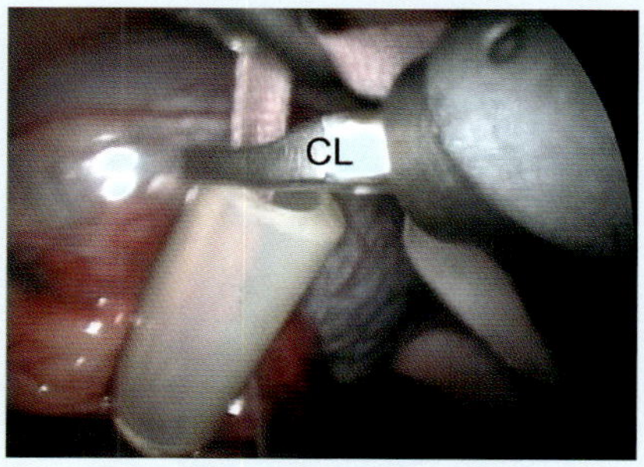

FIGURE 7. The clipper applier (CL) pushes the latex tube as it applies two or more clips to promote the temporary occlusion of renal vessels.

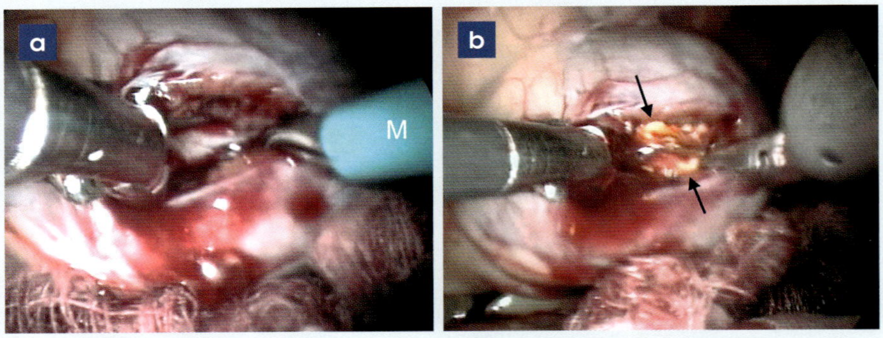

FIGURE 8. a) A short "cold" nephrotomy is performed with Metzenbaum scissors (M), at the midpoint of the convex surface of the kidney. The capsule, cortex, and medulla of the kidney are incised with Metzenbaum scissors. After entering the renal pelvis, the urolith is removed and the pelvis is abundantly irrigated to remove calculogenic matrix and debris. b) After penetrating the renal pelvis, the renal urolith (arrows) is located and removed with Kelly forceps.

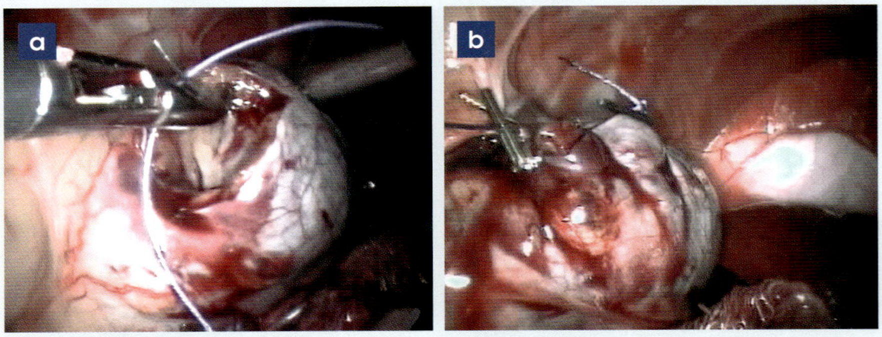

FIGURE 9. a) Intracorporeal nephrorrhaphy with a simple continuous pattern, anchored with b) clips or an intracorporeal knot.

Tips and tricks

- ✓ Place a purse-string suture around the first port, fixing it to the cannula, to prevent CO_2 loss.
- ✓ When using smooth ports, place a segment of latex or the rubber of the hypodermic syringe outside the cannula to prevent it from being pushed too far into the cavity. In order not to dislocate externally, apply a suture from the skin and subcutaneous tissue to the cannula.
- ✓ The tourniquet is made from a silicone tube (about 20 mm in length) with an inside diameter of approximately 6 mm and an outside diameter of less than 10 mm, so that it can pass through the port. An umbilical tape is used to hug the vessels.
- ✓ Occlusion of the tourniquet is achieved by pushing the tube against the vessels and applying two or three clips distributed on the tape without entering the tube.
- ✓ The renal artery and vein are temporarily occluded together, reducing the artery folding inside the tube.
- ✓ Before beginning the vascular occlusion, the suture thread is placed inside the cavity to reduce the time of warm ischemia.
- ✓ The end of the suture should have a robust knot with two clips below it, exempting the need to close the first knot.
- ✓ A sufficiently large (but not very extensive) incision is made to remove the stones and inspect the pelvis, facilitating the renal suture.
- ✓ Large stones are removed from the renal pelvis and kept in the paralumbar fossa, being removed from the cavity once the vascular occlusion is finished.
- ✓ Simple continuous suture is performed, covering a considerable amount of renal tissue, which can be closed with an intracorporeal knot and/or clips (two or three), fixing the thread to the renal capsule.
- ✓ The tourniquet is removed by cutting one end of the tape below the clips. Be very careful so that there is no piece of tape close to the renal vessels.

24.2 NEPHRON-SPARING NEPHROTOMY FOR THE TREATMENT OF *DIOCTOPHYME RENALE* PARASITOSIS

Maurício Veloso Brun

CASE DESCRIPTION

Patients parasitized by *Dioctophyme renale* that have some renal viability, even if reduced, should be submitted to nephrotomy (nephron-sparing surgery) instead of radical nephrectomy.

Key points

- Port placement, introduction, and fixation as well as patient positioning are similar to those described in the previous clinical case.
- The renal capsule, cortex, and medulla are incised (about 1 cm) with Metzenbaum scissors. Using Kelly forceps, the medullary layer is dissected and the pelvis is punctured.
- Nephrorrhaphy is performed with a cross mattress suture pattern.
- The release of the tourniquet and the removal of material from the cavity follow the indications of the previous clinical case.

PORT PLACEMENT

The first port (T1) is placed using a modified Hasson technique, lateral to the inguinal fold at the midpoint between the iliac tuberosity and the costal margin. Two other ports (T2, T3) are placed lateral to T1, in a triangulated fashion.

The patient is positioned in lateral recumbency on the side contralateral to the affected kidney, with flank elevation (e.g., using a rolled towel).

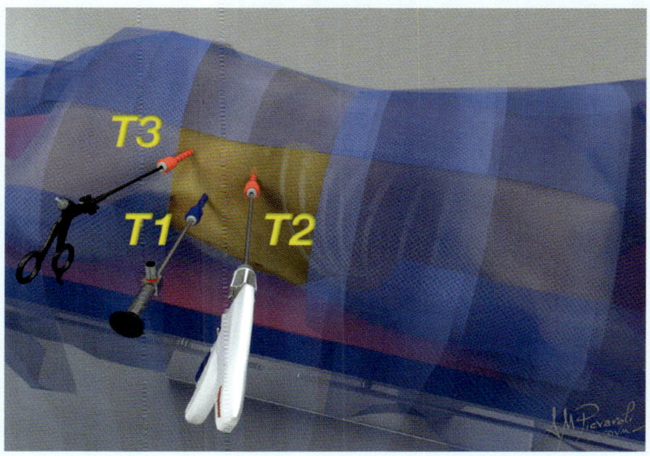

PROCEDURE

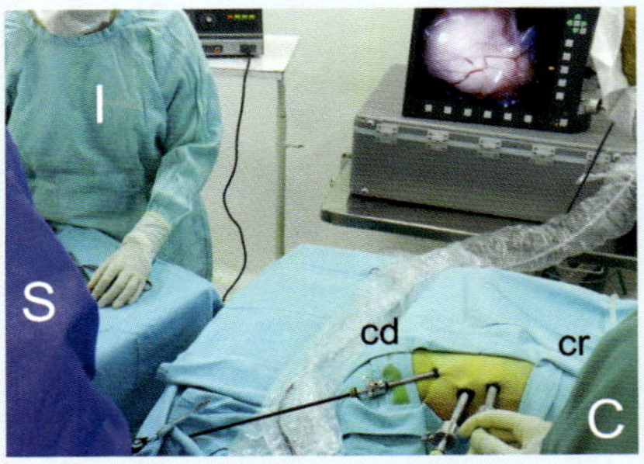

FIGURE 1. Position of surgical team, patient, monitor, and ports. The ports are placed on the flank associated with the parasitized kidney (generally, the right kidney). C, camera; cd, caudal; cr, cranial; I, surgical technologist; S, surgeon.

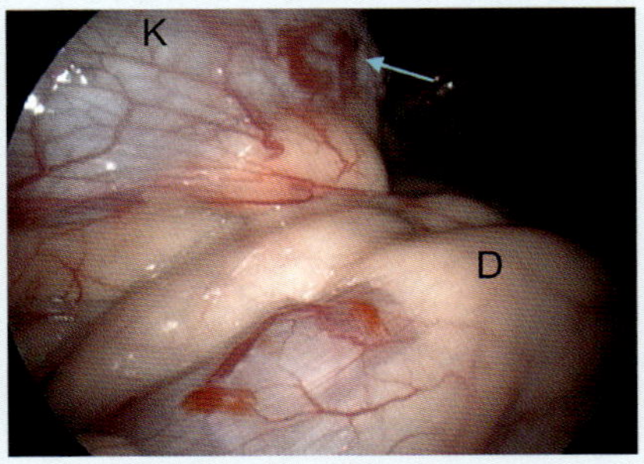

FIGURE 2. The parasitized kidney (K) is examined. The blue arrow indicates the possible penetration site of the parasite. After examination, the dissection of the vessels and the application and temporary maintenance of the Rummel tourniquet follow the same principles outlined in the previous clinical case. Warm ischemia must be no longer than 30 minutes (preferably less than 20 minutes). D, duodenum.

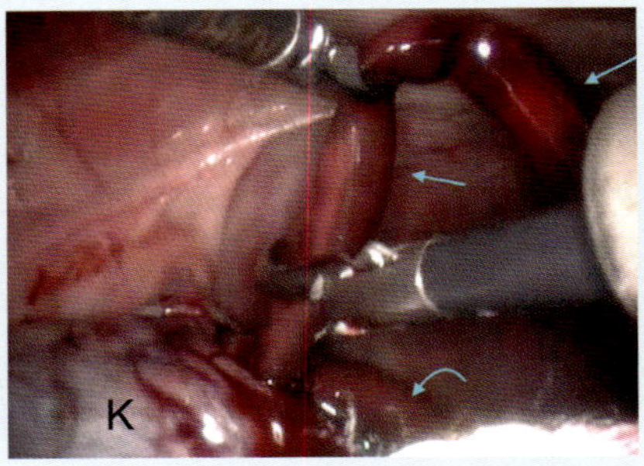

FIGURE 3. The parasites are removed from the renal pelvis by laparoscopic mininephrotomy, picking them up blindly with Kelly forceps. The blue arrows indicate a large *Dioctophyme renale* parasite. K, kidney.

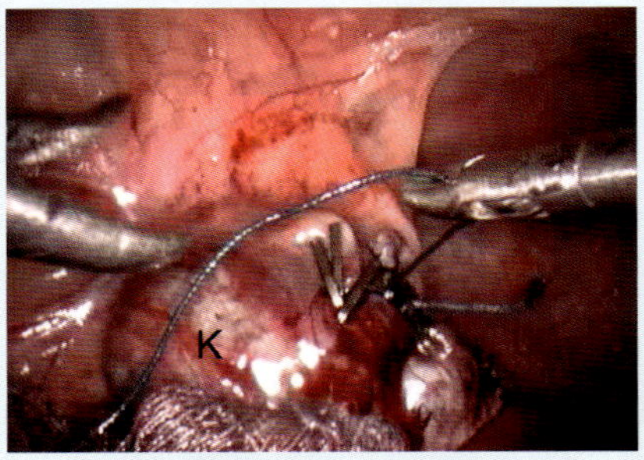

FIGURE 4. Nephrorrhaphy is performed using intracorporeal knots plus clips to gain time during warm ischemia. K, kidney.

Tips and tricks

- ✓ The placement and fixing of the ports, the production and application of the Rummel tourniquet, and the preparation/introduction of the suture are similar to those described in the previous clinical case.
- ✓ Once warm ischemia begins, a mininephrotomy is performed on the midpoint of the convex surface of the kidney.
- ✓ The parasite is removed through the trocar, keeping trocar's valve open or disassembling the instrument, since parasites are usually extensive.
- ✓ A cross mattress suture is placed in the kidney, which can be closed with an intracorporeal knot and/or two or three clip, securing the thread to the renal capsule.
- ✓ When performing nephrorrhaphy with clips, the ends of the thread can be jointed with an intracorporeal knot to reinforce the suture after releasing the tourniquet to reduce ischemia time.
- ✓ Before occluding the cavity, pneumoperitoneum drainage and transoperative ultrasound should be performed to make sure that all parasites have been removed.

25 LAPAROSCOPIC APPROACH TO URETEROLITHIASIS

J. Gutiérrez del Sol, F. J. Pérez Duarte, M. A. Sánchez Hurtado

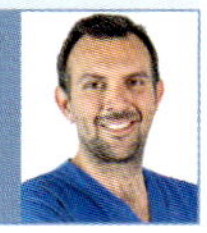

Indications	Contraindications
■ Removal of one or two ureteroliths in the same location ■ In cats there must be some dilatation of the ureter; otherwise, handling and suturing the ureter is very difficult due to its small diameter ■ The size of the ureterolith should be at least 3 mm, since smaller calculi are very difficult to identify laparoscopically	■ Multiple calculi in the same ureter ■ A single urolith in the ureter but multiple nephroliths ■ Severe hydronephrosis ■ Coagulopathy

In recent years there has been an increase in the incidence of ureteral obstructions in small animals caused by urinary calculi, with a higher prevalence in certain breeds. Ureteroliths usually originate in the renal pelvis and can cause problems in the kidneys, ureters, bladder, or urethra, depending on their permanent location.

Delay in diagnosing and treating ureterolithiasis may result in irreversible loss of renal function, as renal blood flow and the glomerular filtration rate (GFR) are decreased in ureteral obstruction. Therefore, if there is complete or incomplete ureteral obstruction, immediate treatment is recommended.

The physiological response to ureteral obstruction is very complex both before and after its resolution. The longer the ureter remains obstructed, the more damage occurs and may be irreversible, depending on the severity and duration of the obstruction. In a study conducted on healthy dogs, it was found that after 7 days of obstruction, the GFR permanently decreased by 35%, and when the obstruction lasted for 14 days, the GFR decreased by 54%. These results were obtained in a canine model with complete obstruction, without preexisting azotemia, chronic interstitial nephritis, or chronic obstructions. Therefore, the extrapolation of a worse outcome in dogs and cats with previous obstruction could be expected, making it imperative to undertake rapid intervention. This study also showed that it took more than 4 months to achieve return to maximum renal function. In contrast, partial obstructions allowed for a greater recovery of renal function after resolution of the obstruction.

Clinical findings in dogs with ureteral obstruction include difficulty urinating, dysuria, stranguria, pollakiuria, polyuria, and hematuria. These patients present with postrenal uremia, which can cause anorexia, depression, abdominal pain on palpation, vomiting, and dehydration. Because urolith formation is often accompanied by urinary infection, signs of pyelonephritis may appear. Obstruction of both ureters at the same time occurs very rarely, thus these patients rarely present with oliguria and anuria.

Ureteral calculi represent the most common cause of ureteral obstructions in dogs and cats. These obstructions sometimes require special diagnostic techniques as well as different treatment modalities, equipment, and specific surgical skills.

Diagnostic imaging methods for detecting uroliths are varied and have improved in accuracy in recent years. Conventional radiography can be a good diagnostic tool for large and radiopaque calculi, being even able to identify the dilation of the ureter. This diagnostic technique has limitations in cases of radiolucent stones or small stones with no ureteral dilation. Excretory urography provides more information than conventional radiography. Ultrasound is used in the assessment of the dilatation of the ureters in the site of obstruction and the renal pelvis, as well as the renal condition, to differentiate a total from a partial obstruction. CT is the diagnostic method of choice in human medicine. In veterinary medicine, it can help determine the number and position of the stones with greater accuracy. Renal scintigraphy is a good tool to assess the GFR and therefore the viability of the kidney where the obstruction is found.

If medical treatment for urolith dissolution is ineffective, or if the stones do not mobilize spontaneously, they must be surgically removed or bypassed to allow urine to flow. In recent years, veterinary medicine has advanced rapidly by incorporating urological techniques from human medicine. The trend in veterinary practice is to reduce the invasiveness and morbidity associated with traditional surgical techniques. Both interventional radiology and endoscopy provide the veterinarian with several options for the treatment of ureteral obstructions caused by calculi. Some of these techniques are retrograde intracorporeal lithotripsy using ureteroscopy, ureteral stents, percutaneous nephrostomy tube placement, subcutaneous ureteral bypass (SUB) devices, and, of course, laparoscopic ureterotomy. In general, ureteral calculi not responding to medical treatment or that are not passively expelled should be removed or voided by one of the aforementioned procedures, to allow a correct flow of urine. Ureterotomy with primary repair has been one of the most accepted techniques in conventional surgery, and in the laparoscopic approach, the same surgical steps are followed. A critical aspect of the success of this surgery is the preservation of the small vessels that nourish the ureter. The laparoscopic approach provides the surgeons the advantage of magnifying these structures and being more delicate with the tissues. The decision-making process for when a case should undergo surgery, as well as the optimal treatment modality that should be used for renal decompression, remains controversial. However, in general, it is considered that immobility of a ureterolith associated with recurrent urinary tract infection is an indication for surgical intervention.

Although there are little references in veterinary surgery, laparoscopic ureterotomy in human surgery has a long history for the treatment of ureterolithiasis when other minimally invasive techniques have not yielded results. This approach began to be used in humans for the treatment of some ureteral and kidney stones. Methods such as ureterorenoscopy, percutaneous nephrolithotomy, or extracorporeal lithotripsy, developed in the 1980s, allowed limiting the indications for surgery, being reserved for complex situations or when the minimally invasive techniques mentioned above failed. The main handicap found in daily clinical practice in veterinary medicine is the size of the patient. The authors emphasize that careful case selection is essential to achieve a successful surgery and to minimize intra- and postoperative complications. In addition, it is essential to highlight that laparoscopic ureterotomy is an advanced and complex technique; therefore, the surgeon must have extensive experience in laparoscopic suturing.

The first reference of laparoscopic ureterotomy in veterinary medicine was presented by the authors of this chapter at the Evendoc Congress held in Lithuania in 2017, and later in 2018 at the VII Convegno Nazionale SICEV, in Prato (Italy). A series of 9 dogs and 3 cats were presented in oral communication.

PATIENT PREPARATION AND POSITIONING

The abdomen is widely clipped and disinfected, as in conventional nephrectomy; therefore, in case of conversion, the surgical field is already prepared (as a rule for all laparoscopic procedures). The surgical clip should extend from the last rib, throughout the paralumbar fossa, to the coxal tuberosity.

The patient is placed in lateral recumbency, right lateral recumbency to approach the left ureter and left lateral recumbency to approach the right ureter. Lumbar elevation using rolled drapes or towels under the patient may be useful to better visualize the kidney and helps to clear the surgical field from the rest of the nearby abdominal viscera. This is not always necessary and depends on the ureteral obstruction site. The most important anatomical landmarks in left-sided cranial obstructions are the kidney, ureter, aorta, renal artery and vein, and colon (**Fig. 1**). In caudal obstructions on this side, special

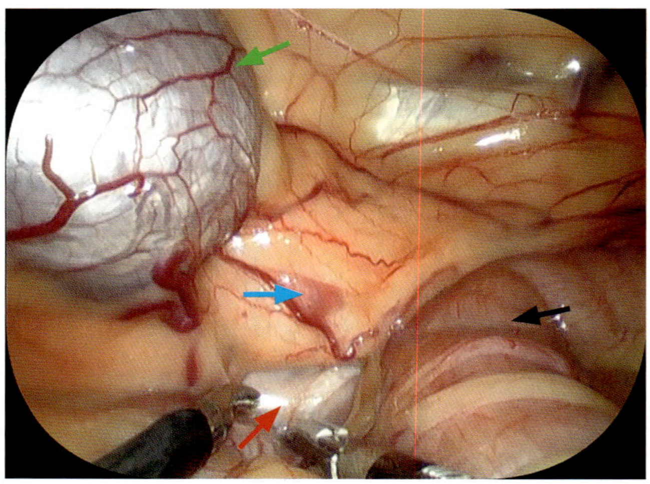

FIGURE 1. Anatomical structures prior to performing left-side laparoscopic ureterotomy: kidney (green arrow), ureter (blue arrow), aorta (red arrow), and colon (black arrow).

consideration should be given to the iliac vessels, colon, and bladder. On the right side, the landmarks are almost identical, with the vena cava instead of the aorta and the duodenum and pancreas instead of the colon.

OPERATING ROOM LAYOUT

The main surgeon and the camera assistant position themselves on one side of the operating table, in front of the patient's abdomen (right or left depending on the ureter to be approached). The endoscopy tower is placed opposite to the surgeons. The anesthesia machine is placed at the head of the operating table, while the instrument table is placed at the foot of the table (**Fig. 2**).

PORT PLACEMENT (FIG. 3)

The trocars are placed using the open technique, thus reducing the risk of injuring the internal organs and the great vessels of the abdomen.

- T1, on the midline at the level of the umbilicus, or slightly lateral to the midline on the side of the obstruction
- T2, caudal and dorsal to T1, in the hemiabdomen of the obstructed ureter
- T3, cranial and dorsal to T1, in the hemiabdomen of the obstructed ureter

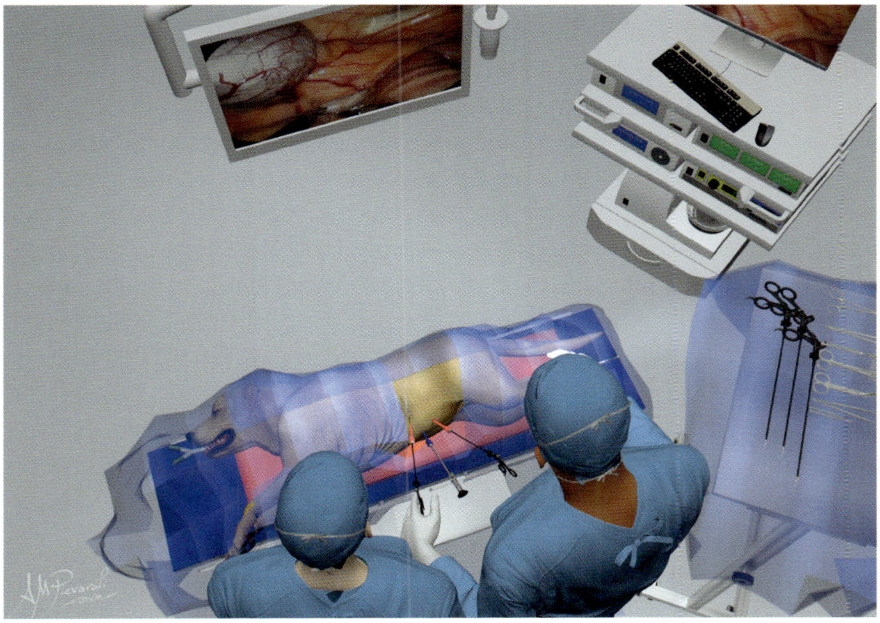

FIGURE 2. Operating room layout for laparoscopic ureterotomy.

Instruments

On the table:

- Standard surgery set
- Telescope 5 mm – 30°
- Three trocars (one 10 mm and two 5 mm, or three 5 mm, or two 5 mm and one 3 mm)
- 5 mm laparoscopic instruments (needle holder, scissors, Maryland dissector, atraumatic grasping forceps)
- 3 mm laparoscopic instruments are not mandatory but can be very useful for cats and small dogs
- 5/0, 6/0 suture
- Extraction bag

Ready to use:

- Bipolar or advanced coagulation system (e.g., LigaSure, Cayman)
- Endoscopic cannula for aspiration/irrigation
- Another trocar or minilaparoscopic device in case retraction maneuvers or tissue separation are needed

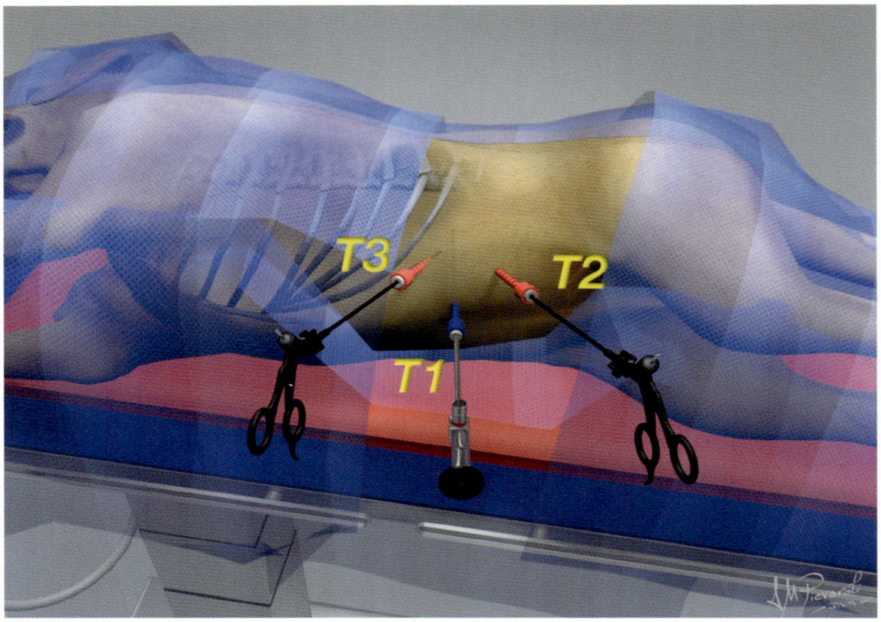

FIGURE 3. Port placement for laparoscopic ureterotomy.

PROCEDURE

- The first trocar is placed using the Hasson entry technique (minilaparotomy open) and the pneumoperitoneum achieved.
- The patient is placed in lateral recumbency and the 5 mm telescope is inserted through T1 to explore the abdominal cavity.
- Once the kidney is visualized, the second and the third trocars are inserted under direct vision, with correct triangulation to facilitate the posterior intracorporeal suture maneuvers as much as possible. Three or four trocars are usually needed for the procedure, although the Teleflex MiniLap device can be used as a suspension element, avoiding the need of a fourth trocar.
- The ureter is then visualized through the peritoneum. In some patients, careful dissection of the perirenal fat is necessary to visualize the ureter (**Fig. 4**).
- Dissection of the ureter is performed with a Maryland dissector and an atraumatic grasping forceps. Sometimes, advanced sealing-coagulation (LigaSure) may be necessary in order to prevent excessive bleeding from the fat surrounding the ureter. It is very important, when possible, to dissect the periureteral vessels rather than coagulate and cut them. The dissection of the ureter should not be extensive, so as to preserve vascularization and prevent suture dehiscence (**Fig. 5**).
- In the dissection maneuvers of the right ureter when the obstruction is close to the renal pelvis, special care should be taken with the vena cava or even the renal vein. These vessels can be closely adhered to the ureter in chronic cases.
- Once the ureterolith has been identified and the ureteral obstruction site dissected, a careful incision of the ureter is made until the mucosa is identified (**Fig. 6**). There are several methods to perform the ureterotomy. In most cases, the authors prefer to cross-section the ureter because, in a laparoscopic approach, this is easier than a longitudinal section. It is important to have the aspirator ready to aspirate possible urine leaks, especially if infection has not been ruled out by urine culture. Once the ureter is open, it is gently pressed with atraumatic forceps to facilitate ureterolith removal (**Fig. 7**). If there are two ureteroliths in close proximity, the incision is made close to the most distal one. Fluid therapy can be increased to promote diuresis and, in this way, help the proximal ureterolith to descend towards the incision. Prior to the cut, a piece of sterile gauze is introduced through the 10 mm trocar and placed just below the area where the ureterotomy will be performed. If there is profuse bleeding when cutting the ureter, it is very important to avoid coagulation; hemostasis is performed by applying pressure on the site with the piece of gauze for several minutes (**Fig. 8**). The removed calculi are introduced in a glove finger for extraction (**Fig. 9**).

- Laparoscopic suturing of the ureter is performed with 6/0 monofilament suture and a circular needle. Two to four stitches are sufficient, depending on the size of the ureterotomy (**Fig. 10**). The suture pattern should always be transverse to preserve the lumen of the ureter. In small dogs and cats it is recommended to place a pigtail stent under fluoroscopy guidance to prevent postoperative ureteral stenosis.

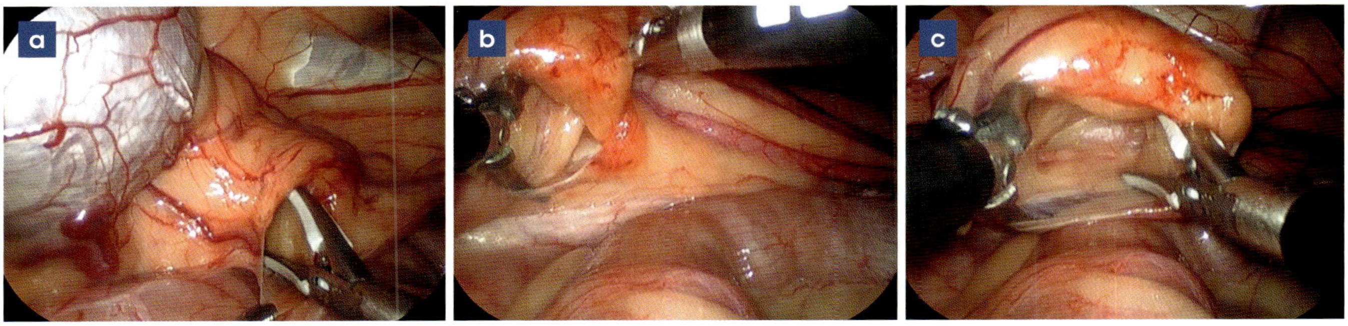

FIGURE 4. a,b) Dissection of periureteral fat with Maryland vessel-sealing device and atraumatic forceps. c) Generally, due to the obstruction, the periureteral fat presents adhesions in the site of obstruction.

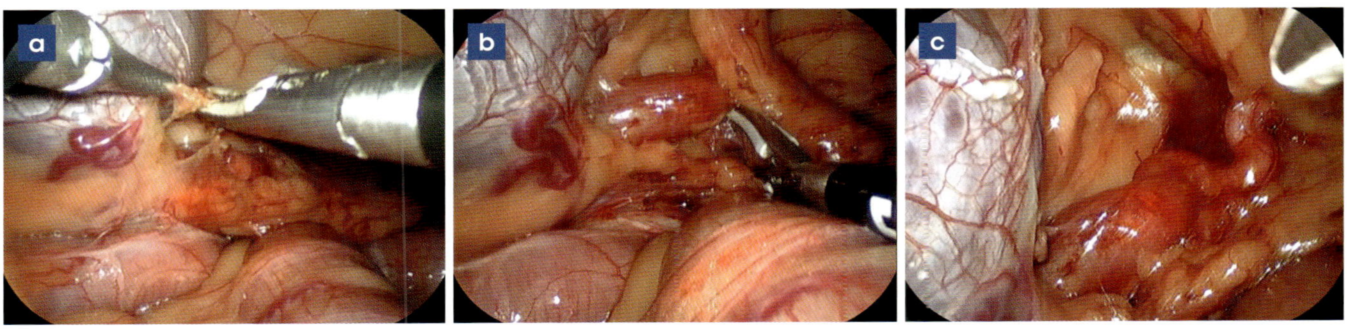

FIGURE 5. a) It may be necessary to coagulate the peritoneum or the periureteral fat with the vessel-sealing device. b) Once near the ureter, blunt dissection is performed to preserve most of the ureteral vascularization. c) Final aspect of the dissected obstructed ureter.

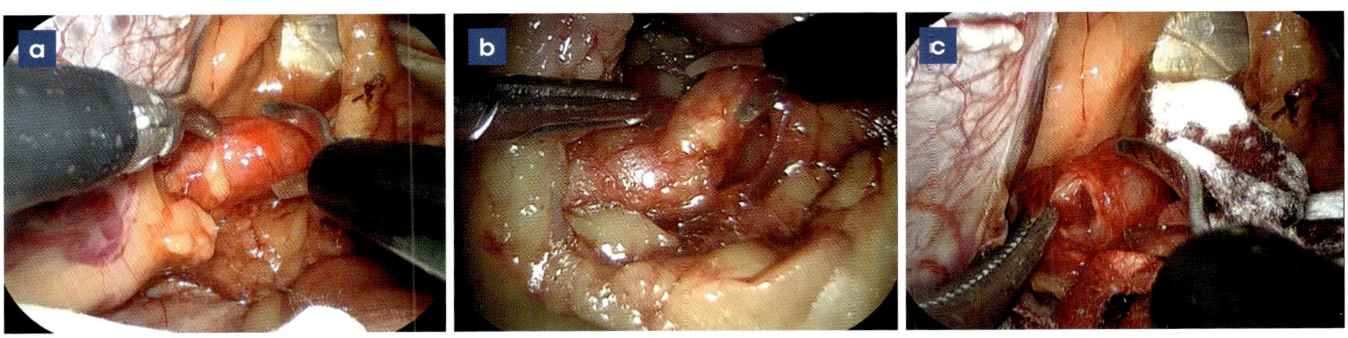

FIGURE 6. a) The position of the scissors prior to cutting must be tangential to the ureter. b) Right ureterotomy; image prior to cutting the ureter in the site of obstruction. c) Left ureterotomy; image showing the different layers of the ureter.

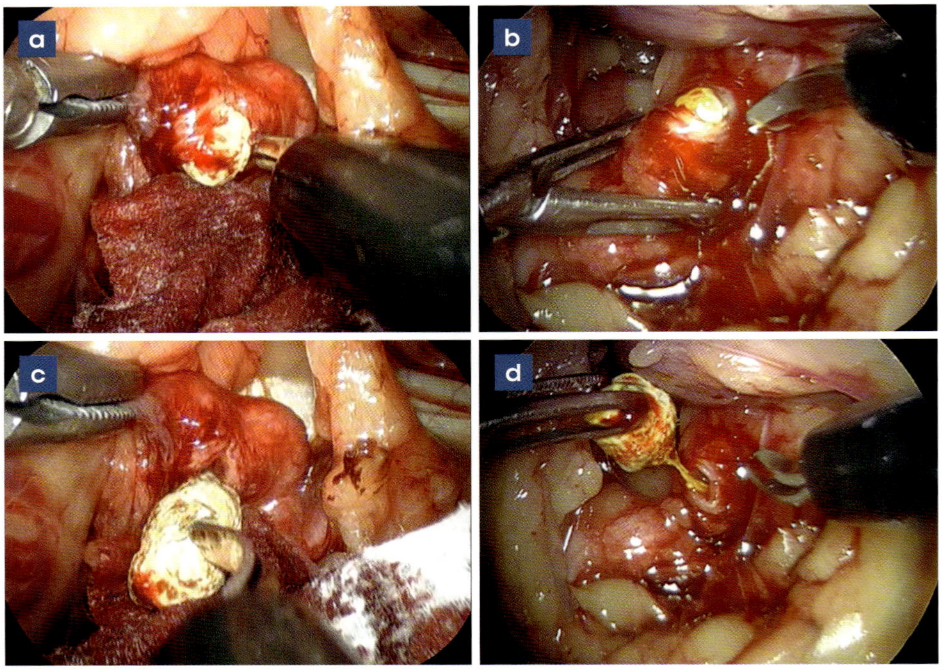

FIGURE 7. a) Left ureterotomy; the ureter is gently pressed using atraumatic forceps to extract the ureterolith. b) Right ureterotomy; pressure maneuver for ureterolith extraction. c) Left ureterotomy; ureterolith extraction. A piece of gauze is prepared to contain the possible leakage of urine. d) Right ureterotomy; ureterolith extraction.

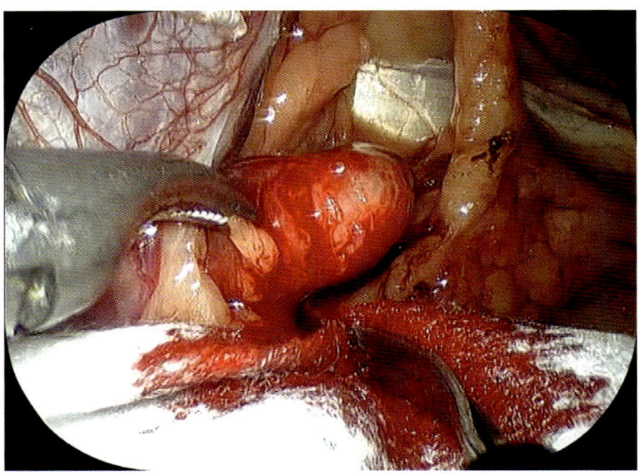

FIGURE 8. Before cutting the ureter, a piece of gauze is placed to control possible bleeding and urine leakage.

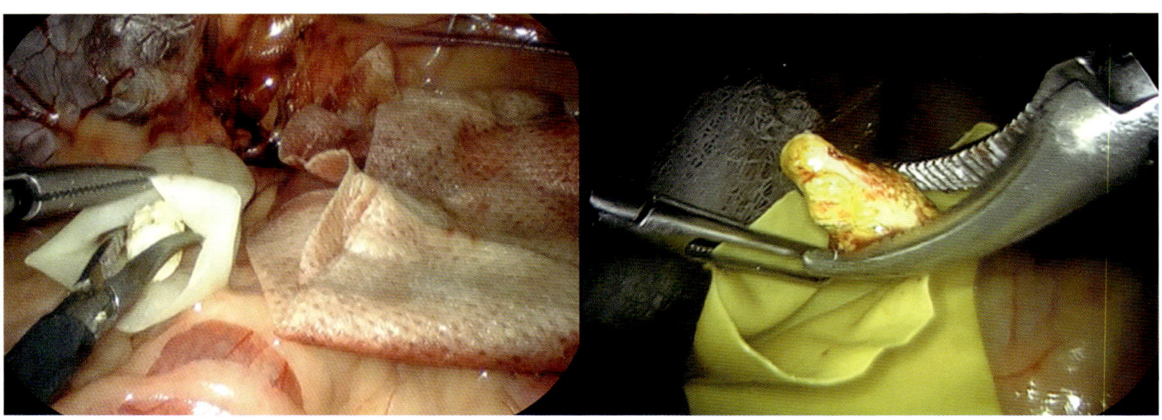

FIGURE 9. Introduction of ureteroliths in the finger of a sterile powder-free glove.

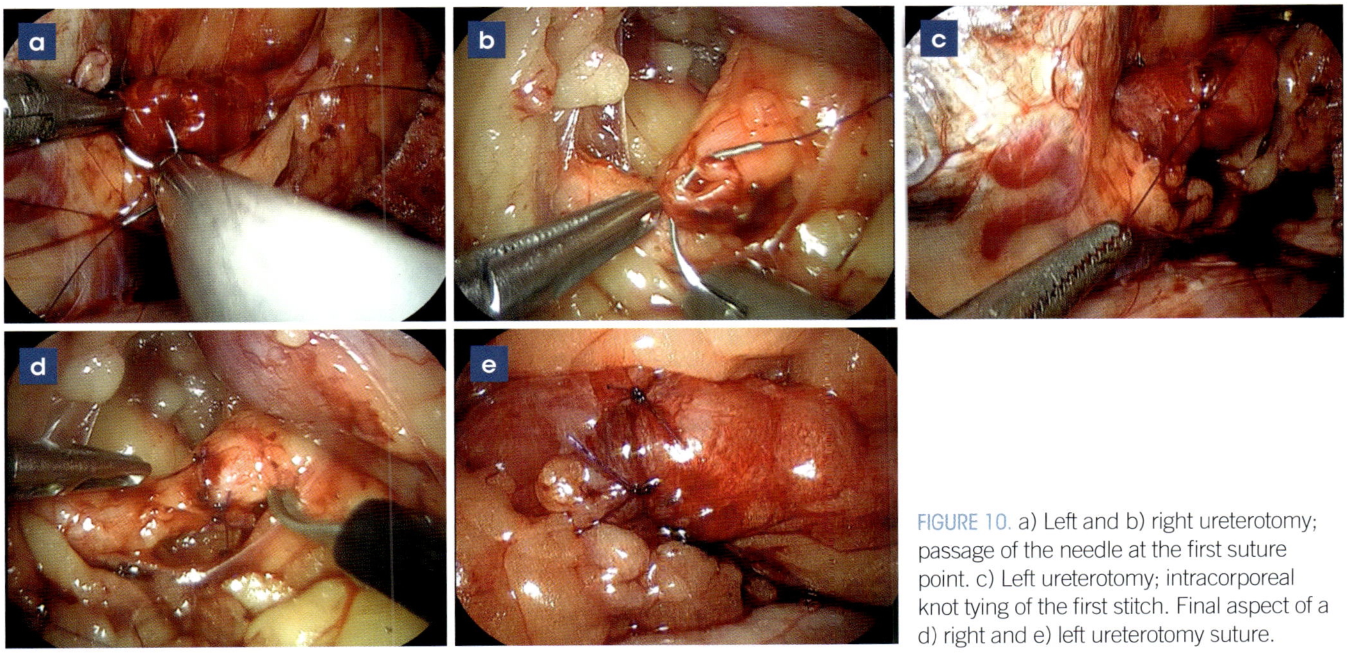

FIGURE 10. a) Left and b) right ureterotomy; passage of the needle at the first suture point. c) Left ureterotomy; intracorporeal knot tying of the first stitch. Final aspect of a d) right and e) left ureterotomy suture.

POSTOPERATIVE MANAGEMENT

- Monitoring of kidney function is of vital importance in these patients.
- Possible urine leaks should be controlled and ultrasound follow-up in the following days is essential if there is suspicion of bleeding or leakage.
- Electrolyte and acid–base abnormalities should be monitored and corrected postoperatively.
- Postoperative analgesics should be given as needed.
- Nonsteroidal anti-inflammatory drugs should be avoided in these patients.

Complications of laparoscopic ureterotomy

- The main complications are those that are general to any laparoscopic procedure (e.g., conversion to open surgery, lacerations to adjacent organs during entry, subcutaneous emphysema, port-site infection).
- Iatrogenic damage to the ureter during its dissection and manipulation.
- Excessive bleeding during dissection and cutting of the ureter.
- Stenosis of the ureter in the suture area, with subsequent kidney damage due to the inability to pass urine.
- Urine leaks.

Key points

- It is essential to identify the location of the ureterolith using diagnostic imaging methods before surgery, in order to dissect the shortest path of ureter possible.
- Arrange T2 and T3 in a triangulated fashion toward the area of the ureter where the ureteromy is to be performed to facilitate the suturing maneuver as much as possible.
- Perform blunt dissection and cold cutting for as long as possible during the procedure to preserve the small vessels that supply the ureter.

SUGGESTED READINGS

CLINICAL CASES

25.1 URETEROTOMY FOR STONE REMOVAL

David García Rubio

CASE DESCRIPTION

A 6-year-old male Czechoslovakian Wolfdog was presented with a 2-week history of apathy, hyporexia, and fever. The patient's rectal temperature was 40°C and he was severely dehydrated. Blood analysis showed moderate neutrophilic leukocytosis and monocytosis and a slight increase in creatinine.

An abdominal ultrasound scan was performed and showed a large number of hyperechogenic particles in suspension inside the bladder and dilation of the right renal pelvis and proximal right ureter. Following the course of the dilated ureter, a hyperechogenic object 1 cm in length with a marked acoustic shadow was noted, corresponding to a ureteral stone.

A diagnosis of ureteral obstruction with associated pyelonephritis was made and a laparoscopic ureterotomy was proposed.

Key points

- The patient should be treated with antibiotics prior to surgery to prevent secondary infections due to contamination caused by an escape of urine following the ureterotomy.
- Each case should be analyzed carefully, assessing the number of stones, their location, and other complications that may advise against surgical intervention and advocate other techniques (e.g., use of a subcutaneous ureteral bypass—SUB—device, ureteral stent).
- It is essential to pinpoint the location of the ureterolith using imaging techniques (ultrasound, CT, radiography) prior to surgery. The lack of sense of touch during the procedure will hinder stone localization.

PORT PLACEMENT

Three 5 mm trocars were used. The patient was placed in dorsal recumbency and the optical trocar was inserted in an umbilical position. Then, the patient was placed into a left lateral recumbency to approach the right renal area. The two other trocars were placed to the right and left of the optical trocar, slightly further forward to the left side.

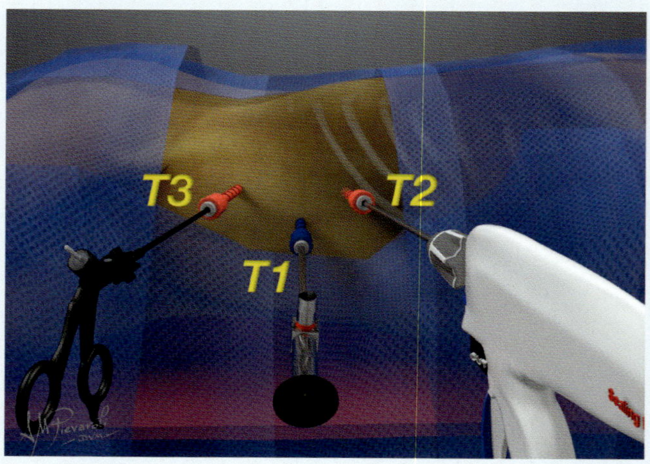

PROCEDURE

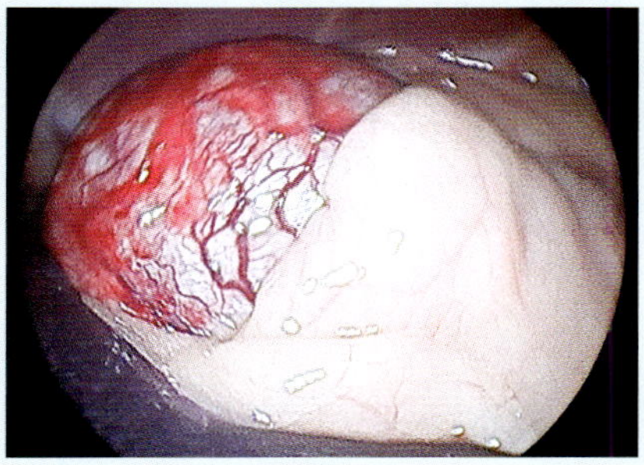

FIGURE 1. View of the kidney affected by the ureteral obstruction. Note its marked engorgement.

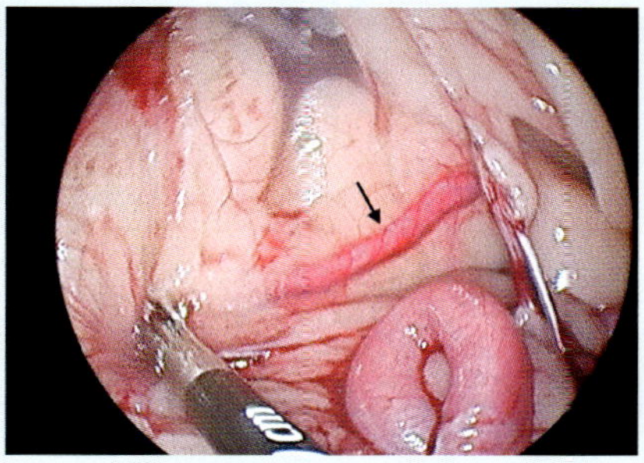

FIGURE 2. Localization and dissection of the ureter (arrow) along its abdominal length towards the bladder.

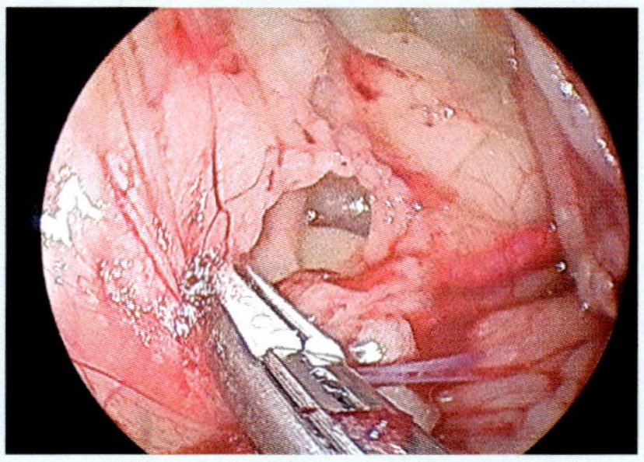

FIGURE 3. Dissection must be performed carefully so as to minimize lesions to the vessels supplying the ureter.

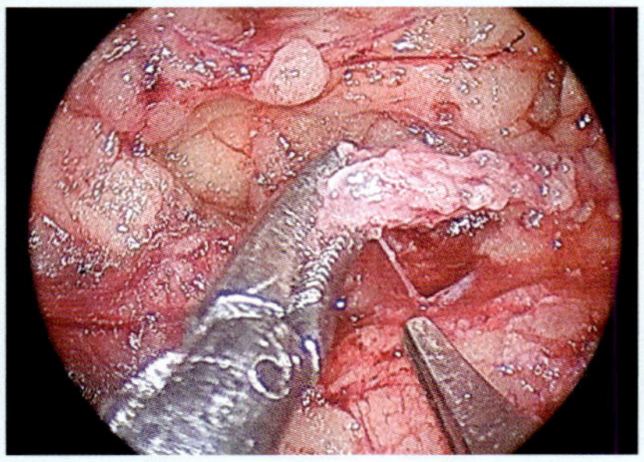

FIGURE 4. Localization of the ureterolith via delicate palpation/compression of the ureter.

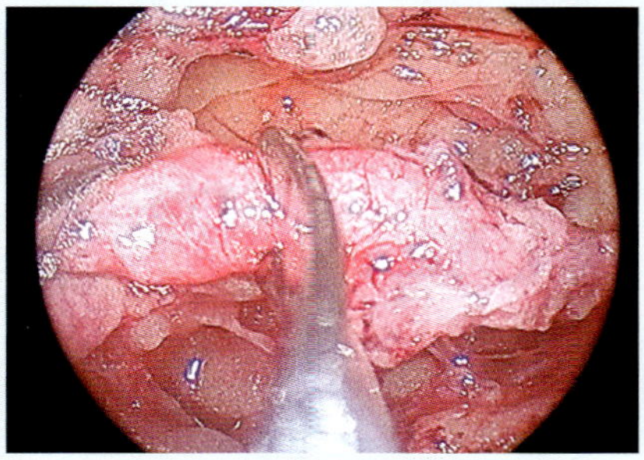

FIGURE 5. The cold knife technique and scissors are used to cut the ureter cross-sectionally in the area cranial to the stone.

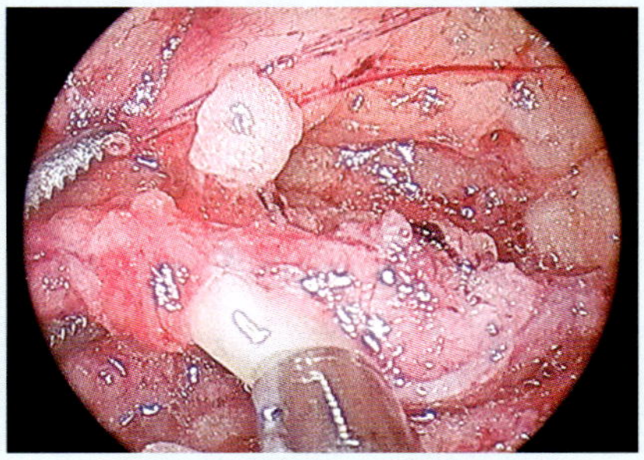

FIGURE 6. Immediate vacuuming of the retained ureteral and renal content to prevent subsequent infections.

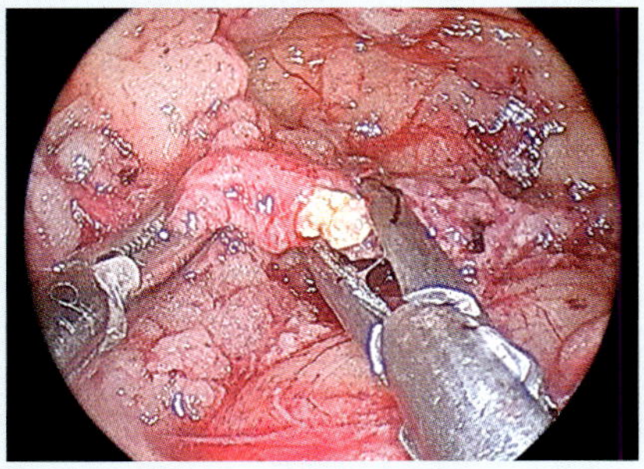

FIGURE 7. Delicate extraction of the ureteral stone and collection for subsequent analysis.

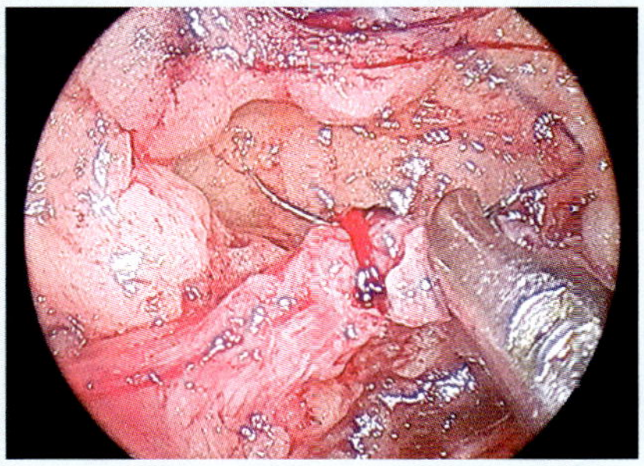

FIGURE 8. Closure of the incision using a single stitch of absorbable 5/0 material and a round-tip needle.

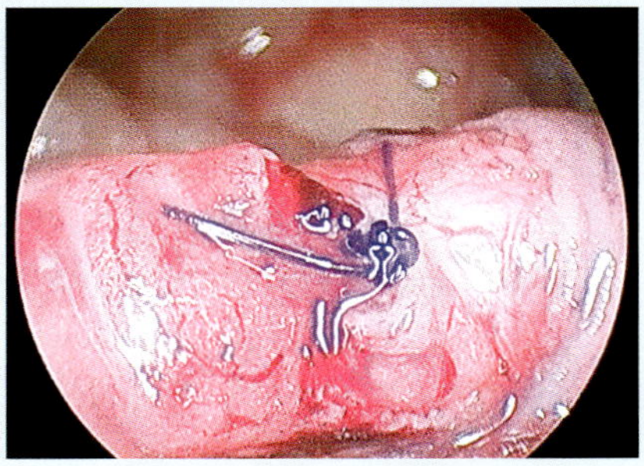

FIGURE 9. Detailed close-up view of the single stitch. If any urine escaped to the abdomen, the area should be lavaged with warmed saline solution.

Tips and tricks

✓ Given the absence of touch sensation, the ureteral stone must be located via transparent visualization and delicate compression of the ureter until resistance is noted.

✓ Avoid or minimize lesions to the vascularization of the ureter. For this, blunt dissection is recommended and avoid using heat sources close to the ureter. In addition, fixing and traction of the ureter must be done delicately using atraumatic forceps whenever possible.

✓ Occasionally, it is useful to insert a temporary double J ureteral stent to encourage wound healing without stenosis.

26 LAPAROSCOPIC NEOURETEROCYSTOSTOMY

Felipe Lillo

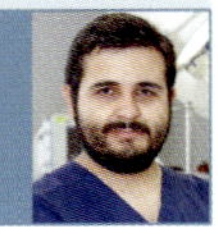

Indications	Contraindications
■ Impassable caudal ureteral obstruction (e.g., inadvertent ligatures, tumors, stenosis, or strictures) ■ Cystoureteral reflux due to extramural ectopic ureter	■ Urinary tract infection ■ Afunctional hydronephrosis ■ Intramural ureteral ectopia ■ Metastatic cancer ■ Adhesions due to previous surgery ■ Strictures that can be resolved with ureteral stents

Ureteral obstructions can be caused by many underlying pathologies. Uroliths are one of the possible causes and can be managed by surgery, laser lithotripsy, or bypassing the obstruction (subcutaneous ureteral bypass, SUB). Nevertheless, other clinical entities that cause distal ureteral obstruction or dysfunction manifest with hydroureter, pyelectasia, or hydronephrosis.

Extramural ureteral ectopia causes urinary reflux and is usually associated with chronic or recurrent urinary tract infections. In these cases, laser wall ablation is not suitable because an endoscopic attempt will lead to urinary rupture and urine leakage to the peritoneal or retroperitoneal cavity.

Inadvertent ligation of the ureter is common in developing countries with low-standard sterilization programs for dogs and cats. Although distal ureteral neoplasias and/or operable tumors in the bladder trigone are less frequent, they are serious obstructive diseases in which the excision of the tissue could be an attempt of curative treatment.

In general, these kinds of ureteral obstruction or dysfunction may be managed through reimplantation of the affected ureter in a healthy portion of the bladder (i.e., neoureterocystostomy). The classical technique described in veterinary medicine involves a cystotomy and a transfixion of the bladder wall with the distal end of the sectioned ureter. Terminal to lateral anastomosis is accomplished intravesically. A laparoscopic version of the open procedure would require very challenging surgical steps, an extensive cystotomy, and percutaneous stay sutures to expose the mucosa of the bladder. Furthermore, since this surgical plan does not prevent cystoureteral reflux, the dysfunction could persist postoperatively.

The Lich–Gregoir technique is a widely used method to prevent urinary reflux in humans and can be performed through a laparoscopic approach. The laparoscopic Lich–Gregoir surgical plan is a good alternative in dogs and cats with nonlithic obstruction or dysfunction of the distal ureter.

> The modern (modified) Lich–Gregoir technique was described in pediatric patients in 1998 by Lapointe et al.

DESCRIBED SURGICAL PROCEDURES

The traditional technique in small animals is a long procedure associated with an extensive incision and a cystotomy. The terminal-lateral anastomosis does not ensure complete avoidance of cystoureteral reflux.

The Lich–Gregoir technique is a nonregurgitating procedure, which is achieved with a two-layer suture pattern. The first pattern is the anastomosis between the previously spatulated ureteral end and the mucosa of the bladder in the surgically created defect. The bladder iatrogenic defect must have 2 cm of seromuscular incision and, in its distal part, a mucosal incision just enough to match the ureter. After the ureter–mucosa anastomosis is complete, a simple running suture is made to close the seromuscular incision, leaving a portion of the ureter between the mucosa and the seromuscular layer, mimicking the intramural course of the ureter that is responsible for the unidirectional emptying of urine into the bladder.

The laparoscopic approach is associated with all the benefits of minimally invasive surgery, such as lower pain perception, less hospitalization time, and limited postsurgical complications.

Tips

It is strongly recommended to place a pigtail catheter to prevent urinary leakage or stenosis of the suture plane.

PATIENT PREPARATION AND POSITIONING

Before surgery, it is imperative to confirm that urine cultures are negative and to assess the functionality of the affected kidney.

The affected side of the abdomen is widely clipped, with the epaxial muscles line as the lateral margins of trichotomy. The contralateral margin is the inguinal longitudinal line, in case conversion is necessary. The patient is placed in lateral recumbency and the table is set in a slight Trendelenburg position (10°). The Trendelenburg position can be delayed until the beginning of the surgery; however, the surgeon should test this position before draping.

The skin is aseptically prepared in the usual fashion. After the installation of surgical drapes and towels, a sterile urinary catheter is placed.

OPERATING ROOM LAYOUT

Both the surgeon and the assistant position themselves on one side of the operating table, ventral to the patient. The monitor is placed caudal or dorsal to the patient. The assistant is to the left of the surgeon. The instrument table is placed in front of the surgeon or the assistant depending on the affected side (**Fig. 1**).

PORT PLACEMENT (FIG. 2)

- T1, 10 cm lateral to the umbilicus
- T2, on the ventral axillary line, 4–6 cm caudal to T1
- T3, on the longitudinal trochanteric line, 3–5 cm caudal to the last rib

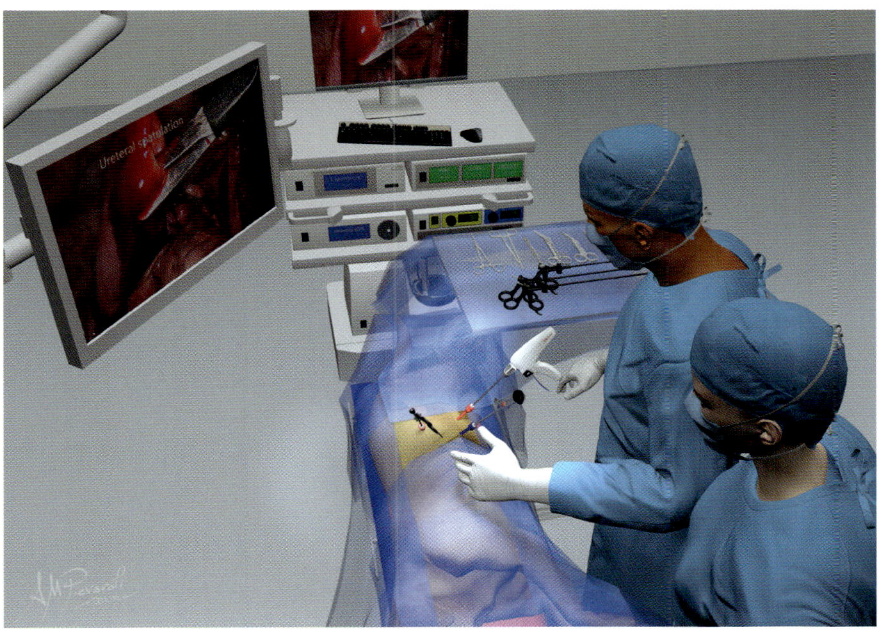

FIGURE 1. Operating room layout for laparoscopic neoureterocystostomy.

Instruments

On the table:

- Standard surgery set
- Telescope 5 or 10 mm – 30°
- Three 5 mm cannulas (or two 5 mm + one 10 mm)
- Grasping forceps
- Maryland forceps
- Laparoscopic needle driver
- Laparoscopic scissors
- Aspiration/irrigation cannula for laparoscopy
- Ultrasonic laparoscopic scalpel or vessel-sealing device
- Ureteral stent set for percutaneous installation (pigtail catheter)
- Endoscopic clip applier (polypropylene, steel, or titanium)

PROCEDURE

- After the first port has been placed and the pneumoperitoneum achieved, the 5 or 10 mm telescope is inserted in T1 and a first exploration of the abdomen is performed to check for any evidence of iatrogenic trauma caused by placement of the first cannula.
- Under endoscopic vision, the other two cannulas, for the operative instruments, are inserted.
- The affected ureter is identified, dissected from the retroperitoneal space, and ligated as caudal as possible but proximal to the obstruction (**Fig. 3**). Sutures, titanium staples, or polypropylene clips (Hem-o-lok) can be used for ligation.
- The bladder is suspended using a straight needle suture inserted percutaneously (**Fig. 4**). A 10–20 mm incision is made in an unscathed region of the bladder. The anastomosis site must be selected carefully to avoid any tension.
- The ureter is sectioned proximal to the ligation and the ureteral end is spatulated to enlarge its circumference (**Fig. 5**). A 5–10 mm longitudinal incision is sufficient. With the empty bladder suspended, the seromuscular incision is made vertically, and the mucosal defect should be limited to just the upper part of the incision.
- The ureter–mucosa anastomosis is made using two absorbable monofilament sutures knotted together (**Fig. 6**). First, with one thread, the lateral wall of the anastomosis is sutured from 12 to 6 o'clock position (**Fig. 7**). Then, the pigtail catheter is passed to the bladder and the kidney (**Fig. 8**). The medial wall of the anastomosis is completed with the other suture and needle (**Fig. 9**). Finally, when both sutures meet, the threads are tied together at 6 o'clock position to complete the anastomosis (**Fig. 10**).
- The seromuscular incision is closed with a running suture to leave an intramural section of the ureter (**Fig. 11**).
- A leaking test without suspension must be performed before finishing the surgery.

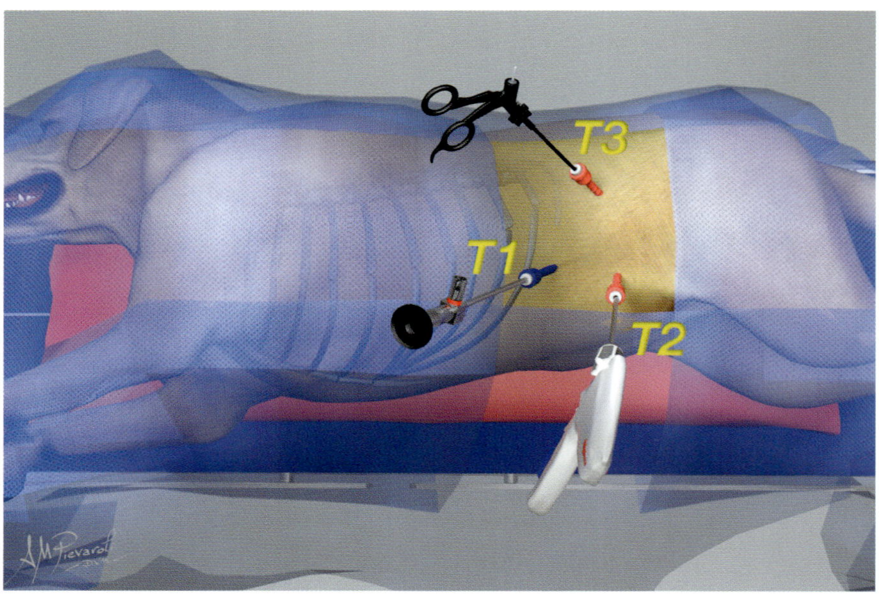

FIGURE 2. Port placement for laparoscopic neoureterocystostomy.

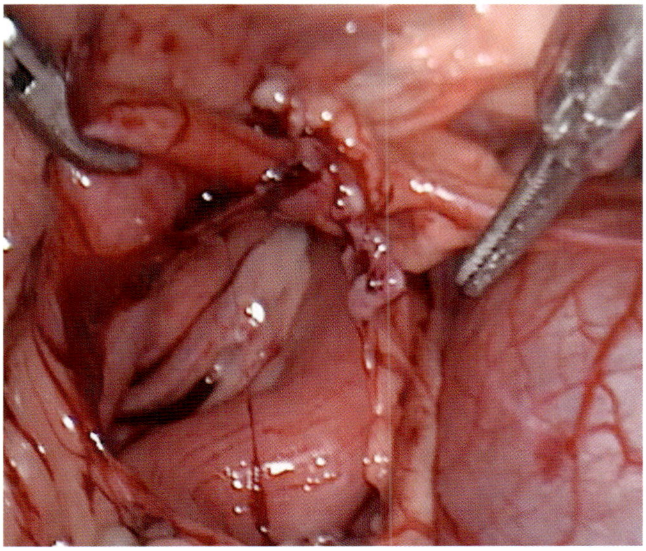

FIGURE 3. The affected ureter is identified and dissected from the retroperitoneal space.

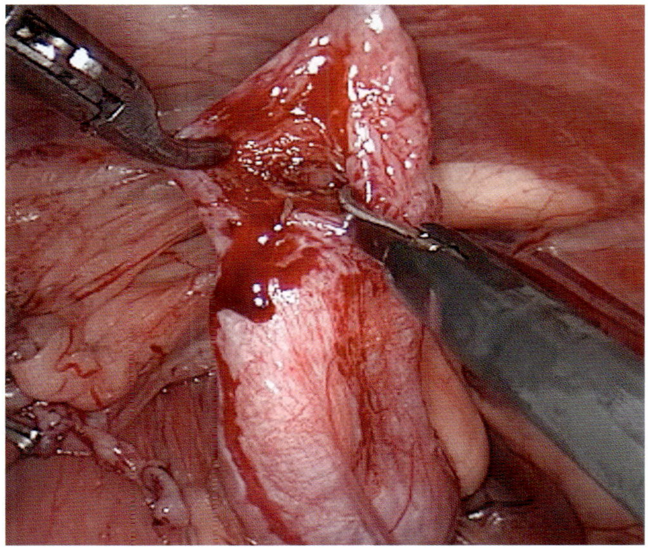

FIGURE 4. The bladder is suspended percutaneously.

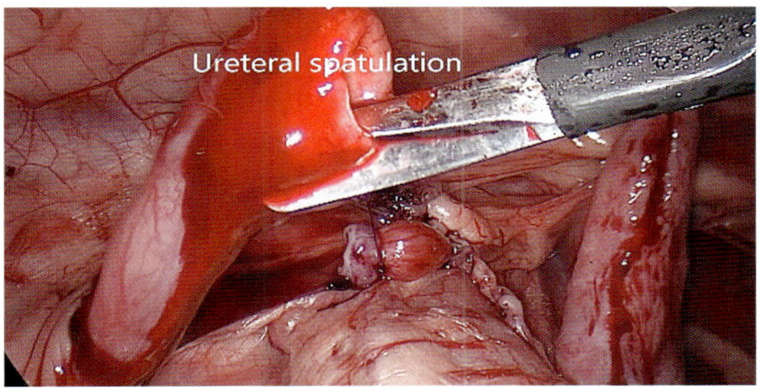

FIGURE 5. The ureter is sectioned proximal to the ligation and the end is spatulated.

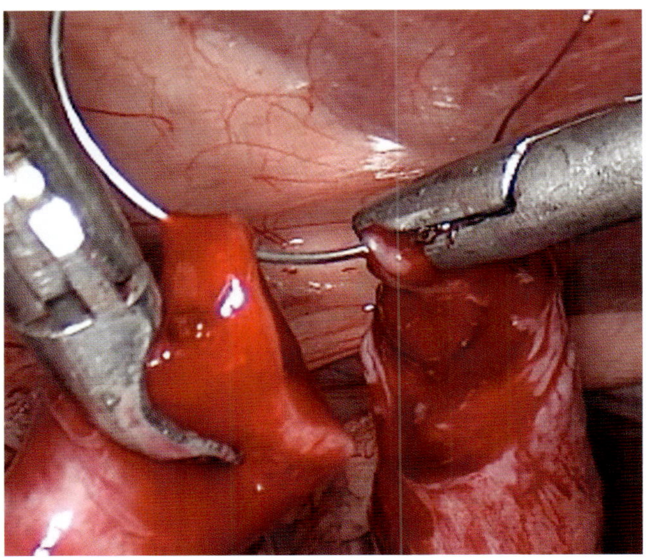

FIGURE 6. Ureter–mucosa anastomosis.

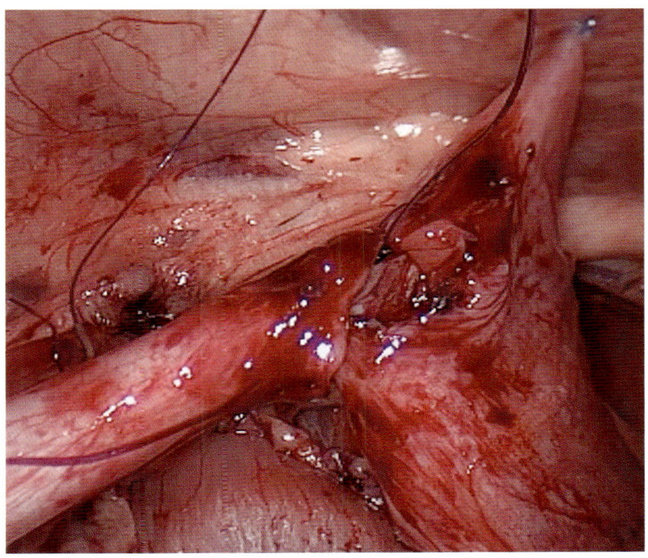

FIGURE 7. Suture from 12 to 6 o'clock position.

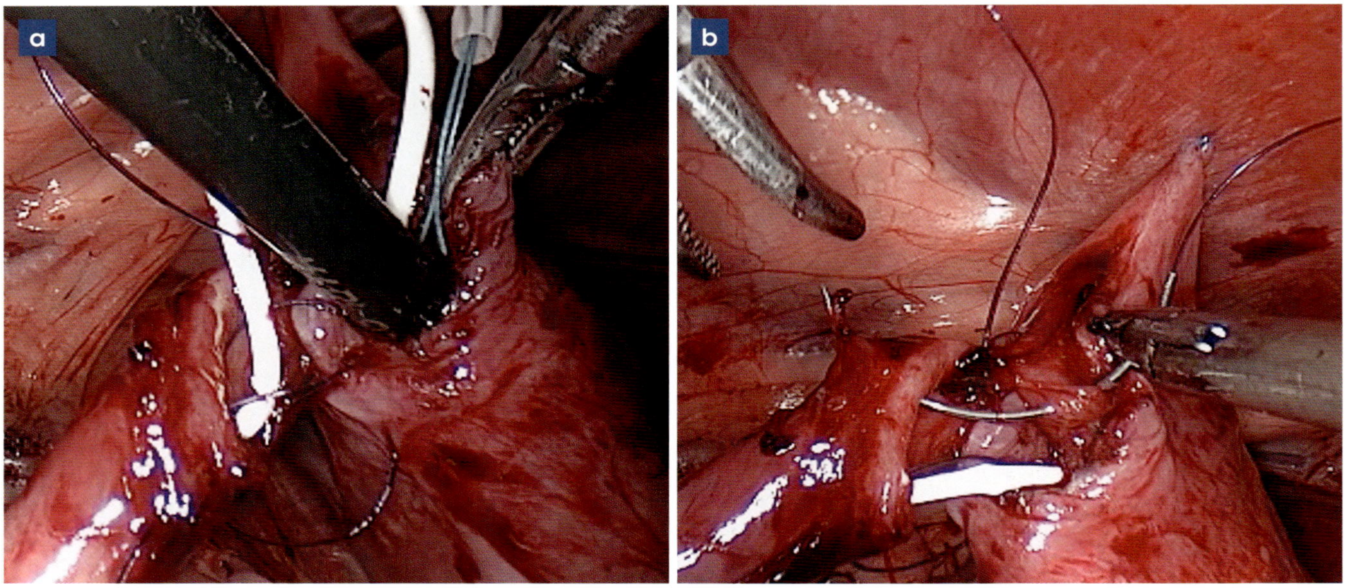

FIGURE 8. a) Introduction of the pigtail catheter end into the bladder. b) Medial edge suture between the ureter end and bladder mucosa over the pigtail catheter (or ureteral stent).

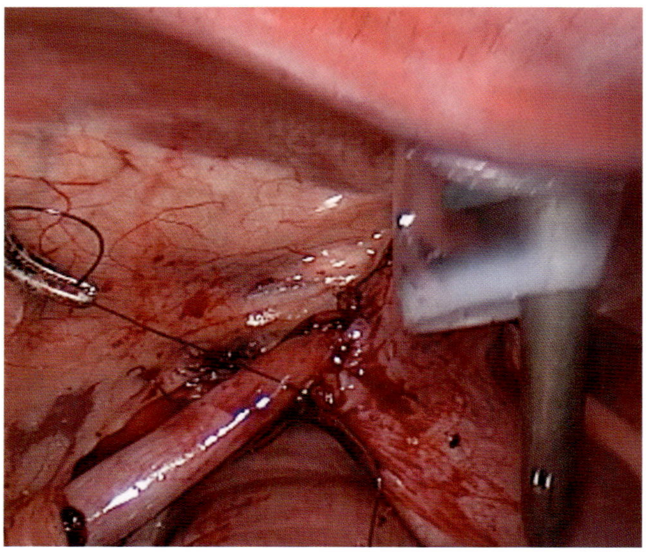

FIGURE 9. The medial wall of the anastomosis is completed with the other suture and needle.

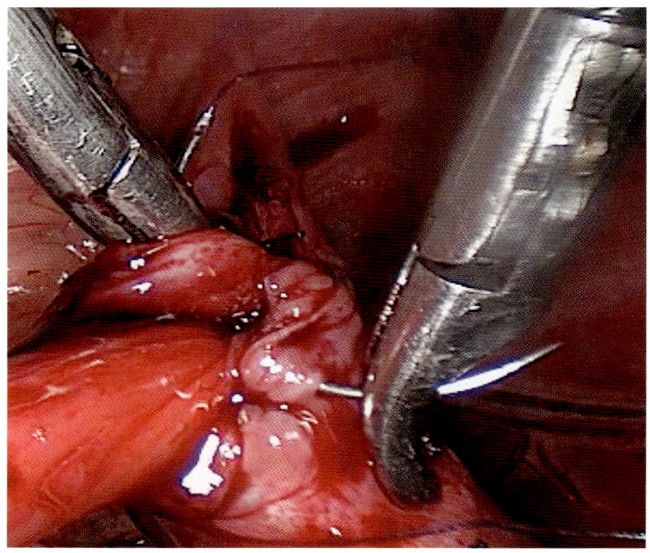

FIGURE 10. Both threads are knotted together at 6 o'clock position to complete the anastomosis.

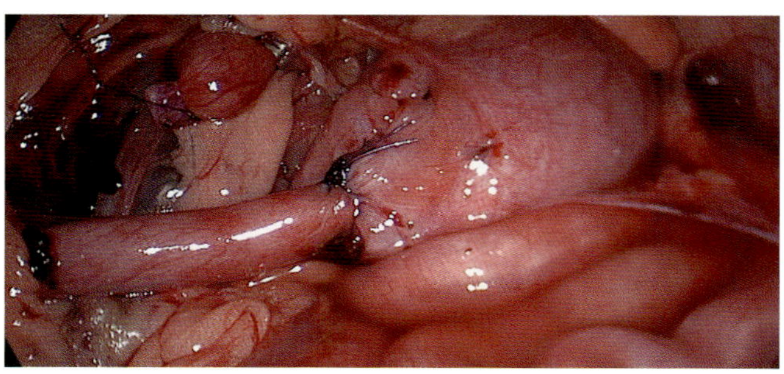

FIGURE 11. Seromuscular incision.

POSTOPERATIVE MANAGEMENT

- Urinary leakage and peritonitis surveillance are indicated for the first 2 days using regular ultrasonography (AFAST). The presence of hematuria is considered normal up to 72 hours after surgery, after which a new exploration is recommended.
- The pigtail catheter must be kept in place for at least 2 months. After this time, it is recommended to perform a cystoscopy to extract the ureteral stent and explore the ureteral neopore. Additionally, a retrograde urography with high pressure can be used to evaluate the presence of urinary reflux.

Complications of laparoscopic neoureterocystostomy

- Urinary leakage and peritonitis
- Ureteral stenosis or strictures
- Blocked pigtail catheter
- Hematuria
- Cystoureteral reflux

Key points

- Bring the ureter to the selected area of the bladder before starting the anastomosis to make sure there will not be too much tension.
- The bladder must be partially filled with saline until the incision is made to better understand the distances and result.
- Periureteral dissection must be minimized, just enough to bring the ureter to the bladder. Extensive detachment could lead to ischemia and/or necrosis of the ureter.

SUGGESTED READINGS

CLINICAL CASES

26.1 LAPAROSCOPY-ASSISTED CUTANEOUS URETEROSTOMY (LACU) IN A CANINE PATIENT WITH PROSTATIC CARCINOMA

Giovanni Allevi

CASE DESCRIPTION

A 9-year-old castrated male mixed-breed dog weighing 8.6 kg was referred for dysuria and hematuria. The CT scan revealed prostatic enlargement (size 4.5×3×3.5 cm) (**Fig. 1**). The prostate gland had an irregular profile that extended up to the urinary bladder neck and trigone. The centripetal compression of the pelvic urethra and the dorsal displacement of the rectum were significant. Multiple and diffuse pulmonary cavitary lesions were detected. Multifocal nodules affecting the spleen and liver were also found. These findings were suggestive of metastasis. Biopsy of the prostate gland confirmed a diagnosis of carcinoma. The owner refused surgical treatment involving total prostatectomy. Laparoscopic bilateral ureteral skin diversion was proposed and accepted.

Each ureter was catheterized with a 4 Fr 130 mm long tom cat catheter during the procedure and for 10 days postoperatively. Wound care included frequent diaper change (every 6–8 hours) and local application of zinc oxide paste. Adjuvant chemotherapy with carboplatin (300 mg/m^2) was given in the postoperative period. The owner reported that the dog showed normal activity and good quality of life. Euthanasia was performed 2 months and 10 days after surgery due to development of respiratory signs, likely related to a metastatic neoplastic process.

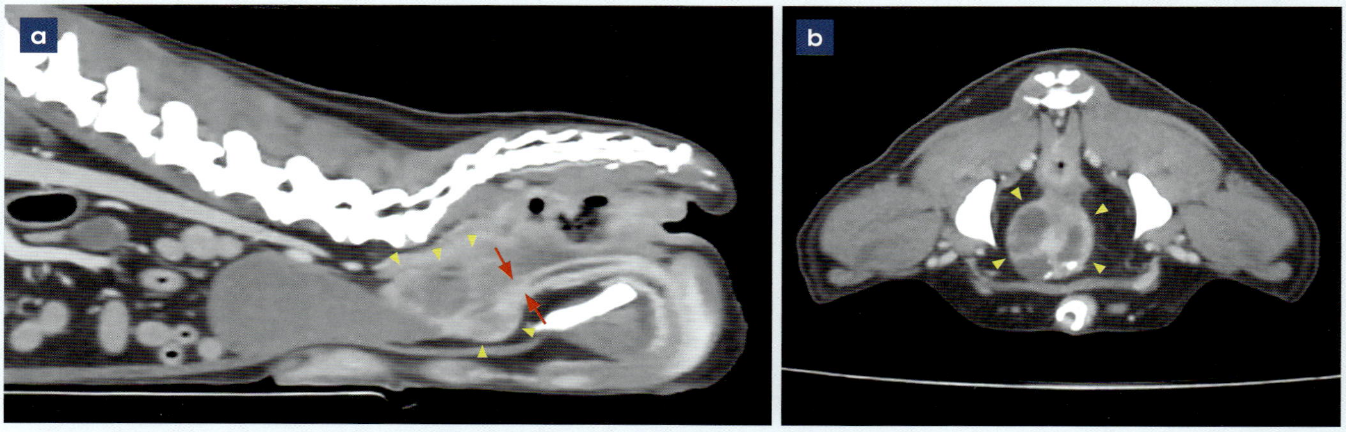

FIGURE 1. Postcontrast CT scan; a) multiplanar sagittal reconstruction and b) transverse section. The prostate gland shows marked enlargement and heterogeneous enhancement (yellow arrowheads) with multiple dotted calcifications. The prostate gland has a close relation with the bladder and the ventral wall of the rectum. A compression of the pelvic urethra caused by the prostatic enlargement is detectable (red arrows).

Key points

- CT angiography is essential for correct patient staging and to decide the best surgical approach.
- Laparoscopy-assisted ureterostomy can be considered a safe procedure to perform as a palliative technique in selected patients with obstruction of the lower urinary tract.

PORT PLACEMENT

The dog was placed in dorsal recumbency for setting up the operating field. A three-port technique with three 5 mm trocars was used (VersaPort, Covidien, Medtronic Italia, Milan, Italy). The first port (T1) was placed caudal to the umbilicus and the abdominal cavity was insufflated with CO_2, maintaining a pressure of 10 mmHg (Karl Storz Veterinary Endoscopy). A 5 mm, 0° laparoscope camera (Karl Storz Veterinary Endoscopy) was inserted and two working ports (T2, T3) were placed caudally, in triangulation with the first port.

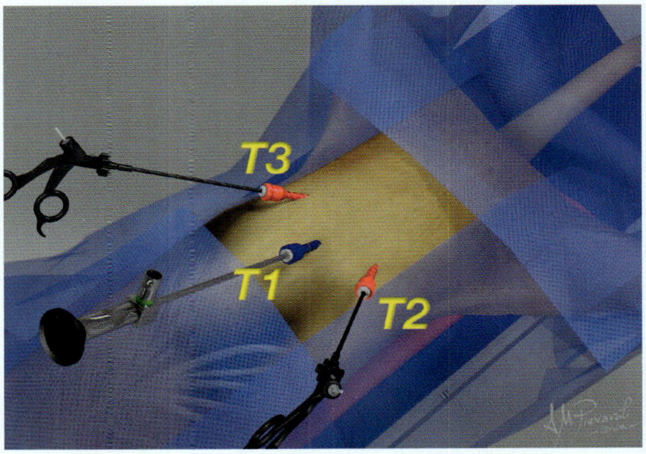

PROCEDURE

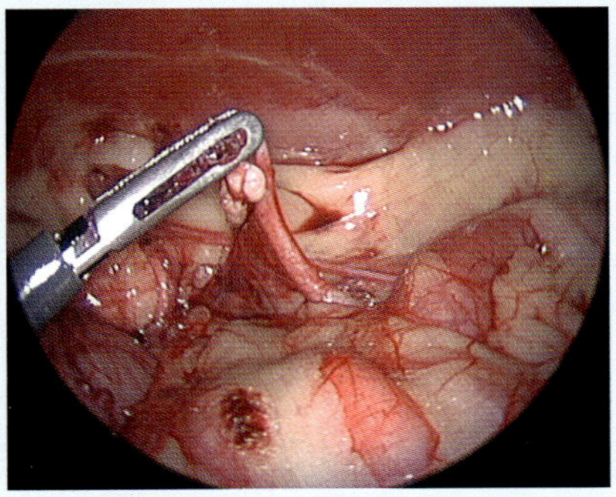

FIGURE 2. The right ureter is isolated and dissected distally, close to its insertion on the bladder.

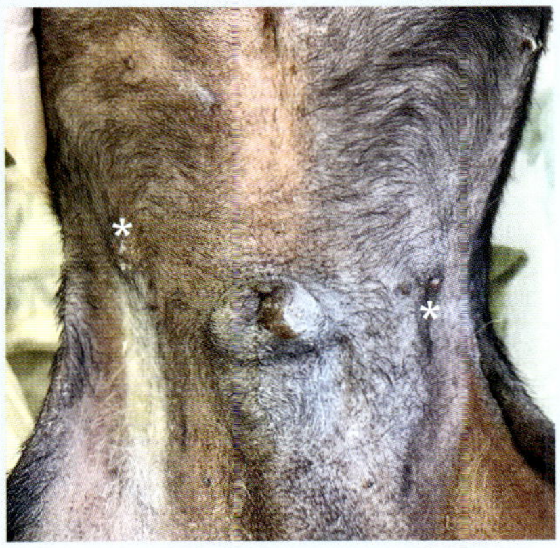

FIGURE 3. Ureterostomy is performed via an open technique. The ureters are anastomosed to the ventrolateral abdominal skin to create a ureterocutaneous stoma (asterisks) using a simple interrupted suture (Ethicon Monocryl 5/0).

Tips and tricks

✓ The owner of the dog preferred laparoscopic surgery over open surgery. The psychological impact of minimally invasive surgery sometimes allows us to perform procedures that otherwise would have been rejected.

27 LAPAROSCOPIC ARTIFICIAL URETHRAL SPHINCTER (AUS) IMPLANTATION

F. J. Pérez Duarte, Maurici Batalla, M. A. Sánchez Hurtado, J. Gutiérrez del Sol

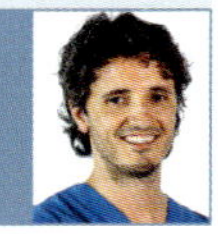

Indications

- Animals with urethral sphincter mechanism incompetence, congenital or acquired, that do not respond to medical treatment.
- Animals with ureteral ectopia in which urinary incontinence persists after corrective surgery of the ectopic ureter.
- Animals in which other surgical techniques for the treatment of urethral sphincter mechanism incompetence have failed.

Contraindications

- The main contraindication is incontinence caused by recurrent cystitis or urinary tract infections. In these cases, the infection should be treated and the AUS implanted only if incontinence persists after a negative urine culture has been obtained.
- In animals with incontinence due to ureteral ectopia, the ectopic ureter should be surgically corrected first and the AUS implanted only if incontinence persists after surgery.
- As for any laparoscopic procedure, patients that are hemodynamically unstable or at high anesthetic risk are not good candidates.

Urinary incontinence in dogs is a relatively common pathology that leads to a decrease in the quality of life of the animal, as well as a significant inconvenience for the owner. A constant and involuntary loss of urine over a prolonged period of time causes the skin around where it is excreted to be always wet. This induces the animal to lick the area to try to clean it, which, together with the irritant effect of urine, causes dermatitis, ulcers, and skin infections. Likewise, ascending urinary tract infections are also favored. For the owners, urinary incontinence is also a serious and even sanitary problem, since they constantly have to clean the areas where their pet's urine losses take place.

Urethral sphincter incompetence is the main cause of incontinence in female dogs, with an incidence of 5%–20% after gonadectomy, since estrogens play an important role in the tone of the urethral sphincter. Some animals with ureteral ectopia also have concomitant urethral sphincter incompetence, so that in many cases incontinence persists even after surgical correction of the ectopia.

Medical treatment of urinary incontinence with alpha-adrenergic agonists or estrogens, directly or indirectly, increases urethral sphincter tone, achieving continence in 60%–90% of cases. However, there is still a significant percentage of animals refractory to medical treatment. In addition, these drugs cause undesirable side effects, such as inappetence, gastrointestinal discomfort, lethargy, or aggressiveness.

In cases that are refractory to medical treatment or when the owners refuse long-term medical therapy, a surgical approach may be used. Several traditional surgical techniques have been used for the treatment of urinary incontinence, such as colposuspension, cystourethropexy, transpelvic sling, or urethral intussusception. The aim of these procedures is to increase the pressure around the urethra by direct compression or by cranially repositioning the bladder sphincter to a more cranial position within the abdomen. The long-term results of these techniques are very variable, achieving continence in 14%–70% of cases, so that a high percentage of animals remain incontinent or require continued medical treatment. For this reason, the use of devices or implants such as the transobturator vaginal tape, the injection of bulking agents (collagen or Teflon), or the implantation of an artificial urethral sphincter (AUS) have been recently described. Injection of collagen into the urethral submucosa has shown very good short-term results, but most animals experience relapses in less than 2 years and necessitate repeat procedures. With the transobturator vaginal tape continence is achieved in 40% of treated animals and in 80% of cases if combined with medical therapy.

The AUS is a silicone device that is surgically placed around the urethra and can be gradually inflated postoperatively through a subcutaneous port. In this way, progressive compression of the urethra is performed until continence is achieved. Several studies involving the implantation of this device by open surgery have shown very good results in the medium to long term, with minimal complications. However, there is only one study on AUS placement by laparoscopic approach. This study was performed on 10 cadaveric female dogs and describes and demonstrates the feasibility of the laparoscopic approach for AUS placement. In 2018, the authors' group presented a case report at the VES Congress 2018 (Lisbon) on the laparoscopic placement of an AUS in a live patient. Since then, the authors have performed this technique in a larger number of patients, although the results have not yet been published in any specialized journal. In this chapter, the surgical technique for laparoscopic AUS placement in living patients is described.

> The placement of an AUS in a live patient by open surgery was first described in 2009 by Rose et al. in four female dogs with urinary incontinence.

PATIENT PREPARATION AND POSITIONING

The patient should be fasted of solids for 12 hours prior to surgery. The abdomen is draped and aseptically prepared as if it were an open surgery.

The animal is placed in dorsal recumbency and a Trendelenburg position of 20°, thus displacing the bowels cranially to obtain more space in the pelvic cavity. At the beginning of the surgery, the urinary bladder should be exposed, with the medial ligament of the bladder and its two lateral ligaments. In some patients, depending on the amount of fat they have, the iliac vessels and the ureters can also be identified. It is advisable to also locate the colon and, in female animals, the uterus or uterine stump.

Once the visceral fascia of the pelvis has been opened, the urethra and periurethral tissue, the bladder trigone, and the entrance of both ureters into the bladder should be identified (**Fig. 1**).

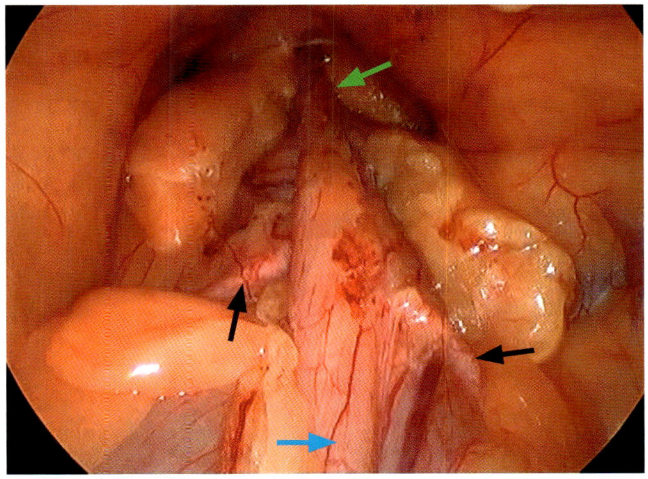

FIGURE 1. The most important anatomical landmarks in laparoscopic AUS implantation are both ureters (black arrows), the bladder (blue arrow), and the urethra (green arrow).

OPERATING ROOM LAYOUT

The laparoscopy tower is placed at the foot of the operating table. The surgeon and the assistant position themselves on the left and right side of the patient, respectively (**Fig. 2**).

Instruments

On the table

- Standard surgery set
- Telescope 5 mm – 30°
- Four cannulas (one 10 mm cannula + two 5 mm cannulas + one 3 mm cannula)
- Vessel-sealing device
- Grasping forceps
- Maryland dissector
- Right-angle dissector
- Needle holder
- Scissors

Ready to use:

- Endoscopic cannula for aspiration/irrigation

PORT PLACEMENT (FIG. 3)

- T1, on the midline at the level of the umbilicus, or slightly lateral to the midline to avoid the falciform ligament
- T2, on the right abdomen, caudal to the umbilicus
- T3, on the left abdomen, caudal to the umbilicus
- T4, on the right abdomen, lateral to T2

PROCEDURE (VIDEO 1)

- The trocars are introduced using the open technique, thus reducing the risk of injuring the internal organs and great vessels of the abdomen. After the first cannula has been placed (T1) and the pneumoperitoneum achieved (CO_2 8–10 mmHg), the 5 mm telescope is inserted.

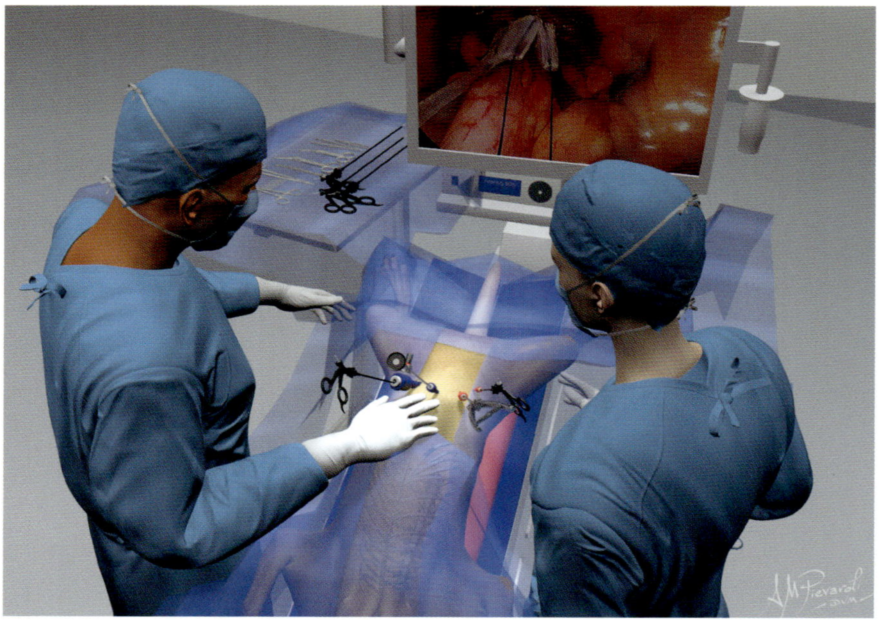

FIGURE 2. Operating room layout for laparoscopic AUS implantation.

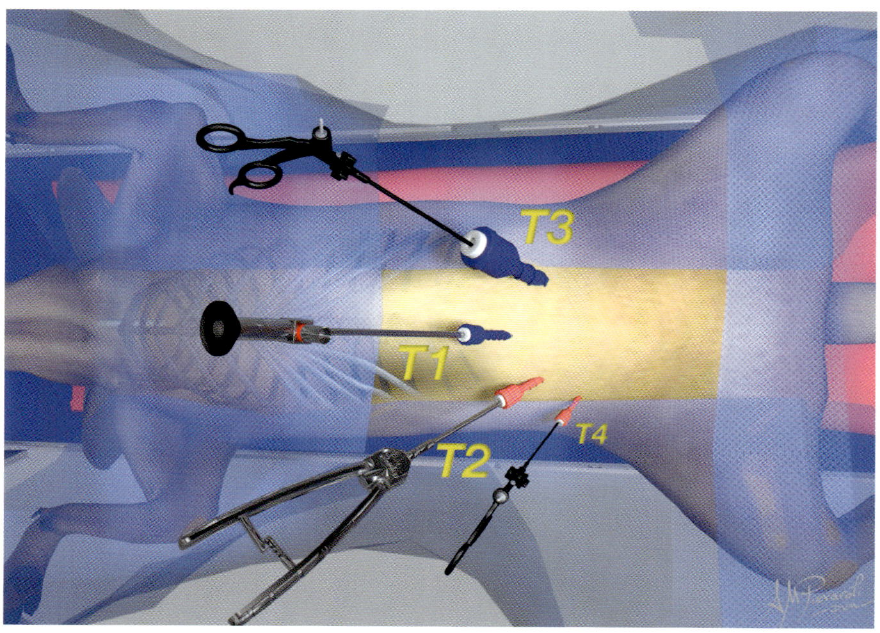

FIGURE 3. Port placement for laparoscopic AUS implantation. Using three trocars may be sufficient, but the authors recommend placing a fourth trocar to retract the bladder cranially during the procedure.

- Under laparoscopic guidance, two further trocars are placed symmetrically on the right (T2, 5 mm) and left (T3, 10 mm) abdominal wall, caudal to the umbilicus and in a triangulated fashion with respect to T1.
- The fourth cannula (T4, 3 mm) is placed on the right abdomen, lateral to T2. This fourth port will be used to introduce a 3 mm grasper to retract the bladder cranially, improving the visualization of the urethra.
- The medial ligament of the bladder is incised using a vessel-sealing device or monopolar scissors until the proximal urethra is exposed, and the bladder is retracted cranially with the 3 mm grasper (**Fig. 4**). Before beginning the dissection of the urethra, it is essential to identify the entrance of the ureters in the bladder trigone to prevent inadvertent ureteral injury.
- In some patients, it is necessary to dissect the fat around the trigone area in order to clearly identify the ureters and bladder trigone. The proximal urethra, caudal to the ureters, is isolated by blunt dissection of the periurethral connective tissue with scissors, Maryland dissector, and right-angle dissector. Thus, a 2 cm window is created circumferentially around the proximal urethra caudal to the ureters and trigone, taking care to avoid trauma to the urethra or vagina during dissection (**Fig. 5**).
- To choose the correct implant size, the outer urethral circumference is estimated by measuring the length of a suture wrapped around the urethra (**Fig. 6**). The AUS should be slightly oversized to the outer urethral circumference, so that it only exerts compression when the cuff is inflated. AUS occluder catheters are available in different lumen diameters (4, 6, 8 10, 12, 14 and 16 mm) and two cuff widths (11 and 14 mm). There are two ways to select the correct AUS size. The first one is by dividing the urethral circumference measurement by 50% (e.g., if the circumference of the urethra is 20 mm, a 10 mm device is chosen). The second one is by comparing the suture that was passed around the urethra with the AUS cuff length, to ensure that the cuff has a circumference equal or larger than that of the pelvic urethra.
- Out of the patient, a 2-0 polypropylene or nylon suture is threaded through the preexisting AUS cuff eyelet closest to the junction with the actuator tubing. The 10 mm trocar is then removed and the AUS occluder catheter is introduced into the abdomen through the trocar incision. The 10 mm trocar is placed again and the pneumoperitoneum reestablished. Using atraumatic grasping forceps, the free end of the AUS cuff is passed around the urethra through the previously created window (**Fig. 7**). During this maneuver, it is helpful to retract the bladder cranially and laterally with the 3 mm grasper in order to better visualize the urethral window.
- The cuff is then closed around the urethra by passing the free end of the suture through the opposite side of the cuff eyelet, from caudal to cranial (**Fig. 8**). The thread is secured by the application of two endoclips and intracorporeal knot tying to prevent slippage of the clips (**Fig. 9**). In the authors' opinion, this is probably the most challenging part of the procedure because the eyelet diameter is narrow in comparison with the suture, and it is very difficult to achieve a good angle with the instruments to introduce the suture through

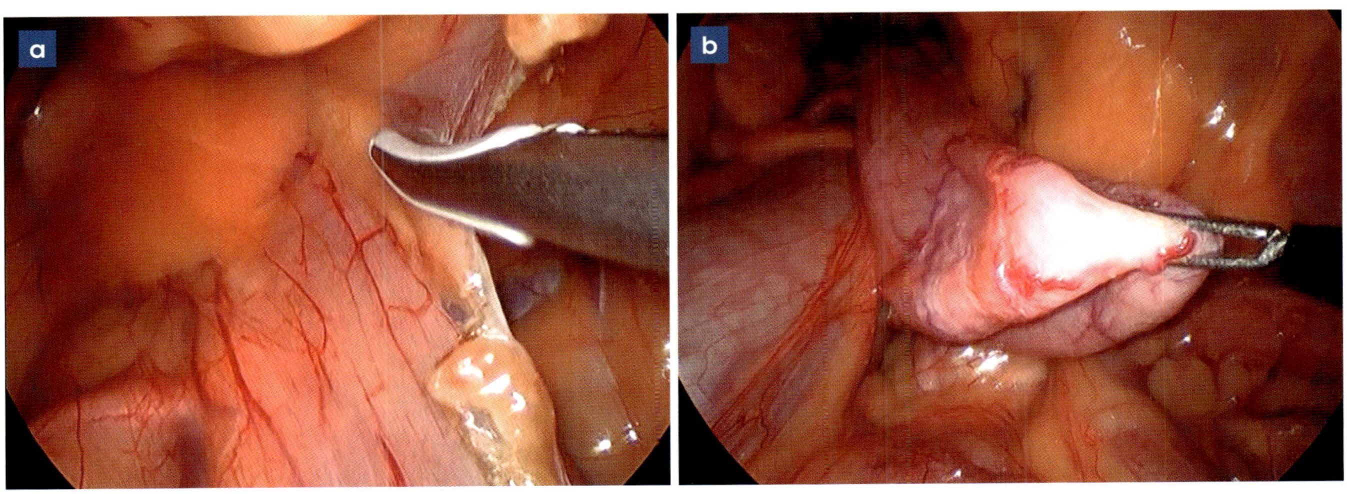

FIGURE 4. a) The medial ligament of the bladder is incised with electrocautery or vessel-sealing device to expose the proximal urethra. b) During the procedure, the bladder should be retracted cranially using a 3 mm grasper in order to improve the visualization of the pelvic urethra.

the eyelet in a caudal to cranial direction. Another way to perform this maneuver easily involves passing, outside the patient, two 2-0 polypropylene or nylon independent sutures through each of the eyelets of the cuff. Once the cuff has been passed around the urethra, both threads are secured by the application of two endoclips and intracorporeal knot tying to prevent slippage of the clips (**Fig. 10**).

- The free end of the actuator tubing is then retrieved from the abdominal cavity through the 10 mm trocar incision, which was extended 4–5 cm (**Fig. 11**). The body wall lateral to this incision is bluntly dissected between the subcutaneous tissue and ventral muscle fascia, creating a pocket for the injection port to one side so that the port septum does not lie directly beneath the skin incision line.
- The actuator tubing is cut to an appropriate length so there is no tension or tube twisting (**Fig. 12**), and the AUS system is primed with sterile saline (0.9% NaCl) to remove all air. This is performed by inserting a long 22-gauge catheter into the lumen of the actuator tubing and retrogradely filling the tubing with the saline solution. The subcutaneous port is also primed to remove all air by flushing sterile saline using a Huber-point needle. The end of the tubing is connected to the barbed connector of the infusion port covering this junction with the blue silicone boot supplied by the manufacturer of the port. This boot reinforces the connection of the port and AUS occluder catheter to prevent kinking, leakage, or disconnection. Finally, the infusion port is anchored to the superficial fascia of the abdominal wall with a 2-0 monofilament nonabsorbable suture using all suture holes around the perimeter of the port, and the trocars incisions are closed routinely. It is recommended to not inflate the device at the time of surgery.

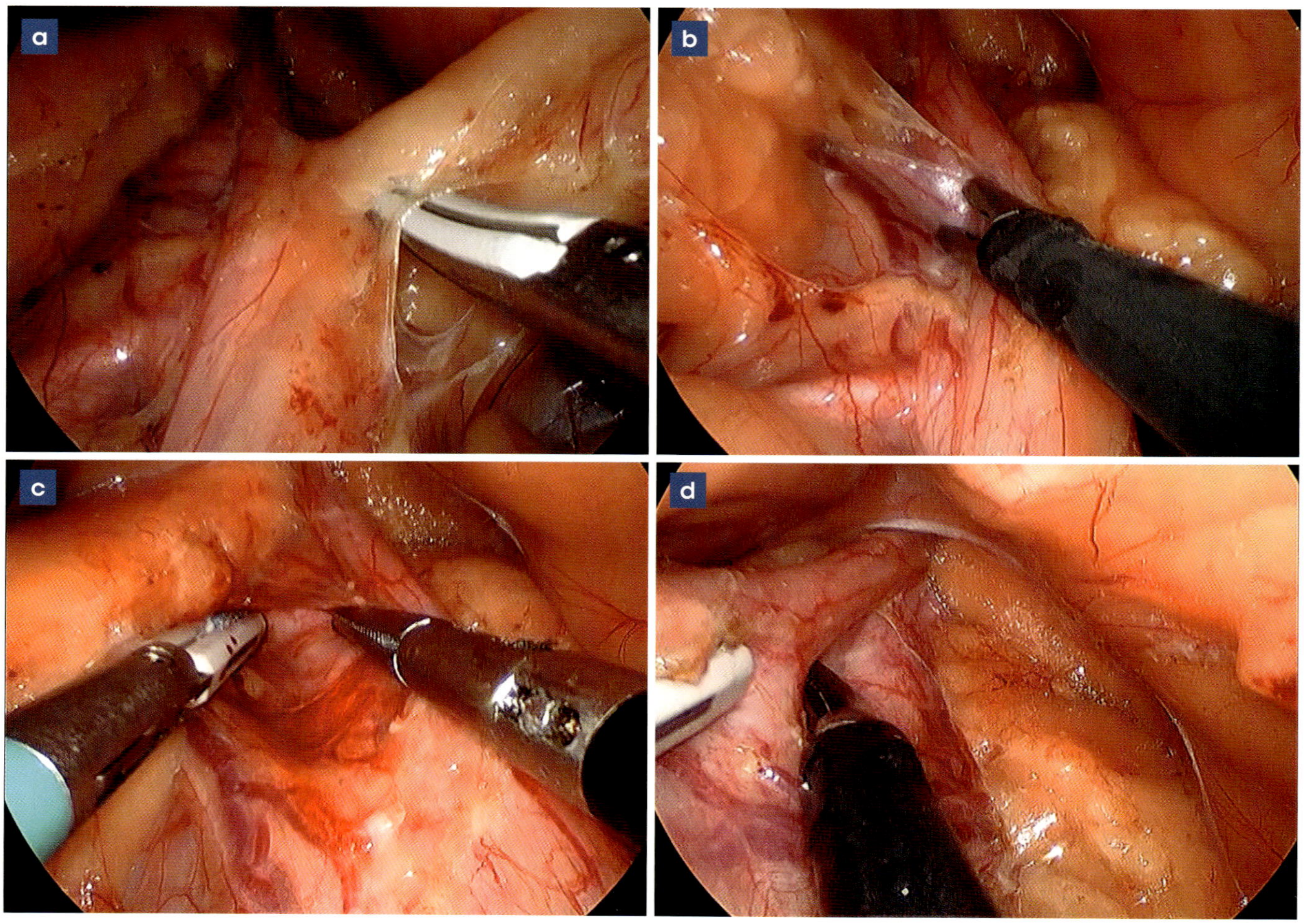

FIGURE 5. a) The fat around the bladder trigone is dissected to clearly identify the ureters and trigone. b,c) The proximal urethra, caudal to the ureters, is dissected and isolated. d) A 2 cm window is created around the proximal urethra caudal to the trigone.

VIDEO 1. Laparoscopic AUS placement.

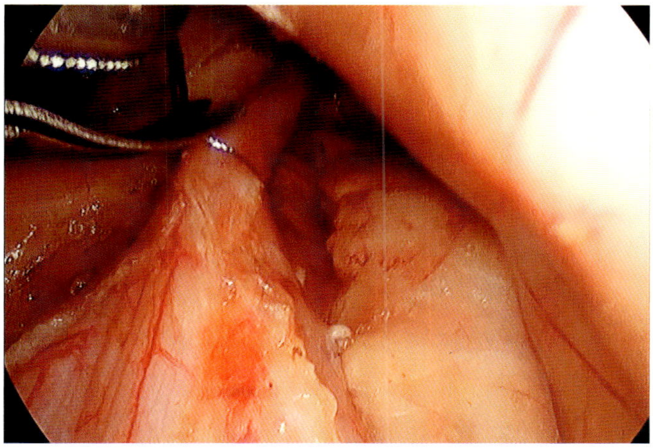

FIGURE 6. The outer urethral circumference, estimated by measuring the length of a suture wrapped around the urethra, is used to choose the correct implant size.

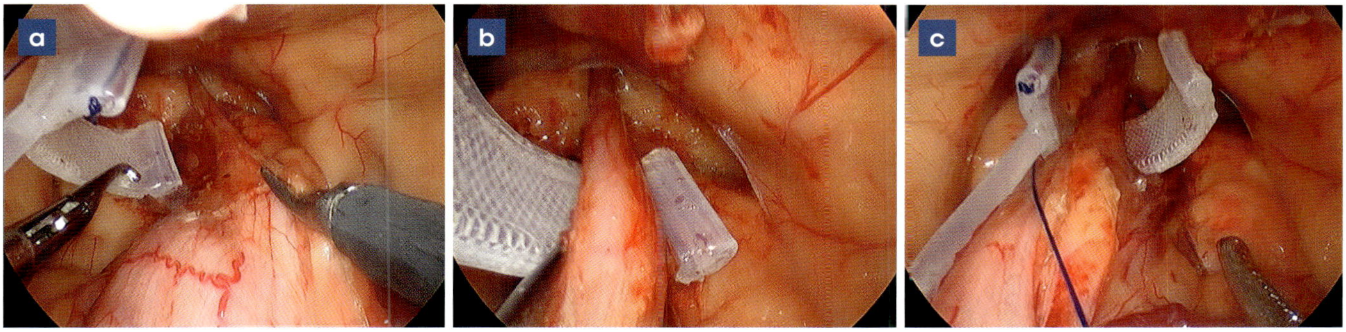

FIGURE 7. With the bladder cranially retracted, the free end of the AUS cuff is passed around urethra through the previously created window.

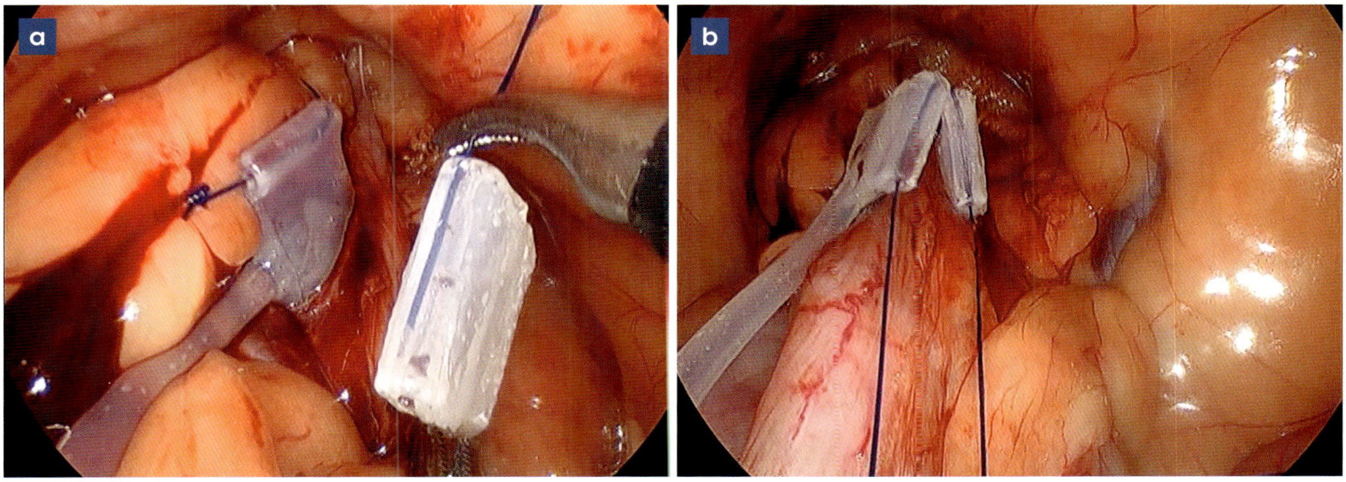

FIGURE 8. a) The free end of the suture is passed through the opposite side of the AUS cuff eyelet, from caudal to cranial. b) This way, the cuff is closed around the urethra.

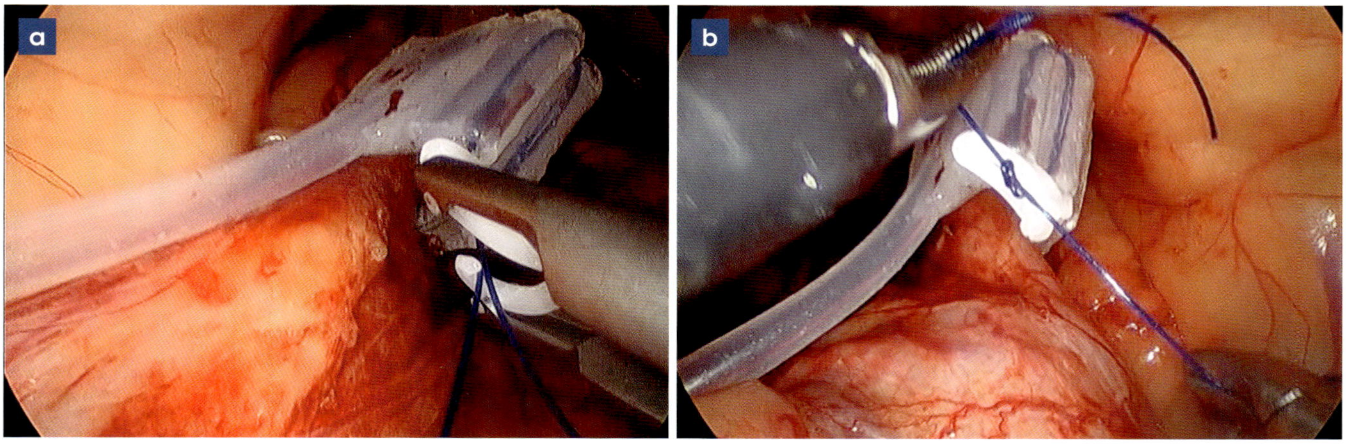

FIGURE 9. a) The AUS is kept closed around the urethra by placing two endoclips across the suture. b) Intracorporeal knot tying is performed to prevent slippage of the clips.

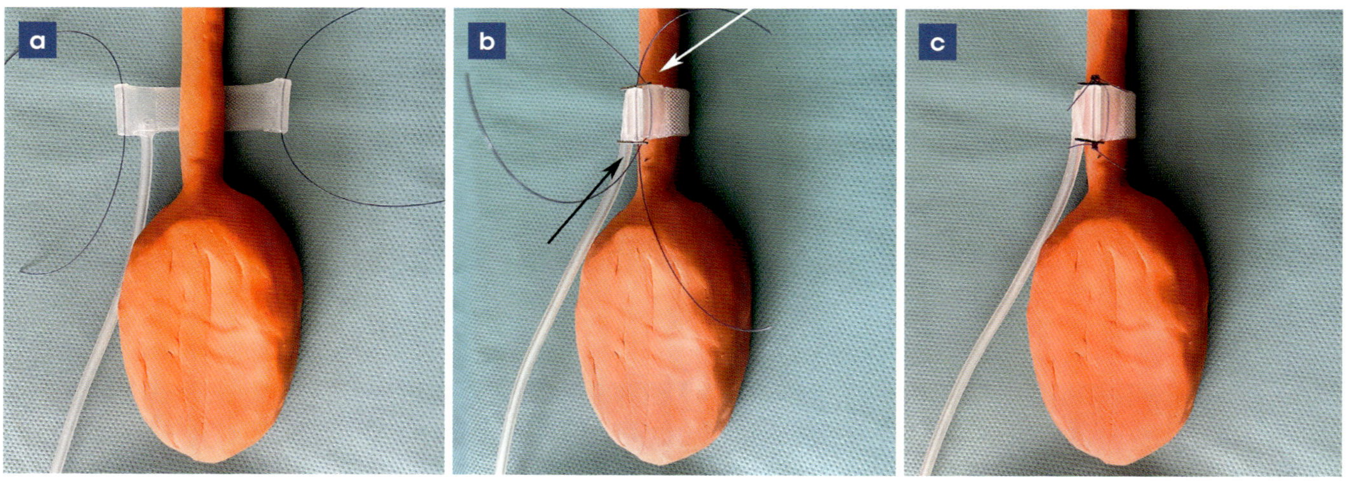

FIGURE 10. a) Outside the patient, two 2-0 independent sutures are passed through each eyelet of the AUS cuff. b) Two endoclips are applied across both caudal threads (white arrow) and the same maneuver is then performed in the cranial sutures (black arrow). c) Intracorporeal knot tying is performed to prevent slippage of the clips.

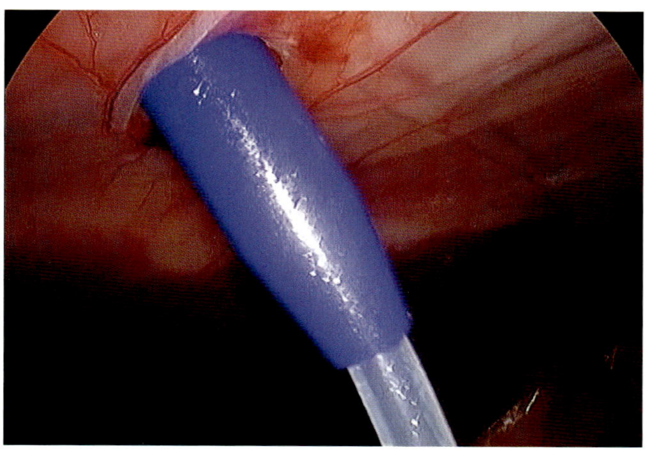

FIGURE 11. The free end of the actuator tubing is retrieved from the abdominal cavity through the 10 mm trocar incision.

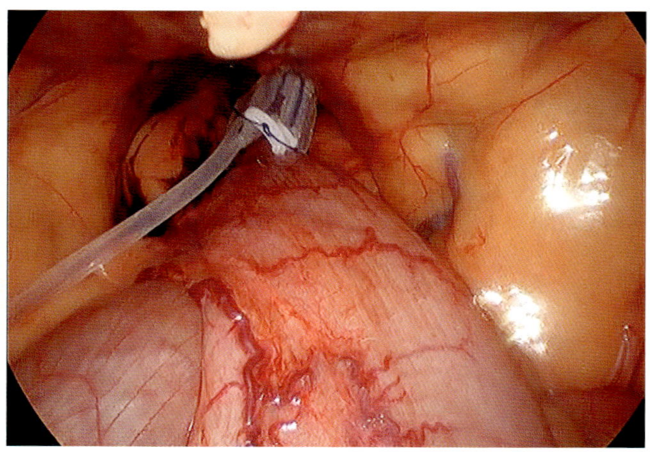

FIGURE 12. The AUS should wrap the urethra with no tension or twisting of the actuator tubing.

POSTOPERATIVE MANAGEMENT

- Adequate analgesia must be provided. Opioids such as methadone, buprenorphine, or hydromorphone can be used every 6–12 hours for the first 24 hours after surgery, depending on the degree of pain presented by the patient.
- The animal should be hospitalized and attention should be paid to the appearance of signs of urethral obstruction.
- The device should not be inflated in the immediate postoperative period to allow revascularization of the dissected periurethral tissue and thus reduce the incidence of urethral atrophy.
- At 24 hours postoperatively, if no complications have occurred, the patient is discharged with analgesics for 3–5 days (tramadol hydrochloride or meloxicam) and antibiotics (amoxicillin–clavulanic acid) for 5–7 days.
- If there are no complications, the patient is reevaluated 6 weeks after surgery. Optionally, patients can be revised at 2–3 weeks and those in which continence has not been achieved are started on medical treatment for incontinence (phenylpropanolamine and/or diethylstilbestrol).
- In patients in which continence has been achieved, only periodic examinations should be performed. In those that continue to have incontinence 6 weeks after surgery, a urine culture should be performed and, in case of a positive result, specific antibiotic therapy should be established until the infection is resolved. If the urine culture is negative, the device is progressively inflated with saline solution. To do this, the skin over the subcutaneous port is aseptically prepared by instilling saline into the port with a Hubber non-coring needle and a 1 mL syringe. The volume of saline to be instilled can be calculated in various ways, generally being 0.1–0.2 mL. Before sending the animal home, the patient should be monitored until they can urinate voluntarily. AUS inflations are repeated, again using volumes of 0.1–0.2 mL, usually at weekly intervals until continence is achieved or signs of urethral obstruction occur. Typically, the total volume of saline needed is 0.4–0.5 mL (range 0.1–0.9 mL) in 3 inflations (range 1–8 inflations).

Complications of laparoscopic AUS implantation

- The main major complication is the development of urethral obstruction, which occurs in 5%–17% of the patients. This problem is usually resolved by removing or replacing the AUS, but sometimes it is necessary to perform serial urethral dilatations or to place a self-expanding metallic urethral stent.
- Minor complications are more frequent and include urinary tract infections, temporary worsening of incontinence within the first 14 days postoperatively, seroma formation or infections in the injection port area, and mild stranguria or hematuria. These complications usually resolve within the first month after surgery.

Key points

- Before beginning the dissection of the urethra, it is essential to identify the entrance of the ureters in the bladder trigone in order to prevent inadvertent ureteral injuries.
- The AUS must be slightly oversized to the outer urethral circumference, so that it only exerts compression when the cuff is inflated.
- Passing the suture laparoscopically through the cuff eyelet can be very challenging. Alternatively, to reduce the difficulty of the maneuver, it is possible to pass two independent sutures through each of the eyelets of the cuff outside the patient.
- The AUS device should not be inflated at the time of surgery.

SUGGESTED READINGS

28 LAPAROSCOPIC PROSTATECTOMY

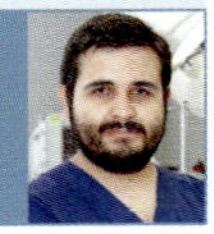

Felipe Lillo, Francesco Collivignarelli

Indications

- Confirmed high-risk prostatic cancer (several biopsies plus imaging evidence and correct clinical setting)

Contraindications

- Advanced and metastatic disease
- Urethral, bone, or deep rectal invasion
- Urinary tract infection
- Very large tumors
- Other cancer o major comorbidity

Prostatic cancer is a catastrophic disease in dogs and humans. Advanced stages are associated with morbidity and less survival. In veterinary practice, orchiectomy is very popular in male dogs; this, among other factors, may determine a relatively low prevalence (0.2%–0.6%) of prostatic cancer. However, this same context could be associated with an increase in the incidence of castration-resistant prostatic cancer, a more aggressive and high-risk form of the disease.

Large prostatic tumors cause fecal constipation, dysuria, hematuria, and urinary tenesmus. Prostatic adenocarcinoma (90% of the cases) usually invades the surrounding tissues and metastasizes through the lymphatic system, affecting regional lymph nodes before distant colonization (e.g., lungs).

Numerous therapeutic approaches have been described as palliative strategies in these cases, while only radical prostatectomy plus coadjuvant therapies are curative.

Open radical prostatectomy has not been demonstrated to be effective in veterinary medicine (median survival time of 200 days). The laparoscopic approach was a good evidence-based alternative in humans in the past; now, the standard of care is evolving toward robotic-assisted techniques.

Laparoscopic radical prostatectomy has become an alternative to treat locally and locally advanced prostatic cancer in dogs as a curative attempt. Patient selection and the owner's commitment are crucial for success. Imaging and histopathological diagnosis must be carefully confirmed before submitting a patient to surgery. If the dog is intact, castration must be performed before laparoscopic radical prostatectomy, to act as hormone therapy due to testosterone deprivation.

Tips

Patient selection is key to a successful surgery.

The first mention of a laparoscopic approach for radical prostatectomy in dogs was at the Veterinary Endoscopy Society Scientific Meeting in 2016, over 30 years after the description of the open partial technique.

DESCRIBED SURGICAL PROCEDURES

Many partial prostatectomy techniques have been described in the past. The general objective was to debulk the tumor, even with very advanced instruments such as ultrasonic aspirators. Nevertheless, the radicality of the technique favors curative intent in most cancers treated surgically. Total excision of the prostate gland should be accompanied by regional lymphadenectomy to reduce the probability of relapse due to lymphatic micrometastasis.

Laparoscopic radical prostatectomy is a challenging procedure in which the surgeon needs to cut the urethra immediately cranial and caudal to the prostate gland; in some cases, the proximal section involves the bladder neck. The urethrovesical anastomosis is performed by intracorporeal suturing, which adds to the difficulty of the technique because advanced skills are needed to maneuver in a limited working space.

In locally advanced prostatic cancer, laparoscopic radical prostatectomy, combined with androgenic deprivation and chemotherapy, is the only curative option.

PATIENT PREPARATION AND POSITIONING

Before surgery, it is imperative to confirm that urine cultures are negative and to prepare the colon with enemas and dietary modifications.

All the abdomen is widely clipped, including the medial aspect of the femoral, inguinal, and perianal regions. The patient is placed in supine recumbency and secured firmly to the operating table with atraumatic straps, and the table is set in a Trendelenburg position (**Fig. 1**). The Trendelenburg position can be delayed until the beginning of the surgery; however, the surgeon should test a 20° position before draping.

The skin and preputial cavity are aseptically prepared in the usual fashion. After the installation of surgical drapes and towels, a sterile urinary catheter is placed.

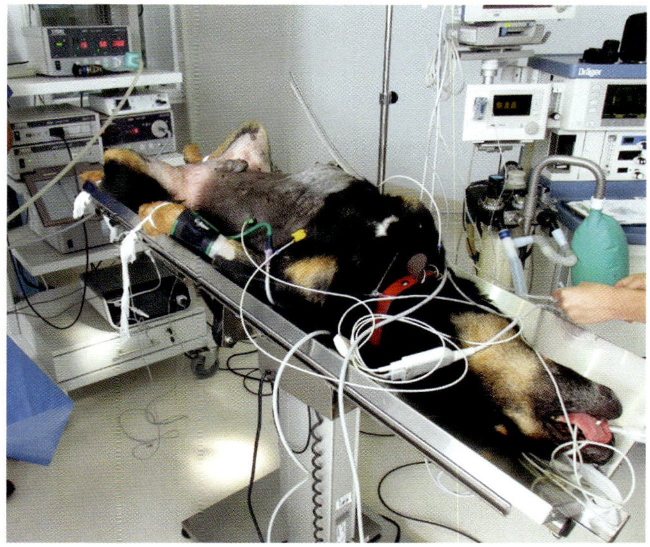

FIGURE 1. Patient in dorsal recumbency and Trendelenburg position.

OPERATING ROOM LAYOUT

Depending on the patient's size, the surgeon positions themselves at the head or on the left side of the operating table. If the surgeon is right-handed, the assistant is to the left of the surgeon. The laparoscopic tower is placed caudal to the patient, the instrument table in front of the assistant, and the anesthesia machine behind the surgeon or next to the laparoscopic tower (left side) (**Fig. 2**).

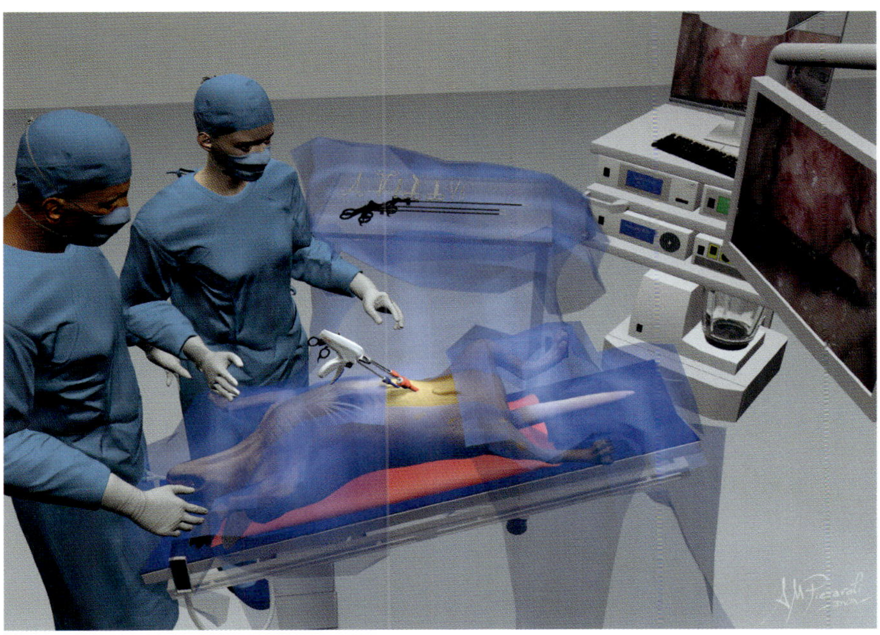

FIGURE 2. Operating room layout for laparoscopic radical prostatectomy.

Instruments

On the table:

- Standard surgery set
- Telescope 5 or 10 mm – 30°
- Two 5 mm cannulas + one 10 mm cannula (or one 5 mm cannula + two 10 mm cannulas if using a 10 mm telescope)
- Grasping forceps
- Maryland forceps
- Laparoscopic needle driver
- Laparoscopic scissors
- Aspiration/irrigation cannula for laparoscopy
- Laparoscopic tissue retrieval bag
- Ultrasonic laparoscopic scalpel or vessel-sealing device

PORT PLACEMENT (FIG. 3)

- T1, on the midline, 1–2 cm caudal to the umbilicus
- T2, immediately medial to the left mammary line, 4–6 cm caudal to T1
- T3, immediately medial to the right mammary line, 4–6 cm caudal to T1
- Optionally, T4 and T5, immediately medial to the inguinal line (left and right), 4–6 cm caudal to T2 and T3, respectively

PROCEDURE

- After the first port has been placed and the pneumoperitoneum achieved, the 5 or 10 mm telescope is inserted in T1 and a first exploration of the abdomen is performed to check for any evidence of iatrogenic trauma caused by placement of the first cannula. The pelvic cavity is explored and the external iliac arteries and common iliac veins are identified.
- Under endoscopic vision, the other two cannulas (T2 for 10 mm right-hand instruments and T3 for 5 mm left-hand instruments) are inserted.
- Using the ultrasonic scalpel, the median vesical ligament is severed as close to the abdominal wall as possible (**Fig. 4**). When the vesicoabdominal peritoneal recess is reached, the caudal peritoneum is opened and the incision extended to the right and dorsally and to the left and dorsally, making a trapezoid-shaped incision in the peritoneum.
- Ventral and lateral periprostatic dissection is made using the ultrasonic scalpel and by divulsion with the Maryland forceps. The surgeon should make sure that the dissection is performed as close as is possible to the tumor to spare the nerves responsible for urinary control (**Fig. 5**).
- The proximal urethra is incised after pushing the prostate gland caudally (away from the bladder neck). When the scalpel reaches the urethral lumen, the urinary catheter can be exteriorized and used as a grasping point (**Fig. 6**). After sectioning the urethra, both vasa deferentia should be visible and are sectioned as well. Using forceps, the vas deferens

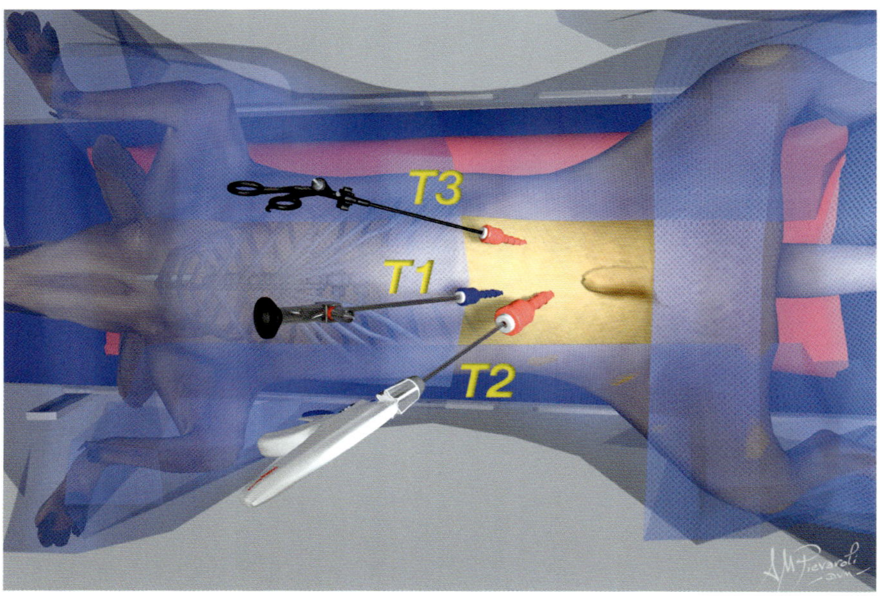

FIGURE 3. Port placement for laparoscopic radical prostatectomy.

stump is grasped to mobilize and elevate the prostate in order to dissect the dorsal aspect of the gland.

- The distal urethra is severed and the tumoral prostate is bagged and saved in the abdomen. The assistant may advance the urinary catheter to identify the urethral lumen. Intracorporeally, a single stitch is made between the rectal-urethral muscle and the dorsal aspect of the bladder neck; this, called the Rocco stitch in human medicine, is used to apposition the urethra to the bladder and dissipate tissue tension.
- Urethrovesical anastomosis can be performed using a separate simple pattern or a double-needle continuous suture pattern. The authors recommend the use of the van Velthoven technique, a running suture pattern. Two threads of absorbable monofilament with half-circle round-body needles are knotted together, and each thread is used to achieve each aspect, dorsal and ventral, of the anastomosis. The dorsal plane is sutured from 3 to 9 o'clock position, stitching from serosa to mucosa on the bladder (**Fig. 7**) and from mucosa to serosa on the urethra (**Fig. 8**), all the way to the

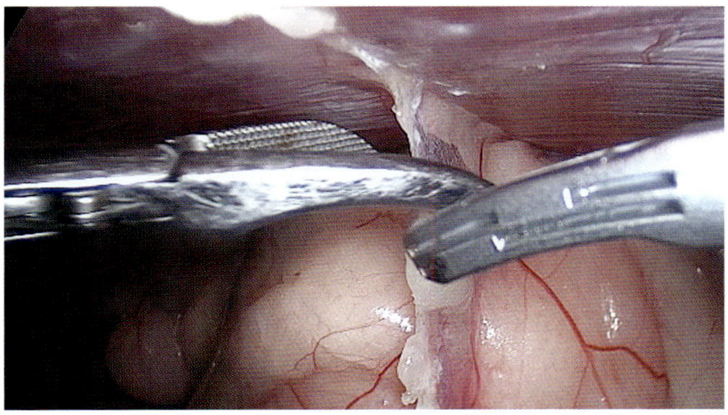

FIGURE 4. The median vesical ligament is severed.

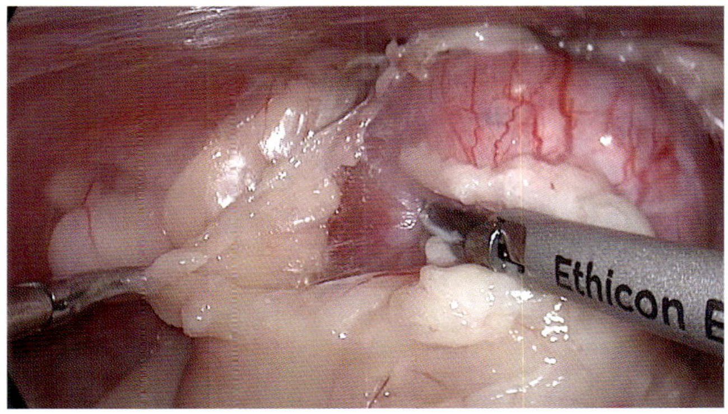

FIGURE 5. The ventral and lateral aspects of the prostate gland are dissected from the peritoneum, as close as possible to spare nerve structures.

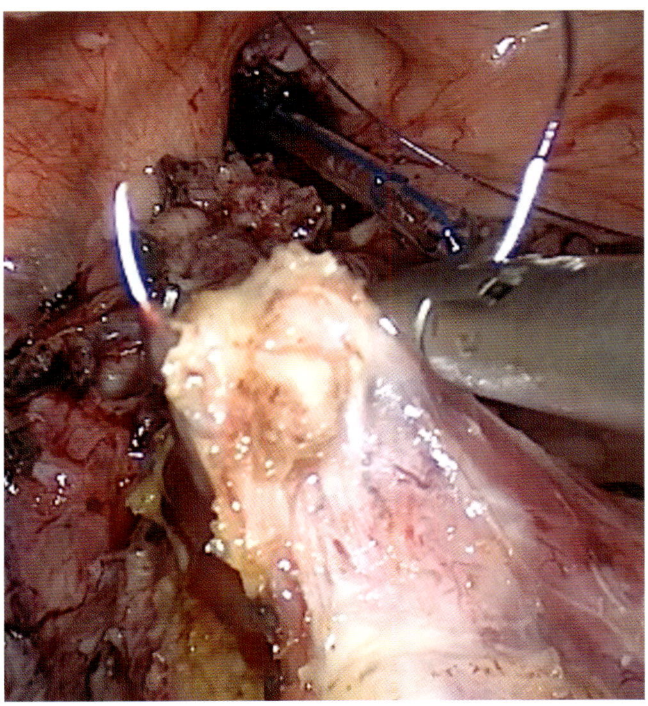

FIGURE 6. The urinary catheter is exteriorized.

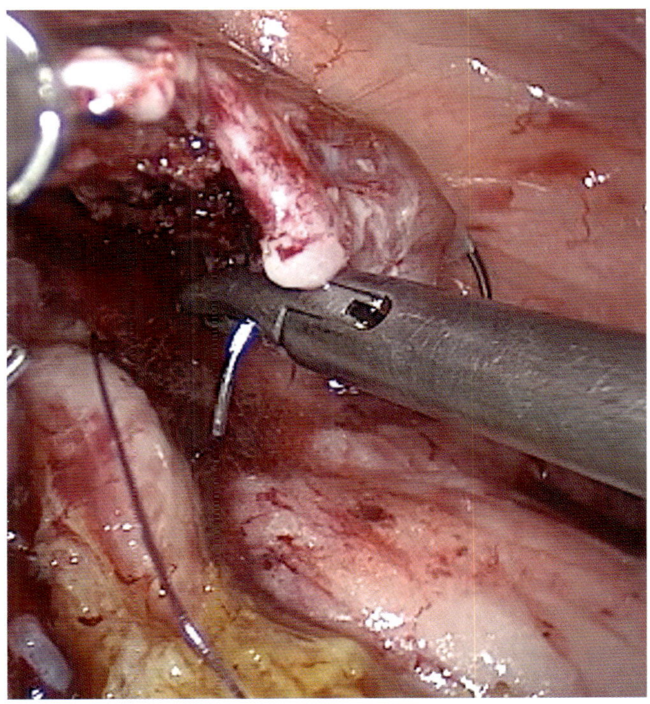

FIGURE 7. The dorsal plane is sutured from 3 to 9 o'clock position, stitching from serosa to mucosa on the bladder.

left angle (**Fig. 9**). The surgeon must be aware of the proximity of both iliac vessels and the rectum on the other side of the suture plane.

- Once the floor of the anastomosis is completed, the assistant inserts the urethral catheter into the bladder to avoid accidental obliteration of the lumen and to facilitate suturing of the ventral plane (**Fig. 10**). Using the other needle, the ventral continuous suture pattern is performed, stitching from serosa to mucosa on the urethra (**Fig. 11**) and from mucosa to serosa on the bladder neck. When the ventral plane suture is completed, both needles are cut off and the sutures are tied and knotted together intracorporeally to finish the urinary reconstruction (**Fig. 12**).
- After profuse lavage and aspiration of the field, a leak test is made to ensure the watertightness of the urethrovesical anastomosis. The test is conducted by filling the bladder with saline solution and observing if there are any signs of saline flow (**Fig. 13**). If there are no leaks, regional lymphadenectomy is performed, the bagged tumoral specimen extracted, the pneumoperitoneum evacuated, and the incisions closed.

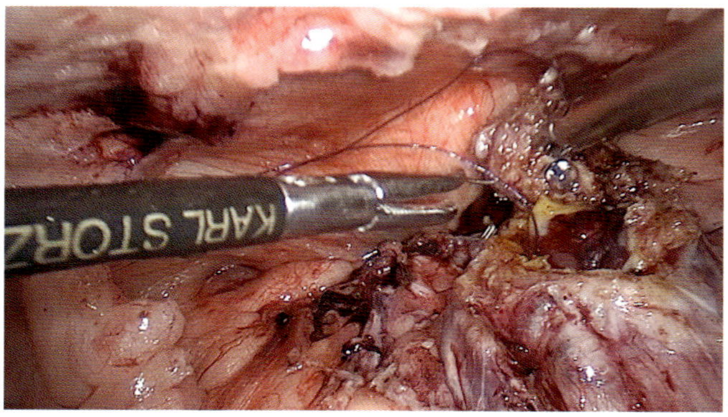

FIGURE 8. Suture from mucosa to serosa on the urethra.

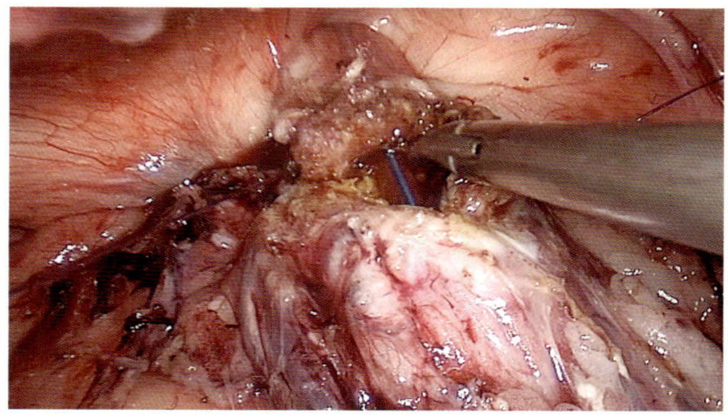

FIGURE 9. Terminoterminal vesicourethral anastomosis.

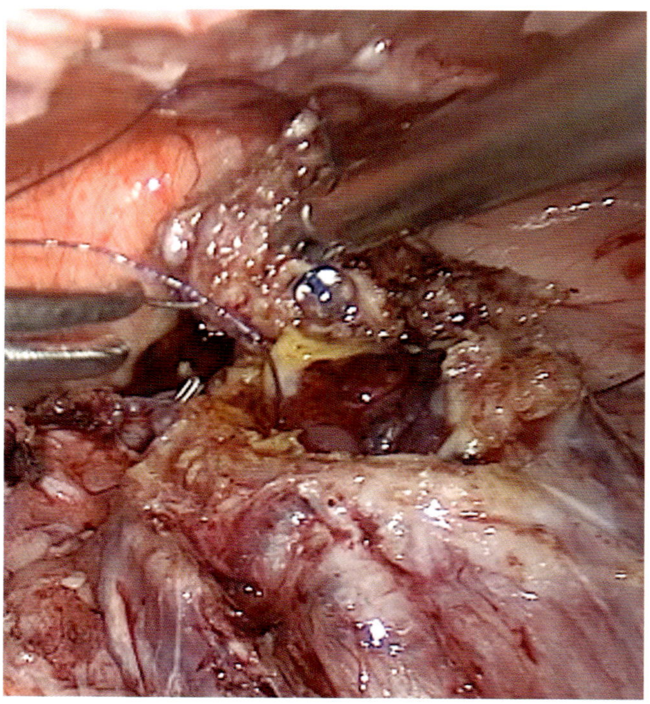

FIGURE 10. The assistant inserts the urethral catheter into the bladder.

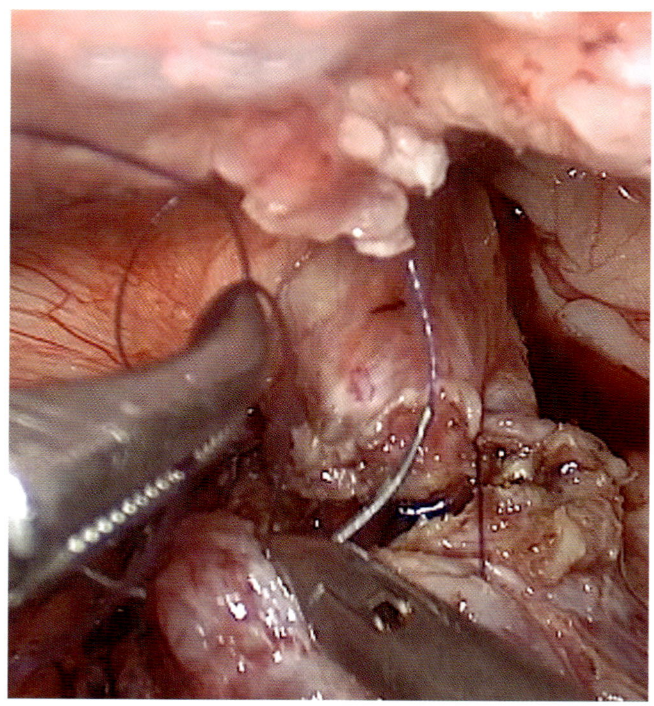

FIGURE 11. Ventral continuous suture pattern, stitching from serosa to mucosa on the urethra.

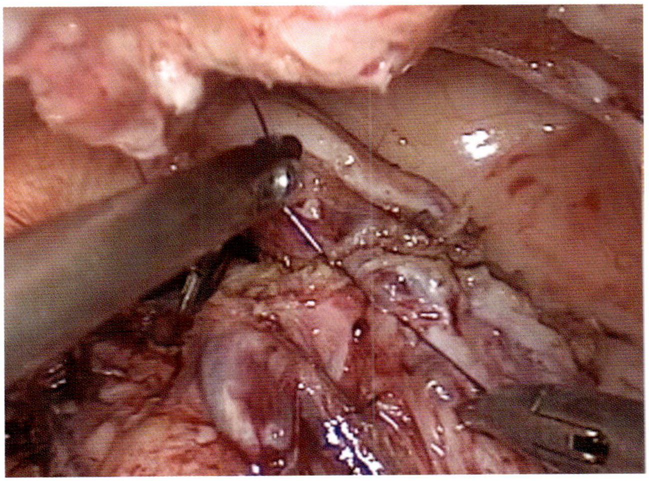

FIGURE 12. Completed urinary reconstruction.

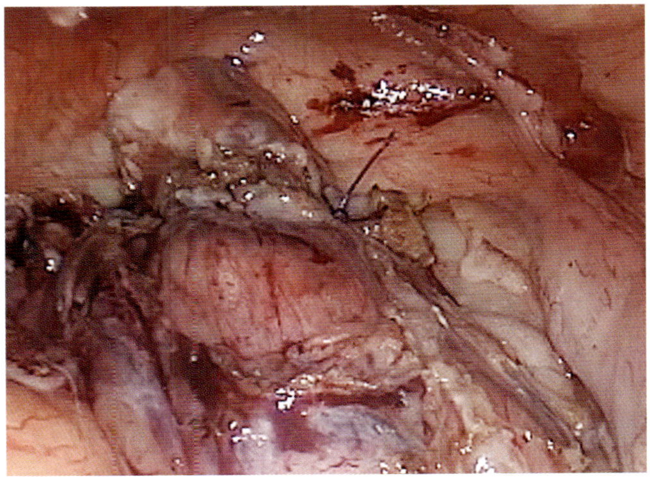

FIGURE 13. The leak test is conducted by filling the bladder with saline. No leaks are noted.

POSTOPERATIVE MANAGEMENT

- Urinary leakage to the peritoneal cavity and urethral obstruction are the most important surgical concerns during the first hours after surgery. The urinary catheter (ideally a Foley catheter) must be maintained for at least 74 hours. Then, the catheter can be changed regularly until the 15th day after surgery.
- Ultrasonographic follow-up (AFAST) every 6 hours for 2 days is used to early detect any leakages.
- Postsurgical analysis of electrolytes and a kidney biochemical panel are recommended.
- Pain must be carefully evaluated and controlled.

Complications of laparoscopic radical prostatectomy

- Early complications include urinary leakage, urethral obstruction, infections, and peritonitis. The general suggestion is to reoperate in the presence of the former two situations, while partial obstructions can be solved using urethral stents.
- The most frequent long-lasting complication described in the literature is urinary incontinence; between 33% and 100% of the patients suffer any form of this condition after surgery. If the nerve-sparing technique has been performed properly, continence can be completely or partially recovered by the 90th day postoperatively.

Key points

- Make sure to avoid injury to the lateral ligaments of the bladder and ureters.
- When performing the urethrovesical anastomosis, use the urinary catheter as guidance. The assistant may actively move the catheter to facilitate needle passage and to avoid inadvertently suturing the catheter to the urethra.
- Delay the extraction of the tissue specimens until the end of the surgery.

SUGGESTED READINGS

29 LAPAROSCOPIC OMENTALIZATION OF PARAPROSTATIC CYSTS

Andrea M. Pievaroli

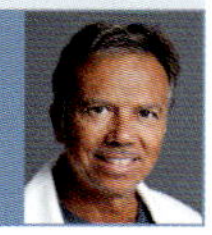

Indications

- Video-assisted drainage of prostatic cysts
- Total/partial resection of discrete prostatic cysts
- Omentalization of discrete prostatic cysts
- Prostate needle aspiration and biopsies

Contraindications

- Extensive adhesions to surrounding tissues
- Presence of purulent material in the cysts; in the case of a laparoscopic approach, abundant laparoscopic abdominal lavage is necessary
- Cardiovascular and pulmonary disease

The general term prostatic cyst refers to those fluid-filled cavity formations that affect the prostate gland or are connected to it. Different terminologies can be found in the literature to identify prostate cysts based on their origin and location.

Small prostatic cysts—or microcysts—located within the prostate tissue are almost always associated with benign prostatic hypertrophy (BPH). Their formation is due to the dysfunctional flow of prostatic secretions. These microcysts are rarely of clinical importance, and if correlated with BHP, castration surgical treatment is successful in most cases.

Discrete prostatic cysts are larger fluid-filled vesicles that develop separately from the prostate gland but have some attachment to the capsule. The fluid aspect is pale yellow to orange to brownish-red. Some authors distinguish discrete prostatic cysts into two categories: prostatic retention cysts and paraprostatic cysts.

Prostatic retention cysts seem to be an evolution of prostatic microcysts that increase significantly in volume due to obstructions of the ducts within the gland parenchyma. Paraprostatic cysts do not have structural communications with the prostate gland or the urethra. The causes of their origin are still controversial; one of the hypotheses is that paraprostatic cysts may originate from the uterus masculinus, an embryonic structure derived from the Müllerian duct system.

Prostate cysts are usually asymptomatic, but as they increase in size, they may extend into the abdomen or the perineal fossa. In this case, they determine the symptomatology linked to compressive phenomena on the adjacent structures. The patient may therefore present with pain and abnormal urination, including stranguria, dysuria, and hematuria. It is also possible to find abnormal defecation, perineal swellings, depression, and inappetence. Patients are generally afebrile unless they result in abscessation due to ascending bacterial infection from the urethra. Cystic lesions may become infected in 50% of the cases; for this reason, early diagnosis and treatment are recommended.

In addition to the clinical signs, a definitive diagnosis is obtained with an ultrasound examination (**Fig. 1**). It is also necessary to perform laboratory investigations and cytological and chemical analysis of the prostate tissue material and the content from the cysts obtained through needle aspiration.

First-choice surgical treatment of discrete prostatic cysts consists of castration combined with ultrasound-guided cyst drainage. In most cases, after a short period of improvement, there is recurrence with a volume increase of the cysts. In this case, a surgical resection of the cysts, associated with omentalization, is necessary. It is preferable to perform a partial resection to reduce the risk of damaging the surrounding structures and minimize the risk of urinary incontinence. The omentum acts as a physiological drain, being a source of vascularization and lymphatic supply. It has angiogenic and phagocytic properties and minimizes the formation of postoperative adhesions.

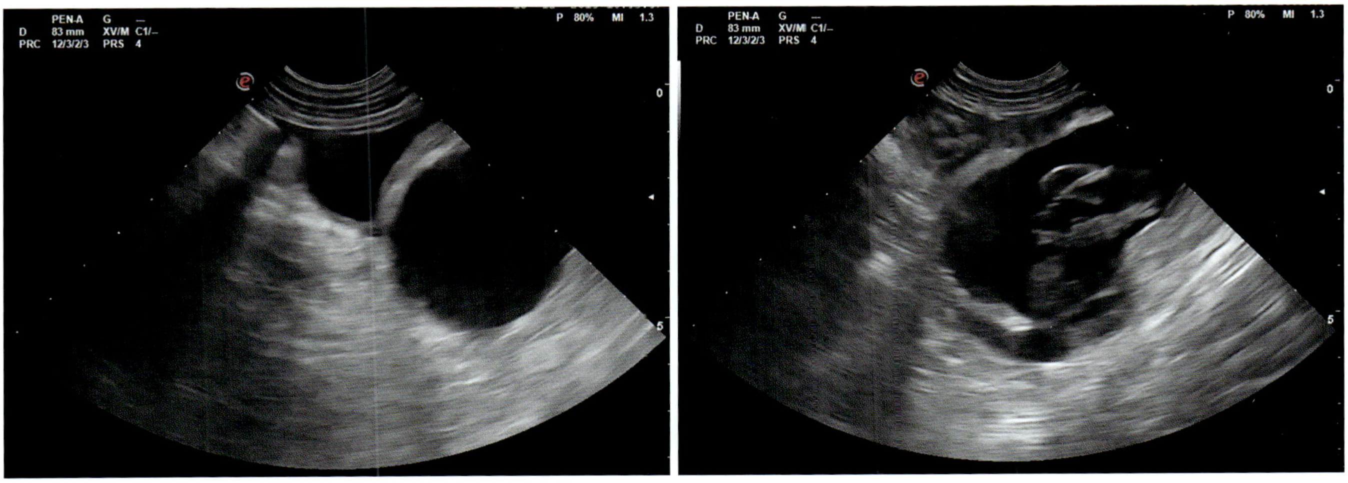

FIGURE 1. Ultrasound images of paraprostatic cysts.

This procedure can also be performed in laparoscopy to reduce invasiveness for the very caudal position of the prostate gland and prostatic cysts.

> Although this procedure has been reported as a personal experience by various authors, the first description in the veterinary literature was notified in 2021 by N. Comas Collgós, et al.

PATIENT PREPARATION AND POSITIONING

The patient should be fasted for 10–12 hours before surgery. It is preferable to start antibiotic therapy before surgery, to minimize the risk of intraoperative infections during the incision and drainage of prostatic cysts. The ventral abdomen is widely clipped, extending caudally to the perineal area. The patient is placed in dorsal recumbency, and the skin is aseptically prepared, including an aseptic wash of the prepuce.

It could be helpful to tilt the table in a Trendelenburg position (20°–30°) to allow the abdominal organs to move away from the pelvic region, improving visualization of the prostate gland and its cysts. It is mandatory to catheterize the bladder to drain the urine and to identify the prostatic urethra during the procedure.

In some cases, the laparoscopic approach has proved effective for treating large paraprostatic cysts. This procedure is described in the veterinary literature only in a few abstracts for presenting clinical cases. It has been reported as a personal initiative by some authors who perform minimally invasive surgery.

VIDEO 1. Laparoscopic omentalization of paraprostatic cysts.

The technique is performed with three ports placed in the caudal region of the abdomen. The author prefers threaded cannulas to prevent slippage from within the peritoneum. The procedure consists of aspirating the contents of the cysts, removing part of the wall, and performing the omentalization as described in the open technique. The passage of the omentum around the prostatic urethra is not always feasible. In this case, the omentum is fixed inside the cavities of the remaining portions of the prostate cysts.

OPERATING ROOM LAYOUT

Because the procedure is performed in the caudal abdomen, the monitor (or the scope tower) is placed at the caudal end of the table, leaving enough space for the surgeons to move during the procedure. The anesthesia machine is placed near the patient's head. The instrument table is set caudolateral to the table, on the same side as the surgeon. The surgeon chooses the right or the left side of the patient depending on the localization of the cysts or according to their personal preferences (right- or left-handed). The assistant positions themselves to the opposite contralateral side. It is preferable to tilt the table to a Trendelenburg position (**Fig. 2**).

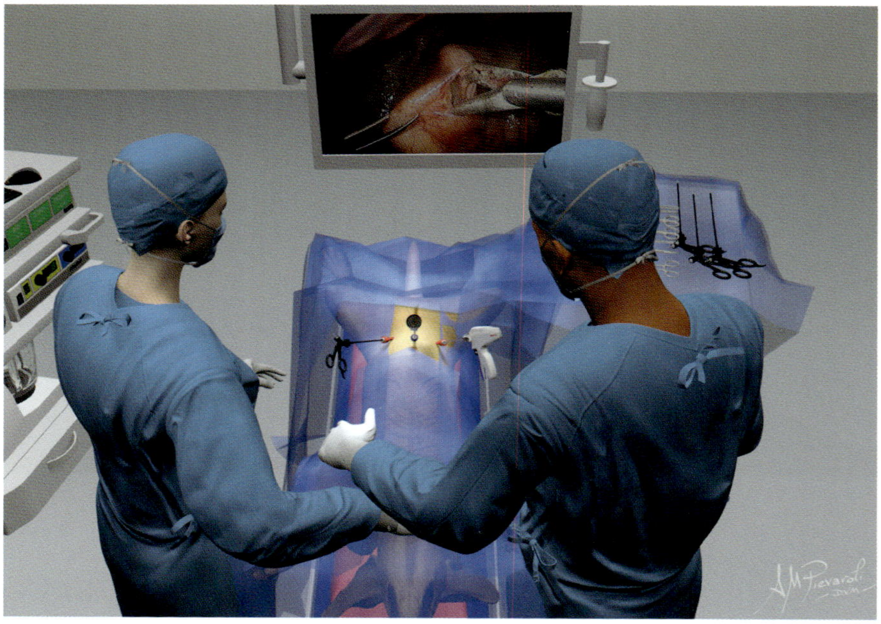

FIGURE 2. Operating room layout for laparoscopic omentalization of paraprostatic cysts.

Instruments

On the table:

- Standard surgery set
- Telescope 5 mm – 30°
- Three 5 mm threaded cannulas/trocars (or 10 mm for larger instruments)
- Grasping forceps
- Sealing device/harmonic scalpel
- Clip applier
- Endoscopic cannula for aspiration/irrigation
- Endoscopic scissors

Ready to use:

- Forth cannula to add a port if necessary
- Laparoscopic needle holder
- Endoscopic retrieval bag

PORT PLACEMENT (FIG. 3)

The technique involves using three ports oriented to the caudal region of the abdomen. Only 5 mm trocars may be sufficient for this type of surgery without using special larger-sized instruments. Pneumoperitoneum is determined according to individual preferences. The author prefers to use the Ternamian technique or a modified Hasson technique, using threaded cannulas as ports (Storz Endotip) because they are more stable once positioned in the patient. The orientation of the cannulas is chosen to allow optimal visualization of the caudal region.

The telescope port (T1) is introduced through the midline caudal to the umbilicus. The operative ports (T2, T3) are positioned laterally to the right and left paramedian lines, on the same line, or in a more caudal position to obtain the correct triangulation. Inserting a fourth operative port (T4) may be necessary during the procedure to introduce additional instruments to the right or left lateral position.

- T1, on the midline, 1–3 cm caudal to the umbilicus
- T2, on a right paramedian position on the same line or caudal to T1
- T3, on a left paramedian position on the same line or caudal to T1
- T4, optional

PROCEDURE

- After the first port placement (T1), caudally to the umbilicus and pneumoperitoneum, has been achieved, the 5 mm telescope is inserted, and the first exploration of the abdomen is performed to make sure no injuries to the organs were caused during the introduction of the first cannula.
- Often, the falciform ligament can be found in this area of the peritoneum, which could prevent correct vision and cloud

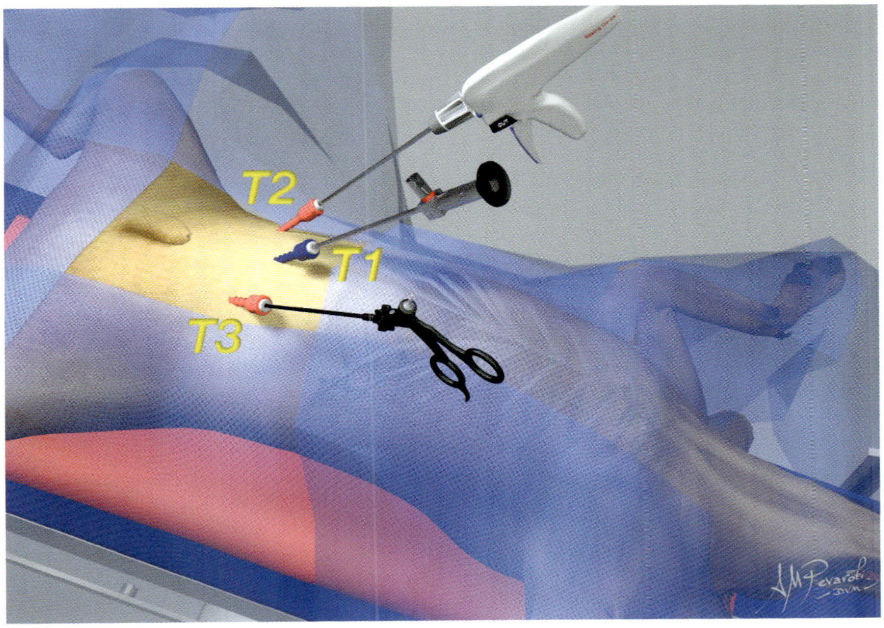

FIGURE 3. Port placement for laparoscopic omentalization of paraprostatic cysts.

the telescope lens. It is necessary to screw deeper to find the proper inclination to overcome the ligament.

- Under endoscopic vision, the other two cannulas for the operative instruments—T2 and T3—are inserted in a paramedian position on the right and left sides.
- An exploration of the region is performed for an initial evaluation of the prostatic cysts. Using a blunt probe and atraumatic forceps (**Fig. 4**) is advisable to manipulate tissues correctly.
- For better visualization of the pelvic region, it is advisable to complete the emptying of the bladder (through the catheter) and resect the ventral bladder ligament (median ligament) using a sealing device or a harmonic scalpel (**Fig. 5**).
- Paraprostatic cysts are not always directly visible because they can be surrounded by adipose tissue. In this case, it is advisable to perform a centesis under direct vision through the abdominal wall before starting the dissection to confirm

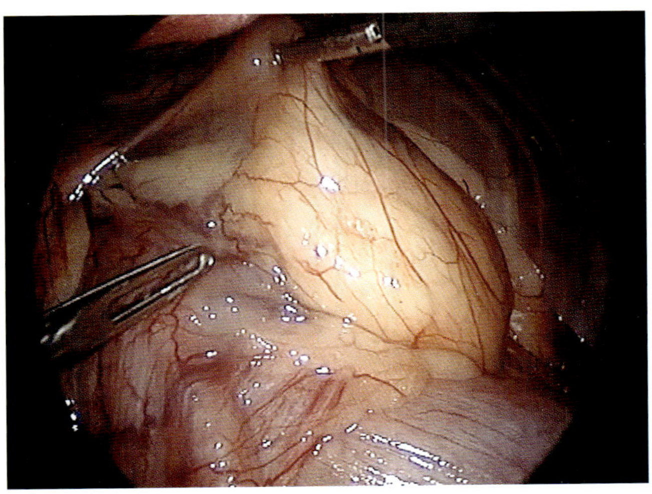

FIGURE 4. A blunt probe and atraumatic forceps for correct manipulation of the tissues must be used. The bladder and intestine need to be moved to visualize the prostate gland area.

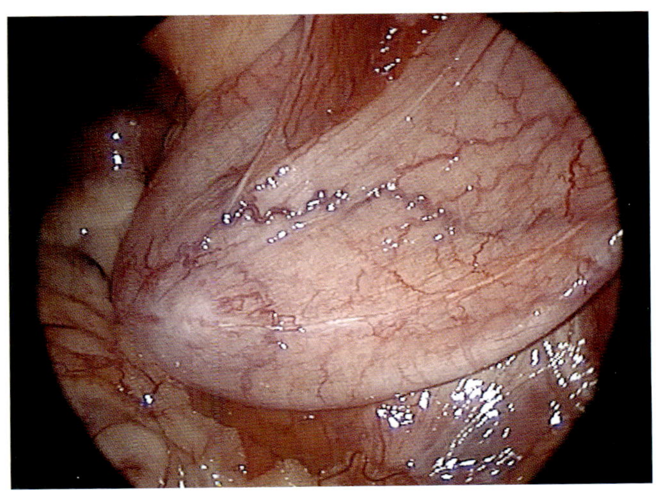

FIGURE 5. The bladder is emptied (through the urethral catheter), and eventually, the ventral bladder ligament is resected (median ligament) for better visualization of the pelvic region.

the location of the cyst, which can affect both the right and the left sides (**Fig. 6**).

- If present, dissection of the covering adipose tissue is performed until the wall of the paraprostatic cyst is identified. With the aid of scissors or a sealing device, the wall is partially incised (**Fig. 7**). The residual fluid content is aspirated to reduce the contamination of the abdomen (**Fig. 8**).
- The opening of the paraprostatic cyst is then continued by removing part of the external wall. Care must be taken not to extend the resection of the cystic wall to the prostate gland or the bladder region to minimize the risk of damage to neurovascular structures (**Fig. 9**).
- Adhesions in the cavity are debrided using a blunt probe or with the tip of the cannula during aspiration and washing.
- Some dissection is performed on the contralateral side if the paraprostatic cyst is present (**Fig. 10**).
- Using two atraumatic forceps, a leaf of omentum is grasped, moved caudally, and packed into the cystic remnant (**Figs. 11 and 12**). It is secured with some clips to the cystic wall (extracapsular technique) (**Fig. 13**). In some cases, an attempt can be made to pass the omentum around the

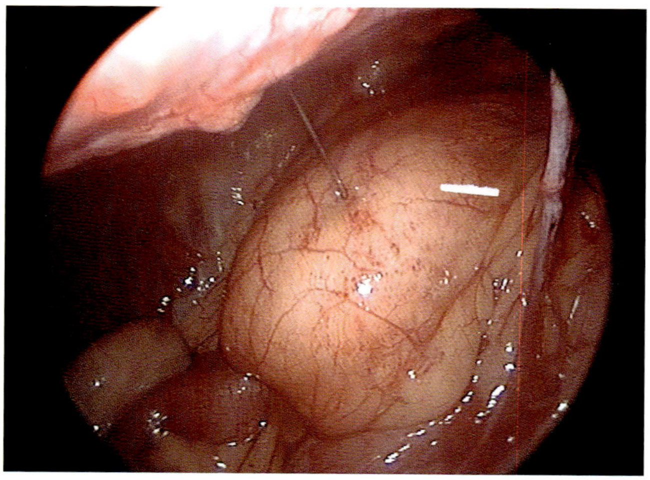

FIGURE 6. A centesis is performed under direct vision through the abdominal wall to confirm the cyst's location, surrounded by adipose tissue.

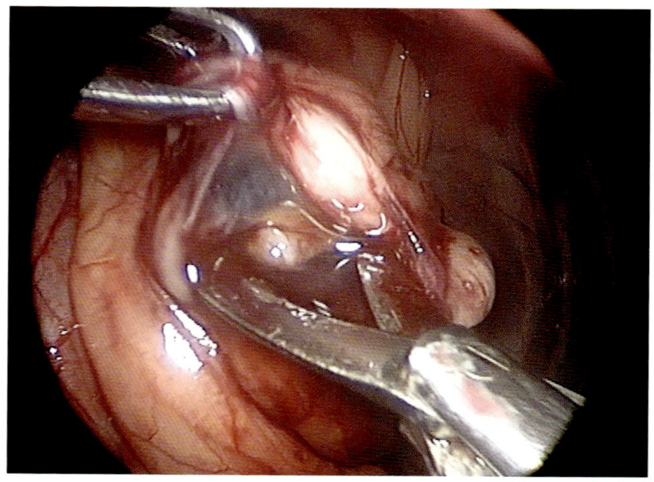

FIGURE 7. Partial incision and dissection of the cyst wall with endoscopic scissors and forceps.

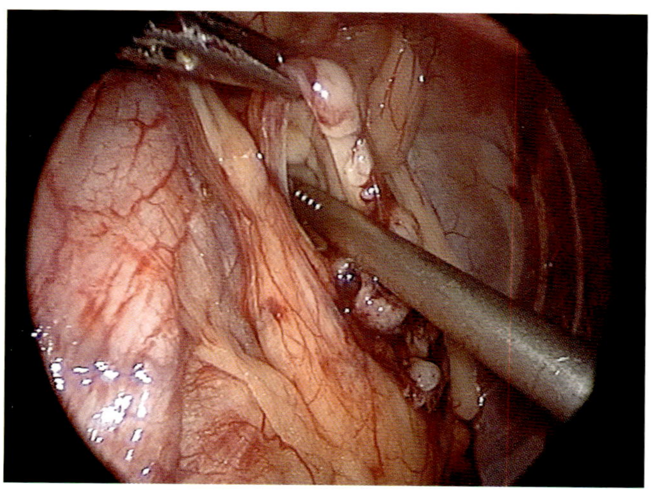

FIGURE 8. Aspiration of the residual fluid content also reduces the contamination of the abdomen.

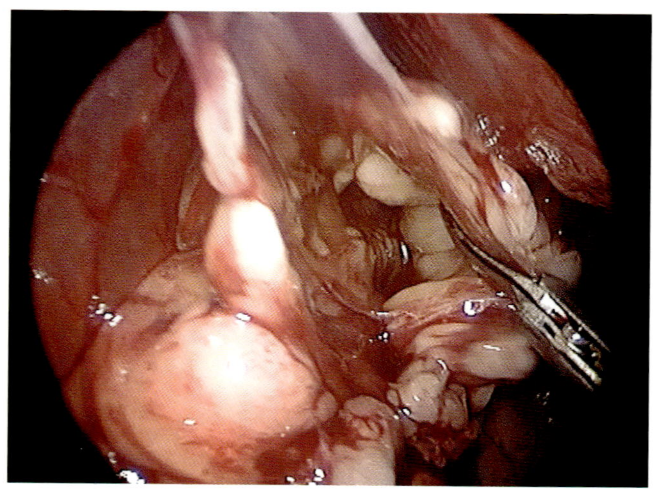

FIGURE 9. Opening of the paraprostatic cyst. Part of the external wall is removed, taking care not to extend the resection of the cystic wall in the prostate gland or the bladder regions to minimize the risk of damage to neurovascular structures.

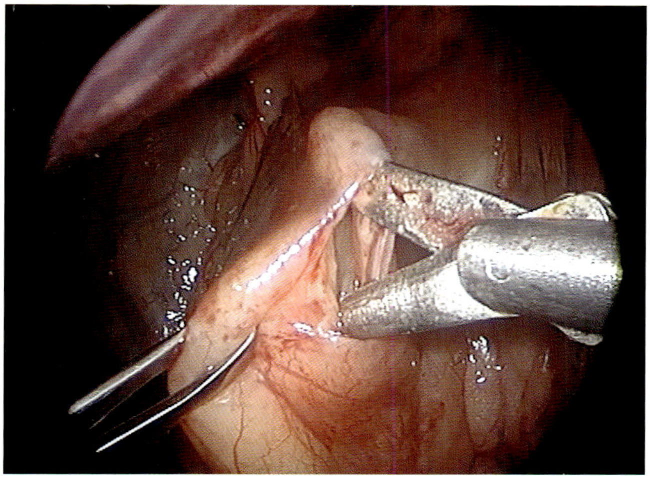

FIGURE 10. Incision and dissection performed on the contralateral side.

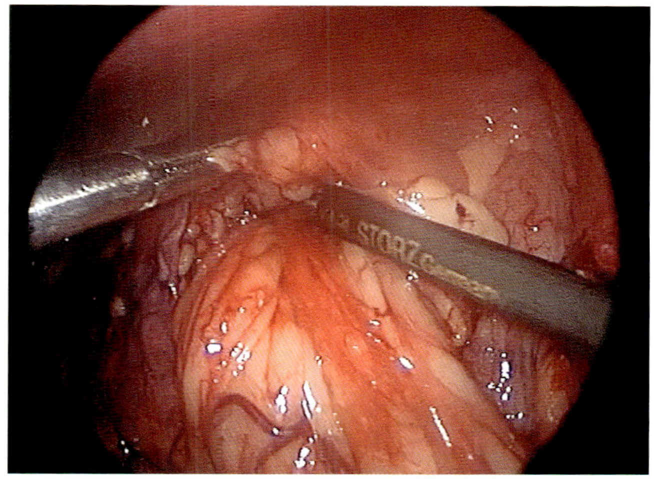

FIGURE 11. With two atraumatic forceps, a leaf of the omentum is grasped, moved caudally, and brought into the cyst cavity.

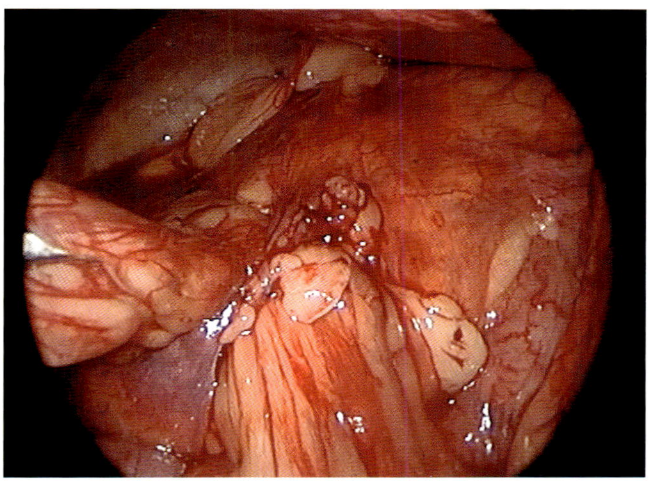

FIGURE 12. Leaf of omentum packed into the cystic remnant.

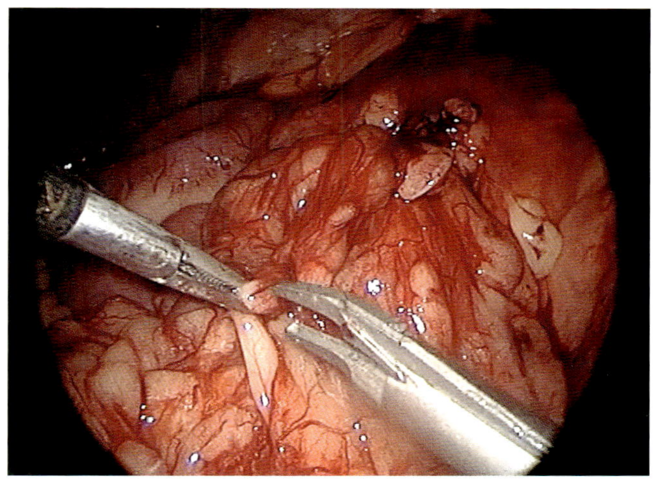

FIGURE 13. The omentum is secured with clips to the cystic wall (extracapsular technique).

urethra in the contralateral cyst, return to the entry incision and suture to itself (intracapsular technique). This second technique, described in open surgery, is more difficult to perform through laparoscopy.

- Before removing the cannulas, the fluids still present in the abdomen are aspirated and washed with warm saline solution (**Fig. 14**). The urinary catheter is removed.
- Intact dogs should also be castrated.

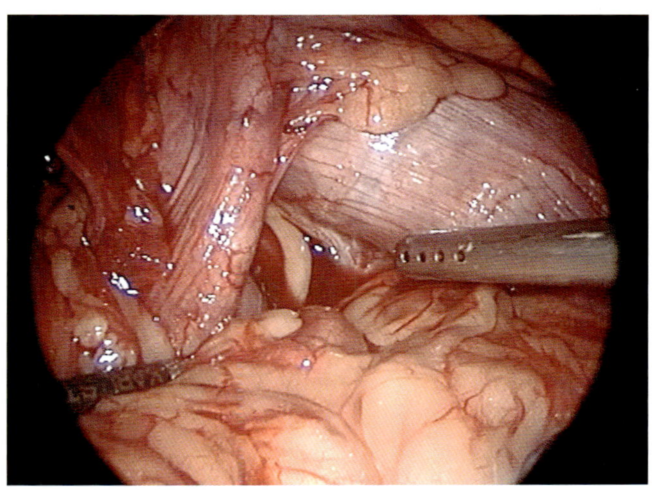

FIGURE 14. Aspiration of fluids still present in the abdomen and washing with warm saline solution.

POSTOPERATIVE MANAGEMENT

- Patients are usually discharged from the hospital within a few hours of the procedure.
- Antibiotic therapy is indicated in the days following surgery.
- Supportive care is given if necessary; multimodal analgesia is continued for at least 1 week.
- Ultrasonographic evaluation of the prostate gland is recommended at set intervals after surgery.

Complications of laparoscopic omentalization of paraprostatic cysts

- Cysts may recur if insufficient omentum is used.
- Urinary incontinence is a frequent sign due to injury of neuronal supply to the bladder and urethra. It may last for some weeks after surgery. If this persists, medical treatment may be necessary (bethanechol/phenylpropanolamine) to restore urinary continence.

Key points

- Preoperative evaluation is important to determine the content type of the cyst. In the case of purulent content, a careful evaluation must be made on whether to perform the laparoscopic approach of a prostatic abscess.
- During the incision or resection of the cyst, care must be taken to preserve the dorsal aspect of the prostate gland, where innervation and vascularization are located.
- The Trendelenburg position, eventually associated with cranial bladder traction, could improve visualization of the prostate gland.
- If the patient is an intact male, it must be neutered to reduce the risk of recurrence.

SUGGESTED READINGS

CLINICAL CASES

29.1 OMENTALIZATION OF A PROSTATIC ABSCESS

David García Rubio

CASE DESCRIPTION

A 12-year-old intact male Pomeranian with episodes of fever, diarrhea, abdominal pain, and purulent discharge from the urethral opening was presented.

The examination of the patient showed a rectal temperature of 39.5°C and pain upon palpation of the caudal abdomen. A rectal examination showed evidence of an enlarged, painful prostate gland. The blood analysis was normal, except for moderate leukocytosis. An ultrasound scan showed an enlarged, heterogeneous prostate gland with multiple small cysts and a large cavity on the dorsocranial aspect with hypoechoic content and swollen walls.

The patient was diagnosed with a prostatic abscess; for this reason, it was decided to perform surgery via laparoscopy to drain and omentalize it.

Key points

- The laparoscopic approach is highly useful in treating single, large abscesses or cysts, but it may not be the best option in cases with multiple interconnected cavities.
- Ensure a sample of the purulent content is taken in advance so that it may be cultured at the laboratory.
- Treatment of the prostate gland is complicated, given its intrapelvic location. Forced Trendelenburg positions help, but the anesthetist must carefully monitor the patient, given the pressure the viscera exert on the diaphragm and the negative effect this causes on the airflow.
- Following surgery, if there was purulent discharge, wash and vacuum several times using tempered saline solution.

PORT PLACEMENT

The patient is placed in dorsal decubitus and a Trendelenburg position at an angle of 20°–25°. Three 5 mm trocars are used. The first is inserted in a supraumbilical position using the open entry technique, and after checking its correct positioning, a pneumoperitoneum is established with CO_2 at 10 mmHg. Two further 5 mm trocars are inserted into more caudal positions aside from the first one, triangulating the prostatic area.

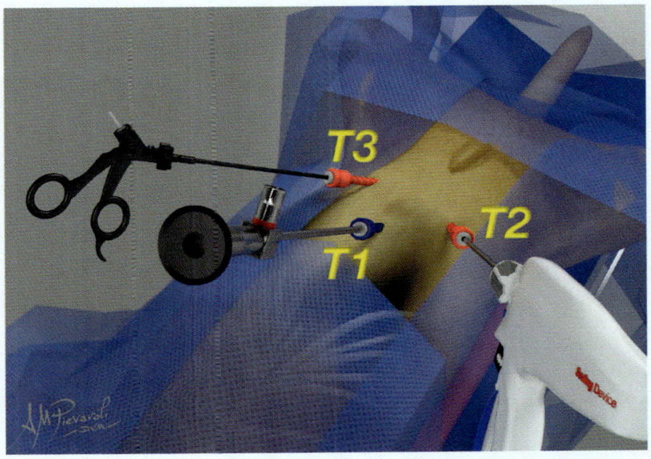

PROCEDURE

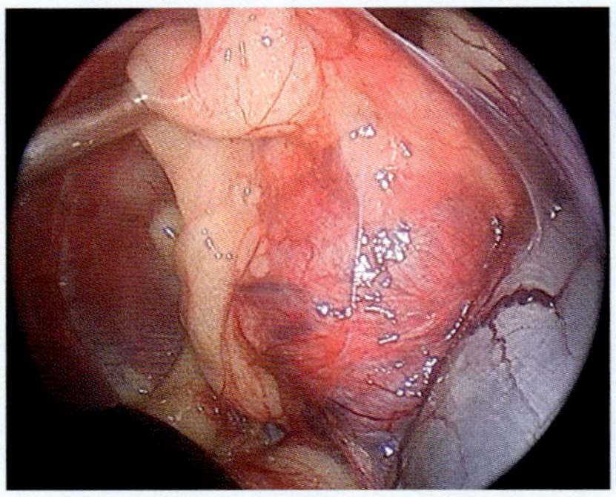

FIGURE 1. Laparoscopic view of the patient's caudal abdomen, with the prostate gland in the center of the image. The bladder can be seen in the lower left area in a blue color.

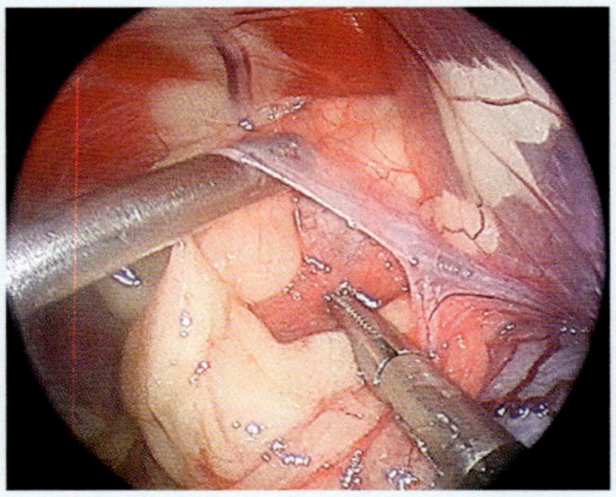

FIGURE 2. Location of the area corresponding to the prostatic abscess via the application of pressure using a dissector.

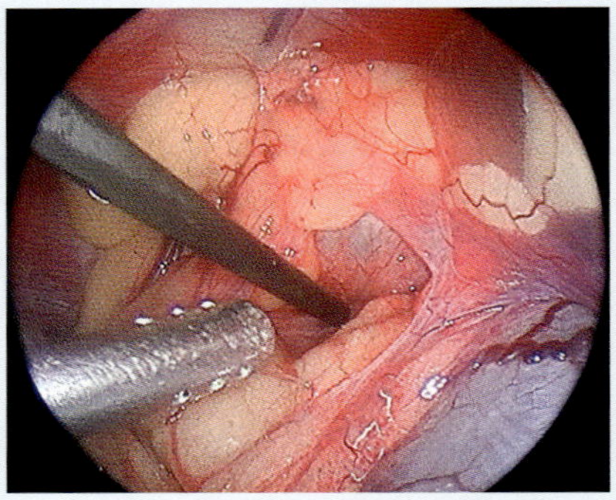

FIGURE 3. In this case, the sharp end of an unopened MiniLap forceps (Teleflex, Morrisville, USA) is used to create a first orifice in the prostatic abscess. A laparoscopic vacuum is always ready at the left port.

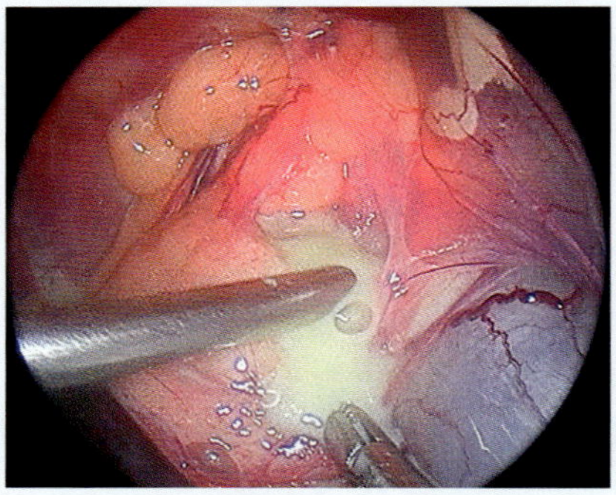

FIGURE 4. Detailed view of the purulent content from the abscess while being vacuumed after expanding the initial orifice using a Maryland dissector.

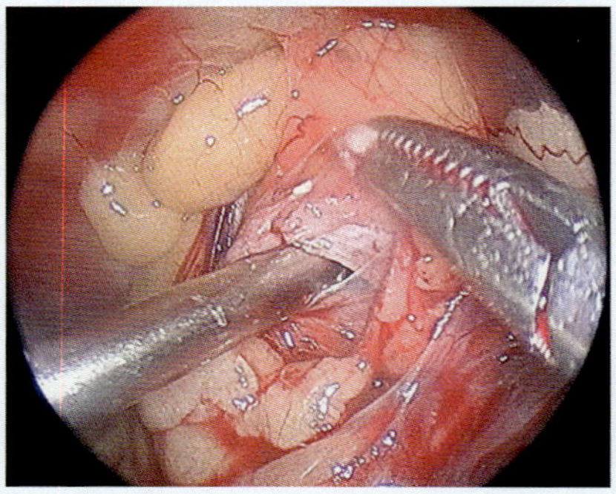

FIGURE 5. When the entry point is sufficiently large, the vacuum is inserted inside the abscess, and all pus is drained.

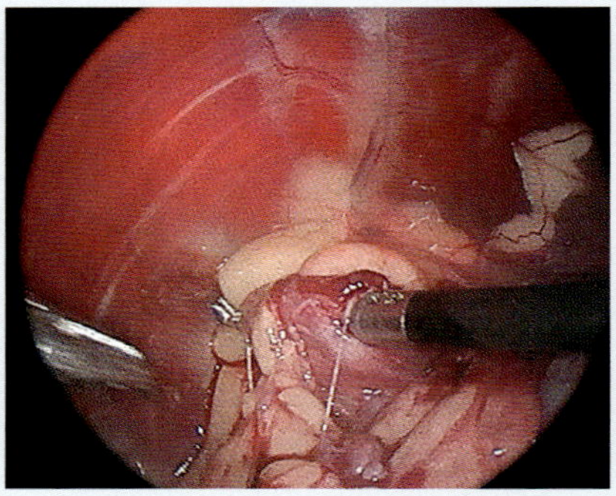

FIGURE 6. Once the contents have been drained, the dissector is inserted and fully penetrates the abscess to perforate the abscess wall from the other side, pushing the instrument through to the outside.

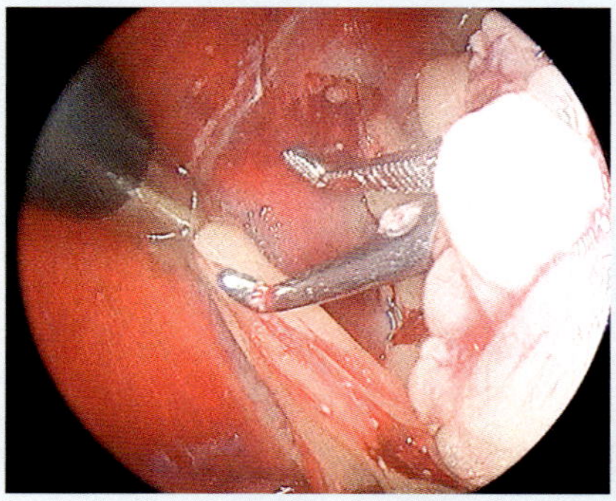

FIGURE 7. Using forceps with the left hand (if the surgeon is right-handed), the greater omentum is located and moved closer to the dissector, which is penetrating the abscess.

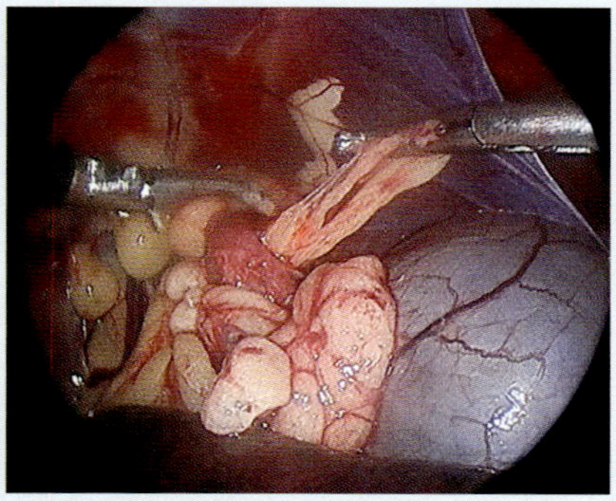

FIGURE 8. The dissector is extracted with the right hand using traction and rotating maneuvers, leaving the largest amount of the omentum possible inside the abscess. This will act as a natural drainage, preventing the abscess from forming again.

Tips and tricks

- ✓ Use touch and resistance to pressure when trying to locate the abscess.
- ✓ Omentalization can often be complemented by partial resection of the abscess ceiling using bipolar coagulation/cutting forceps, thus increasing the drainage zone.

29.2 OMENTALIZATION OF A PARAPROSTATIC CYST IN A DOG

Massimo Barilli

CASE DESCRIPTION

This clinical case concerns a 5-year-old Boxer who underwent abdominal ultrasound examination following episodes of recurrent hematuria. The ultrasound examination revealed a paraprostatic cyst of about 5 cm in diameter to the right of the prostate gland. It was decided to treat this cyst with a laparoscopic approach. The goal was to empty the cyst of its contents, remove the cyst wall, and omentalize the part of the cyst adhering to the prostate gland. Orchiectomy was also performed.

Key points

- Empty the cyst.
- Remove the cyst wall.
- Securely fix the omentum to the cystic wall.

PORT PLACEMENT

The telescope port (T1) is introduced on the midline 1–2 cm caudal to the umbilicus. The operative ports (T2, T3) are positioned more caudally and laterally in a paramedian line to the same side of the cyst (right side in the case). T3 is placed 5–6 cm caudal to T1, and T2 is placed caudal to T3 in a parapreputial position.

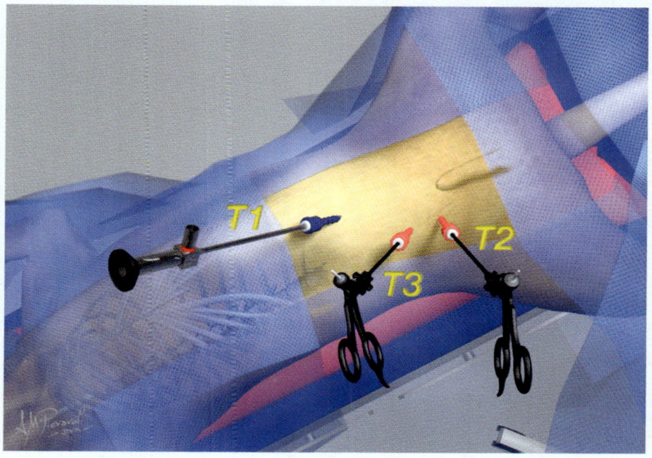

PROCEDURE

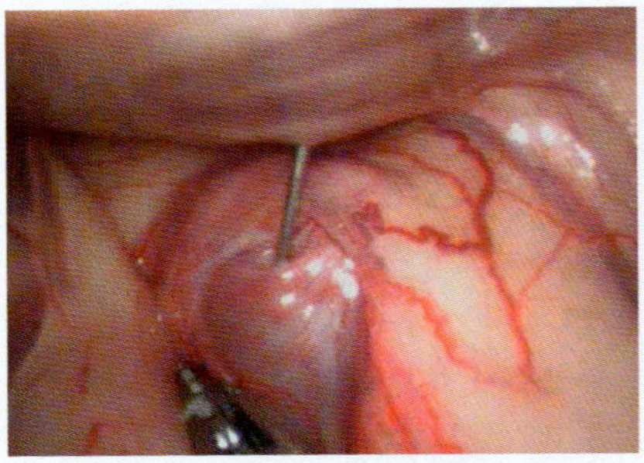
FIGURE 1. Transparietal aspiration of the right paraprostatic cyst.

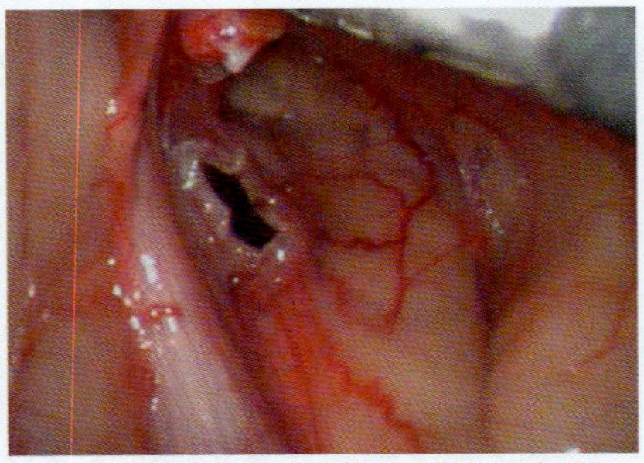
FIGURE 2. Opening the paraprostatic cyst with scissors.

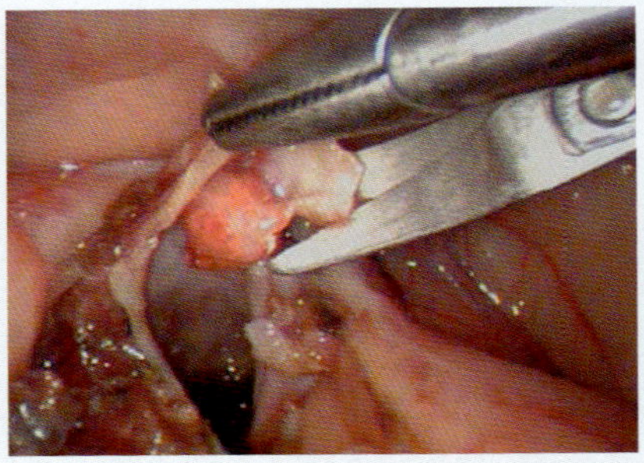
FIGURE 3. Removal of the wall of the paraprostatic cyst.

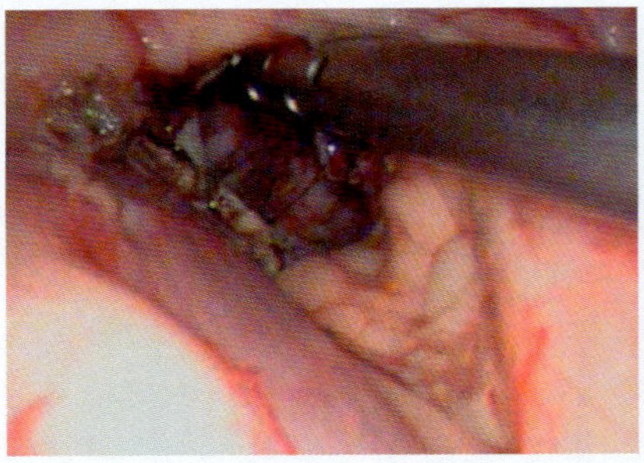
FIGURE 4. Visualization of the cyst bottom.

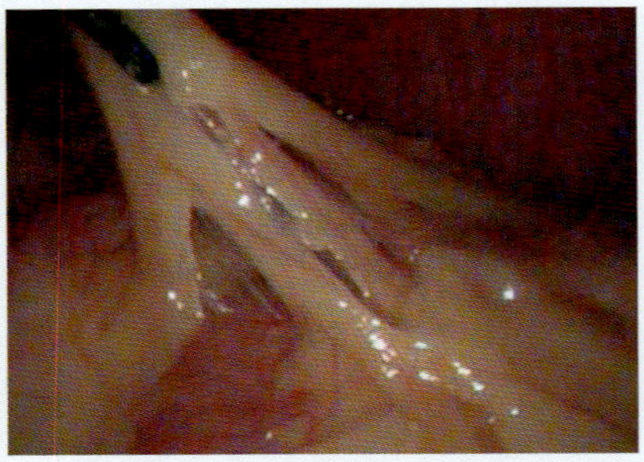
FIGURE 5. Omentum preparation for cyst omentalization.

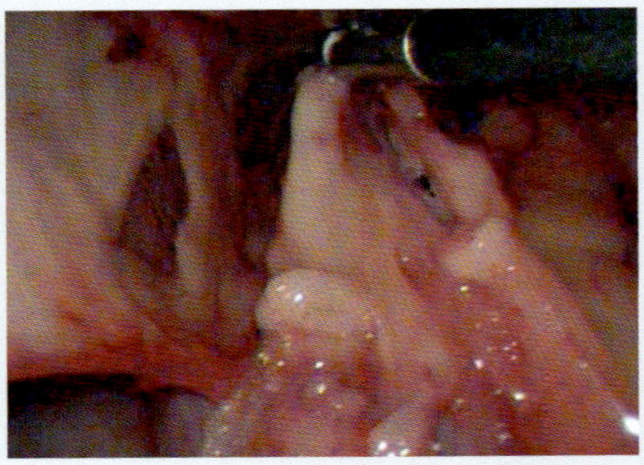
FIGURE 6. Positioning of the omentum into the cyst.

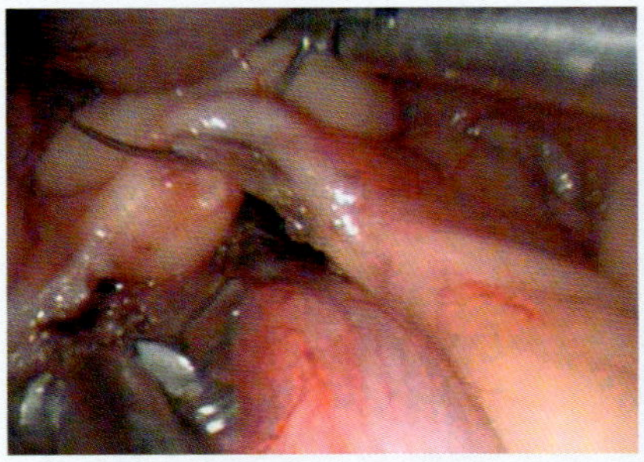
FIGURE 7. Suture of the omentum into the cyst.

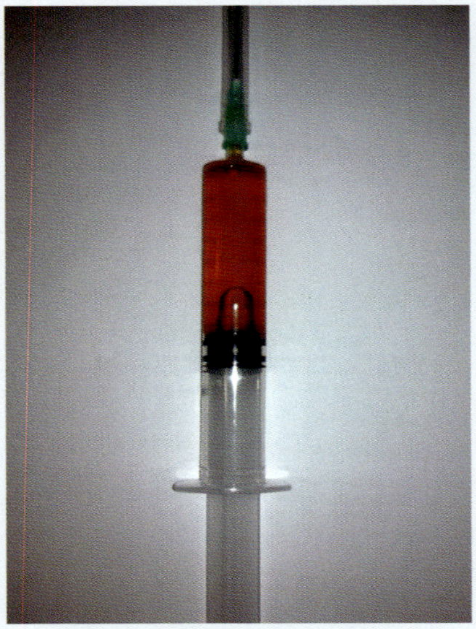
FIGURE 8. Paraprostatic cyst content.

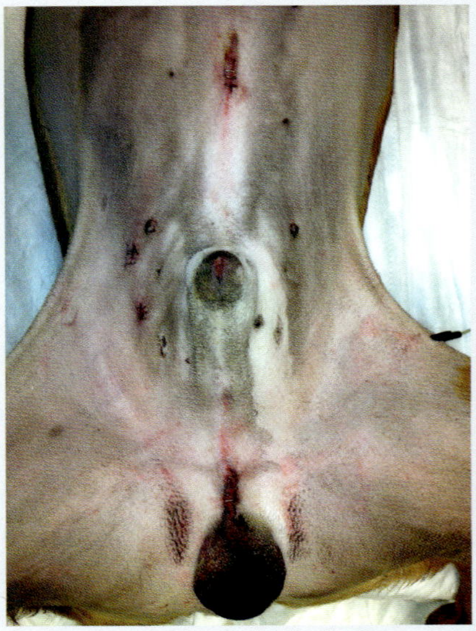
FIGURE 9. Operating field after the surgery.

Tips and tricks

✓ Remove as much cyst capsule as possible.

30 LAPAROSCOPIC GASTROPEXY AND LAPAROSCOPIC-ASSISTED GASTROPEXY

J. Brad Case, Roberto Properzi

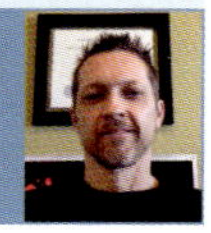

Indications	**Contraindications**
■ Dog breeds at increased risk of gastric dilatation with volvulus ■ Dogs who have undergone splenectomy	■ Cardiovascular unstable dogs ■ Immature or underdeveloped dogs ■ Dogs not at risk of gastric dilatation with volvulus

Gastric dilatation with volvulus (GDV) is a complex disease mostly seen in large and giant deep-chested dogs, although any dog may be affected. It causes a myriad of pathophysiologic consequences, including hypovolemic shock that develops because of a severely dilated and twisted stomach that compresses the caudal vena cava and portal venous structures. If left untreated, mortality is almost certain. Prophylactic gastropexy can virtually eliminate the possibility of GDV development.

Recently, an increasing number of breeders and owners have become aware of the benefits of prophylactic gastropexy.

> Many techniques have been developed to perform gastropexy, but laparoscopic surgery, having very low levels of morbidity and invasiveness, fits well with the concept of prevention.

Over the past 20 years, several laparoscopic gastropexy techniques have been described, but intracorporeal techniques using barbed suture have become the standard of care. Intracorporeal techniques minimize tissue trauma (and pain) compared to "assisted" techniques by eliminating the need for abdominal muscle dissection. However, intracorporeal suturing (specifically knot tying) is challenging and associated with a significant learning curve. The advent of barbed suture has helped to overcome this hurdle and has paved the way for intracorporeal laparoscopic gastropexy to become the preferred method for most minimally invasive surgeons.

Any stable dog at risk of GDV is a candidate for preventative laparoscopic gastropexy. While many risk factors have been associated with an increased incidence of GDV in general, a number of breeds appear to have an inherent risk. Some examples include Great Dane (40%), German Shepherd (24%), Irish Setter (25%), Standard Poodle (25%), and Weimaraner (20%). Additionally, dogs who have undergone splenectomy may also be at an increased risk for GDV, and laparoscopic gastropexy is reasonable in some of these dogs.

The risk of significant complications associated with laparoscopic gastropexy is virtually zero in an experienced surgeon's hands. Additionally, the prognosis for successful treatment is nearly guaranteed, assuming a well-performed incisional gastropexy is made. This chapter will describe the multiport intracorporeal technique for laparoscopic gastropexy, focusing on the important details to ensure a successful outcome.

DESCRIBED SURGICAL PROCEDURES

Laparoscopic-assisted gastropexy was initially described using a two-port technique. With the advent of single-incision laparoscopic surgery ports, a number of single-port "assisted" approaches were described. More recently, multiport, totally intracorporeal techniques have become the preferred approach by many surgeons.

The following procedures are described below:

A. Intracorporeal laparoscopic gastropexy I (B. Case)
B. Intracorporeal laparoscopic gastropexy II (R. Properzi)
C. Laparoscopic-assisted gastropexy
D. Single-port laparoscopic gastropexy (J. Runge and J. Becker)

A INTRACORPOREAL LAPAROSCOPIC GASTROPEXY I

J. Brad Case

Laparoscopic gastropexy is performed with the multiport, intracorporeal sutured procedure using barbed suture. Three 5.5 mm ports are placed on the midline to establish triangulation around the proposed gastropexy site.

Instruments

On the table:

- Standard abdominal surgical pack
- High-definition video camera
- Telescope 5 mm – 30°
- Three 5 mm threaded cannulas
- Two 5 mm laparoscopic needle drivers
- 5 mm laparoscopic Metzenbaum scissors
- 5 mm laparoscopic right-angle dissector
- 5 mm laparoscopic DeBakey forceps
- 5 mm laparoscopic suture scissors
- L- or J-hook monopolar electrosurgical scalpel
- Two 2-0 barbed sutures

OPERATING ROOM LAYOUT

The dog is positioned with its hind end at the foot of the operating table, and the anesthesia circuit and staff are positioned at the head of the operating table. The instrument table and monitors are positioned at the end of the operating table. The surgeon and surgeon's assistant stand to the left side of the dog. The monitor or monitors are placed on the right side near the dog's head (**Fig. 1**).

PORT PLACEMENT (FIG. 2)

- T1, on the midline, 2 cm caudal to the umbilicus
- T2, on the midline, 4 cm cranial to T1
- T3, on the midline, 4 cm cranial to T2

PROCEDURE

- After port placement and pneumoperitoneum have been achieved, the 5 mm telescope is inserted in T1, and an initial exploration of the abdomen is performed.
- Subsequent ports (T2, T3) are then placed under optical guidance, ensuring to avoid the falciform fat (**Fig. 3**). The position of the stomach is assessed. In some cases, the omentum will need to be retracted caudally from the parietal gastric surface. The position of the gastropexy site is then selected, typically at the level (cranial to caudal) of the 13th rib and (medial to lateral) midway between the apex of the 13th rib and the midline. The position can be confirmed intracorporeally by pressing a finger inward at the proposed site while visualizing with the laparoscope. Landmarks to be aware of include the diaphragm muscle, the transversus abdominus muscle, and the 12th costal arch. It is critical to ensure that the gastropexy is performed well caudal of the diaphragm insertion, which lies along the 12th rib (**Fig. 5**).
- A 2-0 monofilament suture is passed transabdominally at the level of the gastropexy site. A laparoscopic needle driver is used to grasp the needle, and the needle is then passed through the gastric antrum and transabdominally back outside the abdomen. The suture is then pulled tightly to place the gastric antrum in contact with the transversus abdominus muscle (**Fig. 5**). The antrum should be able to be retracted somewhat comfortably without excessive force. In some cases, the gastropexy site will need to be altered or the insufflation pressure reduced (sometimes down to 6 mmHg) to facilitate proper positioning of the gastric antrum. Infiltration of the proposed gastropexy site with bupivacaine is then accomplished.
- Under endoscopic visualization, a laparoscopic L-hook electrosurgical wand is inserted into T2 specifically and then used to create a 3–4 cm long wound in the transversus muscle, and a matching wound in the seromuscular portion of the gastric antrum (**Fig. 6**). Laparoscopic Metzenbaum scissors and right-angle dissecting forceps are then used to create a window between the submucosa and seromuscular layers of the antrum.

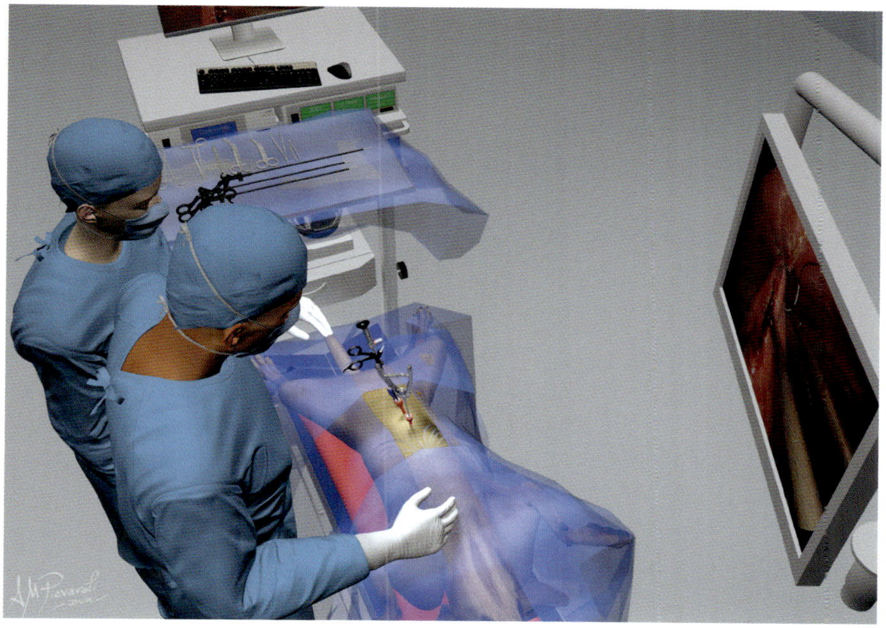

FIGURE 1. Operating room layout for laparoscopic gastropexy.

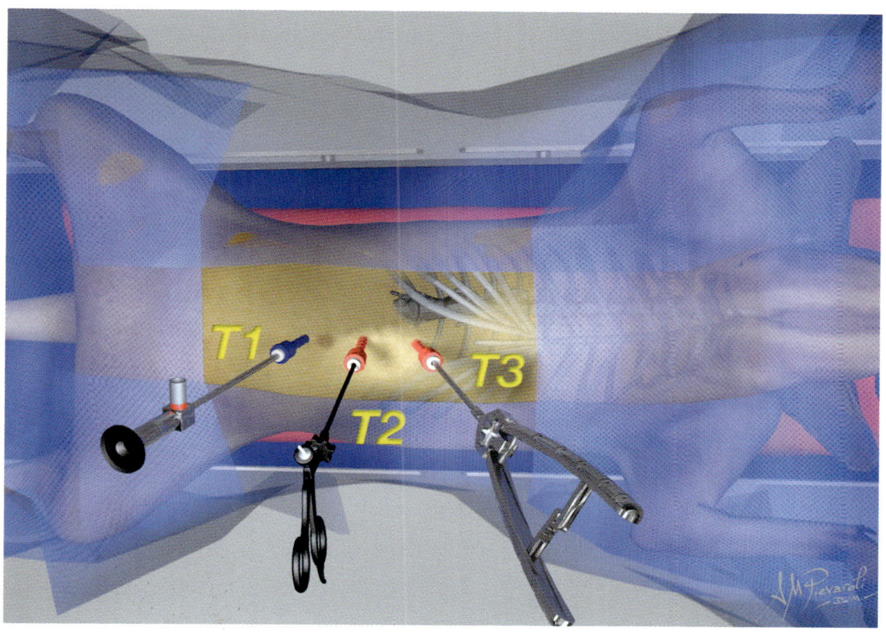

FIGURE 2. Port placement for intracorporeal gastropexy (Brad Case).

- A 2-0, 12 cm long, barbed suture is introduced (transabdominally or via a cannula) and passed from the craniolateral aspect of the gastric antral incision; and then, through the transversus incision to anchor in the suture in place (**Fig. 7**). A simple continuous, full-thickness (transversus muscle to seromuscular gastric antrum) pattern is used to suture the craniolateral incisions together completely. This generally requires five or six passes to suture the first side of the incisional gastropexy completely. It is critical that the last pass of the barbed suture line is backward or 180° from the orientation of the continuous line (**Fig. 8**). This is referred to as a "back stitch" and is important to prevent the pullout of the barbed suture line. Once the backstitch is placed, and the first incision is closed, the needle is cut from the suture strand and removed from the abdomen.

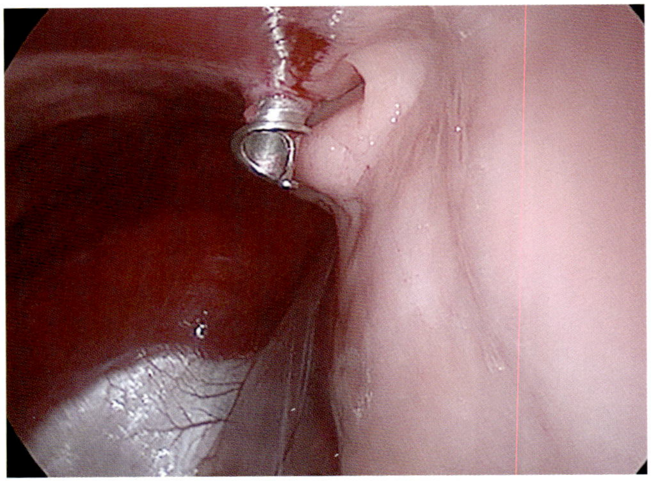

FIGURE 3. Falciform fat can interfere with ports and instrumentation. It is advised to place ports immediately lateral to the falciform ligament.

- A second 2-0, 12 cm long, barbed suture is introduced into the abdomen, and the caudal aspect of the gastropexy is closed in a similar manner as the cranial. The gastropexy is then assessed to ensure that there is no exposed gastric submucosa and that both the cranial and caudal incisions are sutured completely (**Fig. 9**).
- The abdominal cavity is decompressed by removing the T1 and T2 ports while visualizing the stomach to examine its final position within the abdominal cavity.
- The T3 port is removed, and incisions are closed routinely.

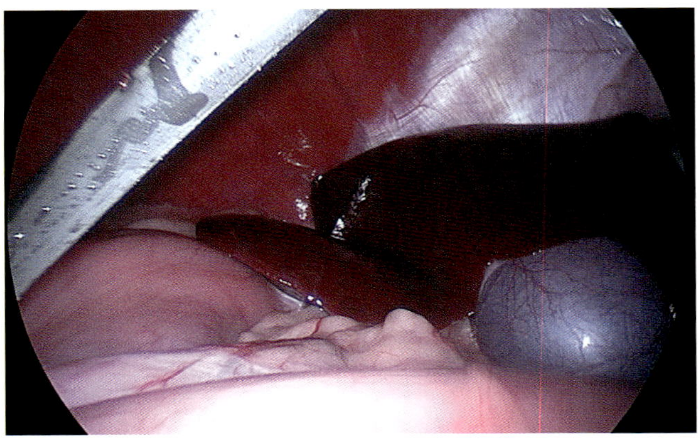

FIGURE 4. Pyloric antrum.

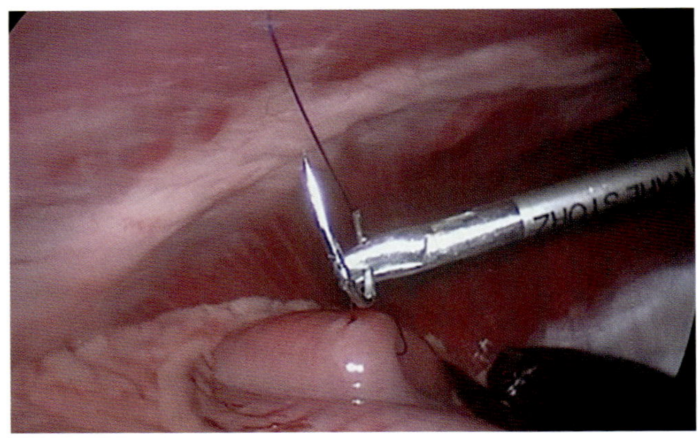

FIGURE 5. Stay suture used to attach the pyloric antrum to the transversus muscle to facilitate the intracorporeal gastropexy.

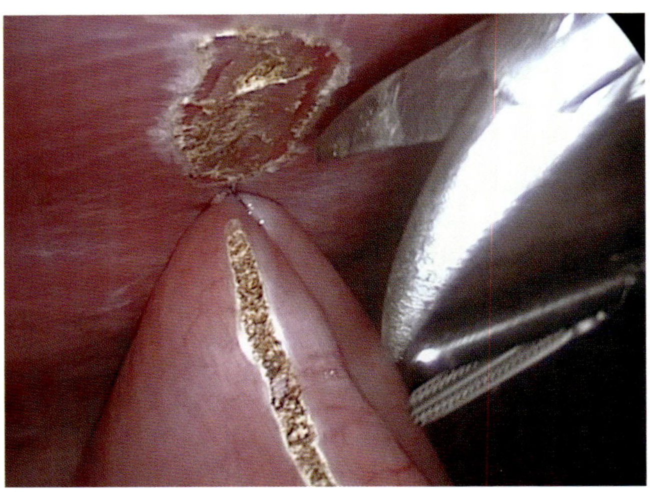

FIGURE 6. Matching incisions in the seromuscular layer of the pyloric antrum and the transversus abdominus muscle.

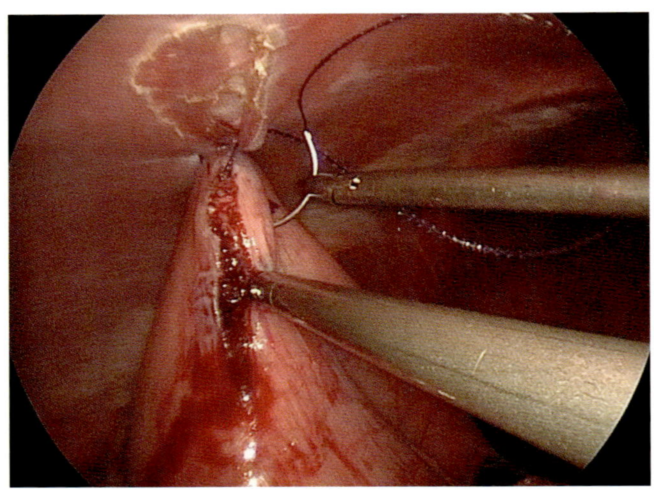

FIGURE 7. Intraoperative image of the initial suture row during intracorporeal gastropexy.

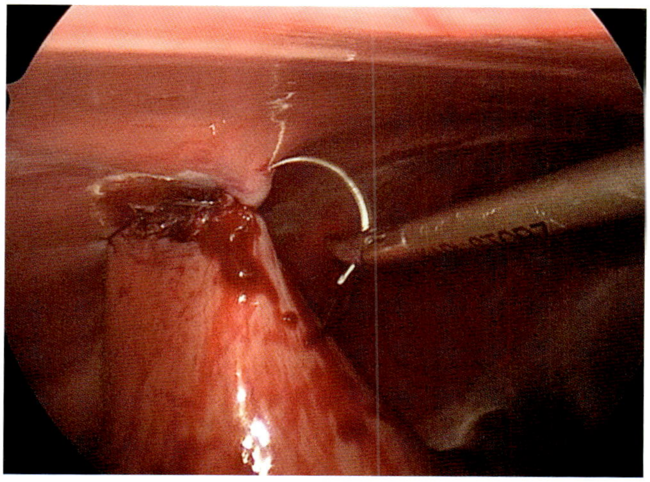

FIGURE 8. A backstitch suture bite is used to terminate the continuous suture pattern when using barbed suture.

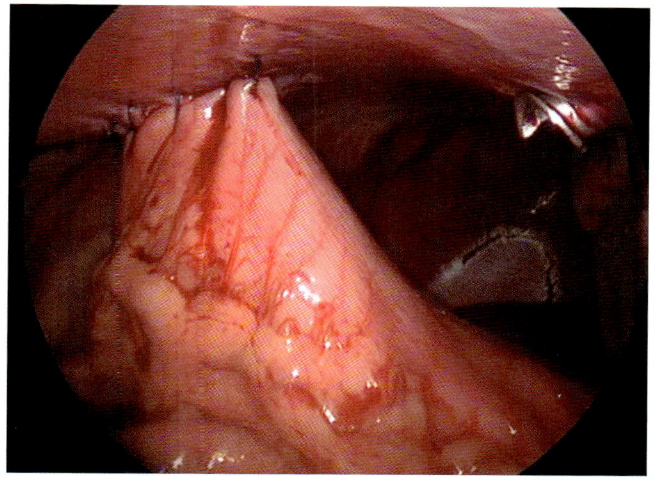

FIGURE 9. Intraoperative image of a completed intracorporeal gastropexy.

B INTRACORPOREAL LAPAROSCOPIC GASTROPEXY II

Roberto Properzi

Instruments

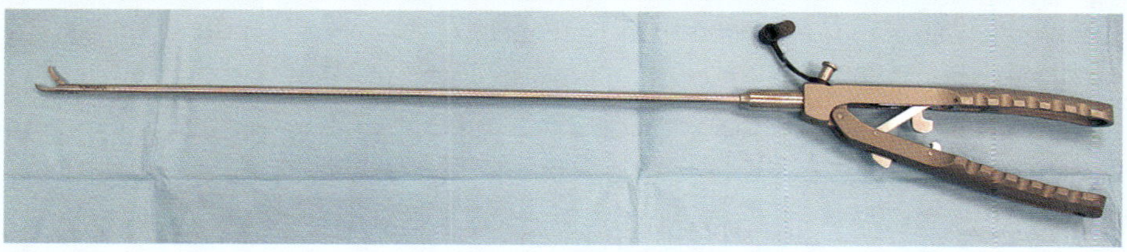

FIGURE 10. Laparoscopic needle holder.

On the table:

- Standard abdominal surgical pack
- High-definition video camera
- Telescope 5 mm – 30°
- Two 5 mm threaded cannulas
- One 12 mm threaded cannula
- Two 5 mm laparoscopic needle holders (**Fig. 10**)
- 5 mm laparoscopic DeBakey forceps
- 5 mm laparoscopic suture scissors
- One 0 USP barbed suture with a 36 mm needle (**Fig. 11**)

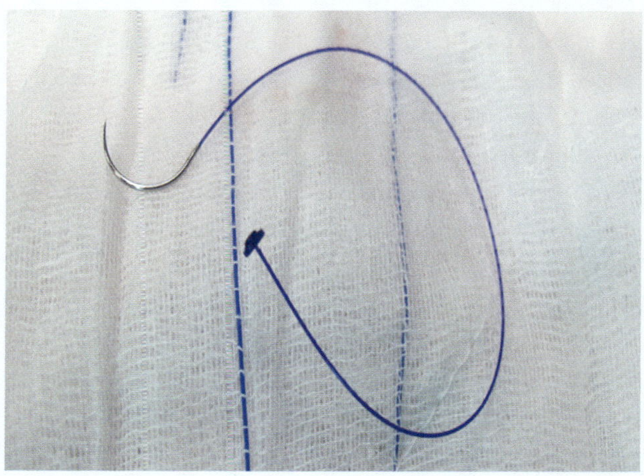

FIGURE 11. Filbloc barbed suture.

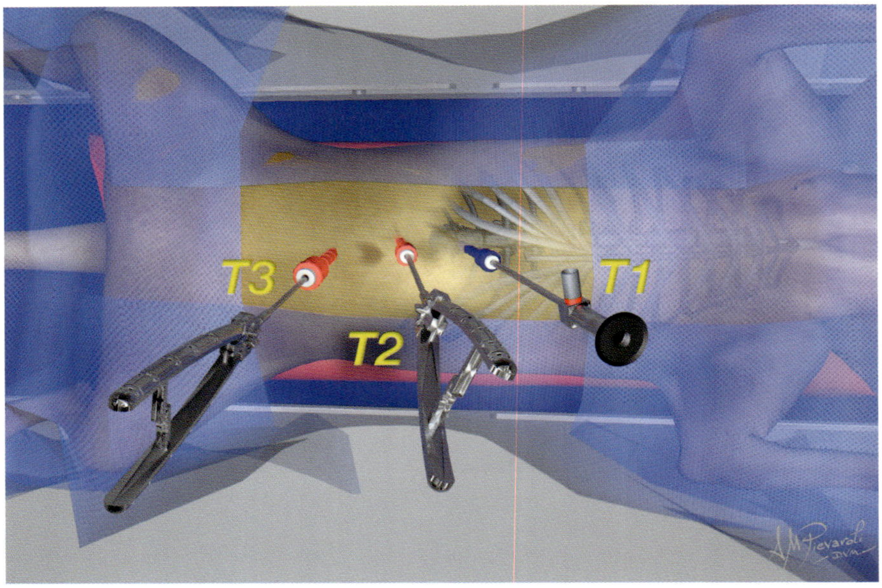

FIGURE 12. Port placement for intracorporeal gastropexy.

PORT PLACEMENT (FIG. 12)

- T1, in the right paramedian position, 2–3 cm caudal to the xiphoid process of the sternum
- T2, in the right paramedian position, between T1 and T3
- T3, on the midline, 2–3 cm caudal to the umbilicus

PROCEDURE (VIDEO 1)

- The dog is positioned in dorsal recumbency. Using the open (Hasson) technique, a 5 mm cannula (T1) is inserted 2–3 cm caudal to the xiphoid process of the sternum in the right paramedian position to create pneumoperitoneum using CO_2 with an automatic insufflator with a pressure of 8–10 mmHg and to insert a 30° telescope measuring 5 mm in diameter. A 12 mm cannula (T3) is inserted 2–3 cm caudal to the umbilicus on the midline under endoscopic guidance. Then, a 5 mm cannula (T2) is inserted between T1 and T3 in the right paramedian position (**Fig. 13**).
- An approximately 3 cm gastropexy is performed via intracorporeal suturing with unidirectional barbed suture without incising both the seromuscular layer of the stomach and the abdominal wall.
- The self-locking 0 polydioxanone monofilament barbed suture is inserted into the abdomen with a laparoscopic needle holder through T3. A second needle holder is inserted into the abdomen through T2 (**Fig. 14**).
- At first, the suture is started between the greater and lesser curvatures of the stomach at 2–3 cm from the pylorus (**Fig. 15**), and the stomach is anchored with the first two bites at the abdominal wall in a right paracostal position 1–2 cm caudal to the 13th rib (**Figs. 16 and 17**).
- The barbed suture passed through the seromuscular laver of the antrum and through the abdominal wall. Subsequent bites are taken 3–5 mm apart. After each bite, the suture is pulled tight to anchor the barbs in the tissue, and the simple continuous suture is completed. The suture is reinforced with an endoclip (**Fig. 18**).

VIDEO 1. Prophylactic laparoscopic gastropexy by total intracorporeal suturing.

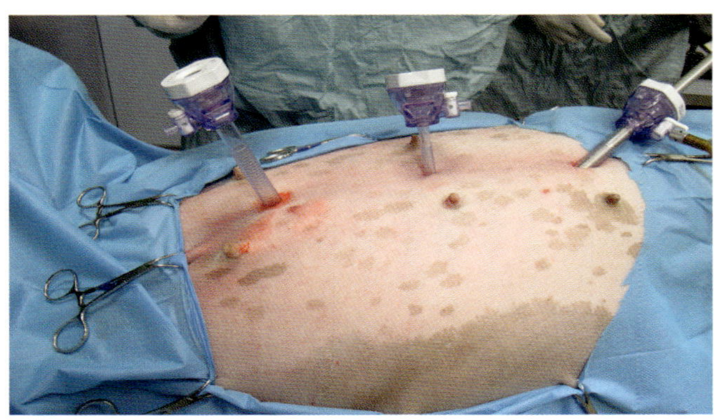

FIGURE 13. Image of the patient, indicating the port placement.

- The redundant end of the barbed suture is cut using laparoscopic hook scissors, which are introduced through T2; the needle is removed through T3, and the telescope is used to evaluate the gastropexy (**Fig. 19**).

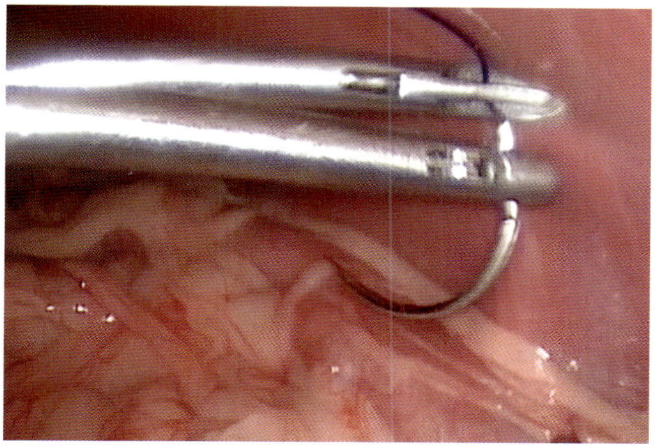

FIGURE 14. Two needle holders are necessary to perform the intracorporeal suture.

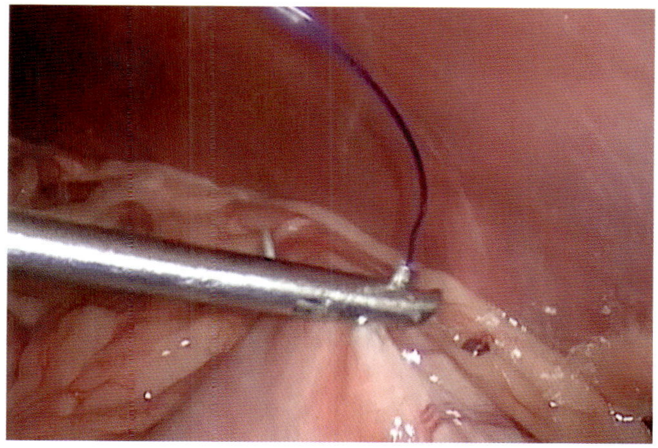

FIGURE 15. The first suture is placed in the seromuscular layer of the stomach.

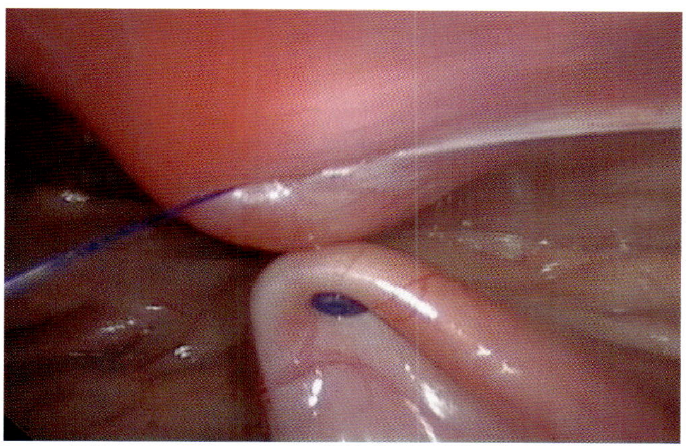

FIGURE 16. Close view of the first suture stitch.

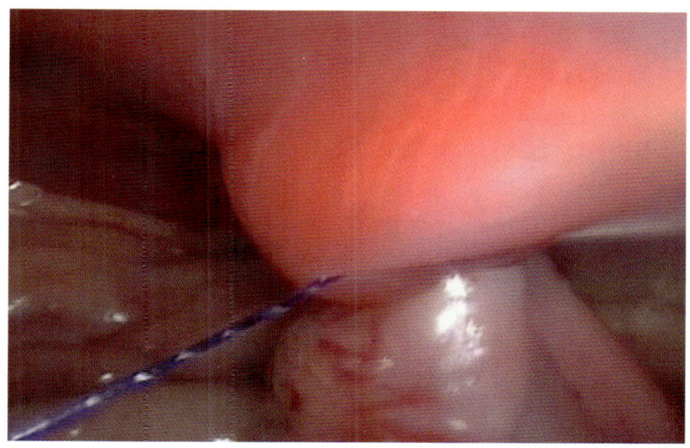

FIGURE 17. Close view of the second suture stitch.

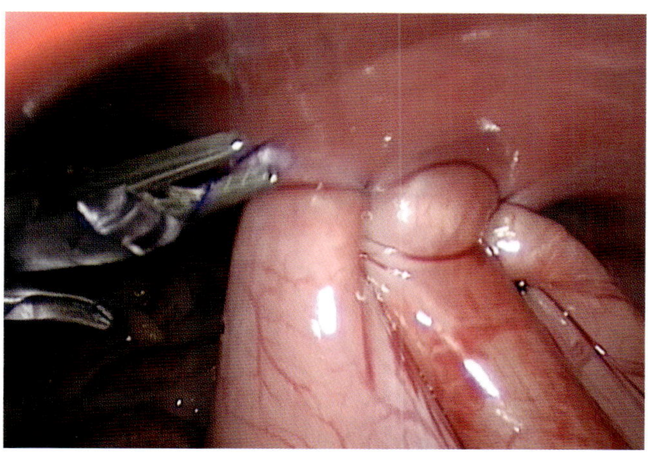

FIGURE 18. At the end of the suture, an endoclip is generally used to reinforce the suture itself.

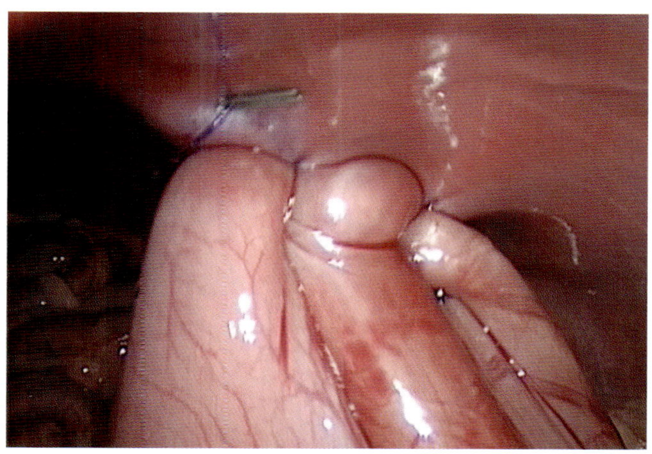

FIGURE 19. Final vision of the gastropexy.

C LAPAROSCOPIC-ASSISTED GASTROPEXY

Instruments

- Standard abdominal surgical pack
- High-definition video camera
- Telescope 5 mm – 30°
- Two 5 mm threaded cannulas
- 5 mm laparoscopic DeBakey forceps
- One absorbable 1 USP suture with ⅜ 46 mm needle

PORT PLACEMENT (FIGS. 20 AND 21)

- T1, in the right paramedian position, 2–3 cm caudal to the xiphoid process of the sternum
- T2, on the midline, 2–3 cm caudal to the umbilicus

PROCEDURE

- The dog is positioned in dorsal recumbency. Using the open (Hasson) technique, a 5 mm cannula (T1) is inserted 2–3 cm caudal to the xiphoid process of the sternum in the right paramedian position to create pneumoperitoneum using CO_2 by an automatic insufflator with a pressure of 8–10 mmHg and to insert a 30° telescope measuring 5 mm in diameter.
- A 5 mm cannula (T2) is inserted 2–3 cm caudal to the umbilicus on the midline under endoscopic guidance.
- A 5 mm laparoscopic DeBakey forceps is then introduced through the right instrument port. The ventral gastric wall proximal to the pylorus and cranial to the attachment of the greater omentum is grasped and lifted towards the right ventral abdominal wall. The appropriate peritoneal area is located about 3 cm caudal to the 13th rib and 3–4 cm lateral to the right rectus abdominis muscle.
- A skin incision (about 3 cm long) is made along this area, at the point where it is possible to easily put the stomach towards the abdominal wall (**Fig. 22**). The needle (triangular, 46 mm, ⅜ circle) of a 4 metric adsorbable suture handled extracorporeally is passed through the abdominal wall, through the seromuscular layer of the stomach and back through the abdominal wall and skin incision (**Figs. 23 and 24**). Two other sutures are placed along the line, and all are tied extracorporeally with the knots buried in the subcutaneous tissue (**Figs. 25 and 26**).
- The telescope is used to evaluate the gastropexy (**Fig. 27**).
- The abdomen is deflated, and all the incisions are closed routinely (**Fig. 28**).

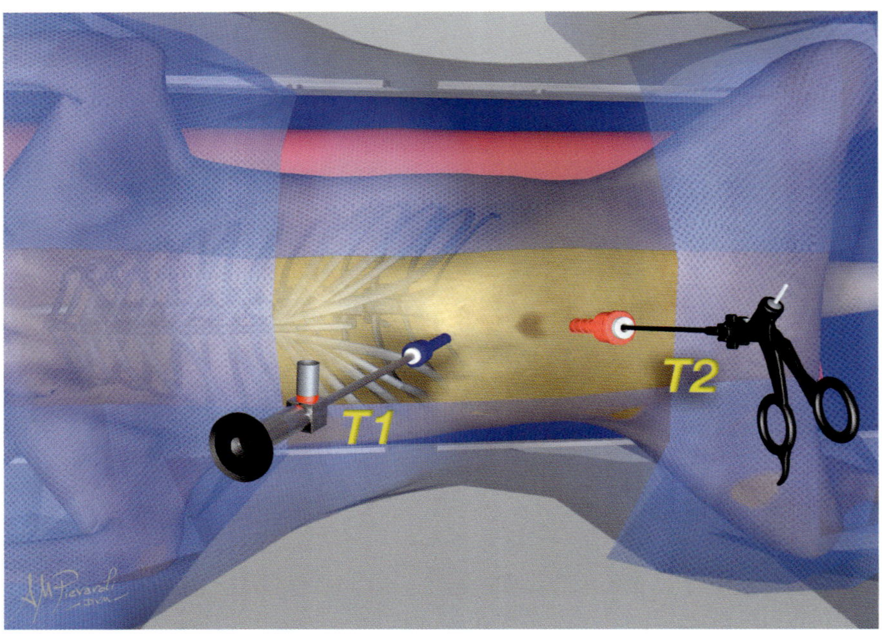

FIGURE 20. Port placement for laparoscopic-assisted gastropexy.

Key points

- Gastropexy should be 3–4 cm, depending on the dog's size.
- Do not pull the stomach too much to avoid an esophageal hiatus laceration resulting in pneumothorax.
- Pneumoperitoneum desufflation can help to put the stomach in the appropriate peritoneal area where the gastropexy is done.

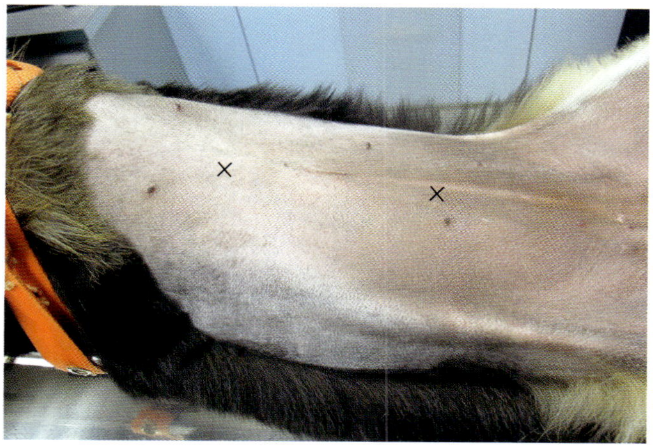

FIGURE 21. The crosses indicate the port placement points.

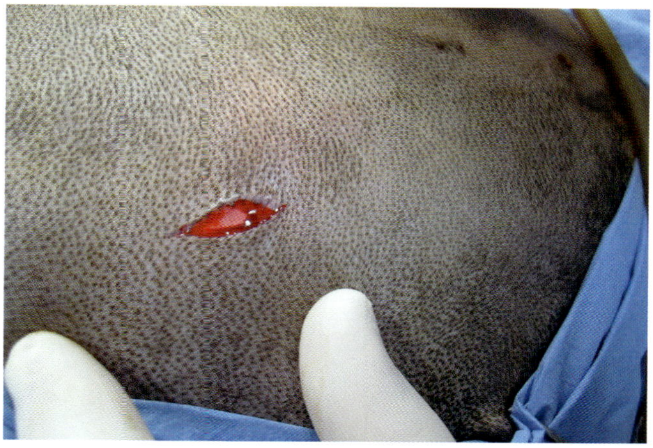

FIGURE 22. Skin and subcutis incision.

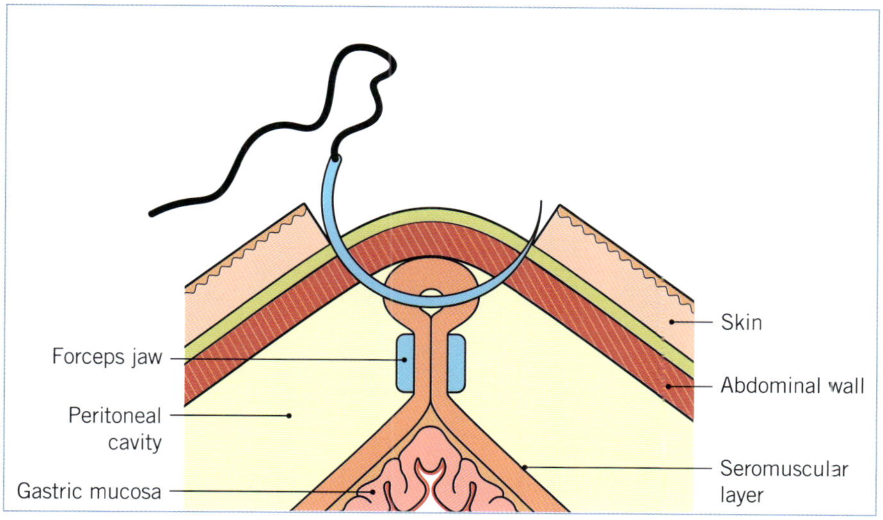

FIGURE 23. Scheme of the suture between the gastric and the abdominal wall.

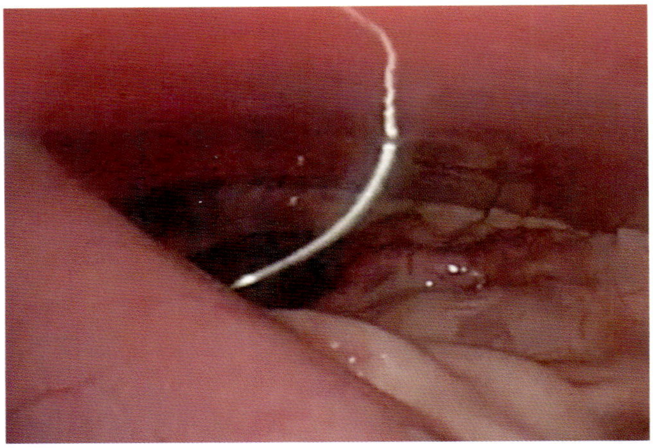

FIGURE 24. The needle is passing through the stomach (intracorporeal image).

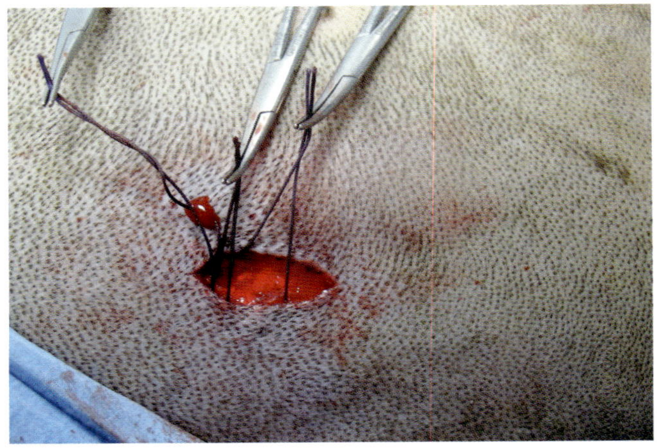

FIGURE 25. Two other sutures are placed along the line.

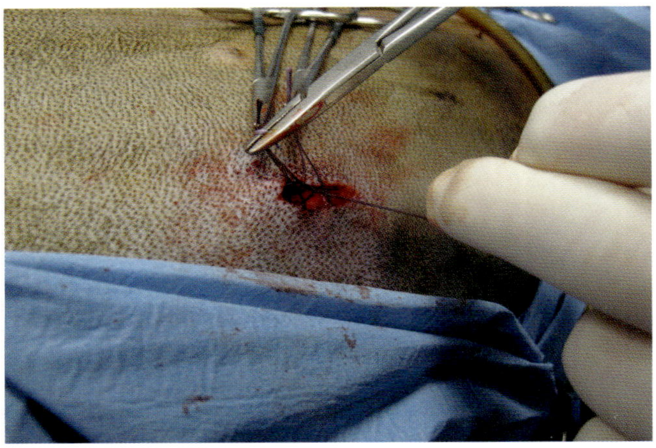

FIGURE 26. All the knots are tied in the subcutis.

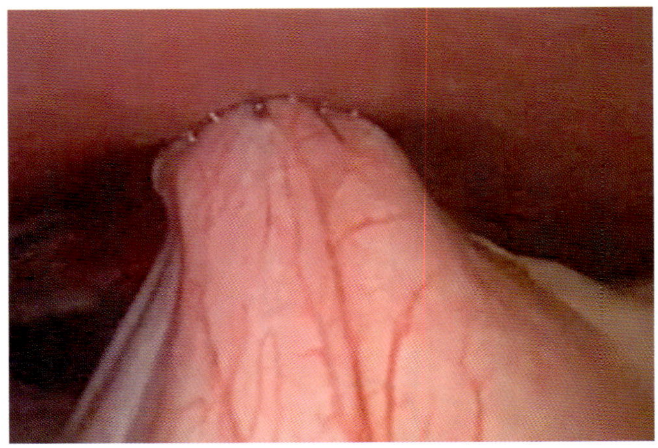

FIGURE 27. Final evaluation of gastropexy done from the internal of the abdomen.

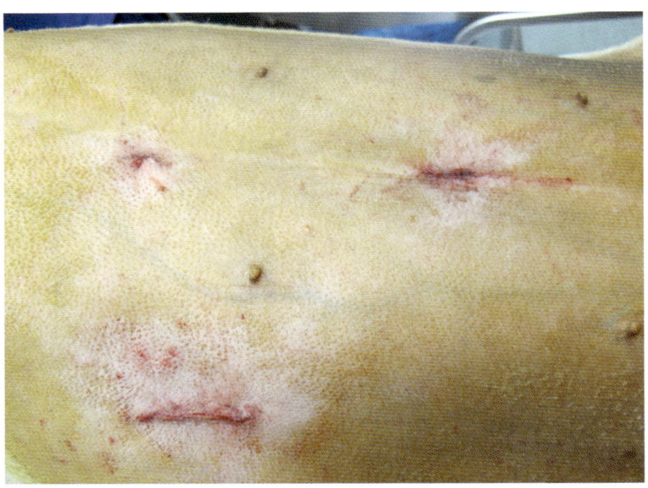

FIGURE 28. All the incisions are closed routinely.

D SINGLE PORT LAPAROSCOPIC-ASSISTED INCISIONAL GASTROPEXY

Jeffrey J. Runge, Joshua G. Becker

OPERATING ROOM LAYOUT

The surgeon should be positioned on the dog's right side with the laparoscopic monitor on the opposite side of the patient (**Fig. 29**).

PORT PLACEMENT (FIGS. 30 AND 31)

- A 2–3 cm skin incision is made starting lateral to the rectus abdominis and approximately 2–5 cm caudal to the right 13th rib.
- Dissection through the oblique and transverse abdominal musculature is continued using a combination of monopolar electrosurgery and sharp dissection.
- Stay sutures are placed in the cauterized or cut edges of the transversus abdominis muscle, and the port is inserted in standard fashion.
- This technique has been primarily described using the SILS port device, although the other single-port devices described in Chapter 7 of this book can also be used.

Instruments

- Standard surgery set
- Telescope 5 mm – 30°
- Single-incision port device
- Standard rigid 10 mm DuVall forceps

PROCEDURE

- After port placement and pneumoperitoneum have been established, the scope is inserted, and a limited abdominal survey is performed in standard fashion, checking for both anatomical landmarks and ensuring that the gross visible anatomy appears within normal limits. Care must be taken to avoid and check for evidence of iatrogenic trauma secondary to port placement.
- The table is tilted in reverse Trendelenburg position for better exposure of the greater curvature of the stomach.
- Standard rigid 10 mm DuVall forceps are inserted toward the antrum of the stomach.
- A relatively avascular region midway between the greater and lesser curvature of the stomach should be identified and grasped atraumatically to be used as the site for incisional gastropexy.

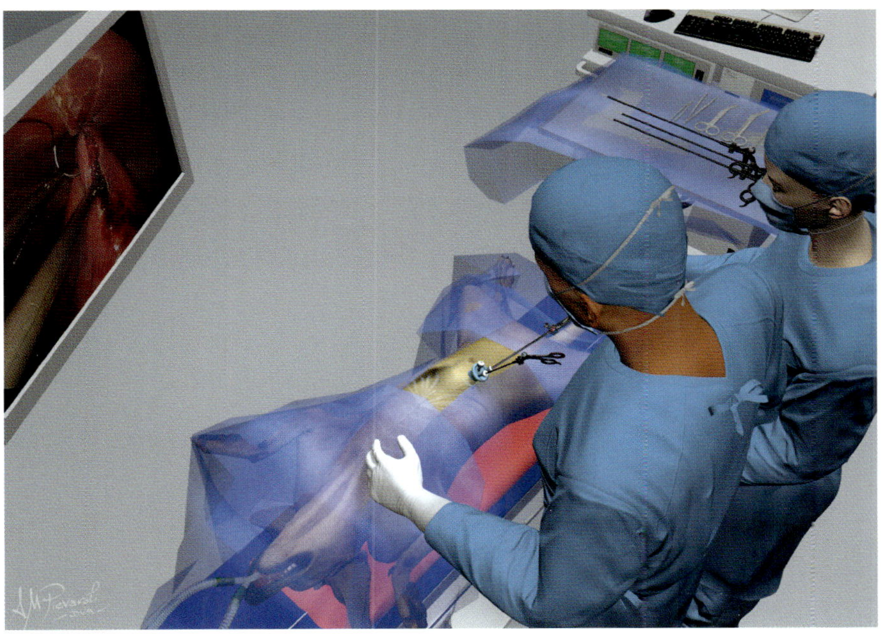

FIGURE 29. Operating room layout for single-port laparoscopic-assisted gastropexy.

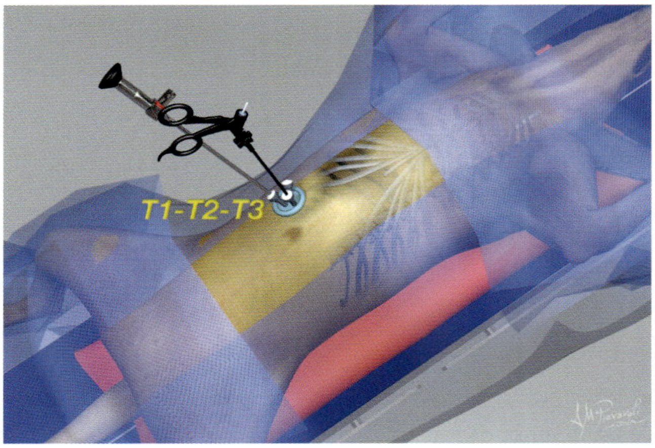

FIGURE 30. Single-port placement for laparoscopic-assisted gastropexy.

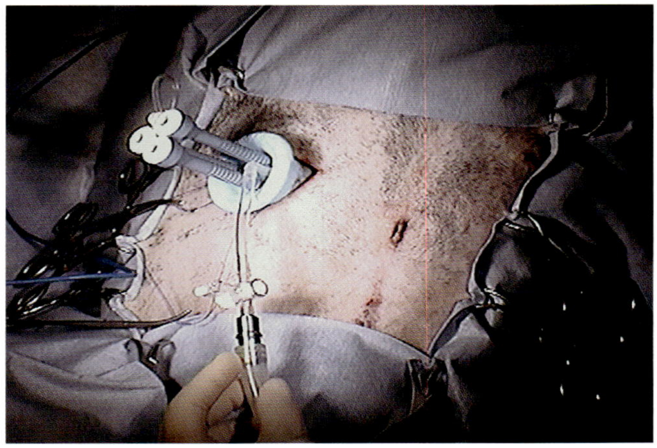

FIGURE 31. Location of SILS port placement for laparoscopic-assisted gastropexy. From this location, one can also combine with ovariectomy or cryptorchid procedures.

- While maintaining a gentle but firm hold of the site, the stomach is carefully exteriorized while removing the port. The stomach is exteriorized through the abdominal incision.
- Stay sutures are placed to maintain the orientation of the stomach axis.
- A 2–5 cm incision (depending on the patient's size) is made through the seromuscular layer of the antrum along the long axis of the stomach. Care should be taken to avoid prominent vasculature emerging from the greater and lesser curvatures.
- The submucosa is dissected from the seromuscular layer to ensure that the sutures are not placed into the gastric lumen.
- Two simple continuous lines of absorbable 2-0 or 0 monofilament suture are placed to appose both margins of the seromuscular layer in the antrum to the transversus abdominis.
- Before closure, the stay sutures that were placed are removed.
- Transected abdominal oblique musculature is closed with interrupted or continuous absorbable suture material.
- The remainder of the incision is closed in a routine fashion.

POSTOPERATIVE MANAGEMENT

- Analgesia following laparoscopic gastropexy is typically minimal and may include 2–3 days of a nonsteroidal drug and an oral, synthetic opioid such as tramadol.
- Food and water can be offered 8–12 hours after surgery.
- Subdivision of the daily food ration into five or six small meals per day for 1 week.
- Activity restriction should be enforced for 2 weeks following surgery to allow for early healing of the gastropexy site. Excessive activity early on may lead to failure of the gastropexy.

Complications of laparoscopic and laparoscopic-assisted gastropexy

- Complications are scarcely reported following intracorporeal laparoscopic gastropexy.
- Suture breakage is the most notable complication that the authors have witnessed and results from grasping the suture line with forceps or by pulling hard on the needle, thereby dislodging the suture from the swaged needle. Suture breakage may go unnoticed and could be a cause of gastropexy failure.
- Surgical site infections have not been reported following laparoscopic gastropexy in dogs, and the risk is likely low.

SUGGESTED READINGS

CLINICAL CASES

30.1 TOTAL LAPAROSCOPIC SUTURELESS GASTROPEXY WITH ABSORBABLE STRAPS IN DOGS

Luca Lacitignola

CASE DESCRIPTION

A prophylactic gastropexy with an absorbable fixation device (Ethicon SecureStrap) was performed in six Neapolitan dogs. The dogs were positioned in dorsal recumbency. Pneumoperitoneum was created by inserting a Veress needle at a maximum pressure of 8 mmHg of CO_2.

The dogs were discharged on the same day of the surgery. Feeding was allowed 8 hours after recovery from anesthesia, and the total food for each day was split into four feedings for at least 7 days after surgery. Robenacoxib (1 mg/kg) was administered orally once a day for 5 days after surgery. Owners were advised to keep their dogs rested and not to allow them to exercise for at least 7 days postoperatively. Skin wounds were covered with sterile dry dressings, and the application of 2% chlorhexidine solution every 3 days was recommended for disinfection. The owners were instructed to return to the hospital for clinical evaluation at 7, 30, and 90 days post-surgery. No intraoperative complications were reported during the surgeries. The total duration of surgery was 25.8 minutes (range, 19–39 minutes; SD, 6.7 minutes), and the time to complete the gastropexy was 10.1 minutes (range, 7–19 minutes; SD, 3.9 minutes). The median number of straps used to complete the gastropexy was 9 (range, 7–11 straps; interquartile range, 1.75 straps). No wound healing complications, vomiting, anorexia, lethargy, diarrhea, or episodes of gastric dilatation were recorded at any follow-up examinations. All dogs appeared healthy upon physical examination and showed no gastrointestinal signs during the follow-up. The ultrasound examination showed no sliding of the stomach from the abdominal wall.

Key points

- One advantage of laparoscopic gastropexy with an absorbable fixation device, which contributes to the decreased duration of surgery, is the elimination of the need to tie intracorporeal knots, resulting in a lower technical skill requirement and less extensive training.
- Ultrasound imaging showed adhesion of the stomach and body wall layers during follow-up assessments.
- The advantages of absorbable fixation devices are essentially the efficiency and simplicity of the application of the straps, which allow for a complete gastropexy to be performed in ≈10 minutes.

PORT PLACEMENT

Three 6 mm stainless steel reusable cannulas (Karl Storz Endoskope) were placed. The central cannula (T1) was placed on the telescope (5 mm laparoscopic 30° telescope, Karl Storz Endoskope) at the level of the umbilicus. Another cannula (T2) was positioned in the left cranial abdomen lateral to the rectus abdominis, just caudal to the third left mammary gland. The last cannula (T3) was placed in the right caudal abdomen lateral to the rectus abdominis, just caudal to the fourth right mammary gland. The monitor was placed on the right side of the patient. The surgeons worked on the right side of the patient.

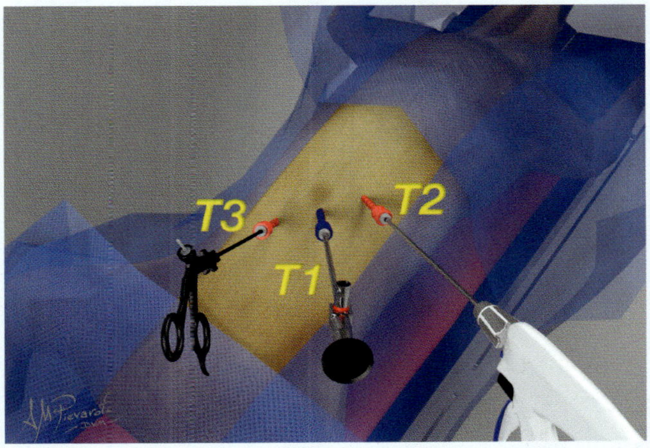

PROCEDURE

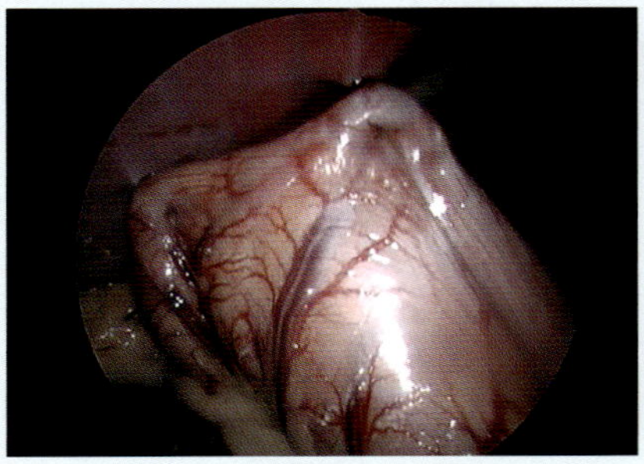

FIGURE 1. Preliminary apposition of the stomach to the abdominal wall with straps. Once the pyloric antrum was visualized, the stomach was grasped with a 5 mm grasper and moved to the right abdominal wall at the paracostal level (12th rib) to locate the exact area for stomach fixation.

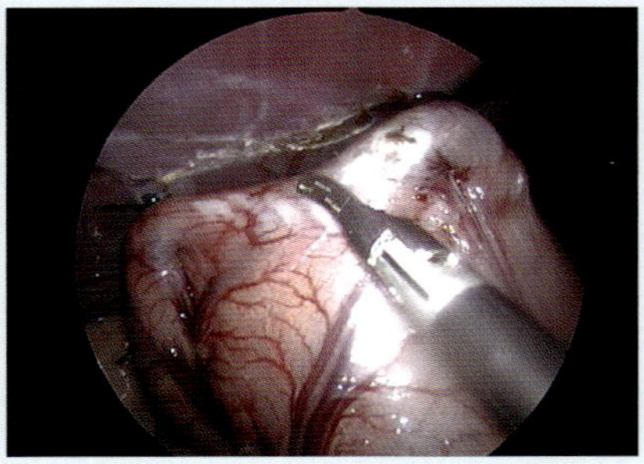

FIGURE 2. Serosa cauterization. The right instrument was removed, and the Ethicon Securestrap applicator was inserted to suspend the stomach to the abdominal wall with a cranial and caudal strap application. Then, a Harmonic scalpel (Ultracision ACE, Ethicon) was inserted to create cauterization lines on the abdominal wall and stomach serosa, according to an ideal line along the longitudinal axis of the stomach with a length of 4–5 cm.

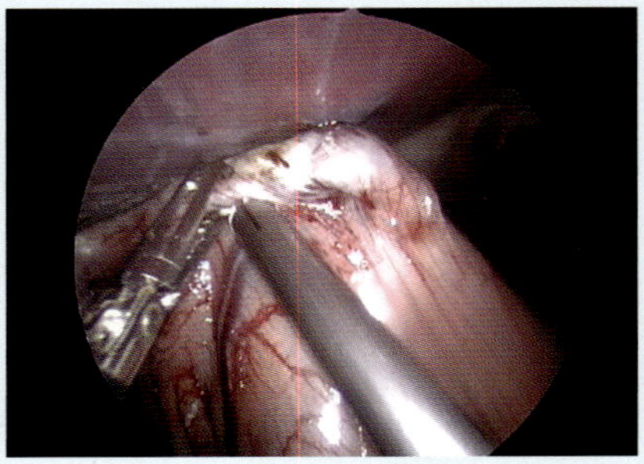

FIGURE 3. Fixation of the stomach was completed by applying the appropriate number of straps to cover the cauterization line and maintaining the apposition by manually pulling the stomach. The pneumoperitoneum was interrupted at the end of the procedure, the abdomen was deflated, and the cannulas were removed. The ports were closed with two layers of absorbable interrupted horizontal mattress pattern sutures (Polyglactin 910).

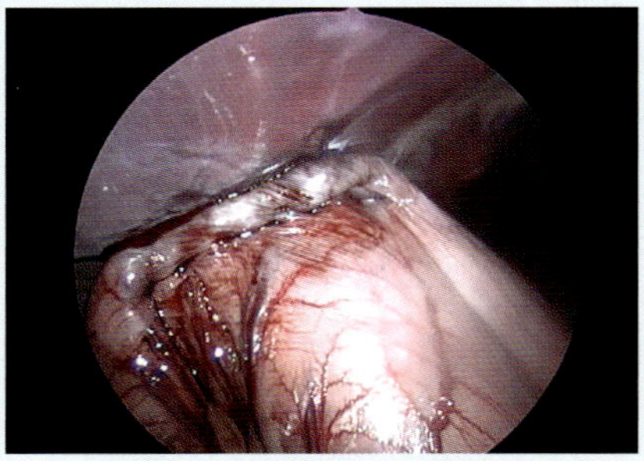

FIGURE 4. Stomach fixation completed.

Tips and tricks

- ✓ In cases with angles between the straps' applicator and abdominal wall presumably less than 60°, an assistant gently pressed the abdomen externally by hand to modify the angle.
- ✓ Serosa debridement promotes strong adhesion between the gastric and abdominal walls.
- ✓ Use 5 mm Babcock grasping forceps to create a seromuscular plica of the stomach to ensure that the absorbable fixation devices only penetrated the seromuscular layer for the constructs of the present study.

30.2 INTRACORPOREALLY SUTURED LAPAROSCOPIC GASTROPEXY USING AN ABDOMINAL WALL INCISION MADE AT RIGHT ANGLES TO THE ROTATION DIRECTION OF THE SUTURING NEEDLE

Motoki Kondo

CASE DESCRIPTION

The patient was a 1-year-old intact Great Dane with a body weight of 60 kg. The patient's owner visited the hospital for total intracorporeal gastropexy. Various preoperative examinations were performed, followed by elective intracorporeally sutured laparoscopic gastropexy.

Key points

- The axis of rotation of the needle holder.
- Relationship between the abdominal wall incision and the surgeon's right-hand port.
- Suture needle movement.

PORT PLACEMENT

A 5 mm trocar was placed along the linea alba at a subumbilical site with respect to the telescope port (T1). The surgeon's right-hand 5 mm port (T2) was placed on the caudal side of the xiphoid process. The surgeon's left-hand 5 mm port (T3) was placed so that it made an angle of 30°–60° to the line connecting the gastroabdominal wall stay suture and the telescope port.

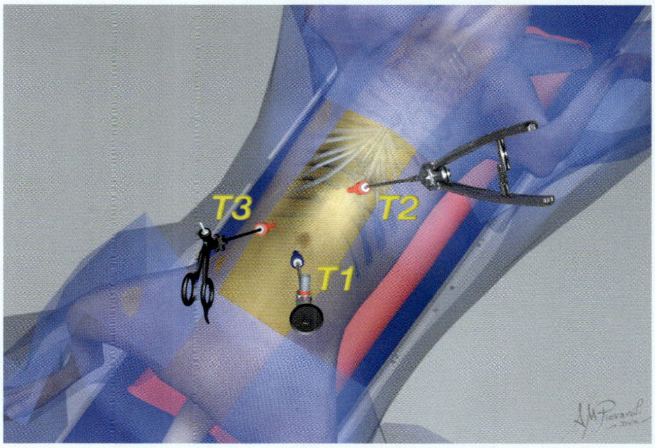

PROCEDURE

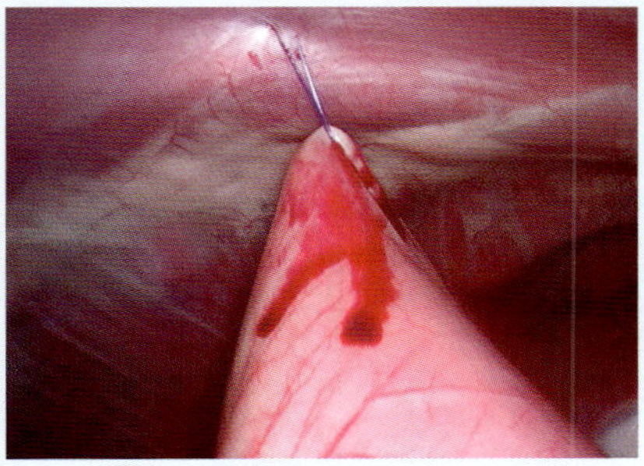

FIGURE 1. A 2-0 PDSII (Ethicon Inc.) suture was inserted percutaneously into the abdominal cavity, into the gastric wall of the pyloric antrum, removed from the body cavity again, and fixed with forceps. This suture was used as a "stay suture" to bring the stomach wall closer to the abdominal wall and was removed after completion of the gastropexy.

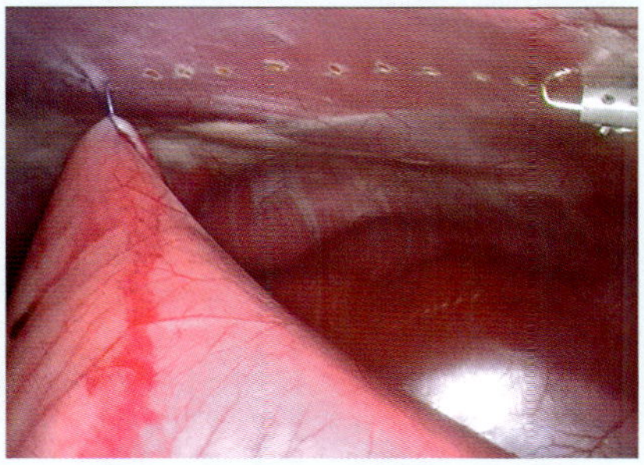

FIGURE 2. The planned incision line was straight and 4–5 cm long and directed toward the surgeon's right-hand port, starting proximal to the stay suture. Creating an incision along this line ensures that the incision can be made at right angles to the rotation direction of the suturing needle.

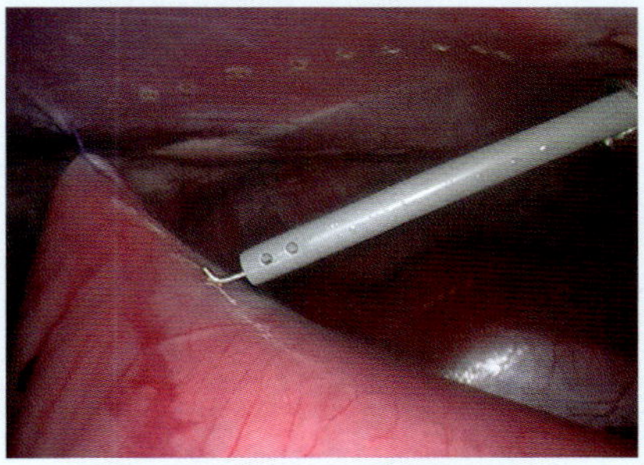

FIGURE 3. A similar incision line was made on the stomach wall to match the incision line on the abdominal wall.

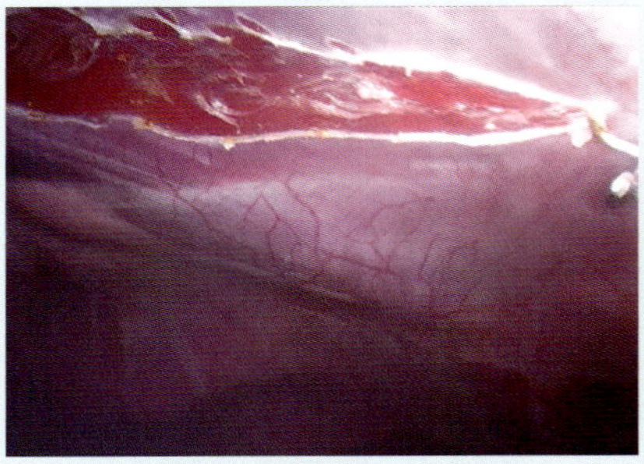

FIGURE 4. The peritoneum of the abdominal wall and the serosa of the gastric wall were incised following the planned incision line.

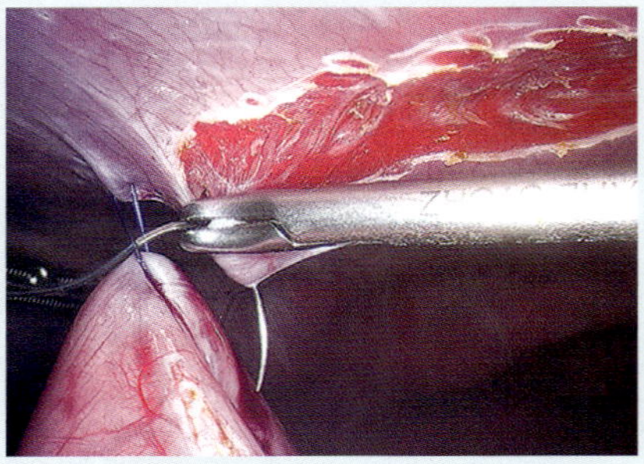

FIGURE 5. A barbed suture (V-Loc180, 3-0, 15 cm, Covidien) was introduced into the abdominal cavity from the outside. As seen in the image, the needle can be easily moved toward the incision by grasping the suture needle at a right angle to the needle holder and rotating the needle holder clockwise. The suture needle inserted through the abdominal wall incision penetrates the serosa.

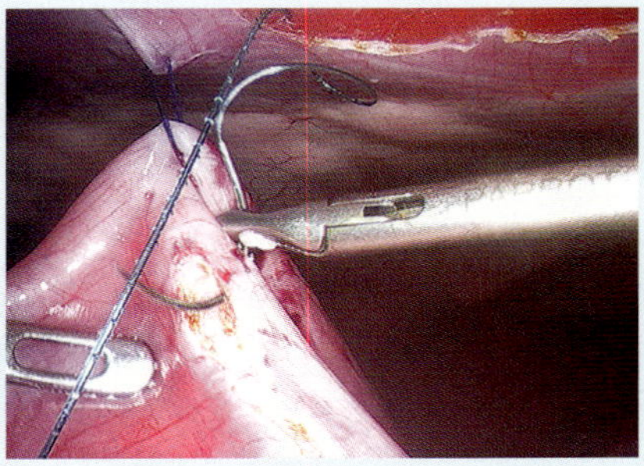

FIGURE 6. Subsequently, the V-Loc was inserted into the incision from the serosal surface of the stomach wall, and the needle holder was rotated clockwise to allow the suture needle to penetrate the stomach wall.

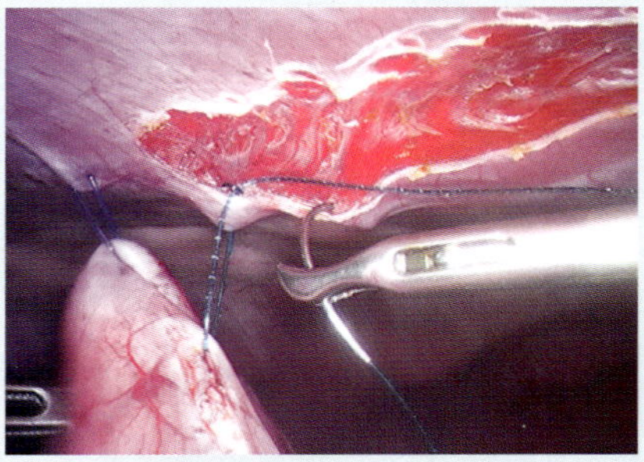

FIGURE 7. A suture needle penetrating the stomach wall was passed through a loop attached to the end, and the initial part of the suture was fixed without ligation. This is the starting point of the posterior wall suture for gastroabdominal wall fixation. Subsequently, the same needle movements used for the first needle were repeated for the abdominal and stomach walls.

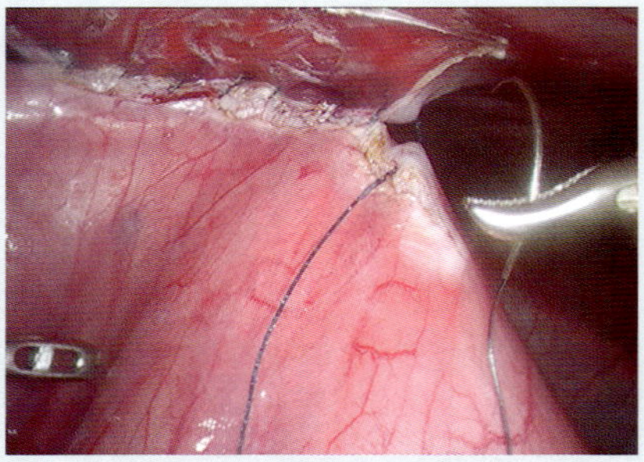

FIGURE 8. The barbed suture does not loosen when tightened; thus, the abdominal and stomach walls can be kept in close contact. The posterior wall was sutured continuously from the distal to the proximal wall, as shown in the image.

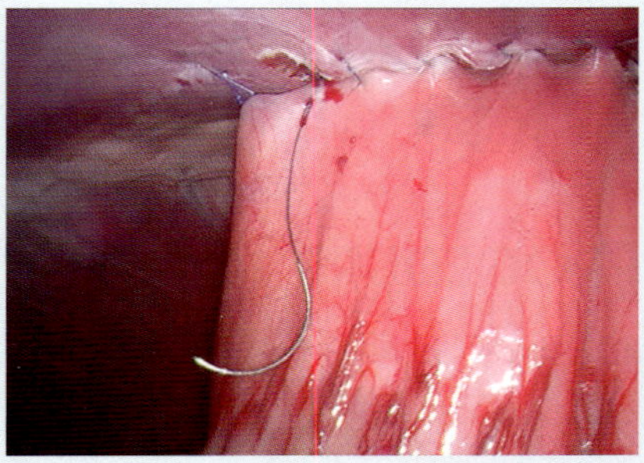

FIGURE 9. The anterior wall was also sutured from the proximal to the distal wall while maintaining tension. The end of the suture was not ligated, and the needle part was cut, leaving one suture end behind. The suture needle was removed from the body through the abdominal wall.

Tips and tricks

- ✓ Suturing becomes difficult if the abdominal wall incision is made parallel to the ribs, as in the case of laparotomy.
- ✓ The use of barbed sutures makes gastric fixation easier because the stomach wall does not separate from the abdominal wall due to gravity during suturing.
- ✓ It is easier to rotate the grasping forceps by turning it in the hand in a slightly exaggerated manner.
- ✓ It is difficult to suture the front wall if it is close to the sutured part of the back wall. If the incision is widened by extending it sufficiently along the stomach wall, the anterior wall can be easily sutured.

30.3 LAPAROSCOPIC GASTROPEXY IN A DOG

Antoine Adam

CASE DESCRIPTION

Offering gastropexy during laparoscopic spay or alone for big dogs or breeds at risk is common. In the author's experience, it does not add morbidity to the other procedures or in a very limited number of cases. The author recommends adding about 20–30 minutes to the laparoscopic spay itself. Based on the dog and the surgeon, it can be done with three cannulas or with a one-port device access.

Key points

- Do not place the cranial T3 port before knowing the stomach location; otherwise, this port can be placed too cranial or often too caudal.
- The dog is tilted to the right side but half tilted. Abdominal pressure is then reduced to 8 mmHg.
- Sometimes, the pressure is even reduced to 6 mmHg if there is too much tension on the stomach to make the gastropexy.
- Take care to stay caudal to the attachment of the diaphragm (which is usually a white line near the last ribs region).
- Start the surgery by punctioning the stomach first, away from the pyloric region (mean 5 cm).

PORT PLACEMENT

- T1, 5 mm camera port approximately 2–3 cm caudal to the umbilicus, on the ventral midline
- T3, 5 mm instrument port approximately 1–2 cm cranial to the umbilicus, on the ventral midline
- T2, 13 mm port for ovariectomy (before gastropexy). It can be a 5 mm port if gastropexy alone.

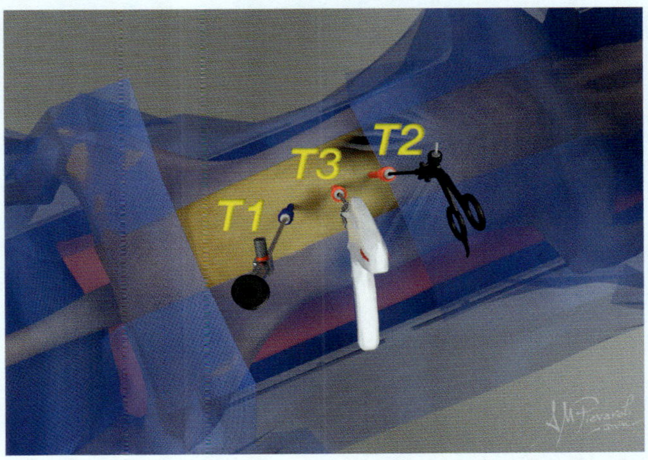

PROCEDURE

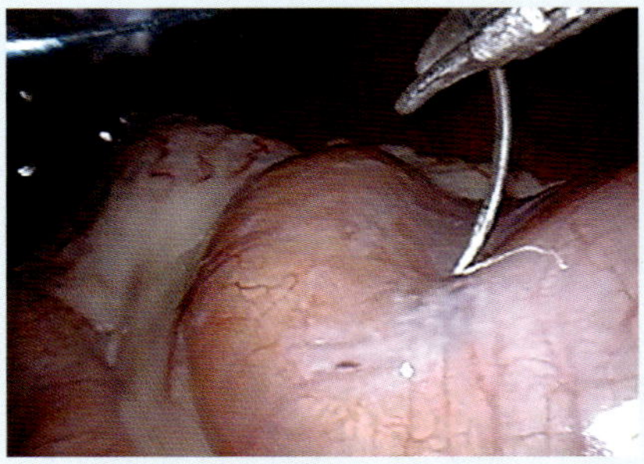

FIGURE 1. First, suture on the stomach a few centimeters away from the pyloric region (mean 5 cm). The author uses a V-Loc 180 2-0 wire. Most of the time, a 15 cm and a 23 cm for giant dogs are used.

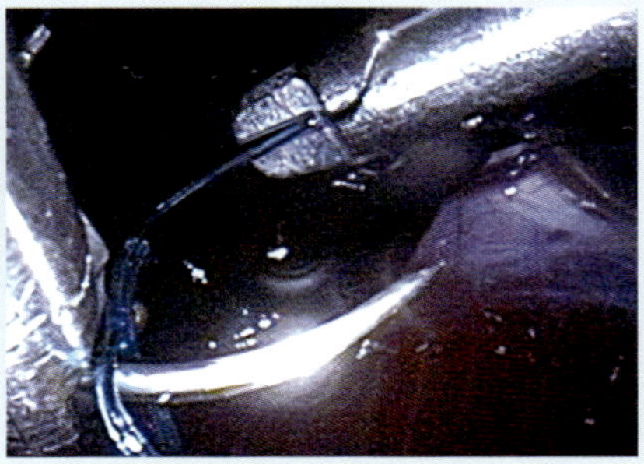

FIGURE 2. Pass the needle inside the loop of the extremity of the V-Loc. Holding the scope as close as possible helps to visualize the hole in the wire. Using flexible forceps also helps.

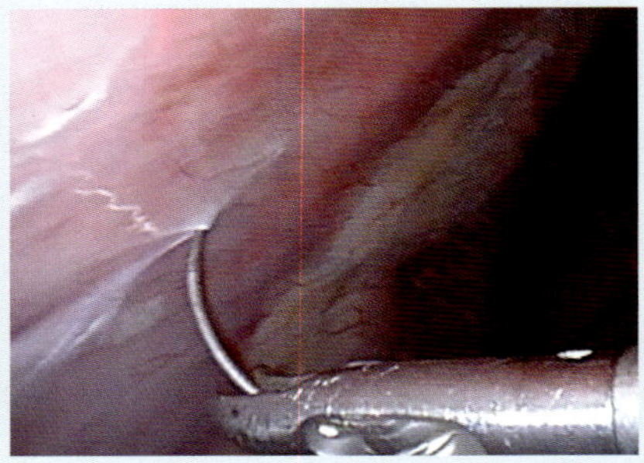

FIGURE 3. First suture of the peritoneal wall. Pass the abdominal wall where the pexy is aimed. (Take care to stay caudal to the attachment of the diaphragm, which is usually a white line near the last ribs region.)

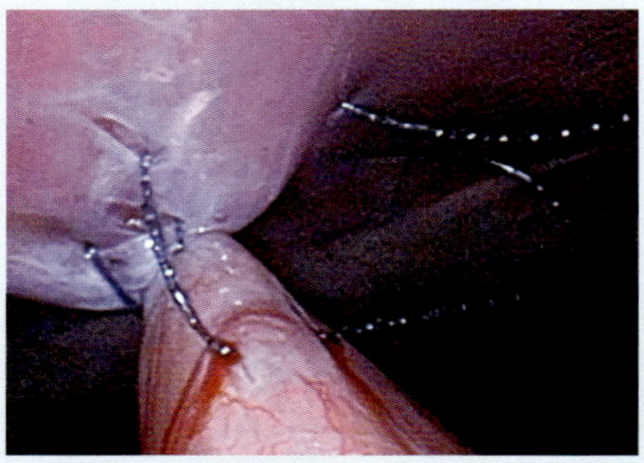

FIGURE 4. Stomach gastropexy. Make between 5 to 10 bites always in the same way and direction: the suture line is perpendicular to the dog's body or in the axis of the great curvature of the stomach. In the end, a last bite can be made in the abdominal wall in the opposite direction.

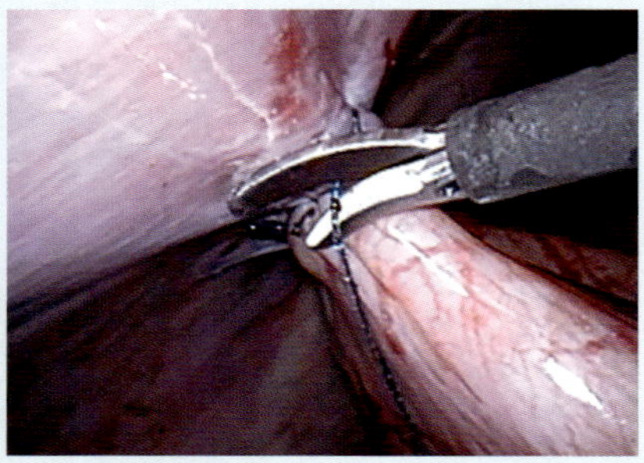

FIGURE 5. Cutting the wire. Insert a scissor to flush cut the wire, grab the distal end of the wire, and pull it inside the cannula. The needle will go in the right direction by pulling the wire instead of the needle itself.

Tips and tricks

- ✓ Take care to try to put the cannula to the right side of the falciform ligament. It is much better for visualization and wire manipulation.
- ✓ Use a Deam Steerable forceps to hold the stomach and for needle manipulation. It helps to put the needle in the right position.
- ✓ Insert and remove the needle through a 13 mm cannula.
- ✓ To remove the needle, hold the wire and pull it through the 13 mm cannula.
- ✓ Use a 15 cm wire; use only a 23 cm for a giant dog.

30.4 TOTAL LAPAROSCOPIC GASTROPEXY (TWO-PORT TECHNIQUE USING ENDOSTITCH)

Justin B. Ganjei

CASE DESCRIPTION

A 1-year-old intact male Great Dane presented for prophylactic gastropexy to prevent gastric dilatation and volvulus due to being an at-risk breed. The patient was healthy otherwise, and preoperative blood work was unremarkable.

Key points

- Placing a percutaneous stay suture in the stomach is essential for this procedure to be completed using a two-port technique.
- There is no need to create a partial thickness incision through the seromuscular layer of the stomach; only an abrasionplasty is needed.

PORT PLACEMENT

- T1, 5 mm telescope trocar, 2 cm caudal to the umbilicus
- T2, 10 mm instrument trocar, 4 cm caudal to the xiphoid process

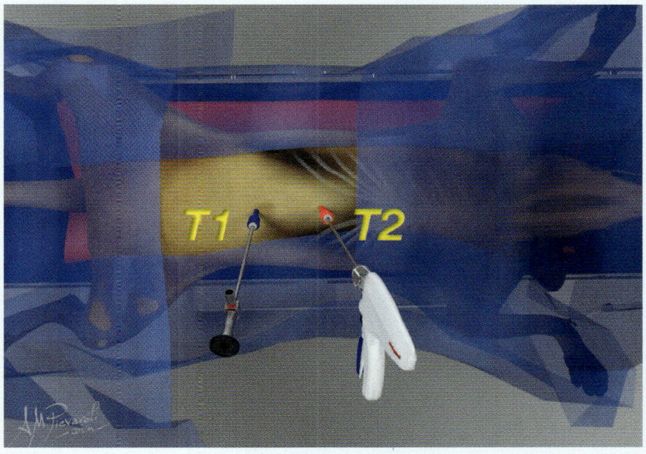

PROCEDURE

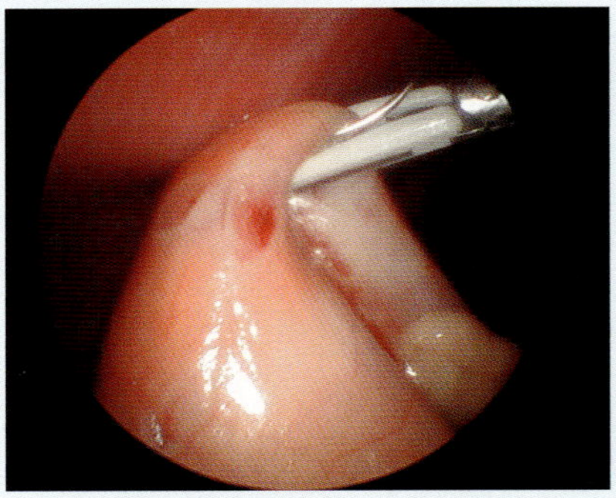

FIGURE 1. Laparoscopic image of a percutaneous suture being used to temporarily secure the pyloric antral region of the stomach to the right ventrolateral body wall. A 0.5 cm incision was made 2 cm caudal to the umbilicus, and a 5 mm balloon trocar was placed using a modified Hasson approach (T1). The abdomen was insufflated to 10 mmHg with CO_2. A 5 mm 0° telescope was introduced. A second port was placed, utilizing a 10 mm balloon trocar 4 cm caudal to the xiphoid process under direct visualization of the telescope (T2). The pyloric antral region of the stomach was identified and grasped using 10 mm laparoscopic Babcock forceps. The stomach was then retracted to the right ventrolateral abdomen 2 cm caudal to the last rib and 5 cm lateral to the linea alba.

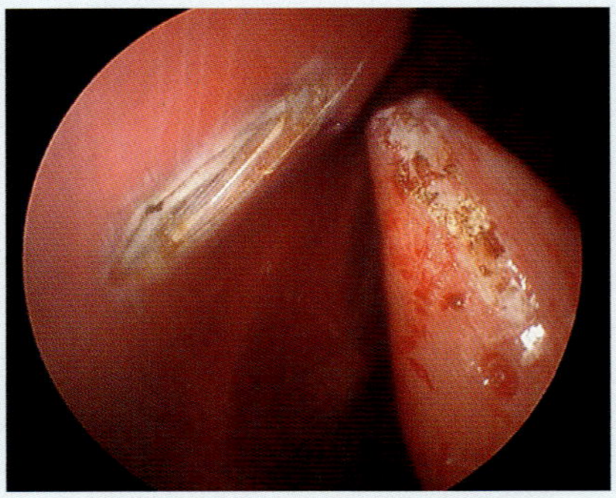

FIGURE 2. Laparoscopic image of the full-thickness seromuscular incision made at the right ventrolateral body wall and the abrasionplasty made in the ventral pyloric antrum using the J-tip electrocautery device. The stomach was then temporarily secured to this position via percutaneous monofilament suture on a taper needle. A 5 mm laparoscopic J-tip electrocautery was then used to perform an 4 cm abrasionplasty of the gastric serosa and an identical length, full-thickness incision through the transversus abdominus in this region.

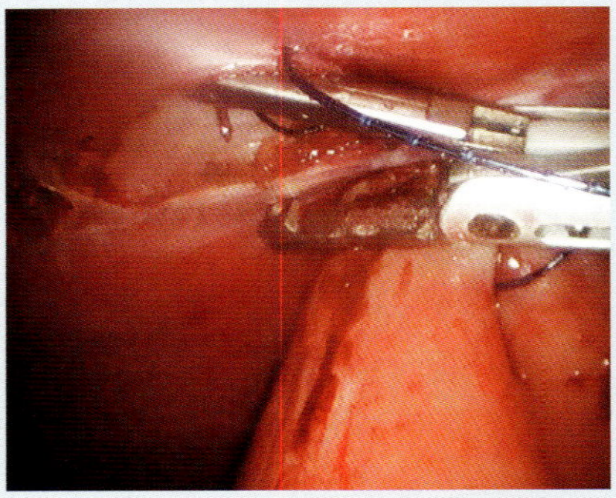

FIGURE 3. Laparoscopic image showing the Endostitch device taking a bite from both sides of the seromuscular incision. An Endostich suture preloaded with a 0 V-Loc was then placed through the instrument port and used to perform an incisional gastropexy. The gastropexy was initiated at the cranial aspect and continued caudally. Approximately 1 cm length of suture line was left as a tag prior to being transected using laparoscopic Metzenbaum scissors.

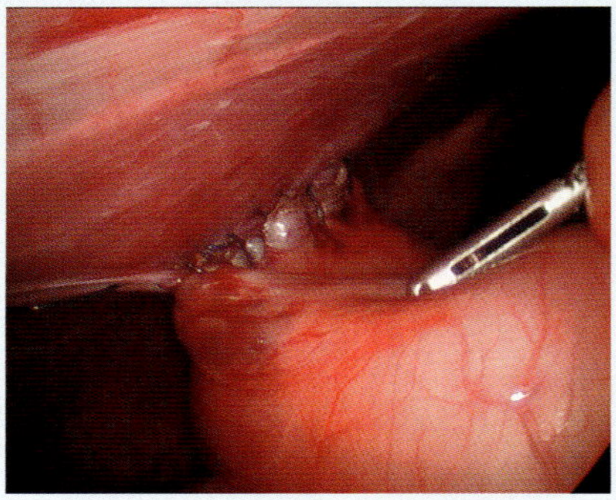

FIGURE 4. Laparoscopic image of the use of Babcock forceps to test the strength of the completed gastropexy. Following completion, the gastropexy site strength was tested by grasping the stomach with Babcock forceps and retracting. The abdomen was evacuated of all CO_2, and port sites were apposed in a standard multilayer fashion. Bupivacaine was infused around all port sites.

Tips and tricks

- ✓ Taking individual bites through each side of the transversus abdominus incision makes it easier to ensure an appropriate amount of tissue is being grasped.
- ✓ The J-tip electrocautery can be inserted through the 10 mm port without losing insufflation.
- ✓ Having an assistant depressing the body wall can help achieve bites through the transversus abdominus.
- ✓ Tension can be applied to the suture line by retracting the Endostitch device through the port.
- ✓ Decreasing capnoperitoneum pressure can facilitate the gastropexy procedure by reducing tension between the stomach and the body wall.

30.5 TREATMENT OF LOWER ESOPHAGEAL SPHINCTER INCOMPETENCE IN A CAT USING TOTAL LAPAROSCOPIC GASTROPEXY

Roberto Giaconella, Veronica Giaconella

CASE DESCRIPTION

A 10-month-old shorthair domestic cat was presented because it had been vomiting and regurgitating for 6 months, was dehydrated, and in poor condition. Despite various attempts at medical treatment, the cat continued regurgitating after each meal.

The term "hiatal pathology" indicates numerous pathologies that affect the lower esophageal sphincter (LES) or the esophageal hiatus of the diaphragm, which in most cases lead to reflux esophagitis. In cats, hiatal pathology may result from:

- defects in the embryonic development of the esophageal hiatus (congenital form)
- factors that alter the pressure of the LES (hiatal hernia, chronic vomiting, delayed stomach emptying, general anesthesia, Trendelenburg surgery, insertion of a nasogastric and pharyngostomy tube)
- abdominal trauma causing a sudden increase in intra-abdominal pressure.

In this case, the LES incompetence was diagnosed endoscopically and was surgically treated by total laparoscopic gastropexy. Fundic gastropexy was performed on the left side. This procedure may be a viable option for cases of severe LES incompetence unresponsive to medical treatment.

Key points

- Vomiting and regurgitation are always present.
- It is very important to understand the underlying cause of LES incompetence.
- Gastropexy is performed on the left side.

PORT PLACEMENT

- Dorsal recumbency
- T1, 1 cm caudal to the umbilicus
- T2, on the right side, 3 cm cranial to the umbilicus in a paramedian position
- T3, on the right side, 2 cm cranial to T2

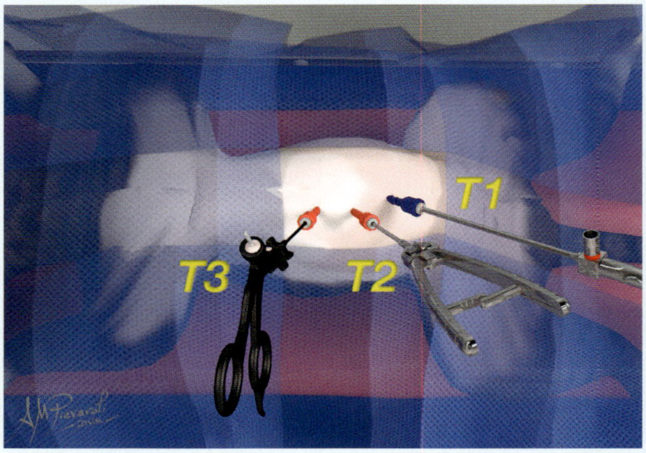

PROCEDURE

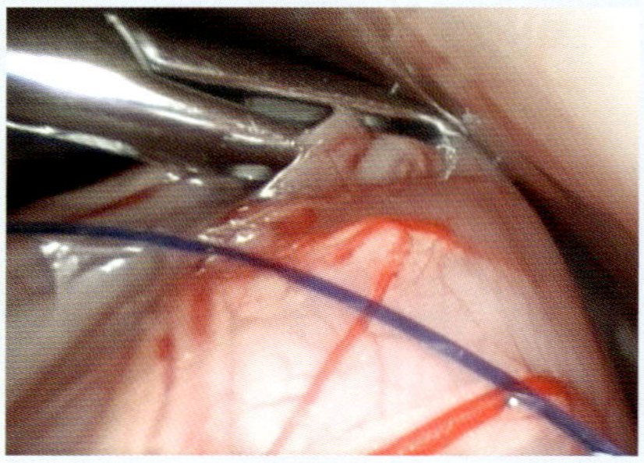

FIGURE 1. Laparoscopic image of the apposition of the stomach to the abdominal wall.

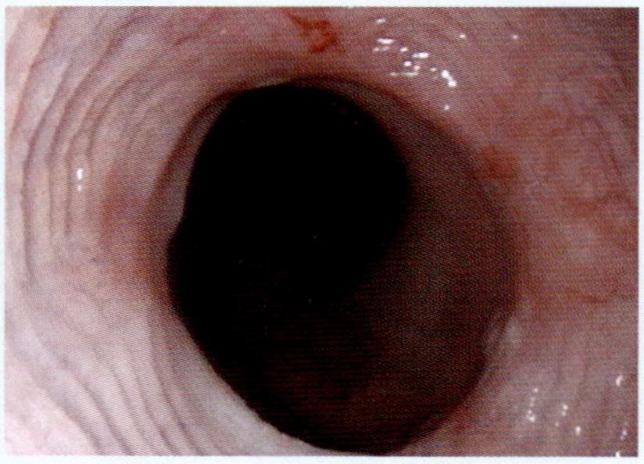

FIGURE 2. Endoscopic image of the lower esophageal incompetent sphincter.

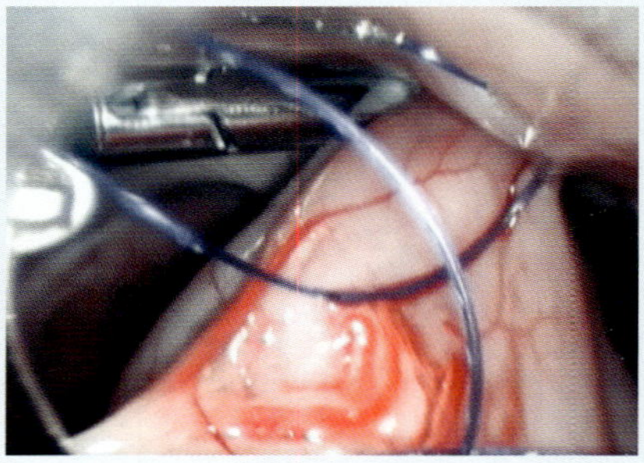

FIGURE 3. Execution of the gastropexy with a self-retaining knotless unidirectional barbed suture (3-0 Filbloc, 15 cm).

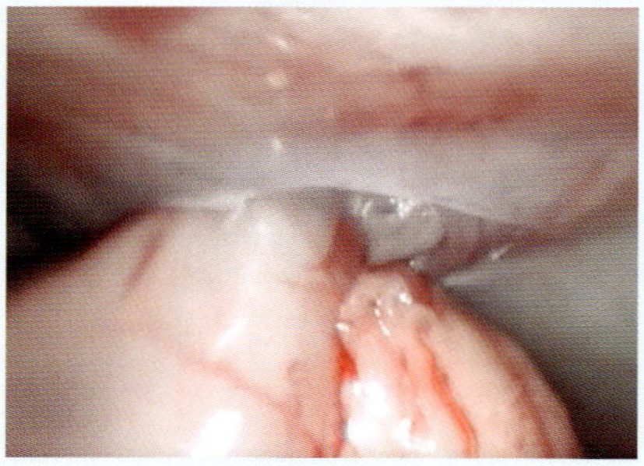

FIGURE 4. Laparoscopic checkup 2 months after surgery.

Tips and tricks

✓ Use barbed suture to perform the gastropexy.
✓ Esophagoscopy performed during surgery is useful to guide the surgeon during the procedure.
✓ Adequate fluid therapy must be administered before and after surgery, and a semiliquid diet for at least 1 week after surgery.
✓ Feed the cat from an elevated position, with multiple small meals during the day.

31 LAPAROSCOPIC-ASSISTED GASTROTOMY

Andrea M. Pievaroli

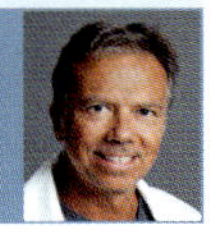

Indications	**Contraindications**
■ Gastric foreign body removal ■ Intraoperative conversion of ineffective flexible endoscopy ■ Access to the stomach for the diagnosis or treatment of pathologies	■ Gastric (or intestinal) perforation with septic peritonitis ■ Cardiovascular and pulmonary disease

This laparoscopic procedure is mainly indicated for removing foreign bodies that cannot be removed through flexible endoscopy. Anamnesis and preoperative investigations are important to identify the type, shape, and size of the foreign body in the stomach and choose the most appropriate technique for the patient. In some selected cases, especially for small objects that cannot cause lesions to the esophagus, induction of emesis must be considered.

Flexible gastroscopy is considered the minimally invasive technique of choice for removing foreign bodies from the stomachs of dogs and cats and is generally decisive in most cases. On the other hand, when gastrotomy is indicated, the laparoscopic-assisted technique is a valid alternative to the open technique, offering the advantages of less invasiveness, lower risk of abdominal contamination, and a faster recovery in the postoperative period.

In the veterinary literature, a total laparoscopic gastrotomy technique was also described in one study performed on 20 dogs. The intracorporeal suture of the gastric wall was performed using both sutures and stapler without significant complications in the postoperative period.

Lew M., Jałynski M., and Brzeski W. published an article in 2005 about the laparoscopic removal of gastric foreign bodies in dogs.

PATIENT PREPARATION AND POSITIONING

Patient preparation also depends on the clinical status at the time of presentation. A preoperative workup is important before performing the surgical procedure. Patients must be carefully evaluated and stabilized for surgery. They could be debilitated, dehydrated, have electrolyte disturbances from repeated episodes of vomiting and may need fluid therapy and other types of investigations before undergoing anesthesia. It is preferable also to give antibiotic therapy before surgery, to minimize the risk of intraoperative infections during the incision of the stomach. The ventral abdomen is widely clipped, extending cranially beyond the xiphoid process. The patient is placed in dorsal recumbency, the skin is aseptically prepared, and a large sterile drape is used to prevent exposure to the table during tilting.

During the procedure, the reverse Trendelenburg position could be helpful to allow the stomach to move more caudally. Also, lateral table tilting could be necessary to make the displacement of the spleen easier and to visualize the stomach better.

The following procedures are described below:

A. Two-port laparoscopic-assisted gastrotomy

B. Single-port laparoscopic-assisted gastrotomy (J. Runge and J. Becker)

A TWO-PORT LAPAROSCOPIC-ASSISTED GASTROTOMY

The laparoscopic-assisted gastrotomy can be performed with basic laparoscopic equipment. It is a mixed technique that consists of a first access step in laparoscopy and a second step of open surgery with standard instruments. The technique is performed with two ports placed in the midline. Alternatively, a single multiport access can be used. The surgeon performs the laparoscopic access to locate the stomach, grasps the area of the gastric wall where the gastrotomy will be performed, brings the stomach close to the abdominal wall, and withdraws it after widening the incision of the same port of the forceps. The surgery continues with a standard open technique in the second part of the procedure. In a cranial and caudal aspect, two stay sutures are placed on the stomach wall to sustain the organ during the gastrotomy. After the gastric wall incision, grasping tools are introduced to extract foreign bodies from the stomach. During the procedure, the telescope is useful for inspecting the stomach and ensuring the removal of foreign bodies. Then, the gastric incision is closed routinely, the stomach is repositioned in the abdomen, and the small incision of the abdominal wall is sutured.

OPERATING ROOM LAYOUT

For laparoscopic-assisted gastrotomy, the surgeon and assistant should stand on the right and left sides of the patient, respectively. If a ceiling or boom-mounted monitor is used, this is placed at the head of the table with the scope tower positioned laterally or caudally. Alternatively, the mobile equipment cart with a monitor is positioned on the right or left side of the table. A second monitor in the contralateral position is recommended. The anesthesia machine is placed near the patient's head. The instrument table is set caudolateral or at the foot of the table (**Fig. 1**).

Instruments

On the table:

- Standard surgery set
- Telescope 5 mm – 30°
- Two 5 mm threaded cannulas/trocars (or 10 mm size for larger instruments)
- Grasping forceps (Duval, Babcock)
- Surgical suction pump

Ready to use:

- Different types of grasping forceps, not necessarily for laparoscopy use
- Endoscopic cannula for aspiration/irrigation

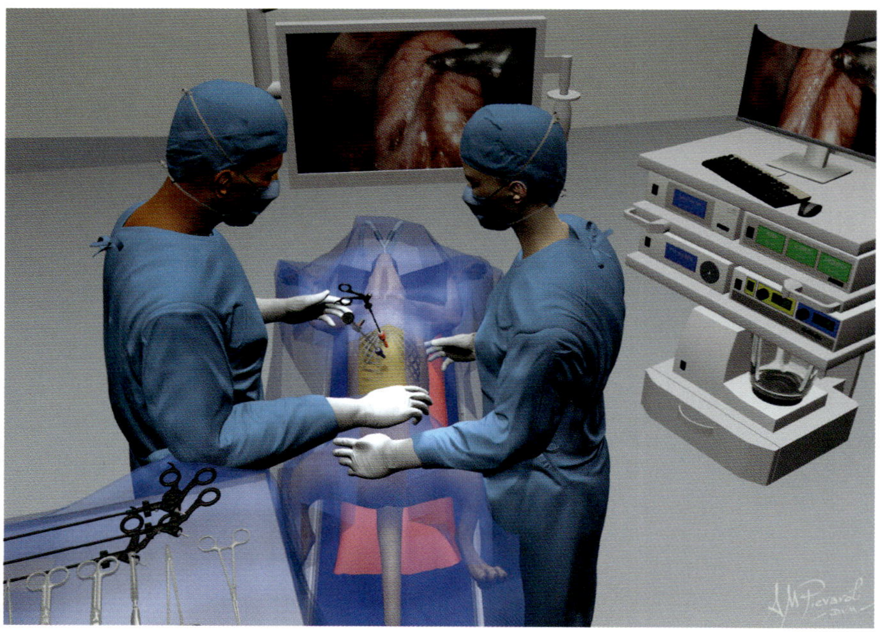

FIGURE 1. Operating room layout for laparoscopic-assisted gastrotomy.

PORT PLACEMENT (FIG. 2)

Two ports or a single multiport device can be used for this procedure. The 5 mm cannulas/trocars may be adequate without using special larger-sized instruments. Pneumoperitoneum is established according to individual preferences. The author prefers to use the Ternamian technique or a modified Hasson technique, using threaded cannulas as ports (Storz Endotip) because they are more stable once positioned in the patient.

The first port (T1) is introduced on the midline, a few centimeters cranial to the umbilicus. After a first abdominal exploration with the scope, the second port (T3) is placed on the midline, usually in a more cranial position than the previous one. Generally speaking, the abdominal wall incision will be approximately midway between the umbilicus and the caudal xiphoid process.

- T1, on the midline, 1–3 cm cranial to the umbilicus
- T3, on the midline, a few centimeters cranial to T1

PROCEDURE

- After the first port placement (T1) cranially to the umbilicus and pneumoperitoneum has been achieved, the 5 mm telescope is inserted, and the first exploration of the abdomen is performed to ensure no injuries to the organs were caused during the introduction of the first cannula.
- In this area of the peritoneum, the falciform ligament can often be found, which could prevent correct vision and cloud the lens of the telescope. It is necessary to screw deeper to find the correct inclination to overcome the ligament.
- The stomach is visible slightly cranial to the port (**Fig. 3**).
- Under endoscopic vision, the second cannula (T3) is inserted on the same midline, a few centimeters cranially to the first one.
- The first (T1) or second port (T3) can be used indifferently to introduce the telescope. The other port will be used for the forceps (**Fig. 4**)
- An exploration of the region is performed for an initial evaluation. For a correct manipulation of the tissues, it is advisable to use a blunt probe and atraumatic forceps.
- After identifying the area of the stomach where to perform the gastrotomy (generally the midbody of the stomach), the Babcock or Duval forceps are introduced to grasp the gastric body gently (**Fig. 5**).
- The scope is removed, and its cannula is withdrawn. Also, the second cannula is elevated along the forceps, and the skin and abdominal wall incision in the midline is started. The initial cut length must include the entry points of the two ports. It is preferable to limit the incision to 3–4 cm. It will be enlarged if necessary, depending on the size of the foreign body to be extracted.
- After cutting the subcutaneous tissue and the abdominal wall, according to the standard surgical technique, there is a rapid desufflation of the peritoneal cavity. This will facilitate the approach of the stomach to the abdominal wall.

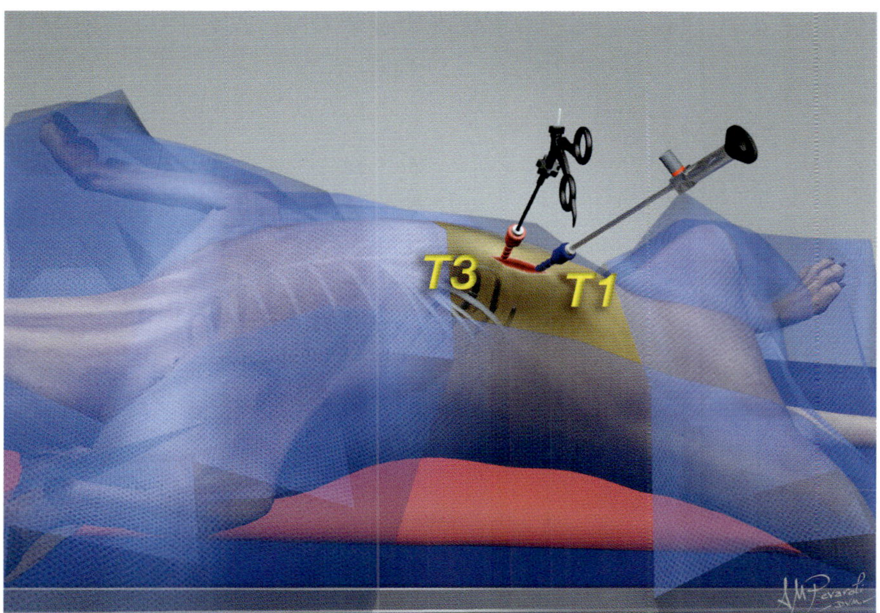

FIGURE 2. Port placement for laparoscopic-assisted gastrotomy.

- At this point, two first stay sutures are placed cranially and caudally in the stomach, and the endoscopic forceps is removed. These sutures are held by small forceps and are tractioned to withdraw the portion of the stomach to be incised (**Fig. 6**). A Gelpi retractor could also be used to retract the abdominal wound.
- Moistened sponges are placed around the wound to prevent the introduction of material into the abdomen. Then a stab incision is made into the stomach wall between the two stay sutures. If necessary, additional stay sutures can be placed in the middle of the incision to visualize the gastric cavity better.
- If fluid is present in the stomach, an aspirator is used to remove most of it. The risk of contamination of the abdcminal cavity and surrounding tissues must be minimized.
- The scope is introduced to inspect and identify the foreign body (**Fig. 7**). Then, by using endoscopic forceps (5–10 mm Babcock) or another type of standard surgery forceps, the single foreign object or multiple parts of it can be extracted (**Figs. 8 and 9**). The scope is used for a last inspection before closure.
- The gastrotomy incision is closed routinely with monofilament sutures, according to the surgeon's personal preferences.

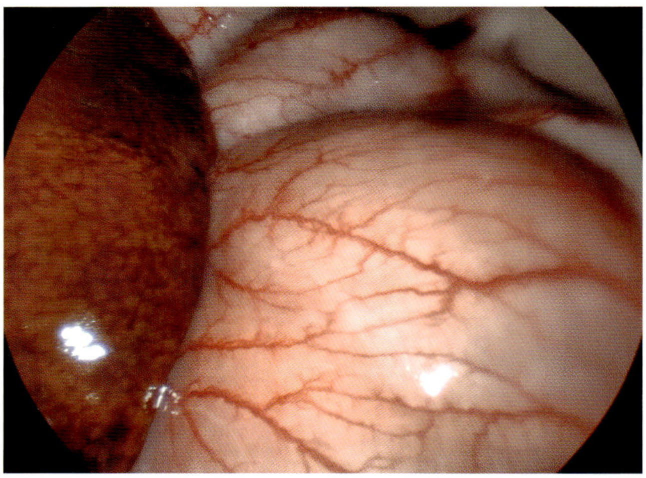

FIGURE 3. After the first port placement (T1), a first exploration of the abdomen is performed. The stomach is visible below slightly cranial to the port.

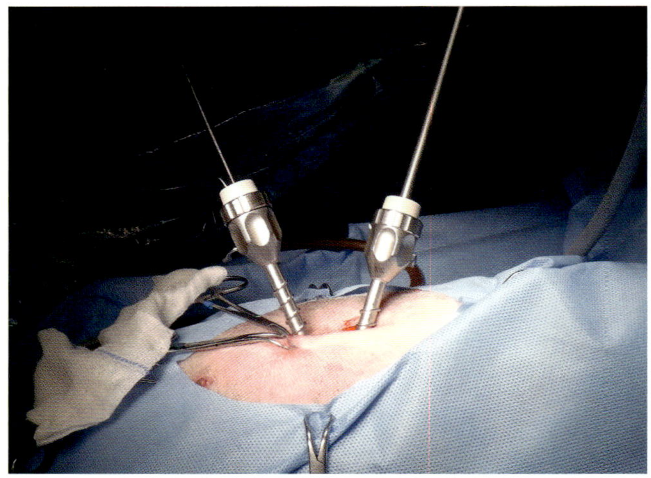

FIGURE 4. Image of the operating field for laparoscopic-assisted gastrotomy.

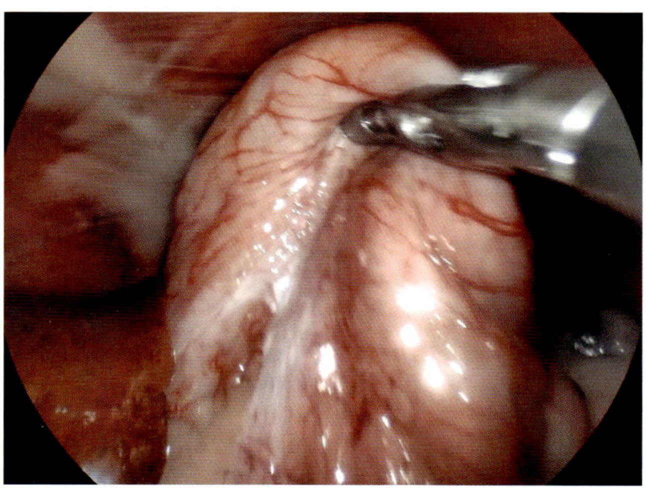

FIGURE 5. A Babcock, a Duval, or other atraumatic forceps are used to gently grasp the gastric body in the area where to perform the gastrotomy.

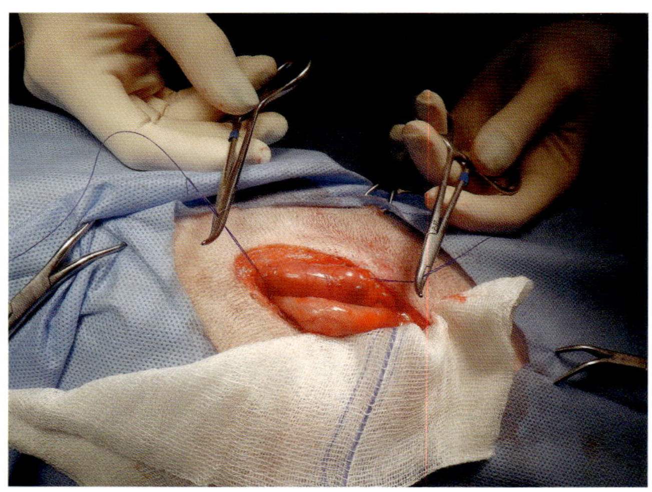

FIGURE 6. Two stay sutures are placed cranial and caudal, held by small forceps. These sutures are tractioned to withdraw the portion of the stomach to be incised.

Before releasing the stomach into the abdomen, a lavage of the gastric incision with saline solution is made, removing the sponges and the stay sutures.

- The body wall and the skin are closed routinely.

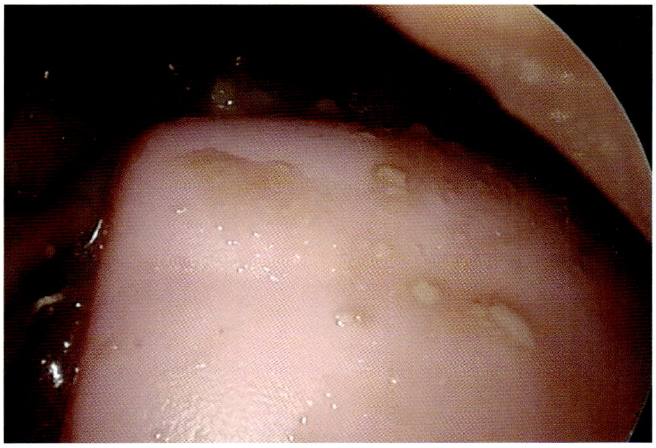

FIGURE 7. Inspection of the gastric lumen with the telescope to look for the foreign body (in the image, the pink silicon object).

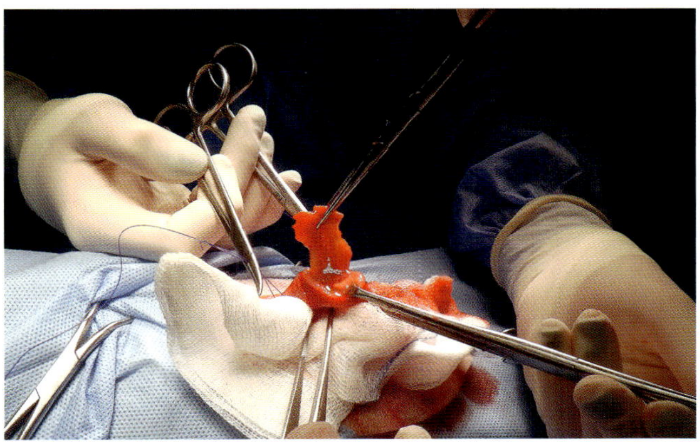

FIGURE 8. Extraction of the foreign body (plastic fragments) using a long standard open surgery Klemmer forceps.

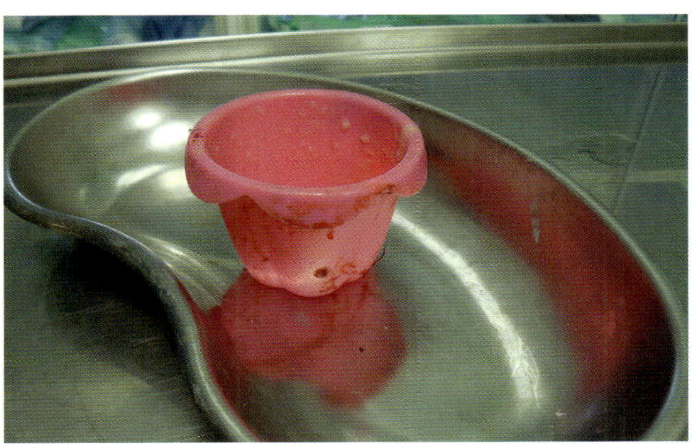

FIGURE 9. Foreign object (silicon) removed from the stomach.

B SINGLE-PORT LAPAROSCOPIC-ASSISTED GASTROTOMY

Jeffrey J. Runge, Joshua G. Becker

Instruments

- Standard surgery set
- Telescope 5 mm – 30°
- Single-incision port device
- Alexis wound retractor or Gelpi
- Straight or articulating forceps
- A blunt palpation probe or fan retractor
- Biopsy instruments (if indicated)
- Thoracoabdominal, gastrointestinal anastomotic, or endogastrointestinal anastomotic staplers (as needed for stapled anastomosis)

OPERATING ROOM LAYOUT

The surgeon may stand to the left or to the right of the patient toward the foot of the table. The surgeon may need to work from both the left and right sides of the patient. There should be enough space in the operating room to allow the surgeon to move safely between both sides of the patient.

If multiple video monitors are available, they are positioned at the head of the table on the right and left sides. A single monitor is acceptable as long as it can easily be moved to the opposite side of the surgeon; ceiling or boom-mounted monitors are preferable. The instrument table is best placed at the foot of the table to avoid interference with the anesthetist/anesthesiologist.

An extra-large patient drape is recommended to prevent exposure of the patient and operating table during patient manipulation/tilting.

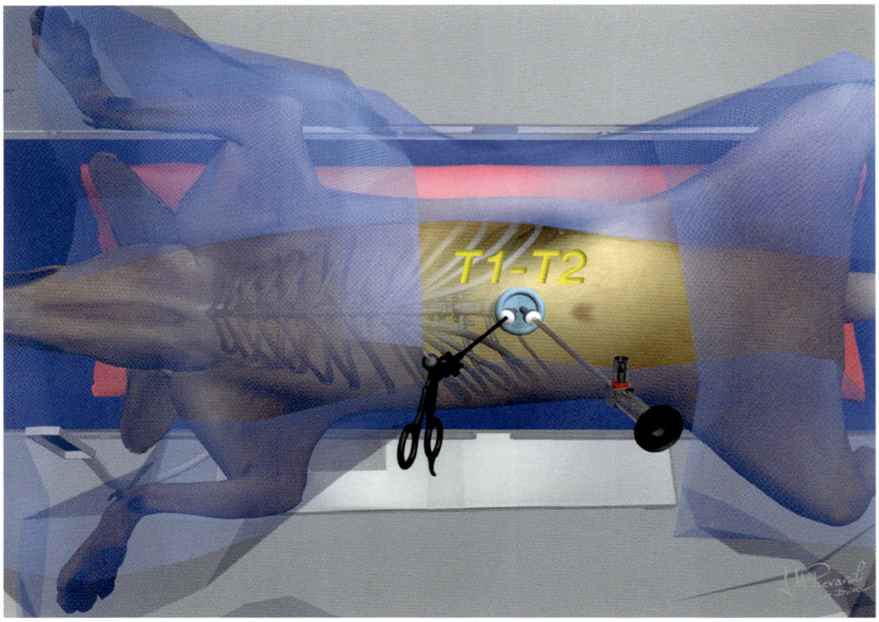

FIGURE 10. Port placement for single-port laparoscopic-assisted gastrotomy.

PORT PLACEMENT (FIG. 10)

The port is placed on the midline, approximately midway between the umbilicus and the xiphoid process.

PROCEDURE

- After port placement and pneumoperitoneum have been established, the scope is inserted, and the abdomen is surveyed in standard fashion, checking for anatomical landmarks and ensuring the gross visible anatomy (body wall, viscera, etc.) appears within normal limits. Care must be taken to avoid and check for evidence of iatrogenic trauma secondary to port placement.
- A 5 mm laparoscopic Debakey or Babcock forceps is inserted and used to grasp the body of the stomach, which is then elevated ventrally.
- The endoscope and inner cannulas (SILS port) or the bulkhead of the EndoCone are removed while the grasp on the gastric body is gently but firmly maintained—the abdomen will desufflate rapidly.
- The port is removed, and the laparoscopic DeBakey or Babcock forceps are used to extracorporealize the stomach.
- Stay sutures are placed in the stomach.
- A small Gelpi or Alexis wound retractor is used to maintain retraction of the abdominal incision, and the laparotomy sponges are used to pack off the stomach. Minimal enlargement of the abdominal incision is usually required depending on the patient's size and the foreign material to be removed.
- An extracorporeal gastrotomy is performed using the standard open technique. 5 or 10 mm endoscopic Babcock forceps can be used to retrieve foreign bodies from the gastric lumen. The endoscope can be used as a gastroscope to guide and ensure the complete removal of the gastric foreign material. Still, it should not be used again for laparoscopy because of contamination of the endoscope.
- After removing all foreign material, the gastrotomy site can be closed in a standard simple-continuous single-layer or two-layer fashion using an appropriate absorbable monofilament suture material (this author prefers a two-layer closure). A knotless suture can also be used to close the gastrotomy and may provide a faster closure time with similar results to standard closure using a normal suture.
- The abdominal incision site can be closed in a standard fashion.

POSTOPERATIVE MANAGEMENT

- Local analgesics at the time of incision site closure are recommended.
- Depending on the medical condition prior to surgery, the patient could be discharged from the hospital within a few hours of the procedure or be hospitalized to continue supportive care and therapy.
- Nonsteroidal anti-inflammatory drugs are typically contraindicated in patients after gastrointestinal surgery out of concern for interference in gastrointestinal wound healing.
- Antibiotic therapy is indicated in the days following surgery.
- The overall necessity of these can be case-dependent, but most are generally recommended for at least 24 hours after surgery as important prophylactic measures: antacids (e.g., proton pump inhibitors), antiemetics (e.g., maropitant, ondansetron), prokinetics (e.g., metoclopramide), appetite stimulants (e.g., capromorelin).
- It has become a common practice to encourage a return to enteral feeding as quickly as possible postoperatively, often as early as 6–8 hours after surgery if no evidence of vomiting or nausea is noted. This is likely linked to a study on a captive Beagle population that strongly suggests that early enteral feeding plays a significant role in stimulating or accelerating gastrointestinal wound healing and surgical site strength.
- Exercise is restricted for 2 weeks until skin sutures are removed.

Complications of gastrotomy

- Gastrotomy leakage or dehiscence.
- Septic peritonitis.

Key points

- Reduce the abdominal CO_2 pressure to facilitate the approach of the stomach to the abdominal wall.
- Before performing the stomach wall incision, apply laparotomic gauze around the area to be incised to reduce the risk of contamination of the abdominal cavity.
- Make a short stomach incision, then lengthen the incision just enough to extract the foreign body.
- Perform lavages of the incision site before repositioning the stomach into the abdomen.

SUGGESTED READINGS

32 SINGLE-PORT LAPAROSCOPIC-ASSISTED INTESTINAL SURGERY

Jeffrey J. Runge, Joshua G. Becker

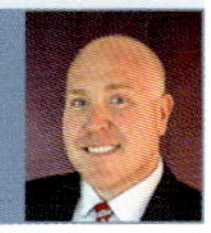

Benefits

- Reduced surgical time
- Smaller incisions
- Reduced number of incisions as compared to multiport laparoscopy
- Ability to extract larger areas of tissue
- Ability to combine total laparoscopic procedures with laparoscopic-assisted procedures
- Reduced incisional morbidity (e.g., splenic laceration)
- Incisional utility (i.e., common/consistent point of entry, improving familiarity of the approach and potentially reducing risks of complication)

Challenges

- A single surgical point of entry results in reduced working space, limited field of view, decreased exposure, altered principles of triangulation, and increased potential for instrument collision
- Requires additional purchase of equipment (wound retractor and SILS device)
- A learning curve is present

The single-incision approach to laparoscopic-assisted intestinal surgery, including procedures such as enterostomy tube placement, intestinal biopsy, and resection and anastomosis, may offer some advantages compared with traditional laparotomy and multiple-port techniques. Incision size is predetermined and may be large enough in small dogs to allow unrestricted exteriorization of the small intestine. A potential disadvantage of multiple ports and port enlargement is increased soft tissue injury and loss of ability for further laparoscopic exploration or intervention. Recently, single-incision laparoscopic surgery and EndoCone ports have become available to veterinary surgeons.

> In human medicine, the first publication on the treatment of intestinal penetrating wounds and strangulated hernias was made by B. Travers in 1812.

PATIENT PREPARATION AND POSITIONING

The patient is placed in dorsal recumbency and the skin is aseptically prepared. The abdomen should be prepared for an open approach in case conversion or additional port placement is required. The front and rear limbs should be secured for the procedure. Tilting the operating table laterally and in a Trendelenburg or reverse Trendelenburg position may be very helpful in perioperative visualization, depending on the patient's size.

OPERATING ROOM LAYOUT

The surgeon positions themselves on the left or right side of the patient, toward the foot of the table. Since the surgeon may need to work from both the left and right sides of the patient, there should be enough space for the surgeon to move safely from one side of the table to the other. If multiple video monitors are available, they are positioned at the head of the table on the right and left sides. A single monitor is acceptable as long as it can easily be moved to the opposite side of the surgeon. Ceiling or boom-mounted monitors are preferable. The instrument table is placed at the foot of the table to avoid interference with the anesthetist/anesthesiologist. An extra large patient drape is recommended to prevent exposure of the patient and operating table during patient manipulation/tilting (**Fig. 1**).

Instruments

- Standard surgery set
- Telescope 5 mm – 30°
- Single-incision port device
- Alexis wound retractor or Gelpi retractor
- Straight or articulating forceps
- A blunt palpation probe or fan retractor
- Biopsy instruments
- Thoracoabdominal, gastrointestinal anastomotic, or endo gastrointestinal anastomotic staplers (as needed for stapled anastomosis)

PORT PLACEMENT (FIG. 2)

- Depending on the port used and the location of the lesion/area of interest, the port can be inserted either at the level of the umbilicus or more caudally as necessary (**Fig. 3**).
- The port should not be placed farther caudal than midway between the umbilicus and the pubis—otherwise, extracorporeal evaluation of the small intestine would be restricted.

PROCEDURE

- After the port has been placed and a pneumoperitoneum established, the telescope is inserted and the abdomen is surveyed in standard fashion, checking for anatomical landmarks and assessing gross anatomy. Care must be taken to avoid and check for evidence of iatrogenic trauma secondary to port placement.
- After intracorporeal evaluation is completed, a portion of jejunum is exteriorized from the peritoneal cavity, and the small intestine is run in standard fashion (**Fig. 4**).
- The extraction incision may need to be slightly enlarged to facilitate exteriorization and prevent strangulation of the mesenteric vasculature.
- A small Gelpi retractor or Alexis wound retractor is used to maintain retraction of the abdominal incision during extracorporeal enterotomy, and the affected bowel is isolated and

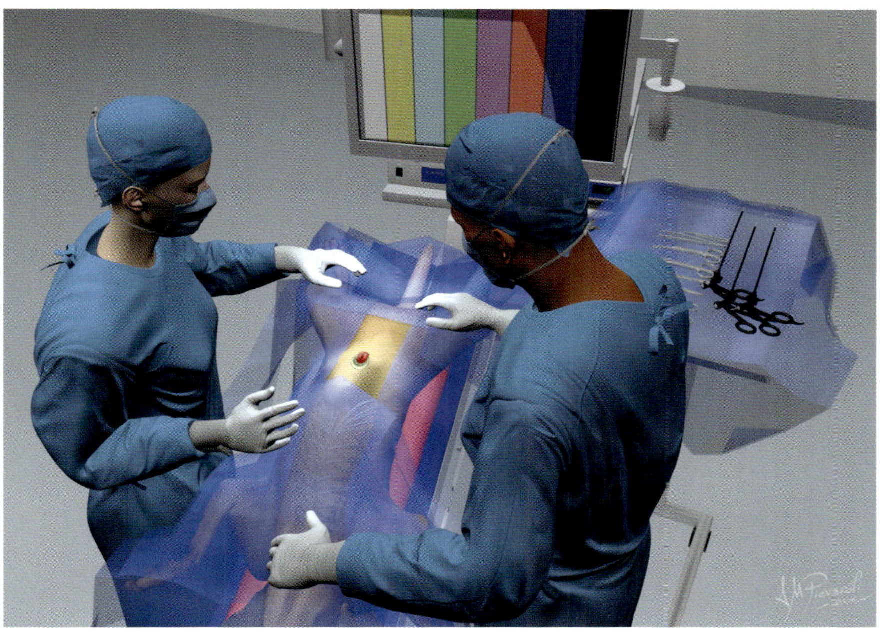

FIGURE 1. Operating room layout for single-port laparoscopic-assisted intestinal surgery.

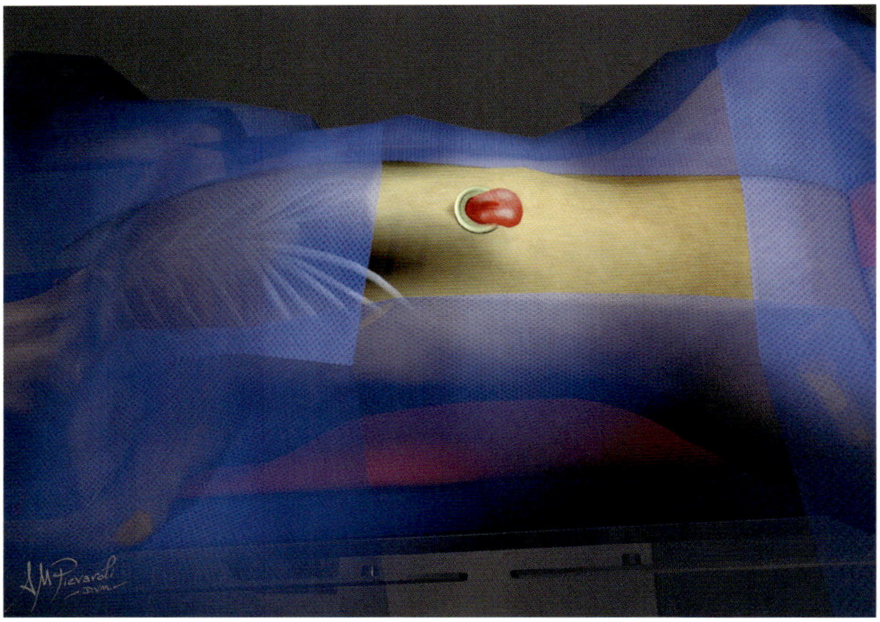

FIGURE 2. Port placement for single-port laparoscopic-assisted intestinal surgery.

packed off using laparotomy sponges. Use of a polyurethane wound retractor is advisable in cases of suspected or documented gastrointestinal neoplasia to minimize the risk of port-site metastasis.

- The bowel segment of interest is extracorporeally isolated.

For foreign body removal:

- An antimesenteric enterotomy is performed aborad to the site of the intestinal foreign body to avoid incising compromised intestinal tissue.

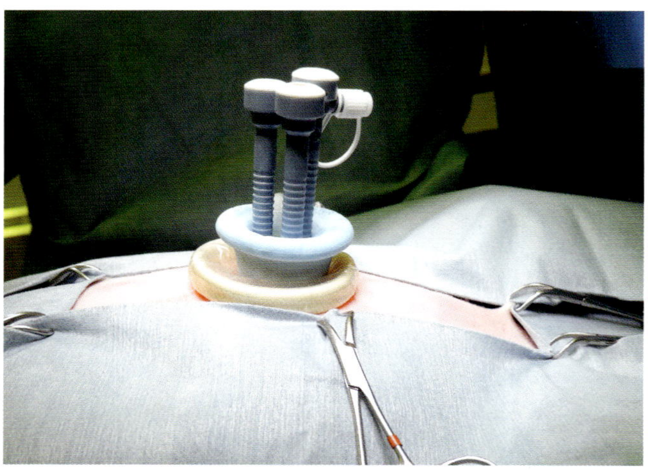

FIGURE 3. SILS port placed through a wound retractor on the ventral midline just cranial to the umbilicus. This enables access to the stomach and intestines.

For intestinal biopsy:

- The enterotomy is made in an elliptical fashion using a scalpel blade or in a circular manner using a 4–5 mm biopsy punch (**Fig. 5**).

Enterotomy closure:

- The enterotomy site can be closed in either a transverse or longitudinal orientation depending on the concern for luminal compromise.
- The site should be closed in a single-layer appositional pattern to minimize tissue eversion and mucosal necrosis.
- A continuous or interrupted pattern can be used.
- A knotless suture can also be used for enterotomy closure.

For intestinal resection and anastomosis:

- Care must be taken to prevent strangulation of the mesenteric vasculature when exteriorizing the intestines.
- Case selection for resection and anastomosis should be considered carefully and, as with all minimally invasive procedures, the surgeon should be prepared for conversion to open surgery.

Omentalization: Intracorporeal or extracorporeal gastrointestinal omentalization can be performed.

- Extracorporeal:
    - The greater omentum is typically easy to exteriorize with the enterotomy or anastomosis site.

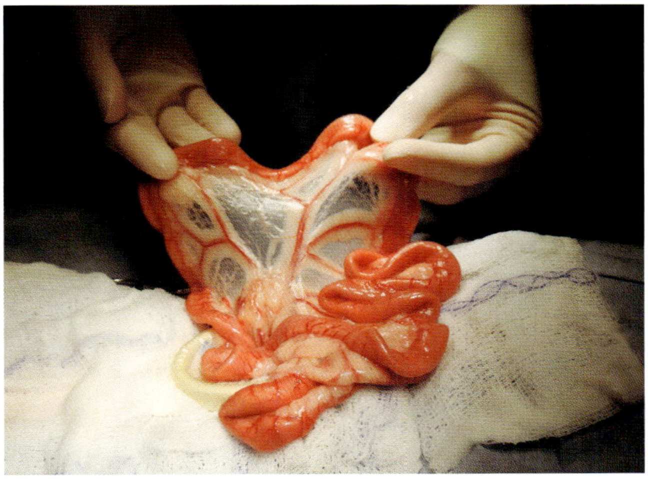

FIGURE 4. A portion of jejunum is exteriorized from the peritoneal cavity.

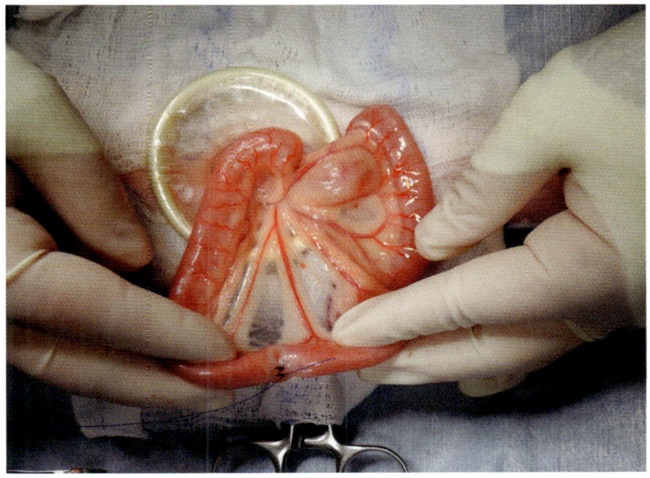

FIGURE 5. An intestinal loop is pulled through the wound retractor for full-thickness intestinal biopsy.

    - The omentum can then be wrapped around the circumference of the bowel, and some surgeons prefer to tack it in place with one or two seromuscular sutures.
- Intracorporeal: It can be performed in patients in which the original extraction incision has not been enlarged too much to prevent reinsertion of the port.
    - The port is reinserted and the peritoneum examined to identify the surgery site.
    - The greater omentum is grasped using laparoscopic Babcock forceps and wrapped around the site. One or two seromuscular sutures can be placed.

Closure:

- The abdominal incision site is closed in standard fashion.

POSTOPERATIVE MANAGEMENT

- Local analgesics at the time of incision site closure are recommended.
- Injectable analgesics during the immediate postoperative period are also indicated, typically until the patient is eating and drinking.
- The patient can be discharged with a short course of additional medications for pain control.
- Nonsteroidal anti-inflammatory drugs are typically contraindicated in patients after gastrointestinal surgery out of concern for interference in gastrointestinal wound healing.
- The overall need for gastrointestinal modification therapy is case dependent, but it is generally recommended for at least 24 hours after surgery as an important prophylactic measure:
    - antacids (e.g., proton pump inhibitors)
    - antiemetics (e.g., maropitant, ondansetron)
    - prokinetics (e.g., metoclopramide)
    - appetite stimulants (e.g., capromorelin).
- It has become common practice to encourage a return to enteral feeding as quickly as possible after surgery, often as early as 6–8 hours postoperatively if no evidence of vomiting or nausea is noted.
- Mild sedatives can be used as needed depending on the patient's anxiety and temperament.

Complications of single-port laparoscopic-assisted intestinal surgery

- Enteral site dehiscence
- Septic peritonitis
- Aspiration pneumonia
- Gastrointestinal ileus
- Incorrect port placement
- Conversion to open laparotomy
- Iatrogenic trauma to peripheral organs
- Hemorrhage
- Incisional complications (e.g., seroma, bruising, infection, dehiscence)

Key points

- Enteral feeding is very important for early hospital discharge.
- Laparoscopic-assisted intestinal surgery is contraindicated in cases of linear foreign bodies, septic peritonitis, and in the presence of adhesions.
- Adequate knowledge of gastrointestinal anatomy and physiology is mandatory.
- The surgeon must be ready for conversion to traditional laparotomy, if needed.

SUGGESTED READINGS

33 LAPAROSCOPIC-ASSISTED COLOPEXY

Massimo Barilli

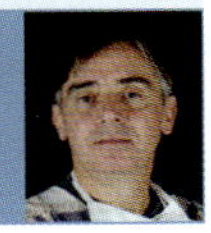

Indications

- Reduction of rectal sacculation in perineal herniation
- Management of rectal prolapse

Contraindications

- Intracranial disease
- Cardiovascular and pulmonary diseases
- Coagulopathy

The fixation of the colon to the abdominal wall, colopexy, is indicated for the management of severe or recurrent prolapse of viable rectal tissue. Colopexy can also be used to reduce rectal sacculation before or after perineal herniorrhaphy, and colopexy without herniorrhaphy has been reported as a viable option in the management of perineal herniation. Colopexy can be performed at a separate surgery or during the herniorrhaphy procedure.

In a study, colopexy, cystopexy, vasopexy, castration, and perineal hernia repair were performed under the same operative time with minimal postoperative complications.

A laparoscopic approach for colopexy has been described experimentally in dogs, and there are some reports of laparoscopic or laparoscopic-assisted colonic procedures in dogs and cats.

PATIENT PREPARATION AND POSITIONING

The patient's abdomen is clipped and aseptically prepared from the xiphoid process to the pubic brim. Prophylactic perioperative antibiotics are recommended (cefazolin 22 mg/kg IV). For laparoscopic-assisted colopexy, the patient is placed in dorsal recumbency with the front and rears limbs secured for the procedure. The patient is put in a Trendelenburg position (with the head lower than the abdomen) and the operating table is tilted to the right.

OPERATING ROOM LAYOUT

The cannulas are placed in a triangulated fashion, with the surgeon facing caudally (**Fig. 1**).

The following procedures are described below:

A. Two-port laparoscopic-assisted colopexy
B. Three-port laparoscopic-assisted colopexy and vasopexy

A TWO-PORT LAPAROSCOPIC-ASSISTED COLOPEXY

Instruments

- Standard surgery set
- Telescope 5 mm – 30°
- Two 5 mm cannulas
- Grasping forceps

PORT PLACEMENT (FIG. 2)

- T1, on the midline, 1–2 cm caudal to the umbilicus
- T3, on the left lateral abdominal wall

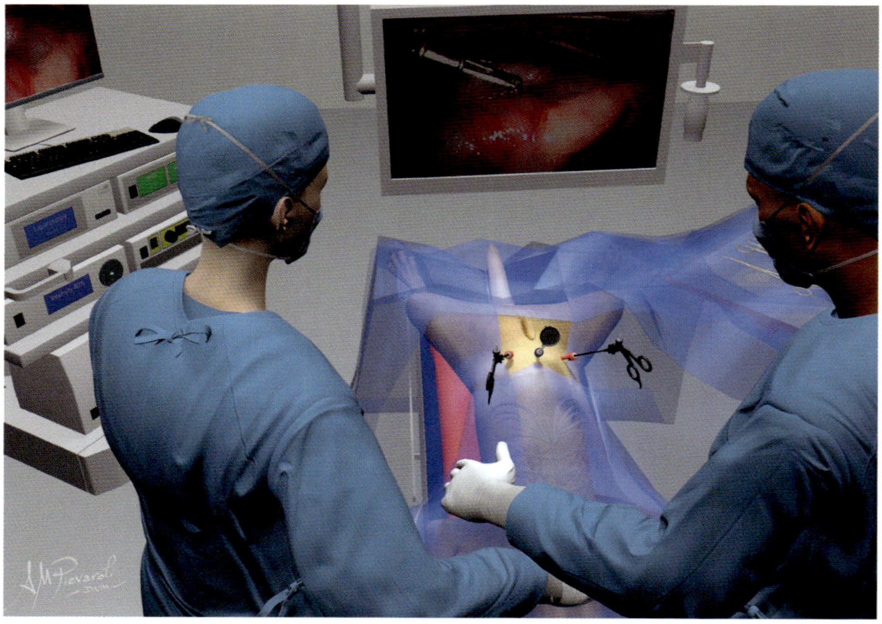

FIGURE 1. Operating room layout for laparoscopic-assisted colopexy.

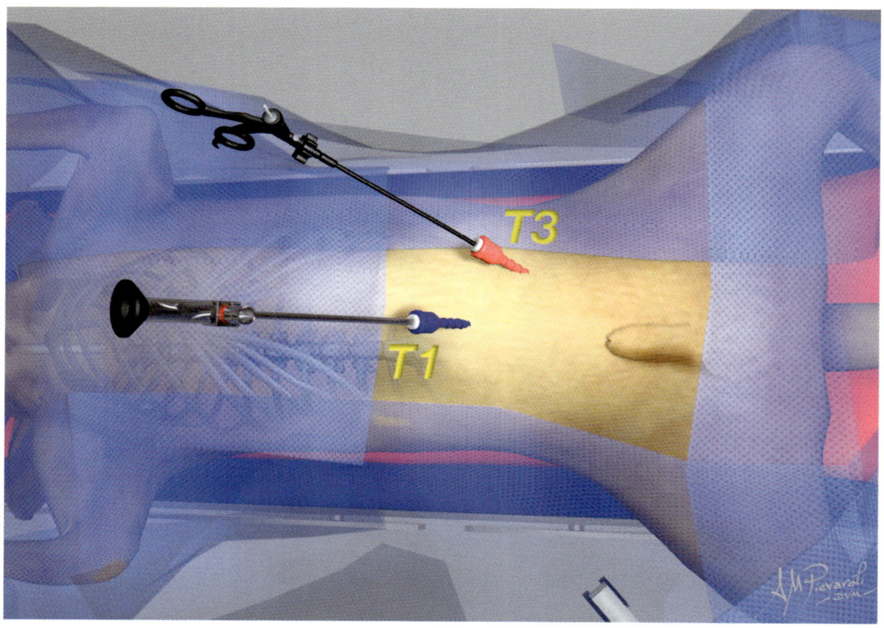

FIGURE 2. Port placement for two-port laparoscopic-assisted colopexy.

PROCEDURE

- After the ports have been placed and the pneumoperitoneum achieved (**Fig. 3**), the 5 mm telescope is inserted in T1 and a first exploration of the abdomen is performed to check for any evidence of iatrogenic trauma caused by placement of the first cannula.
- The grasping forceps are inserted in T3, the descending colon is grasped with the forceps, and gentle traction is cranially applied to the colon (**Fig. 4**). The site from where the colon is grasped is the location for the incisional colopexy (**Fig. 5**).
- After the colon has been firmly grasped, the pneumoperitoneum is evacuated. The forceps and colon are exteriorized by removing the cannula (T3) and extending the port incision longitudinally to 4–5 cm (**Fig. 6**).

- Two stay sutures can be placed on the antimesenteric border of the colon (**Fig. 7**).
- A partial-thickness incision (3–4 cm) on the antimesenteric border of the colon is made and, with an appositional technique, interrupted sutures of 3-0 or 2-0 polydioxanone or polyglyconate are placed through the colon wall and through the left lateral abdominal wall musculature.
- Care should be taken not to penetrate the lumen of the colon.
- Before closure, the stay sutures are removed and the pneumoperitoneum is briefly reestablished through T1. The colopexy is examined laparoscopically to ensure that optimal positioning has been achieved and that excessive hemorrhage is not present (**Fig. 8**).
- After evacuating the remaining pneumoperitoneum, the subumbilical midline cannula is removed and the port-site incisions are closed in routine fashion.

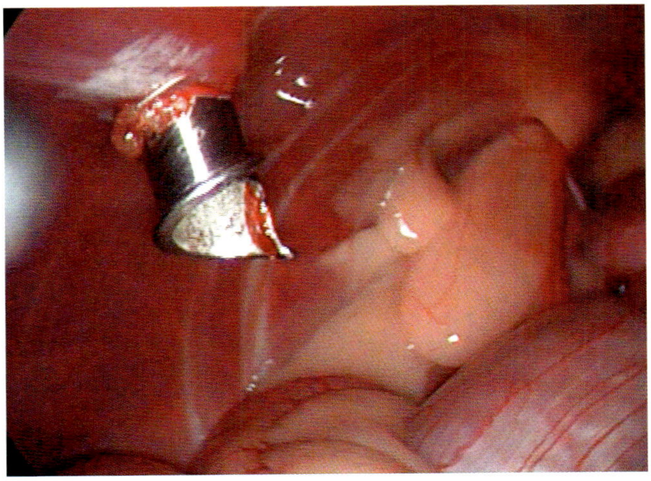

FIGURE 3. Port placement (T3).

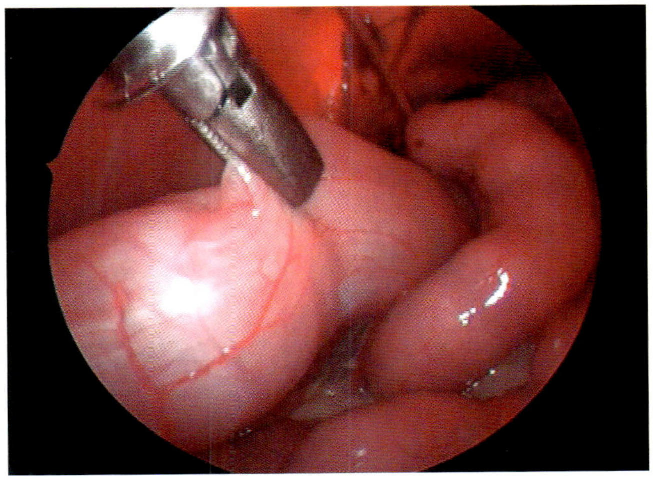

FIGURE 4. Cranial traction of the colon.

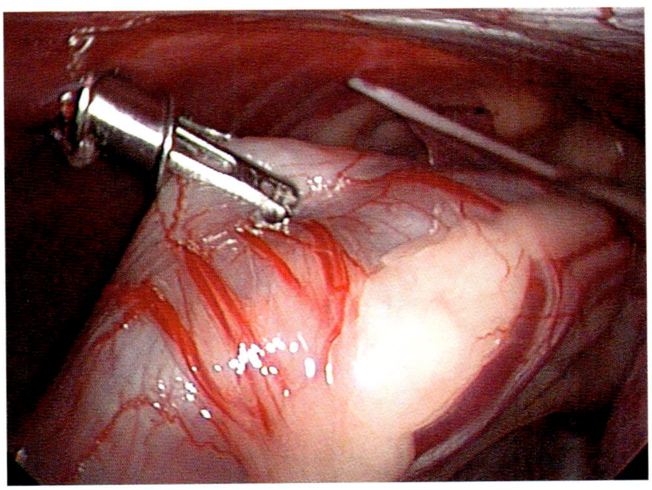

FIGURE 5. Site of colon grasping.

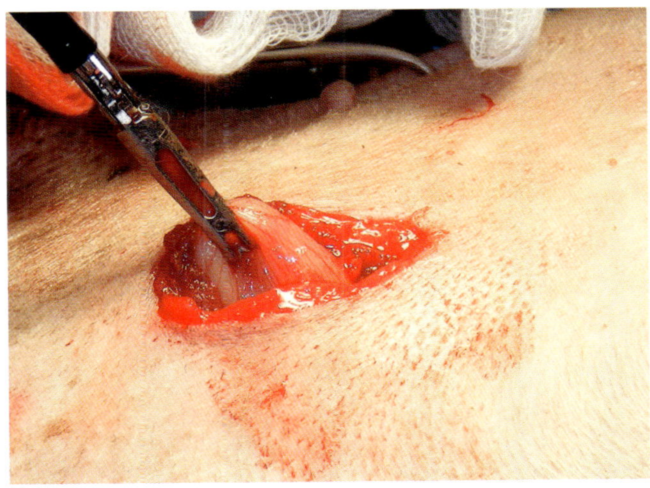

FIGURE 6. Exteriorization of the colon.

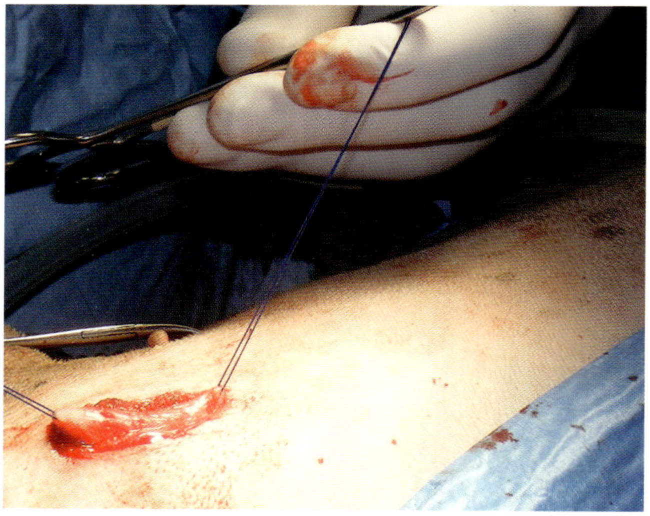

FIGURE 7. Placement of stay sutures.

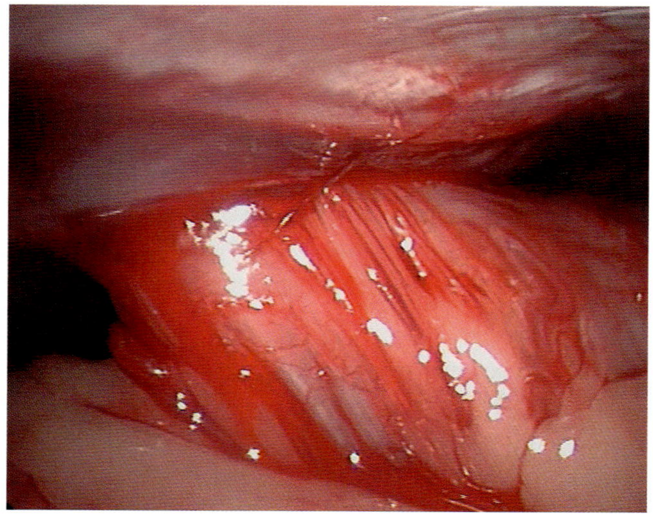

FIGURE 8. Laparoscopic visualization of colopexy.

B THREE-PORT LAPAROSCOPIC-ASSISTED COLOPEXY AND VASOPEXY

Instruments

- Standard surgery set
- Telescope 5 mm – 30°
- Three 5 mm cannulas
- Grasping forceps

PORT PLACEMENT (FIG. 9)

- T1, on the midline, 1–2 cm caudal to the umbilicus
- T3, on the left lateral abdominal wall
- T2, on the right lateral abdominal wall

PROCEDURE

- Before vasopexy, intact dogs should be castrated with an open technique, with the testicular artery and vein ligated separately from the vas deferens.
- After the ports have been placed and the pneumoperitoneum achieved, the 5 mm telescope is inserted in T1 and a first exploration of the abdomen is performed to check for any evidence of iatrogenic trauma caused by placement of the first cannula.
- The vasa deferentia are identified in the inguinal canals on each side.
- Using the grasping forceps inserted in T2, the right vas deferens is grasped and retrieved from the right inguinal canal by applying gentle cranial traction.
- The same maneuver is repeated on the left vas deferens using a grasping forceps inserted in T3.
- A small skin incision is made 3–4 cm caudal to T2 and a straight mosquito forceps is inserted through the abdominal wall into the abdominal cavity. The mosquito forceps are used to grasp the left vas deferens and pull it out through the abdominal incision.
- A small skin incision is performed 3–4 cm caudal to T3, and the same maneuver is repeated to pull the right vas deferens out of the abdominal cavity.
- After vasopexy, laparoscopic-assisted colopexy is performed.
- The pneumoperitoneum is evacuated and each vas deferens is sutured to the external muscle fascia of the abdominal wall using one or two monofilament sutures in an interrupted pattern.
- Before skin closure, the pneumoperitoneum is reestablished through T1 and the vasopexies are examined laparoscopically to ensure that optimal positioning has been achieved and that excessive hemorrhage is not present.
- After evacuating the remaining pneumoperitoneum, all the cannulas are removed and the port-site incisions are closed in routine fashion.

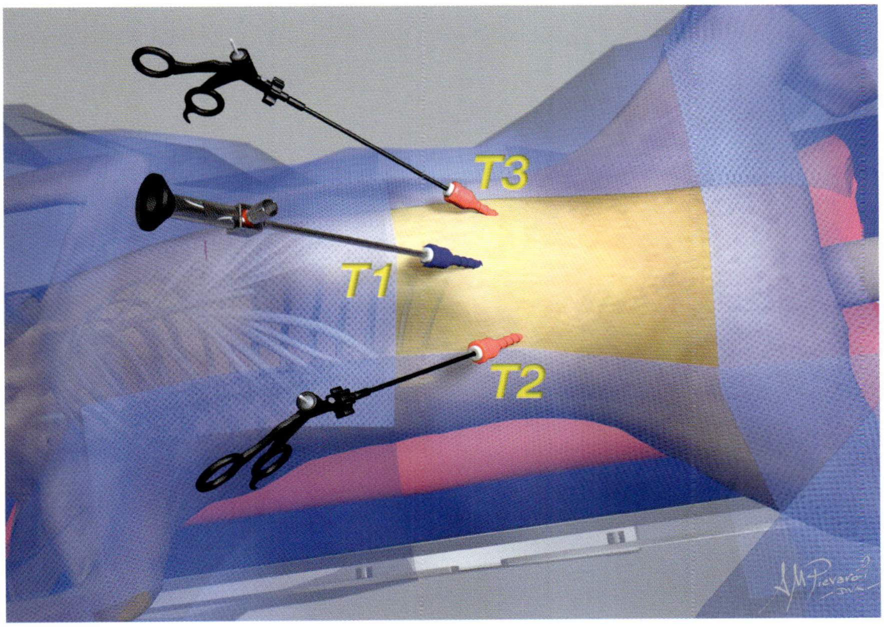

FIGURE 9. Port placement for three-port laparoscopic-assisted colopexy and vasopexy.

POSTOPERATIVE MANAGEMENT

- Immediate postoperative management focuses on pain control.
- Hospitalization is recommended for 1 day after surgery to manage pain and monitor for signs of intestinal issues.
- The patient should be discharged with an E-collar and instructions for 14 days of activity restriction to allow proper healing of the skin and colopexy site.
- If colopexy integrity is in question, focal abdominal ultrasonography can be performed 2–6 months after surgery.

Complications of laparoscopic-assisted colopexy

- In the hands of expert laparoscopic surgeons, intraoperative complications are rare; however, access-related issues are complications in any laparoscopic surgery.
- Complications include colon perforation during dissection, splenic lesion on cannula introduction, incorrect port placement, residual subcutaneous emphysema, incisional fistula, and incisional infections.
- Postoperative complications include tenesmus, colitis, constipation, rectal prolapse, and signs of stranguria.

Key points

- Consider colopexy for recurrent rectal prolapse not responding to other treatments.
- Care should be taken not to penetrate the colon lumen.

SUGGESTED READINGS

CLINICAL CASES

33.1 TOTALLY LAPAROSCOPIC COLOPEXY IN A CAT

Andrea M. Pievaroli

CASE DESCRIPTION

A 1-year-old male cat was presented with recurrent episodes of rectal prolapse. Previous repeated conservative treatments, such as purse-string reduction and supportive medical therapies, had failed. A totally laparoscopic colopexy was elected, using a 2.7 mm telescope and 3 mm instruments designed for minilaparoscopy. Rectal prolapse no longer occurred in the weeks following surgery. At the check-up 10 months postoperatively, no clinical signs were observed.

Key points

- The surgeon must have a minimum skill in intracorporeal laparoscopic suturing.
- Be careful not to perforate the intestinal mucosa with the needle.

PORT PLACEMENT

The patient was placed in dorsal recumbency, in an oblique position slightly tilted to the right. The first port (T1) was placed on the midline, 2–3 cm caudal to the umbilicus. The second port (T2) was placed on the midline, 2–3 cm caudal to T1. The third port (T3) was placed 1 cm to the left, in a paramedian position at the level of the umbilicus.

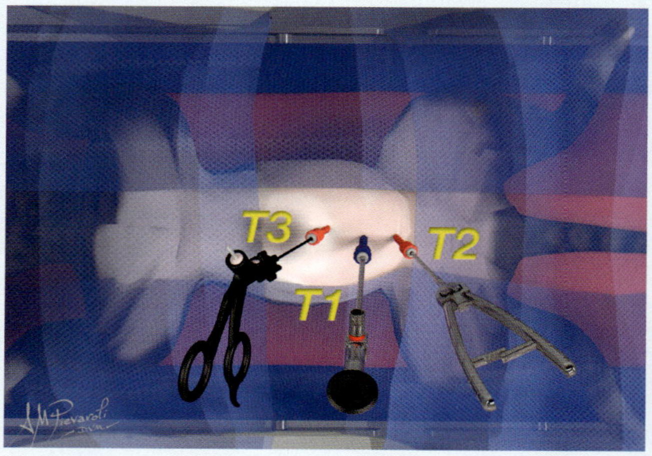

PROCEDURE

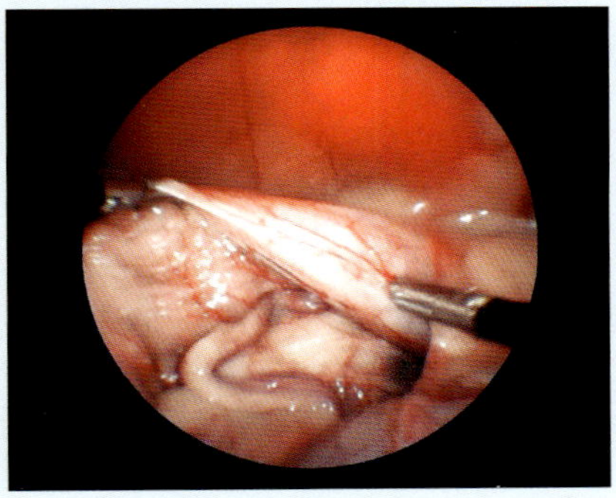

FIGURE 1. The colon is located (rectal prolapse has been reduced preoperatively) and traction is performed in a cranial direction.

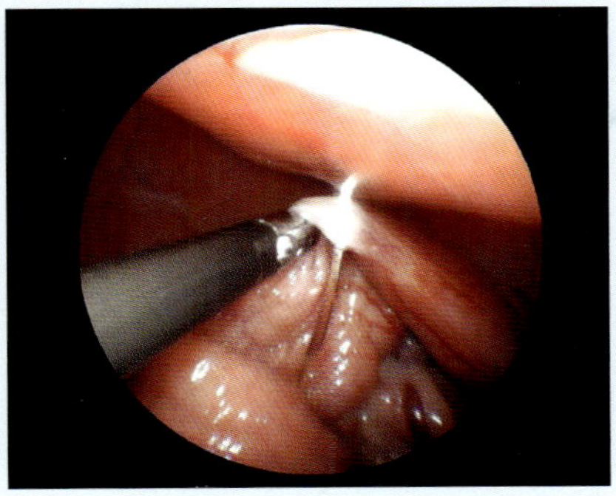

FIGURE 2. To keep the colon in place and extended cranially, it is helpful to insert a temporary suture percutaneously and pass it through the seromuscular layer.

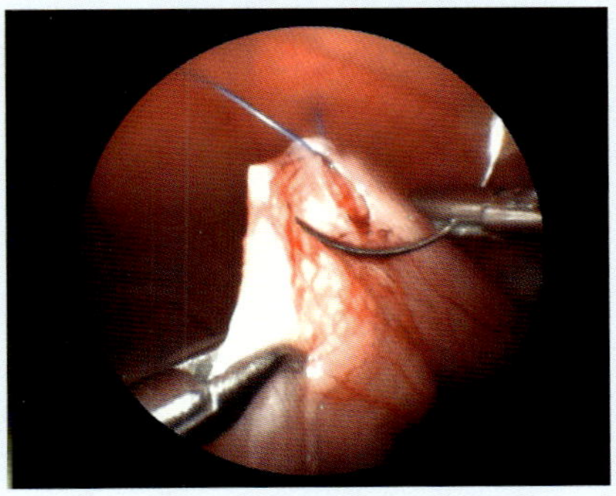

FIGURE 3. A monofilament suture (e.g., polydioxanone or poliglecaprone) with a taper-point needle is used to perform the colopexy.

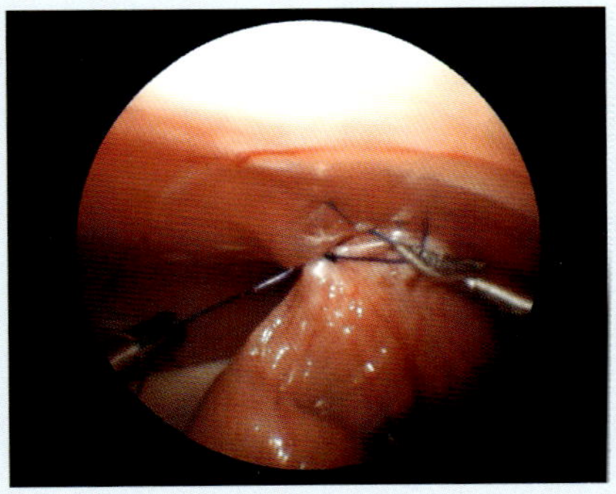

FIGURE 4. Using a laparoscopic needle holder, the colopexy is performed suturing the seromuscular layer to the abdominal wall with a simple interrupted pattern.

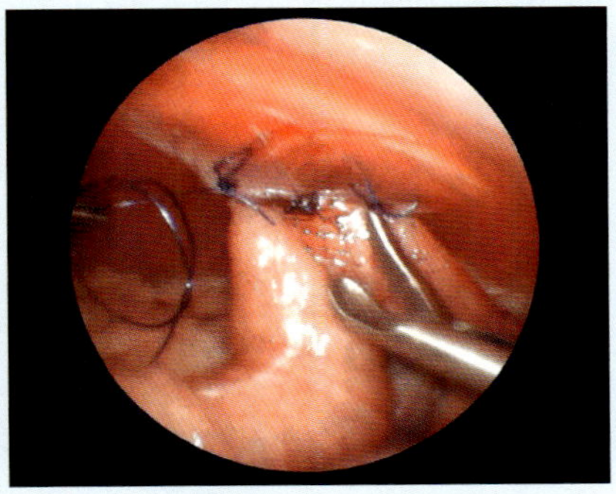

FIGURE 5. To ensure good resistance to traction, at least four or five knots should be applied for a length of 2–3 cm.

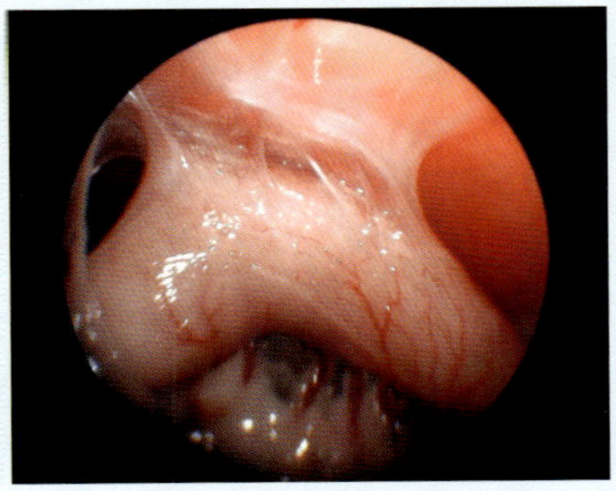

FIGURE 6. Follow-up at 10 months of colopexy. The adhesion between the colon and the peritoneum is clearly visible.

Tips and tricks

- ✓ Place a temporary percutaneous suture to keep the colon reduced cranially.
- ✓ Use monopolar electrocautery or scissors to create a 3–4 cm longitudinal line in the peritoneum to promote adherence.

33.2 LAPAROSCOPIC COLOPEXY AND OVARIECTOMY IN A DOG

Christopher B. Thomson

CASE DESCRIPTION

A 3-year-old intact female Boston Terrier dog was presented with recurrent rectal prolapse following recent whelping. Previous attempts at conservative management via purse-string reduction and stool softeners had failed. The owners were also interested in having their pet ovariectomized. The physical examination and preoperative diagnostics (complete blood count, serum chemistry, urinalysis) were unremarkable. Following surgery, the prolapse was no longer observed clinically and the physical examination was normal at a 9-month postoperative check-up.

Key points

- Colopexy is indicated for severe or recurrent rectal prolapse if conservative management fails.
- A partial-thickness incision is created in the body wall. No incision is made in the colon.
- Reduction can be assessed intraoperatively by a nonsterile assistant via digital rectal examination.
- A delayed absorption suture (V-Loc 180, Medtronic, Salem, MA) was used to allow formation of the adhesion.

PORT PLACEMENT

A commercial SILS port (T1, T2, T3) was used in a subumbilical position. Roughly 5 cm caudal to the SILS port, a single 5 mm threaded Ternamian endoport (T4) was used for intracorporeal suturing.

The patient was initially placed in dorsal recumbency for port placement. Following insufflation, the patient was tilted to right lateral recumbency for ovariectomy (left sided) and colopexy. Tilting to left lateral recumbency was then performed for right ovariectomy.

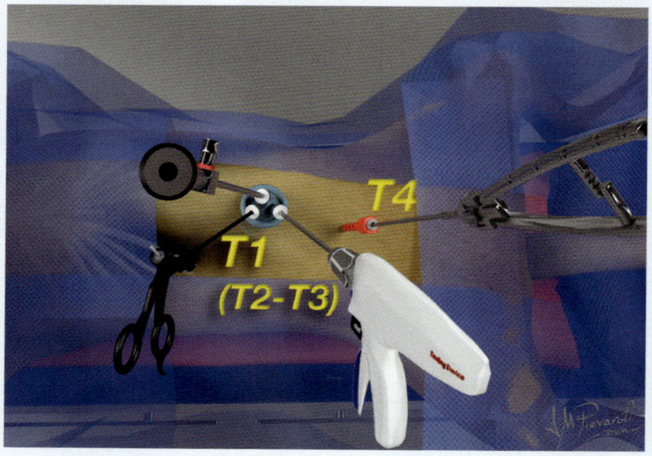

PROCEDURE

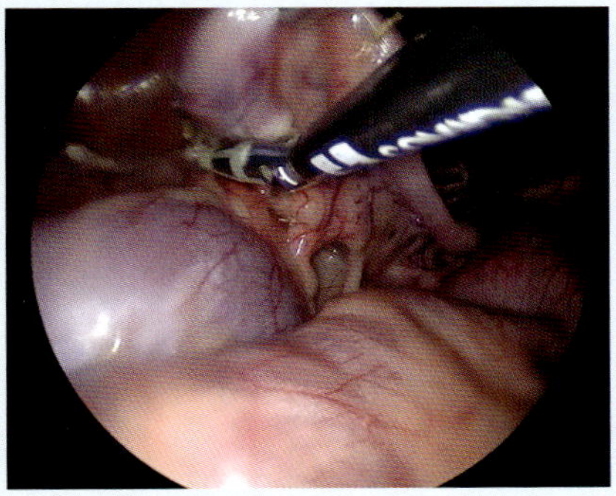

FIGURE 1. Left ovariectomy is performed in standard fashion using a vessel-sealing device prior to colopexy.

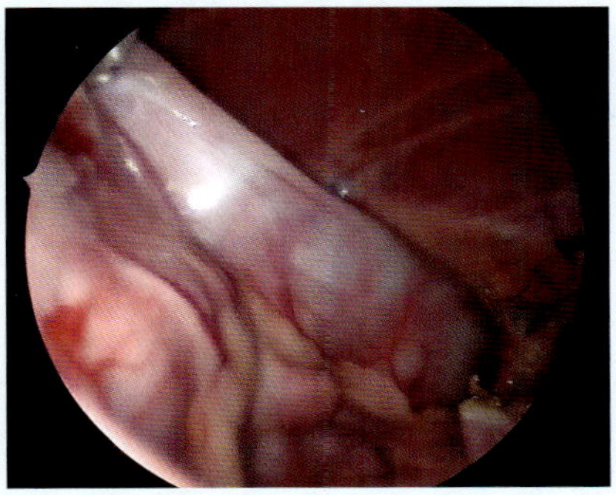

FIGURE 2. The rectum is reduced via gentle cranial retraction of the colon using laparoscopic Babcock graspers.

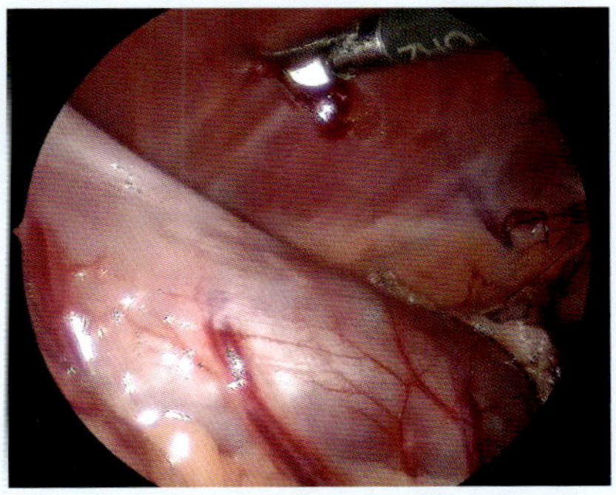

FIGURE 3. An incision is made in the peritoneum and underlying musculature of the left body wall using laparoscopic Metzenbaum scissors.

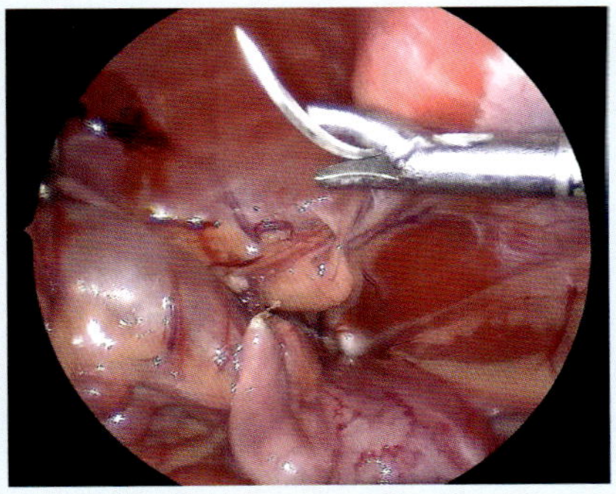

FIGURE 4. A barbed knotless suture is passed percutaneously through the body wall.

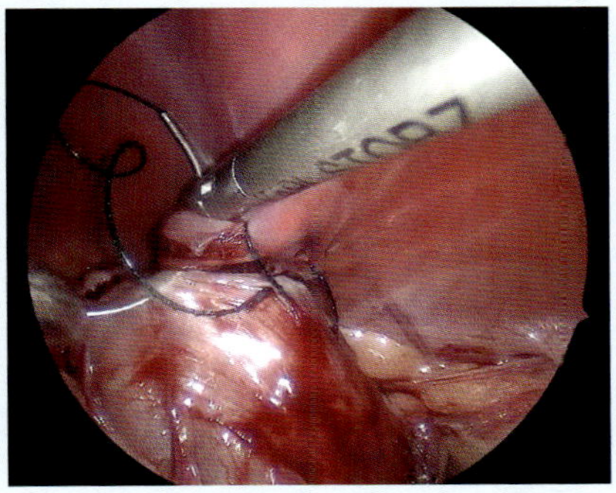

FIGURE 5. Starting in a caudal-to-cranial direction, intracorporeal suturing is performed via an appositional simple continuous pattern. Suture bites engage the transversalis fascia on the body wall side and are partial thickness in the colon.

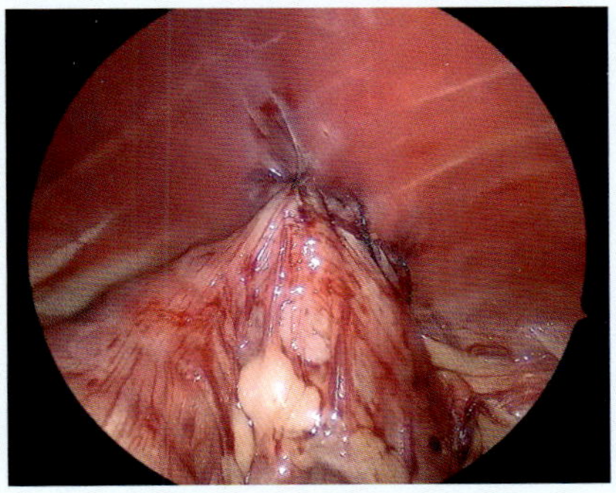

FIGURE 6. After completing the colopexy, the suture is passed into the transversalis fascia in opposing directions to lock the pexy site, and it is then completely passed through the body wall for the needle to be cut.

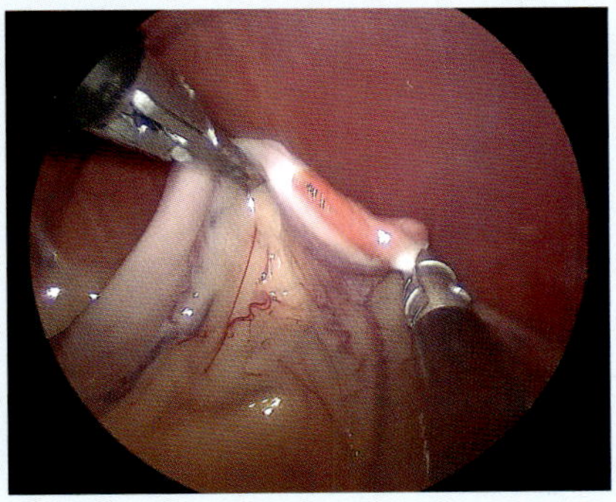

FIGURE 7. Following colopexy, the patient is rotated into left lateral recumbency and a standard right sided ovariectomy is performed.

Tips and tricks

- ✓ Left ovariectomy is performed first so that the colopexy does not obstruct visualization.
- ✓ A single cranially located interrupted stay suture can be placed to facilitate retraction during suturing if a three-port technique is used (instead of the SILS port described above).
- ✓ The use of a barbed knotless suture eases suturing, but other types of sutures can be used.

34 LAPAROSCOPIC LIVER SURGERY

David García Rubio, Edoardo Poggi, Luciano Borghetti

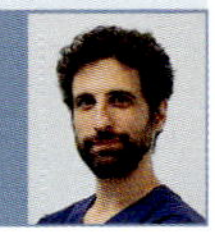

Indications

- Localized liver tumors
- Liver abscesses or cysts
- Traumatic liver hemorrhage
- Arteriovenous fistulas

Contraindications

- Large, multiple masses or masses close to the hepatic hilum
- Coagulopathies
- Other pathologies that make major surgery inadvisable

Laparoscopic liver surgery has become the standard therapy in human surgery due to its benefits as compared with laparotomy (e.g., less pain, fewer complications, shorter hospital stays, and better cosmetic results). It is, however, a modality yet to be developed in veterinary surgery, with only one recent article evaluating laparoscopic liver resection in cadavers and a few clinical cases. This may be partly due to the fact that not many cases of liver disease benefit from a minimally invasive approach. The late development of clinical signs in cases with hepatic neoplasms means that these are usually very large and extensive at the time of diagnosis, making the laparoscopic approach inadvisable. Nevertheless, thanks to improvements in diagnostic imaging systems, these pathologies are being detected earlier and earlier, and if the size, location, and extent of the pathology allow it, the laparoscopic approach will provide all the advantages of minimally invasive procedures mentioned above.

Anatomically, the liver is made up of six lobes: the left medial and lateral lobes, the quadrate lobe, the caudate lobe (with the papillary and caudate processes), and the right medial and lateral lobes. The lobes are usually grouped into divisions to facilitate surgical assessment, with the left division consisting of the left medial and lateral lobes, the central division consisting of the right medial and quadrate lobes, and the right division consisting of the caudate lobe and the right lateral lobe. While the left lobes are generally separated from each other and from the central division, the lobes of the other two divisions show a less distinct separation, with interlobular fusions of varying degree. When performing a total or partial lobectomy, this must be taken into account, together with other factors related to the pathology, in order to achieve the best surgical success possible.

In the dog, the hepatic artery subdivides into branches to each of the divisions after it crosses the hepatoduodenal ligament. The portal vein in turn divides at the hepatic hilum into a right branch (which supplies the right division) and a left branch (which supplies the central and left divisions). Each lobe is ultimately supplied by a branch of the hepatic artery and one to three lobar portal veins. In the cat, the portal vasculature is divided into three main branches leading to each of the divisions (left, right, and central).

The authors' experience in case selection is in line with the selection criteria used in human surgery and those seen by Michael A. E. et al. for laparoscopic liver lobectomies: masses smaller than 5 cm in diameter, isolated, located in peripheral areas, with the central and left divisions being the most accessible for resection.

A total or partial lobectomy can be performed, depending on the pathology to be treated and its location. Laparoscopic surgical techniques are similar, typically with the use of advanced vascular sealants (radiofrequency such as LigaSure or ultrasound such as harmonics) or mechanical sutures.

The first published laparoscopic hepatectomy in veterinary medicine, carried out in 12 cadaveric and 6 live canine patients, was reported in 2021 by Michael A. E., Case J. B., et al.

PATIENT PREPARATION AND POSITIONING

The entire abdomen is clipped and aseptically prepared, from the xiphoid process to the pubic brim, including at least 10 cm of the costal arch. The patient is placed in dorsal recumbency and in a reverse Trendelenburg position to better visualize the liver.

OPERATING ROOM LAYOUT

The endoscopy tower and the monitor are placed at the patient's head. The surgeon and the assistant position themselves caudally, depending on the lobe to be resected (e.g., for left hepatectomy, surgeon on the patient's right side and assistant on the patient's left side) (**Fig. 1**).

The following procedures are described below:

A. Right medial hepatectomy in a cat using a bipolar sealing device
B. Laparoscopic partial left lateral hepatectomy
C. Laparoscopic partial left medial hepatectomy

A RIGHT MEDIAL HEPATECTOMY IN A CAT USING A BIPOLAR SEALING DEVICE

Instruments

On the table:

- Standard surgery set
- Telescope 5 mm – 30°
- Two 5 mm cannulas + one 10 mm cannula
- Laparoscopic atraumatic grasping forceps
- Laparoscopic dissector forceps with monopolar electrocautery
- Vessel-sealing device (Ligasure, Medtronic, Minneapolis, MN)
- Gauze

Ready to use:

- Suction and irrigation laparoscopic device
- Additional 5 mm cannula
- Palpation probe or laparoscopic retractor
- Hemostatic gelatin sponge (Gelfoam) or regenerated cellulose (Tabotamp)

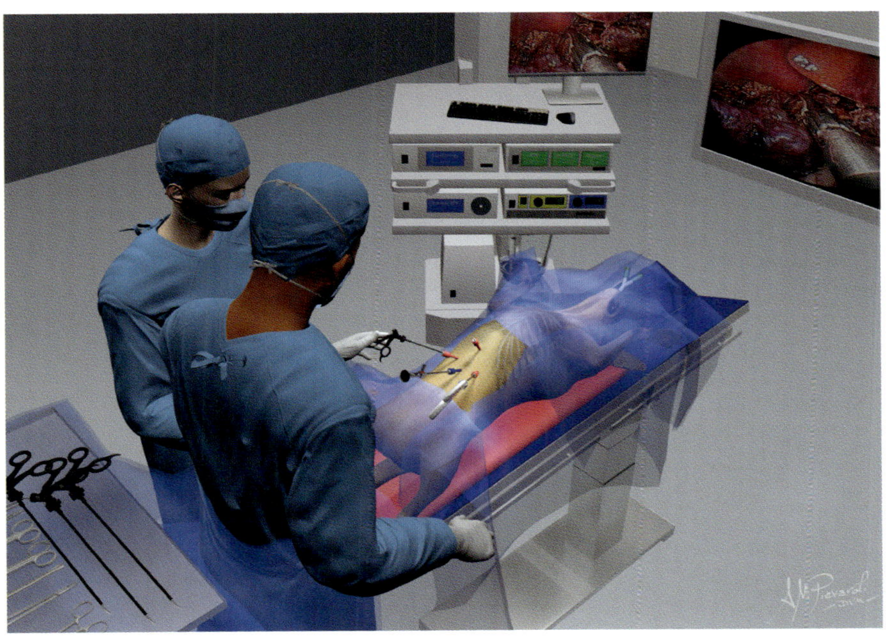

FIGURE 1. Operating room layout for right medial hepatectomy using a bipolar sealing device.

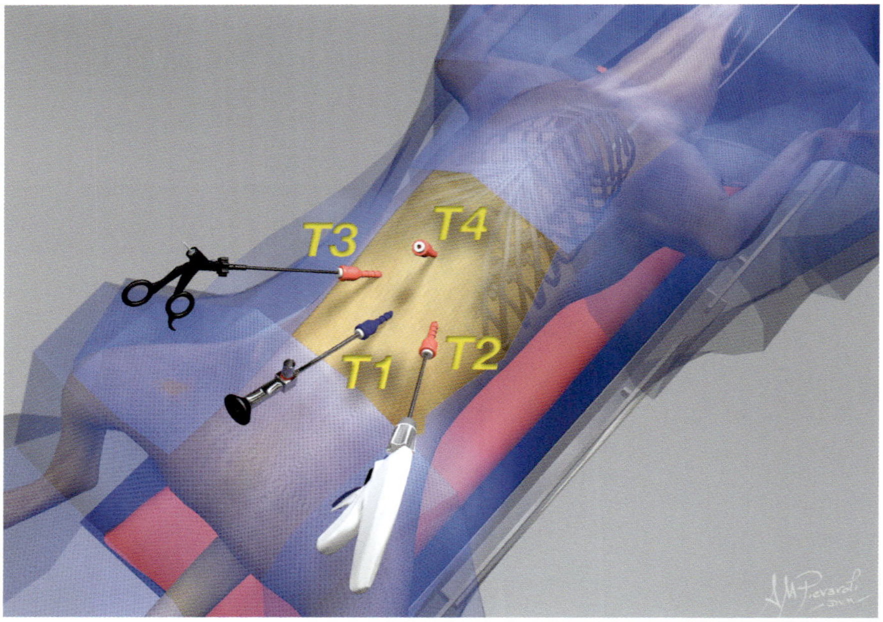

FIGURE 2. Port placement for right medial hepatectomy using a bipolar sealing device.

PORT PLACEMENT (FIG. 2)

- T1, on the midline, 4–6 cm caudal to the umbilicus
- T2, on the patient's left side, 2–3 cm cranial to T1
- T3, on the patient's right side, 2–3 cm cranial to T1
- T4 (optional), on the midline, 2–3 cm caudal to the xiphoid process

PROCEDURE

- After the first port has been placed and the pneumoperitoneum achieved (CO_2 at 6 mmHg), the 5 mm 30° telescope is inserted and a first exploration of the hepatic lobes is performed. The two lateral ports are then placed.
- The falciform ligament, which could prevent correct vision, is found in this area. In large or obese patients, the authors recommend resecting it using a bipolar sealing system to make surgery more comfortable.
- The mass is identified and its extent and size assessed (**Fig. 3**). The possible presence of metastases in other lobes should also be investigated.
- In this case, the tumor (biliary cystadenoma in a cat) is located in the apical part of the right medial lobe, and a partial lobectomy is performed.
- First, the gallbladder is freed from its attachments to the right medial lobe (**Fig. 4**).
- Since the junction of this lobe with the quadrate lobe is quite intimate, the resection area can be marked on the liver surface using a monopolar instrument to facilitate subsequent excision (**Fig. 5**).
- Then, the liver parenchyma is dissected and the bile vessels and ducts ligated using a bipolar sealing device (**Figs. 6 and 7**).

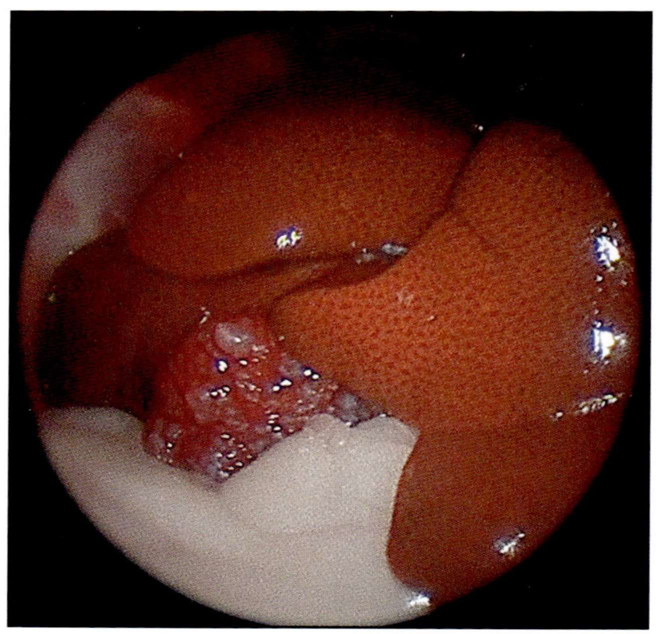

FIGURE 3. Visualization of the hepatic mass.

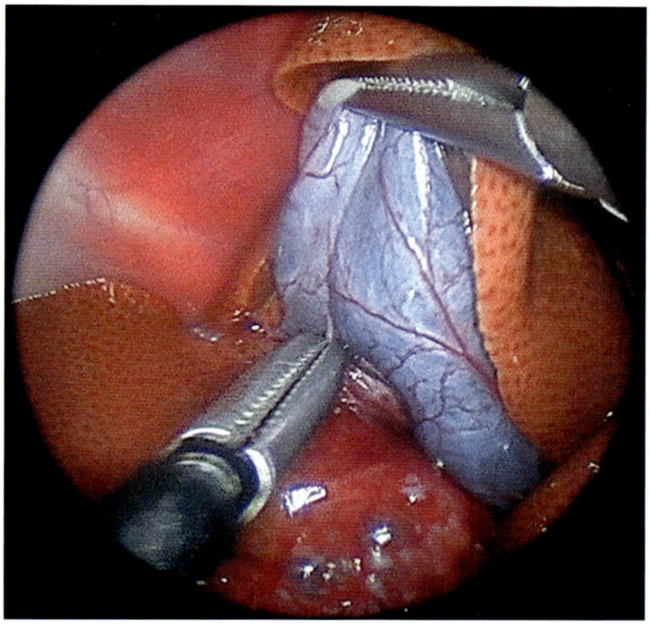

FIGURE 4. The gallbladder is dissected from the right medial lobe.

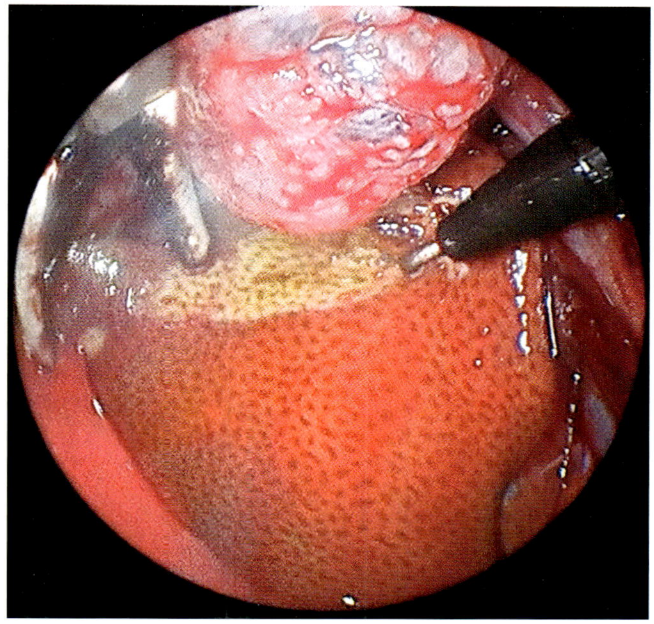

FIGURE 5. Using a monopolar instrument, the resection area is marked on the liver surface.

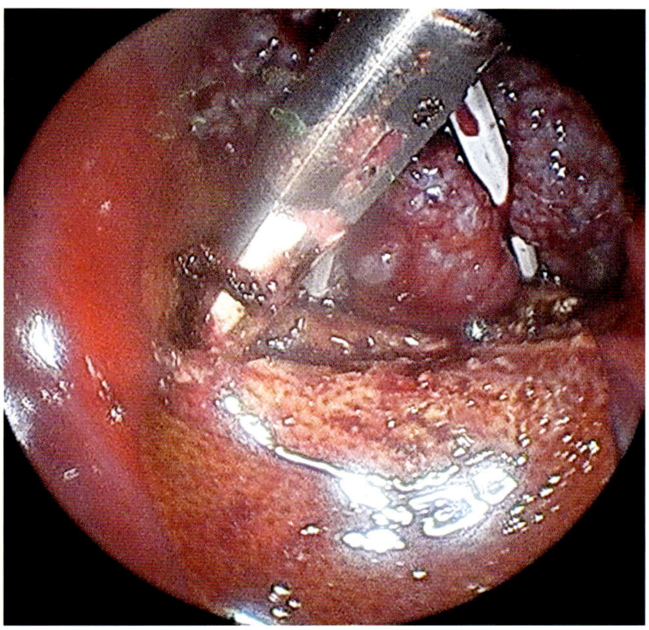

FIGURE 6. Bipolar dissection of the affected liver parenchyma.

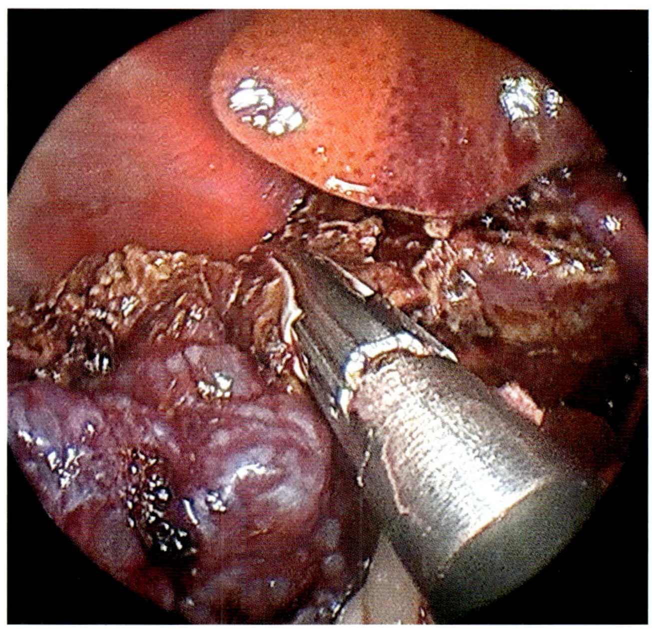

FIGURE 7. Dissection continues until the entire area is resected.

- Once the part of the affected lobe has been completely removed, the surgical field is checked for any bleeding or bile leakage (**Fig. 8**).
- The tumor is retrieved using an extraction bag (**Fig. 9**), and the incisions are closed routinely.

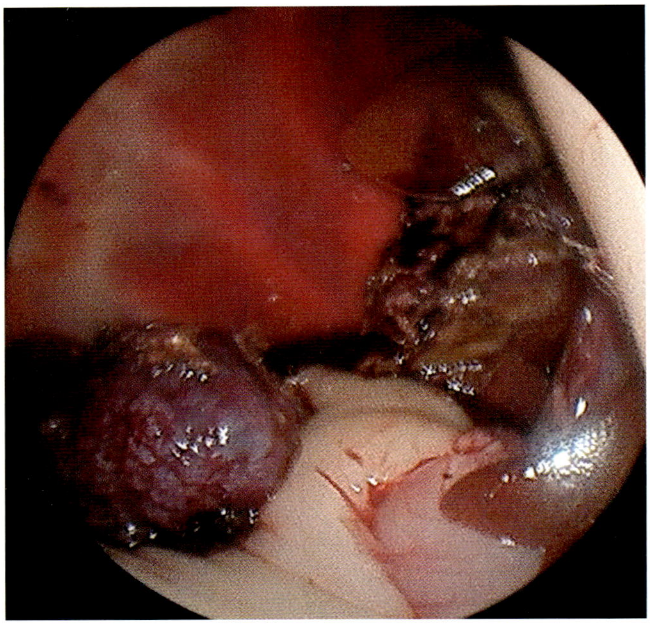

FIGURE 8. Bleeding control after tumor resection.

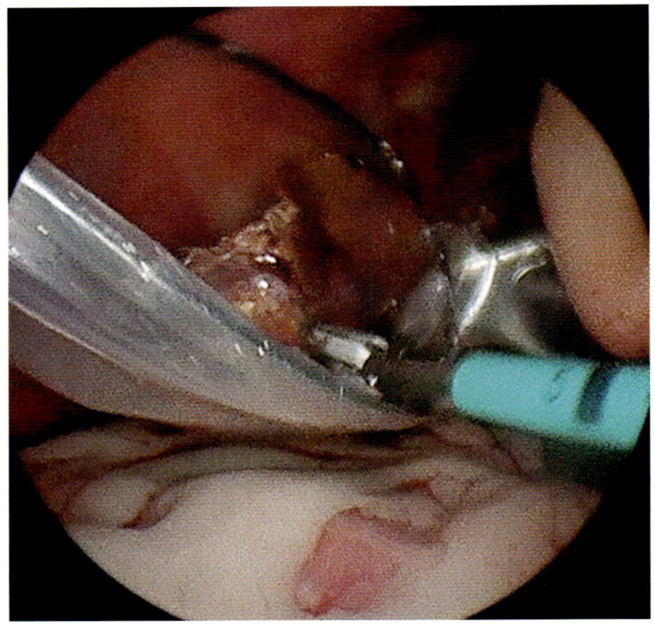

FIGURE 9. Use of an extraction bag to remove the tumor.

B LAPAROSCOPIC PARTIAL LEFT LATERAL HEPATECTOMY

Instruments

On the table:

- Standard surgery set
- Telescope 5 mm – 30°
- Three 5 mm cannulas (or two 5 mm cannulas + one 10 mm cannula)
- Laparoscopic atraumatic grasping forceps
- Laparoscopic grasping forceps
- Laparoscopic dissector forceps with monopolar electrocautery
- Vessel-sealing device (ultrasonically activated scalpel) or laparoscopic mechanical stapler device
- Gauze

Ready to use:

- Suction and irrigation laparoscopic device
- Additional 5 mm cannula
- Palpation probe or laparoscopic retractor
- Hemostatic gelatin sponge (Gelfoam) or regenerated cellulose (Tabotamp)

PORT PLACEMENT (FIG. 2)

- T1, on the midline, 2–3 cm caudal to the umbilicus
- T2, in the left cranial quadrant of the abdomen, 2–3 cm cranial to T1
- T3, in the right cranial quadrant of the abdomen, at the same level as T2
- T4 (optional), on the midline, 2–3 cm caudal to the xiphoid process

PROCEDURE (VIDEO 1)

- A three-port technique can be used to approach the liver laparoscopically, as in the case of the dog presented here. Abdominal access is obtained using a sutureless modified Hasson technique. After a 5 mm incision has been made in the skin and subcutaneous tissues 2–3 cm caudal to the umbilicus, a 5 mm laparoscopic cannula (T1) is introduced into the abdomen and the abdominal cavity is insufflated with CO_2 at an intra-abdominal pressure of 7 mmHg.
- The liver is then explored laparoscopically with the 5 mm 30° telescope (**Fig. 10**).
- Under laparoscopic visualization, the second (T2) and the third (T3) ports (two 5 mm cannulas) are placed in the left and right cranial quadrants of the abdomen, respectively, in a triangulated fashion around the left lateral lobe.

- Using the laparoscopic grasping forceps, a piece of gauze is placed under the affected liver lobe to protect the surrounding structures during cauterization of the hepatic parenchyma (**Fig. 11**).
- The liver parenchyma is initially divided using the ultrasonically activated scalpel (Ultracision Harmonic Scalpel) at a power level of 3 (75% of full power) in the knife mode (**Fig. 12**).
- After complete resection of the mass, the surgical site is checked for hemostasis while lavaging and aspirating the fluid with a suction and irrigation device (**Fig. 13**).
- At this point, the piece of gauze is removed and the mass is placed into the specimen retrieval device.
- All the cannulas are withdrawn from the body wall and the specimen retrieval bag is exteriorized after enlarging the incision. The port sites are closed routinely.

VIDEO 1. Laparoscopic partial left lateral hepatectomy with an ultrasonically activated scalpel.

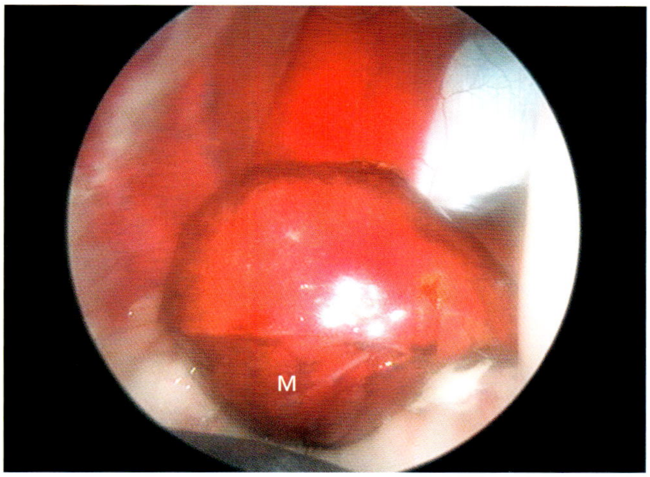

FIGURE 10. Visualization of the hepatic mass (M).

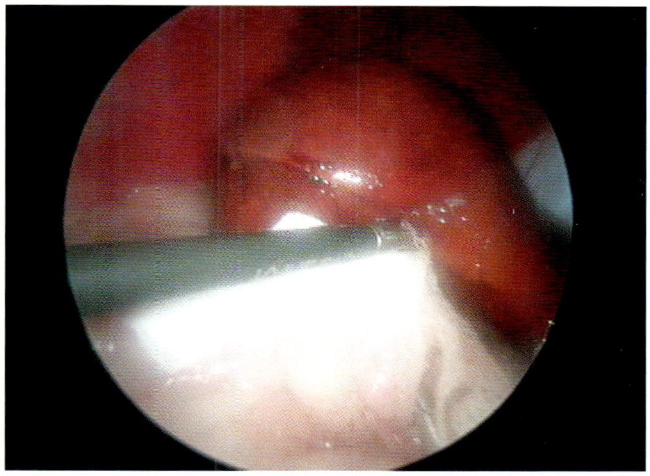

FIGURE 11. A piece of gauze is placed under the hepatic mass using the laparoscopic grasping forceps.

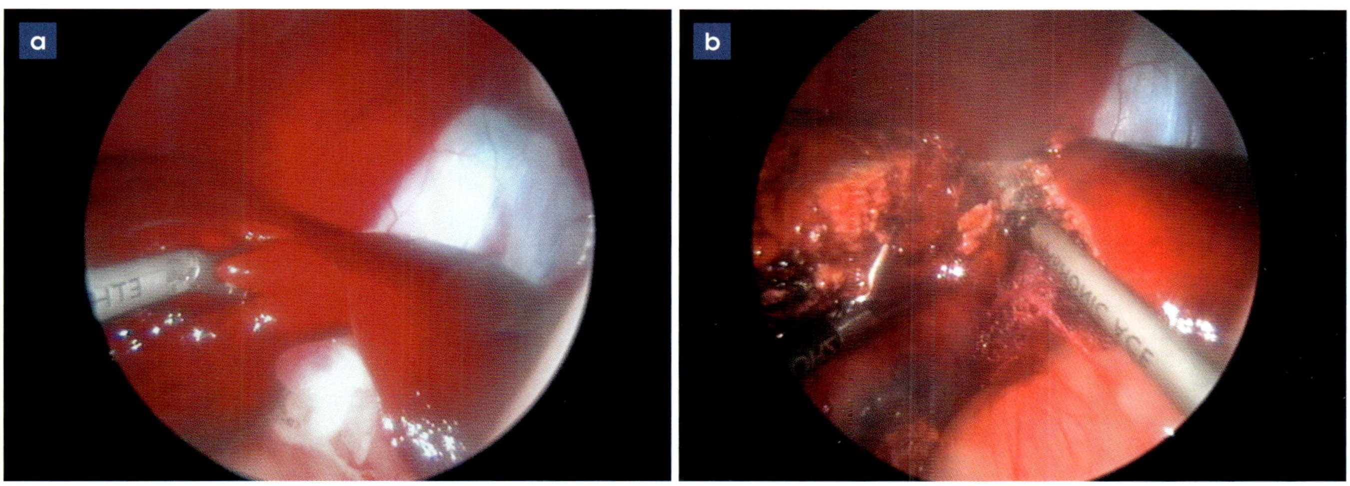

FIGURE 12. Dissection of the hepatic parenchyma around the mass using the ultrasonically activated scalpel.

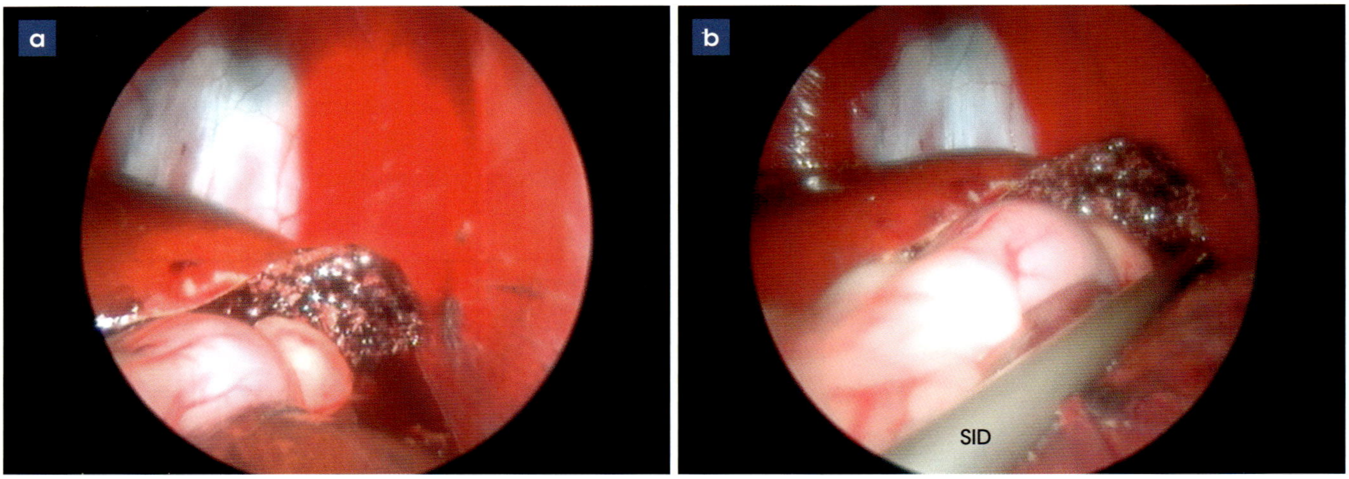

FIGURE 13. a) Final visualization of the dissected parenchyma to check for hemostasis. b) Irrigation of the surgical site with sterile fluid and aspiration using a suction and irrigation laparoscopic device (SID).

C LAPAROSCOPIC PARTIAL LEFT MEDIAL HEPATECTOMY

Instruments

On the table:

- Standard surgery set
- Telescope 5 mm – 30°
- Three 5 mm cannulas (two 5 mm cannulas + one 10 mm cannula)
- Laparoscopic atraumatic grasping forceps
- Laparoscopic grasping forceps
- Laparoscopic dissector forceps with monopolar electrocautery
- Vessel-sealing device (ultrasonically activated scalpel) or laparoscopic mechanical stapler device
- Gauze

Ready to use:

- Suction and irrigation laparoscopic device
- Additional 5 mm cannula
- Palpation probe or laparoscopic retractor
- Hemostatic gelatin sponge (Gelfoam) or regenerated cellulose (Tabotamp)

PORT PLACEMENT (FIG. 2)

- T1, on the midline, 2–3 cm caudal to the umbilicus
- T2, in the left cranial quadrant of the abdomen, 2–3 cm cranial to T1
- T3, in the right cranial quadrant of the abdomen, at the same level as T2
- T4 (optional), on the midline, 2–3 cm caudal to the xiphoid process

PROCEDURE

- A three-port technique can be used to approach the left medial lobe of the liver laparoscopically, as in the case of the dog presented below. After the camera port has been placed 2–3 cm caudal to the umbilicus using a modified Hasson technique, a 5 mm laparoscopic cannula (T1) is introduced into the abdomen and the abdominal cavity is insufflated with CO_2 at an intra-abdominal pressure of 8 mmHg.
- The liver is then explored laparoscopically with the 5 mm 30° telescope (**Fig. 14**).
- Under laparoscopic visualization, the second (T2) and the third (T3) ports (two 5 mm cannulas) are placed in the left and right cranial quadrants of the abdomen, respectively, in a triangulated fashion around the left medial lobe.
- If there are adhesions between the mass and the falciform ligament, they should be removed first with the ultrasonically activated scalpel (**Fig. 15**).

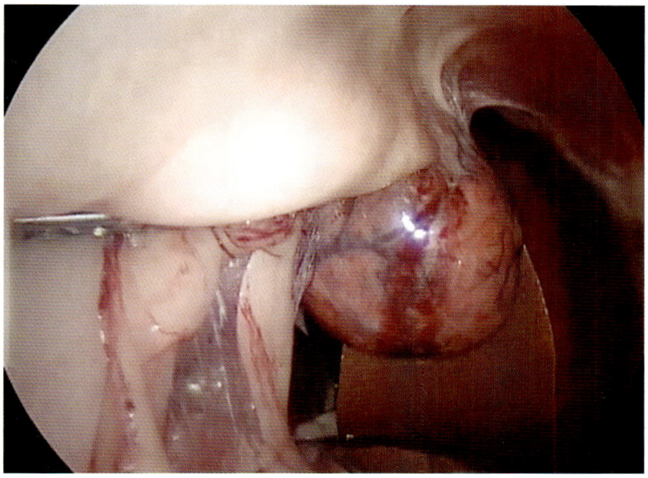

FIGURE 14. Visualization of the hepatic mass.

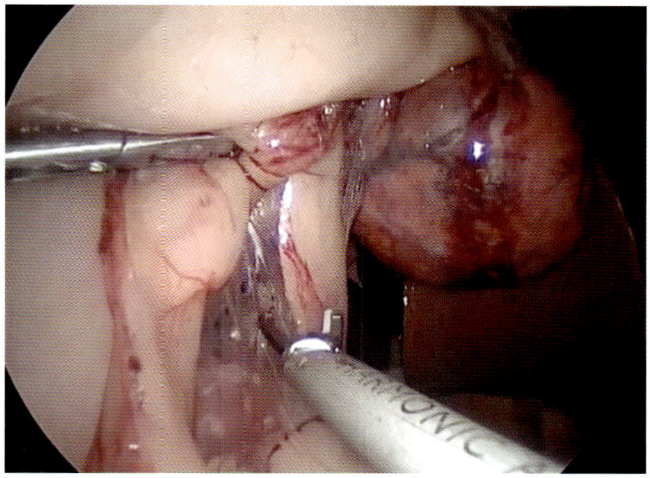

FIGURE 15. Dissection of the adhesions between the mass and the falciform ligament using the ultrasonically activated scalpel.

- Using the laparoscopic grasping forceps, a piece of gauze is placed under the affected liver lobe to protect the surrounding structures during cauterization of the hepatic parenchyma (**Fig. 16**).
- The liver parenchyma is initially divided using the ultrasonically activated scalpel (Ultracision Harmonic Scalpel) at a power level of 3 (75% of full power) in the knife mode (**Fig. 17**).
- After complete resection of the mass, the surgical site is checked for hemostasis while lavaging and aspirating the fluid with a suction and irrigation device.
- Two cellulose absorbable hemostats (Tabotamp) are placed over the dissected parenchyma for 5 minutes to promote hemostasis (**Fig. 18**). Then, following the removal of the cellulose absorbable hemostats and the piece of gauze, a further check for hemostasis is performed.
- At this point, the mass is placed into the specimen retrieval device (**Fig. 19**).
- After removing the cannulas and evacuating the pneumoperitoneum, the specimen retrieval bag is exteriorized through a small enlargement of the incision. The port sites are closed routinely.

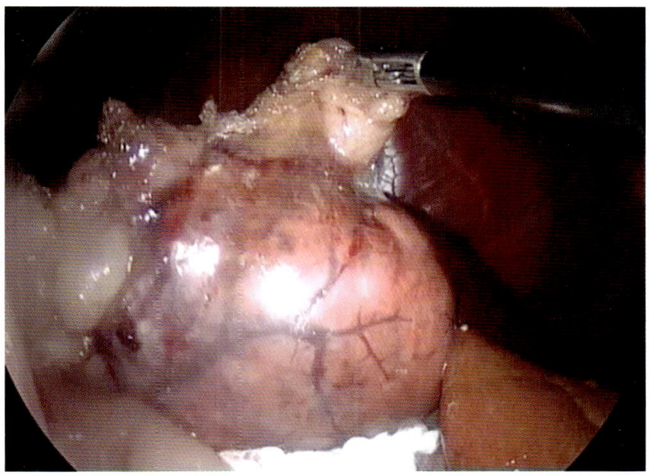

FIGURE 16. A piece of gauze is placed between the hepatic mass and the surrounding tissues using the laparoscopic grasping forceps.

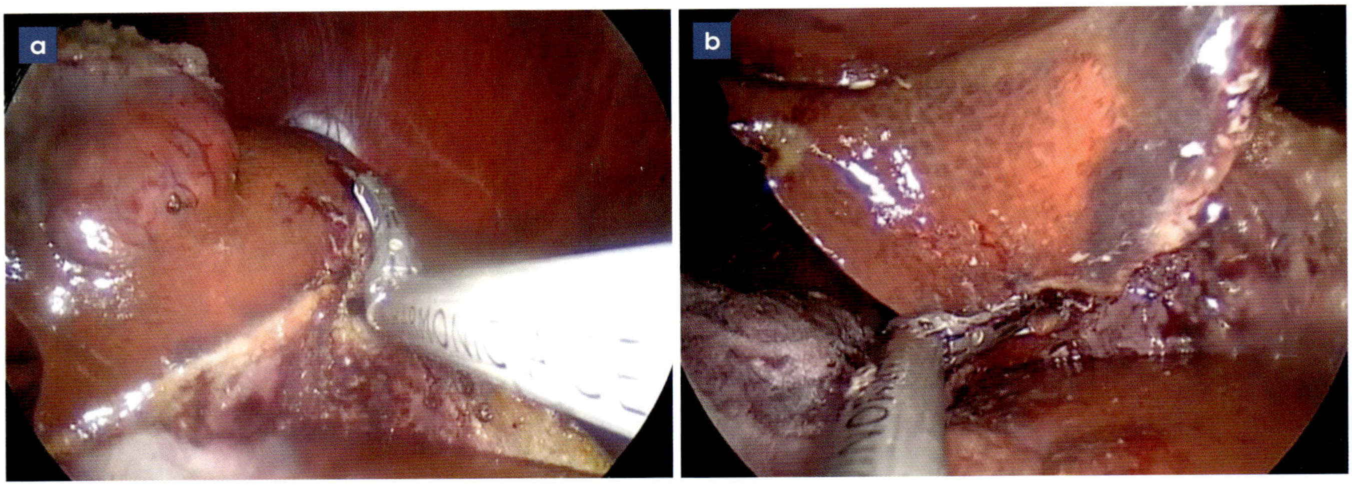

FIGURE 17. Dissection of the hepatic parenchyma around the mass using the ultrasonically activated scalpel.

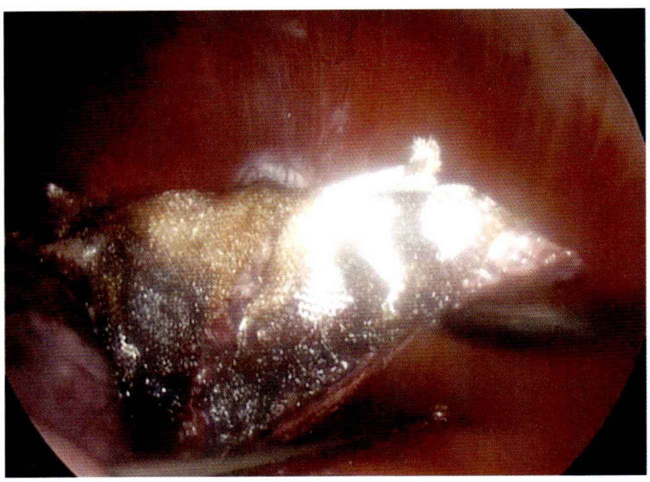

FIGURE 18. Two cellulose absorbable hemostats (Tabotamp) are temporarily placed on the dissected parenchyma, and the surgical site is irrigated with sterile fluid and aspirated with a suction and irrigation laparoscopic device.

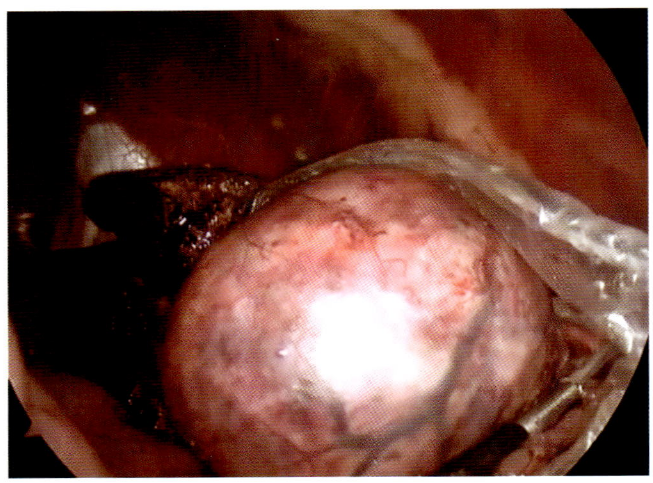

FIGURE 19. The mass is placed in a specimen retrieval bag using the laparoscopic grasping forceps.

POSTOPERATIVE MANAGEMENT

- Postoperative pain management includes the administration of an opioid drug and/or a nonsteroidal anti-inflammatory drug.
- The possible presence of hemoabdomen and/or bile leak should be evaluated by ultrasound.
- Biochemistry panels in the postoperative period may show a long-lasting increase in liver enzyme activity.

Complications of laparoscopic liver surgery

- Intraoperative hemorrhage. Bleeding from the hepatic parenchyma is mild and can be stopped by compression or cauterization. Bleeding can be severe if the major vessels have not been ligated properly.
- Bile leak is a typical problem in liver resection, because of incomplete sealing of the bile ducts in the parenchyma. If it is not severe, it is self-limiting in most cases.

Key points

- If the falciform ligament is very thick and bulky, retract it using a percutaneous suture to create more working space.
- Before starting liver dissection, place a piece of gauze under the mass to prevent damage to the surrounding tissues.
- It is helpful to delineate the plane of dissection using a harmonic scalpel or a monopolar device before starting to cut the parenchyma.
- An ultrasonically activated harmonic scalpel (Ultracision Harmonic Scalpel) is utilized to dissect the hepatic parenchyma around the affected lobe. An Endo GIA stapler can also be used to perform a liver lobectomy.
- Hemorrhage is the most frequent complication of liver lobectomy. It can be controlled with a monopolar or bipolar device.
- To promote hemostasis on the dissected hepatic parenchyma, pieces of hemostatic gelatin sponge (Gelfoam) or regenerated cellulose (Tabotamp) can be used.

SUGGESTED READINGS

CLINICAL CASES

34.1 LAPAROSCOPIC EXCISIONAL LIVER BIOPSY IN A DOG

Przemysław Prządka, Bartłomiej Liszka, Joanna Tunikowska, Stanisław Dzimira, Dariusz Patkowski

CASE DESCRIPTION

A 14-year-old male Miniature Schnauzer weighing 8 kg was evaluated for treatment of a liver tumor. The tumor, 2.7×2.3×1.3 cm in size, was located in the left medial lobe of the liver. After ultrasound examination and contrast tomography, the patient was qualified for laparoscopic excisional liver biopsy.

Key points

- Accurate preoperative diagnostic imaging allows for proper planning of liver tumor resection.
- In cases of extensive or unfavorably located tumors, laparoscopic biopsy of the liver lesion should be performed prior to resection.

PORT PLACEMENT

A three-port technique was performed. An optical trocar (T1) was introduced into the peritoneal cavity, on the midline and caudal to the umbilicus, using the Hasson technique. After establishing the pneumoperitoneum and examining the viscera and abdominal wall, two trocars for instruments (T2, T3) were placed on either side of T1 in a triangulated fashion.

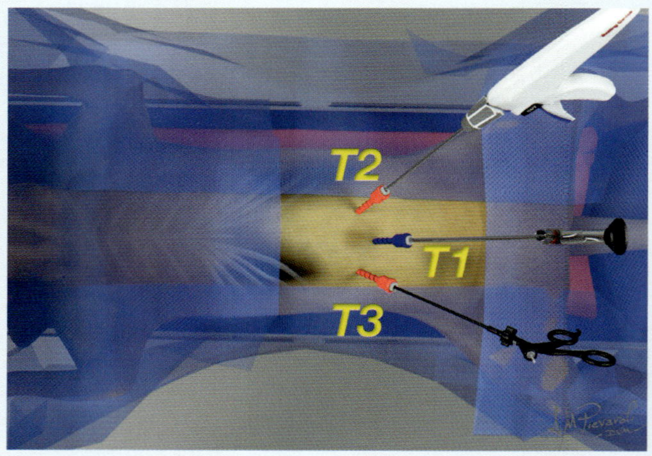

PROCEDURE

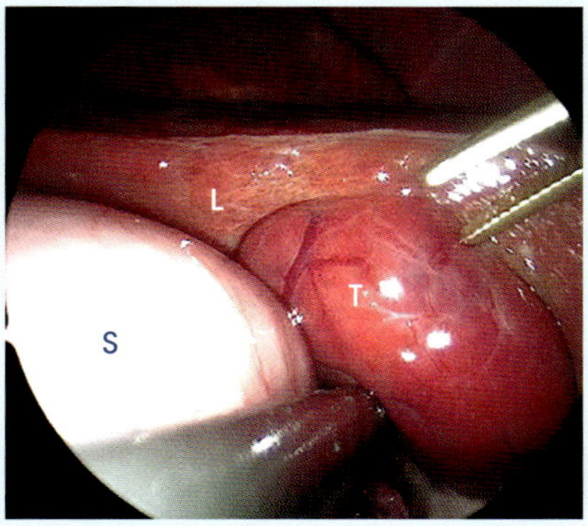

FIGURE 1. Laparoscopic view of the liver tumor. L, liver; S, stomach; T, tumor.

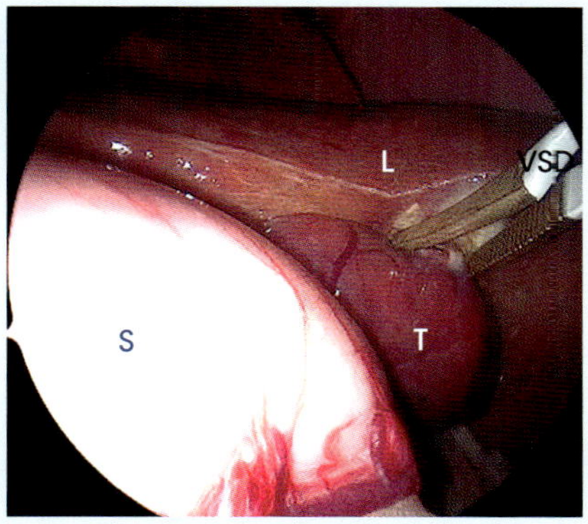

FIGURE 2. The tumor (T) is dissected using a vessel-sealing device (VSD) and laparoscopic forceps. The coagulated tissues are cut off using laparoscopic scissors. L, liver; S, stomach.

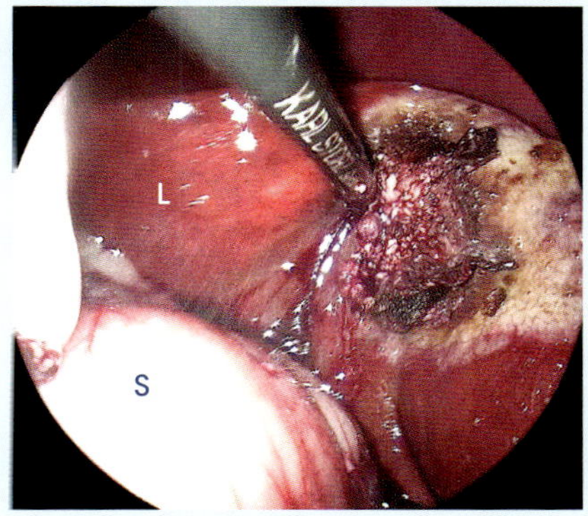

FIGURE 3. Laparoscopic view of the site of the removed tumor. The dissected mass is placed inside the thumb of a sterile glove and retrieved from the abdominal cavity through T1, after enlarging the incision. L, liver; S, stomach.

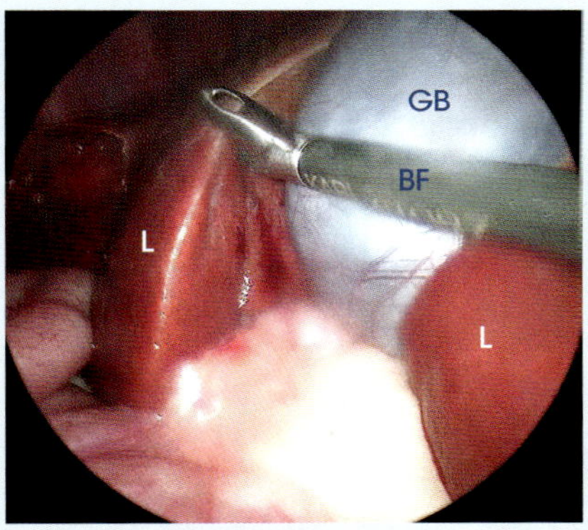

FIGURE 4. Additional samples from other parts of the liver are collected using laparoscopic biopsy forceps (BF). GB, gallbladder; L, liver.

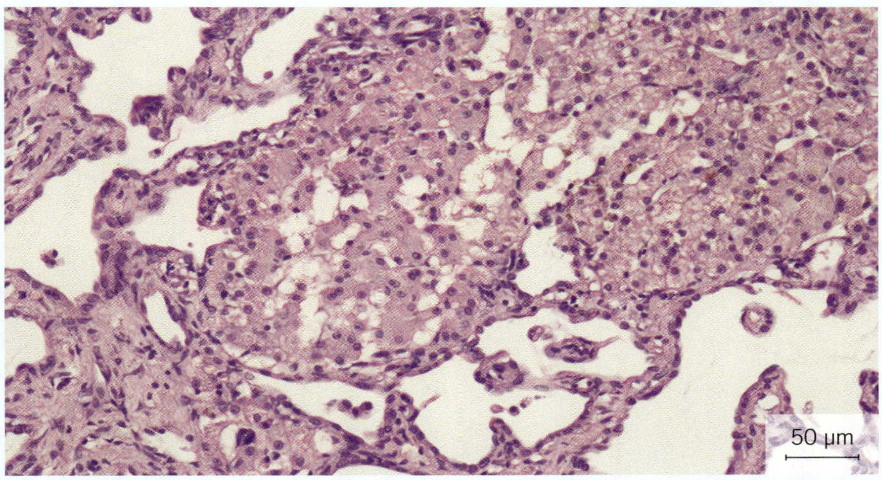

FIGURE 5. Histopathological image showing chaotic hepatocellular proliferation, partially with fatty degeneration and microcellular cirrhosis (hematoxylin–eosin, ×200).

Tips and tricks

- ✓ The use of a vessel-sealing device is very helpful in controlling intraoperative bleeding.
- ✓ Correct trocar placement provides adequate visibility and access to the resected part of the liver. It may be necessary to introduce a fourth trocar to improve surgical access.

34.2 LAPAROSCOPIC EXCISION OF A HEPATIC CYST AND OMENTOPEXY IN A PERSIAN CAT

Giovanni Allevi

CASE DESCRIPTION

An 8-year-old neutered male Persian cat was presented for a second opinion on the diagnosis of a hepatic cyst. The physical examination revealed abdominal distension. Routine hematologic analysis and serum biochemistry showed an increase in AST (288 IU/L; range 15–35), ALT (244 IU/L; range 32–87), and TBIL (0.39 mg/dL; range 0–0.26). A CT scan revealed small single cysts in both kidneys, a pancreatic cyst, and multiple hepatic cysts, the largest in the right liver lobe. The latter cyst was surgically excised through a laparoscopic approach. At a 6-month follow-up after surgery, abdominal ultrasonography revealed no recurrence of the liver cyst.

Key points

- Performing a CT scan is essential for patient staging before surgery.
- Laparoscopic resection and omentalization of hepatic cysts can be considered a safe minimally invasive procedure.

PORT PLACEMENT

The patient was placed in dorsal recumbency under general anesthesia. A three-port technique was used: the first port (T1) was placed 3 cm caudal to the umbilicus using a modified Hasson technique. After establishing the pneumoperitoneum, the other two 5 mm ports (T2, T3) were placed 3 cm lateral and 3 cm cranial to T1.

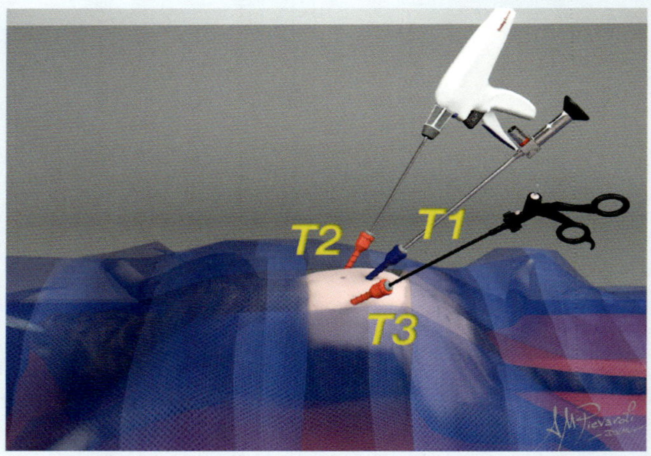

PROCEDURE

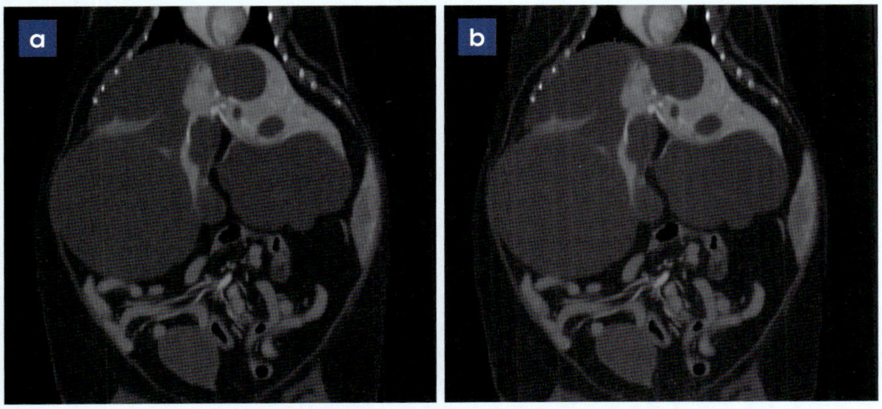

FIGURE 1. CT scan images of the hepatic cysts.

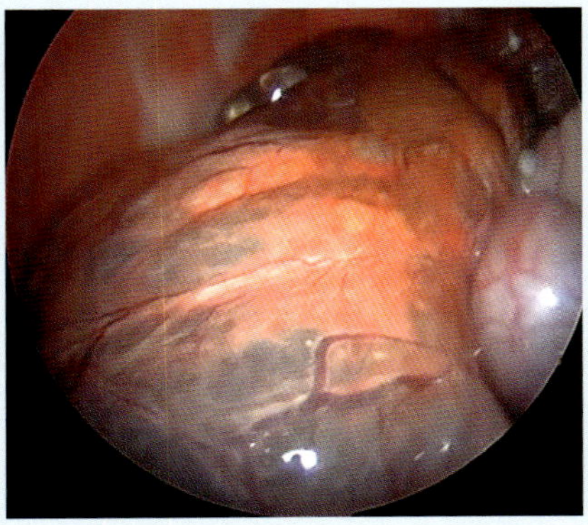

FIGURE 2. A large hepatic cyst originating from the right medial liver lobe is identified in the right cranial abdomen during laparoscopic exploration of the abdominal cavity. Other small liver cysts were also seen.

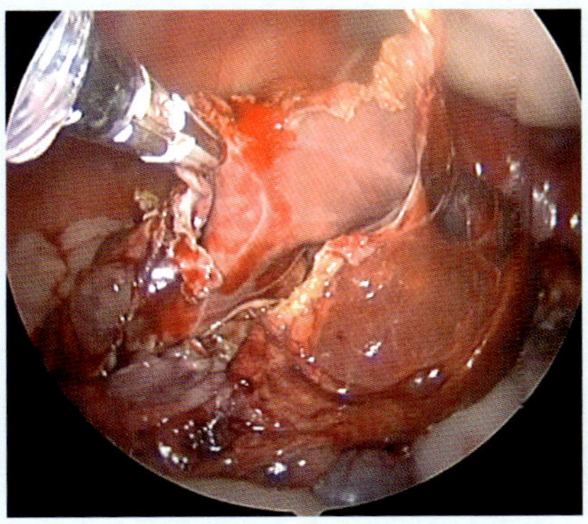

FIGURE 3. After draining the large cyst using a transabdominal needle, the cyst wall is dissected with a 5 mm laparoscopic vessel sealer/divider device. The same procedure is performed on the smaller liver cysts.

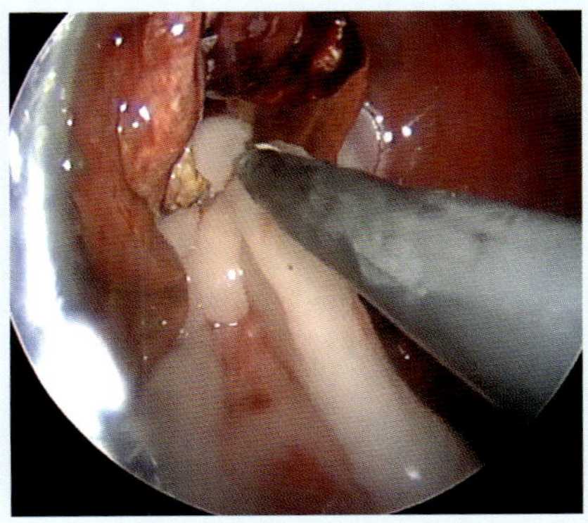

FIGURE 4. Omentopexy of the cystic wall by coagulating the omentum to the wall of the cyst using LigaSure. This avoids intracorporeal suturing and thus reduces surgical time. Only the larger cyst was omentalized.

Tips and tricks

✓ Cyst omentalization can be performed by sealing the omentum to the cystic wall. This decreases surgical length, which is especially helpful in those patients that need a short duration of anesthesia.

35 LAPAROSCOPIC MICROWAVE ABLATION OF THE LIVER

J. Brad Case, Beau B. Toskich

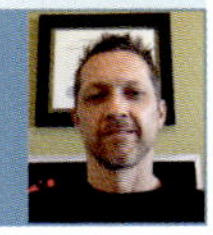

Indications

- Precise criteria for microwave ablation of hepatic lesions in dogs have not been determined
- Well-defined lesions smaller than 3 cm that do not abut hepatic ducts or main portal vein branches are reasonable targets for microwave ablation

Contraindications

- Large (>5 cm) or ill-defined neoplastic lesions
- Neoplastic lesions affecting the hilum
- Unstable patients that will not tolerate capnoperitoneum
- Cases in which laparotomy and resection is determined to be safer

Laparoscopic thermal ablation is commonly performed in humans for malignant conditions such as hepatocellular carcinoma (HCC) and colorectal liver metastasis. Although a number of thermal ablation modalities exist, microwave ablation (MWA) has become the dominant modality for most hepatic ablations. The major advantages of MWA include minimal heat sink effect, larger and more consistent ablation zone formation, ability for multiple synchronous ablations, and more rapid ablation cycles. In humans, the benefits of laparoscopic thermal ablation over laparotomy and resection include liver remnant preservation, reduced hospitalization time, lower analgesic requirements, and fewer complications.

MWA has become the preferred treatment for HCC measuring less than 2 cm in human patients who are not liver transplant candidates. Laparoscopic MWA and MWA via laparotomy of hepatic neoplasia has been previously described in two and five dogs, respectively. In this report, laparoscopic MWA of an HCC in one dog and multiple sarcomas in another dog was performed without operative complications. Although incomplete ablation was suspected in one dog with HCC, no significant regrowth occurred and the patient survived for more than 3 years following the procedure with no disease progression or return of clinical signs. Multiple subsequent cases have been performed demonstrating complete ablation and no recurrence after more than 1 year of follow-up including CT imaging.

Currently, explicit guidelines for laparoscopic MWA of liver neoplasia in dogs do not exist. However, multiple clinical scenarios may lead the surgeon to consider this option. One such scenario is for the treatment of patients with nonresectable neoplasia; nodular HCC or recurrence of HCC following previous liver lobectomies are two examples. This chapter serves as a general overview of laparoscopic MWA for hepatic neoplasia in dogs. To perform laparoscopic MWA safely and effectively, specific training and experience using microwave technology are required prior to use in clinical patients.

> The first clinical report of laparoscopic microwave ablation in dogs was published in 2019 by Alberto Oramas et al.

DESCRIBED SURGICAL PROCEDURES

As long as a thorough laparoscopic evaluation of the liver is performed, multiple port orientations are possible for MWA. The orientation of the microwave probe is determined based on cautious and accurate pre- and intraoperative assessment.

A two-port laparoscopic approach for complete exploration of the liver has been previously described and is recommended. The first port is placed at, or just caudal to, the umbilicus. The second port is placed at approximately one-third of the distance between the umbilicus and the xiphoid cartilage. The use of a SILS port for the umbilical port facilitates the utilization of a 12 mm inner cannula, which is necessary for the laparoscopic ultrasound probe. Depending on the surgeon's preference and any other procedures being performed, additional ports may be added.

Microwave probes are placed percutaneously after exploration and identification of the lesions to be ablated. The position of the probe varies, but accurate placement of the probe within the lesion should be achieved. Because the size and morphology of individual lesions are variable, accurate preoperative planning based on CT imaging as well as intraoperative imaging with laparoscopic ultrasound is strongly recommended. Additionally, understanding the three-dimensional size and shape of the ablation zone created by the microwave probe is essential. The exact orientation of the probe also depends on the shape and size of the lesion and on locoregional anatomy. Probes may be placed either within the center of mass in small (<2 cm) tumors or in bracket fashion for larger or irregularly shaped lesions.

The energy profiles (i.e., power and duration) for destruction of quantified volumes of tissue have been developed and tested preclinically in specific tissues in multiple species (including canine) over the past few decades. These studies demonstrate consistent and complete zones of ablation and are the basis for manufacturer power/duration recommendations to create specific-sized zones of ablation. Specifically, the length, diameter, axial area, and length beyond the probe tip of an ablation zone are known based on power and duration settings. Most modern MWA units utilize a power setting of between 45 and 65 watts and between 3 and 5 minutes per cycle. Again, preoperative CT is deemed necessary by the authors if considering thermal ablation for curative intent of a neoplastic lesion in a clinical case.

The exact location and morphology of the lesion as well as the desired margin need to be considered when planning the ablation. Discrete lesions less than 2 cm in diameter can be effectively ablated with a single probe and ablation cycle creating an ablated zone roughly 3.5–4 cm in diameter. As lesion size increases (and therefore the desired zone of ablation), multiple probe insertions (synchronized or performed sequentially) are required. Again, because of the risk of incomplete ablation and hepatic abscessation, the authors consider lesions larger than 5 cm in diameter to be contraindicated for MWA.

PATIENT PREPARATION AND POSITIONING

A physical examination, blood panel (complete blood count, serum biochemistry, clotting profile), and CT scan of the abdomen should be performed prior to considering laparoscopic MWA for hepatic neoplasia. Although abdominal ultrasound is commonly used for preoperative assessment of liver disease, CT is recommended for preoperative planning and to determine the role (staging and biopsy, or potentially for liver resection or ablation) laparoscopy may play in the diagnosis and treatment. Additionally, fine needle aspiration cytology can be useful in determining a tentative preoperative diagnosis, which may influence the surgical procedure and approach.

In general, the dog should be fasted for at least 8 hours prior to anesthesia and have an IV catheter placed for fluid and medication therapy during the procedure. The urinary bladder should be drained with a urinary catheter (if possible) at the time of anesthesia induction. Premedications that result in splenic enlargement, such as acepromazine, should be avoided. Perioperative analgesia may include opioid medications. Local anesthesia with bupivacaine is recommended at individual port sites prior to incision.

The dog is placed in dorsal recumbency, and the abdomen is clipped from the xiphoid process to the pubis and dorsally past the level of the 13th rib. If a hydraulic float table is available, the patient may be positioned directly on the operating table and the hydraulic function used to create about 30° of reverse Trendelenburg as well as lateral positioning as needed. The reverse Trendelenburg position can also be accomplished with a traditional operating table and the patient can be gently shifted on the table to acquire a lateral oblique position. Due to the lobar nature of the canine liver (**Fig. 1**), alteration of position is usually required to evaluate the entire organ. The skin is aseptically prepared as for traditional laparotomy. This ensures that adequate preparation and quick conversion to laparotomy can be performed if needed.

OPERATING ROOM LAYOUT

The dog should be positioned with his hind end at the foot of the operating table and the anesthesia machine and staff positioned at the head of the table. The instrument table is placed at the patient's foot, but the patient drape should not be attached to the instrument table. This allows alteration of patient position without pulling on the instrument table or exposing the sides of

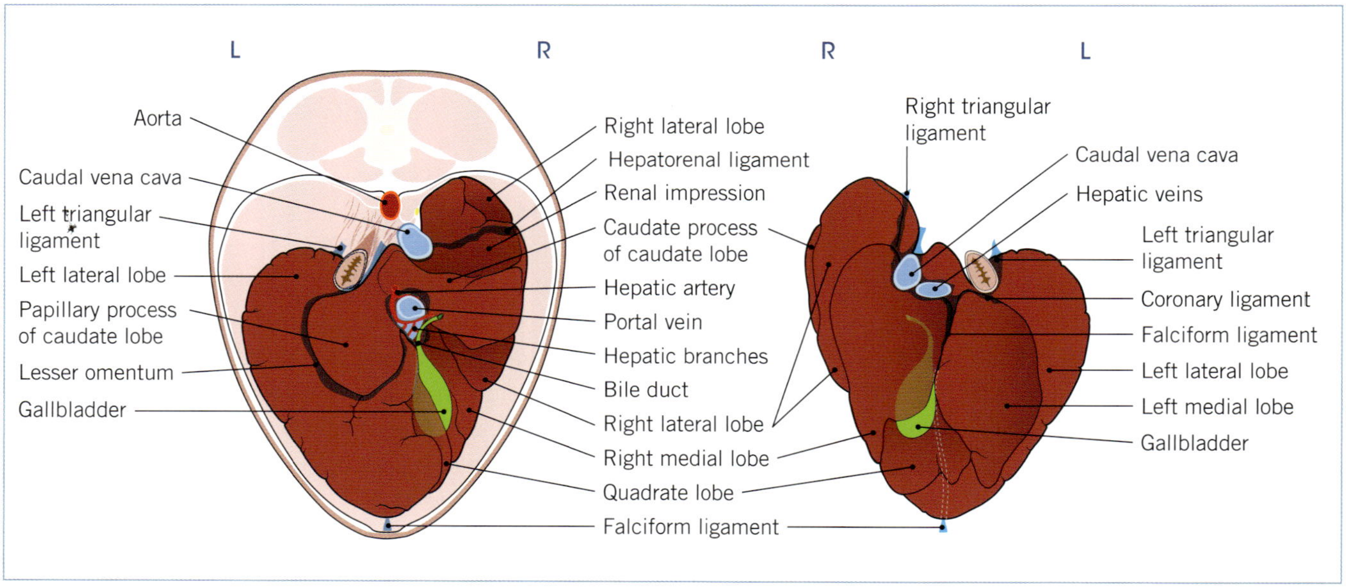

FIGURE 1. Anatomical diagram of the canine liver. Note the fissured lobar anatomy, which makes complete evaluation with laparoscopy challenging. Alteration of patient position (lateral and reverse Trendelenburg) is often required, especially for lateral lobes such as the right lateral lobe.

the patient. Alternatively, the instrument table can be placed over the patient's head as long as the anesthesia staff has adequate room for monitoring. The monitors are placed towards the patient's head so that they can be viewed easily, and in line, while exploring the liver. The surgeon and the assistant position themselves on opposite sides of the patient and can switch sides as needed. In general, for lesions of the central and left division, it is preferable for the surgeon to be located on the patient's right side, while for right division lesions the surgeon should be positioned on the patient's left side. The ultrasound and MWA units can be on either side of the patient but positioned more towards the patient's head (**Figs. 2 and 3**).

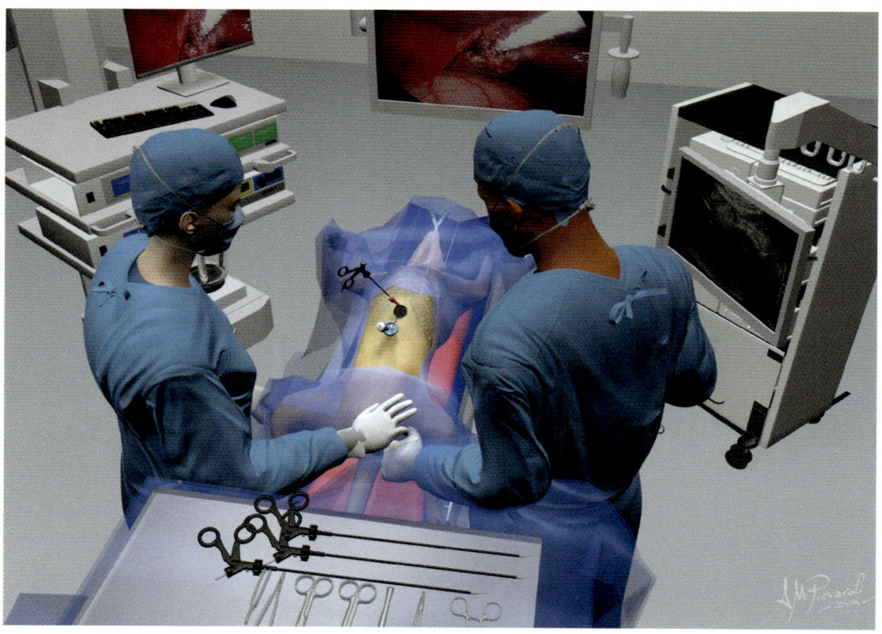

FIGURE 2. Operating room layout for laparoscopic ultrasound examination of the liver and MWA of neoplastic lesions.

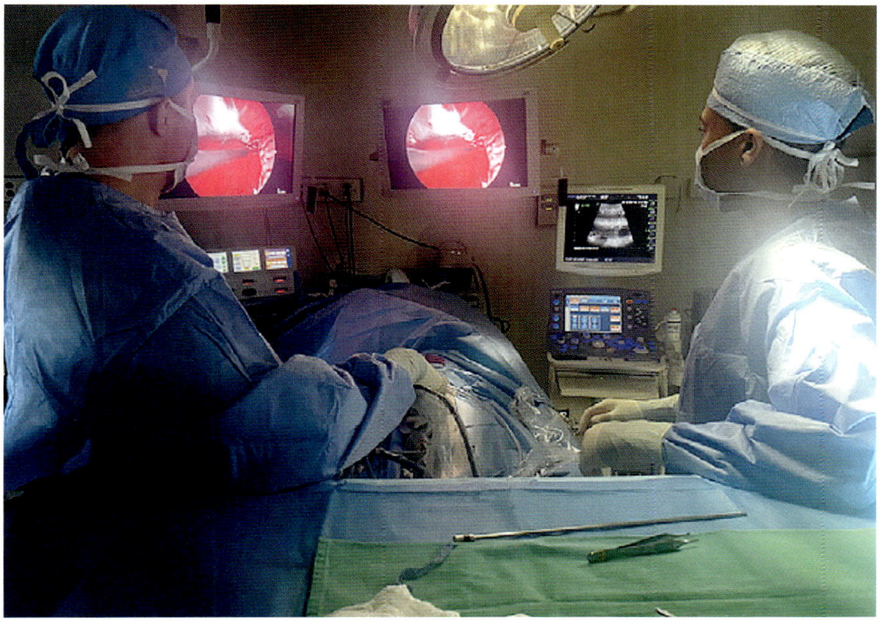

FIGURE 3. Intraoperative image of the operating room layout during laparoscopic ultrasound examination of the liver.

Instruments

On the table:

- Standard abdominal surgical pack
- High-definition video camera
- Telescope 5 mm – 30°
- Three 5 mm threaded cannulas and a SILS port
- 12 mm cannula for laparoscopic ultrasound
- Laparoscopic blunt probe, straight 5 mm
- Ultrasound unit with laparoscopic probe (**Fig. 4**)

Ready to use:

- Microwave ablation generator and probe (**Fig. 5**)

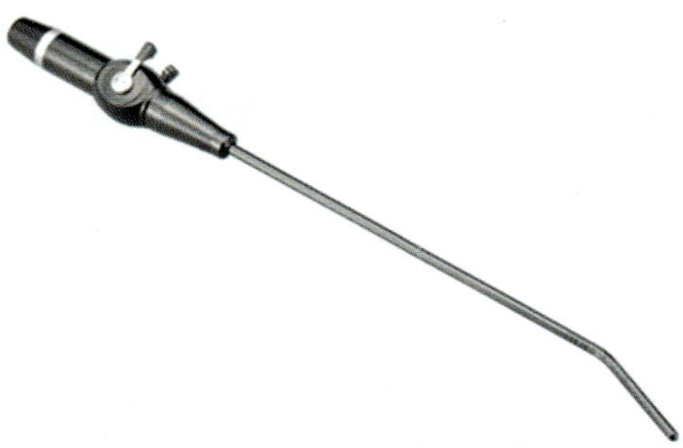

FIGURE 4. Laparoscopic ultrasound probe.

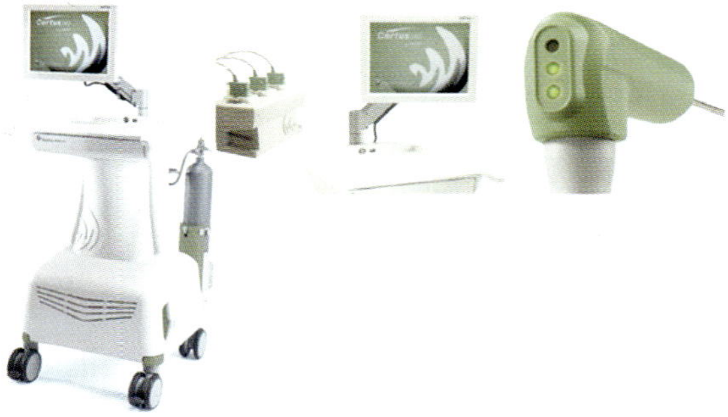

FIGURE 5. Microwave ablation unit including a generator, settings display monitor, and CO_2-cooled microwave ablation probe.

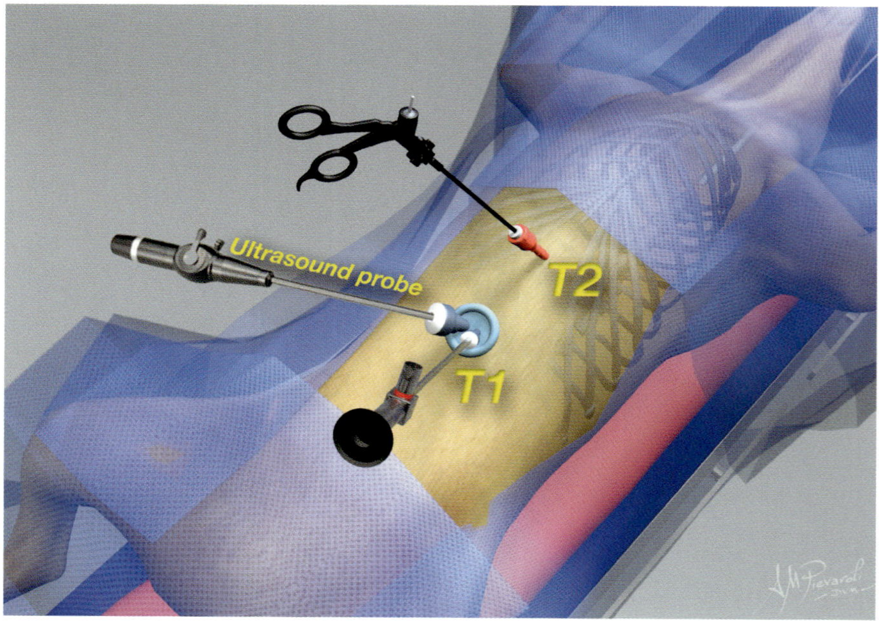

FIGURE 6. Port placement for laparoscopic ultrasound examination of the liver and MWA of neoplastic lesions.

PORT PLACEMENT (FIG. 6)

- T1 (SILS), on the midline, at the level of the umbilicus
- T2, on the midline, one-third the distance between the umbilicus and the xiphoid cartilage
- Microwave probe, variable depending on the lesion

PROCEDURE

- After the first port has been placed and the pneumoperitoneum achieved, the 5 mm telescope is inserted and a first exploration of the abdomen and liver is performed.
- The second port is then placed under optical guidance.
- The lesion of interest is identified and a laparoscopic ultrasound examination is performed (**Figs. 7 and 8**). The size and morphology of the mass are assessed. Important regional structures (e.g., major portal veins, viscera) are identified. In some cases, alteration of patient position may be necessary to identify and assess lesions.
- Once the lesion of interest has been evaluated laparoscopically and ultrasonographically, the ablation plan is designed. The orientation and trajectory of the MWA probe is determined and ultrasound used to guide accurate positioning within the mass. The ablation energy profile (power and duration) is confirmed. Additionally, the need for multiple serial or synchronous ablations is assessed based on the size, shape, and location of the mass lesion. It is often necessary to use a laparoscopic retractor or blunt probe to elevate the affected liver lobe away from adjacent viscera, such as the stomach, prior to ablation (**Fig. 9**).
- Once the ablation cycle is initiated, the laparoscopic ultrasound probe is removed from the mass to avoid thermal injury to the probe. The lesion is observed closely throughout the entire ablation cycle to ensure that the probe maintains accurate position within the mass, that no adjacent viscera or regional anatomical structures are in contact with the lesion or probe, and to assess the gross change in the tissue. Typically, hepatic tissue takes on a charred appearance when it is ablated (**Fig. 10**). Although, both primary and secondary mechanisms of tissue death occur following MWA, any neoplastic tissue that remains pink to red following ablation is at risk for incomplete ablation and recurrence.
- When the ablation cycles have been completed, laparoscopic ultrasound assessment is performed. Generally, lesions become hypoechoic or hypoattenuating to the surrounding parenchyma on CT (**Fig. 11**), and no blood flow should be observed within the ablated zone via Doppler. If regions of concern for incomplete ablation are identified, additional ablation cycles can be performed. However, caution should be exercised when performing additional ablations, as extending the ablation zone may increase the risk for complications such as hepatic abscess formation (**Fig. 12**).
- A biopsy of the margin is then obtained for histopathology to assess neoplastic viability.
- Finally, the ports are removed and incisions closed routinely.

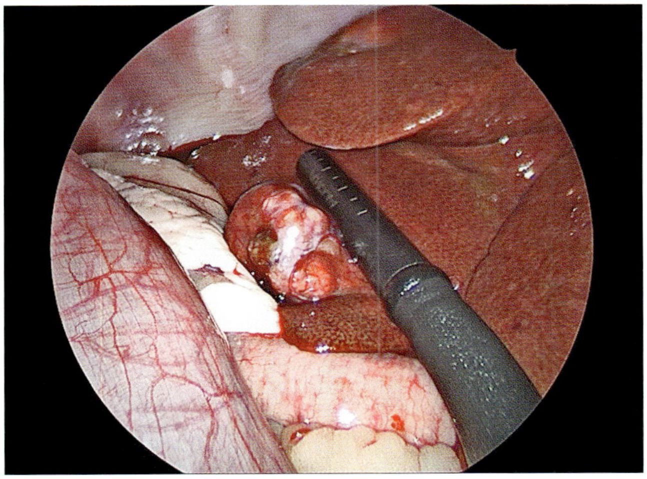

FIGURE 7. Intraoperative view of an HCC in the caudate lobe of a dog undergoing laparoscopic ultrasound assessment prior to MWA.

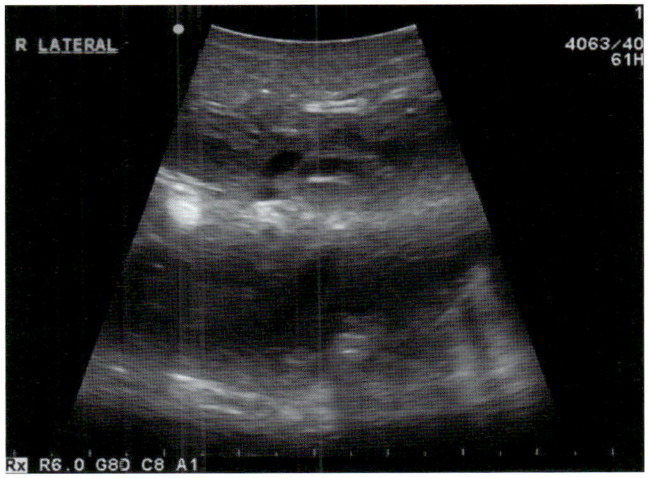

FIGURE 8. Laparoscopic ultrasound image of the liver.

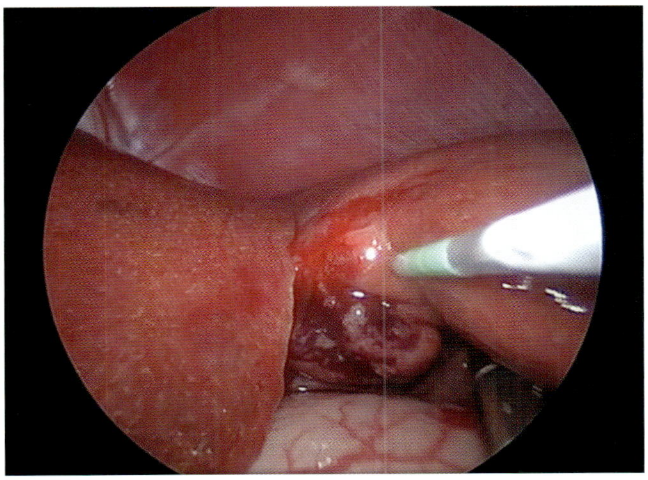

FIGURE 9. A blunt probe is used to elevate the lesion away from the visceral gastric surface.

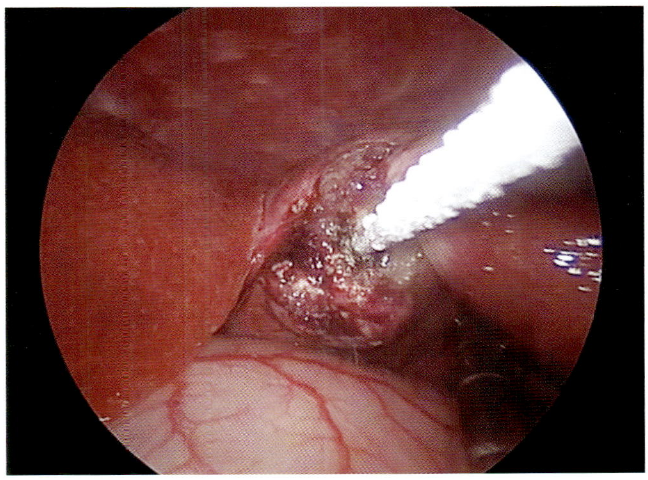

FIGURE 10. The lesion develops a characteristic charred appearance as the end of the ablation cycle nears.

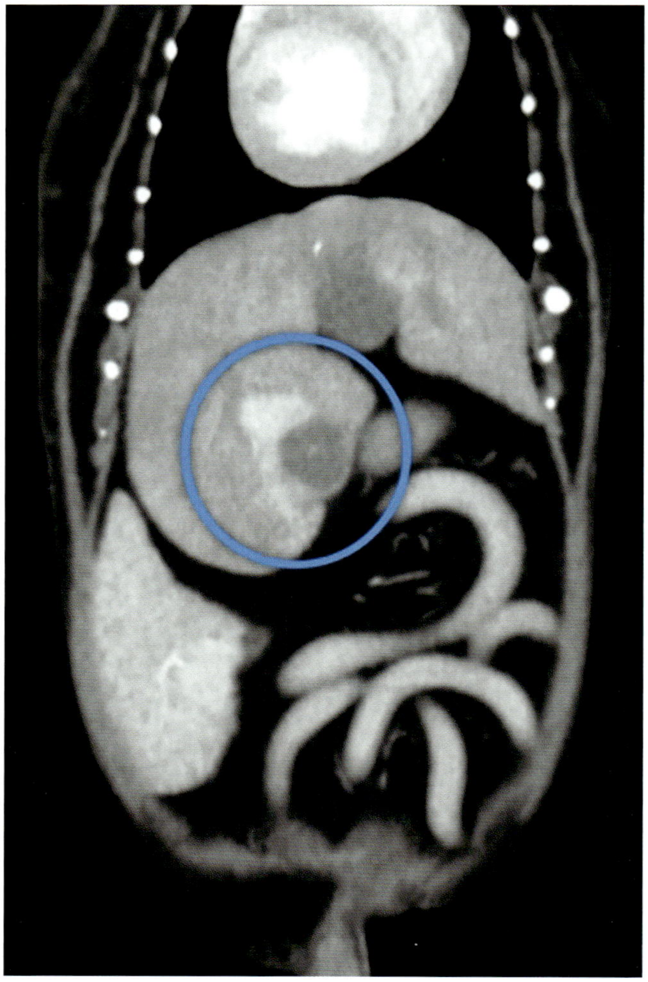

FIGURE 11. Frontal plane CT image acquired 6 months after laparoscopic MWA of a 5 cm mass in a dog. Note the region of hypoattenuation with contrast enhancement on the periphery (circle). The hypoattenuating region is consistent with previous ablation, while the contrast enhancement is evidence of recurrence.

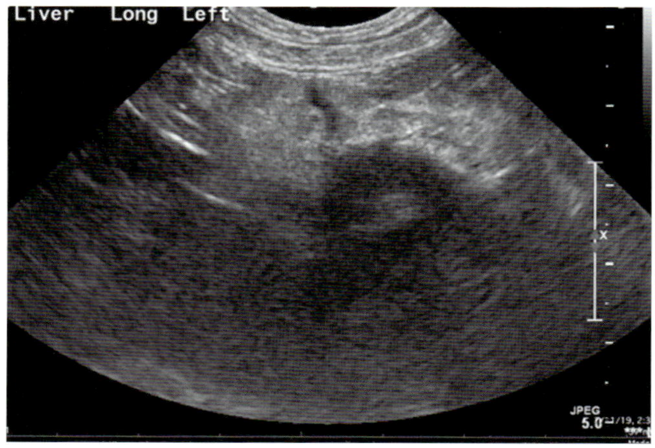

FIGURE 12. Transabdominal ultrasound image of the liver of a dog with a hepatic abscess detected 6 weeks following laparoscopic MWA of an HCC. The abscess resolved after a course of antimicrobial medication.

POSTOPERATIVE MANAGEMENT

- Analgesia requirements following laparoscopic MWA are typically minimal but may include 2–3 days of an oral synthetic opioid, such as tramadol. Nonsteroidal anti-inflammatory drugs are contraindicated in dogs with liver disease. Alternatives to opioids such as gabapentin are also reasonable choices for postoperative analgesia.
- Food and water can be offered ad libitum 8–12 hours after surgery as long as no contraindications exist.
- Because MWA creates tissue necrosis, it is recommended that dogs be prescribed antimicrobial prophylaxis for 3–4 weeks to reduce the risk of abscessation. Amoxicillin with clavulanic acid is a reasonable choice.
- Dogs should be monitored for 48–72 hours after MWA for postablation syndrome or early signs of abscessation. Possible signs of postablation syndrome include fever, inappetence, lethargy, and minor abdominal discomfort. Signs should resolve within 3–5 days. If they continue or worsen, or if vomiting and significant abdominal pain are observed, hepatic abscessation should be ruled out.
- A complete blood count and serum biochemistry profile are performed at 24–48 hours, 10–14 days, and 6 weeks after the MWA procedure. ALT levels are expected to increase following MWA, but this should resolve by 4–6 weeks.
- Follow-up transabdominal ultrasound and CT imaging are recommended every 4–6 months after MWA of neoplastic lesions such as HCC. Earlier or later monitoring may be reasonable in some cases, depending on the histopathology and clinical outcome of the patient.

Complications of MWA of hepatic lesions

- Complications are scarcely reported following MWA in dogs. However, hepatic abscess formation has been observed in one dog 6 weeks after surgery. The dog was prescribed 4 weeks of amoxicillin with clavulanic acid and the infection resolved.
- Postablation syndrome is challenging to identify clinically, as the signs occur early, are generally mild, and resolve quickly. Thus, the incidence and significance are hard to determine.
- Surgical site infections have not been reported following laparoscopic MWA in dogs, but bruising and discomfort around the probe site are possible and typically resolve with conservative management.
- Incomplete ablation and recurrence are risks with MWA. Thus, accurate case selection, planning, and application of the technique are critical to minimize this risk.
- Nontarget ablation to adjacent critical organs is rare but a potentially life-threatening complication of ablation.

Key points

- Well-defined neoplastic lesions <3 cm that do not abut hepatic ducts or main portal veins are candidates for MWA.
- Incomplete ablation and recurrence are rare risks with MWA. Accurate case selection, procedural planning, and technique application are critical to minimize this risk.

SUGGESTED READINGS

36 LAPAROSCOPIC CHOLECYSTECTOMY

Eric Monnet

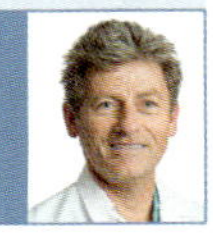

Indications

- Cholecystectomy is indicated for treating gallbladder mucocele, cholangiohepatitis, and gallbladder neoplasia.
- The selection of cases is paramount for the success of this procedure with laparoscopy. It is indicated for cases without common bile duct obstruction.
- It implies that dogs need to have normal total bilirubin and normal bile duct anatomy on ultrasound.

Contraindications

- Dilation of the bile duct on ultrasound is considered a contraindication for the procedure with laparoscopy. If any signs of bile duct dilation are present, a laparotomy is required to evaluate the patency of the common bile duct.
- Laparoscopy might be converted to laparotomy if the cystic or the common bile duct are looking distended or abnormal at the beginning of laparoscopy.

Cholecystectomy is more likely the most common surgery performed in human patients. Cholecystectomy performed before biliary tract obstruction seems to be associated with a better prognosis than when the biliary tract is obstructed in dogs.

PATIENT PREPARATION AND POSITIONING

The patient is placed in dorsal recumbency. The dog can be placed in a slightly oblique position toward the left to allow for better visualization of the gallbladder and cystic duct by moving the falciform ligament and the pyloric antrum away from the surgical field. A reverse Trendelenburg position also helps retract the stomach away from the gallbladder.

OPERATING ROOM LAYOUT

The patient is in dorsal recumbency at the end of the table. The surgeon is standing at the end of the table, and the tower monitor is placed at the head of the dog next to the anesthesia equipment. The table with instruments is set behind the surgeon. An assistant will be standing on the left side of the surgeon to hold the camera and the grasping forceps holding the apex of the gallbladder (**Fig. 1**).

Instruments

- Telescope 5 mm – 0° or 30°
- Four-port technique: three 5 mm cannulas + one 10 mm cannula
- Single-port technique: one single access port + one 5 mm cannula
- 5 mm palpation probe
- Two 5 mm fine teeth grasping forceps
- 5 mm right-angle forceps or 5 mm articulated dissector
- 5 mm vessel-sealing device: Maryland jaw
- J-hook extension for electrocautery
- 10 mm medium/large endoclip
- 5 mm suction/irrigation device
- 10 mm retrieval pouch

PORT PLACEMENT

Four-port placement (**Fig. 2**):

- T1, 5 mm cannula on the midline 1 cm caudal to the umbilicus
- T2, 5 mm cannula on the right side, 2 cm cranial to the umbilicus, and 3–4 cm from the midline

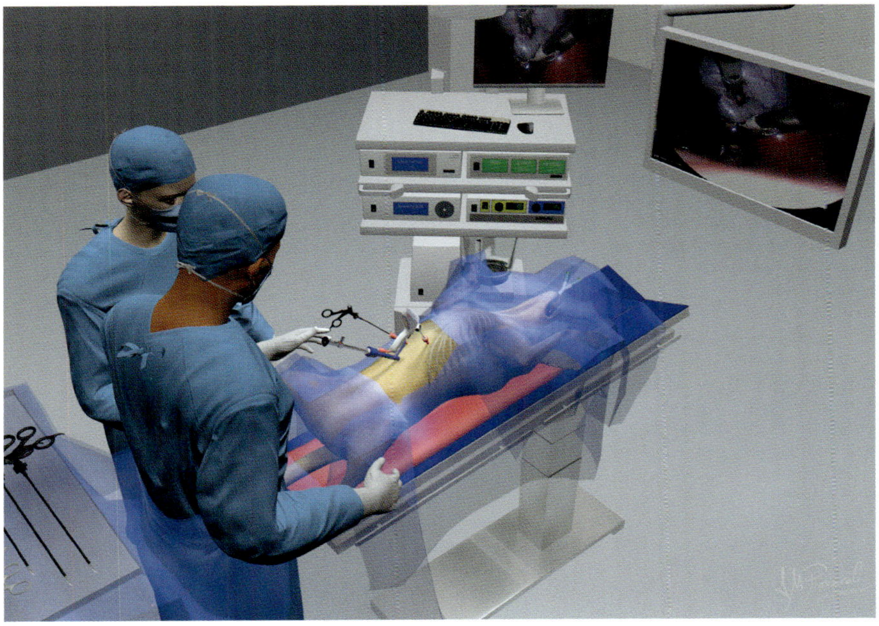

FIGURE 1. Operating room layout for laparoscopic cholecystectomy.

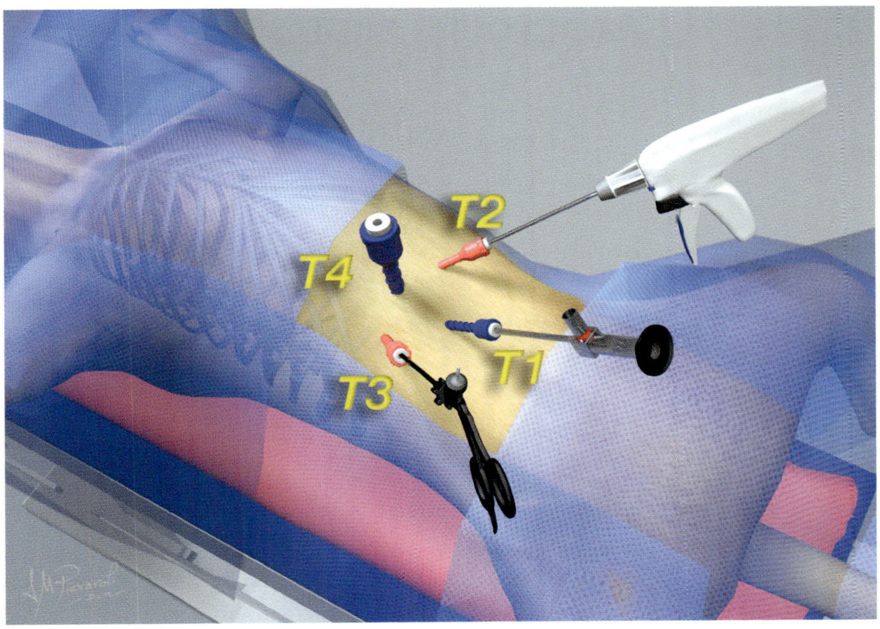

FIGURE 2. Port placement for four-port laparoscopic cholecystectomy.

- T3, 5 mm cannula on the left side, 2 cm cranial to the umbilicus, and 3–4 cm from the midline
- T4, 5 –12 mm cannula on the midline 1 cm cranial to the umbilicus

Four ports (three 5 mm ports and one 5–12 mm port) are most commonly required for surgery. The ports are placed in a triangular fashion around the cranial abdomen. Two ports are placed on the midline with the camera port (T1) 1 cm caudal to the umbilicus. The 5–12 mm port (T4) is placed 1 cm cranial to the umbilicus. This port is used for grasping forceps during the dissection, and then the clip applicator closes the cystic duct and the retrieving pouch to remove the gallbladder. The two other 5 mm ports are placed on the left (T3) and right (T2) sides of the midline, 2 cm cranial to the umbilicus and 3–4 cm from the midline.

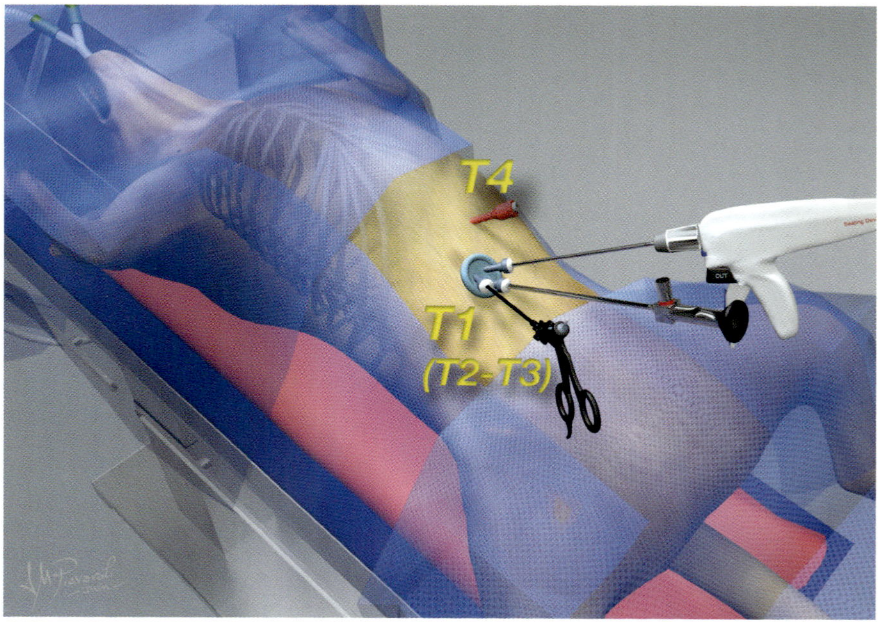

FIGURE 3. Port placement for single-incision port system for laparoscopic cholecystectomy.

Single-port placement (**Fig. 3**).

- T1, T2, T3, on the midline 1 cm caudal to the umbilicus
- T4, 5 mm cannula 2 cm cranial to the umbilicus 3–4 cm from the midline on the left side

The utilization of a single-incision port system on the midline has been described with an extra cannula on the left side of the abdominal cavity. The single-incision port system is placed 1 cm caudal to the umbilicus. Two 5 mm cannulas and one 5-12 mm cannula are placed in the single port access system (T1, T2, T3). An extra 5 mm cannula (T4) is placed 2 cm cranial to the umbilicus 3–4 cm from the midline on the left side. The dissecting forceps is introduced through this cannula during the dissection of the cystic duct.

One port is used for the telescope. Two ports are used to retract the gallbladder during the dissection. Then, curved dissectors or an articulated dissector are used to dissect around the cystic duct. Introducing the curved dissectors or the articulated dissector from the cannula on the right side of the abdomen is better. An electrocautery with a J-hook can be used to dissect the gallbladder from the liver parenchyma. A vessel-sealing device can also be used for dissection. A suction/irrigation unit is needed to clean the surgical field if there is some bleeding from the liver parenchyma during the procedure.

PROCEDURE (VIDEO 1)

The gallbladder is located in the hepatic fossa of the quadrate lobe. The common bile duct and the cystic duct are important anatomical structures that need to be identified during the procedure. The cystic artery in dogs is usually very close to the cystic duct and does not need to be dissected from it for its ligation. Branches of the portal vein can be very superficial in the quadrate lobe and need to be recognized during the surgery.

VIDEO 1. Step-by-step description of laparoscopic cholecystectomy in dogs.

The following procedures are described below:

A. Dissection from the cystic duct
B. Dissection from the apex of the gallbladder
C. Intraoperative cholangiogram

A DISSECTION FROM THE CYSTIC DUCT

- It is preferable to start the dissection at the level of the cystic duct. One fine-tooth grasping forceps is used to retract the gallbladder ventrally and cranially to expose the cystic duct; the other is used to retract the infundibulum of the gallbladder caudally (**Fig. 4**).
- This maneuver opens the angle between the cystic duct and the common bile duct. Using two forceps also helps to retract the edge of the quadrate lobe of the liver, which can interfere with visualization.
- If it is difficult to grab the gallbladder wall because of severe distension. It is possible to insert a needle percutaneously to aspirate it. A Veress needle can also be used to aspirate the content from the gallbladder. It can be difficult if there is a mucocele aspiration of the gelatinous content from the gallbladder.
- Right-angle or articulated forceps are then used to dissect the cystic duct from the quadrate lobe. Usually, the cystic artery is dissected with the cystic duct. The cystic artery is usually very close to the cystic duct in dogs; therefore, there is no need to dissect and ligate the cystic artery separately.

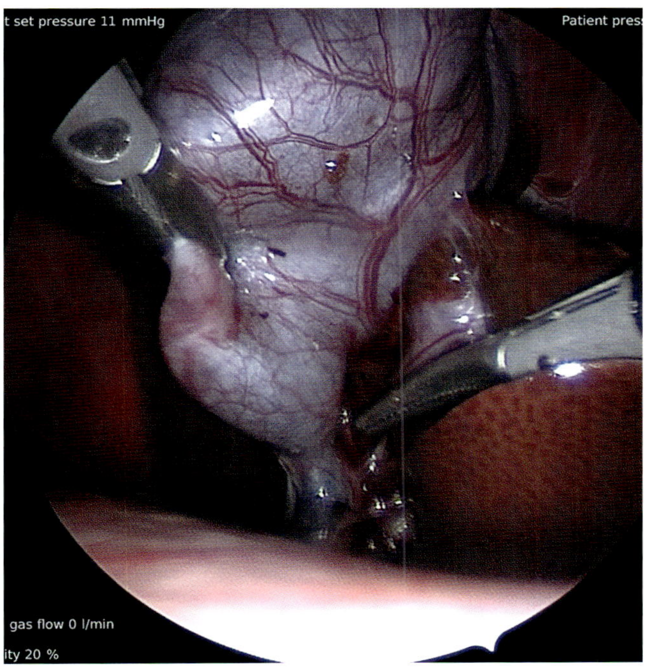

FIGURE 4. Exposure of the cystic duct with one forceps holding the infundibulum and a dissecting forceps starting the dissection 360° around the duct.

- After complete dissection of the cystic duct is done, three large/medium 10 mm endoclips (Endoclips, Medtronic, Minneapolis, MN) are used to ligate the cystic duct (**Fig. 5**). Usually, two clips are placed distally on the cystic duct making sure the common bile duct is not occluded.
- One clip is placed proximally. The cystic duct is then transected between the proximal clip and the two distal clips, trying to leave 0.25 cm of the cystic duct distal to the two clips left on the cystic duct. Large/medium 10 mm clips have been shown to provide a safe cystic duct closure. A vessel-sealing device has been shown to be safe in an in vitro study on canine cadaveric cystic duct. However, it is difficult to know how the cystic duct is healing after using a vessel-sealing device, and we do not know how a diseased cystic duct will behave with a vessel-sealing device.
- Extracorporeal and intracorporeal ligations have also been used to ligate the cystic duct. A linear stapler (EndoGIA, Medtronic, Minneapolis, MN) has also been used on very large cystic ducts. Self-locking polymer clips have been used instead of metallic clips to ligate the cystic duct during laparoscopy.
- After the cystic duct/gallbladder are retracted ventrally, the gallbladder dissection is carried away toward the apex (**Fig. 6**). Two strong attachments are present at the infundibulum of the gallbladder. Those two attachments need to be dissected first with a vessel-sealing device.
- Then, a dissection plane between the gallbladder and the liver parenchyma is identified (**Fig. 7**).

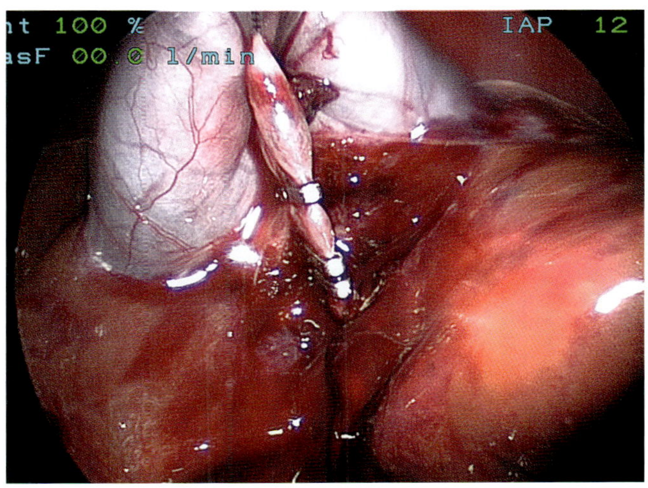

FIGURE 5. Three 10 mm large endoclips have been placed on the cystic prior to its transection.

- The gallbladder should peel away from the liver parenchyma without many attachments or adhesions. Usually, the attachments are on the periphery of the gallbladder along the reflection of the peritoneum. Another strong attachment is present at the apex of the gallbladder.
- The vessel-sealing device is used to dissect and transect all the strong attachments. The electrocautery with a J-hook is also used to facilitate the gallbladder dissection from the liver parenchyma.
- As an alternative technique, the gallbladder dissection from the hepatic fossa can be performed within the gallbladder wall, leaving the gallbladder subserosal surface attached to the liver parenchyma. This technique is supposed to minimize the risk of bleeding from the liver parenchyma (**Fig. 8**).

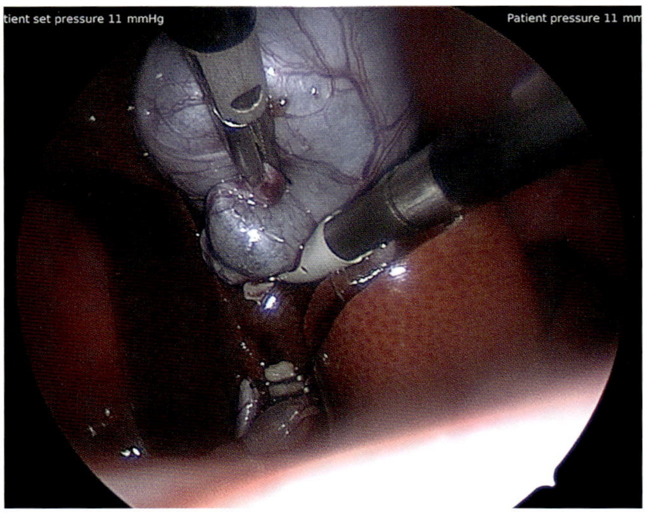

FIGURE 6. The cystic duct has been transected, and the gallbladder dissection is started from the cystic duct with a vessel-sealing device.

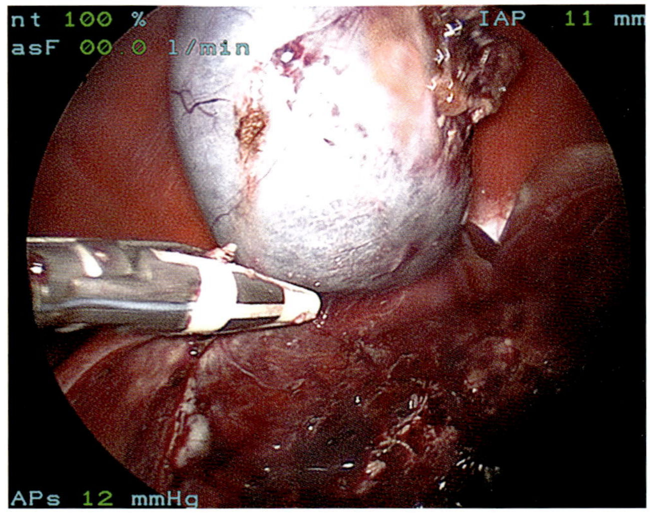

FIGURE 7. The vessel-sealing device is used to transect the last attachment at the apex of the gallbladder.

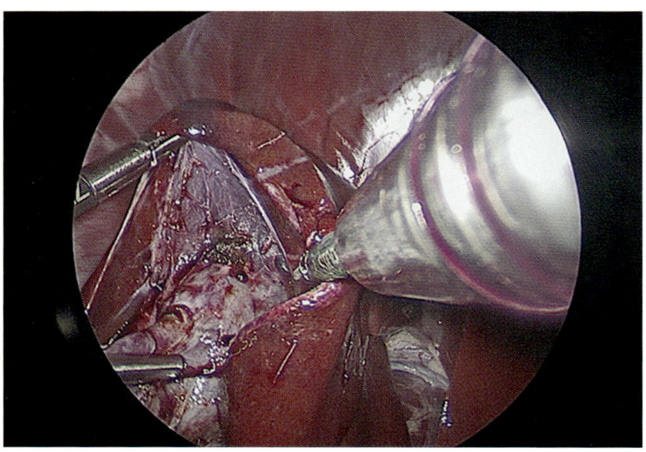

FIGURE 8. The dissection of the gallbladder was carried in a subserosal layer of the gallbladder.

Key points

- Appropriate retraction of the apex and infundibulum of the gallbladder to visualize the cystic duct.
- Utilization of an articulated forceps to dissect the cystic duct.
- Establish a good plane of direction between the gallbladder and the liver parenchyma.
- 10 mm large endoclips are appropriate to ligate the cystic duct.

B DISSECTION FROM THE APEX OF THE GALLBLADDER

- If the cystic duct cannot be visualized because of the gallbladder size, then the dissection is started at the apex of the gallbladder. After cranial retraction of the quadrate lobe, the gallbladder dissection is started (**Fig. 9**).
- A plane of dissection is established between the gallbladder and the liver. It is important not to penetrate the liver parenchyma to minimize bleeding during the procedure.
- After completion of the dissection of the gallbladder, the cystic duct and artery are ligated with 10 mm large/medium endoclips, sutures, or linear stapler.
- The cystic duct is transected. The surface of the liver is inspected for bleeding. If bleeders are present, the electrocautery is used.
- After placing the gallbladder in a retrieving pouch, it is removed from the abdominal cavity after extending a port site on the midline to approximately 5 cm in length. If a single-incision port has been used, the gallbladder is removed through the incision of the port.

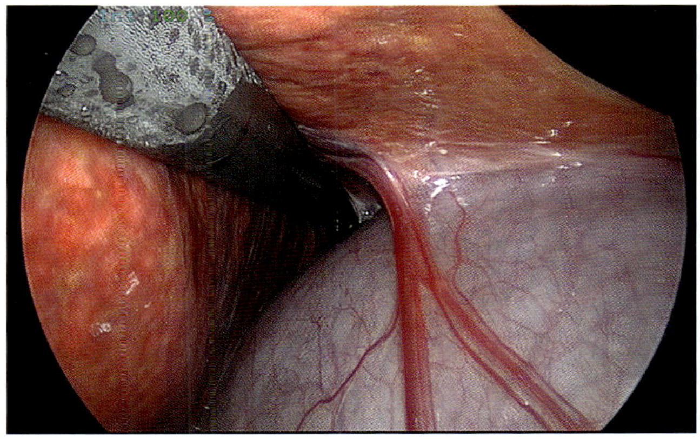

FIGURE 9. The dissection of the gallbladder is started at the apex.

Key points

- Establish a good plane of direction between the gallbladder and the liver parenchyma.
- Follow the curvature of the gallbladder when starting at the apex.

C INTRAOPERATIVE CHOLANGIOGRAM

- Iatrogenic trauma to the common bile duct is the most common complication of laparoscopic cholecystectomy in humans. An intraoperative cholangiogram has been used during laparoscopy to help identify the common bile duct.
- Intraoperative cholangiogram is also used to confirm patency of the common bile duct. Intraoperative cholangiogram requires catheterization of the cystic duct. The cystic duct is partially incised after placing a clip distally, and a catheter is advanced in the proximal part of the duct toward the common bile duct. A contrast agent is then injected under fluoroscopy to visualize the remaining of the biliary system.
- Fluorescent imaging is also used to identify the biliary tract. Indocyanine green is injected intravenously 1 hour before surgery. Near-infrared light is then used during laparoscopy to induce fluorescence of the indocyanine green that is eliminated by the biliary system. This technique has not been well-established in dogs yet.

POSTOPERATIVE MANAGEMENT

- In the postoperative period, the dog should be watched for bile peritonitis and hemorrhage signs.
- It is not unusual to see an elevation of the bilirubin in the first 24–48 hours after surgery because of the manipulation of the bile duct.

Complications of laparoscopic cholecystectomy

- If the gallbladder is punctured during the dissection, a grasping forceps is used to clamp the puncture site and twist it to prevent further bile leakage in the abdominal cavity. The abdominal cavity needs to be flushed at the end of the procedure to eliminate the bile that leaked into the peritoneal cavity.
- Bleeding from the liver parenchyma can develop doing the dissection of the gallbladder from the hepatic fossa. It is usually controlled with compression with a palpation probe or with electrocautery. Hemostatic sponges can also be applied to the liver parenchyma. It is also important to identify branches of the portal veins that can be closely associated with the wall of the gallbladder (**Fig. 10**). The dissection can be carried out between the branches of the portal vein and the gallbladder.
- Occlusion of the common bile duct is another complication that can happen after laparoscopic cholecystectomy. It is usually due to the placement of clips across the common bile duct while ligating the cystic duct.

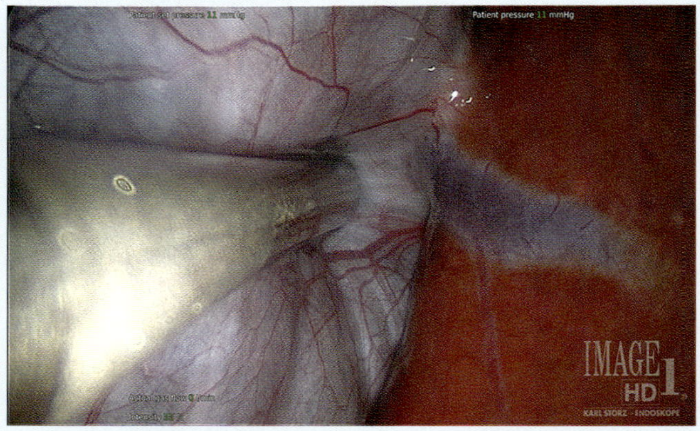

FIGURE 10. Visualization of a superficial branch of the portal vein.

Conversion rate

Conversion rates between 4% and 30% have been reported in dogs for laparoscopic cholecystectomy. The major cause for conversion is related to visualization and difficulty manipulating the gallbladder to expose the cystic duct. Adhesions are common causes of elective conversion (**Fig. 11**). Rupture of the gallbladder does not always indicate conversion. In 2018 Kanai et al. reported a gallbladder rupture rate of 2.6% in their study, and those cases could be treated laparoscopically. Large cystic duct precluding the utilization of clips has been another cause of elective conversion. Utilizing an EndoGIA should eliminate the need for conversion for large cystic ducts.

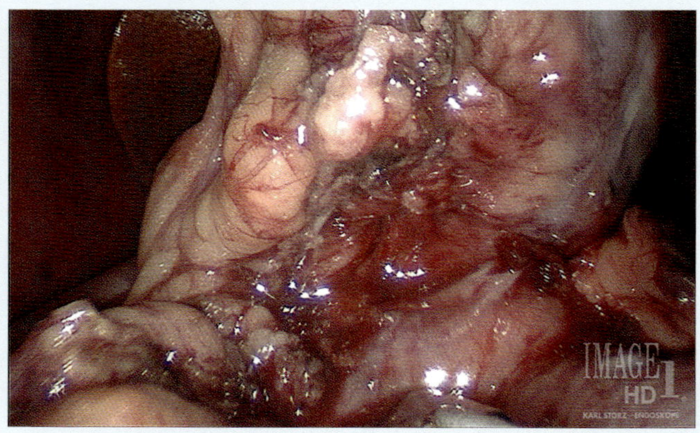

FIGURE 11. Severe adhesions of the omentum over the gallbladder could require conversion because it interferes with the visualization of the cystic duct.

SUGGESTED READINGS

CLINICAL CASES

36.1 SINGLE-PORT LAPAROSCOPIC CHOLECYSTECTOMY TECHNIQUE IN DOGS

Jeffrey J. Runge, Joshua G. Becker

TECHNIQUE DESCRIPTION

Laparoscopic cholecystectomy is only typically recommended in patients with asymptomatic or mildly symptomatic cholelithiasis. There is a dearth of literature on laparoscopic cholecystectomy, and case selection is mainly based on anecdotal reports and individual experience. In dogs with gallbladder mucoceles with extrahepatobiliary obstructions, there is a concern for persistent postoperative obstruction with laparoscopic cholecystectomy. In general, if the total serum bilirubin is significantly elevated, if there is evidence of bile peritonitis, or if there is a concern for any obstructive process, an open approach is strongly advised.

Key points

- Care must be taken to avoid and check for evidence of iatrogenic trauma secondary to port placement. Particular attention should be paid to the liver, gallbladder, and extrahepatic biliary tree, as omental adhesions are common findings in patients with gallbladder disease.
- The presence of bile pigment in the abdomen or around the gallbladder increases the clinical index of suspicion for biliary tract perforation, in which case conversion is advised.
- Any adhesions should be gently dissected with a blunt probe or similar atraumatic device. Conversion to an open approach is advised if adhesions are excessive or obscure visualization and cannot be dissected. For adhesions on the more apical parts of the gallbladder, it may be possible to section them with a vessel-sealing device and complete the procedure without conversion.
- Depending on the surgeon's preference, the gallbladder can be dissected before or after cystic duct dissection, ligation, and sealing. For cystic duct dissection, the gallbladder is elevated ventrally with a retractor to expose the cystic duct.
- Regardless of the technique used, triple ligation of the ducts is advised, with the duct transected between the two most distal ligation sites using laparoscopic scissors.
- Ensuring the tissue is appropriately dissected and firmly grasped with forceps, the gallbladder can often be removed through the incision along with the single-port device. In some cases, exteriorization of the gallbladder may be aided by drainage of the bile from the gallbladder lumen. This can be done by placing the gallbladder into a specimen retrieval bag, closing the bag, removing the port, and then partially exteriorizing the bag through the port incision. The bag is then partially opened, and either the gallbladder is aspirated via a sterile large-gauge needle and syringe or a small incision is made into the gallbladder and is aspirated via surgical suction. Once the gallbladder is appropriately reduced in size, the retrieval bag is closed and removed from the abdomen.
- It is recommended that patients be hospitalized overnight for continued monitoring and postoperative care. This is particularly important in patients with comorbidities, which is not uncommon in patients with gallbladder disease.

PORT PLACEMENT

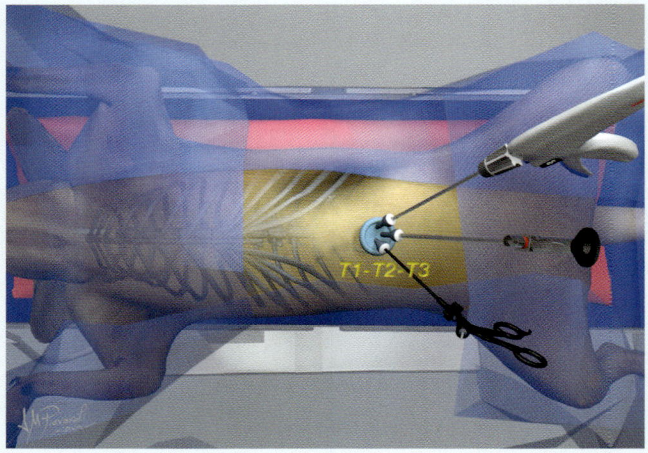

The patient was placed in dorsal recumbency or near the very caudal edge of the operating table. The abdomen should be aseptically prepared for an open approach in case conversion or additional port placement is required. An operating table with the capacity for reverse Trendelenburg position and lateral tilt function can be helpful with perioperative visualization, depending on the patient's size. The surgeon typically stands on the patient's right side to begin, though it will likely be necessary to move to the caudal end of the patient intraoperatively. The endoscopic tower is positioned toward the head of the patient, and the surgical table should be able to move to facilitate surgeon placement at the caudal end of the patient. The port is placed in standard fashion at the level of the umbilicus.

PROCEDURE

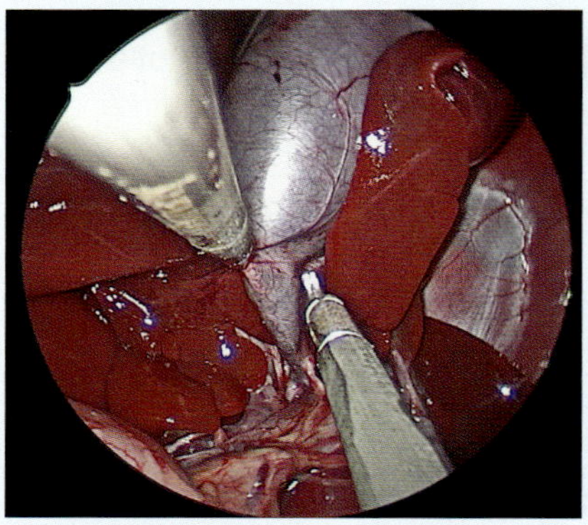

FIGURE 1. View of the cystic duct before dissection and ligation.

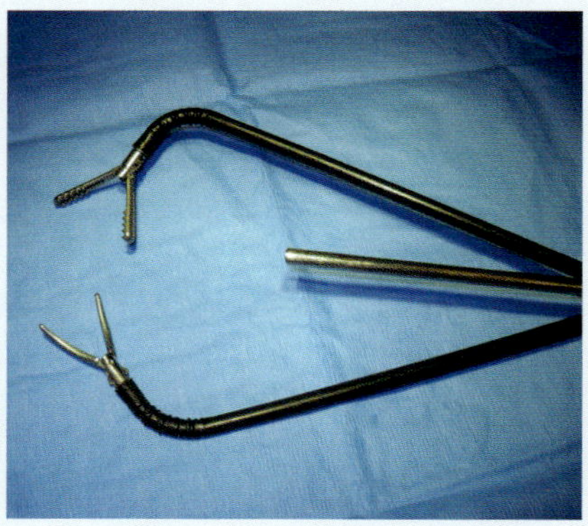

FIGURE 2. Right-angled or articulating Kelly forceps are used to dissect a plane cranial to the cystic duct to free the duct for ligation via a suture, vessel-sealing device, or clip application. The use of articulating Kelly instruments enables cystic duct dissection in a confined space.

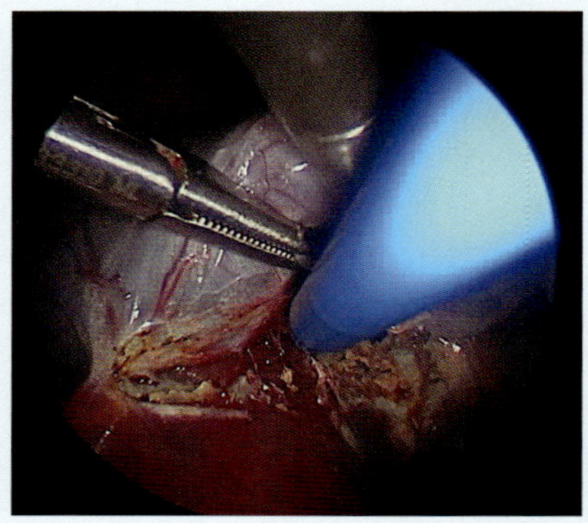

FIGURE 3. Use an extra 5 mm port to insert additional instruments or retractors if necessary. Surgeon frustration can be quickly extinguished by rapidly adding an extra 5 mm port to enable ergonomic dissection and elevation.

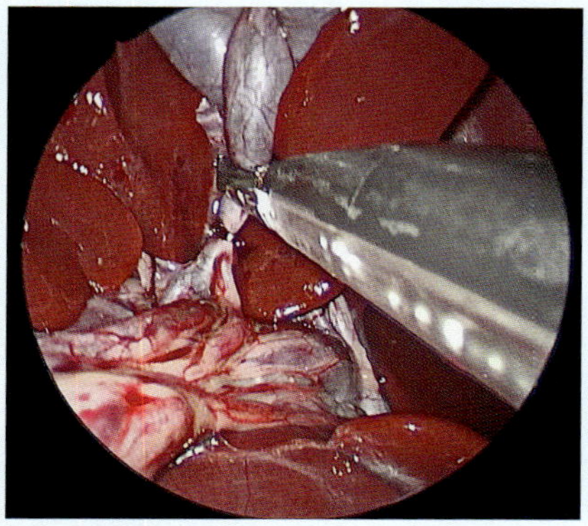

FIGURE 4. Cystic duct being clipped using a 10 mm clip applier.

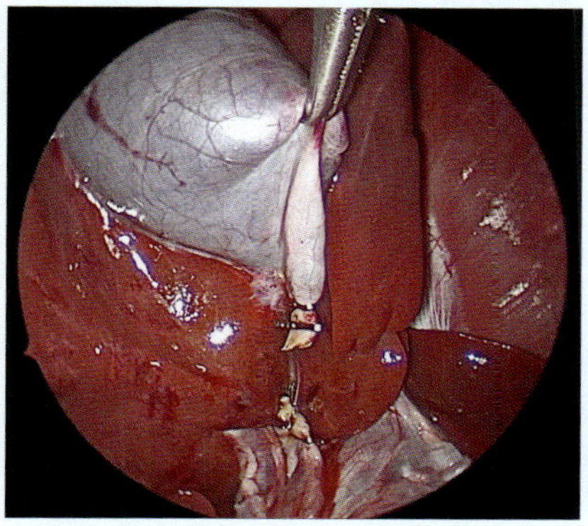

FIGURE 5. Image depicting transection of the cystic duct with elevation of the gallbladder to begin dissection and removal.

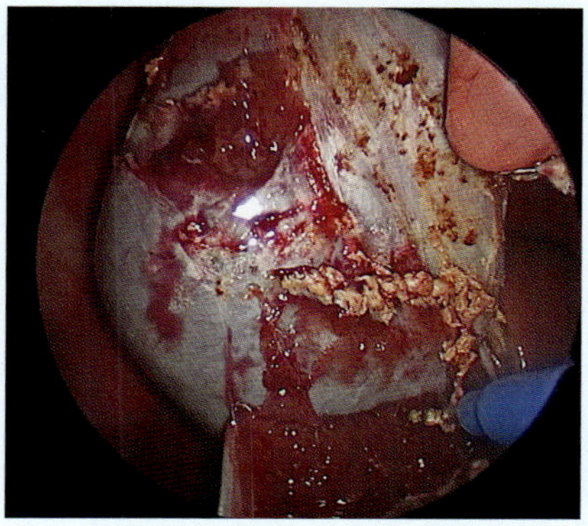

FIGURE 6. A vessel-sealing device or a combination of vessel-sealing and monopolar electrosurgery are recommended for dissection of the gallbladder from the fossa. Hook cautery is being used for gallbladder dissection.

Tips and tricks

- ✓ The use of a transabdominal stay suture is often needed to suspend the gallbladder to achieve this critical view properly. If this is not possible, an additional port is warranted for fan retraction and elevation of the gallbladder.
- ✓ The surgeon can use intracorporeal or laparoscopic extracorporeal suture techniques for suture application. If using an extracorporeal technique, right-angled forceps are used to pass a length of 2-0 to 3-0 absorbable monofilament (polydioxanone is recommended) through the cannula and into position on the duct. A second pair of right-angled forceps is passed around the duct and used to grasp the suture to bring it around the duct. The suture is then withdrawn through the same cannula, a laparoscopic slip knot is prepared extracorporeally, and then positioned on the duct using a knot pusher. Based on the current literature, a 4S-modified Roeder knot is recommended for slipknot application.
- ✓ Although not designed to seal nonvascular luminal structures, vessel-sealing devices have been evaluated for sealing the cystic duct in veterinary medicine. However, there is a concern for increased potential for failure, and caution is heavily advised in their use, particularly in cases where there is a concern for pathologic changes in the cystic ducts.
- ✓ Grasping of the gallbladder wall is discouraged out of concern for gallbladder friability. If the gallbladder is perforated, sealing the perforation via laparoscopic clips can be attempted, but conversion to an open approach is advised with any significant bile leakage.
- ✓ After gallbladder removal, the surgical site at the hepatic fossa should be carefully reevaluated to ensure appropriate hemostatic control and checked for evidence of ongoing biliary leakage. The surgical site can be liberally lavaged, and the fluid aspirated using a suction and irrigation device.

36.2 LAPAROSCOPIC CHOLECYSTECTOMY AND INTRAOPERATIVE BILE DUCT FLUSHING FOR EXTRAHEPATIC BILIARY OBSTRUCTION IN A DOG

Hiroo Kanai

CASE DESCRIPTION

An 11-year-old intact male Chihuahua weighing 3.1 kg was presented for vomiting and abdominal pain. The patient was transferred to the author's hospital because the medical treatment provided by a nearby doctor was ineffective. Extrahepatic biliary obstruction (EHBO) was diagnosed at the author's hospital based on an increase in the jaundice index, a marked increase in hepatic enzyme levels, and findings of gallbladder mucocele and peritonitis on ultrasonography. EHBO surgery was performed laparoscopically.

Key points

- The entire EHBO surgical procedure was performed laparoscopically.
- For diagnosis, intraoperative cholangiography (IOC) was utilized.
- There were significant adhesions of the diaphragm, gallbladder, and stomach.
- The cystic duct was closed via laparoscopic suturing.
- Mirizzi syndrome, already reported in human medicine, was suspected.

PORT PLACEMENT

A 10 mm trocar is placed 1–2 cm to the right of the umbilicus for a camera port (T1). Two additional ports (T2, T3) are placed in a triangulating pattern around the anticipated location of the gallbladder. A fourth port is placed on the right side at the mid-abdominal level (T4). An assistant will use this fourth port to elevate the liver cranially.

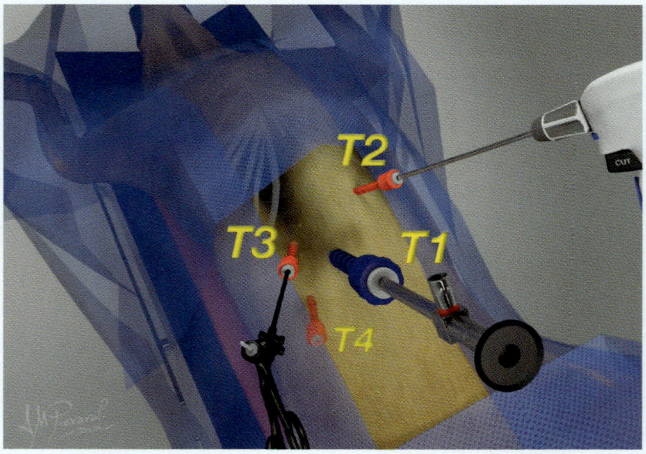

PROCEDURE

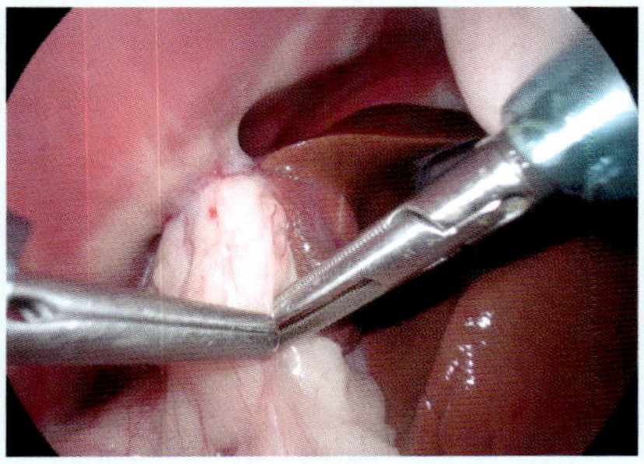

FIGURE 1. The diaphragm, gallbladder, and stomach are severely adhered. Careful detachment of the gallbladder and diaphragm, being careful not to puncture the diaphragm.

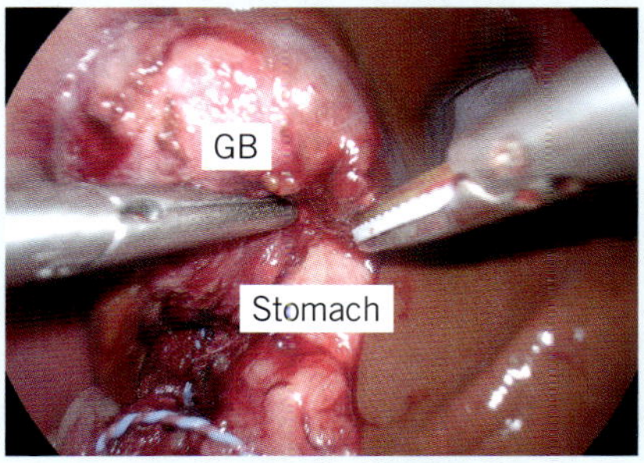

FIGURE 2. The gallbladder (GB) and the stomach are very tightly adhered. When severe adhesions exist around the bile duct, cystic duct dissection can be associated with a higher risk of iatrogenic injury to the hepatic duct, bile duct, cystic artery, and liver.

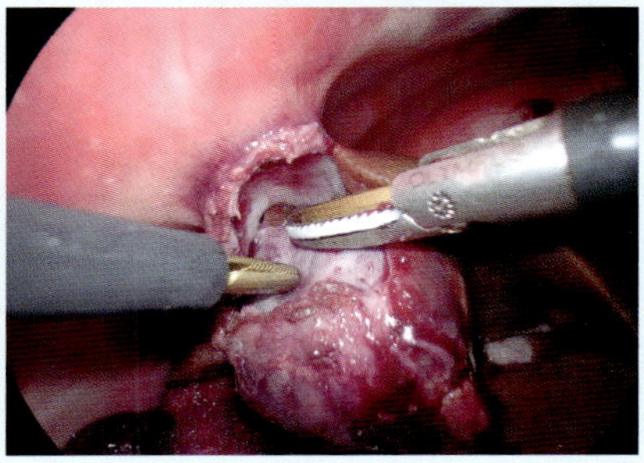

FIGURE 3. Dissection within the subserosal layer of the gallbladder from the gallbladder fundus to the cystic duct prior to cystic duct transection, fundic dissection first (FDF) technique (SAMIT method), is performed. This picture shows the view of the serosal surface of the gallbladder.

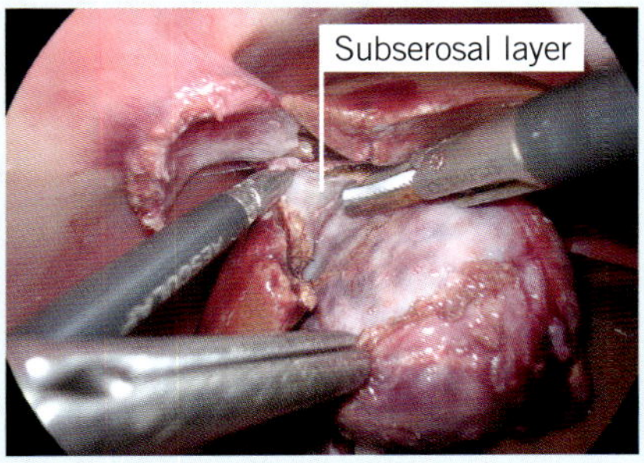

FIGURE 4. A small incision is made in the gallbladder serosa using laparoscopic Metzenbaum scissors. Retraction of the gallbladder serosa by a surgical assistant using forceps in entering within the subserosal layers of the gallbladder.

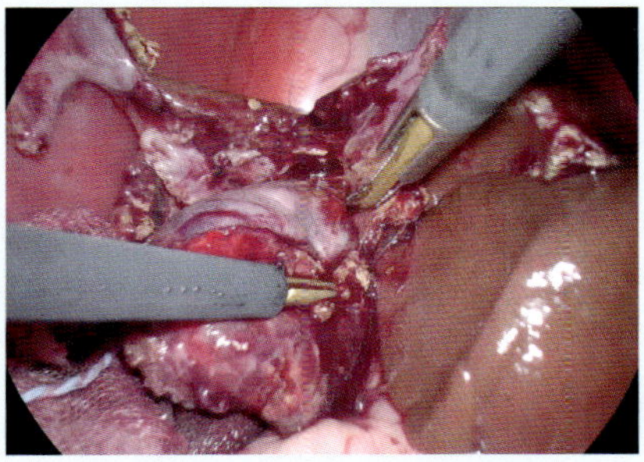

FIGURE 5. While counter traction is applied, dissect within the subserosal layer of the gallbladder from the gallbladder fundus to the cystic duct, then isolate the gallbladder from the liver using an ultrasonic coagulation cutting device. It is important to stay within the subserosal layers.

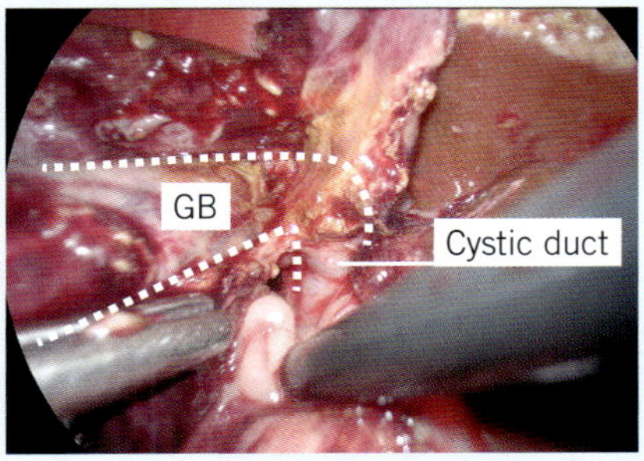

FIGURE 6. Careful dissection is continued, and the cystic duct is visualized. By using the FDF method, the cystic duct can be separated without damaging the liver, hepatic duct, and common bile duct.

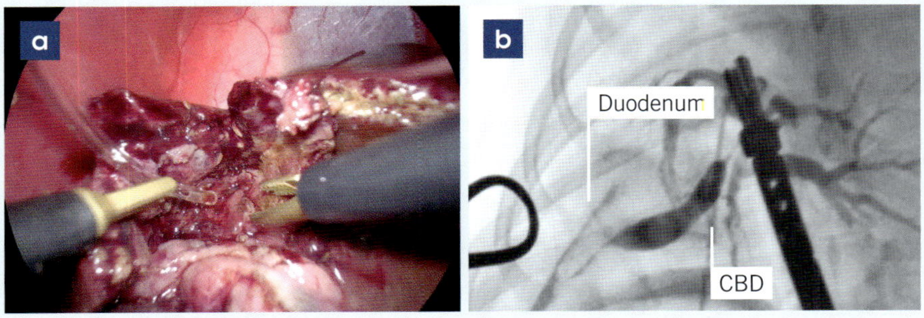

FIGURE 7. a) After cutting the cystic duct, a catheter is inserted from the stump to perform intraoperative cholangiography. b) IOC findings, with no obstruction in the common bile duct (CBD). The cause of jaundice was thought to be adhesions around the cystic duct and common bile duct. This is called Mirizzi's syndrome in human medicine.

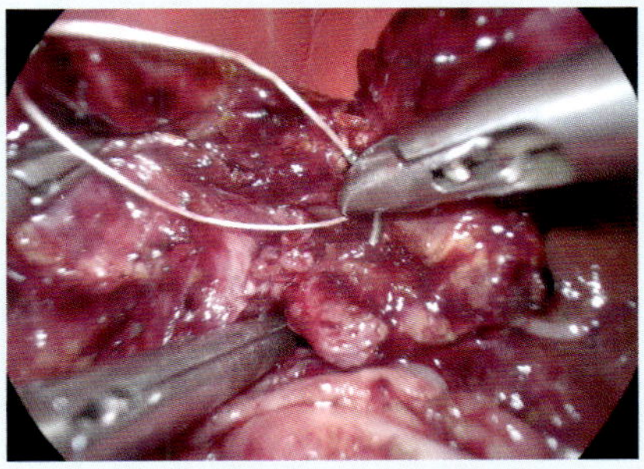

FIGURE 8. The distance from the stump of the cystic duct to the common bile duct is short, so the cystic duct cannot be ligated. Therefore, the cystic duct stump is closed with three simple sutures.

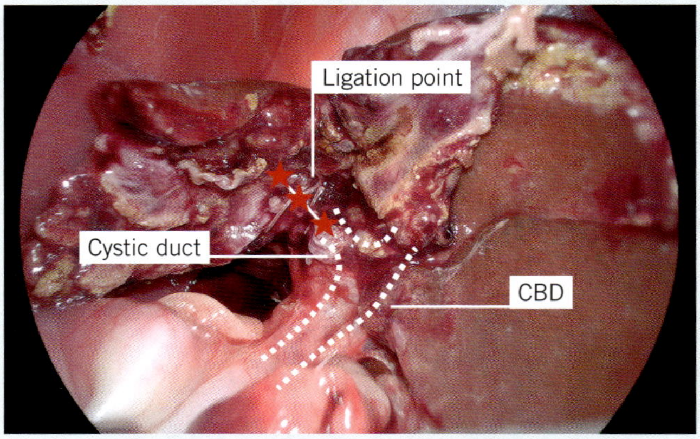

FIGURE 9. This photo shows the anatomy around the cystic duct and common bile duct at the end of surgery. By using the FDF method, EHBO cases could be safely treated without damaging important structures such as the common bile duct and hepatic duct and without bleeding from the liver. This case was discharged 4 days after surgery.

36.3 CHOLECYSTECTOMY AND BILE DUCT FLUSHING

Ikuya Ehara

CASE DESCRIPTION

A 12-year-old neutered female Schnauzer weighing 6.3 kg was presented with loss of appetite and inactivity. Gallbladder mucocele and biliary obstruction were suspected based on liver enzyme elevations and bile stasis findings. The patient underwent laparoscopic cholecystectomy and flushing of the bile duct.

Key points

- One intraoperative complication to be aware of when performing laparoscopic cholecystectomy for gallbladder disease in dogs is injury to the hepatic veins coursing within the liver parenchyma on either side of the gallbladder neck.
- To avoid intraoperative complications, it is important not to stray from the subserosal layer when dissecting out the gallbladder.
- Attention must be paid not to traumatize the hepatic duct of the right medial liver lobe, particularly if there is dilation of the cystic duct and gallbladder neck, which increases the risk of accidentally dissecting the bile duct downstream on the common bile duct side rather than the cystic duct side from its connection with the right medial lobar hepatic duct. Also, the surgeon must be aware that there is a tendency to neglect proper identification of this hepatic duct when there is severe inflammation of the gallbladder rendering its dissection plane to enter the liver parenchyma.
- It is important to be cognizant of the specific location the surgeon is at while dissecting around the gallbladder and the bile duct, even with the use of the dome-down technique.

PORT PLACEMENT

With the patient in true dorsal recumbency, four ports consisting of two to the right (T1, T3) and one in the left abdomen (T2), and one caudal to the xiphoid process (T4) were established. Avoid placing the telescope caudal to the umbilicus if using a telescope with a 30° visual angle.

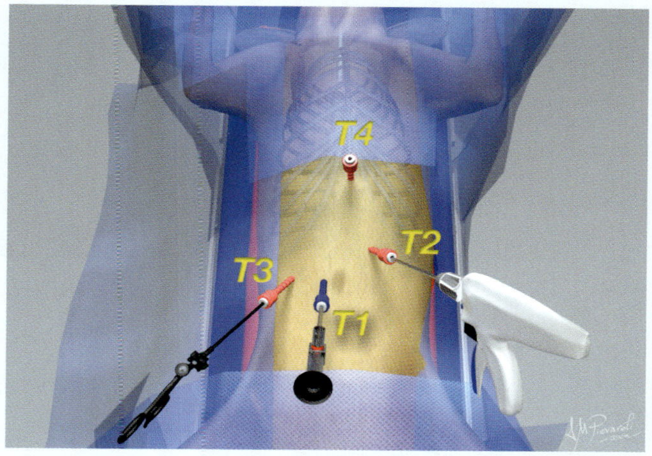

PROCEDURE

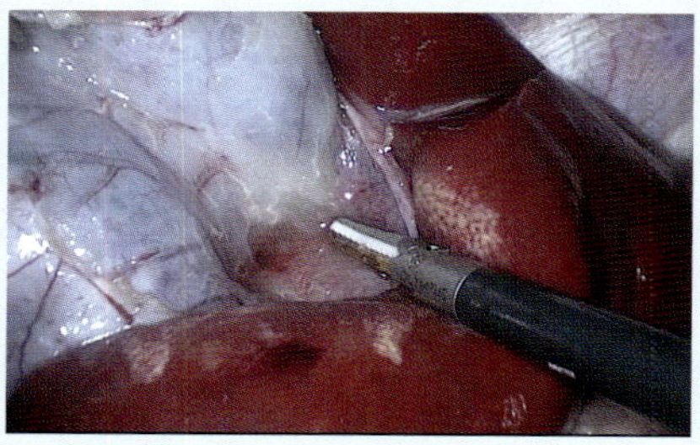

FIGURE 1. The gallbladder is dissected beneath the serosa after creating a small incision with scissors in the serosa. Subserosal dissection can be difficult depending upon the degree of subserosal fibrosis that results from inflammation.

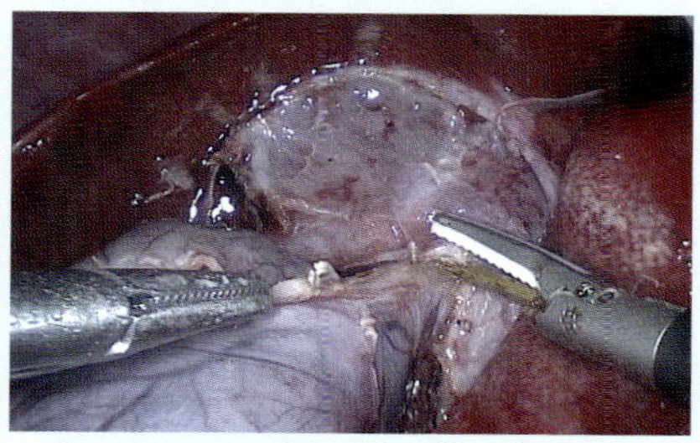

FIGURE 2. After gallbladder dissection, the gallbladder neck and the cystic duct are dissected near the point of right medial lobe hepatic duct entry using monopolar electrocautery, ultrasonic coagulation, and a cutting device.

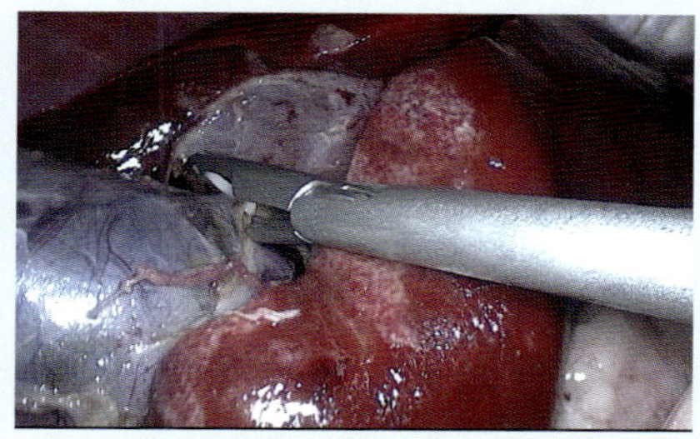

FIGURE 3. For cystic duct transection, the gallbladder side of the cystic duct is closed with a hemoclip (5 mm Hem-o-lok, MK) to prevent leakage from the gallbladder content.

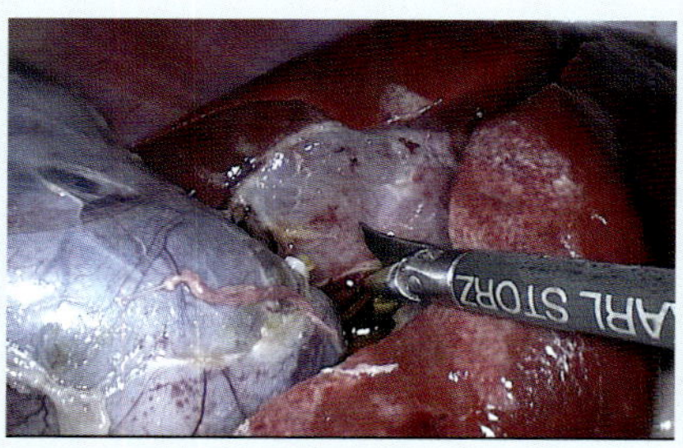

FIGURE 4. The common bile duct side of the cystic duct is transected with scissors after clipping. Care should be taken to avoid hemorrhage from the cystic duct and artery.

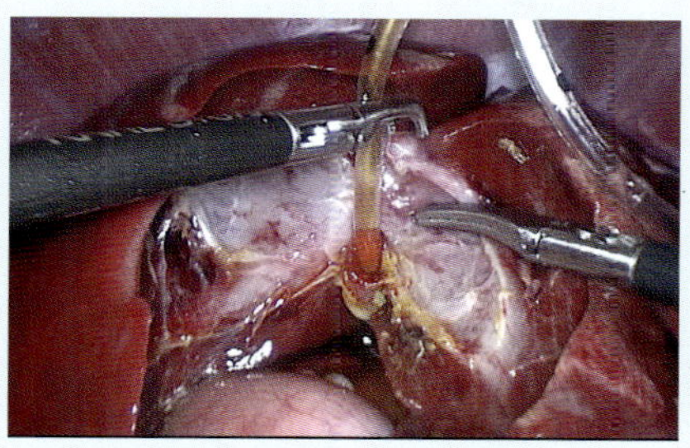

FIGURE 5. A silastic catheter (7 Fr) is inserted into the cystic duct for biliary tract flushing.

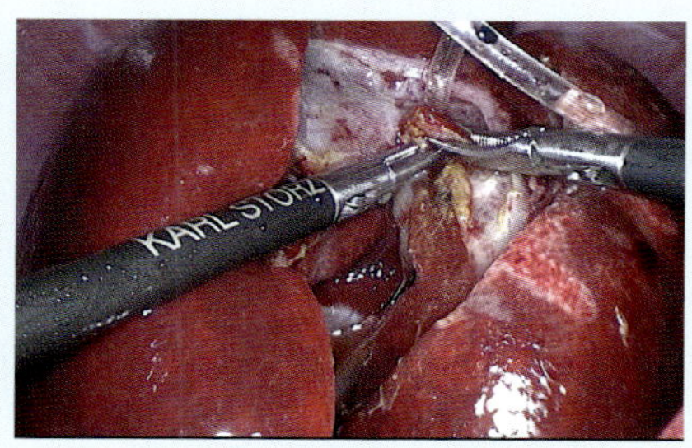

FIGURE 6. Maryland right-angle forceps are placed perpendicular to the cystic duct to prevent leakage of saline during bile duct flushing.

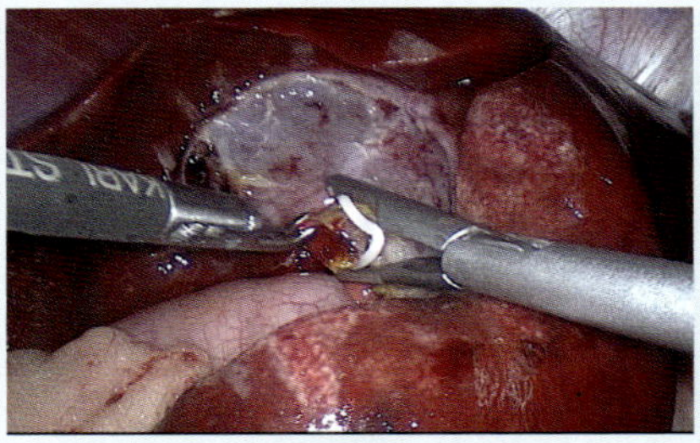

FIGURE 7. The common bile duct side of the cystic duct is closed with hemoclips (5 mm Hem-o-lok, MK) after bile duct flushing.

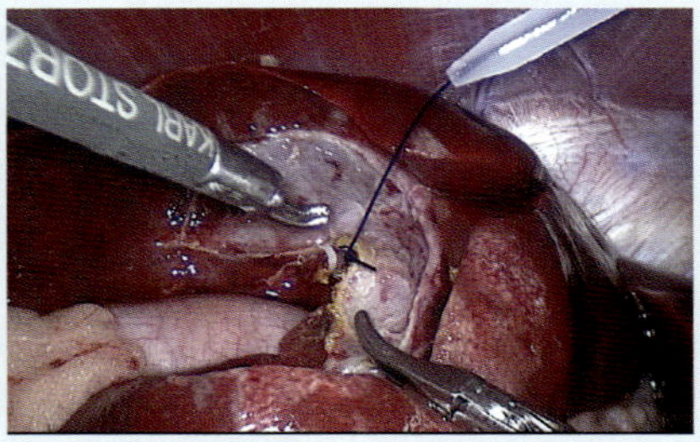

FIGURE 8. A ligating loop (2-0 PDS Endoloop Ligature, Johnson & Johnson) is placed around the cystic duct to secure its closure.

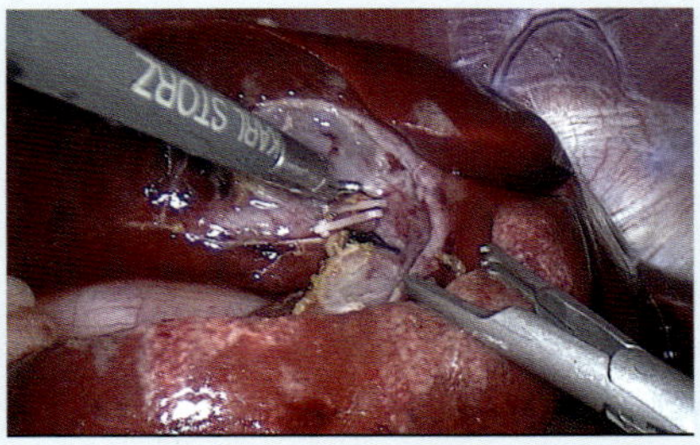

FIGURE 9. Completed cystic duct closure.

Tips and tricks

- ✓ Approach under dorsal recumbency.
- ✓ Dome down technique.
- ✓ Subserosal dissection of the gallbladder.
- ✓ Take care to avoid traumatizing the hepatic vein.
- ✓ Be careful to avoid traumatizing the hepatic duct of the right medial liver lobe.

36.4 LAPAROSCOPIC CHOLECYSTECTOMY IN A DOG USING THE SUBSEROSAL LAYER DISSECTION TECHNIQUE

Motoki Kondo

CASE DESCRIPTION

The patient was a 9-year-old spayed female toy Poodle with a body weight of 2.7 kg. A health examination conducted a few years ago revealed biliary sludging. The liver enzymes appeared elevated 1 year ago, and the animal experienced recurrent vomiting and diarrhea thereafter. Ultrasonography revealed a suspected gallbladder mucocele for half a year. Laparoscopic cholecystectomy was performed because the biliary sludge and gallbladder mucus increased and was refractory to pharmacotherapy.

Key points

- Secure the cystic duct.
- Handle penetrating vessels between the gallbladder serosa and wall appropriately to minimize bleeding.
- Be aware that the subserosa is the appropriate dissectible layer and maintain it during dissection.

PORT PLACEMENT

A 10 mm trocar was placed on the right side of the umbilicus as the camera port (T1). The operator's right-hand port (10 mm) was placed at the left subcostal margin, one-third lateral to the midline (T2). The operator's left-hand port (5 mm) was placed at the right subcostal margin, two-thirds lateral to the midline (T3). An assistant port (5 mm) was placed on the outer caudal side of the operator's left-hand port (T4).

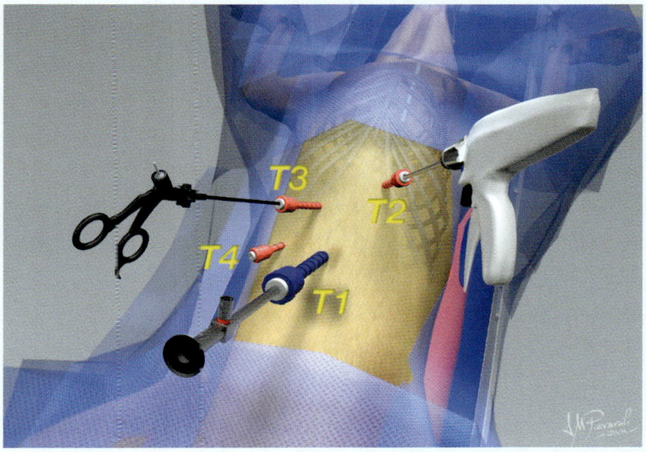

PROCEDURE

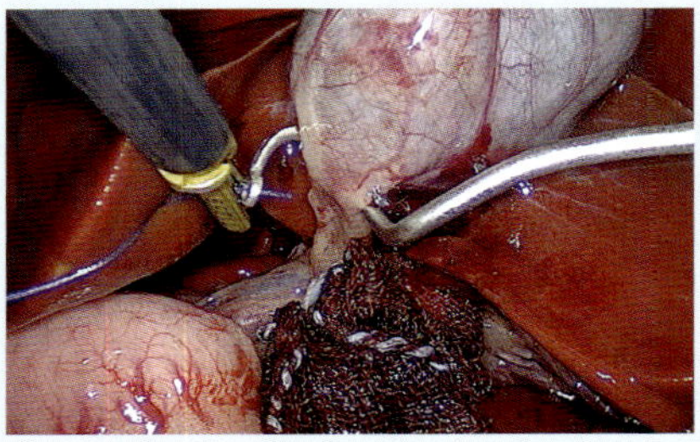

FIGURE 1. Prior to gallbladder dissection, the original threader for endoscopic surgery is rotated around the cystic duct, and a 3-0 Vicryl suture thread, which will be used as a tourniquet, is passed through the ring at the tip.

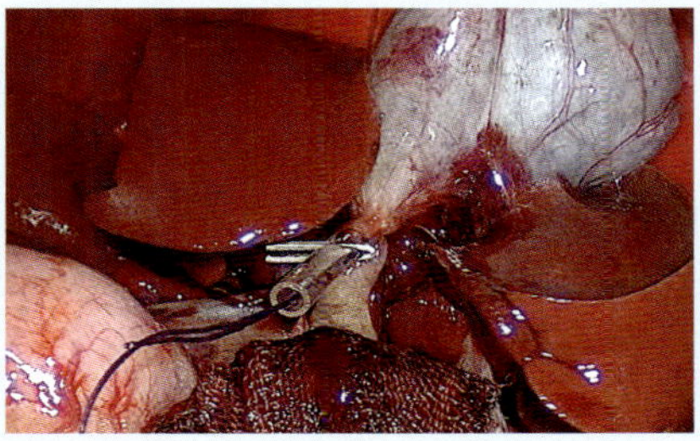

FIGURE 2. The threader is pulled out, and the 3-0 Vicryl suture thread is looped around the cystic duct. The 3-0 Vicryl is tightened with a 7-0 feeding tube cut to 1.5 cm to act as a tourniquet and stop blood flow in the gallbladder artery.

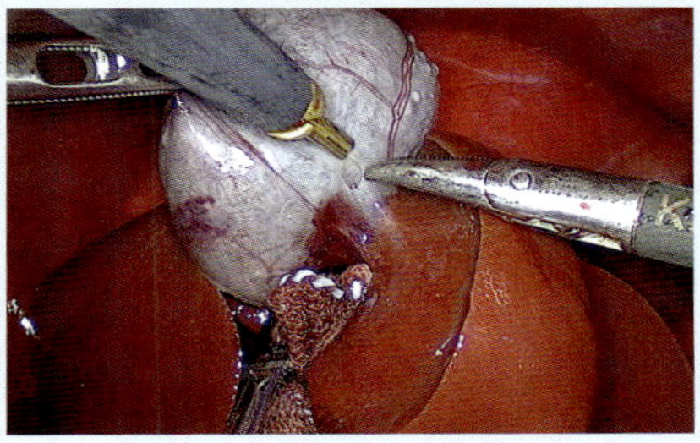

FIGURE 3. The gallbladder serosa is incised with scissors at the 4 o'clock position to expose the subserosal layer of the gallbladder.

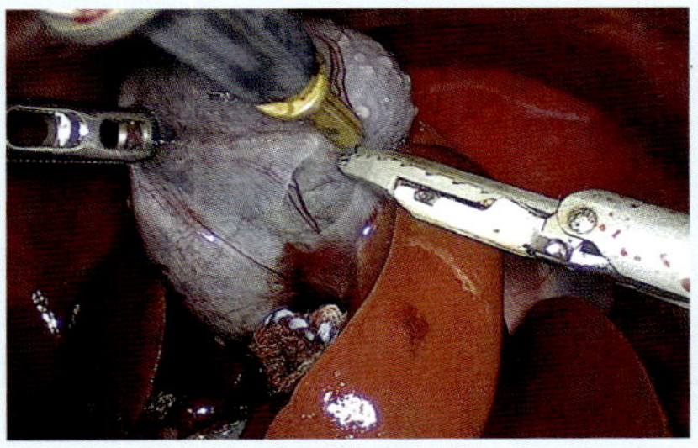

FIGURE 4. The serosal incision is extended circumferentially along the gallbladder–liver attachment using right-angle dissection forceps or an ultrasonic coagulation incision device (Thunderbeat, Olympus).

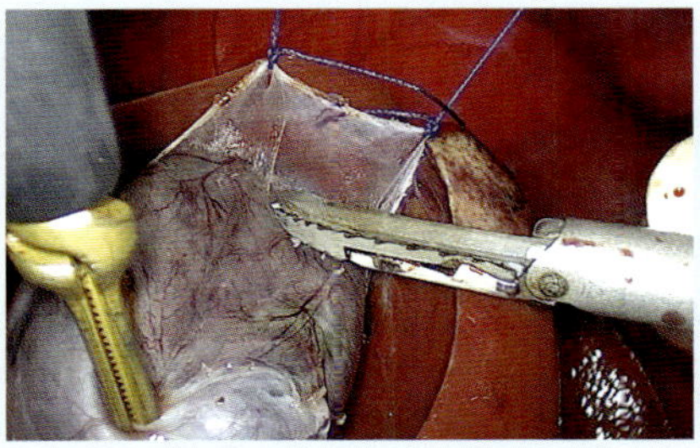

FIGURE 5. At 12 and 2 o'clock positions, sutures are hung on the serosa of the gallbladder and pulled out of the body to be pulled and fixed (marionette method). This provides proper traction to the gallbladder serosa and facilitates the dissection of the subserosal layer. The operator pulls the gallbladder serosa caudally using left-handed Debakey forceps, and the subserosal layer of the gallbladder, which is under traction, is bluntly peeled off using right-handed forceps. If it is the appropriate layer, it can be dissected without resistance.

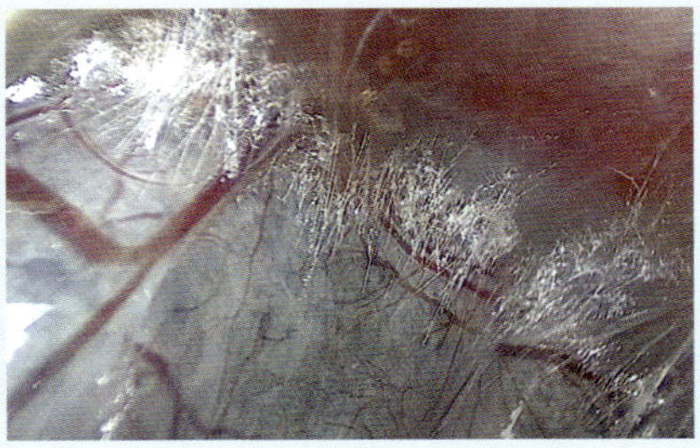

FIGURE 6. Close-up photograph of the appropriate dissectible layer. By maintaining this appropriate dissectible layer (subserosal layer) and carefully treating the blood vessels penetrating from the gallbladder serosa to the gallbladder wall, the gallbladder can be dissected from the serosa with almost no bleeding.

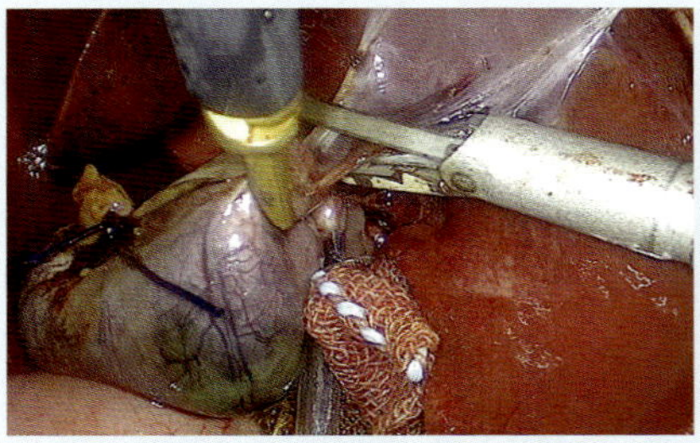

FIGURE 7. After peeling off the subserosal layer up to the cystic duct, the tourniquet is removed and the gallbladder serosa is finally dissected between the subserosal layer and the tourniquet installation layer (the entire gallbladder layer), connecting the two layers.

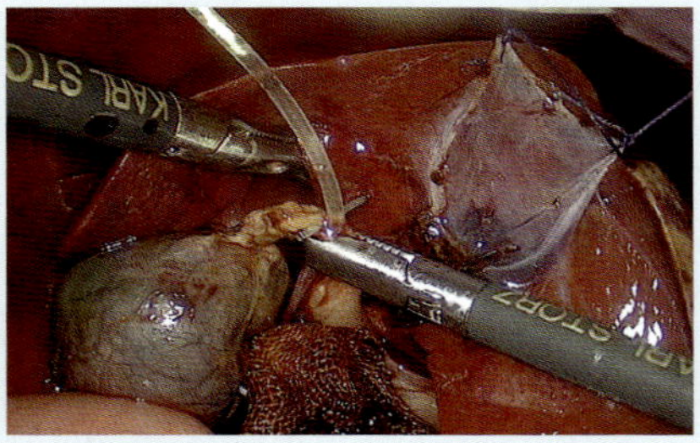

FIGURE 8. After making a small incision in the cystic duct, a 6 Fr feeding tube is inserted and the common bile duct is flushed with saline. It is ensured that there are no residual debris in the common bile duct by checking that the flushing solution flows smoothly.

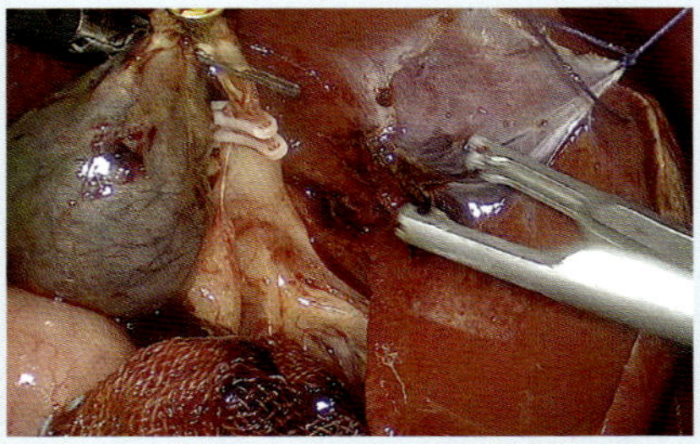

FIGURE 9. Finally, a polymer clip (Hem-o-lok) is double-attached to the cystic duct, and the gallbladder is excised. The excised gallbladder is placed in a collection bag and removed from the body.

Tips and tricks

✓ Appropriate counter traction for blunt dissection.
✓ Avoid bleeding as much as possible.
✓ Look closely at the dissectible layer.
✓ Open the dissected surface three-dimensionally.

36.5 CHOLECYSTECTOMY

David García Rubio

CASE DESCRIPTION

The patient was an 11-year-old Miniature Schnauzer with a history of vomiting, cranial abdominal pain, and increased liver enzymes in blood analyses. An abdominal ultrasound scan showed an extremely enlarged gallbladder with hyperechoic content compatible with gallstones and increased wall thickness. A decision was made to perform a laparoscopic cholecystectomy.

Key points

- The gallbladder is closely attached to the quadrate lobe of the liver and the right lateral lobe, and its arterial supply comes through the cystic artery, which runs alongside the cystic duct in dogs.
- The cystic duct must be tied before it is joined to the hepatic ducts, and care must always be taken to ensure there are no posthepatic obstructions.
- The liver bed may suffer capillary bleeding. Attempt to dissect the peritoneum, rather than wrenching the gallbladder from the bed, although this is sometimes impossible in smaller patients.
- Dissection is simpler if the cystic duct and artery are tied and cut first and, using the stump as a support, dissection is made from proximal to distal.

PORT PLACEMENT

Patient in dorsal decubitus position and anti-Trendelenburg position. The first optical trocar is placed in the mid-infraumbilical position (T1) with two lateral ports for instrumentation (T2, T3). A fourth trocar (T4) may be used to support the vesicle in the right paraxifoid position.

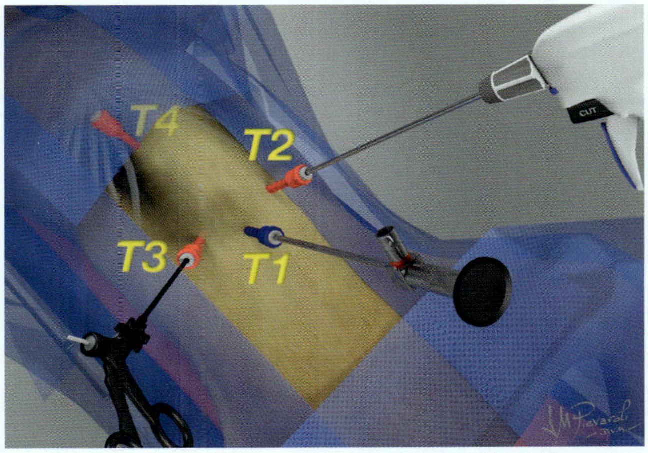

PROCEDURE

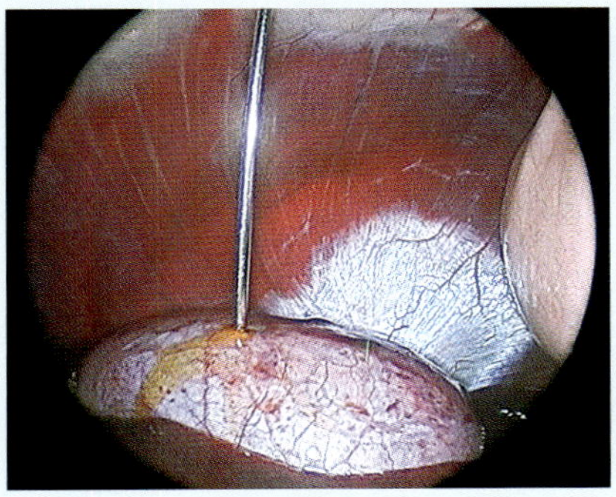

FIGURE 1. Drainage of the content from the gallbladder using a Veress needle.

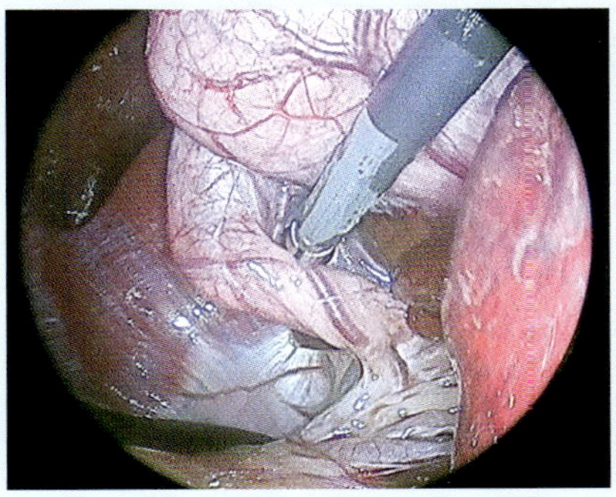

FIGURE 2. Detailed view of the cystic duct with the cystic artery close beside it and dissection of the peritoneum around.

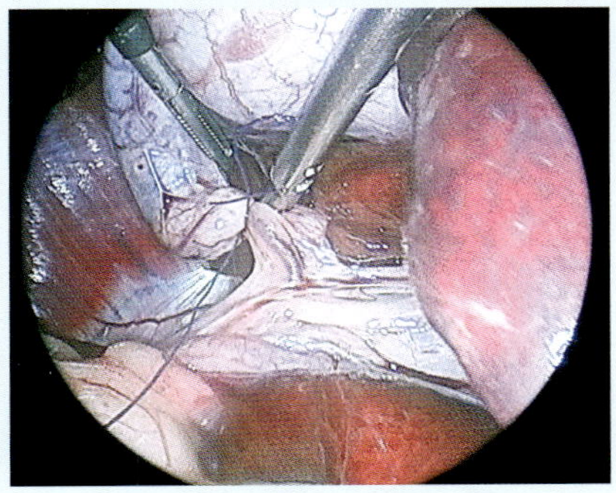

FIGURE 3. In this case, and given the dilation of the cystic duct, ligatures are used for the initial closure, which is then reinforced with hemoclips.

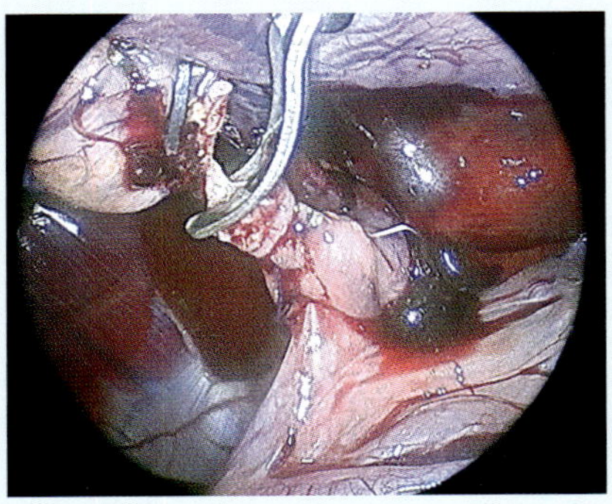

FIGURE 4. Cutting of the cystic duct and artery once both ends have been tied with two sutures/hemoclips.

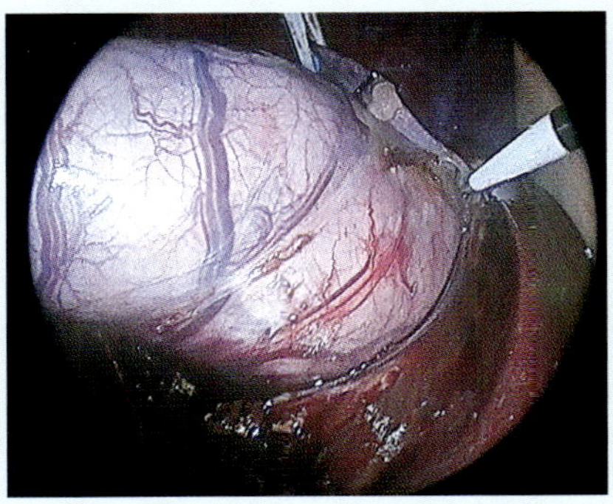

FIGURE 5. Dissection of the gallbladder peritoneum and quadrate lobe of the liver with the help of a monopolar L-hook.

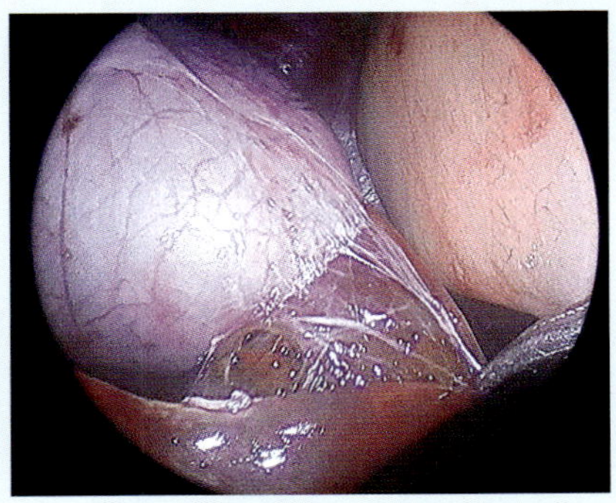

FIGURE 6. Some areas are more easily separated using blunt dissection. Continue until the entire gallbladder is free from liver tissue, fully dissecting the quadrate and right lateral lobes of the liver.

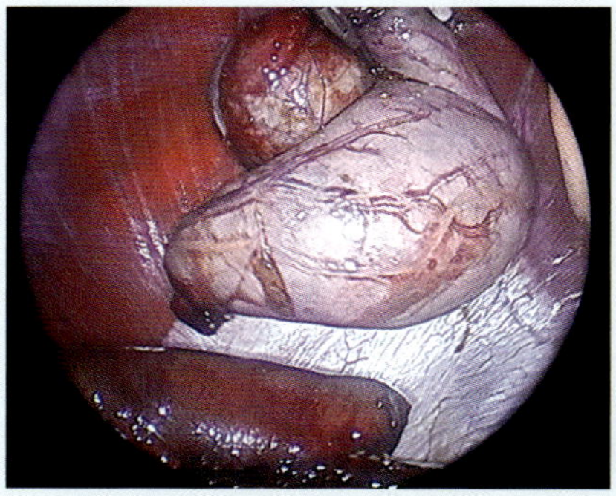

FIGURE 7. Complete separation of the gland for its extraction via collection bag.

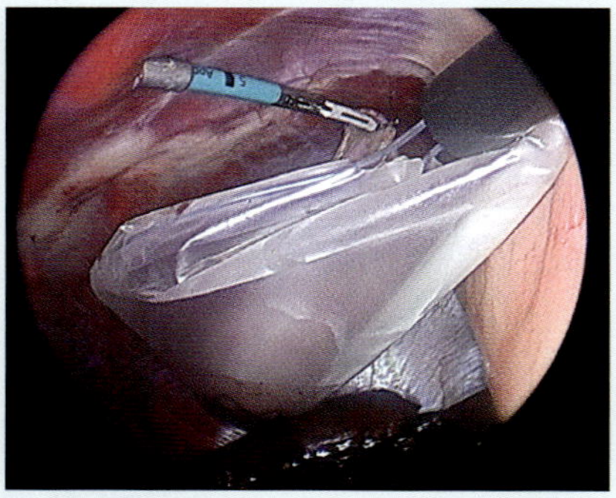

FIGURE 8. Final appearance of the surgical area and check for absence of bleeding.

Tips and tricks

- ✓ Resecting the falciform ligament at the start of surgery is recommended to improve viewing.
- ✓ Emptying very strained and extremely full gallbladders will help clamp and minimize the risk of the same tearing during handling, but it may cause the content from the gallbladder to escape to the exterior.
- ✓ Be prepared for the possible existence of aberrant bile ducts that drain on different levels from the gallbladder.
- ✓ Threading and pulling a suture from the outside, surrounding the cystic duct, may help subsequent placement of the hemoclips.

36.6 CHOLECYSTECTOMY BY THREE-PORT ACCESS AND "COLD" DISSECTION

Maurício Veloso Brun

CASE DESCRIPTION

Cholecystectomy is indicated for patients with cholelithiasis, biliary mucocele, and biliary mud with no response to clinical treatment. After adequate clinical stabilization, the author has routinely performed it by three-port access, without any source of ultrasonic or thermal energy in most cases. This way, the risk of thermal injury is exempted, and liver damage is reduced. As the patient has chronic liver disease routinely, reduced capnoperitoneum is recommended (6 mmHg for dogs; 4 mmHg for cats).

Key points

- For pure cholecystectomy, preoperative imaging studies should demonstrate no occlusion of the duodenal papilla and biliary tree.
- The patient is placed in dorsal recumbency. Depending on the gallbladder size and the amount of fat in the falciform ligament, brief lateralization of the patient to the left will facilitate gallbladder exposure.
- Generally, it is not necessary to use the reversed Trendelenburg position. However, in some cases, this position can facilitate gallbladder exposure.
- Occlusion of the cystic duct will usually involve the hemostasis of the artery and vein together. In some patients, cystic vessels are located only after the cystic duct dissection.
- The scope will be positioned in the lateral port, and the gallbladder will be removed together with the first port at the midline.
- The first port is repositioned, and multiple liver biopsies are performed.

PORT PLACEMENT

The first trocar (T1, 10 mm) is placed on the ventral midline. In females, the port is placed at the midpoint of the distance between the umbilical scar and the edge of the pubis. In males, it is placed in a corresponding position, respecting the limits imposed by the edge of the foreskin. The second port (T2, 5 or 10 mm) is placed next to the surgeon's dominant hand in triangulation with the first and third trocars (T3, 5 mm). Alternatively, the second port can be placed on the ventral midline when working with patients with abundant falciform fat. For this, keeping the animal in dorsal recumbency will be necessary, slightly oblique to the left.

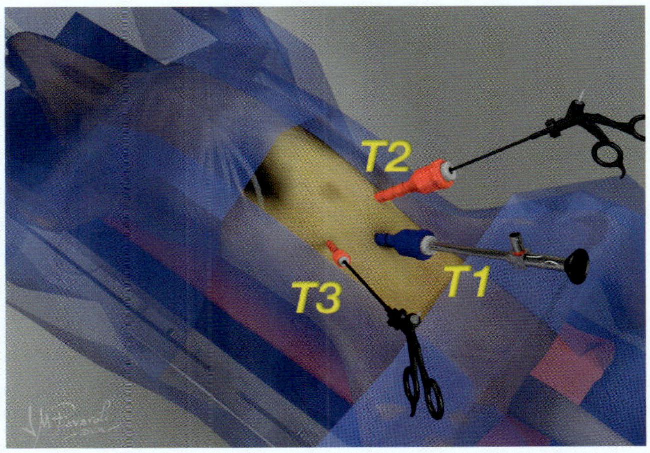

PROCEDURE

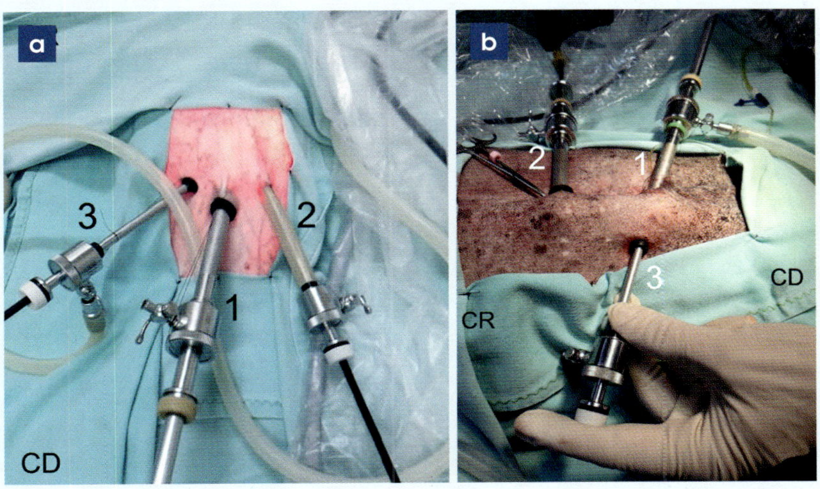

FIGURE 1. a) Placement of the three ports for cholecystectomy. b) Alternatively, in patients with abundant falciform fat, the second portal can be placed on the ventral midline. CD, caudal; CR, cranial.

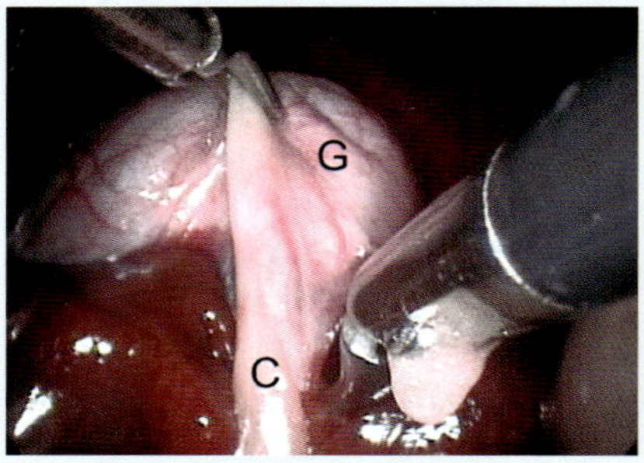

FIGURE 2. With the nondominant hand, the gallbladder neck is pulled with Kelly forceps near the cystic duct. With the dominant hand, the cystic duct is dissected with Kelly, Maryland, and Mixter forceps. Exposure of the cystic duct (C) by apprehension and traction of the gallbladder neck (G) with the nondominant hand.

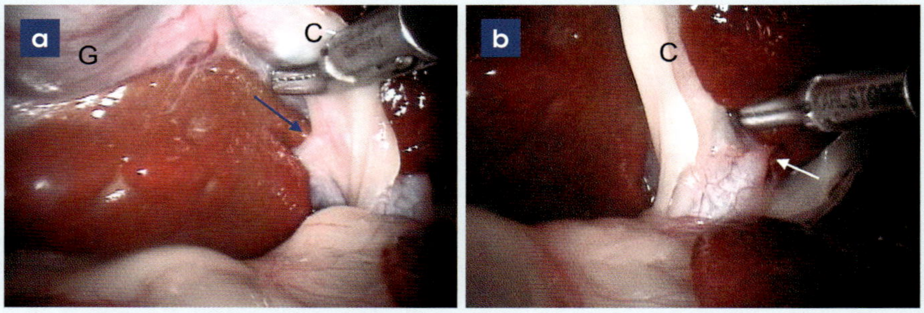

FIGURE 3. Assessment of the gallbladder (G) and biliary tree, defining the safe distance for dissection of the cystic duct (C). The arrows show hepatic ducts close to the cystic duct that drains into the choledochal.

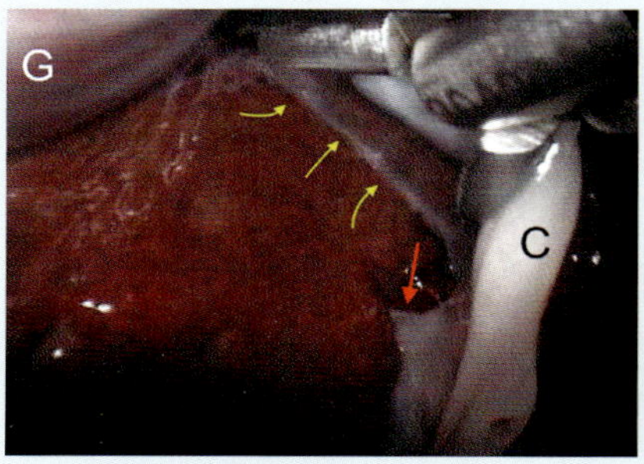

FIGURE 4. Dissection of the cystic duct (C) from lateral to medial on the right side of the gallbladder. Note the adequate dissection plane between the peritoneum layers that cover the cystic duct and the hepatic bed (yellow arrows). The red arrow shows a hepatic duct signaling the distal limit of the dissection.

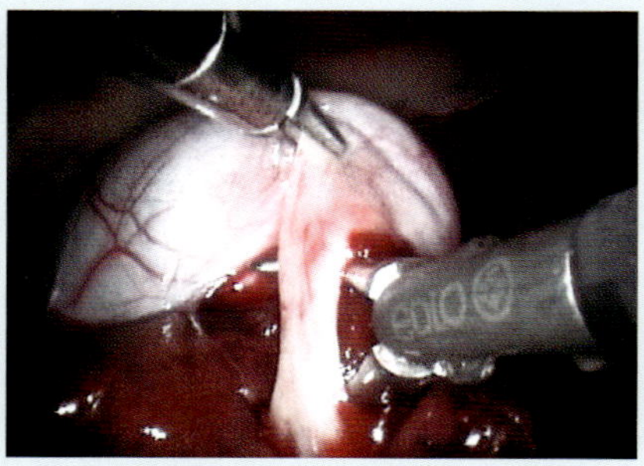

FIGURE 5. Dissection continues behind the cystic duct, from left to right, until the adequate length is obtained for the application of the hemostatic clips.

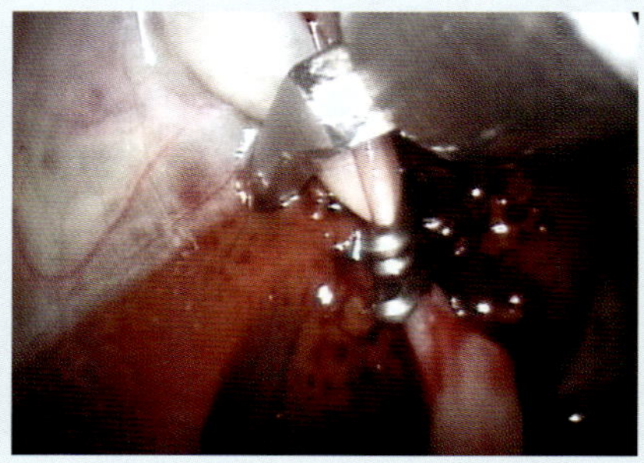

FIGURE 6. Application of hemostatic clips in the cystic duct, proximally and distally to the gallbladder. The cystic duct is clipped, keeping a distance of about 5–10 mm between the last clip of the stump and the first clip that will be removed with the gallbladder.

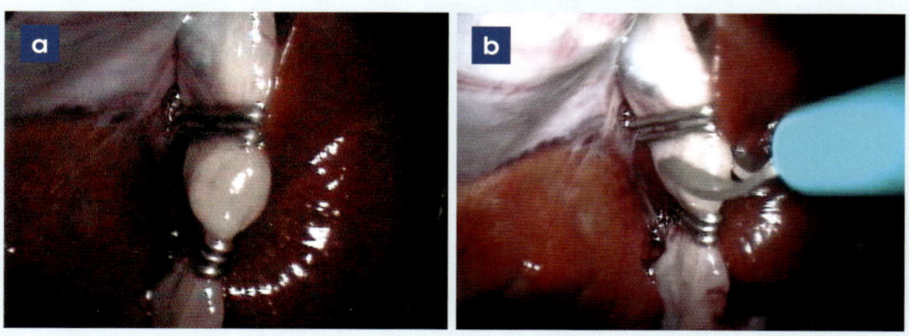

FIGURE 7. a) Adequate distribution of the proximal and distal clips in the cystic duct. b) “Cold” section between the clips with Metzenbaum scissors.

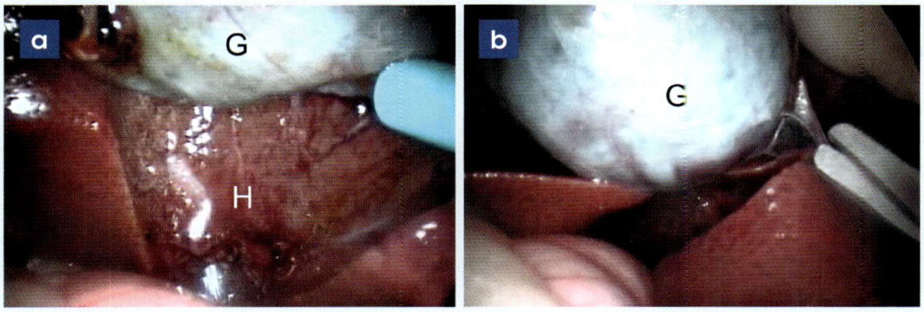

FIGURE 8. a) The correct dissection plane is found between the layers of peritoneum covering the hepatic bed (H) and gallbladder (G). b) Dissection is performed coldly with Metzenbaum scissors, also used to release the gallbladder from the edges of the liver.

Tips and tricks

- ✓ A careful laparoscopic assessment of the biliary tree, cystic duct, and choledochal are necessary before the cystic dissection begins. The limits for applying the clips will be defined before isolating the cystic duct and cystic vessels.
- ✓ If the gallbladder is very full of bile, a video-guided transparietal cholecystocentesis with a fine needle (spinal needle or 20-gauge catheter) is indicated, followed by its partial drainage and occlusion of the puncture site with clips.
- ✓ Dissecting the cystic duct close to the liver is facilitated with a Mixter forceps. The cystic duct dissection should be performed superficially to the liver, reducing bleeding.
- ✓ When using titanium clips, at least three clips on the remaining stump and two clips close to the gallbladder neck are indicated. When using self-blocking polyamide clips, two clips can be used close to the stump and one clip close to the neck.
- ✓ The ideal bladder dissection plane (between the layers of peritoneum of the gallbladder and the liver surface) will generally allow much easier dissection with minimal bleeding.
- ✓ The dissection will be carried out uniformly along the contact surface between the gallbladder and the liver. The vesicle fixation tissue close to the hepatic border will be sectioned with Metzenbaum scissors without electric energy.
- ✓ When the gallbladder is attached by little tissue close to its apex, the final inspection of the hepatic bed will be performed. When the gallbladder is completely released, the hepatic lobes cover this area.
- ✓ The scope is passed to the lateral port to show the gallbladder removal by the ventral midline access. This reduces the inflammatory response seen when the gallbladder is removed through the lateral muscle wound.
- ✓ To avoid extending the middle line access wound, a short segment of the gallbladder neck is externalized. In the gallbladder-exposed segment, the plastic component of the 16-gauge catheter will be introduced to aspirate bile, reducing its volume.

36.7 CHOLECYSTECTOMY IN A DOG

F. J. Pérez Duarte, J. Gutiérrez del Sol, M. A. Sánchez Hurtado

CASE DESCRIPTION

A 7-year-old, 4 kg Miniature Schnauzer dog was presented at the hospital for chronic onset of vomiting, anorexia, and inappetence. A serum biochemical profile showed mild elevations of ALT, ALP, and GGT. Abdominal ultrasonography revealed ultrasonographic evidence of gallbladder mucocele with hyperechoic and organized bile sediment and kiwifruit pattern, with no distended bile ducts. Laparoscopic cholecystectomy was performed as surgical treatment. No complications were noted during the procedure. The animal had minimal postoperative morbidity, and clinical signs improved.

Key points

- Careful patient selection is the key to achieving the best results, discarding animals with signs of bile duct obstruction, overdilated gallbladders, or when biliary perforation is suspected.
- Coagulation tests should always be performed before surgery.
- If there is no clear suspicion of biliary obstruction, the common bile duct should not be catheterized.

PORT PLACEMENT

The first 10 mm port, for telescope, is established in the umbilical area (T1). Lateral and triangulating with this first trocar, two other 5 mm ports are placed (T2, T3). In this way, an optimal working angle between the gallbladder and the instruments is achieved. Finally, a fourth 5 mm trocar is introduced in the left subcostal region to use a retractor or atraumatic grasping forceps to keep the gallbladder suspended (T4).

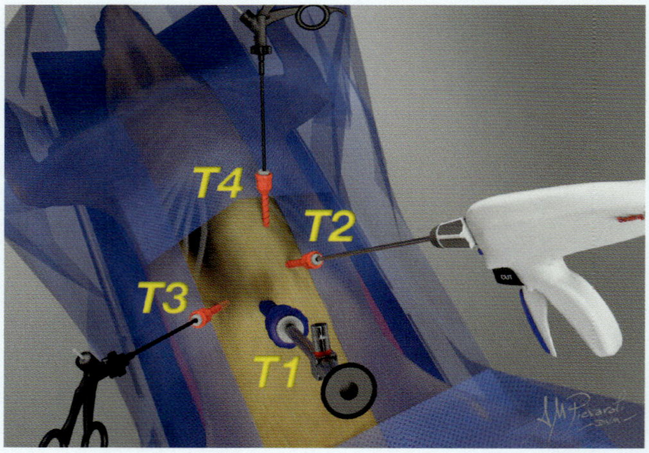

PROCEDURE

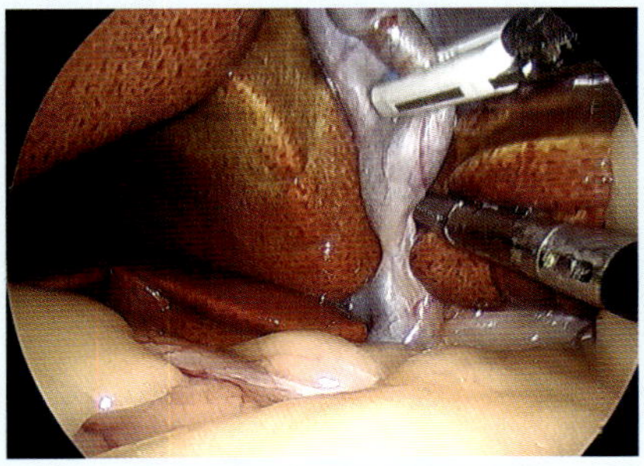

FIGURE 1. Upon entering the peritoneal cavity, the surgery begins with exploring the abdominal cavity and the exposure of the gallbladder and bile ducts.

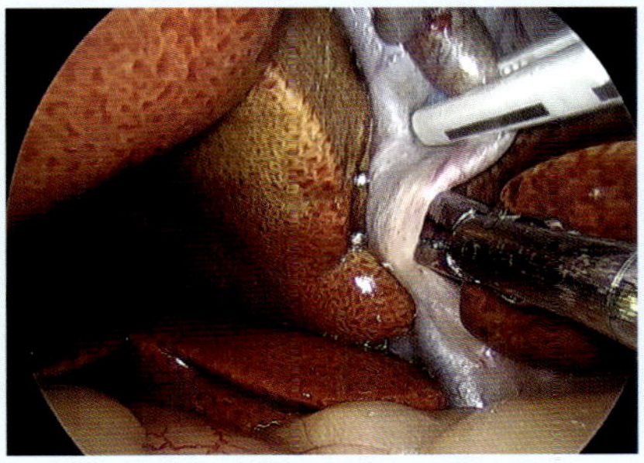

FIGURE 2. The cystic duct is dissected using a coagulation hook and a right-angle dissector, freeing it from its posterior adhesions to the liver.

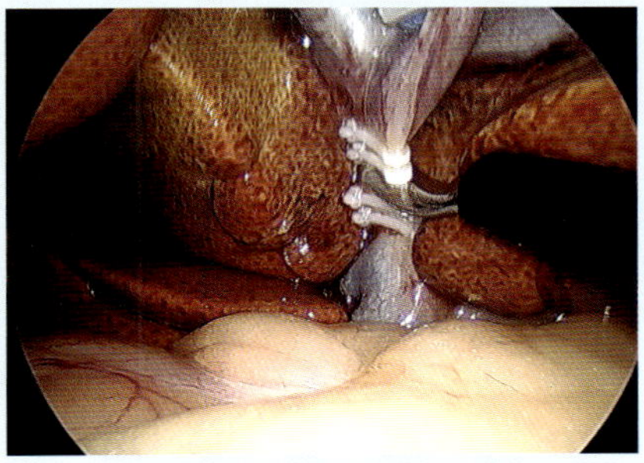

FIGURE 3. Occlusion of the duct is carried out using polymer ligation clips, placing at least two clips in the most proximal portion of the duct and another one in the distal portion.

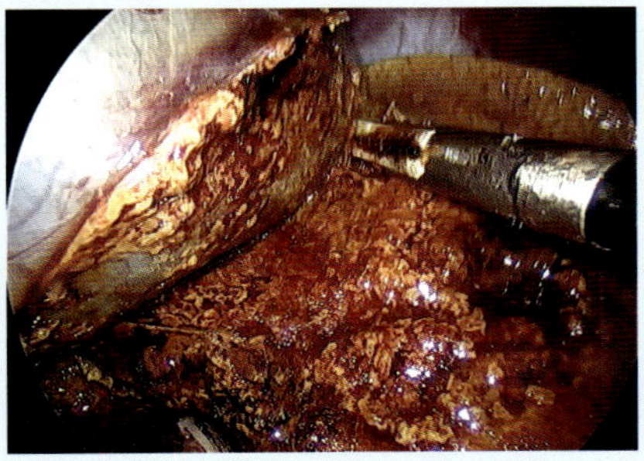

FIGURE 4. Blunt dissection maneuvers and monopolar coagulation carry out the gallbladder release from the hepatic fossa.

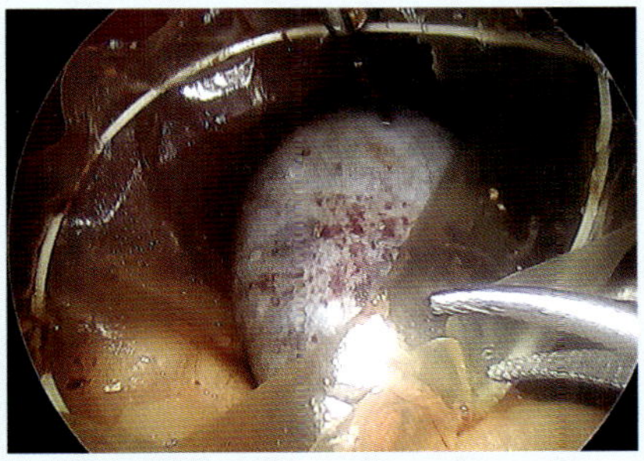

FIGURE 5. After its complete release from the hepatic fossa, the gallbladder is introduced into an extraction bag to retrieve from the abdominal cavity through the 10 mm trocar incision

Tips and tricks

- ✓ Sometimes, three trocars are enough to perform the procedure, but in the author's experience, a fourth trocar is advisable to achieve a good surgical field exposition.
- ✓ Gallbladder dissection is performed alternating blunt dissection maneuvers with monopolar coagulation or a vessel-sealing device, thus minimizing bleeding of the hepatic parenchyma.
- ✓ Surgery usually starts with dissection of the cystic duct, but the antegrade freeing of the gallbladder should be envisaged in complicated cases where the cystic duct is not clearly identified.
- ✓ Allow an intraoperative time out every time prior to dividing and clipping the cystic duct. Only structures traceable to the gallbladder should be divided/clipped.

36.8 LAPAROSCOPIC CHOLECYSTECTOMY IN A DOG

Ivan Jevtic

CASE DESCRIPTION

A dog with clinical signs of apathy, vomiting, food refusal, and changes in the color of feces. Biochemical analysis showed an increase in bilirubin of 146.9 (1.7–10.3) μmol/L; cholesterol 29.7 (3.1–6.5) mmol/L; ALP 3696.7 (10.6–100.7) U/L; ALT 4231.8 (8.2–57.3) U/L; AST 629.9 (8.9–48.5) U/L. After laparoscopic cholecystectomy, the dog was cheerful without pain, the color of the feces normalized, and did not vomit. A biochemical control analysis was performed 10 days after surgery, and a decrease in the value of the examined ALP parameters was observed at 459.2 (10.6–100.7) U/L; ALT 182.8 (8.2–57.3) U/L; AST 37.0 (8.9–48.5) U/L. Histopatholcgical findings corresponded to cholangitis and pericholangitis.

Key points

- Gallbladder mucocele was diagnosed.
- There was no common bile duct obstruction.
- The dog had vomiting and changes in the color of feces.

PORT PLACEMENT

The four-port technique was used. Port T1 for optics was positioned 2 cm below the umbilicus; port T3 was positioned 3 cm cranially from the umbilicus and 5 cm to the left of the midline. Port T2 was positioned 4 cm to the right of the umbilicus, and port T4 was placed 7 cm cranially from the umbilicus and 3 cm to the right of the midline. Ports T1 and T2 were 10 mm, and T3 and T4 were 5 mm.

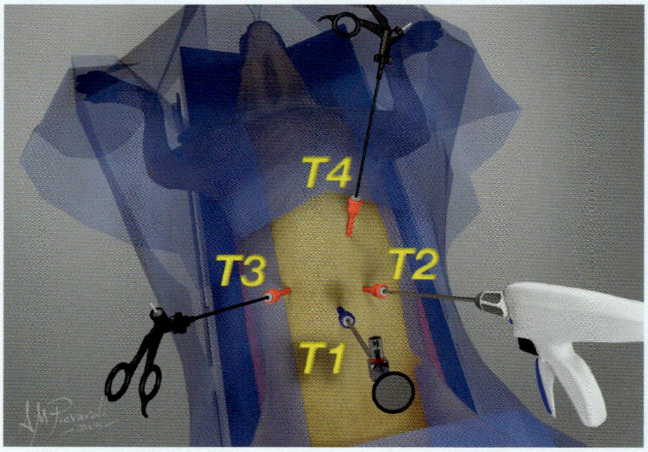

PROCEDURE

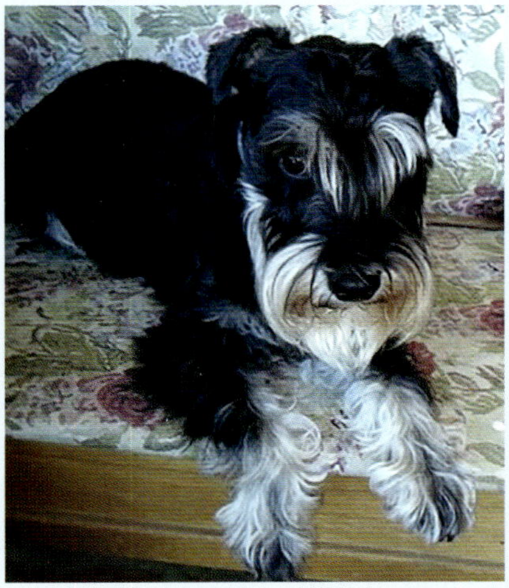

FIGURE 1. 4-year-old male Miniature schnauzer dog, weighing 8.6 kg.

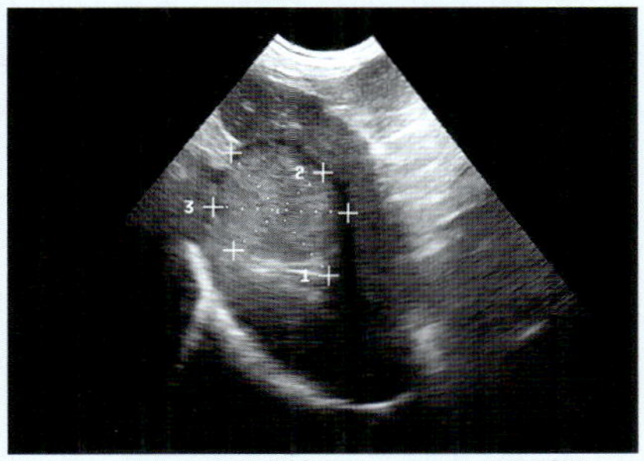

FIGURE 2. Mucocele was diagnosed by ultrasound examination.

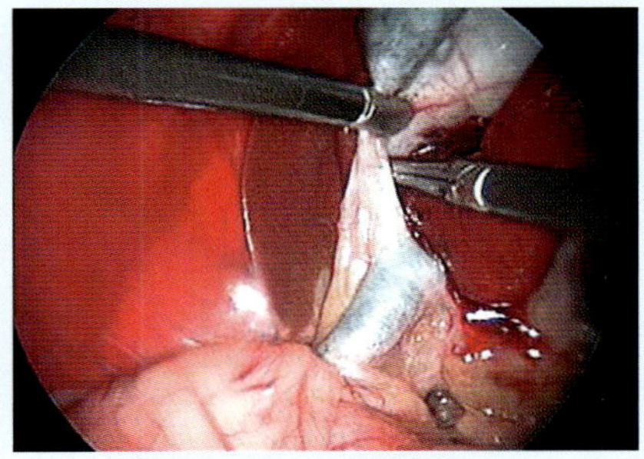

FIGURE 3. The cystic duct was fixed from T2 with a grasper, and a dissector was used to separate the duct from the liver tissue.

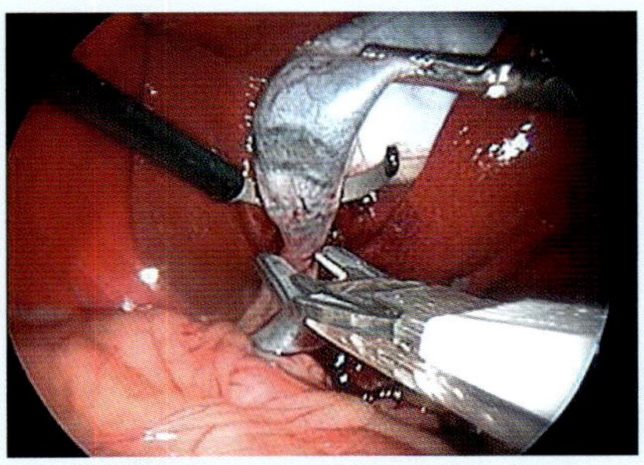

FIGURE 4. The duct was separated from the surrounding tissue with an endo mini retractor to have a better ligation with the endoclip.

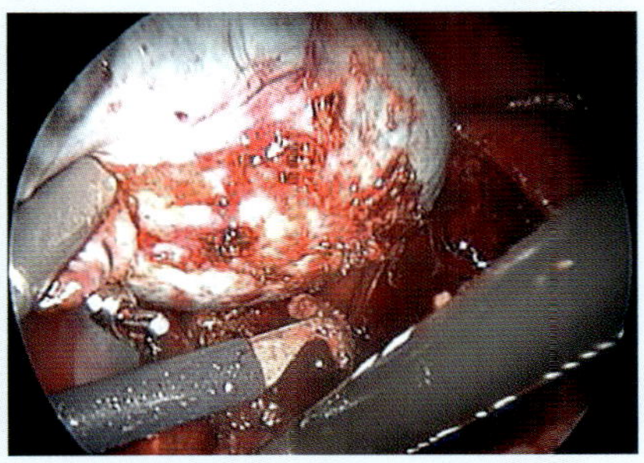

FIGURE 5. After dissecting the cystic duct between the clips, the gallbladder was separated using a monopolar hook.

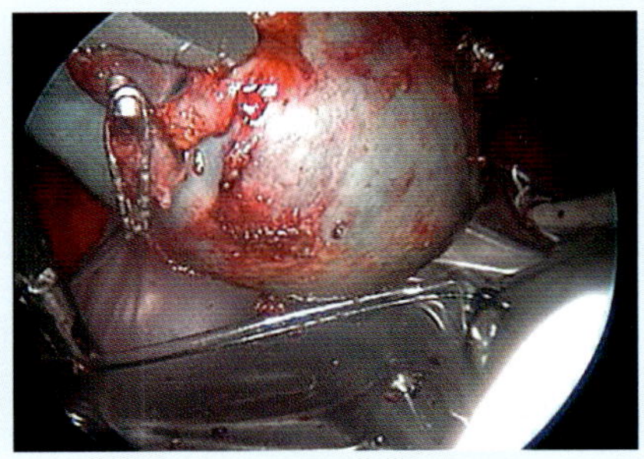

FIGURE 6. The separated gallbladder was extracted from the abdomen with the endobag.

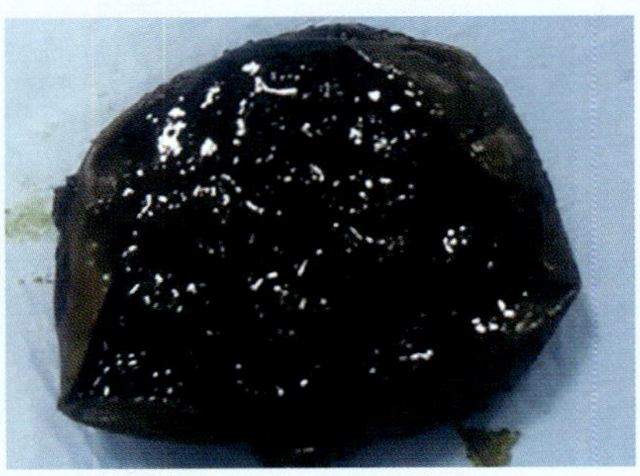

FIGURE 7. By opening the gallbladder, a mucocele was noticed.

Tips and tricks

✓ The use of mini endo retractors enables easier use of an endoclip for cystic duct ligation.

36.9 FUNDUS-FIRST CHOLECYSTECTOMY

Christopher B. Thomson

CASE DESCRIPTION

An 11-year-old neutered male Pomeranian dog was presented for hyporexia and progressive cholestatic liver enzyme elevations. A physical examination identified moderate pain on deep abdominal palpation. Ultrasound identified formed inspissated bile and a thickened and hyperechoic gallbladder wall, suggestive of a forming mucocele. Laparoscopic cholecystectomy and liver biopsy were performed. Histopathology was consistent with a gallbladder mucocele with chronic hepatitis.

Key points

- Fundic first dissection (FDF) has been developed and refined by the Small Animal Minimally Invasive Treatment (SAMIT) group from Japan.
- FDF dissects the gallbladder from the liver first, allowing clear visualization of the cystic duct prior to ligation.
- Identifying the subserosal layer is vital to allow for a clean dissection, minimizing hemorrhage from the liver parenchyma.

PORT PLACEMENT

A commercial SILS port was used at the subumbilical position (T1, T2). Roughly 5 cm cranial to the SILS port was a single, 10 mm threaded Ternamian endoport (T4). A 5 mm threaded Ternamian endoport (T3) was placed on the right of the midline.

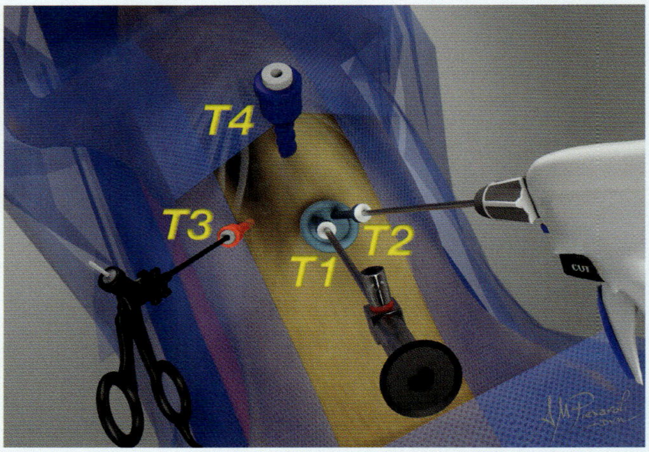

PROCEDURE

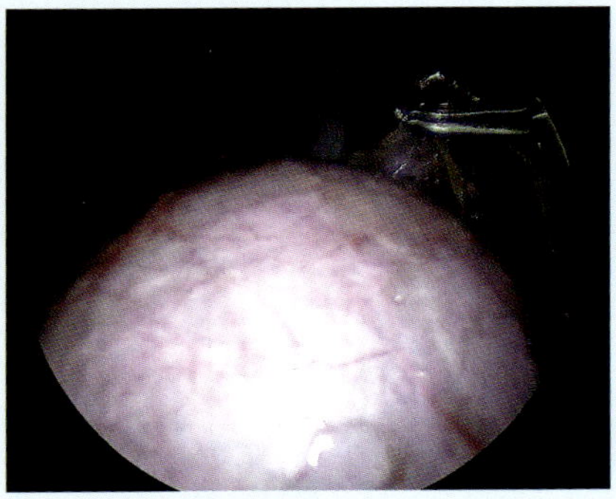

FIGURE 1. After pneumoperitoneum is established, the liver is retracted away from the gallbladder near the juncture of the quadrate lobe and the gallbladder to display the serosal attachments. The serosa is cut with laparoscopic Metzenbaum scissors.

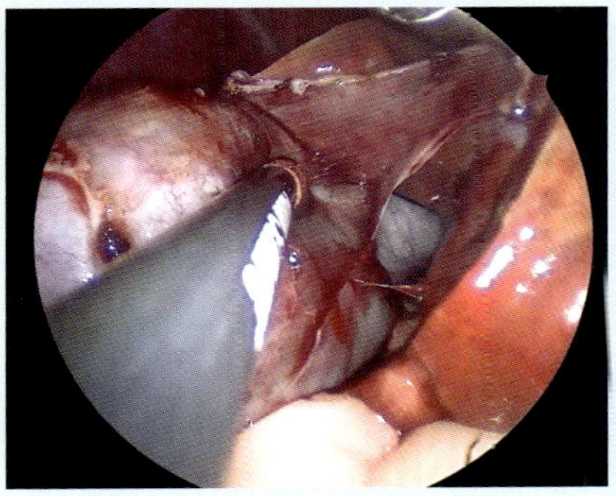

FIGURE 2. This dissection is continued within the hepatic fossa with a combination of blunt dissection via blunt probe, Endo Peanuts (Medtronic, Salem, MA), bipolar or harmonic vessel-sealing devices, and monopolar electrosurgery.

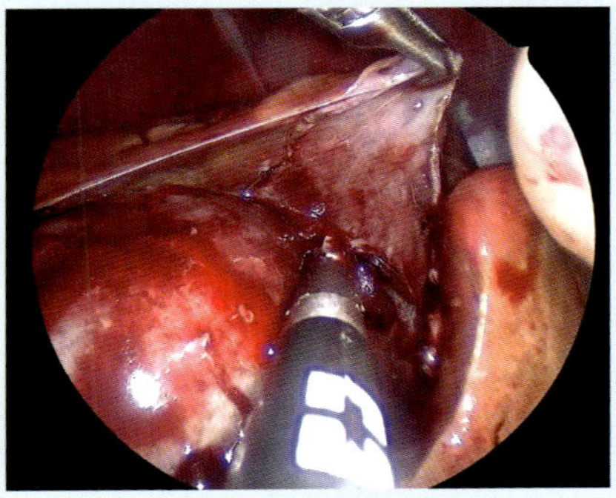

FIGURE 3. The subserosal dissection is finished at the neck of the gallbladder, allowing clear visualization of the cystic duct.

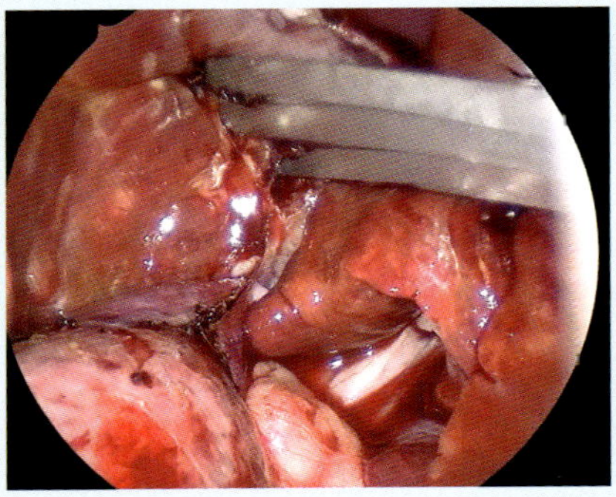

FIGURE 4. Elevation of the liver can be assisted through a fan retractor.

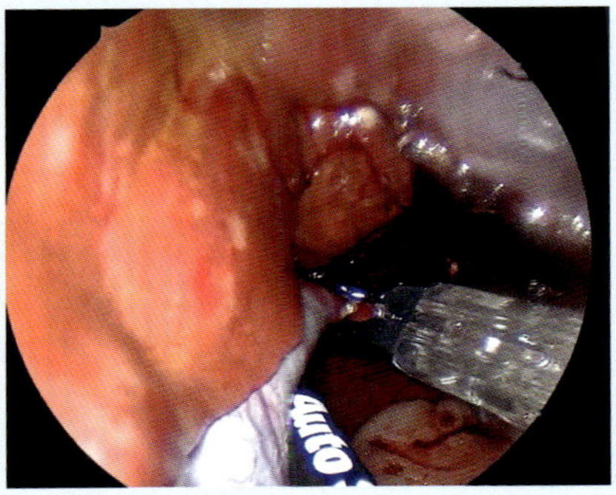

FIGURE 5. The cystic duct is ligated where it merges near the first hepatic duct; pictured is the use of large (10 mm) laparoscopic clips (Endo Clip II 10 mm Medtronic, Salem, MA).

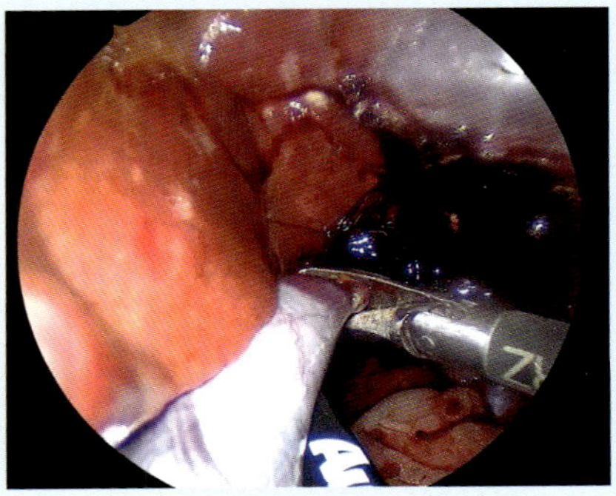

FIGURE 6. The gallbladder is transected with Metzenbaum scissors.

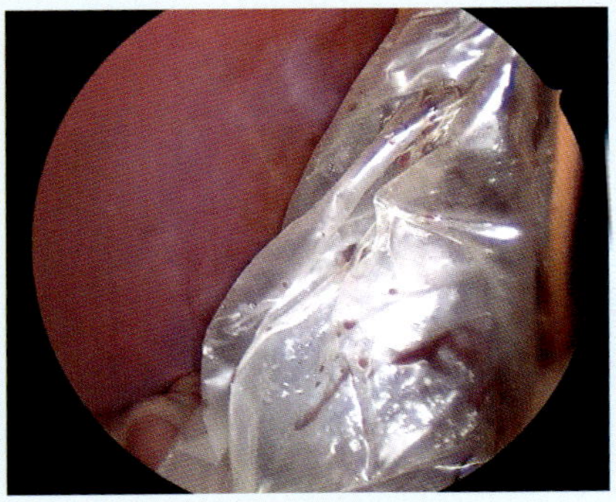

FIGURE 7. Lavage and suction should be performed prior to removal of the gallbladder via a specimen retrieval bag.

Tips and tricks

- ✓ Tension between the liver and the gallbladder allows visualization of the thin white serosal layer.
- ✓ Grasp the quadrate lobe subserosa with an instrument through the right port and right medial lobe subserosa via instrument in the cranial midline port, while dissection is performed via instruments in the caudal midline port.
- ✓ Three clips are placed on the patient's side, one or two on the gallbladder side, prior to transection.

37 LAPAROSCOPIC TREATMENT OF EXTRAHEPATIC PORTOSYSTEMIC SHUNT

Francesco Collivignarelli, Roberto Properzi, Maurício Veloso Brun, Robson Pasquale

A LAPAROSCOPIC TREATMENT OF EXTRAHEPATIC PORTOSYSTEMIC SHUNT WITH CELLOPHANE BAND

Francesco Collivignarelli, Roberto Properzi

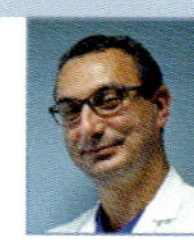

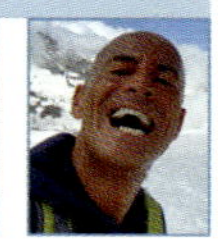

Indications

- Confirmed single extrahepatic portosystemic shunt

Contraindications

- Unstable patient
- Multiple extrahepatic portosystemic shunts
- Intrahepatic portosystemic shunt

During the last 10 years, the diagnostic and therapeutic uses of laparoscopy in surgery have increased dramatically in dogs and cats. Advantages of laparoscopy include the magnified viewing of intra-abdominal structures, decreased surgical morbidity, reduced postoperative pain, and small integumentary scars. Disadvantages include the cost of equipment, specialized training required, and reduced tactile sensation on the surgeon's part.

Portosystemic vascular shunts are congenital defects in the normal venous return of gastrointestinal blood. This abnormal blood flow allows toxins and hepatotropic agents to bypass the liver and enter the systemic circulation, resulting in a milieu of clinical signs such as hepatic encephalopathy and reduced growth. Attenuation of the aberrant vessel can be accomplished by suture ligation, ameroid constrictor application, intravascular coil embolization, or cellophane banding.

The attenuation of extrahepatic portosystemic shunt (PSS) vessels using laparoscopic visualization and laparoscopically placed cellophane bands is described below.

Hematobiochemical disorders associated with extrahepatic PSS

- Microcytosis
- Hypoalbuminemia
- Hypoglycemia
- Hypokalemia
- ALP and ALT increased
- Hypocholesterolemia
- BUN decreased
- Preprandial bile acids normal or increased
- Postprandial bile acids increased
- Preprandial NH_3 normal
- Postprandial NH_3 increased

Clinical findings associated with extrahepatic PSS

- Often, dogs younger than 1 year
- Reduced growth and poor state of nutrition
- Neurological signs (seizures, central blindness, coma)
- Gastrointestinal signs (diarrhea, pica)
- Renal-urinary signs (polyuria-polydipsia, urate uroliths)

PATIENT PREPARATION AND POSITIONING

Encephalopathic patients should be stabilized before surgery. Fluid and electrolyte imbalances should be corrected preoperatively. Perioperative antibiotics are recommended for patients undergoing PSS surgery.

After clipping, the skin is aseptically prepared, and dogs are positioned in dorsal recumbency with no tilt of the operating table. A Veress needle is introduced through a stab incision 1 cm caudal to the umbilicus, and the abdomen is insufflated with carbon dioxide to maintain an adequate pressure measured in mmHg. Alternatively, a modified Hasson technique is used to establish the camera port.

Sites for placement of trocar cannulas are selected to provide adequate visualization of the cranial abdomen and to allow instrumental liver manipulation. Each trocar/cannula unit is inserted through the skin and subcutaneous tissue via a stab incision with a number 15 scalpel blade. Bladeless trocars are then gently pushed through the abdominal musculature or the linea alba to avoid penetrating the underlying organs in the abdominal cavity.

OPERATING ROOM LAYOUT

The operating surgeon and surgeon assistant will stand at the end of the table, so it is important that the dog is positioned with the pelvic limbs at the end of the table. The anesthesia team and laparoscopic tower should be positioned near the front of the table to facilitate room for the surgical team to work. The instrument table is best positioned over the operating table but cranial to the dog's abdomen (**Fig. 1**).

Instruments

On the table:

- Standard surgical pack
- High-definition video camera
- Telescope 5 mm – 30°
- Two 5 mm threaded cannulas + one 12 mm threaded cannula
- Laparoscopic Babcock and Kelly, right-angle forceps, 5 mm
- Laparoscopic cotton-tip (Endopeanuts), blunt dissection probes, 5 mm
- L- or J- hook monopolar electrosurgical tip, 5 mm
- 10 mm titanium endoscopic clips (Endoclip)
- 3–5 cm wound retractor
- Cellophane band

PORT PLACEMENT (FIG. 2)

- T1, 1 cm caudal to the umbilicus
- T2, to the left paramedian abdominal wall, equidistant between the costochondral arches and the umbilicus

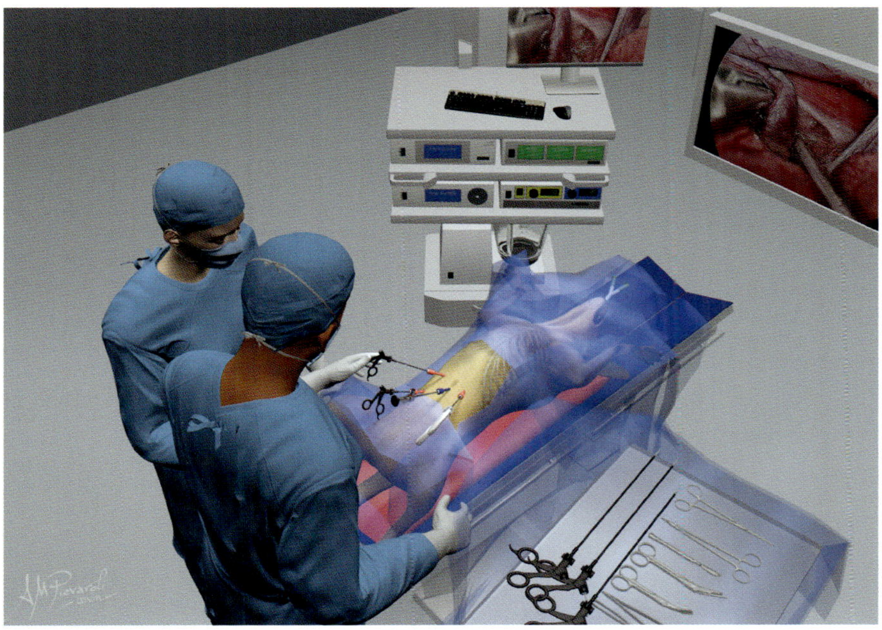

FIGURE 1. Operating room layout for laparoscopic treatment of extrahepatic PSS.

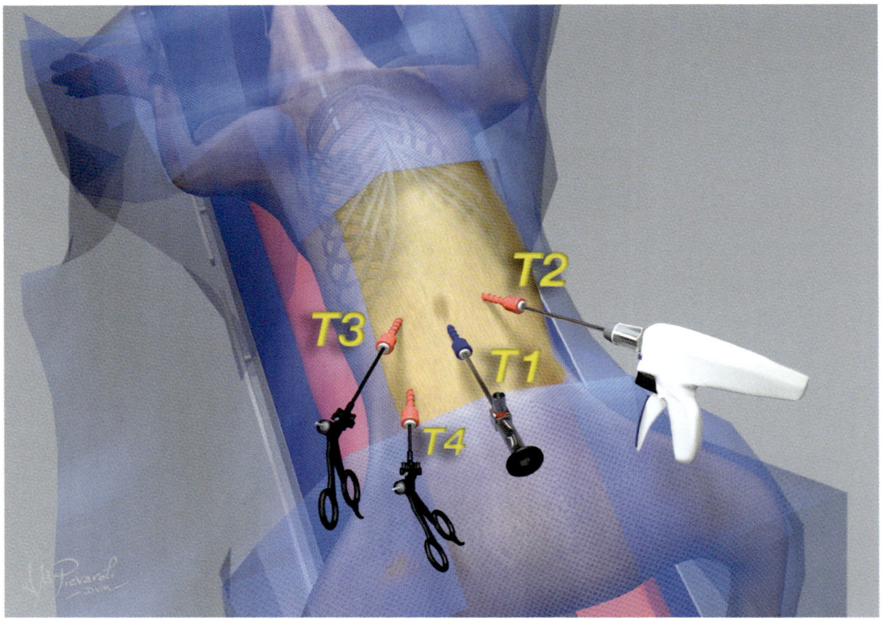

FIGURE 2. Port placement for laparoscopic treatment of extrahepatic PSS with cellophane band.

- T3, to the right paramedian abdominal wall equidistant between the costochondral arches and the umbilicus
- T4, 5 mm cannula placed in the right caudal abdomen equidistant from the umbilicus and pubic bone for laparoscopic Babcock forceps

PROCEDURE

- The abdomen is visually explored with the laparoscope, and an extrahepatic PSS is seen (**Fig. 3**).
- The vessel is dissected from the surrounding tissue using laparoscopic right-angled forceps and Maryland forceps (**Fig. 4**).
- A single cellophane band of 4 mm in width is introduced into the abdomen and positioned around the shunt vessel (**Fig. 5**).
- The vessel is temporarily occluded by grasping both ends of the cellophane band and applying tension.
- The pancreas and jejunum are evaluated visually for any congestion, change in color, or change in motility.
- No gross signs of portal hypertension are observed during the 3-minute observation period.
- The cellophane band is then secured with some hemostatic clips to occlude the shunt vessel (**Fig. 6**) progressively.

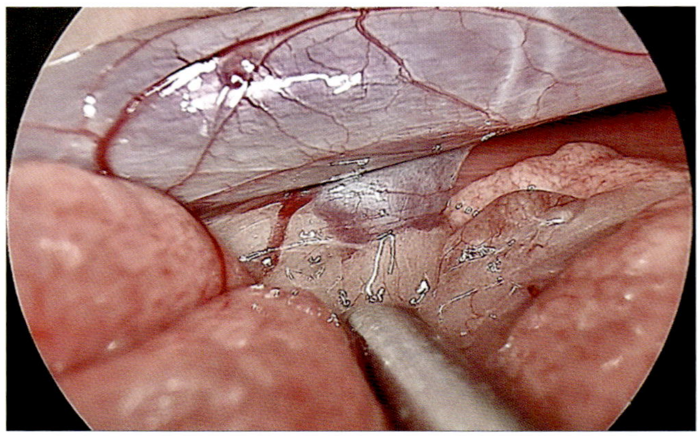

FIGURE 3. Extrahepatic PSS seen during exploratory laparoscopy.

POSTOPERATIVE MANAGEMENT

- Discharge 24 hours after surgery.
- Lactulose and a low-protein diet until normalization of serum bile acids.
- A recheck examination 6 weeks postoperatively is necessary.

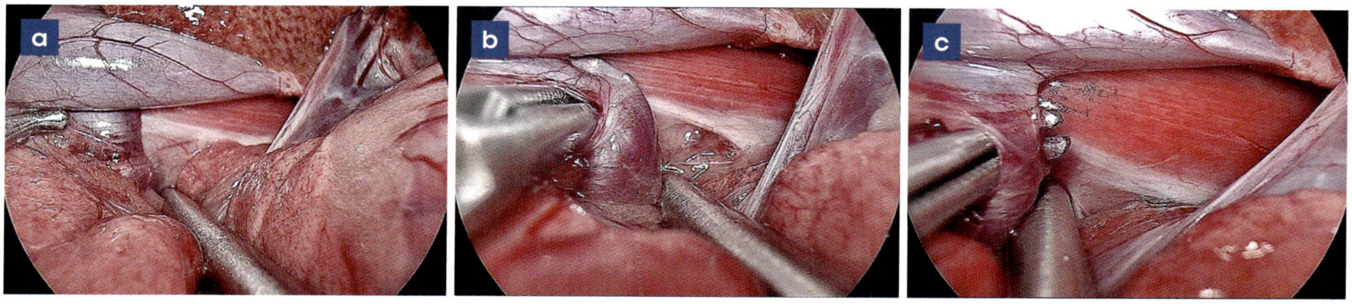

FIGURE 4. The anomalous vessel is dissected using laparoscopic right-angled forceps and Maryland forceps.

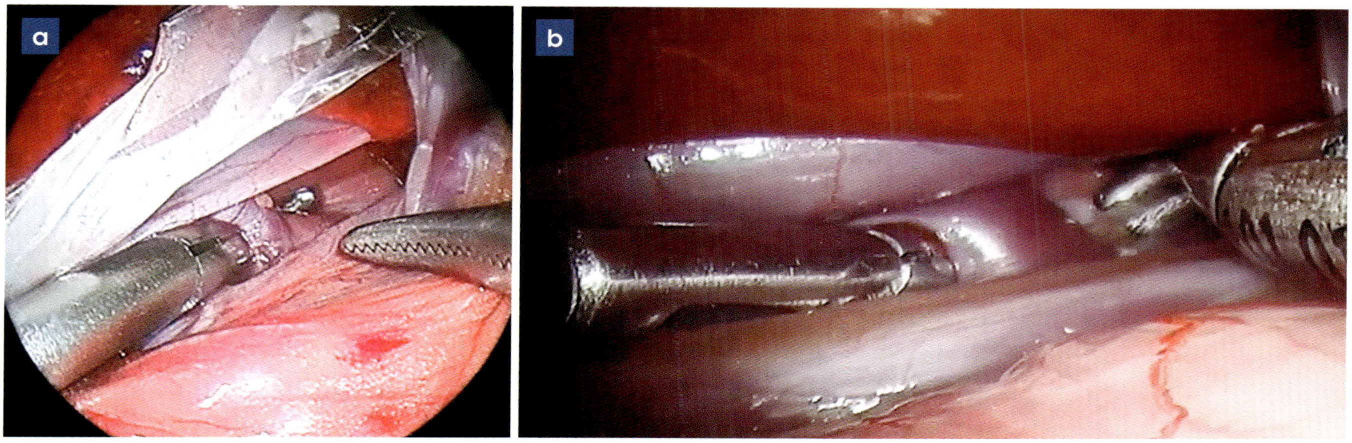

FIGURE 5. A 4 mm wide cellophane band is introduced into the abdomen and positioned around the shunt vessel.

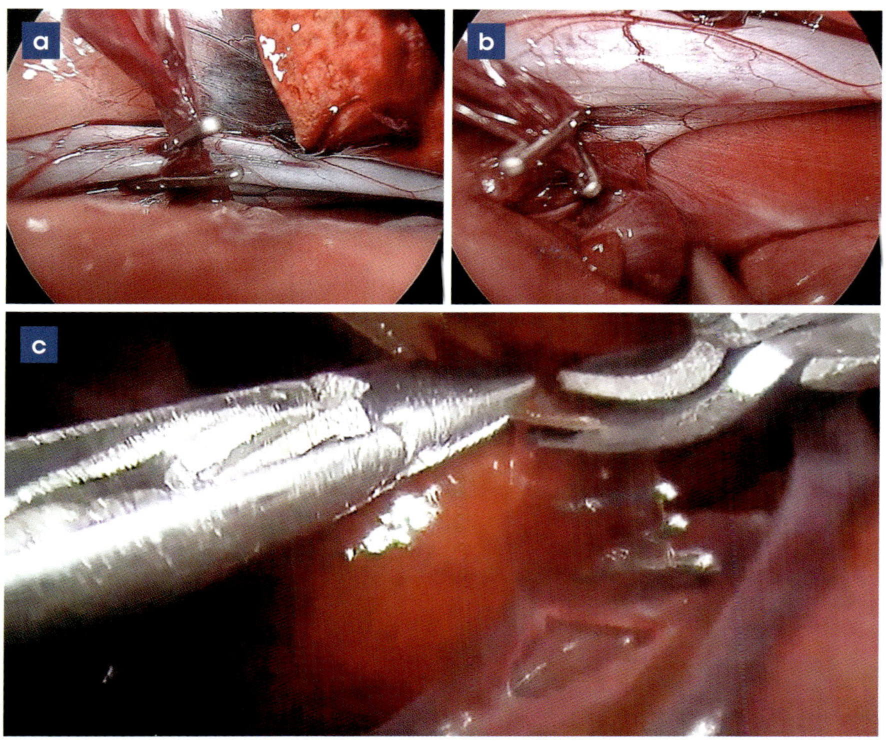

FIGURE 6. The cellophane band is secured with some hemostatic clips.

Key points

- Use a contrast CT scan for the diagnosis.
- Sometimes, it is possible to have the diagnosis also with abdominal ultrasonography.
- Always perform liver function tests before surgery.
- Stabilize the patient at least 2 weeks prior to surgery using metronidazole, lactulose, and a diet containing highly digestible protein.
- After the temporary occlusion of the shunt, evaluate the pancreas and jejunum for any congestion, change in color, or change in motility.
- After placing a cellophane band around the shunt vessel, secure it with three or four hemoclips.
- Eliminating the edges of the cellophane band helps to pass it around the shunt.

B LAPAROSCOPIC TREATMENT OF EXTRAHEPATIC PORTOSYSTEMIC SHUNT WITH AMEROID CONSTRICTOR

Maurício Veloso Brun, Robson Pasquale

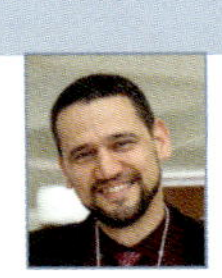

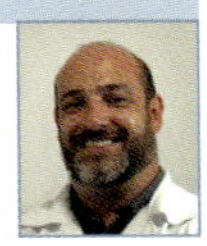

It is very well established in the literature that ameroid ring constrictors are one of the best options available for extrahepatic primary shunt occlusion in small animals. The authors' group was looking for different alternatives to implant it in a minimally invasive approach. In the alternative technique that will be described as follows, the ameroid's passage is occluded with a polypropylene suture that is passed over two holes made in the inner casein ring (**Fig. 7**). Thus, locking the passage of the ameroid ring and keeping the shunt inside the ameroid's internal opening. Furthermore, this approach reduces the volume of implanted material (hemostatic cellulose membrane) that would remain inside the ameroid and in contact with the vena cava.

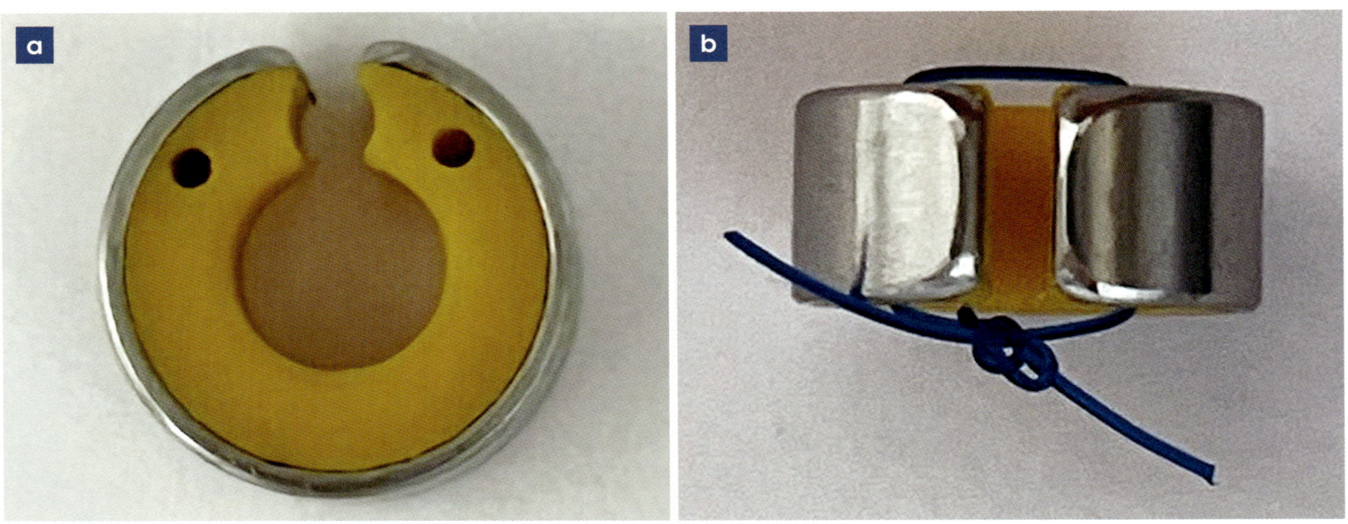

FIGURE 7. Preparation of the ameroid for fully laparoscopic implantation. The casein portion was drilled bilaterally to the pin slot. The suture will be passed in these formed tunnels to close the ameroid.

OPERATING ROOM LAYOUT

The surgeon and surgeon's assistant stand on the side of the patient facing the dog's abdomen, and the endoscopic tower is placed on the contralateral side of the patient (**Fig. 8**).

PORT PLACEMENT (FIG. 9)

- The first port (T1) is positioned using the modified Hasson technique lateral to the inguinal fold at the midpoint between the iliac tuberosity and the costal margin.
- Two other ports (T2, T3) are positioned in triangulation and lateral to the first.

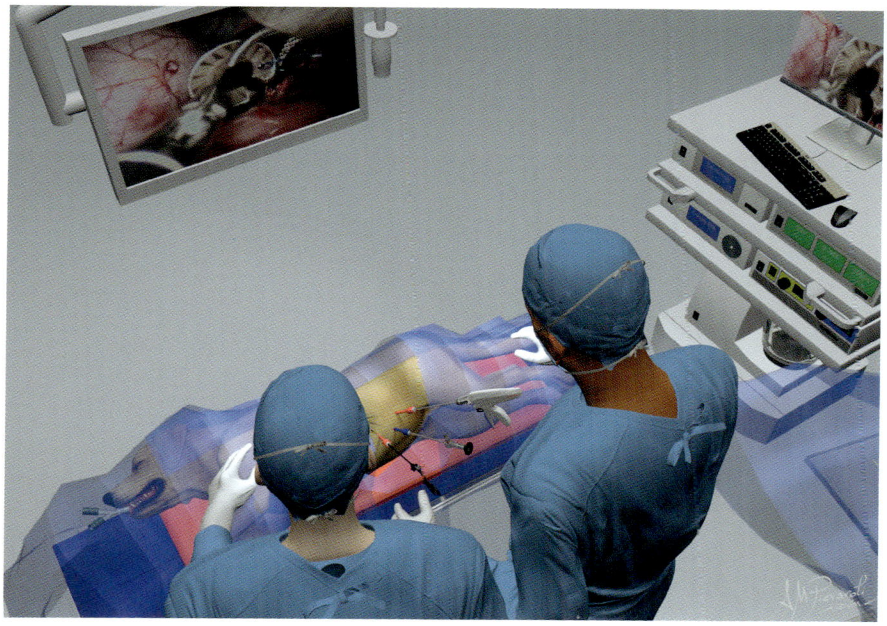

FIGURE 8. Operating room layout for laparoscopic extrahepatic PSS with ameroid constrictor.

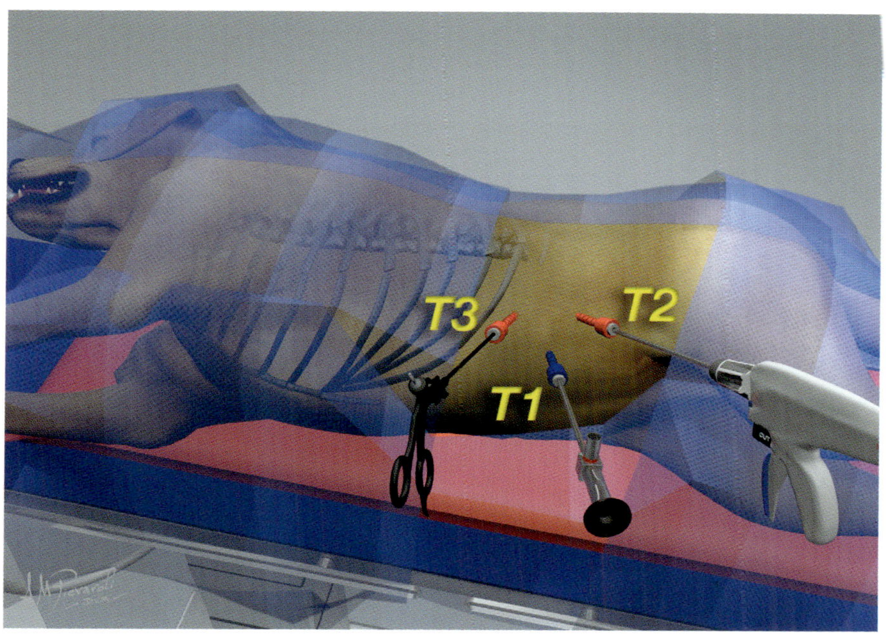

FIGURE 9. Port placement for laparoscopic extrahepatic PSS with ameroid constrictor.

PROCEDURE

- The patient is positioned in left or right lateral decubitus, with the flank elevated. The decubitus must be on the opposite side of the entry point of the shunt into the vena cava.
- An abnormal larger vein is sought, initially in a cranial position to the phrenicoabdominal vessels and draining into the vena cava on the left (**Fig. 10**) since it is a common position for congenital extrahepatic shunts.
- The shunt is bluntly dissected with Kelly, Maryland, or Mixter forceps (**Figs. 11 and 12**).
- The anomalous vessel is positioned inside the ameroid constrictor, keeping its slot facing ventrally (**Figs. 13–15**).
- A shunt-compatible ameroid ring size diameter is chosen, and two 1 mm perforations are performed in the inner casein ring with a micro drill. Each perforation is performed on one of the sides of the slit close to the stainless steel outer ring.
- A segment of 2-0 or 0 polypropylene suture is passed through the two holes, which will be occluded intracorporeally. The occlusion of this interrupted suture through the ameroid ring will create a barrier, consequently locking the

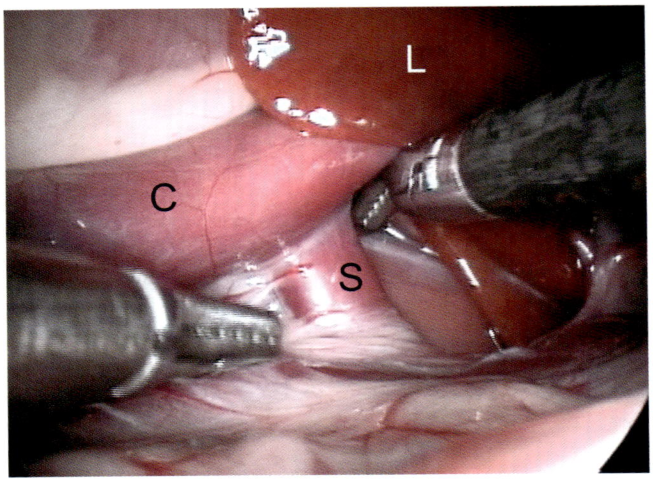

FIGURE 10. Location of the anomalous vessel/shunt (S) draining into the vena cava (C) cranially to the bilateral phrenicoabdominal vessels. L, liver.

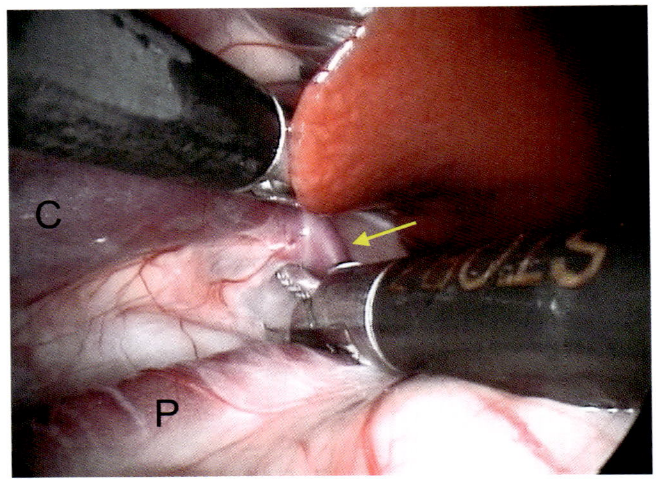

FIGURE 11. Dissection caudally to the shunt (arrow). C, vena cava; P, portal vein.

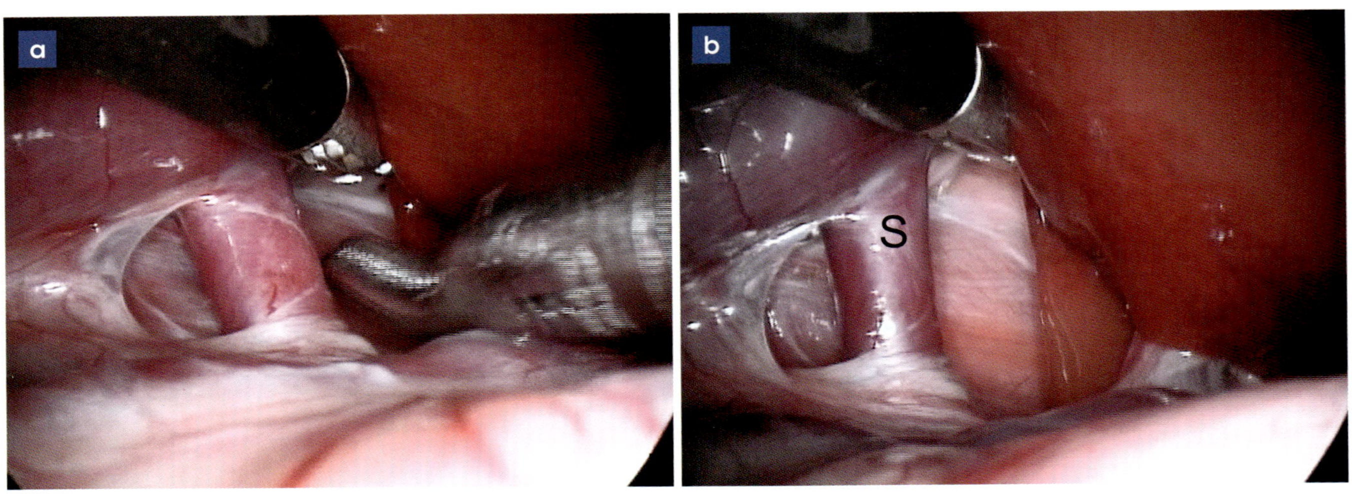

FIGURE 12. a) Dissection of the cranial aspect of the shunt. b) Shunt (S) after dissecting the adjacent tissues for constrictor positioning.

shunt inside the ameroid, thus avoiding the dislodgement through the ameroid's slot.

- The passage of the polypropylene suture tip through the ameroid hole can be a difficult maneuver, as the vena cava tends to project over the ameroid ring; the suture knot to occlude the ameroid ring is performed under the implant (in this perspective), that is, medially to the patient, moving the intracorporeal knot away to prevent contact with the vena cava (**Figs. 16–19**).
- To facilitate the placement of the ameroid over the shunt, a laparoscopic forceps grasper is used to firmly grasp at its midpoint in the contralateral position of the ameroid's slot key (pin); the forceps will push the edges of the ameroid slot against the shunt, positioning it completely inside the ameroid ring.
- After the suture (knot) occlusion is completed, multiple liver biopsies are performed with biopsy forceps (**Fig. 20**).

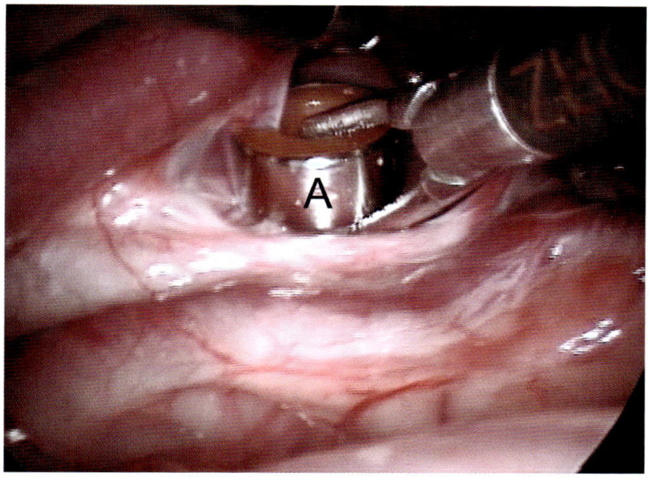

FIGURE 13. Application of the ameroid constrictor (A) directing its slot to the shunt, from cranial to caudal. For proper positioning, the shunt dissection should be slightly larger than the constrictor height.

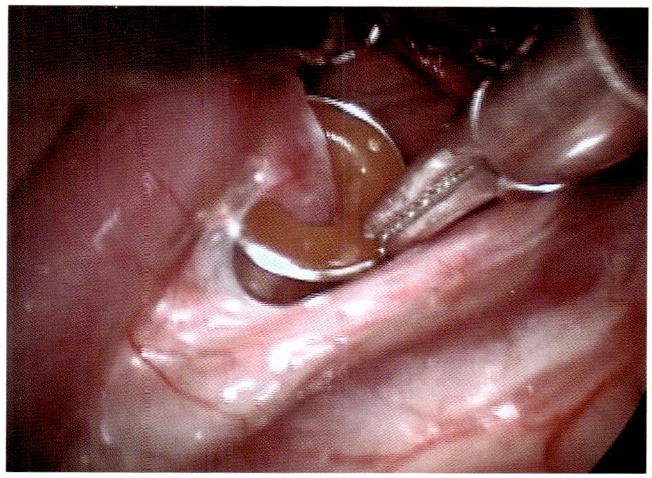

FIGURE 14. Complete shunt imprisonment inside the ameroid constrictor. As the constrictor slot needs to face the scope (ventrally in this perspective), the ameroid will be rotated by the axis of the anomalous vessel with the forceps.

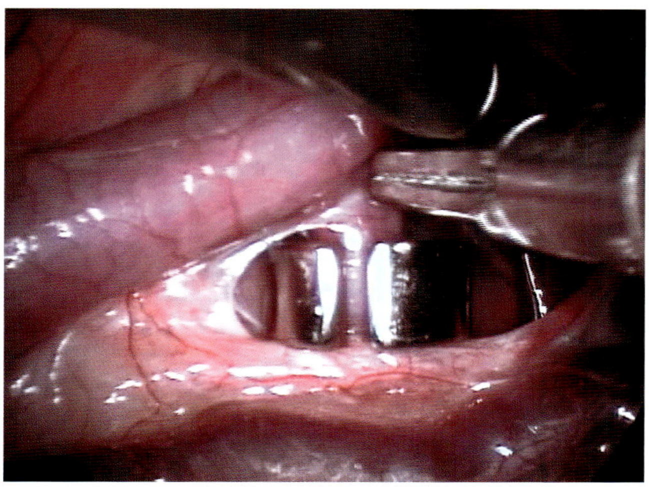

FIGURE 15. Correct positioning of the ameroid constrictor for subsequent closing of its slot, avoiding the risk of displacement.

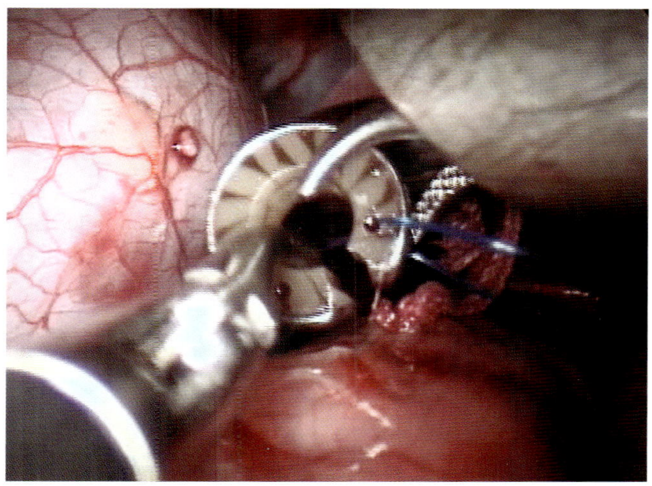

FIGURE 16. View of the polypropylene thread inside the cranial perforation of the ameroid.

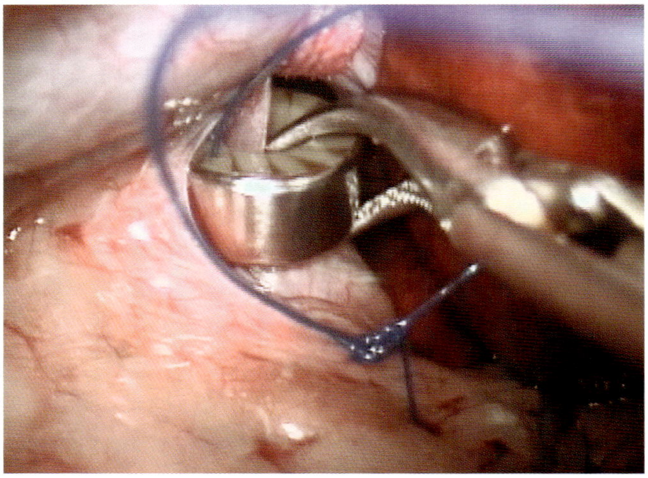

FIGURE 17. Polypropylene thread seized and pulled under (in this perspective) the ameroid.

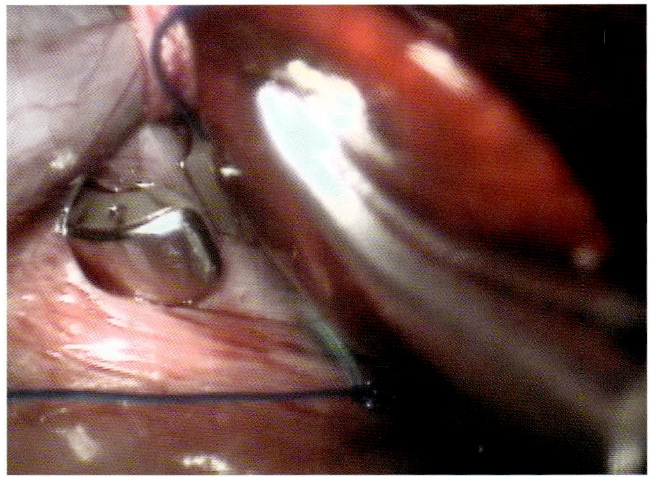

FIGURE 18. Sutures closure under the ameroid to prevent shunt displacement through the pin slot.

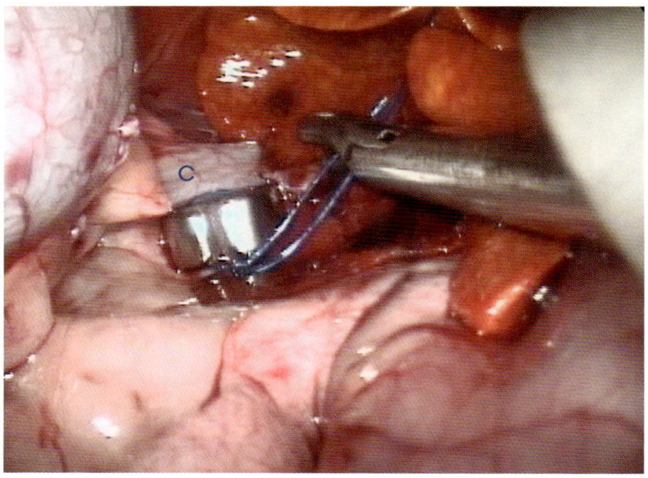

FIGURE 19. Occlusion of the suture under the ameroid so that the knot is not in direct contact with the vena cava (C).

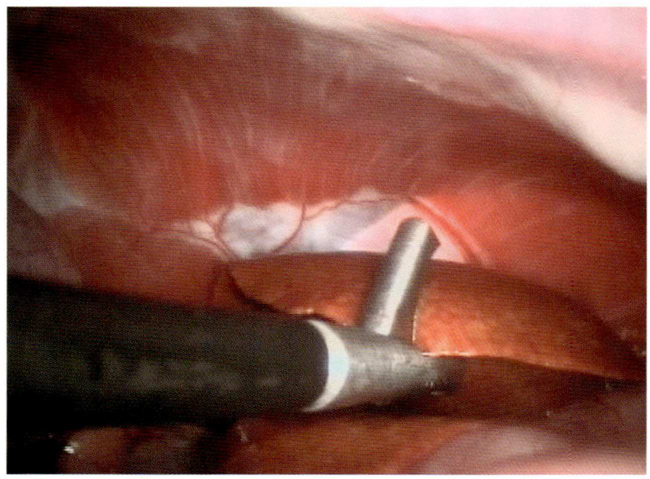

FIGURE 20. At the end of the procedure, multiple liver biopsies are performed with biopsy forceps.

Key points

- The flank approach allows excellent exposure of extrahepatic shunts located cranially to the phrenic-abdominal vessels. The contralateral cavity accesses in relation to the point of entry of the shunt into the vena cava allow better exposure for dissection of the anomalous vessel and facilitate the positioning of the ameroid ring. The shunt will present itself perpendicularly to the vena cava in this position.
- In some cases, a slight dissection of the vena cava, just cranial to the shunt, may be necessary, and it must be repaired with umbilical tape/vessel loop. Its traction will allow better shunt exposure even for dissection and ameroid ring positioning. However, caval traction must be very careful not overly occlude cardiac blood flow.
- Passage of the polypropylene suture through the ameroid holes will be facilitated if the polypropylene suture segment is passed in one of the holes before entering into the abdominal cavity, tying off both ends of the suture segment together and forming a loop.
- Once the shunt is inside the ameroid, the loop is cut, and then the portion of the suture on the top of the ameroid (in this perspective) is passed "from top to bottom" in the contralateral hole.
- Double half knot followed by three single half knots (in the configuration 2=1=1=1) is used to make the suture knot.

Complications of laparoscopic treatment of extrahepatic portosystemic shunt with cellophane band or ameroid constrictor

- Hypoglycemia within 4 hours after extrahepatic PSS attenuation.
- Intraoperative and postoperative hemorrhage.
- Portal hypertension, less common in patients undergoing gradual shunt occlusion.
- Seizures and encephalopathy, mainly in cats and small-breed dogs.
- Persistence or recurrence of clinical signs.

SUGGESTED READINGS

CLINICAL CASES

37.1 SPLENOCAVAL SHUNT

David García Rubio

CASE DESCRIPTION

A canine patient, a 1-year-old Yorkshire terrier weighing 1.8 kg experiencing seizures. Blood analyses only showed a slight increase in ALT and increased four times the normal value for postprandial bile acids.

By performing an abdominal ultrasound and then a CT scan, the existence of an anomalous extrahepatic splenocaval vascular communication was confirmed. After the patient was medically stabilized 2 weeks before surgery, the shunt was progressively closed using a cellophane strip and laparoscopic approach.

Key points

- A prior CT scan and a good working knowledge of the different types of shunts are recommended to plan surgery better.
- The patient should be medically stabilized at least 2 weeks before surgery through metronidazole, lactulose, and a diet containing highly digestible protein.
- It is important to use a pure cellophane strip that does not contain plastic by-products.
- Recent studies have not proven beneficial with the intraoperative attenuation of the shunt at diameters <3 mm.

PORT PLACEMENT

The patient is placed in left lateral decubitus position, and four 5 mm trocars are used. The optical trocar (T1) is inserted in the umbilical position. Two additional ports are inserted; the right (T2) is slightly ahead of the optical trocar, while the left (T3) is inserted at a greater distance, at the medium height of the right flank, such that the shunt may be approached as perpendicularly as possible. Lastly, a fourth trocar (T4) in a more cranial direction is used as a separator.

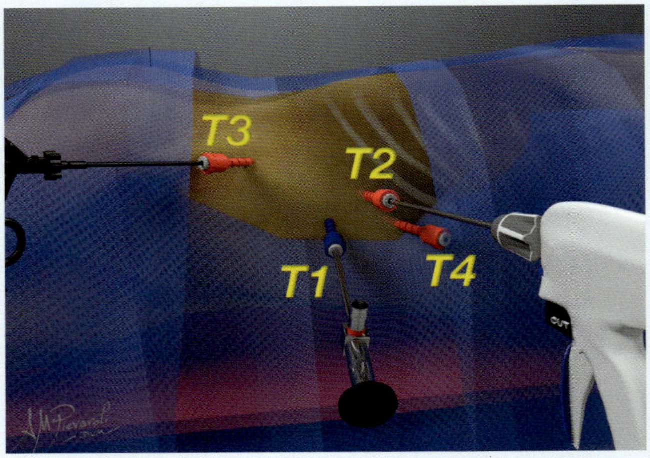

PROCEDURE

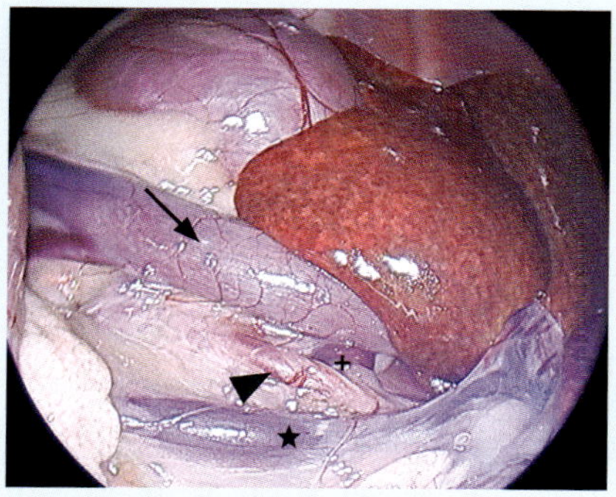

FIGURE 1. General view of the abdomen with the patient in left lateral decubitus: vena cava (arrow), hepatic artery (arrowhead), portal vein (asterisk), and splenocaval shunt (cross).

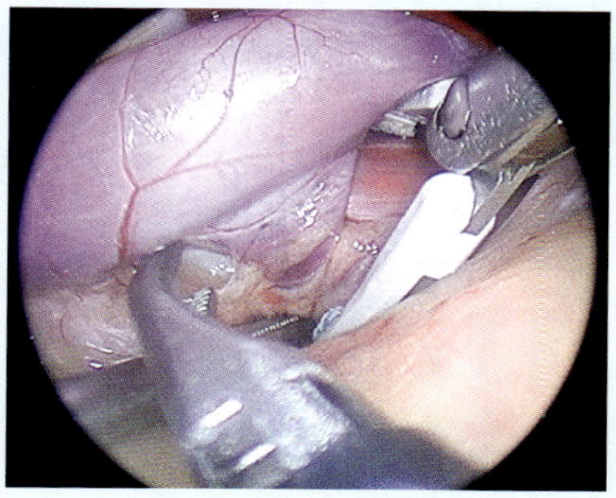

FIGURE 2. After locating the shunt, the surrounding fasciae are carefully dissected as close to the vena cava as possible.

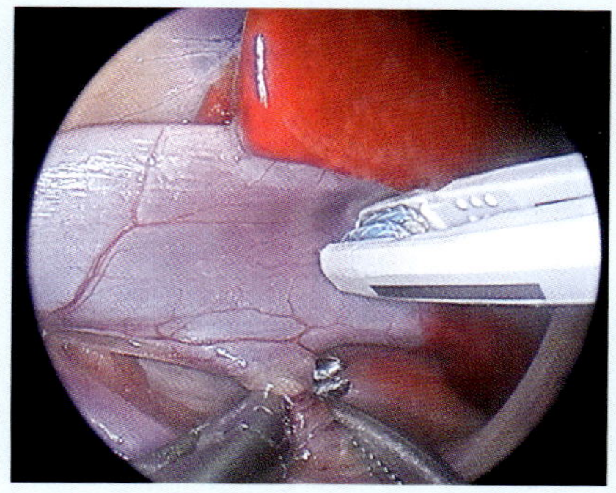

FIGURE 3. Dissection should be sufficiently wide to allow the cellophane strip to pass through without being too loose in order to favor its mobility.

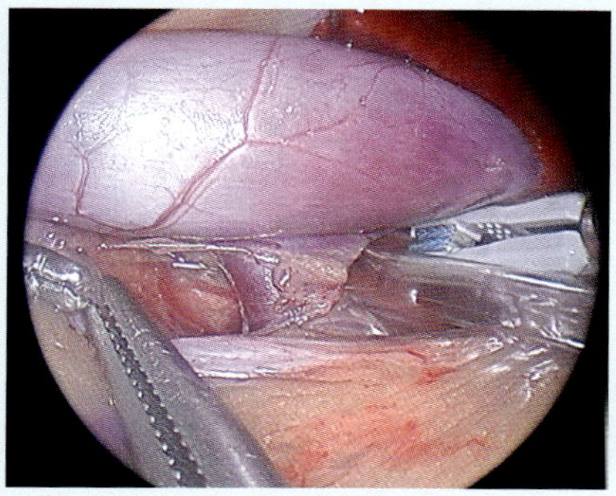

FIGURE 4. Passage of the cellophane strip once the shunt has been dissected. This should be done gently without forcing the vein.

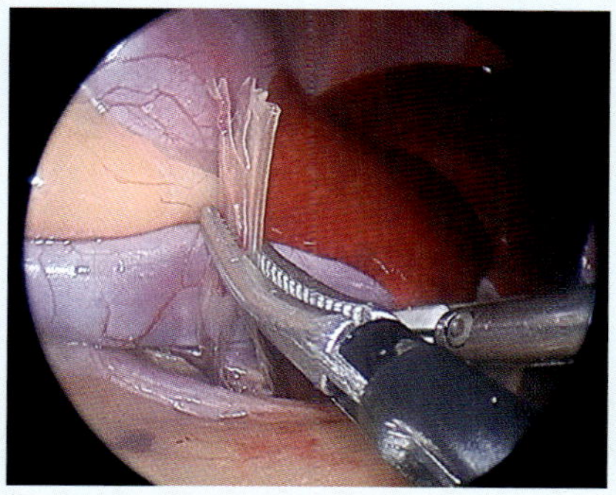

FIGURE 5. Cellophane strip in position, surrounding the shunt without strangulating it.

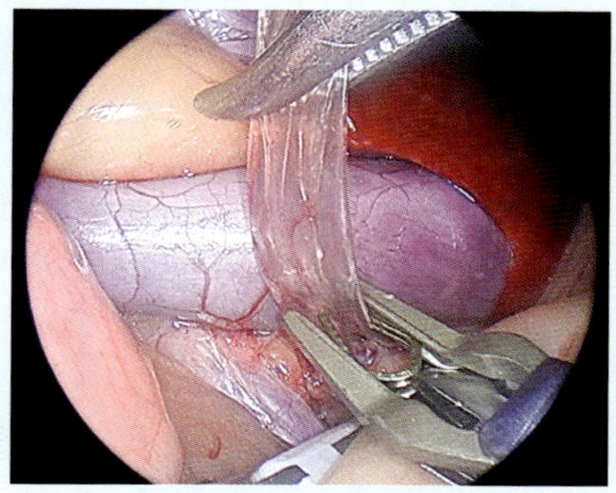

FIGURE 6. Proceed to close the strip around the shunt by using titanium clips.

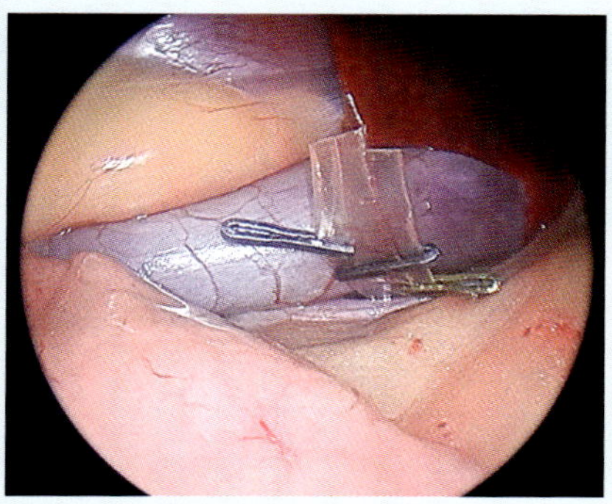

FIGURE 7. Final appearance of the procedure after placing the clips and recutting the excess from the cellophane strip. The clips may be placed in alternate positions to ensure the cellophane strip does not move.

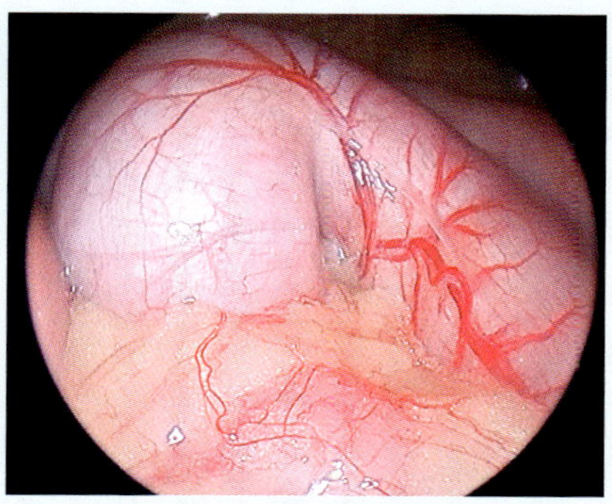

FIGURE 8. After completing the procedure, spend a few minutes observing for possible signs of portal hypertension, such as an increase in intestinal peristalsis, intestinal paleness or cyanosis, or pancreatic edema. If any of these appear, release the cellophane strip and position it, so it is looser.

Tips and tricks

- ✓ In very deep shunts, a right-angle dissector is incredibly useful.
- ✓ To aid in the passage of the cellophane strip, it can be cut into a point at one end, or a suture may be added to facilitate grip.
- ✓ The portal vein is usually above the shunt, so a fourth separation trocar is very useful.
- ✓ Instead of titanium clips, polymer ligatures may be used as these do not create as many image artifacts in ultrasound or CT scans.

37.2 LAPAROSCOPIC ATTENUATION OF A SPLENOPHRENIC SHUNT IN A DOG

Edoardo Poggi, Luciano Borghetti, Francesca Izzo

CASE DESCRIPTION

A 5-year-old male Shi-Tzu dog presented for neurological signs. A serum biochemical profile showed that preprandial bile acids were markedly elevated. A diagnosis of a splenophrenic shunt was made by the use of CT angiography.

Key points

- Diagnosis of a splenophrenic shunt was made using CT angiography; ultrasound is also possible to find the abnormal vessel.
- The patient is positioned in right lateral recumbency with a left lateral approach to improve the visualization and dissection of the shunt vessel.
- If necessary, a fourth (T4) port (5 mm cannula, Kii Advanced Fixation Sleeve, Applied Medical) was placed in the dorsal part of the abdomen to retract the stomach.
- A postoperative CT scan angiography was done to check the correct position of the cellophane band and the mild attenuation of the shunt.
- Serum biochemical profiling revealed nothing remarkable 4 months after the surgery. Bile acid concentrations were near the normal range of preprandial and postprandial bile acids, and by the physical examination, there was no evidence of neurological signs.

PORT PLACEMENT

The patient was positioned in right lateral recumbency for the laparoscopic procedure with a left lateral approach. A modified Hasson technique was used to establish the camera port (T1), 2–3 cm lateral to the umbilicus on the left side. After that, a 5 mm 30° telescope was introduced in the 5 mm cannula, and the abdomen was insufflated with CO_2 to an intra-abdominal pressure of 6 mmHg.

The second (T2) and the third (T3) ports (two 5 mm cannulas) were positioned under laparoscopic visualization: T2 on the mid-abdominal level just caudal to the last rib (the surgeon's left hand) and T3 at the same level of T2 just cranial to the pelvic limb (the surgeon's right hand).

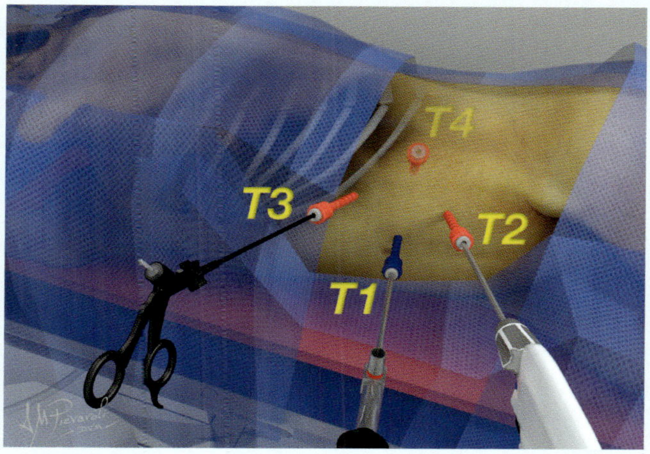

PROCEDURE

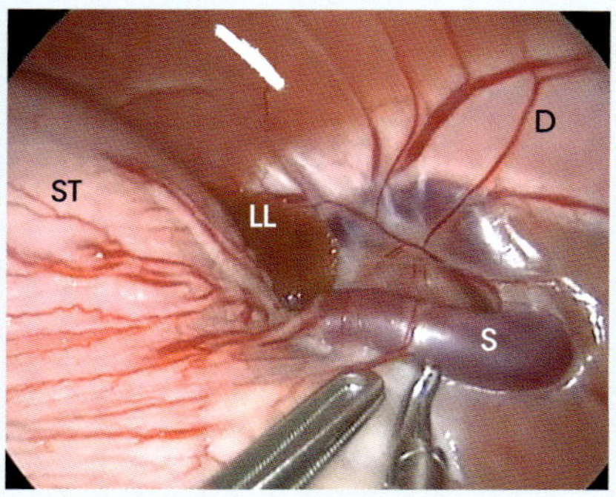

FIGURE 1. Under laparoscopy visualization, a shunt (S) is found, originating from the splenic vein, passing cranial to the liver along the diaphragm (D), and inserting into the caudal vena. Laparoscopic visualization of the shunt vessel and adjacent organs. LL, left liver lobe; ST, stomach.

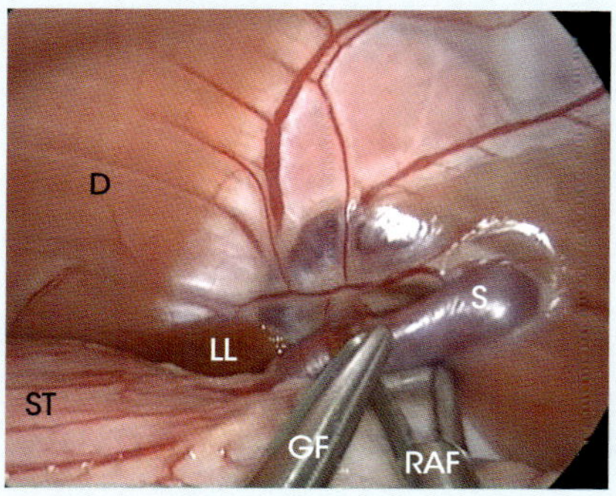

FIGURE 2. The vessel (S) is dissected from the surrounding tissue using a 5 mm laparoscopic right-angle dissection forceps (RAF; Clickline Right-Angled dissecting forceps, Karl Storz, El Segundo, CA) aided with a 5 mm laparoscopic grasping forceps (GF; Clickline Grasping forceps, Karl Storz, El Segundo, CA). D, diaphragm; LL, left liver lobe; ST, stomach.

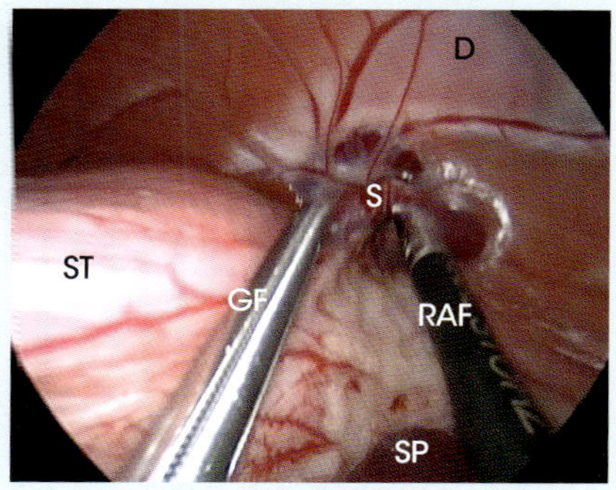

FIGURE 3. Complete dissection of the shunt vessel (S). D, diaphragm; GF, grasping forceps; RAF; right-angle forceps; SP, spleen; ST, stomach.

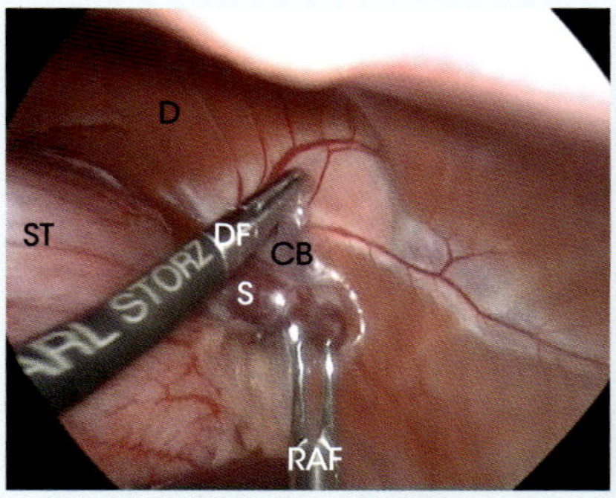

FIGURE 4. Cellophane band (CB) positioning around the shunt vessel (S). D, diaphragm; DF, dissecting forceps; RAF; right-angle forceps; ST, stomach.

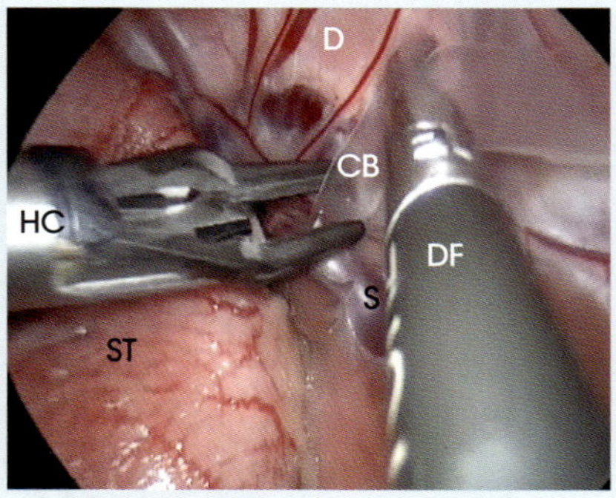

FIGURE 5. The cellophane band (CB) is grasped with a laparoscopic dissecting forceps (DF) and then secured with hemoclips (HC). D, diaphragm; S, shunt; ST, stomach.

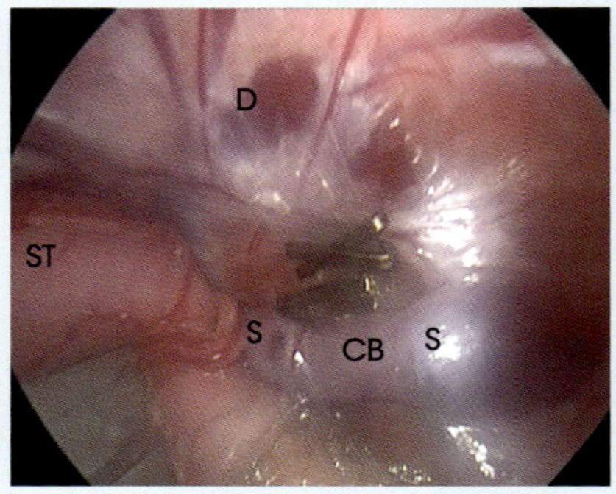

FIGURE 6. After its isolation, a cellophane band (CB) is positioned around the shunt vessel (S), and it is secured with four hemoclips (Epix Universal Clip Appliers 5 mm, Applied Medical). Final view of the attenuated shunt vessel. D, diaphragm; ST, stomach.

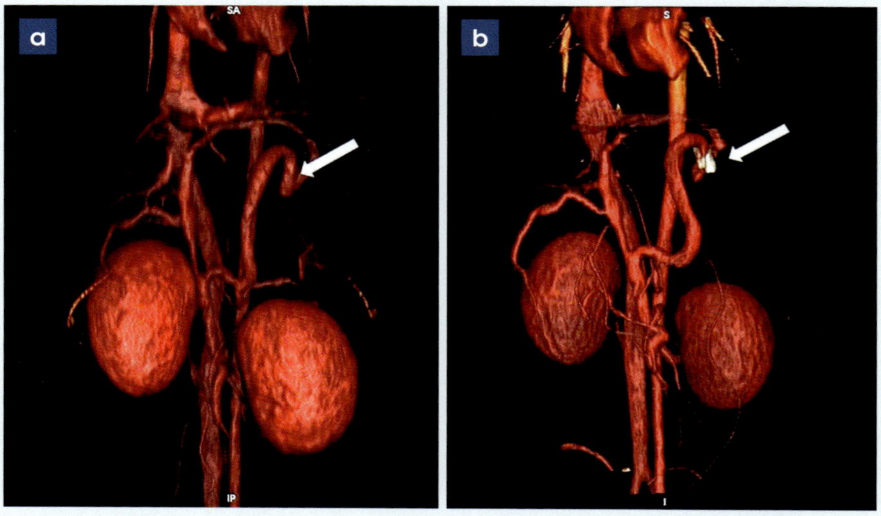

FIGURE 7. Ventrodorsal view of a 3D reconstruction of CT scans of the shunt vessel (white arrow) a) before and b) after attenuation.

Tips and tricks

- ✓ A triangular cushion can be placed under the right lateral side to raise the spine and improve visualization of the shunt.
- ✓ If the stomach is bloated, an orogastric tube can be placed to achieve gastric decompression and to reduce gastric contents.

37.3 LAPAROSCOPIC ATTENUATION OF A SPLENOCAVAL SHUNT IN A DOG

Edoardo Poggi, Francesca Izzo, Luciano Borghetti

CASE DESCRIPTION

A 2-year-old male Yorkshire Terrier was evaluated for acute onset of several clinical signs (vomiting, weakness, disorientation). After physical examination, a serum biochemical profile showed elevated preprandial bile acids. A CT scan angiography revealed the presence of a splenocaval shunt.

Key points

- The patient was positioned in left lateral recumbency with a right lateral approach to improve the visualization and dissection of the shunt vessel with a 5 mm right-angle laparoscopic dissector forceps.
- Finally, the pancreas and jejunum were visually evaluated for congestion change in color, but there were no signs of hypertension.
- A postoperative CT scan angiography was done to check the correct position of the cellophane banding and the correct attenuation of the shunt.
- Serum biochemical profiling revealed nothing remarkable 4 months after surgery. Bile acid concentrations were near the normal range of preprandial and postprandial bile acids, and after physical examination, there was no evidence of neurological signs.

PORT PLACEMENT

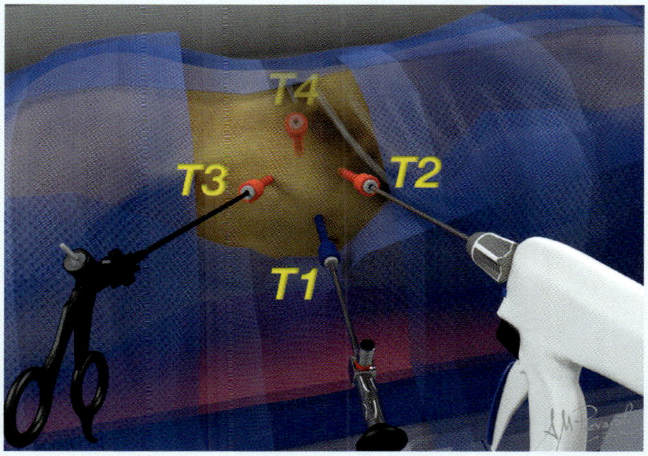

The patient was positioned in left lateral recumbency with a right lateral approach. Abdominal access was obtained using a modified Hasson technique. A 5 mm skin incision was made 2 cm lateral to the umbilicus on the right side, a 5 mm cannula (T1) (Kii Sleeve with Advanced Fixation, Applied Medical) was introduced into the abdomen, and abdominal insufflation with CO_2 was initiated with an intra-abdominal pressure of 6 mmHg. A 5 mm 30° telescope (Hopkins Forward-Oblique Telescope, Karl Storz, Tuttlingen, Germany) was introduced through the 5 mm cannula to explore the abdomen (T1).

The second (T2) and the third (T3) ports (two 5 mm cannulas, Kii Sleeve with Advanced Fixation, Applied Medical) were then placed under laparoscopic visualization, T2 on the mid-abdominal level just a caudal to the last rib (the surgeon's right hand) and T3 at the same level of T2 just cranial to the pelvic limb (the surgeon's left hand). If necessary, a fourth (T4) port (5 mm cannula, Kii Sleeve with Advanced Fixation, Applied Medical) can be placed to retract the liver in the dorsal part of the abdomen.

PROCEDURE

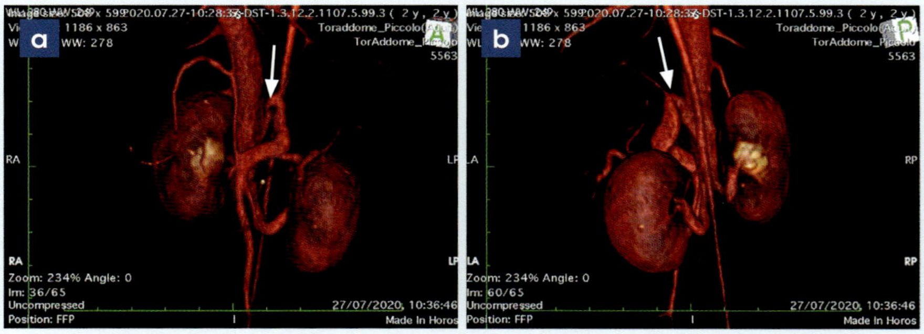

FIGURE 1. Diagnosis of a splenocaval extrahepatic shunt was made by the use of CT angiography. It is also possible to use ultrasound to find the abnormal vessel. a) 3D presurgical CT scan volume rendering of the shunt vessel (white arrow) in a) ventrodorsal and b) dorsoventral view.

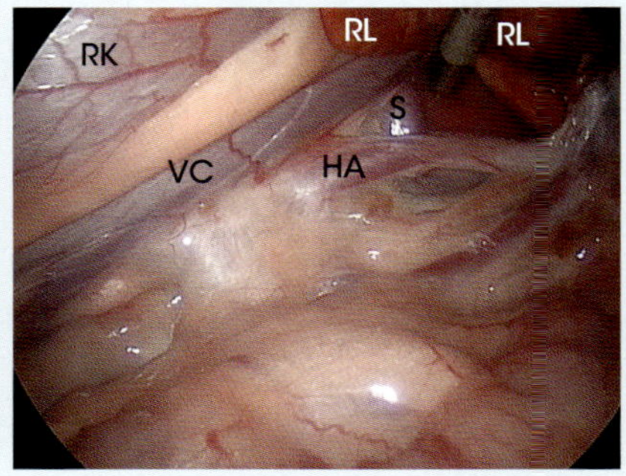

FIGURE 2. After laparoscopic exploration of the abdomen, an abnormal shunt vessel (S) is noted at the epiploic foramen. HA, hepatic artery; RK, right kidney; RL, right liver lobe; VC, vena cava.

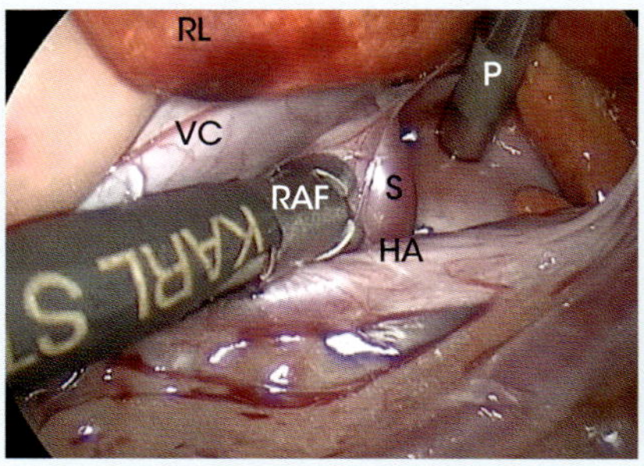

FIGURE 3. The vessel (S) is dissected with a right-angle laparoscopic forceps (RAF; Clickline Right-Angled dissecting forceps, Karl Storz, El Segundo, CA) and aided with a 5 mm laparoscopic palpation probe (P). HA, hepatic artery; RL, right liver lobe; VC, vena cava.

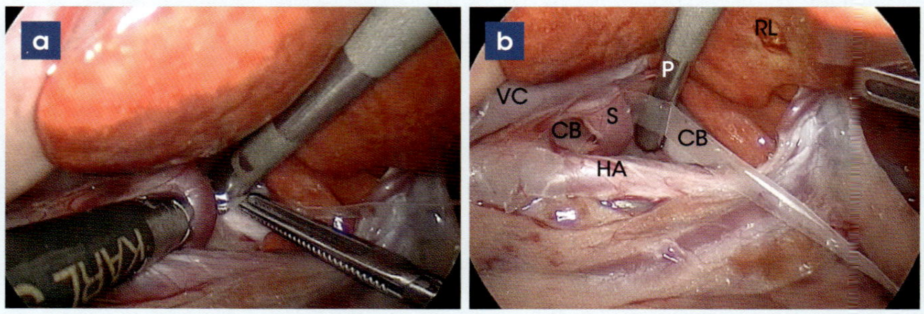

FIGURE 4. A cellophane band (CB) is introduced into the abdomen and placed around the shunt vessel (S). HA, hepatic artery; P, palpation probe; RL, right liver lobe; VC, vena cava.

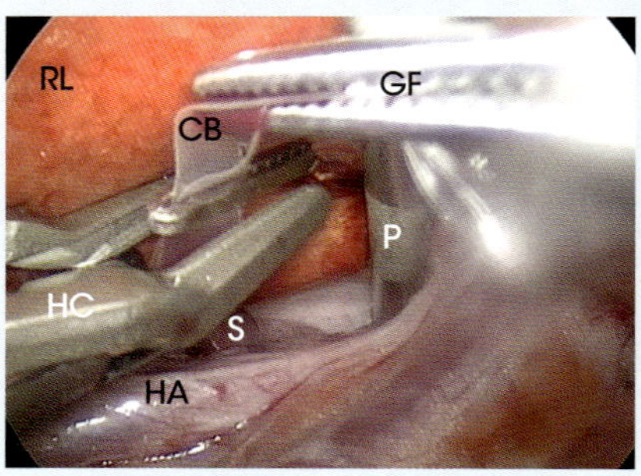

FIGURE 5. The cellophane band (CB) is secured with hemostatic clips (HC; Epix Universal Clip Appliers 5 mm, Applied Medical). GF, grasping forceps; HA, hepatic artery; P, palpation probe; RL, right liver lobe; S, shunt.

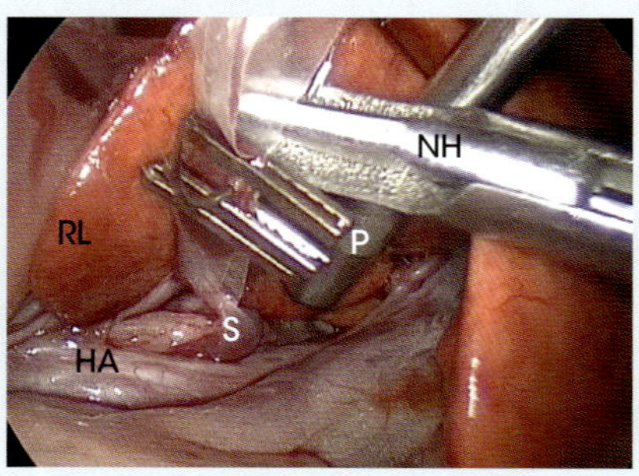

FIGURE 6. The cellophane band is secured with three hemostatic clips (Epix Universal Clip Appliers 5 mm, Applied Medical) and a surgical knot with a 3-0 nonabsorbable nylon suture (Ethicon; Ethicon, Sommerville). HA, hepatic artery; NH, needle holder; P, palpation probe; RL, right liver lobe; S, shunt.

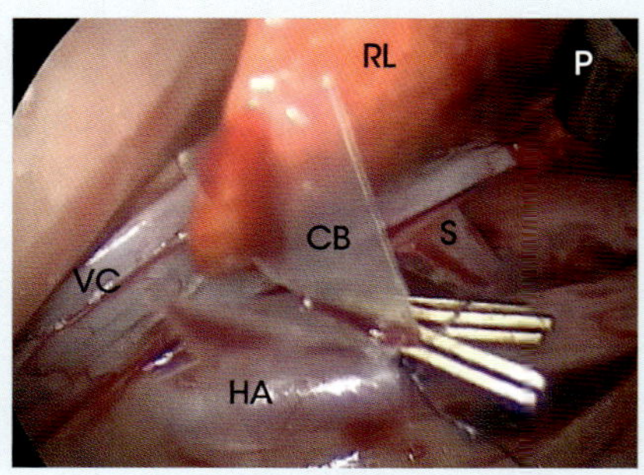

FIGURE 7. Final visualization of the attenuated shunt vessel (S). CB, cellophane band; HA, hepatic artery; P, palpation probe; RL, right liver lobe; VC, vena cava.

Tips and tricks

✓ A triangular cushion can be placed under the right lateral side to raise the spine to improve the visualization of the shunt.

37.4 LAPAROSCOPIC ATTENUATION OF A LEFT INTRAHEPATIC PORTOSYSTEMIC SHUNT IN A CAT

Edoardo Poggi, Filippo Cinti, Francesca Izzo

CASE DESCRIPTION

A 15-month-old female domestic shorthair cat was referred for seizures, vomiting, and lethargy. A serum biochemical profile showed that preprandial bile acids were markedly elevated (151.1 µmol/L) and low amylase (268 U/L), while other parameters were within the normal limit. A diagnosis of a left intrahepatic PSS (portal vein–left hepatic vein) was confirmed by CT angiography.

Key points

- Diagnosis of a left intrahepatic PSS was made using CT angiography. It is also possible to use ultrasound to find the abnormal vessel.
- A postoperative CT scan angiography was performed to check the correct position of the cellophane banding and understand the grade of shunt attenuation.
- Two months after surgery, the clinical condition was improving, and the serum biochemical profiling was within the normal limit with fasting serum bile acids 1.1 µmol/L

PORT PLACEMENT

A four-port technique was used for the laparoscopic procedure. The patient was positioned in right lateral recumbency for left lateral flank approach. A modified Hasson technique was used to establish the camera port (T1) positioned 2–3 cm lateral to the umbilicus on the left side. A 5 mm 30° telescope (Hopkins Forward-Oblique Telescope, Karl Storz, Tuttlingen, Germany) was then introduced in the 5 mm cannula (Kii Sleeve with Advanced Fixation, Applied Medical).

The second (T2) port and the third (T3) port (two 5 mm cannulas, Kii Sleeve with Advanced Fixation, Applied Medical) were positioned under laparoscopic visualization: T3 on the mid-abdominal level just caudal to the last rib (the surgeon's left hand) and T2 at the same level of T3 just cranial to the pelvic limb (the surgeon's right hand).

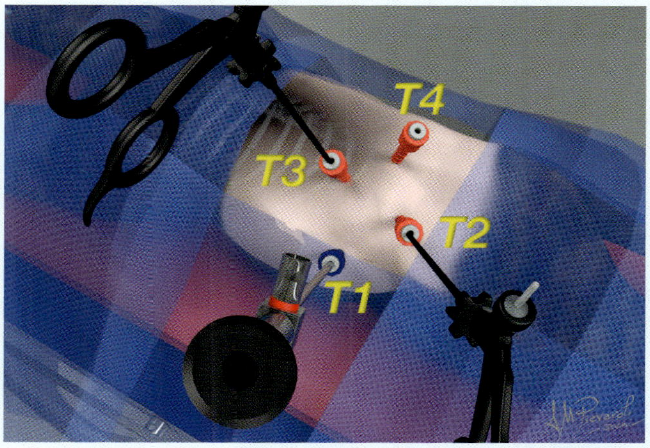

In this case, a fourth (T4) additional port (5 mm cannula, Kii Sleeve with Advanced Fixation, Applied Medical) was placed (3–5 cm cranial to T2 and 3–5 cm caudal to T3) in the dorsal part of the abdomen for stomach retraction.

PROCEDURE

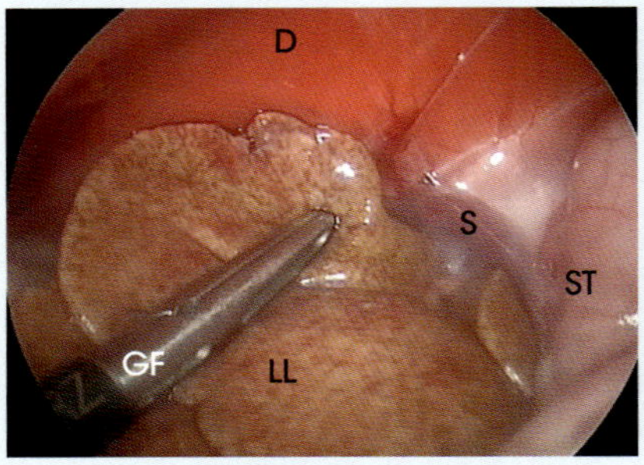

FIGURE 1. The patient is positioned in right lateral recumbency with a left lateral approach to improve the visualization and dissection of the shunt vessel. Laparoscopic visualization of the shunt vessel (S) and adjacent organs. D, diaphragm; GF, grasping forceps; LL, left liver lobe; ST, stomach.

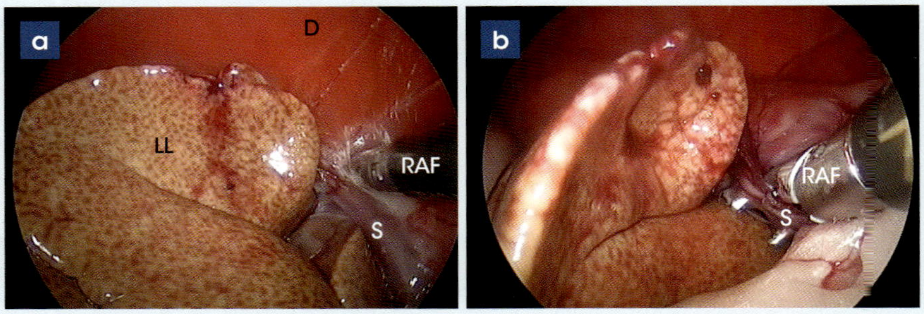

FIGURE 2. Large shunt, originating from the portal vein, passing cranial to the liver along the diaphragm (D), and inserting into the left hepatic vein visualized during laparoscopic abdominal exploration. Dissection of the shunt (S) vessel with a 5 mm laparoscopic right-angle dissection forceps (RAF; Clickline Right-Angled dissecting forceps, Karl Storz, El Segundo, CA). LL, left liver lobe.

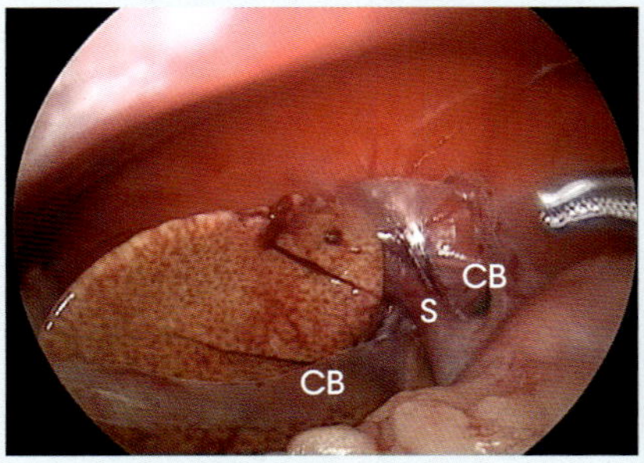

FIGURE 3. After shunt dissection, a cellophane band (CB) is positioned around the abnormal shunt vessel (S).

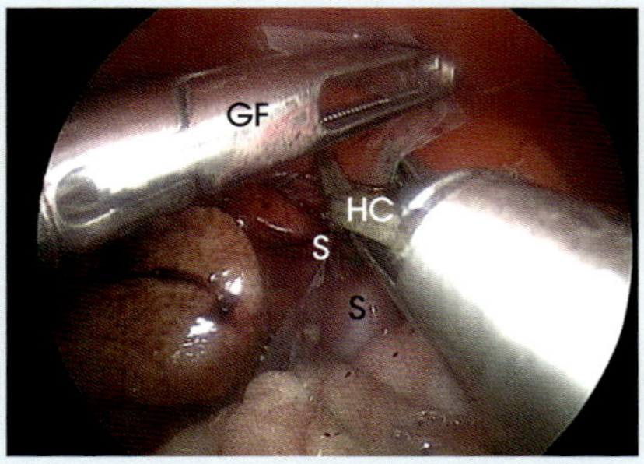

FIGURE 4. The cellophane band is grasped with a laparoscopic grasping forceps (GF) and then secured with hemoclips (HC). S, shunt.

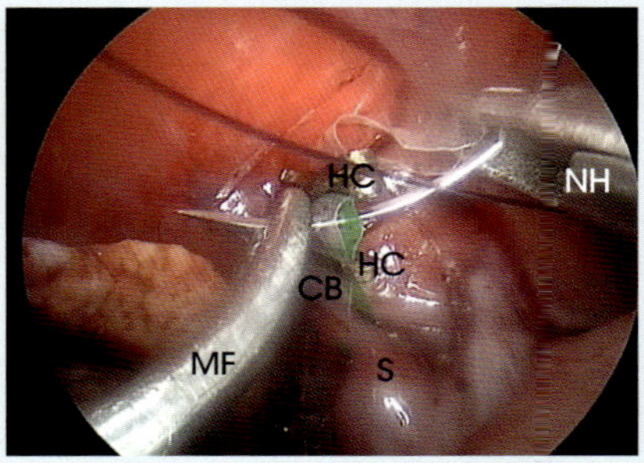

FIGURE 5. Position of a surgical knot with a laparoscopic needle holder (NH) aided with laparoscopic Maryland forceps (MF) to fix the cellophane band (CB), using 3-0 monofilament nonabsorbable nylon suture (Ethilon, Ethicon, Sommerville).
HC, hemoclip; S, shunt.

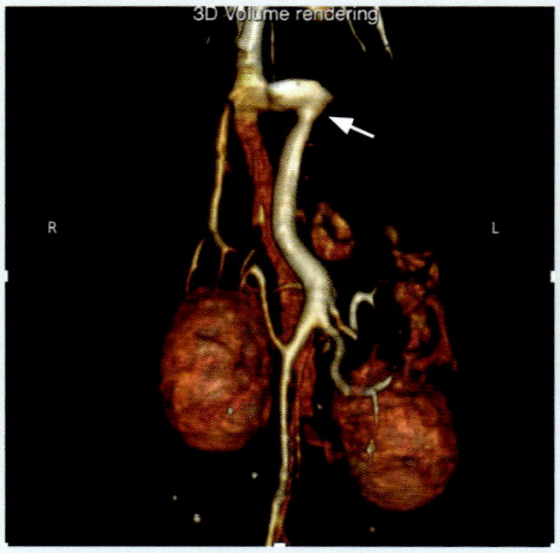

FIGURE 6. 3D presurgical CT scan reconstruction of the shunt vessel (white arrow) in ventrodorsal view.

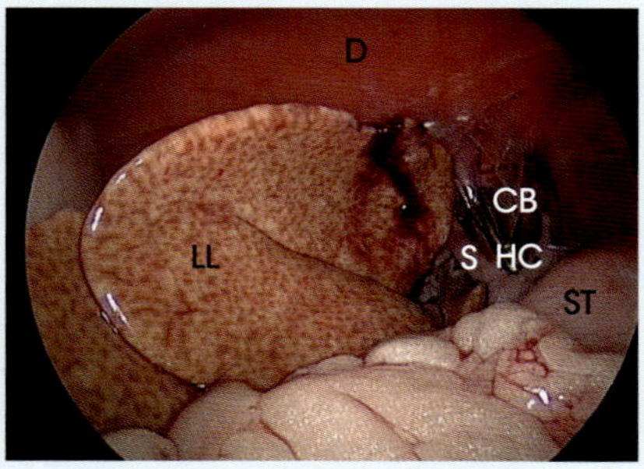

FIGURE 7. Final visualization of the attenuated shunt vessel (S) and adjacent organs. CB, cellophane band; D, diaphragm; HC, hemoclip; LL, left liver lobe; ST, stomach.

Tips and tricks

- ✓ A triangular cushion can be placed under the right lateral side to raise the spine and improve visualization of the shunt.
- ✓ If the stomach is bloated, an orogastric tube can be placed to achieve gastric decompression and reduce gastric contents.

37.5 LAPAROSCOPIC PORTOSYSTEMIC SHUNT ATTENUATION IN A DOG

F. J. Pérez Duarte, J. Gutiérrez del Sol, M. A. Sánchez Hurtado

CASE DESCRIPTION

An 18-month-old, 19 kg mixed-breed dog was presented at the hospital for chronic onset of vomiting, weakness, and weight loss. A serum biochemical profile showed mild elevations in ALT and AST and decreased albumin and globulin levels. Postprandial bile acids were markedly elevated. Abdominal ultrasonography and CT scan revealed a 0.7 mm diameter PSS through the portal vein and left internal iliac vein. Laparoscopic attenuation of the shunt was performed laparoscopically with a cellophane band. The animal had minimal postoperative morbidity, and clinical signs improved.

Key points

- The shunt must be clearly identified by ultrasound or CT before laparoscopic access is considered.
- Be very delicate during the dissection of the shunt to prevent vessel injuries.
- Intraoperative attenuation of the shunt is not necessary and may result in a less favorable outcome.
- Cellophane available from local stores usually is not usually truly cellophane, so only use film bands designed for its use in surgery.

PORT PLACEMENT

The telescope port was established 1–2 cm lateral to the umbilicus on the left side of the abdomen (T1). Two other instrument ports were placed slightly dorsal and lateral to the first trocar (T2 and T3), thus achieving a triangulation between instruments and optics.

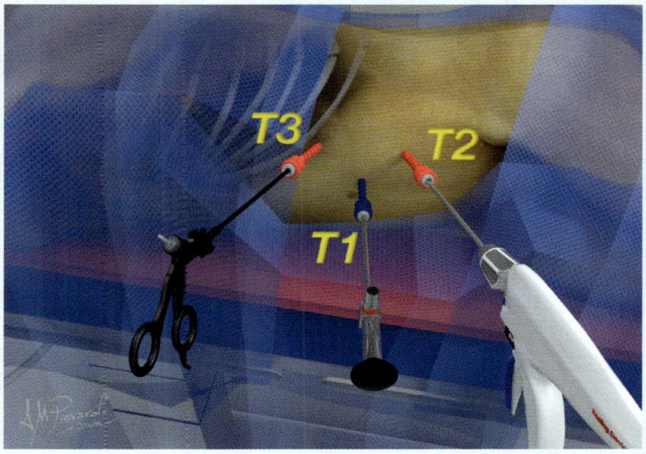

PROCEDURE

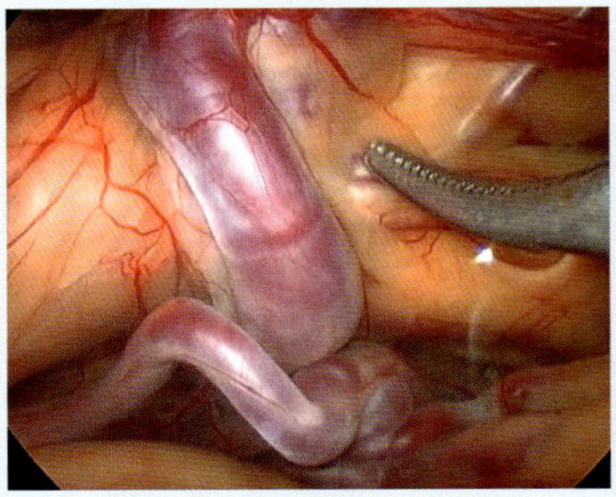

FIGURE 1. Identification of the shunt path between the left kidney and the iliac vein.

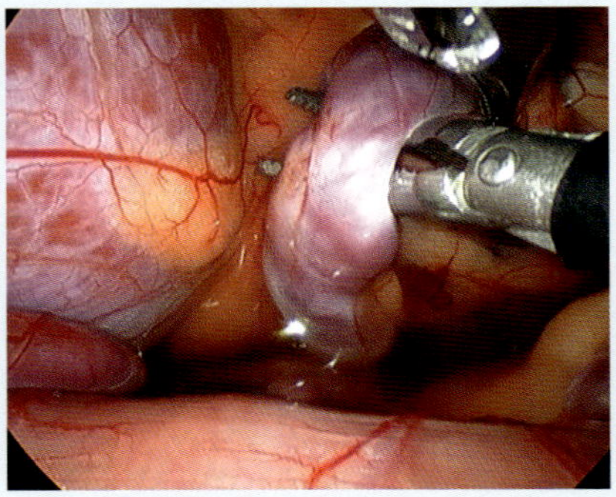

FIGURE 2. Dissection of the shunt is performed, with Maryland and a right-angle dissector, close to its entry into the iliac vein.

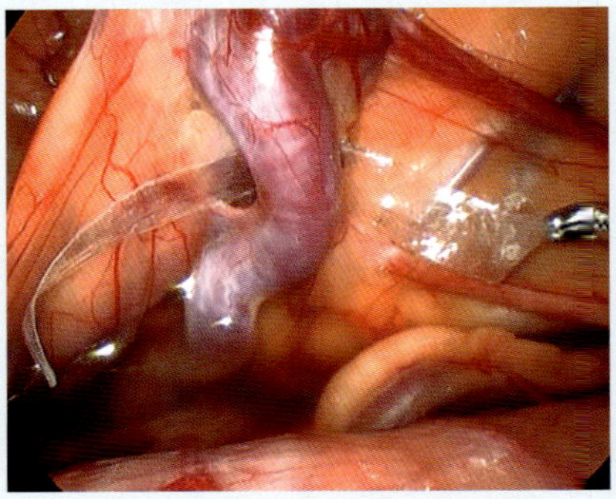

FIGURE 3. Once the shunt has been completely individualized, the cellophane band is passed around it.

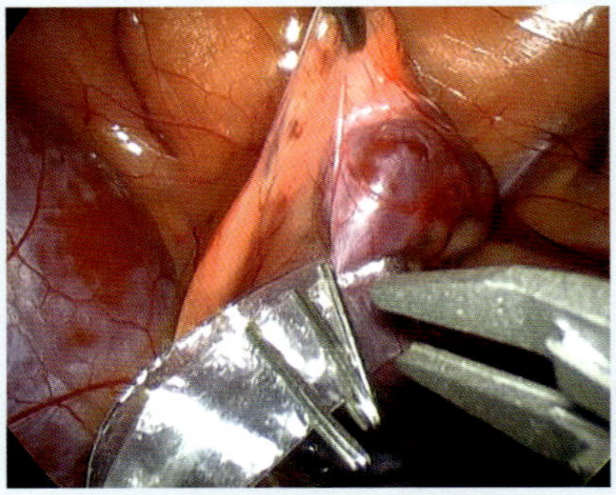

FIGURE 4. The cellophane band is closed with two or three hemostatic clips without attenuating the diameter of the vessel at this point.

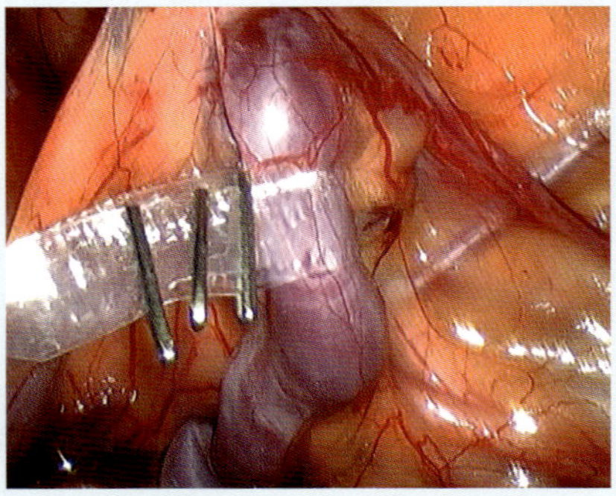

FIGURE 5. Finally, the excess cellophane is trimmed and removed. The intestinal loops should be checked to identify any signs of portal hypertension.

Tips and tricks

- ✓ Due to the small size of some patients, 3 mm instruments are advisable.
- ✓ Usually, three trocars are enough to perform the procedure, but sometimes a fourth trocar or a MiniLap instrument is necessary to achieve a good surgical field exposition.
- ✓ Eliminating the cellophane band's edges helps pass it around the shunt.

38 LAPAROSCOPIC PANCREATIC SURGERY

S. A. van Nimwegen, F. O. Buishand, J. Kirpensteijn

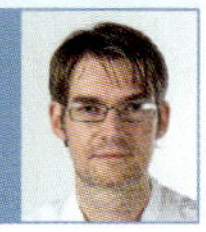

Indications

- Pancreatic biopsy for the identification of pancreatitis
- Excision of isolated pancreatic lesions (masses, pseudocysts, abscesses) in the distal two-thirds of either the right or left pancreatic lobe

Contraindications

- A large pancreatic lesion (larger than one-third of the circumference of the pancreatic lobe) located close to the pancreatic body
- Neoplastic lesions with extensive metastases to abdominal lymph nodes or the liver
- Total pancreatectomy

The use of laparoscopic surgery of the pancreas in companion animals has been limited so far. Several reports on laparoscopic or laparoscopic-assisted pancreatic biopsies have been published, but only two case reports on laparoscopic resection of a canine insulinoma and laparoscopic omentalization of a pancreatic cyst in a cat, respectively. Several large case series in the human field have demonstrated clear advantages of laparoscopic pancreatic surgery over the open approach. Extrapolating this to veterinary medicine provides a rationale for extending the role of laparoscopic pancreatic surgery in companion animals.

DESCRIBED SURGICAL PROCEDURES

The following procedures are described below:

A. Three-port pancreatic biopsy

B. Three-port excision of pancreatic lesions, excluding lesions in the distal left pancreatic lobe

C. Three-port excision of pancreatic lesions in the distal left pancreatic lobe

D. Laparoscopic approach for insulinoma going beyond the pancreas

A THREE-PORT PANCREATIC BIOPSY

According to the literature, a ventral approach using three ports is the most commonly used technique for laparoscopic pancreatic biopsies. It gives full access to the right pancreatic lobe, the corpus, and the proximal part of the left lobe. However, the distal part of the left pancreatic lobe cannot be visualized with this technique. Additionally, sometimes it can be difficult to access the corpus and the left lobe because of their position dorsal to the other abdominal organs. A left flank approach in sternal/oblique recumbence is more suited to reach the distal part of the left pancreatic limb. In case of diffuse pancreatitis, the tip of the right limb of the pancreas is preferably biopsied because it is the most easily accessible. As an alternative, a single-port laparoscopic approach can be considered.

PATIENT PREPARATION AND POSITIONING

Dry food should be withheld 12 hours before surgery, whereas canned food can be fed until 6 hours before surgery. In the case of pancreatitis, attention should be paid to factors that could increase the complication rate, including hypoalbuminemia, disseminated intravascular coagulation, and diabetes mellitus. Any fluid and electrolyte balance abnormalities, coagulation, oncotic pressure, or plasma glucose levels should be corrected preoperatively. The use of prophylactic antibiotics is not generally indicated for laparoscopic pancreatic biopsies.

The abdomen should be clipped ventrally from the xiphoid process to the pubis, and laterally the patient should be clipped to approximately the mid-abdominal level.

The patient should be positioned in dorsal recumbency. Ideally, a (motorized) tilt table is used to allow tilting to the left and to the right, as well as head-up and head-down. For the ventral approach, it is crucial to be able to tilt the patient to the left and to the right. Additionally, a reverse Trendelenburg (head-up) position may improve the visibility of the cranial part of the abdomen. For the flank approach, the dog must be placed in sternal recumbency.

OPERATING ROOM LAYOUT

The surgeon and the assistant stand on the left side of the animal; the assistant is holding the camera and is located a bit behind the surgeon that performs the procedure. The monitor is located on the opposite side of the patient to facilitate a triangulating approach in-line with the monitor (**Fig. 1**). Table position can vary from normal to reversed Trendelenburg, especially for visualization of the corpus and left pancreatic lobe. Left lateral tilt can significantly improve access to the right pancreatic lobe and corpus.

Instruments

On the table:

- Telescope 5 mm – 0° or 30°
- Endoscopic grasping forceps, including Babcock
- 5 mm cup biopsy forceps

Alternatives:

- Pretied loop ligature
- Endoscopic Metzenbaum scissors

PORT PLACEMENT (FIG. 2)

- T1, in the midline, 1 cm caudal to the umbilicus
- T2, on a left paramedian position, lateral to the third mammary gland (if only the right lobe and corpus are accessed, T2 can be placed in the midline, 1–3 cm cranial to the umbilicus, with the patient in left lateral tilt for an easier approach)
- T3, on a right paramedian position, lateral to the third mammary gland
- T4 (optional), based on the intra-abdominal situation

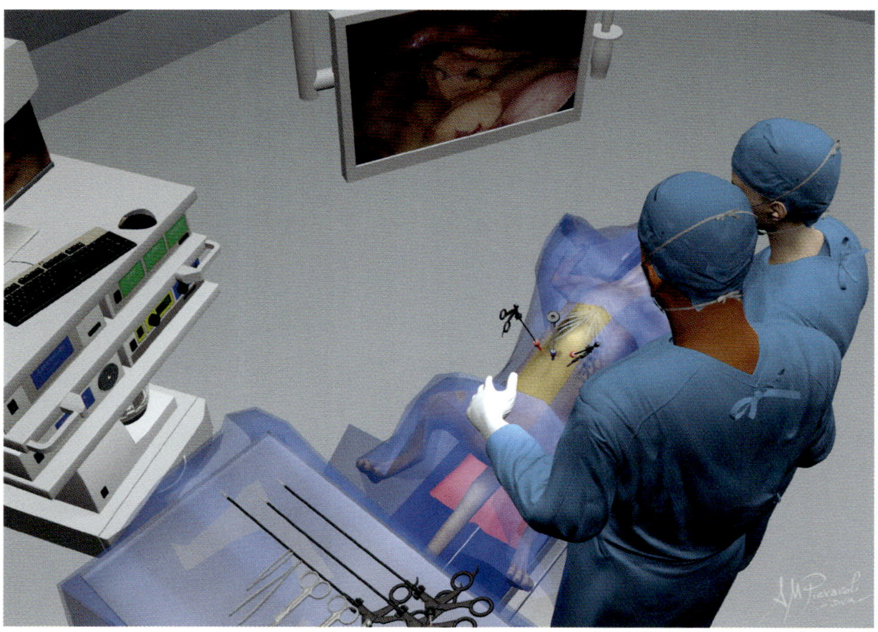

FIGURE 1. Operating room layout for three-port pancreatic biopsy.

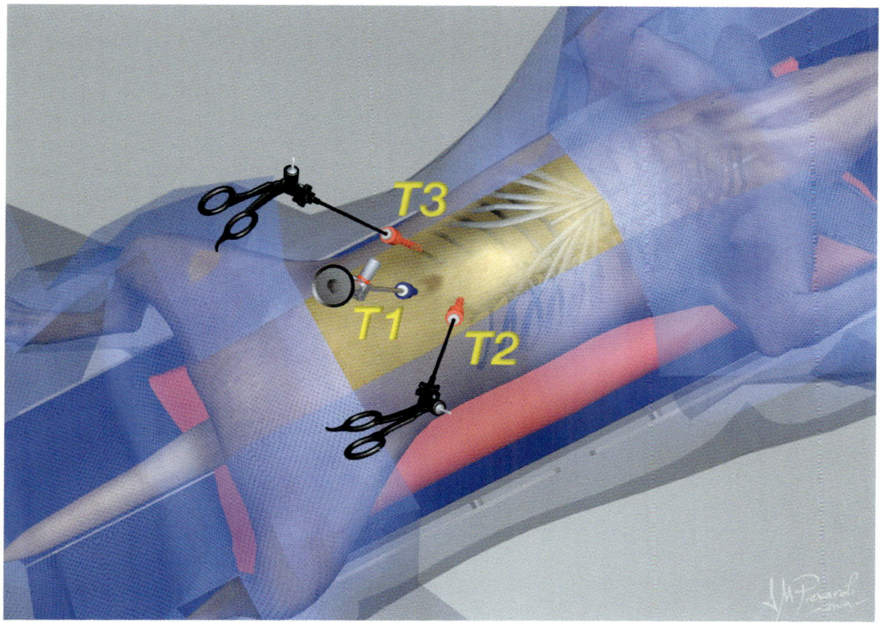

FIGURE 2. Port placement for three-port pancreatic biopsy.

PROCEDURE

- Pneumoperitoneum is established using an open modified Hasson technique with stay sutures in the external rectus sheath and a blunt threaded cannula (T1) for visual guidance of abdominal entry. As an alternative, a Veress needle can be used.
- The other two cannulas, T2 and T3, are placed under visual guidance.
- Lateral tilt of the patient to the left side can significantly facilitate access to the right pancreatic lobe (**Figs. 3a and 3b**).
- Avoid grasping the pancreas directly. Manipulation of the pancreas is preferably done by gently pulling the duodenum towards the left side, further exposing the right lobe's lateral surface. If needed, further manipulation of the pancreatic lobe can be performed by grasping the mesoduodenum just next to the pancreas (**Figs. 3c and 3d**).
- After placing the cup biopsy forceps on the distal edge of the (preferably right) pancreatic lobe, the forceps are closed, and a pause of 10–30 seconds is made to achieve hemostasis (**Fig. 3e**).
- The forceps containing the biopsy are gently tugged away from the pancreas (**Fig. 3f**).
- Alternatively, a pretied loop ligature can be placed and tightened proximal to the biopsy site, and the pancreatic tissue distal to the ligature can be transected using endoscopic Metzenbaum scissors.
- The distal part of the lobe is easily accessible for cup forceps or pretied ligature loop biopsy.

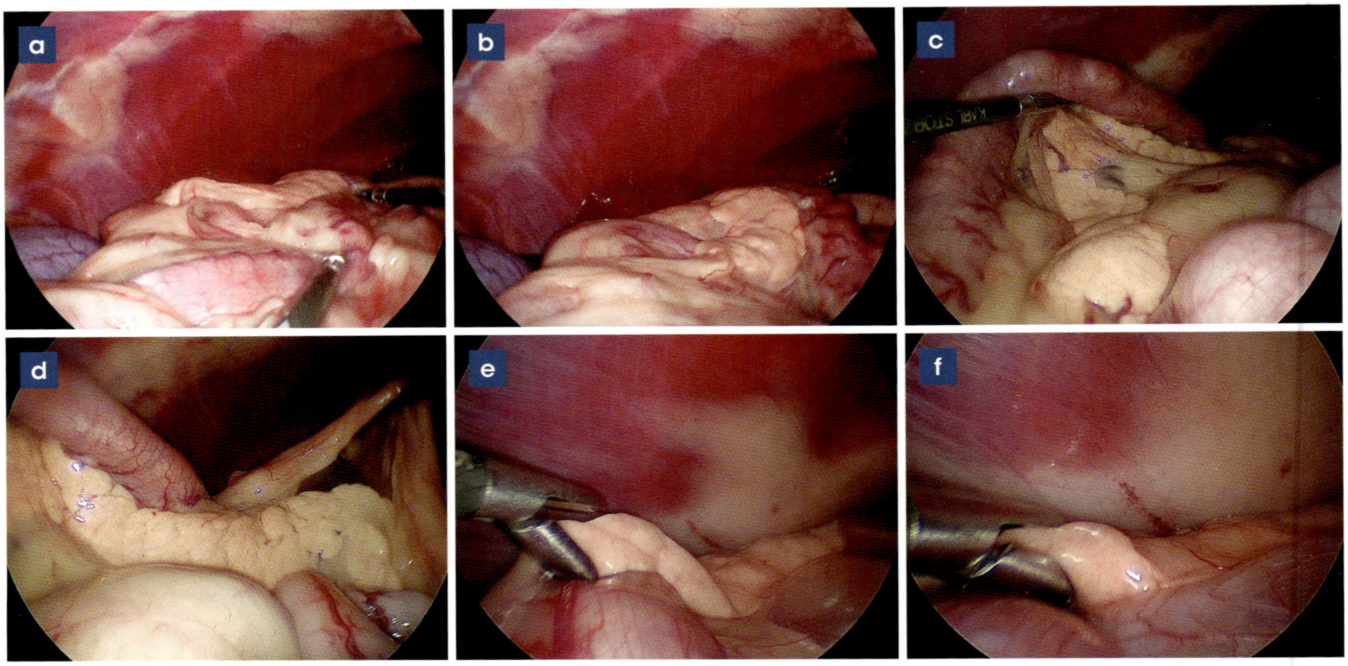

FIGURE 3. Ventral approach to the right pancreatic lobe in dorsal recumbency with 30° left lateral tilt in a 20 kg female mixed-breed dog. a,b) View of the lateral surface of the right pancreatic lobe after retraction of the duodenum to the left side. Especially with some left lateral tilt, the distal part of the lobe can stay in position without further retraction, enabling easy access for biopsy. c,d) View of the medial side of the distal lobe up to the corpus and proximal left lobe of the pancreas. This approach requires continuous upward retraction of the duodenum and/or omentum. e,f) Positioning of cup biopsy forceps on the edge of the distal tip of the right pancreatic lobe.

Key points

- The pancreas should be handled as gently as possible to prevent postoperative pancreatitis. Avoid grasping the pancreas directly for reasons other than the biopsy itself.
- A left lateral tilt can highly improve access to the right pancreatic lobe in dorsal recumbency.
- In case of generalized pancreatic disease, a biopsy of an avascular area of the distal edge of the right lobe is preferred because of easy access and low risk of complications from damage to the ductal system.

B THREE-PORT EXCISION OF PANCREATIC LESIONS, EXCLUDING LESIONS IN THE DISTAL LEFT PANCREATIC LOBE

The corpus, the entire right pancreatic lobe, and the proximal part of the left pancreatic lobe can be approached using either a ventral approach in dorsal recumbency or a right-sided flank approach in sternal/oblique recumbency. Ideally, the patient is positioned on a motorized tilt table so that lateral tilting and (reverse) Trendelenburg can facilitate a good overview of the abdominal cavity. Despite tilting, it can be difficult to use a ventral approach to obtain sufficient visualization of the ventral surface of the corpus and the left pancreatic lobe. A right-sided flank approach may provide better access to the corpus and proximal left lobe. Both approaches are described below.

PATIENT PREPARATION AND POSITIONING

Dry food should be withheld 12 hours before surgery, whereas canned food can be fed up to 6 hours before surgery. Liquid, easily digestible food preparations should be given up to 1–2 hours before surgery in the case of insulinomas and if dogs are clinically hypoglycemic. If clinical signs of hypoglycemia occur in the immediate preoperative period, the dog should be administered 1–5 mL of 50% dextrose intravenously over 10 minutes, based on the clinical effect, to stabilize blood glucose concentrations before surgery. Prophylactic antibiotics are not indicated for laparoscopic pancreas surgery unless the surgical procedure is anticipated to last longer than 90 minutes or there are clinical signs of an active bacterial infection.

In the case of a ventral approach, the abdomen should be clipped from the xiphoid process to the pubis. It is important to perform wide clipping and aseptic preparation because intraoperatively changing the dog's position or converting to an open procedure might be necessary. Therefore, the authors prefer a 360° surgical clip. For a right-sided lateral or a semisternal approach only, the right caudal hemithorax and the lateral abdomen should be clipped and aseptically prepared.

Positioning in dorsal recumbency for a ventral approach should be performed as described for procedure A. To access the right pancreatic lobe, the patient is best tilted over to the left side as far as possible (30° or more). The corpus and the proximal part of the left lobe can be visualized by tilting the dog far to the left side and head up (reverse Trendelenburg position) so that the omentum and spleen move to the left and can be more easily retracted cranially while the intestines move left and caudal.

The patient is placed in sternal or sternal-oblique recumbency for a right-sided flank approach. The sternum and pelvis should be tightly supported using two moldable vacuum or gel-foam cushions, one under the sternum and one between the pelvic limbs supporting the pubis while the abdomen hangs more or less free in between. The patient should be tilted 30°–45° to the left side (sternal-oblique).

Anatomical landmarks

Besides knowledge of the pancreatic anatomy, it is imperative to know the location of the draining lymph nodes of the pancreas in cases of malignant disease. The pancreaticoduodenal, splenic, mesenteric, and hepatic lymph nodes drain the pancreas. Additionally, the colic and gastric lymph nodes most likely also drain the pancreas.

OPERATING ROOM LAYOUT

For the ventral approach, see procedure A (**Fig. 1**). The patient is positioned in sternal and/or left-oblique recumbency for the right-sided flank approach. The surgeon and assistant are located on the right side of the animal; the assistant is holding the camera and standing behind the surgeon performing the procedure. The monitor is located on the opposite side of the patient to facilitate a triangulating approach in-line with the monitor (**Fig. 4**). Up to 30° left lateral tilting improves access to the corpus and proximal left pancreatic lobe.

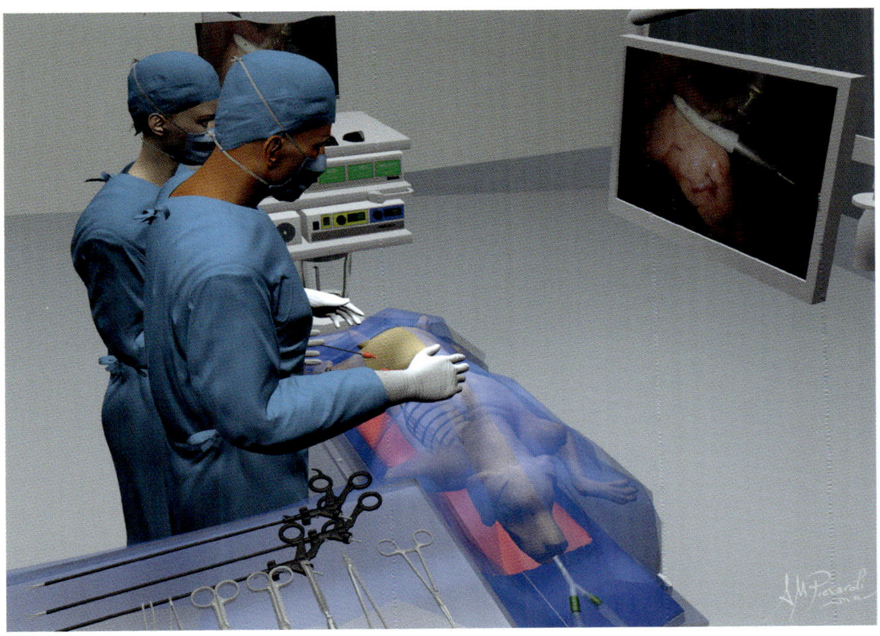

FIGURE 4. Operating room layout for right-sided flank laparoscopic approach to the pancreas.

Instruments

On the table:

- Telescope 5 mm – 0° or 30°
- Endoscopic grasping forceps, including Babcock
- Curved endoscopic dissecting forceps
- Vessel-sealing or ultrasonic device

Alternatives:

- Laparoscopic linear stapler
- Pretied loop ligature

Ready to use:

- Specimen retrieval bag for neoplastic lesions
- Fan retractors
- Endoscopic suction and irrigation instrument
- Endoscopic Metzenbaum scissors

PORT PLACEMENT

Ventral approach (**Fig. 2**):

- T1, T2, T3, similar as described for procedure A
- T4 (optional), placed if needed based on surgeon's preference, for constant retraction of organs

Right-sided flank approach (**Fig. 5**):

- T1, 1–3 cm caudal to the last right rib and 3–5 cm ventral to the transverse spinous processes or epaxial musculature (T1 will turn into T2 if the optic is subsequently positioned between both instruments)
- T2, T3, T4 (optional), placed according to the surgical procedure and intra-abdominal situation, enabling a proper triangulated laparoscopic approach

PROCEDURE

Ventral approach:

- Pneumoperitoneum is established using an open modified Hasson technique using stay sutures in the external rectus sheath and a blunt threaded cannula (T1) for visual guidance of the abdominal entry.
- The other cannulas, T2, T3, and optionally T4, are placed under visual guidance.
- Both sides of the right pancreatic lobe can be inspected by pulling the duodenum ventromedially or grasping and lifting it upward. The dorsal side of the corpus and left lobe can be approached by grasping and elevating the greater omentum and stomach cranially. To visualize the ventral surface of the corpus and left pancreatic lobe, the ventral leaf of the omentum is perforated in an avascular part, and the stomach is pulled cranially in a reverse Trendelenburg position.
- If the lesion is located in the distal right pancreatic lobe, that part of the lobe is grasped using endoscopic grasping forceps, while bipolar vessel-sealing forceps are used to carefully dissect, seal and divide the pancreatic parenchyma proximal to the lesion. The extent of the surgical margin depends on the type of lesion and distance to vital structures,

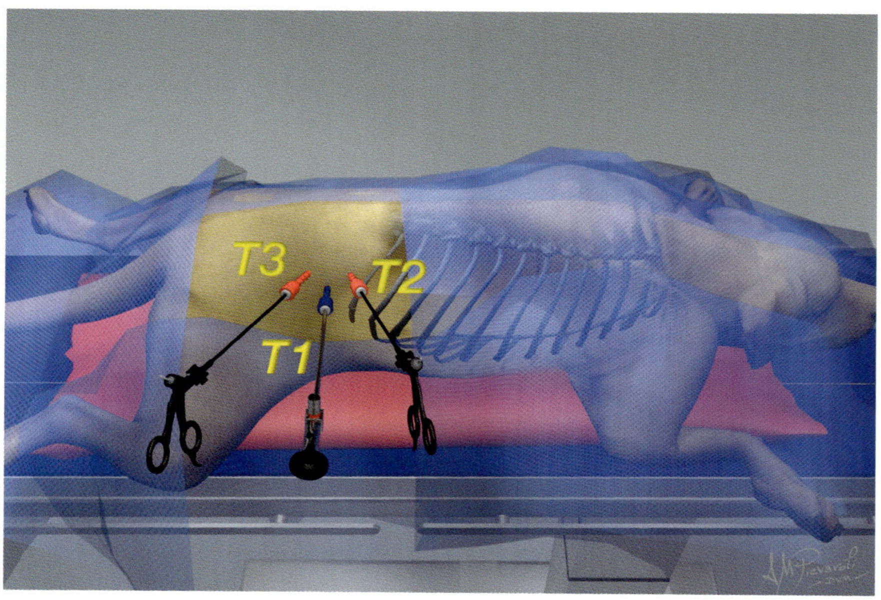

FIGURE 5. Port placement for right-sided flank approach for three-port excision of pancreatic lesions.

including the common bile duct, pancreaticoduodenal artery, and pancreatic ducts.

- Extensive full-thickness excision of the right distal pancreatic lobe may significantly impair duodenal blood supply. When maintaining as much duodenal blood supply as possible in a subtotal (distal) right pancreatectomy and sparing blood supply close to the pancreatic corpus, including the recurrent duodenal arteries arising from the right gastroepiploic artery, the remaining blood supply to the duodenum will usually be sufficient.
- Because the existence of a pancreatic duct in an individual canine patient is uncertain, amputation of the distal right lobe to a level proximal to the accessory pancreatic duct carries an uncertain prognosis.
- Alternatively, a pretied ligature loop, an endoscopic linear stapler, or endoscopic vascular clips can be used for a partial pancreatectomy.
- If the lesion is located close to the pancreatic body, a nodulectomy should be carried out by dissecting closer to the lesion. This is only feasible if the lesion is located at the periphery of the pancreas and is not associated with the larger vessels and pancreatic ducts, and thus comprises only up to one-third of the diameter of the pancreatic lobe.
- Laparoscopic right distal pancreatectomy for treatment of an adhered right ovarian remnant in dorsal recumbency was performed in a Labrador Retriever (**Fig. 6**). The ovarian remnant was closely adhered to and partly encased by the distal pancreatic lobe, covered by adhesions of mesovarial and mesometrial tissues to the distal pancreatic lobe and mesoduodenum. Therefore, it was decided to remove the remnant en bloc with the distal tip of the right pancreatic lobe.

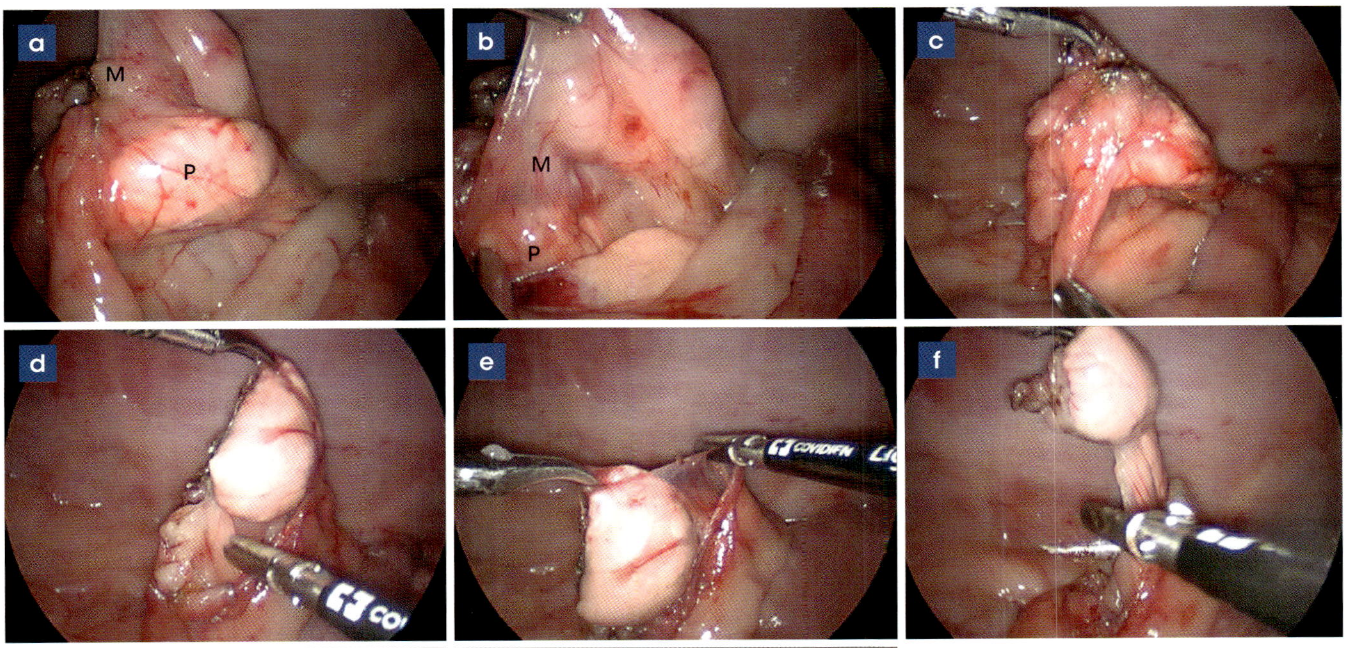

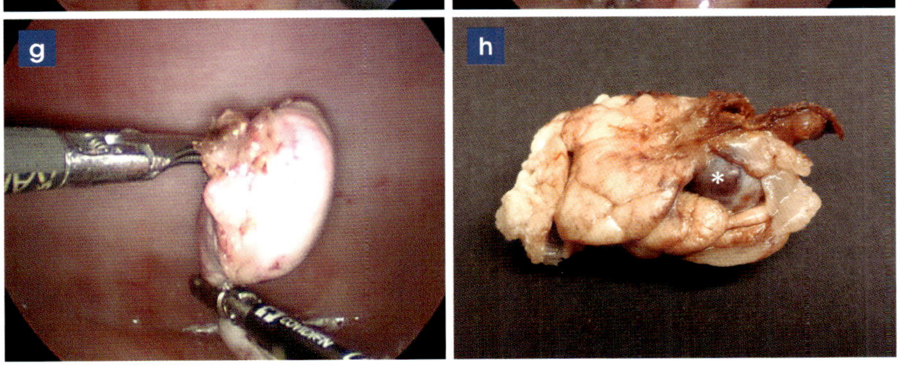

FIGURE 6. Ventral approach to the right pancreatic lobe. a,b) After dissecting adhered mesometrial and omental attachments, the mesovarial adhesions (M) to the distal pancreatic lobe (P) could be visualized. c–e) After dissecting the adhered mesovarial and mesometrial tissues, dissection of the distal pancreatic lobe was commenced, cutting the mesoduodenum close to the pancreatic attachment. f,g) Amputation of the distal tip of the right pancreatic lobe using a vessel sealer/divider instrument. h) Tissue specimen showing the ovarian remnant (*) encased by the adhered pancreatic tissue.

Right-sided flank approach:

- If a Veress needle is used, a towel clamp is used to retract the 13th rib to reduce the risk of puncturing underlying abdominal organs during Veress needle placement. The needle is inserted just caudal to the 13th rib in the right paralumbar fossa. Alternatively, a modified Hasson technique can be used to insert the first port (T1).
- After abdominal insufflation, the other ports, T2, T3, and optionally T4, are placed under visual guidance.
- The lateral surface of the right pancreatic lobe can be visualized and accessed. The proximal part of the right lobe, the corpus, and the proximal part of the left lobe up to the portal vein can be accessed by carefully retracting the liver craniodorsally. The medial surface of the right lobe, the dorsal surface of the corpus, and the proximal part of the left lobe can be approached by lifting the duodenum upward. This approach can also access most of the draining pancreatic lymph nodes.

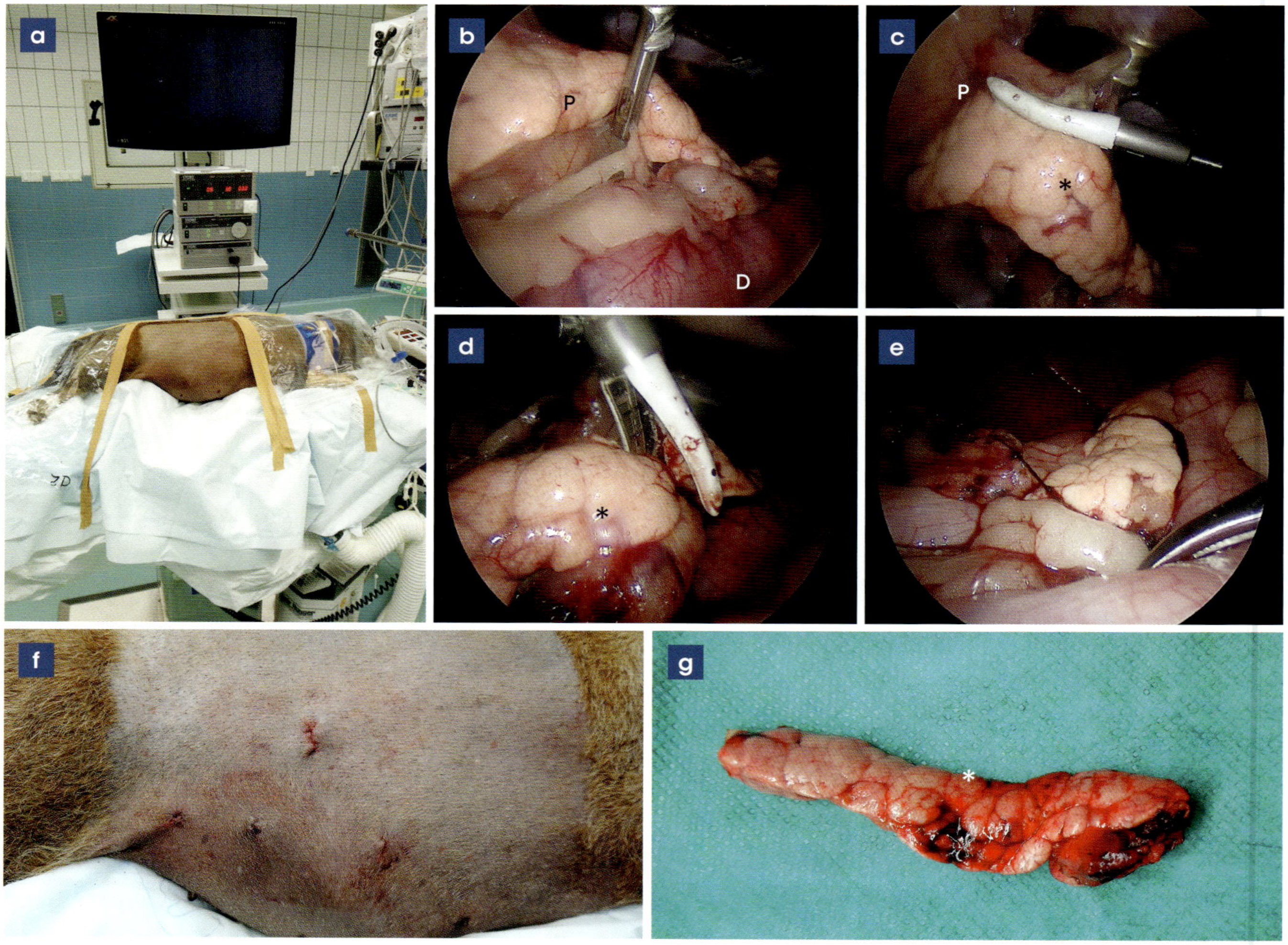

FIGURE 7. Lateral approach to the right pancreatic lobe in a Dachshund. a) The dog was positioned in sternal recumbency with the thorax and pelvis supported and the abdomen hanging freely. The table can be tilted sideways for up to 30°. b) Lateral view of the distal right pancreatic lobe (P) with the relatively small insulinoma (*) located approximately halfway in the right lobe, in the area of the accessory pancreatic duct in close relation to the duodenum (D). c) If possible, the pancreatic lobe distal to the tumor is dissected from its mesoduodenal attachments staying close to the lobe to avoid mesoduodenal blood vessels. Part of the caudal pancreaticoduodenal artery running through the excised part of the pancreatic lobe, together with its branches to the duodenum, are transected. d) Parenchymal transection of the pancreatic lobe just proximal to the insulinoma (*) using a vessel sealer/divider. e) View of the remaining pancreatic lobe after excision of the distal part. f) View of the abdominal wall after surgery. A fourth port was used to gain better access for dissection alongside the distal pancreatic lobe. g) The excised tissue specimen containing the insulinoma (*).

- The partial pancreatectomy or nodulectomy techniques are similar to what has been described for the ventral approach.
- A right distal pancreatectomy to remove an insulinoma in sternal-oblique recumbency was performed (**Fig. 7**). An insulinoma was suspected, and the diagnosis was confirmed after measuring a high plasma insulin level concomitant with hypoglycemia. Triple-phase contrast CT showed a small nodule in the distal half of the right pancreatic lobe without apparent lymphadenopathy or other signs of metastasis. The 1 cm insulinoma was excised en bloc with the distal right pancreatic lobe through a right flank laparoscopic approach in sternal and left-oblique recumbency.

Key points

- The corpus, the entire right pancreatic lobe, and the proximal part of the left pancreatic lobe can be approached using either a ventral or right-sided flank approach.
- Placing the patient in sternal or left-oblique recumbency may improve access to the corpus and proximal left pancreatic lobe using a right lateral approach because less retraction of tissues is needed.
- The pancreatic blood supply should always be identified during surgery, and extreme caution should be taken to prevent damage to the pancreaticoduodenal arteries and the ductal system. However, transection of the caudal pancreaticoduodenal artery running through the right pancreatic lobe is unavoidable when performing distal right pancreatectomies.

C THREE-PORT EXCISION OF PANCREATIC LESIONS IN THE DISTAL LEFT PANCREATIC LOBE

A left-sided laparoscopic flank approach gives access to the dorsocaudal space to the antrum of the stomach, dorsal to the head of the spleen, and ventrolateral to the left kidney and adrenal gland. It will be difficult to access the corpus and proximal section of the left lobe using this approach. Therefore, the authors recommend using this approach exclusively for lesions in the distal part of the left lobe.

PATIENT PREPARATION AND POSITIONING

The patient should be prepared similarly to what has been described for procedure B, and the patient should be placed in sternal recumbency. Refer also to the anatomical landmarks and instruments described in procedure B.

OPERATING ROOM LAYOUT

For a left-sided flank approach in sternal recumbency, both the surgeon and the assistant are to the left of the patient, with the camera holder a bit behind the operating surgeon. The monitor is located on the opposite side of the patient to facilitate a triangulating approach in-line with the monitor (**Fig. 8**). Up to 30° right-lateral tilting may improve access.

PORT PLACEMENT (FIG. 9)

- T1, 1–3 cm caudal to the last left rib and 3–5 cm ventral to the transverse spinous processes or epaxial musculature (T1 will turn into T3 if the optic is subsequently positioned between both instruments)
- T2, T3, T4 (optional), placed according to the surgical procedure and intra-abdominal situation, enabling a proper triangulated laparoscopic approach

PROCEDURE

- If a Veress needle is used, a towel clamp is used to retract the 13th rib to reduce the risk of puncturing underlying abdominal organs during Veress needle placement. The needle is inserted just caudal to the 13th rib in the right paralumbar fossa. Alternatively, a modified Hasson technique can be used to insert the first port (T1).
- After abdominal insufflation, the other ports, T2, T3, and optionally T4, are placed under visual guidance.
- A limited part of the dorsal surface of the left pancreatic lobe can be visualized cranioventrally to the left kidney. After retracting the omentum cranially, a larger part of the lobe can be seen shining through the omentum. The omentum needs to be bluntly perforated in an avascular portion to access the left pancreatic lobe.

- The partial pancreatectomy or nodulectomy techniques are similar to what has been described for procedure B.
- Take care to avoid trauma to the closely related splenic artery and vein during the dissection of the left pancreatic lobe.
- Lateral approach to the left pancreatic lobe (**Fig. 10**). An insulinoma was diagnosed in a Jack Russel Terrier. Triple-phase contrast CT revealed a 2.1 cm tumor situated in the distal part of the left pancreatic lobe without signs of metastasis. A left-sided flank approach in sternal recumbency provided perfect access to the insulinoma without the need for extensive retraction of tissues. The distal part of the pancreatic lobe containing the tumor was excised using a vessel sealer/divider. Blood glucose level increased from 2.2 mmol/L preoperatively to 6.9 mmol/L directly after pancreatectomy. The dog recovered uneventfully and was discharged from the hospital 1.5 days after surgery.

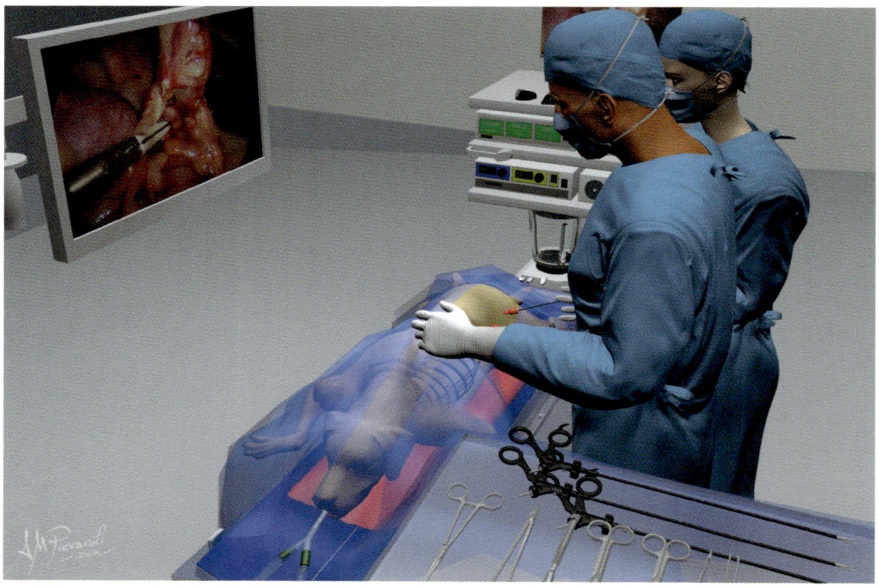

FIGURE 8. Operating room layout for three-port excision of pancreatic lesions in the distal left pancreatic lobe.

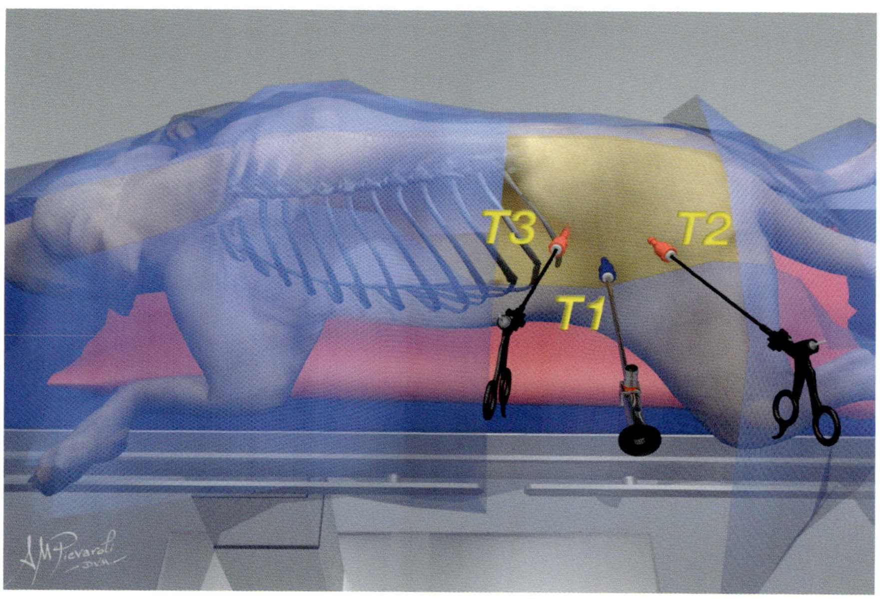

FIGURE 9. Port placement for three-port excision of pancreatic lesions in the distal left pancreatic lobe.

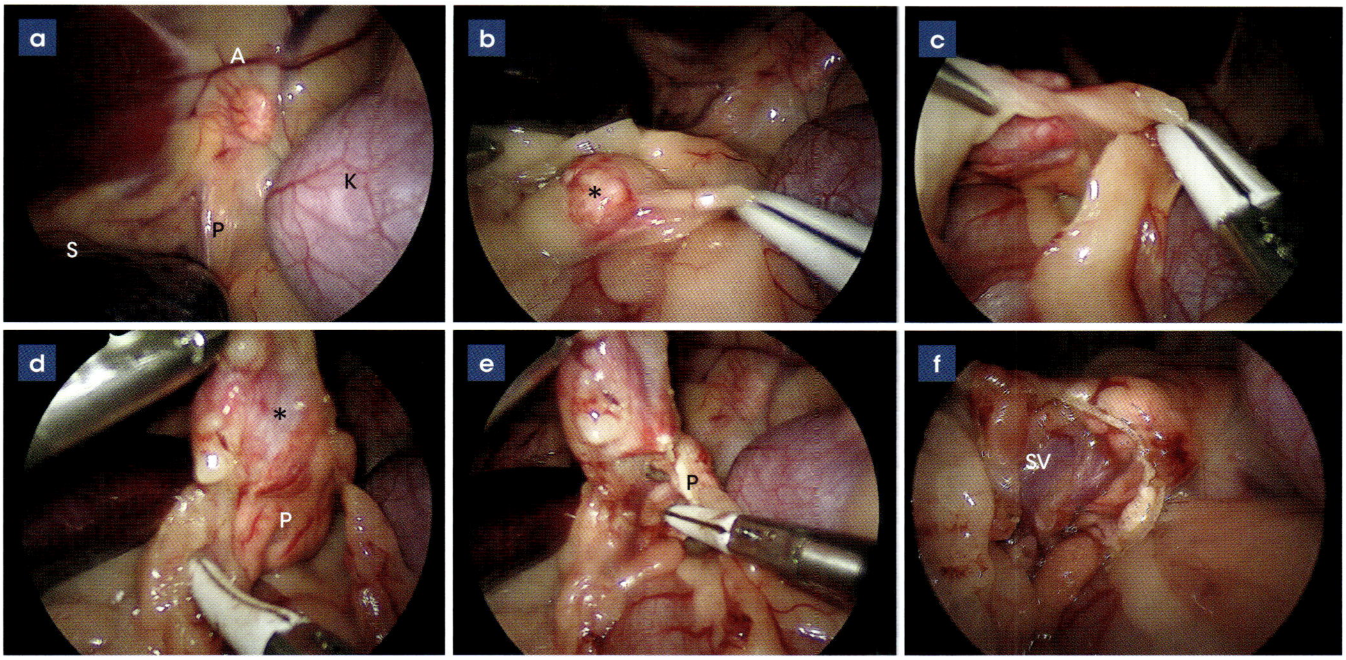

FIGURE 10. a) Overview of the left flank anatomic situation in sternal recumbency, showing the left kidney (K) and adrenal gland (A). The distal tip of the left pancreatic lobe (P) is situated just caudal to the head of the spleen (S) and cranioventrally to the kidney. It can be more or less covered by omentum. b) In this case, the tumor (*) is situated in the distal tip of the left pancreatic lobe and is readily accessible with the left flank approach. c) After creating an opening in the omental leaf close to the pancreas, both sides of the lobe can be observed. d) The tumor (*) and distal lobe (P) are dissected free by transecting the omental attachments, staying close to the lobe to avoid trauma to splenic blood vessels. e,f) The pancreas (P) is transected through normal pancreatic tissue using a vessel sealer/divider. Note the proximity of the splenic vein (SV).

Key points

- The sternal or sternal-oblique position causes passive movement of abdominal organs away from the pancreas.
- The left-sided flank approach should be exclusively used for surgical resection of lesions located in the distal left lobe.
- Lateral traction of the distal part of the left lobe can facilitate access to approximately the distal half of the left lobe in most cases.

D LAPAROSCOPIC APPROACH FOR INSULINOMA GOING BEYOND THE PANCREAS

For successful laparoscopic treatment of insulinomas, several important aspects should be taken into account. Canine insulinomas show a high rate of metastasis to various draining lymph nodes and the liver, and disease staging, as well as postoperative plasma glucose levels, are important prognostic factors for survival time. A complete laparoscopic evaluation of the liver and all possible draining lymph nodes is often laborious and sometimes considered nonfeasible. Furthermore, as discussed, the preferred laparoscopic approach to the pancreas highly depends on tumor location. Therefore, complete preoperative tumor staging should be performed, preferably by triple-phase contrast CT and (fine needle) biopsy of any abnormalities. Any abnormal lymph node on preoperative imaging should be assessed surgically and should thus be taken into consideration when planning a laparoscopic approach. The liver should be inspected during surgery, and any lesions encountered should be biopsied. The authors then suggest doing a quick but thorough laparoscopic evaluation of all visible lymph nodes.

Hyperglycemia and normoglycemia directly after insulinomectomy are associated with better survival. If plasma glucose levels do not increase to at least normoglycemia within 10–20 minutes after insulinomectomy, further dissection of possible draining lymph nodes by laparoscopic or open techniques should be considered. Therefore, it is also advised to locate normal-appearing possible draining lymph nodes on preoperative imaging and preemptively consider the options of surgical excision in your planned surgical approach, should plasma glucose levels stay below the normal range.

POSTOPERATIVE MANAGEMENT

- Direct postoperative constant-rate infusion of fentanyl at an IV dosage of 5–10 µg/kg/h is commonly used for analgesia. One day after surgery, fentanyl is usually discontinued and replaced by 0.2 mg/kg IV methadone every 4 hours or 15–20 µg/kg IV buprenorphine every 8 hours until discharge. In severely painful patients, 3–5 µg/kg/minute IV constant-rate infusion of ketamine can be added.
- Otherwise healthy patients can usually be discharged 2 days after surgery with 2 mg/kg PO carprofen twice a day. Alternatively, tramadol (3–5 mg/kg PO every 6–8 h) and/or gabapentin (5–10 mg/kg PO every 8–12 h) can be used if nonsteroidal anti-inflammatory drugs are contraindicated.
- Offering an easily digestible, balanced, and complete diet right after surgery is well tolerated by most patients. A balanced electrolyte solution should be administered IV if a patient is not consistently eating.
- When patients show clinical signs of pancreatitis that persist for more than 24 hours after surgery, further diagnostics should be performed, including serum lipase activity.
- Patients that demonstrate vomiting and inappetence should be supported with additional therapy that could include maropitant, metoclopramide, omeprazole, and/or ranitidine for several days.
- Blood glucose levels should be closely monitored after insulinoma resection. If severe hypoglycemia (<2 mmol/L) occurs and the patient is not eating and demonstrates clinical signs of hypoglycemia, the patient should be stabilized using a balanced electrolyte solution with 5% dextrose IV. Therapy with diazoxide (5–30 mg/kg twice daily) should also be initiated.
- Some dogs will develop hyperglycemia after insulinoma resection due to atrophy of the normal β cells by feedback inhibition. Hyperglycemia may be transient and resolve with time, but if it is persistent, insulin administration is required. Eventually, the normal pancreatic endocrine function will resume in most cases, although some dogs may require lifelong insulin therapy.

Complications of laparoscopic pancreatic surgery

- Pancreatitis
- Pancreatic fistula
- Persistent bleeding from the pancreatic parenchyma
- Surgical-site infection
- Wound dehiscence

SUGGESTED READINGS

CLINICAL CASES

38.1 PANCREATECTOMY IN A CASE OF INSULINOMA

David García Rubio

CASE DESCRIPTION

A 9-year-old dog was presented with sporadic, spontaneous episodes of weakness. The blood analysis showed hypoglycemia and high insulin serological levels. A CT scan confirmed the presence of an insulinoma on the distal part of the left lobe of the pancreas.

Key points

- An initial CT scan is recommended to rule out metastasis and precisely locate the tumor. In laparoscopic surgery, the option of palpating the pancreas to detect the mass is lacking, which is one of the techniques used in open surgery to locate them; for this reason, prior localization via imaging is essential.
- The difficulty with surgery and the capacity to perform it with minimal invasion will highly depend on the location of the mass, with the apex areas of the pancreas the simplest to operate on.

PORT PLACEMENT

The patient was placed in dorsal recumbency, and the first 5 mm optical trocar (T1) was inserted in the mid-infraumbilical position. Then, the patient was placed in left lateral recumbency, and pneumoperitoneum was established. Two accessory 5 mm trocars (T2, T3) were placed cranial and caudal to T1 and slightly displaced to the left side of the abdomen.

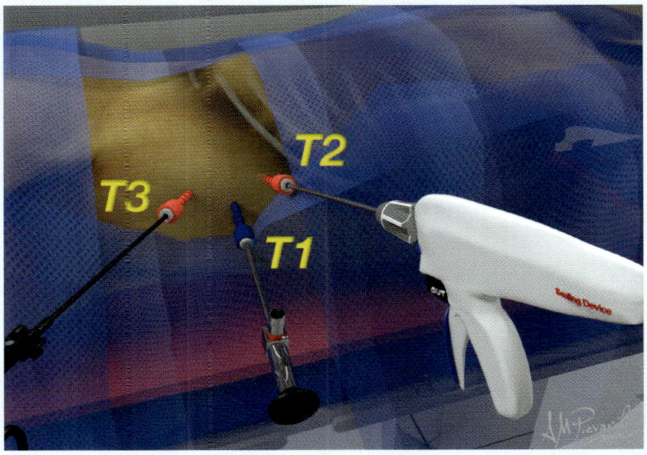

PROCEDURE

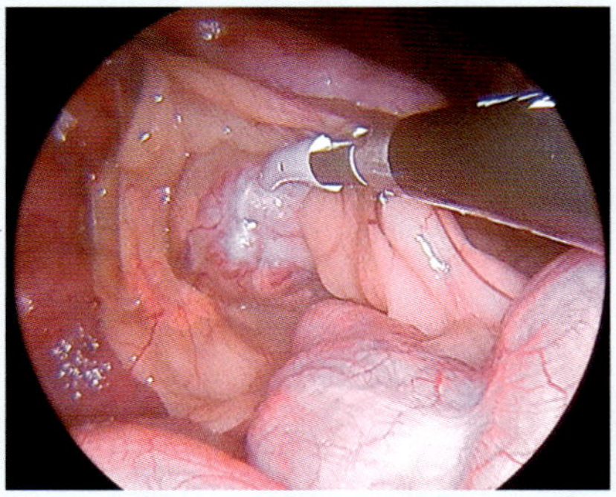

FIGURE 1. Traction of the descending duodenum using atraumatic forceps and localization of the insulinoma, visible as a round mass that is slightly paler than the surrounding pancreatic tissue.

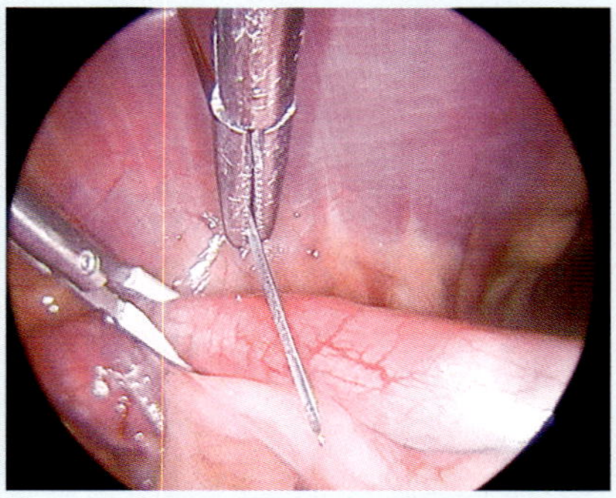

FIGURE 2. Inserting a suture using a straight needle from the outside facilitates the fastening of the duodenum.

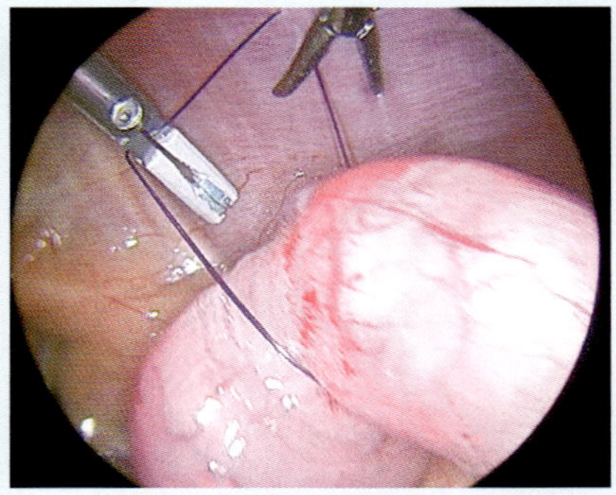

FIGURE 3. After surrounding the duodenum, taking care not to puncture any vessels, the needle is externalized again, and the knot is tightened from the outside. This step is repeated in a more cranial location of the duodenum to fix it at two points, allowing the pancreas to be comfortably explored.

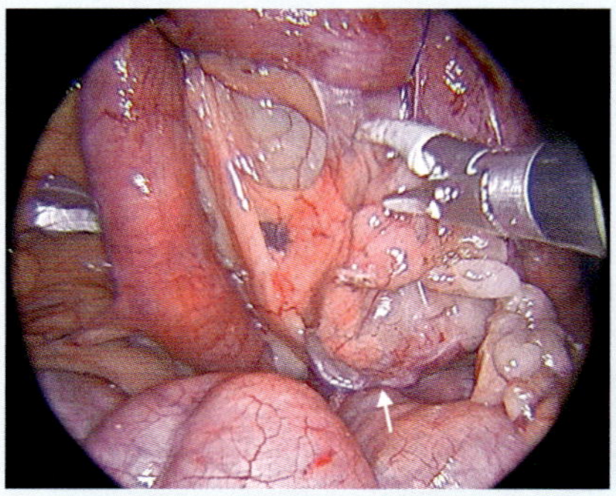

FIGURE 4. Image of the left lobe of the pancreas after extracorporeal fixing. The arrow indicates the neoplasia.

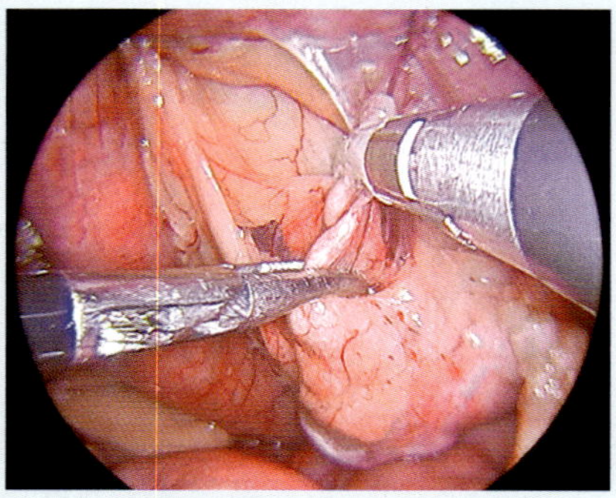

FIGURE 5. Using a bipolar sealing device, the tissues and blood vessels surrounding the area of the pancreas to be removed are cauterized and cut.

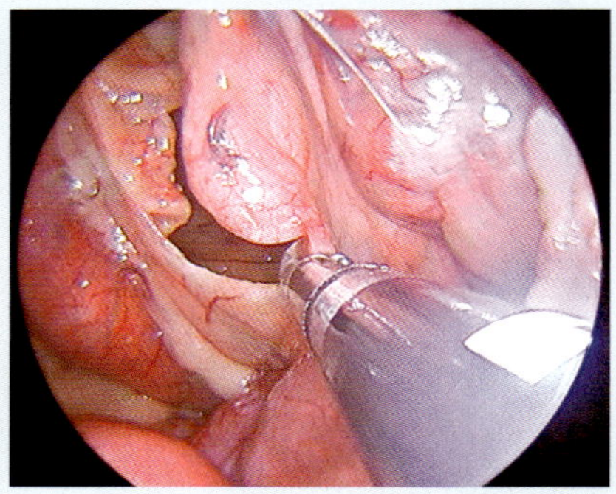

FIGURE 6. Then, dissection is performed, starting with the medial area of the mesoduodenum.

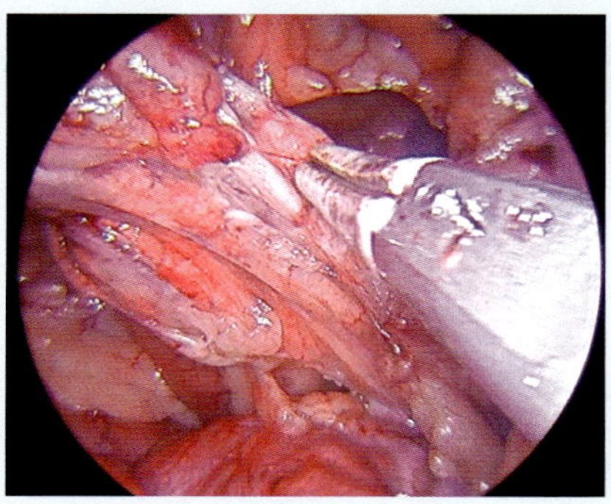

FIGURE 7. Lastly, the separation of the mass from the rest of the pancreas, which continues in a cranial direction, is carried out in the same way. The pancreatic duct can be seen in the image in white, indicated by the tip of the forceps.

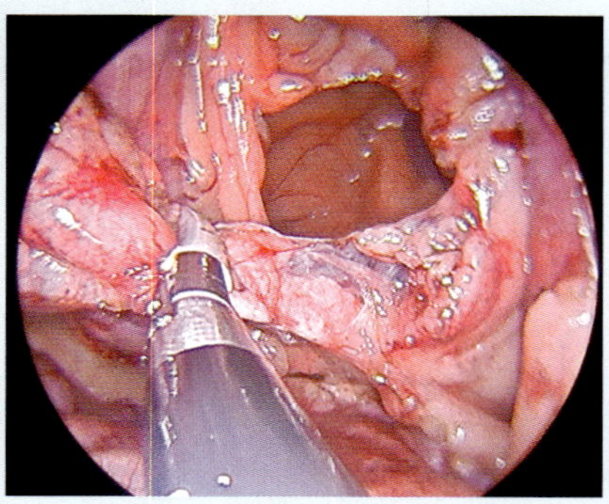

FIGURE 8. Coagulation and cutting of both sections using the bipolar sealing device and complete mass removal.

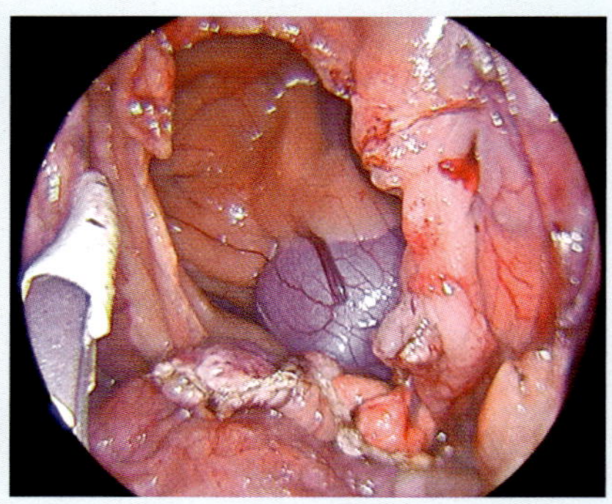

FIGURE 9. Final appearance of the defect following extirpation of the insulinoma.

Tips and tricks

✓ For traction of the duodenum (in left neoplasia) or stomach (in right neoplasia), a fourth trocar or extracorporeal sutures, as in the case described, may be used.

✓ The use of bipolar sealing devices facilitates and really accelerates dissection without bleeding of the adjacent tissue and the pancreatic tissue.

38.2 LAPAROSCOPIC RIGHT LATERAL PANCREATIC LOBECTOMY IN A DOG

Edoardo Poggi, Filippo Cinti, Francesca Izzo

CASE DESCRIPTION

A 6-year-old male Australian Shepherd dog was referred for laparoscopic surgical resection of a right lobe pancreatic mass (1.5 cm), diagnosed with CT scan (**Fig. 1**).

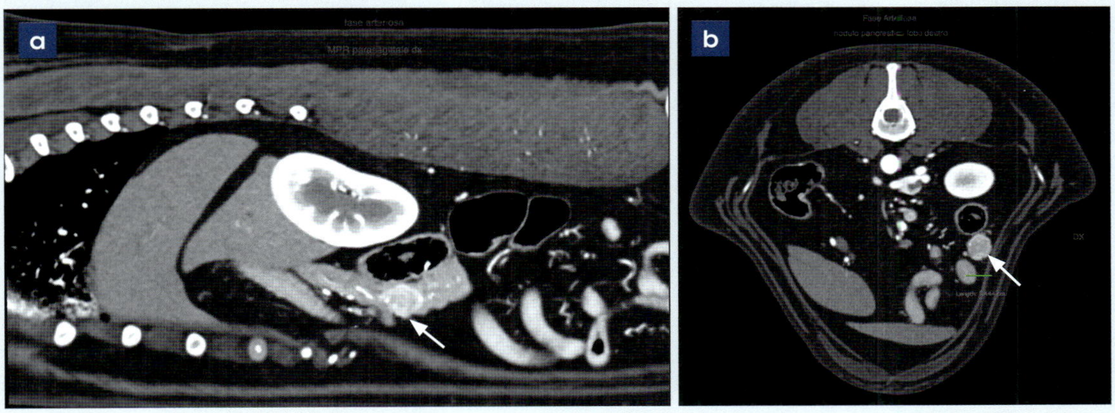

FIGURE 1. a) Sagittal and b) transverse views showing the pancreatic mass (white arrows).

Key points

- CT scan revealed a right lateral pancreatic lobe mass (1.5 cm).
- The dog is aseptically prepared and positioned first in dorsal recumbency to place the primary port (T1). After that, the patient is turned to the left side, and the other instrument ports (T2 and T3) are placed in a triangulated fashion around the mass.
- Before starting with the dissection, the pancreas is grasped with atraumatic laparoscopic grasping forceps.

PORT PLACEMENT

A laparoscopic four-port technique was used to approach the pancreas. The dog was aseptically prepared and positioned in dorsal recumbency to establish the first port with a modified Hasson technique. The patient was then turned into left lateral recumbency, and two ports were placed in the right abdominal flank in a triangulating fashion around the right pancreatic limb. The fourth port was placed dorsally for organ retraction. With the ports in position, the right lobe of the pancreas was visualized laparoscopically with a 5 mm 30° laparoscope.

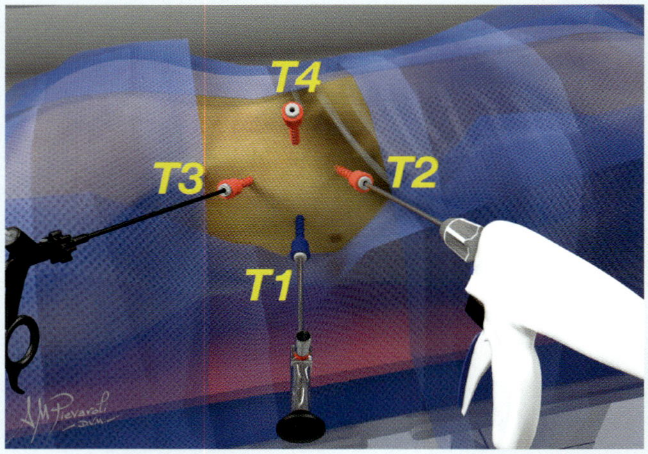

PROCEDURE

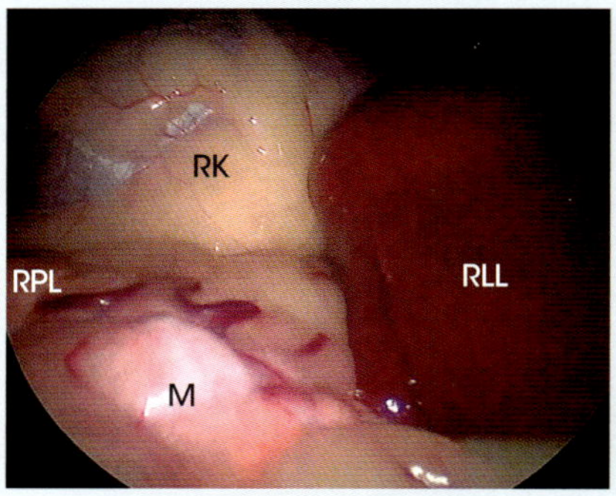

FIGURE 2. Laparoscopic visualization of the mass (M) and adjacent organs. RK, right kidney; RLL, right liver lobe; RPL, right pancreatic lobe.

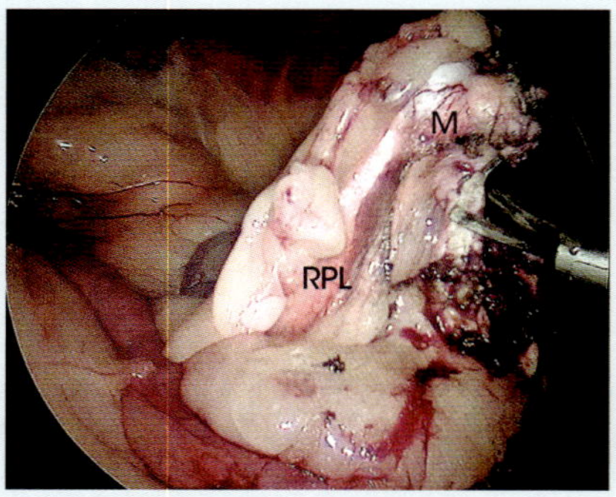

FIGURE 3. After visualization of the mass, the right pancreatic lobe (RPL) is grasped with atraumatic laparoscopic grasping forceps, and the mass (M) is dissected with a ultrasonically activated harmonic scalpel blade.

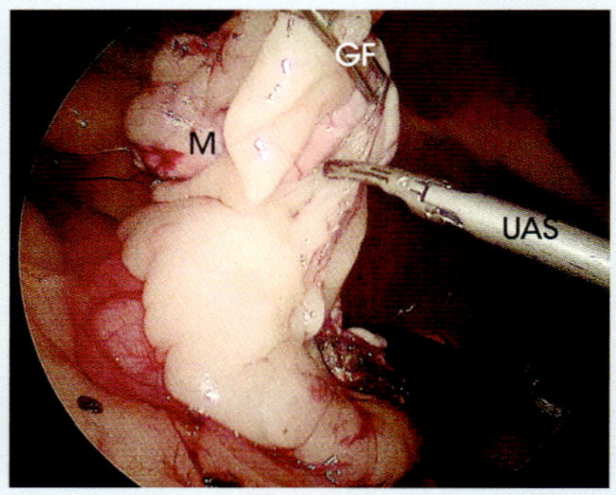

FIGURE 4. The ultrasonically activated scalpel is set up at a power level of 3 (75% of full power) in the knife mode. No massive bleeding or other intraoperative complications are seen. The right limb of the pancreas with the mass (M) is freed from the duodenum with an ultrasonically activated scalpel (UAS) aided with laparoscopic grasping forceps (GF).

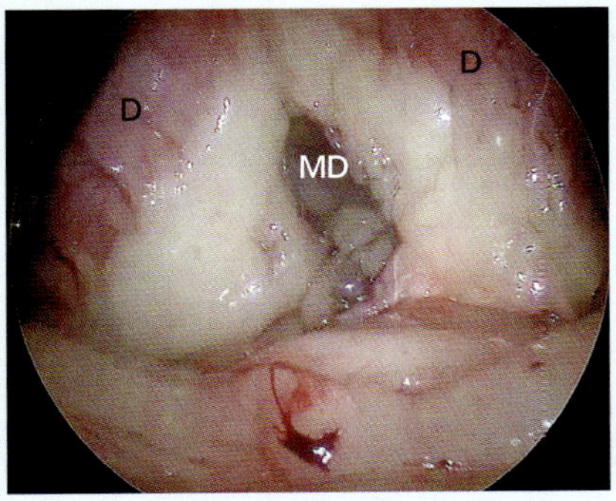

FIGURE 5. A large part of the right pancreatic lobe was resected and dissected from the duodenum and mesoduodenum. Visualization of the duodenum (D) and mesenteric defect (MD).

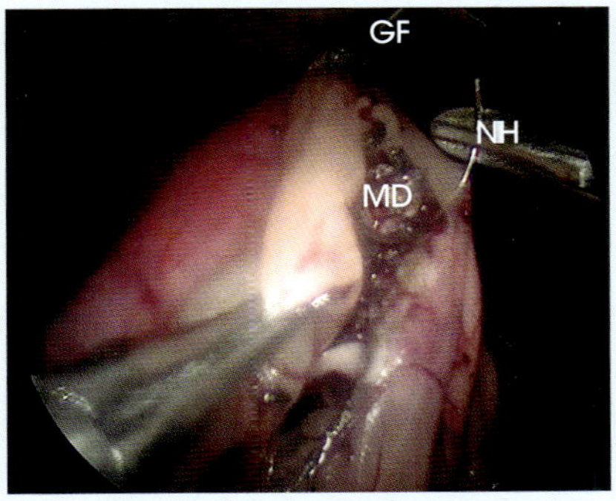

FIGURE 6. After complete resection of the mass, the mesenteric defect is closed with a simple interrupted suture pattern using a 4-0 monofilament absorbable glyconate suture. Beginning of the laparoscopic suture with a laparoscopic needle holder (NH) aided with laparoscopic grasping forceps (GF) to close the mesenteric defect (MD).

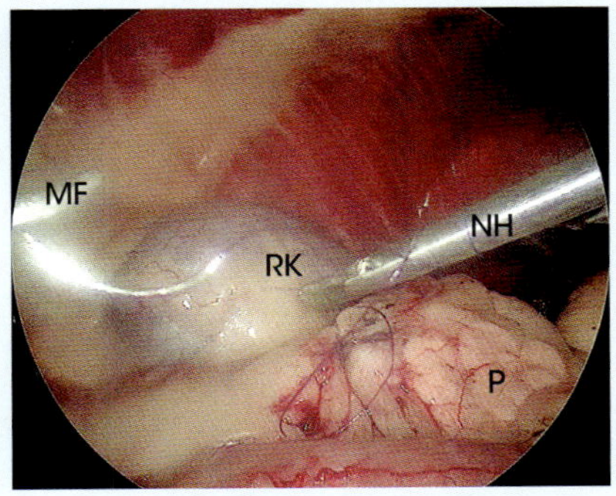

FIGURE 7. Visualization of the last knot of the laparoscopic suture with suture instruments (NH, needle holder; MF, Maryland forceps) and adjacent organs. RK, right kidney; P, pancreas.

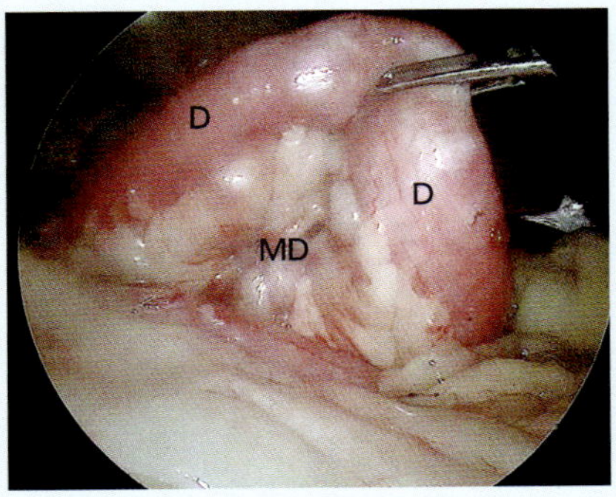

FIGURE 8. The final check shows the duodenum (D) with the sutured mesenteric defect (MD) and a correct hemostasis.

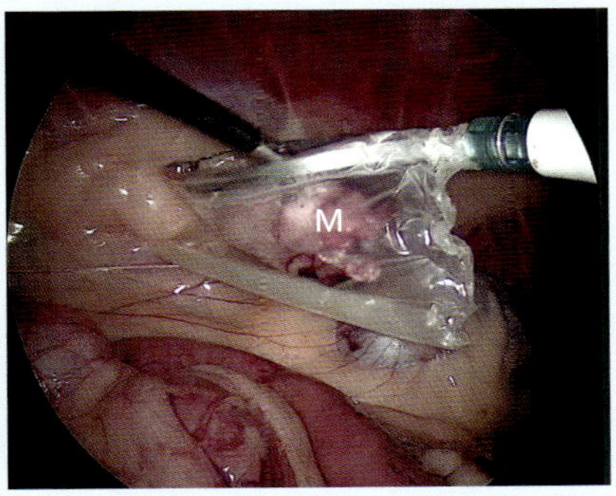

FIGURE 9. The mass (M) is placed into the specimen retrieval bag and the bag containing the mass is exteriorized and then removed through the port incision. At this point, the cannulas are removed after purging of the pneumoperitoneum. The port incisions are closed routinely by placing sutures in the muscular fascia and then closing the skin with an intradermal suture pattern.

Tips and tricks

- ✓ To establish T1, it is easier to put the patient first in dorsal recumbency and then turn it on left lateral recumbency to position the other ports (T2 and T3).
- ✓ To promote hemostasis on the dissected hepatic parenchyma, it is possible to put pieces of hemostatic gelatin sponge (Gelfoam) or regenerated cellulose (Tabotamp).
- ✓ The mesenteric defect was closed with a simple interrupted suture pattern. After that, the mass was put into a specimen retrieval device and finally removed through an enlarged abdominal incision.

38.3 LAPAROSCOPIC OMENTALIZATION OF A PANCREATIC CYST IN A CAT

Michael Brückner

CASE DESCRIPTION

A 15-year-old spayed female domestic shorthair cat was presented with a 1-year history of daily vomiting. Abdominal ultrasound demonstrated a well-defined multilobulated cystic structure located between the spleen and left kidney. Laparoscopic exploration revealed that the cystic structure originated from the left pancreatic limb. With laparoscopic guidance, the structure was percutaneously drained. A partial cystectomy was then performed, with omentalization of the cyst. Clinical signs initially improved, but the patient developed multiple small pancreatic cysts throughout the whole pancreas over the next year.

Key points

- The cyst was drained percutaneously.
- The cyst wall was temporarily suspended from the abdominal wall with a percutaneous needle–suture combination.
- Endoclips were used to avoid intracorporeal suturing.

PORT PLACEMENT

Two 6 mm Endotip trocars were placed, one in the umbilicus (T1, camera port) and one halfway between the umbilicus and the pubic rim (T3).

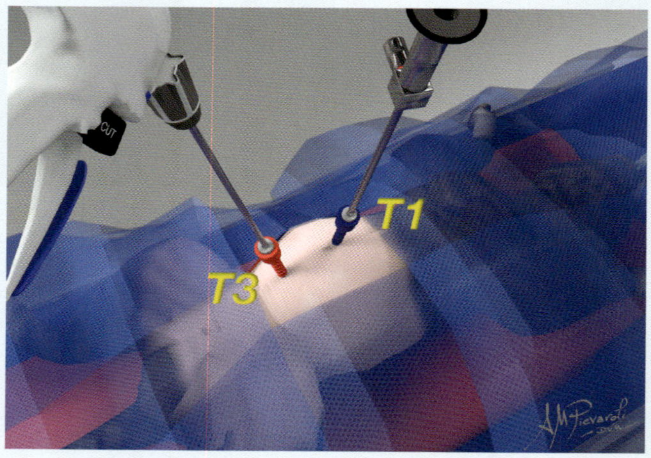

PROCEDURE

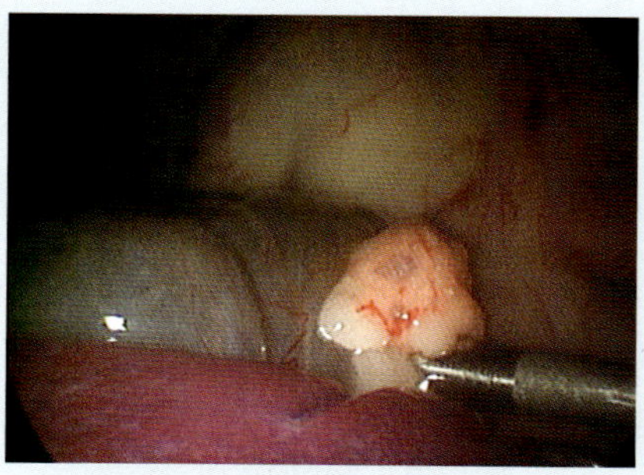

FIGURE 1. The palpation probe is on the tip of the left limb of the pancreas in front of the pancreatic cyst. The spleen is in the bottom left corner.

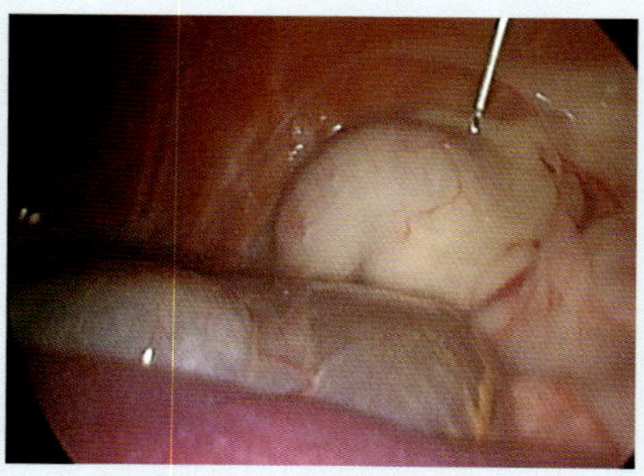

FIGURE 2. A spinous needle is percutaneously inserted to empty the cyst fluid before opening the cyst.

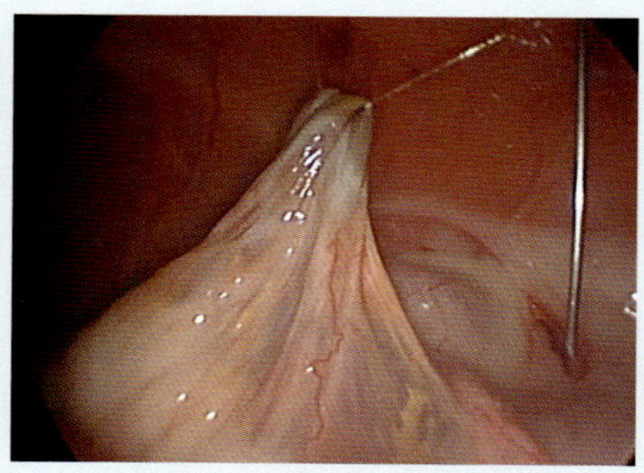

FIGURE 3. The cystic wall is suspended with a percutaneous suture, and the spinal needle is left in place to empty the remaining fluid

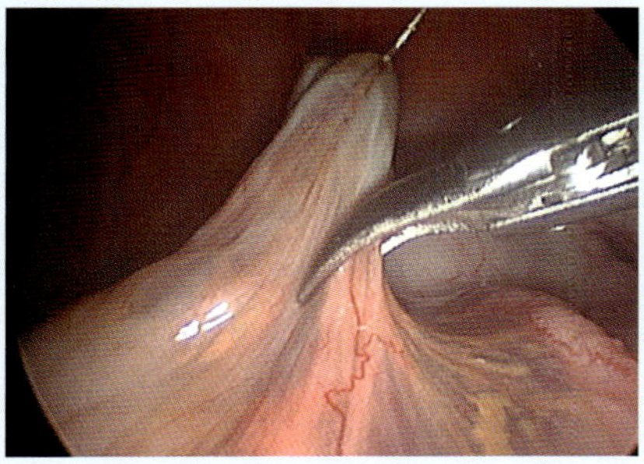

FIGURE 4. Endoscopic scissors are used to incise the capsule before partial cystectomy is performed with a vessel-sealing device. The normal pancreas is visible to the right of the image.

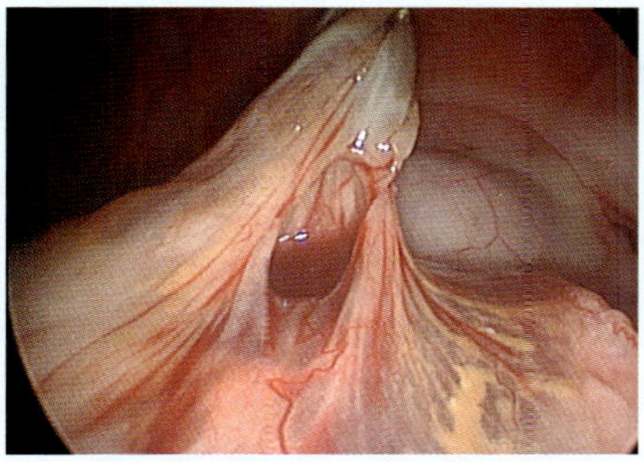

FIGURE 5. The remaining fluid can be removed via the spinal needle under visual guidance through the opening in the cyst wall.

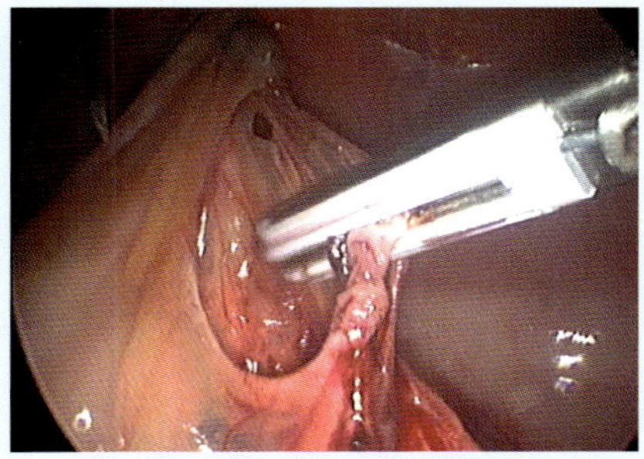

FIGURE 6. The vessel-sealing device is used for partial cystectomy, allowing to retrieve tissue for histopathologic analysis.

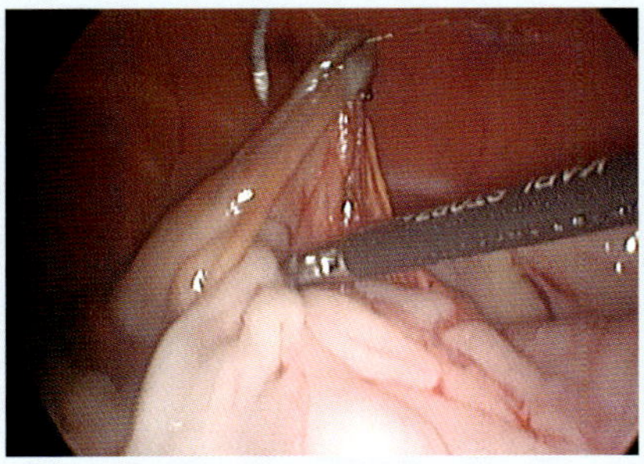

FIGURE 7. Omentum is inserted into the remaining cyst wall with the help of endoscopic grasping forceps.

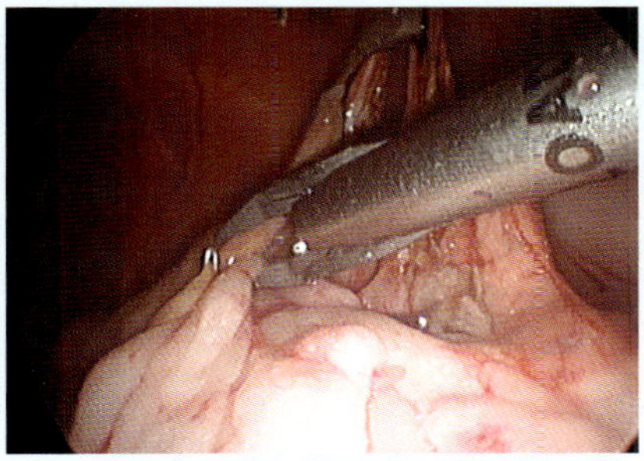

FIGURE 8. An endoclip applier is used to fixate the omentum to the wall of the pancreatic cyst.

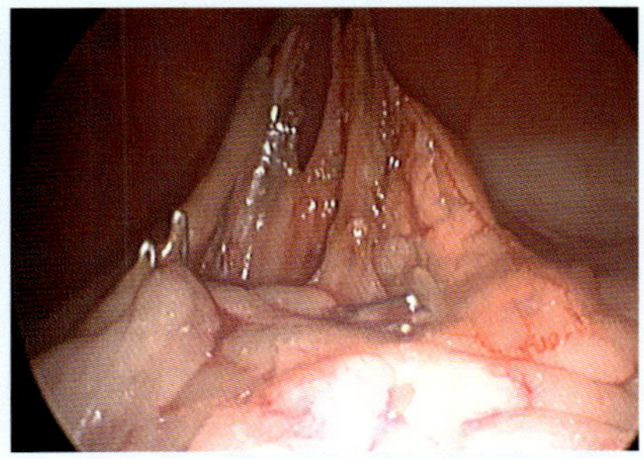

FIGURE 9. Final image after fixation of the omentum with two endoclips on each side of the cystic wall.

Tips and tricks

- ✓ Drain the cyst with a spinal needle inserted percutaneously.
- ✓ Open the cystic wall with scissors.
- ✓ Resect the cyst using a vessel-sealing device.
- ✓ The use of endoclips avoids the need for intracorporeal suturing with barbed sutures.

39 LAPAROSCOPIC SPLENECTOMY

Maurici Batalla

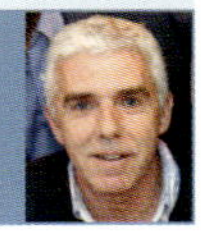

Indications

- Treatment of spleen masses, diffuse neoplasms, hematomas, torsions, traumas, abscesses, and immune-mediated diseases. Hemangiosarcoma is, notably, the most common neoplasm in the spleen of dogs.
- Masses and spleens that are not very large or excessively friable. It is a subjective criterion that depends on the size of the spleen concerning that of the abdomen and on the surgeon's experience in assessing the case.
- In short, it consists of working with a spleen that allows intra-abdominal mobilization without traumatizing it due to its weight or friability, or that its extraction outside of the abdomen does not finally entail an incision as in conventional surgery.

Contraindications

- The size of the splenic mass or spleen may be a contraindication. So are ascites, hemoabdomen (**Fig. 1**), severe splenic trauma, coagulopathy, and portal hypertension.
- Laparoscopic exploration allows for assessing the contraindications related to the visual appearance of the organ.
- An obese patient can be operated on, but if the amount of fat makes it difficult to see the vessels, the intervention must be converted to open surgery.
- In the same way, if adhesions cannot be treated laparoscopically or the blood vessels cannot be correctly identified in a torsion.

Laparoscopic splenectomy is a routine procedure performed by veterinary laparoscopists. Compared to conventional surgery, its advantages are faster patient recovery, less postoperative pain, smaller incisions, and less bleeding.

It is essential to make a good diagnosis to choose the candidate patients with a complete blood test, urinalysis, abdominal ultrasound, thoracic X-ray, and even a CT scan. With all this, enough information is obtained to know if metastasis is seen, what size the spleen is, what shape and location, and if there are adhesions, free fluid, or any alteration in the abdominal organs.

The spleen is located on the left side of the abdomen. The head is between the stomach and the left kidney. The phrenicosplenic ligament supports it from the diaphragm and the gastrosplenic ligament, through which the veins and short gastric arteries run, supporting the splenic hilum with the greater curvature of the stomach. The tail of the spleen is also attached to the omentum and the colon by the splenic-colic ligament with its vascularization, allowing it greater mobility. The main vascularization is in the hilum with the splenic artery and vein.

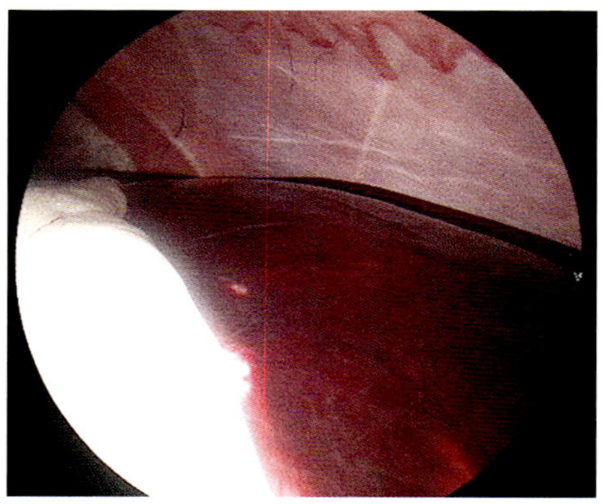

FIGURE 1. Hemoabdomen.

PATIENT PREPARATION AND POSITIONING

As in open surgery, the patient should be fasted for at least 12 hours. The use of perioperative prophylactic antibiotics depends on the patient's age, the existence of concomitant diseases, and the duration of surgery. In healthy animals, they are unnecessary, but they can be administered during the induction of anesthesia and withdrawn in the first 24 hours. To avoid a reduced surgical space, it is advisable to empty the bladder of urine and the stomach of air if it exists and is distending it.

The patient is placed in supine recumbency. The entire abdominal wall is clipped as if it were an open splenectomy. If it was necessary to convert laparoscopy to conventional surgery, it could be done quickly. Finally, the field drapes are placed in an ideal way for this laparoscopy.

OPERATING ROOM LAYOUT

The monitor is placed on the patient's left side, in front of the surgeon and the assistant, who stand on the right side. The anesthesia team is placed cranial to the patient and the instrument table caudal. Using an operating room table with lateral tilting, Trendelenburg, and reverse Trendelenburg options is ideal (**Fig. 2**).

The following procedures are described below:

A. Multiport laparoscopic splenectomy
B. Single-incision laparoscopic splenectomy
C. Laparoscopic-assisted splenectomy
D. Hand-assisted splenectomy

Instruments

On the table:

- Standard surgery set
- Telescope 5 mm – 30°
- Two 5 mm cannulas
- One 10–12 mm cannula
- SILS port
- Atraumatic grasping forceps
- Vessel-sealing device
- Laparoscopic retractors
- Maryland dissector
- Retrieval bag

Ready to use:

- Endoscopic cannula for aspiration/irrigation
- Endoclips

PORT PLACEMENT (FIG. 3)

- T1, 2–3 cm caudal to the umbilicus
- T2, caudal to the umbilicus
- T3, cranial to the umbilicus

Normally, using three ports is necessary, although occasionally, a fourth port or a minilaparoscopic grasper may be necessary for spleens that are difficult to mobilize.

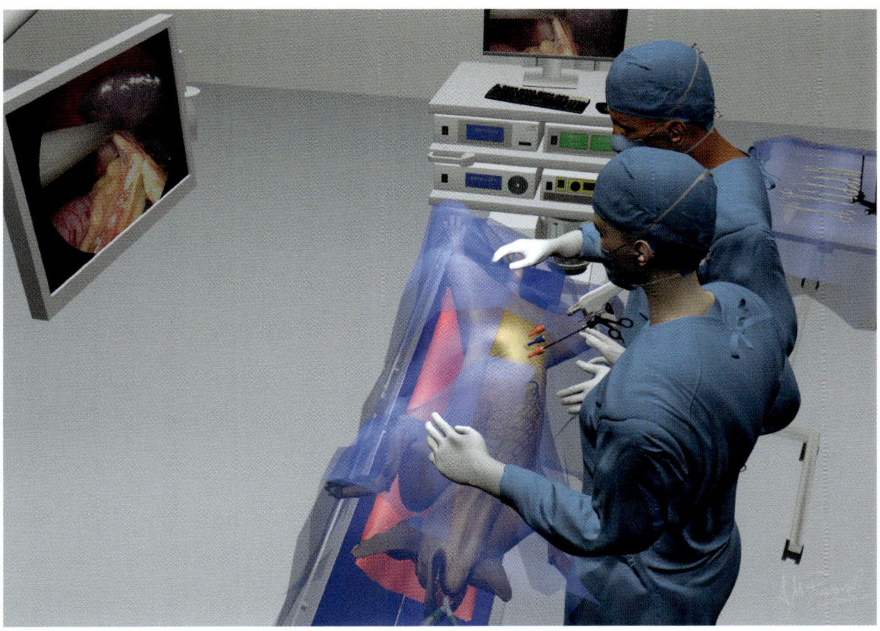

FIGURE 2. Operating room layout for laparoscopic splenectomy.

The first port, the optic port (T1), is placed 2–3 cm caudal to the umbilicus to avoid the falciform ligament. The tail of the spleen is usually located in this area. The second (T2) and the third (T3) ports are introduced caudal and cranial to the umbilicus, respectively. After creating an 8–10 mmHg pneumoperitoneum, an abdominal examination is performed. This allows deciding if a laparoscopic splenectomy is feasible. And, if it is, the right distance between ports to work comfortably. This depends on the size, shape, and location of the spleen. Generally, with a distance shorter than 10 cm between the cranial and caudal ports, it is possible to intervene without a problem. It is recommended that the caudal port be 10–12 mm to be able to insert endoclips or an extraction bag at the end of the procedure.

A MULTIPORT LAPAROSCOPIC SPLENECTOMY

PROCEDURE

- The patient is positioned supine and normally tilted to the right at about 45°. In some patients, it is possible to perform the intervention even in a horizontal position. On the contrary, in some cases, a completely lateral position is necessary to access the most cranial part of the spleen. Ultimately, the inclination depends on the size, morphology, friability, and location of the spleen and its vascularization or adhesions, if any.
- The most important instrument in any surgery is the vessel sealer. This allows for sealing vessels up to 7 mm. In cases where the thickness of the vessels creates doubt about the effectiveness of the sealant, endoclips can be used. Or, better, the surgery can be turned into a laparoscopic-assisted splenectomy.
- The splenic hilum needs to be seen clearly. This is done using a blunt probe or any closed blunt instrument to tilt the spleen about 45° to the left (**Fig. 4**). Its use must be very cautious since it is a very labile organ (splenic masses are even more labile). Sometimes it works well to tilt the patient quickly about 45° to the left and slowly reposition the patient at an angle of 45° to the right. This way, the spleen can be tilted to avoid pressing it with the instruments. But normally, they should be used. The spleen must be appropriately positioned so the area to be intervened can be correctly visualized.
- The ideal process would be to seal the hilar vessels first, which are those that provide the greatest vascularization (**Fig. 5**). Then, the short gastric vessels with the gastrosplenic ligament that frees the cranial part of the spleen to mobilize it better (**Fig. 6**). Finally, the rest of the omentum, ligaments, and vascularization (**Fig. 7**). Reality does not always allow these steps (e.g., either because adhesions or fat make it difficult to see the hilum, or because a very large central mass in the spleen makes it difficult to lift the spleen to access the

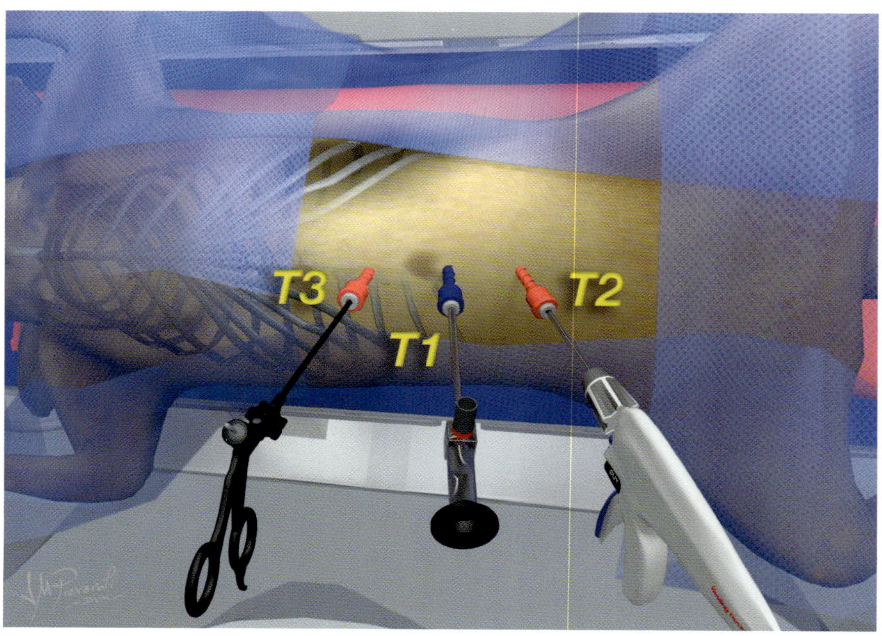

FIGURE 3. Multiport placement for laparoscopic splenectomy.

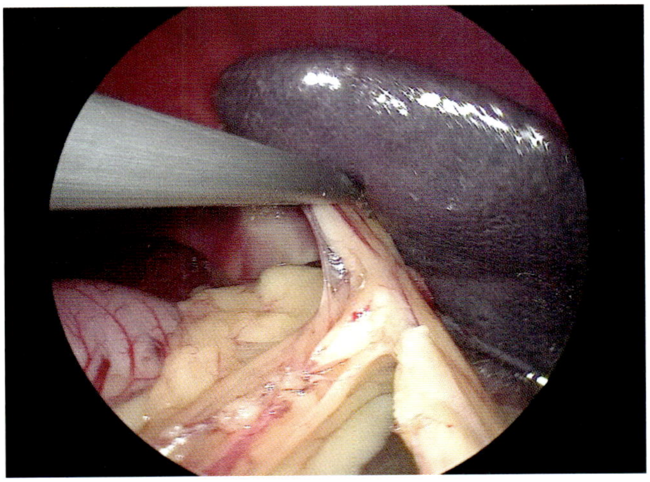

FIGURE 4. Tilting of the spleen.

hilum). In this case, it is best to start with the head and tail to release tension and facilitate the tilting of the spleen. Therefore, any unforeseen situation forces to decide the order of the steps in each intervention. Sometimes there are adhesions or the omentum surrounding the spleen. Before mobilizing it, all adhesions must be dissected and resected, and all its vessels sealed (**Fig. 8**). Once the entire organ is correctly visualized, it is time to tilt the spleen to seal its vessels.

- Once the entire spleen is released, an extraction bag is introduced where the spleen is placed. There are oversized pouches for large but not always manageable spleens in a dog's abdomen. According to the author, it should be used only if the spleen is easily inserted into the bag or if it is easily deployed. If not, gentle manual removal with a suitable

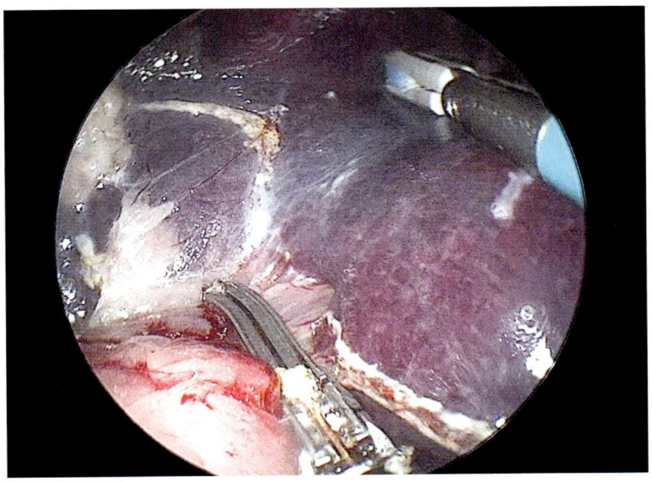

FIGURE 5. Sealing of the hilar vessels.

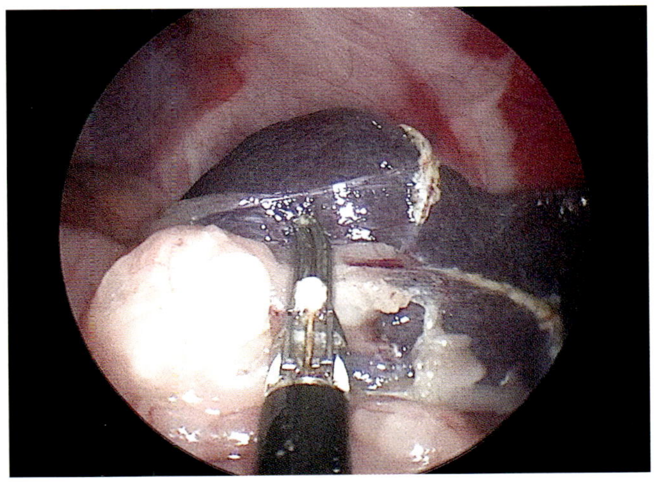

FIGURE 6. Sealing of the short gastric vessels.

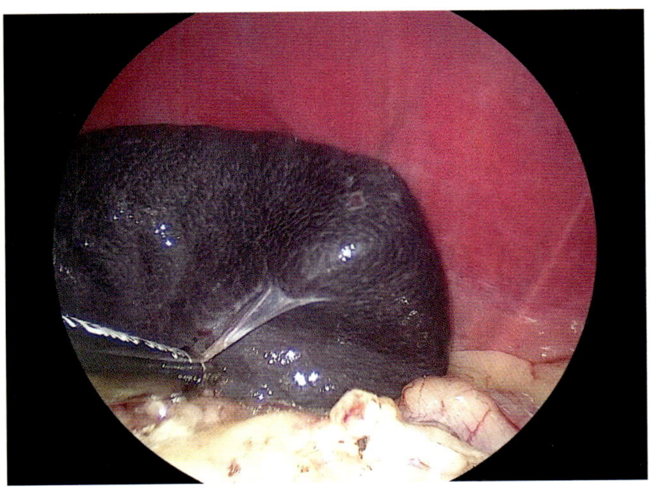

FIGURE 7. Ligament and vascularization of the tail of the spleen.

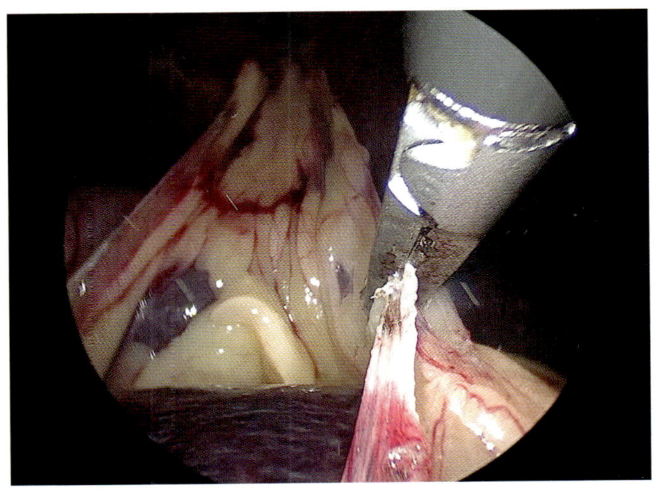

FIGURE 8. Resection of the omentum and vessels.

incision allows the spleen to be removed safely. There is more risk of splenic rupture or seeding of attempting to insert a large or fragile spleen into the bag than to remove it manually.

- Finally, the two free cannulas are extracted, and the caudal cannula of the bag is maintained. An incision is made from the caudal port towards the cranial ones as wide as is necessary to extract the spleen.

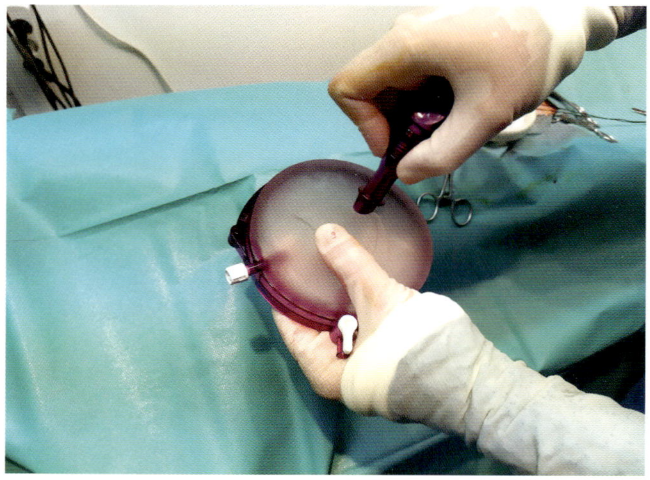

FIGURE 9. GelPOINT.

B SINGLE-INCISION LAPAROSCOPIC SPLENECTOMY

PROCEDURE

- There are different types of SILS ports. The Covidien SILS device is the most widely used. It is easy to insert into the abdomen with a 2.5 cm incision. But the proximity of long instruments and the optics can make the surgeon's job difficult.
- Another system, much more comfortable, according to the author, is the GelPOINT (**Fig. 9**). It has different advantages. The first is three sizes for incisions from 1.5 cm to 7 cm. If the appropriate size is chosen for each spleen, widening the incision to remove the spleen is unnecessary. It has a gel cap much wider than the incision. This means that the distance between the instruments is sufficient to avoid unwanted contact between them. In addition, it can introduce them through ports that are placed anywhere in the gel. Also, its location can be changed at any time. Finally, the device has an Alexis retractor that protects the wound and spleen during extraction.
- These devices are inserted just caudal to the umbilicus (**Fig. 10**), always trying to avoid the falciform ligament. A medium or large size GelPOINT can be centered on the umbilicus since the same Alexis separator (**Fig. 11**) totally or partially separates the ligament.
- The procedure is the same as above. The port incision is enlarged according to the port size. If a GelPOINT of a suitable diameter for the spleen is used, it is not necessary to widen the incision. The Alexis separator protects the abdominal wall and the spleen, thus facilitating the extraction of the spleen.

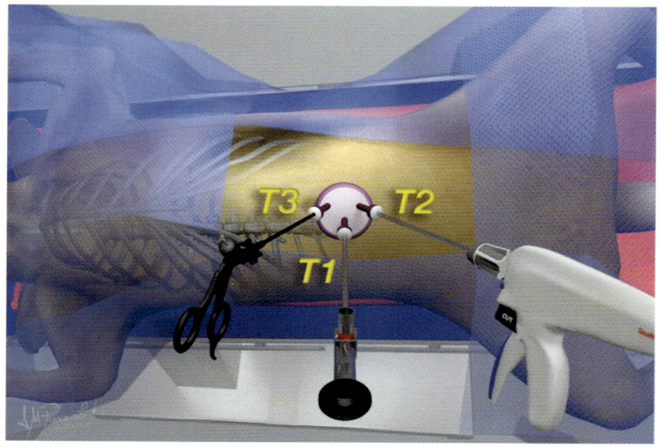

FIGURE 10. Single-port placement with GelPOINT.

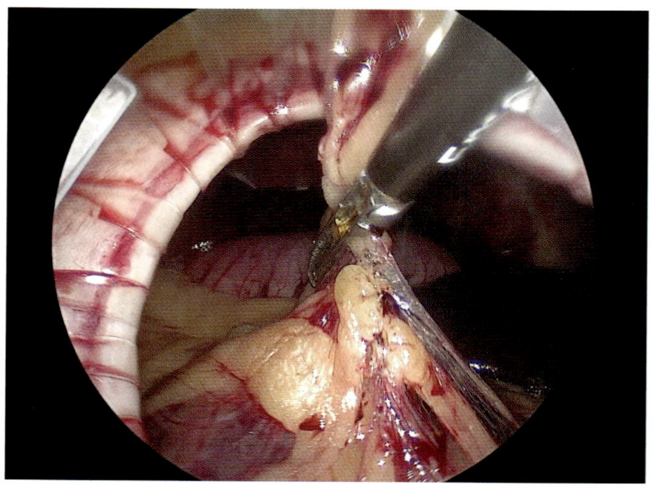

FIGURE 11. View of the Alexis separator during resection of the omentum and vessels.

C LAPAROSCOPIC-ASSISTED SPLENECTOMY

PROCEDURE

It can be performed with either the multiport or the single-incision technique. There are two types of procedures:

- The first consists of performing a laparoscopy to explore the state of the abdomen and see the location, size, and abnormalities of the spleen. The best site for the abdominal incision to remove the spleen and perform the external splenectomy is then determined.
- The second tries to facilitate the exteriorization of the spleen to finalize the intervention outside. In this way, a smaller abdominal incision than in the first case is made. The cranial and caudal ligaments are divided, and the short gastric vessels are sealed. At this time, the spleen is sufficiently released to extract it outside the abdomen, where the hilum vessels and any other splenic vessels have yet to be sealed, as well as remnants of omentum or ligaments.

D HAND-ASSISTED SPLENECTOMY

GelPort is a system like GelPOINT, but the hand is introduced instead of introducing some ports. In the center of the gel on the cap, there is an incision through which the hand can be inserted without losing the pneumoperitoneum. This is prevented by the gel that adheres closely to the wrist. An abdominal incision of up to 9 cm can be made. The cap has a diameter of 12 cm, so a hand that is not very large can be well inserted.

The introduction is also in the umbilical zone. It is necessary to place two ports, one cranial and one caudal, in the device for optics and instruments.

PROCEDURE

- This technique only makes sense in very large patients with a large, heavy, or fragile spleen to be mobilized with laparoscopic instruments. The device and the hand are too large to be used on a small or medium patient. The hand would occupy a good part of the abdomen, and the incision would be much larger than necessary to extract the spleen.
- The hand is inserted through the GelPort (**Fig. 12**) to elevate the spleen. The optics are introduced through one port and the sealer through the other. The spleen is placed with the hand in the best way to seal the vessels. Once released, the cap of the device is opened, and the hand with the spleen is removed. The Alexis retractor protects the incision and spleen.

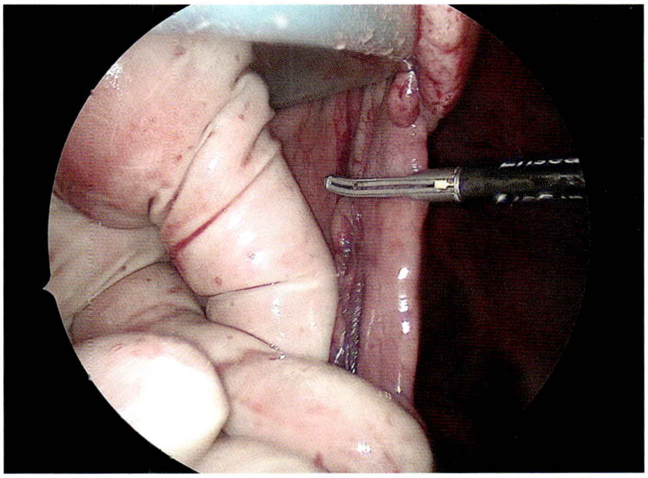

FIGURE 12. The hand is inserted through the GelPort to elevate the spleen.

- The procedure is uncomfortable for the surgeon since the hand is very compressed in the gel, hindering its mobility. Despite this, it could be an interesting technique in very specific cases.

POSTOPERATIVE MANAGEMENT

- Overnight postoperative hospitalization is recommended for pain management and monitoring, though some patients can be discharged the same day if postoperative recovery is swift.
- Local analgesics at the time of incision site closure are recommended.
- The literature has described the use of μ-agonist opioids every 4 hours during the first 12 hours after the operation and subsequently oral tramadol (2–4 mg/kg every 8–12 h) and/or carprofen (2 mg/kg every 12 h). The owner can administer oral analgesics if necessary.
- The main treatment for malignant neoplasms is splenectomy, but add-on chemotherapy may lengthen survival time.
- Follow-up of the patient is the same as with conventional surgery. The histopathological result will tell if image control is necessary over time. With the use of abdominal ultrasound, chest radiography, or CT, studies will be carried out in the cases that require it. This would be the case of malignant neoplasms such as hemangiosarcoma.

Complications of laparoscopic splenectomy

- The most important intraoperative complication is hemorrhage. This is due to injury to the spleen at the time of introduction of the first trocar or Veress needle, the rupture of the spleen during its mobilization, its friability, excess pressure of the instruments on the spleen, or a poor sealing of the vessels during the procedure. If bleeding is severe, it should be converted to open surgery.
- Incorrect port placement.
- The difficulty of a certain complex intervention or the surgeon's lack of experience during the procedure becomes a complication that implies the conversion to conventional surgery.
- Septic complications can be a risk in immunosuppressed animals.
- Incisional complications (e.g., seroma, bruising, infection, dehiscence).

Key points

- Laparoscopic splenectomy is already a routine procedure performed by veterinary laparoscopists.
- Its advantages, compared to conventional surgery, are the faster recovery of the patient, less postoperative pain, smaller incisions, and less bleeding.
- It is indicated for masses and spleens that are not very large or excessively friable.
- There are different ways to do it: multiport laparoscopic splenectomy, single-incision laparoscopic splenectomy, laparoscopic-assisted splenectomy, or hand-assisted splenectomy.
- The inclinations of the patient and the table are essential to achieve correct positioning. In this way, unnecessary movements with the laparoscopic instruments that could injure the spleen are avoided.

SUGGESTED READINGS

CLINICAL CASES

39.1 LAPAROSCOPIC SPLENECTOMY IN A SMALL DOG

Andrea M. Pievaroli

CASE DESCRIPTION

An 8-year-old male Shih Tzu dog (weight 7 kg) was referred to perform a laparoscopic splenectomy for the presence of neoplasia of 2.5 cm in diameter. Considering the small size of the lesion, the three-port technique was performed. The spleen was extracted with a bag to limit the risk of neoplastic cells spreading. The result of the histological examination indicated a lymphoid splenic nodular hyperplasia. The dog recovered quickly and was discharged the day after surgery.

Key points

- Preoperative imaging to measure the dimensions of the neoplasia and adopt the most appropriate technique considering the dog's size.
- Use of a vessel-sealing device.

PORT PLACEMENT

- Patient in dorsal recumbency, slightly tilted to the right
- T1, 1 cm cranial to the umbilicus, 2 cm on a right paramedian line
- T2, on the midline, 2–3 cm caudal to T1
- T3, on the midline, 2–3 cm cranial to T1

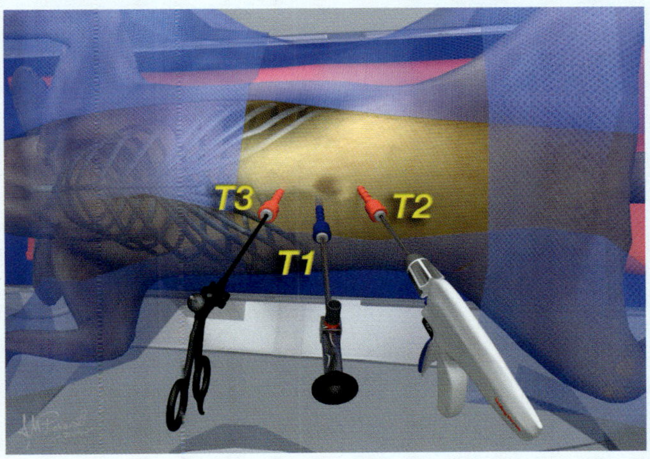

PROCEDURE

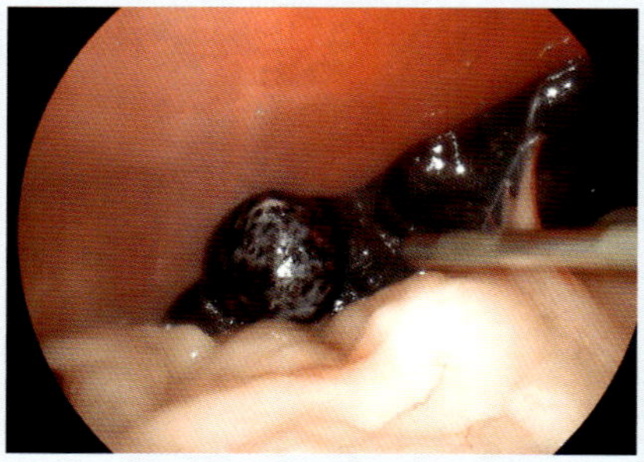

FIGURE 1. The neoplasia located is clearly visible in the cranial aspect of the spleen.

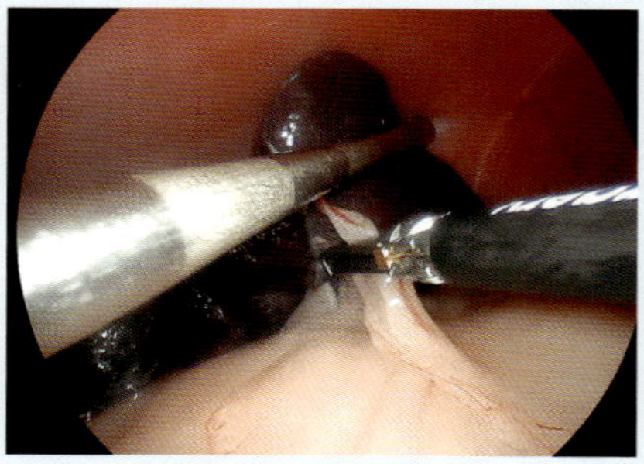

FIGURE 2. A blunt probe and a vessel-sealing device are used to dissect the vessels. In this case, the author starts from the caudal portion.

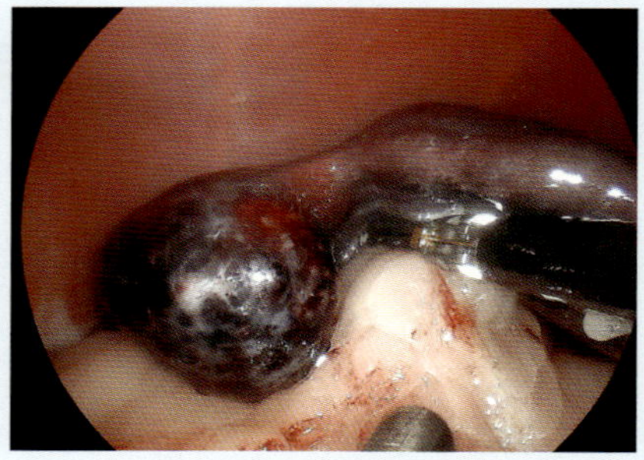

FIGURE 3. The vessel-sealing device is essential for coagulating the vessels and being sure that there is no bleeding.

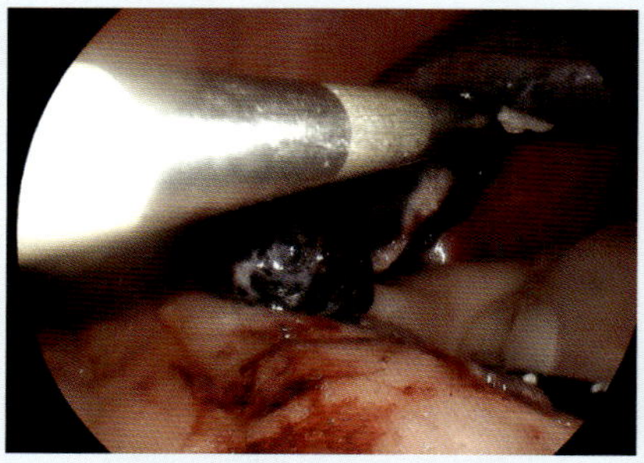

FIGURE 4. The dissection of the vessels is completed, and the spleen is ready to be removed.

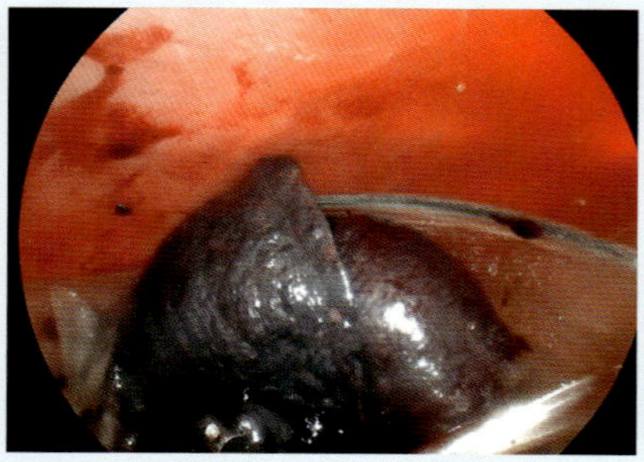

FIGURE 5. The spleen is placed in an endoscopic retrieval bag to reduce the risk of rupture with consequent spreading of neoplastic cells.

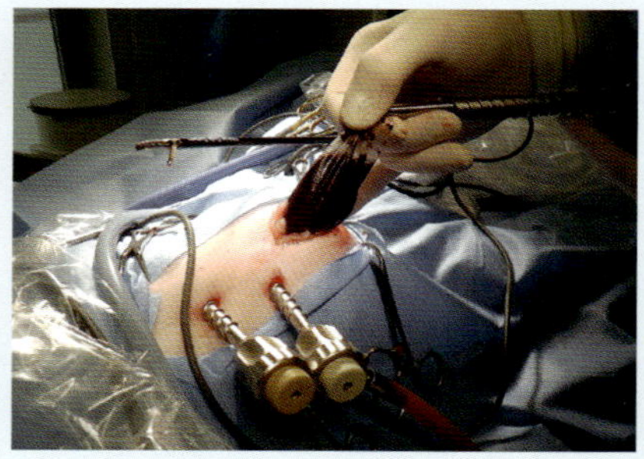

FIGURE 6. The caudal port is removed, and the incision is enlarged just enough to let the bag come out.

Tips and tricks

- ✓ Be careful to manipulate the spleen and use a blunt probe to reduce the risk of rupture.
- ✓ A wound retractor can also be used to extract the spleen.

39.2 SPLENECTOMY

D. L. Casas García

CASE DESCRIPTION

A 12-year-old female Schnauzer was presented with a history of apathy and abdominal pain. The abdominal ultrasound revealed the existence of a 4×5 cm focal lesion with a mixed pattern in the spleen without associated lymphadenopathies or splenomegaly. The thoracic X-rays discarded the existence of alterations. An exploratory laparoscopy and splenectomy were scheduled for the patient.

Key points

- Image studies, especially abdominal ultrasound, are essential before prescribing a splenectomy by minimally invasive techniques.
- A large spleen or a large mass, as well as hemoabdomen, are described as the main contraindications for laparoscopic splenectomy.
- Intraoperative hemorrhage is the main complication described in laparoscopic splenectomy in small animals.

PORT PLACEMENT

From a minimally invasive point of view, splenectomy in small animals can be carried out by multiport laparoscopic surgery, single-port laparoscopic surgery, and the assisted laparoscopic technique. In this case, three 6 mm ports were placed: T1 (telescope), T2 (right-hand port), and T3 (left-hand port).

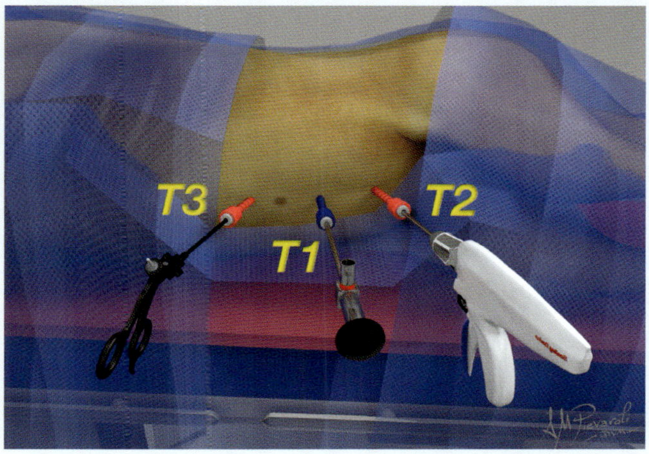

PROCEDURE

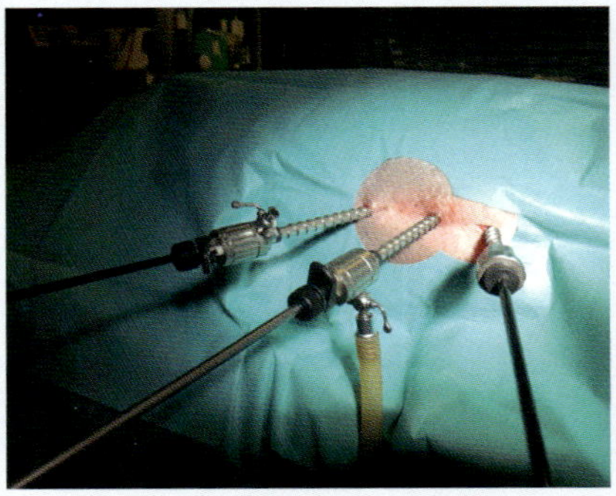

FIGURE 1. The multiport technique was chosen for the splenectomy using three 6 mm ports.

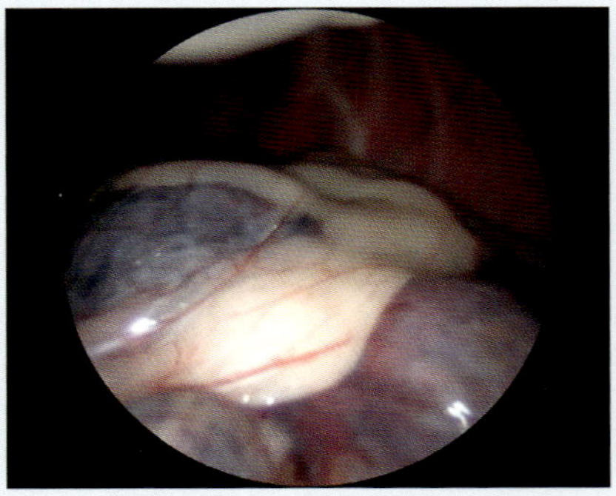

FIGURE 2. During the laparoscopy, the affected part of the spleen is identified, avoiding trauma to the spleen to avoid abdominal expansion.

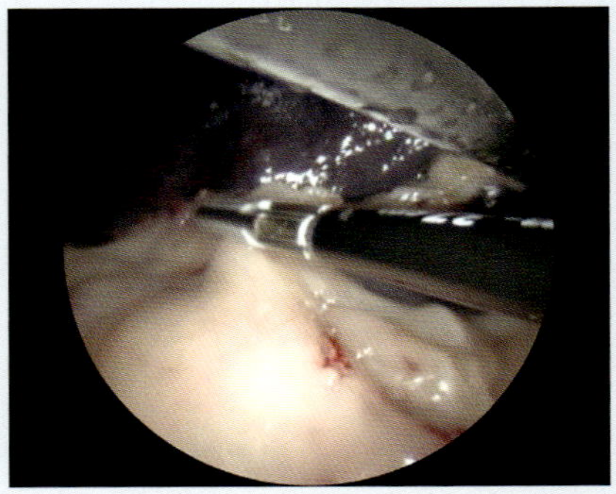

FIGURE 3. With the animal placed in right lateral recumbency, exposing the splenic hilum to start the vascular seal in the ventrodorsal direction is easier.

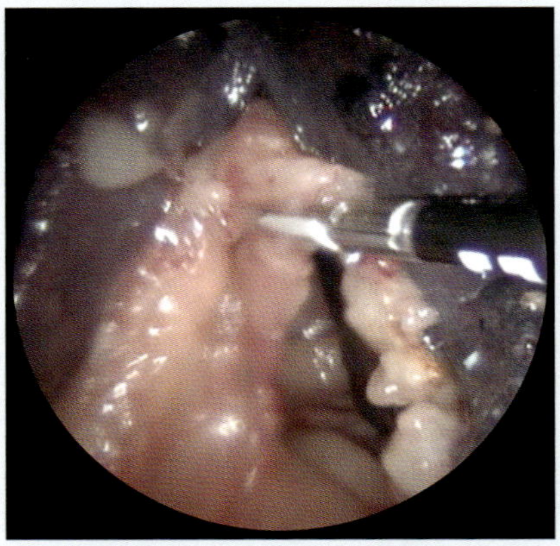

FIGURE 4. While doing the vascular sealing of the splenic hilum, suspending the spleen with nontraumatic forceps can be useful.

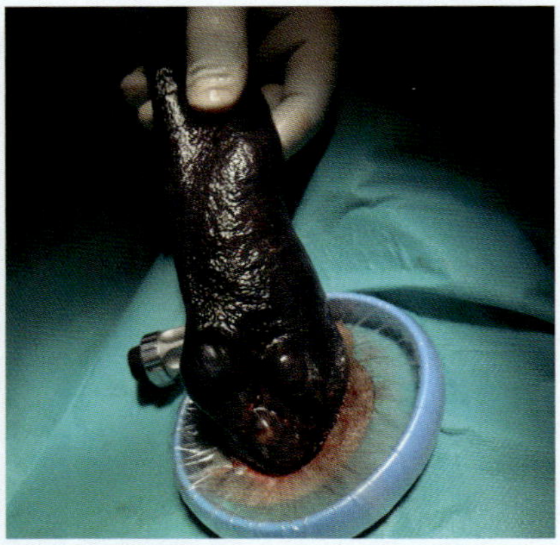

FIGURE 5. Once the vascular sealing of the splenic hilum is finished, using a tissue retractor can help for a safe spleen extraction to avoid tumor seeding.

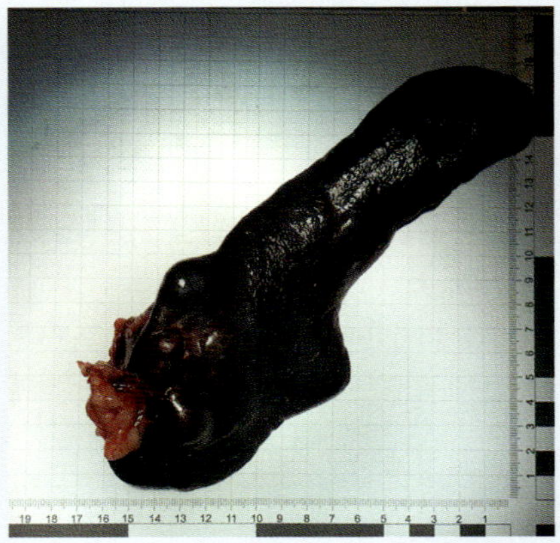

FIGURE 6. Once the spleen has been exteriorized, it is prepared to be sent to the laboratory for histopathological examination.

Tips and tricks

- ✓ Strict patient fasting is recommended because an increased intestinal volume can diminish the laparoscopic field and complicate the surgery when trying to move the spleen.
- ✓ Positioning the patient in right lateral recumbency helps to have good access to the splenic hilum.
- ✓ In the multiport technique joining the incisions of the two most caudal ports is enough to remove the spleen.
- ✓ The use of tissue retractors can avoid the risk of metastasis because of neoplastic seeding during spleen removal.
- ✓ The use of tissue retractors allows the spleen to cross the abdominal wall more smoothly, avoiding breaking the splenic capsule during the removal maneuver.

39.3 LAPAROSCOPIC SPLENECTOMY FOR HEMANGIOSARCOMA

Fabien Collard

CASE DESCRIPTION

A splenic hemangiosarcoma was diagnosed by ultrasound-guided fine-needle aspiration in an 11-year-old crossed-breed dog. The neoplasia consisted of a single 3 cm diameter mass located in the splenic tail. The table was positioned in a slightly reversed Trendelenburg position.

Key points

- A fan retractor to mobilize the spleen.
- A laparoscopic sealing device to seal and divide vessels.
- A specimen plastic bag to remove the spleen.

PORT PLACEMENT

The patient was placed in dorsal recumbency for placement of the first port (T1, optic) through the umbilicus. Then, the dog was partially rotated (45°) and the second port (T3) was inserted 1 cm cranial to the prepuce. Afterwards, the dog was replaced in dorsal recumbency to insert the third port (T2) 10 cm laterally and 2 cm caudally to the second port.

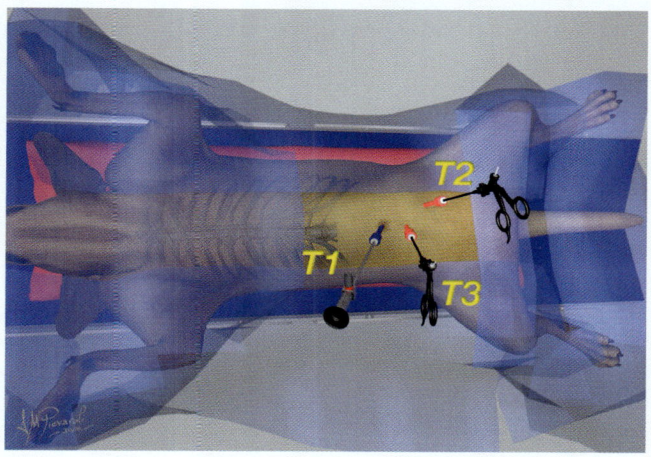

PROCEDURE

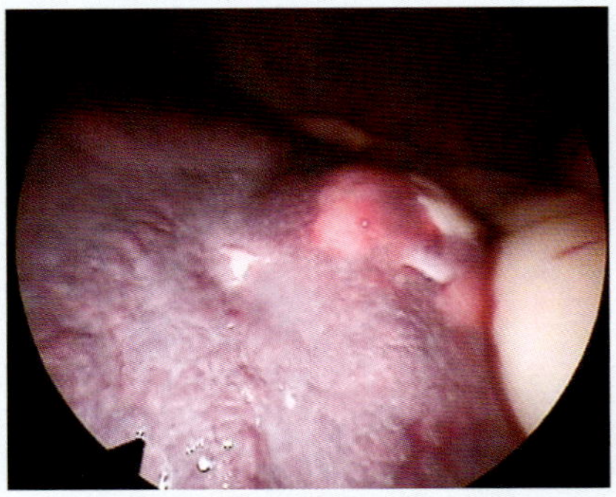

FIGURE 1. Image of the splenic mass. After establishing a pneumoabdomen with a Veress needle and port insertion, an abdominal exploration is performed, and the splenic mass is located.

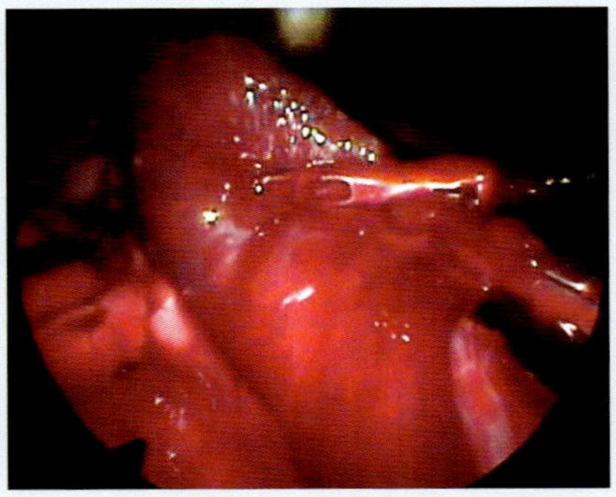

FIGURE 2. The spleen is grasped with a forceps to enable the visualization of its ventral aspect. A fan retractor should be used to avoid splenic laceration and bleeding.

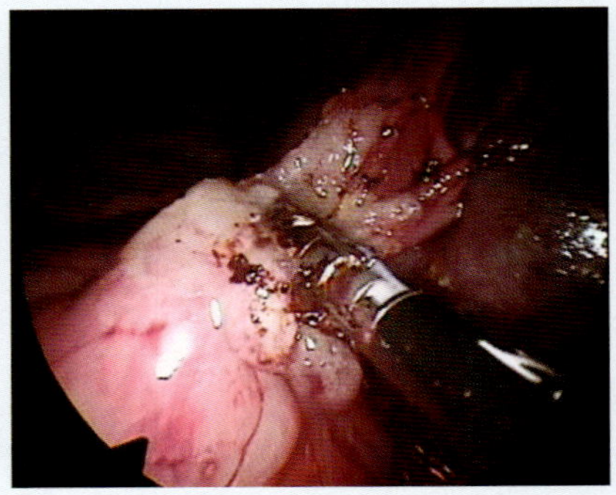

FIGURE 3. Dissection of splenic attachments started at the caudal aspect of the spleen. A LigaSure V is introduced through T3 and used to seal vessels and omental insertion as close as possible to the spleen.

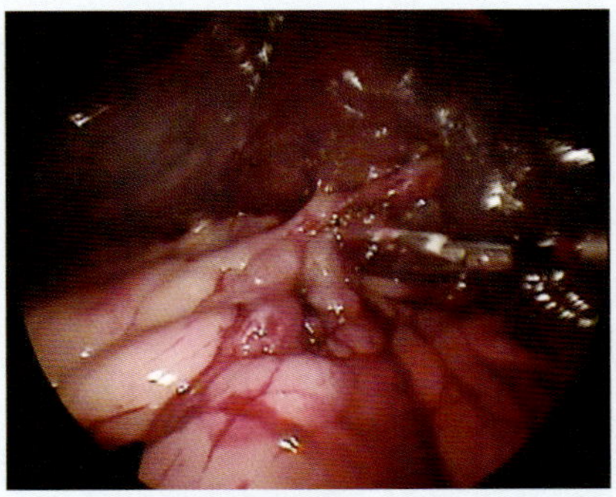

FIGURE 4. The splenic artery and vein are identified and sealed. Dissection is progressed cranially. Splenic attachments are grasped with forceps to allow spleen retraction and avoid splenic laceration and bleeding.

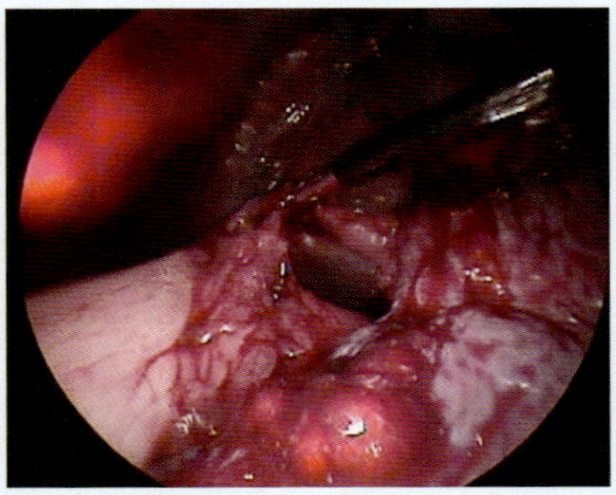

FIGURE 5. After having detached the tail of the spleen, a LigaSure V is placed through T2. The second half of the spleen is detached. Cranially, short gastric arteries are sealed and divided to release the spleen totally.

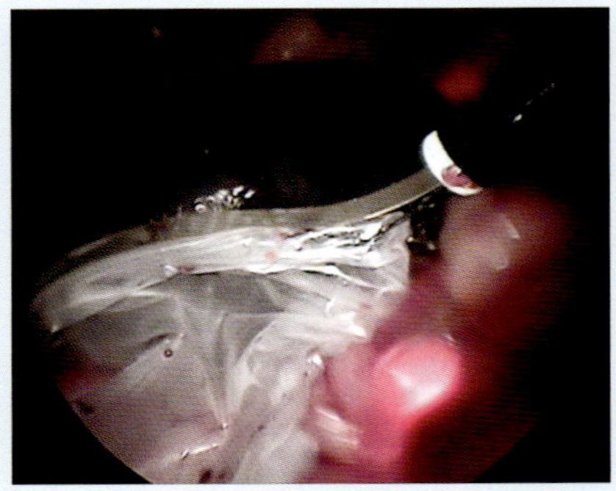

FIGURE 6. The spleen is placed in a plastic specimen bag and removed from the abdomen. If the spleen is too large, part of the spleen with the mass may be placed in the bag to minimize the risk of bleeding and seeding into the abdominal cavity. The spleen is removed after the enlargement of one port incision.

Tips and tricks

✓ T2 must be positioned caudal to the splenic tail.

✓ If a fan retractor is not available, the splenic attachment should be grasped with forceps to mobilize the spleen.

40 LAPAROSCOPIC ADRENALECTOMY

Francesco Collivignarelli, Felipe Lillo

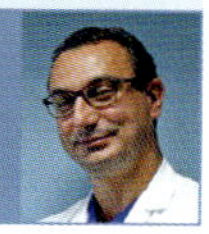

Indications

- Animals with functional tumors up to 5 cm in diameter that do not exhibit vascular invasion
- Case selection for laparoscopic adrenalectomy is key to success

Contraindications

- Animals that may be poorly tolerant of pneumoperitoneum (e.g., with severe cardiorespiratory disease or diaphragmatic herniation)
- Insufficient training and experience with the technique
- Lack of the appropriate instrumentation

Adrenalectomy is traditionally viewed as one of the most challenging interventions in soft tissue surgery, no matter the surgical approach used. Approaches used in the past include ventral celiotomy, a paracostal approach, and, more recently, transperitoneal laparoscopic resection.

Endocrine testing for functionality and diagnostic imaging are critical components of the preoperative workup for adrenal masses and form the basis for deciding whether surgical resection is warranted and, if so, which surgical approach is preferred.

> Adrenal surgery has a long history, with the first planned adrenalectomy performed in 1914 by Sargent. Mayo performed the first flank approach for pheochromocytoma in 1927, although he was unaware of the entire disease process involved at the time of surgery.

ENDOCRINE TESTING

Preoperative medical treatment is a vital component for successfully managing these tumors. Functional adrenocortical tumors are administered trilostane (2.5–5 mg/kg PO twice daily) for 2–3 weeks before surgery. Supplementation with corticosteroids before initiation of surgery to avoid a hypoadrenocortical episode in the recovery period is important. Suitable choices include dexamethasone (0.1–0.2 mg/kg IV), prednisolone sodium succinate (1–2 mg/kg IV), or hydrocortisone (2 mg/kg IV). If pheochromocytoma is suspected, pretreatment with an α-adrenergic blocker, such as phenoxybenzamine (escalating dose up to 1–1.5 mg/kg PO twice daily), should be considered for several weeks preoperatively until the animal is normotensive.

Phenoxybenzamine has been shown to improve the outcome in dogs undergoing adrenalectomy. In cats with functional adrenocortical tumors, it has been suggested that treatment with trilostane should be initiated until the skin abnormalities accompanying the condition in this species resolve. Cats with aldosterone-secreting tumors should have their metabolic and electrolyte disturbances corrected before surgery.

DIAGNOSTIC IMAGING

Ultrasonography and contrast-enhanced computed tomography (CECT) are often used for preoperative imaging. Ultrasonography has been shown to have a sensitivity and specificity of 80% and 90%, respectively, for detecting vascular invasion and tumor thrombus. In one study, the sensitivity and specificity of CECT for detecting tumor thrombus were reported to be 92% and 100%, respectively. In the author's institution, all potential candidates for adrenalectomy generally undergo ultrasonography as a screening test to provide noninvasive prognostic information for owners. If adrenalectomy is recommended based on the findings of ultrasound, all dogs have a CECT scan recommended to rule out vascular invasion, to define the extent of any thrombi present, and to evaluate the anatomical margins of the tumor. Approximately 20%–48% of adrenal neoplasms exhibit vascular invasion into the vena cava, phrenicoabdominal veins, or renal vasculature, with pheochromocytomas more prone to invade than adrenocortical tumors. If detected preoperatively, vascular invasion into the vena cava should be considered an indication for an "open" approach at this point, but invasion into the phrenicoabdominal vein alone (**Fig. 1**) does not rule out a laparoscopic approach at our institution, as the phrenicoabdominal vein is ligated/sealed at its entry point into the caudal vena cava, theoretically removing any risk of embolization.

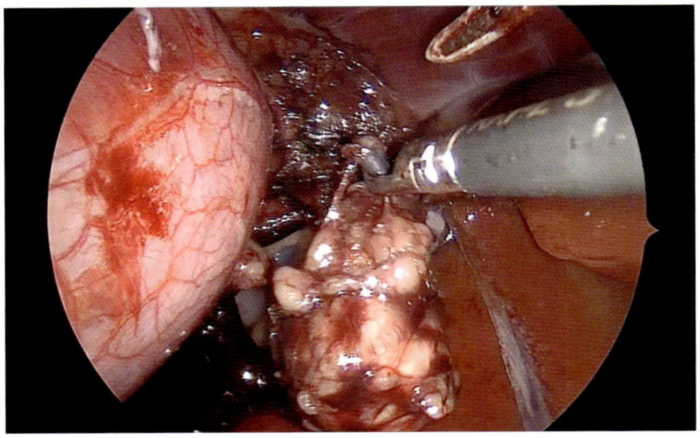

FIGURE 1. Invasion into the phrenicoabdominal vein alone.

DESCRIBED SURGICAL PROCEDURES

The laparoscopic approach to adrenalectomy has been performed in humans since the early 90s and has now been described in small numbers of veterinary patients. This approach combines the best aspects of both the paracostal and ventral celiotomy approaches. Positioning the animal in lateral or sternal recumbency provides excellent visualization of the gland and surrounding structures without the pain and morbidity associated with the paramedian muscle incision. Unlike the celiotomy approach, extensive retraction and compression of surrounding organs are unnecessary.

The following procedures are described below:

A. Adrenalectomy in sternal recumbency
B. Adrenalectomy in lateral recumbency
C. Retroperitoneal adrenalectomy

A ADRENALECTOMY IN STERNAL RECUMBENCY

Laparoscopic adrenalectomy performed with the patient in sternal recumbency has the advantages of allowing gravitational displacement of the abdominal organs, better visualization of the adrenal gland, and a shorter surgical time than conventional laparoscopy or open adrenalectomy.

PATIENT PREPARATION AND POSITIONING

The caudal aspect of the hemithorax and the lateral abdomen on the affected side is clipped and prepared for aseptic surgery. The patient is placed in sternal recumbency supported by two inflatable or gelatin cushions. One cushion is placed between the pelvic limbs extending no further cranial than the pubis to support the pelvis, and the other cushion is placed under the sternum to elevate the chest. The patient is secured to allow table rotation during adrenalectomy, and care is taken to avoid compression of the ventral aspect of the abdomen from the operating table.

OPERATING ROOM LAYOUT

The video monitor is placed on the contralateral side of the affected adrenal gland (**Fig. 2**). A 5 mm, 0° or 30° laparoscope (Storz, Tuttlingen, Germany) is connected to a video camera, and a light source and images are recorded.

Instruments

On the table:

- Standard surgical pack
- High-definition video camera
- Telescope 5 mm – 30°
- Two 5 mm threaded cannulas + one 12 mm threaded cannula
- Laparoscopic Babcock, Kelly, right-angle forceps, 5 mm
- Laparoscopic cotton-tip (Endopeanuts), blunt dissection probes, 5 mm
- L- or J-hook monopolar electrosurgical tip, 5 mm
- 10 mm titanium endoscopic clips (Endoclip)
- Specimen retrieval bag
- Bipolar vessel-sealing systems (LigaSure, Covidien, Mansfield, MA; or Enseal, Ethicon Endosurgery, Cincinnati, OH)
- Ultrasonic vessel sealers (Harmonic, Ethicon Endosurgery)
- Self-retaining retractor

PORT PLACEMENT (FIG. 3)

The ports are placed in a semicircular line extending from the 13th rib to the iliac crest.

- T1, central trocar in the flank
- T2, cranial to the iliac crest
- T3, caudal to the last rib

PROCEDURE

- The Veress needle is inserted just caudal to the last rib in the paralumbar fossa ipsilateral to the affected side, or a modified Hasson technique is used to insert the first port. After abdominal insufflation with CO_2 (intra-abdominal pressure 8–10 mmHg), two or three 5 mm ports are placed just caudal to the kidney in the paralumbar fossa.
- Exposure and dissection of the adrenal glands are performed differently on the right and left sides because of anatomic differences. To achieve full exposure of the right adrenal gland, the right lateral hepatic lobe is retracted cranially, and the kidney is retracted caudally (**Fig. 4**). Whereas on the left side it is only necessary to retract the kidney caudally for sufficient exposure (**Fig. 5**).

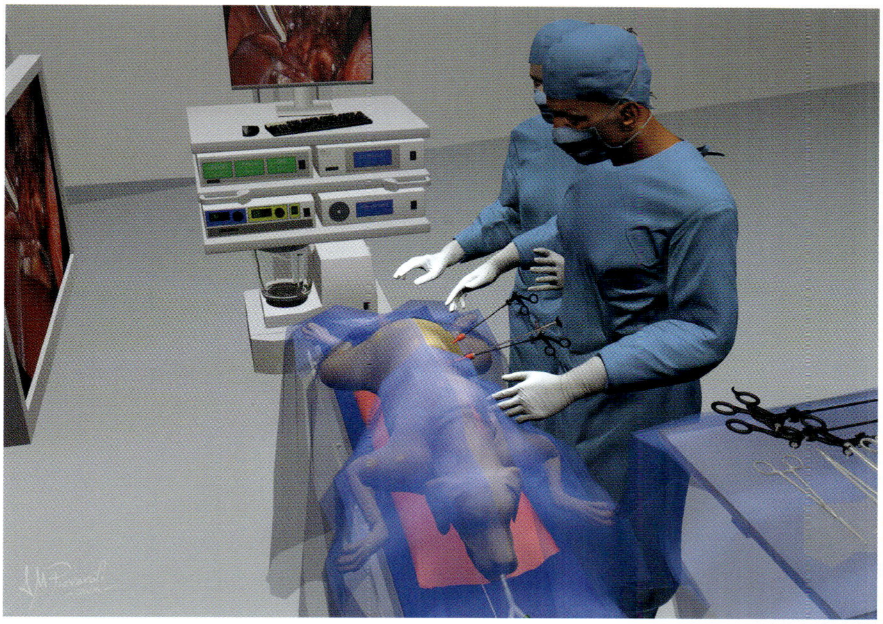

FIGURE 2. Operating room layout for laparoscopic adrenalectomy in sternal recumbency (supported by two inflatable or gelatin cushions).

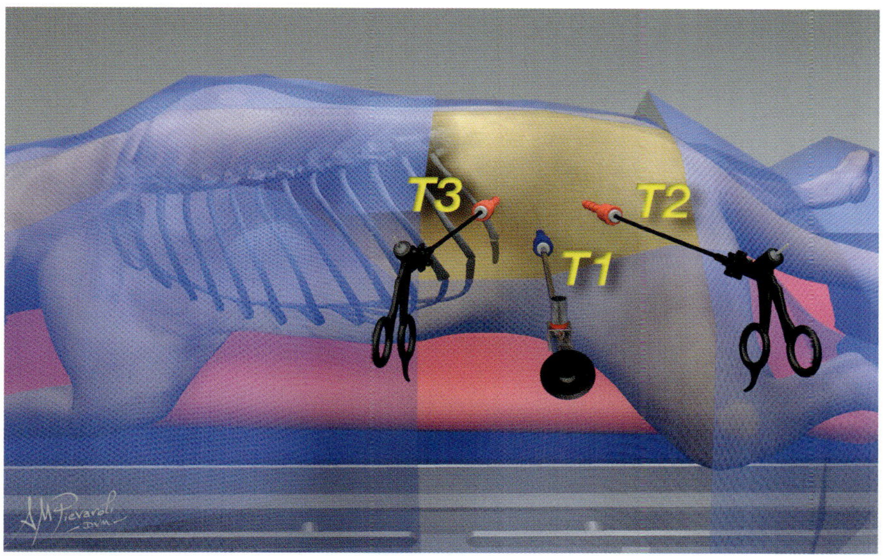

FIGURE 3. Port placement for laparoscopic adrenalectomy in sternal recumbency.

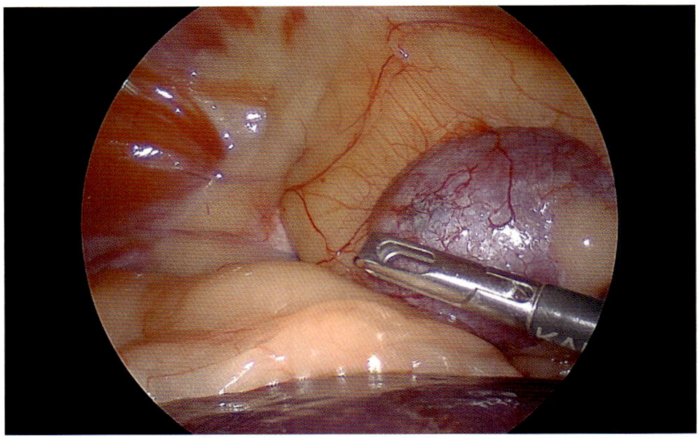

FIGURE 4. The right lateral hepatic lobe is retracted cranially, and the kidney is retracted caudally.

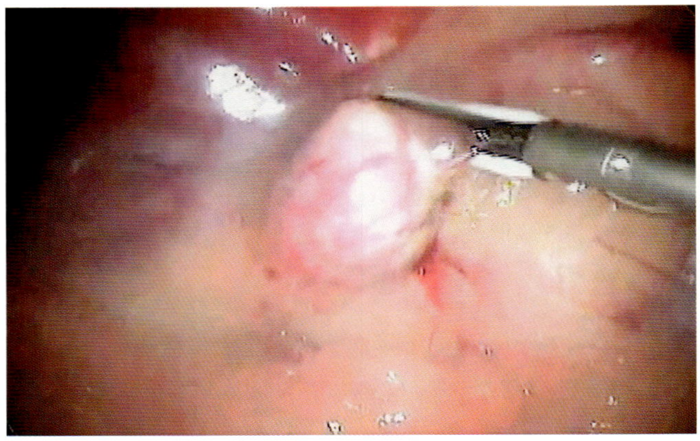

FIGURE 5. On the left side, it is only necessary to retract the kidney.

- Circumferential dissection of the adrenal gland is performed using dissecting forceps and the vessel-sealing and dividing device (**Figs. 6 and 7**).
- The approach is extended first dorsally by sealing or clipping the dorsal phrenicoabdominal vessel (**Fig. 8**).
- The adrenal gland is carefully dissected from its attachments to the fibrous tissue formed between it and the aorta, laterally and caudally to the adrenal gland (**Fig. 9**).
- After the final dissection plane is established, the adrenal gland is attached on the ventral side to the remaining structures, including the vena cava (**Fig. 10**).
- With careful manipulation and dissection, the ventral phrenicoabdominal vessels are isolated, and either sealed or a hemoclip is applied.

Tips

The periadrenal tissue should be grasped as little as possible to minimize the risk of capsular rupture.

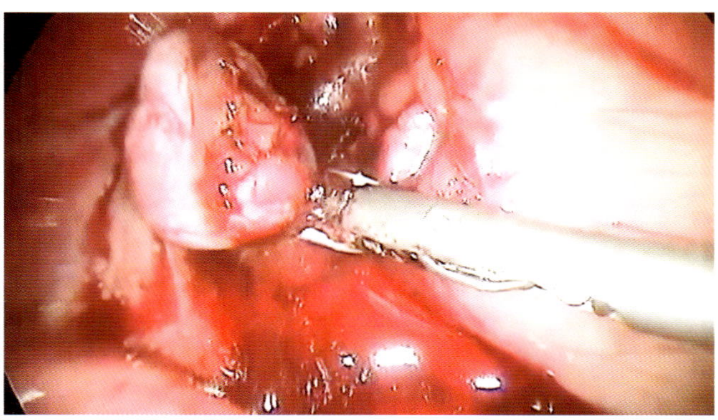

FIGURE 6. Circumferential dissection of the adrenal gland.

- After dissection of the adrenal gland, either a retrieval bag or a finger from a surgical glove is used for gland removal to prevent abdominal wall contamination.
- The abdomen is decompressed after inspection for hemorrhage, and the laparoscopic port sites are sutured.
- The adrenal tissue is submitted for histopathologic examination.

Key points

- To minimize the risk of capsular rupture, the periadrenal tissue should be grasped as little as possible.
- The quality of the supportive care available for the postoperative period.

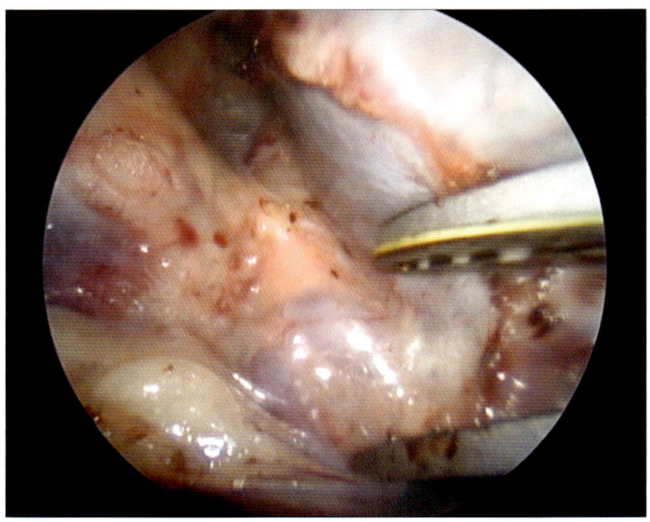

FIGURE 7. Dissection of the adrenal gland.

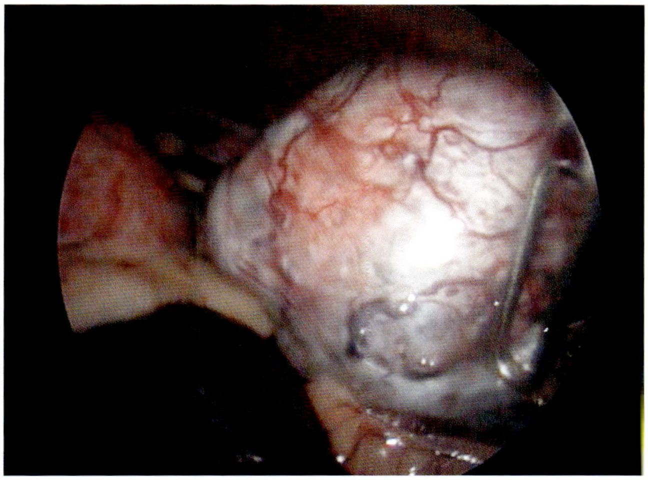

FIGURE 8. Dorsal dissection by sealing or clipping the dorsal phrenicoabdominal vessel.

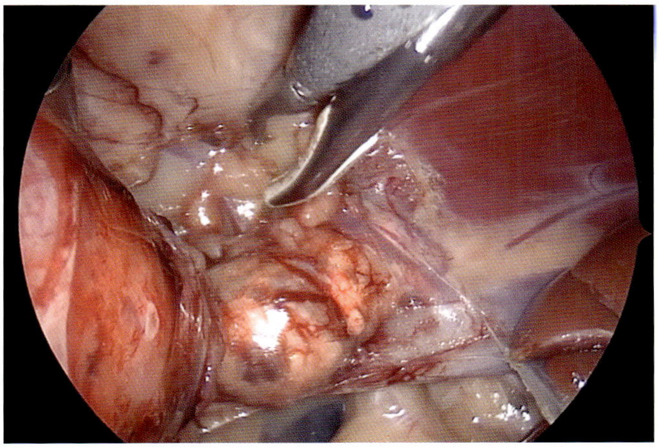

FIGURE 9. Adrenal gland dissection from its attachments to the fibrous tissue.

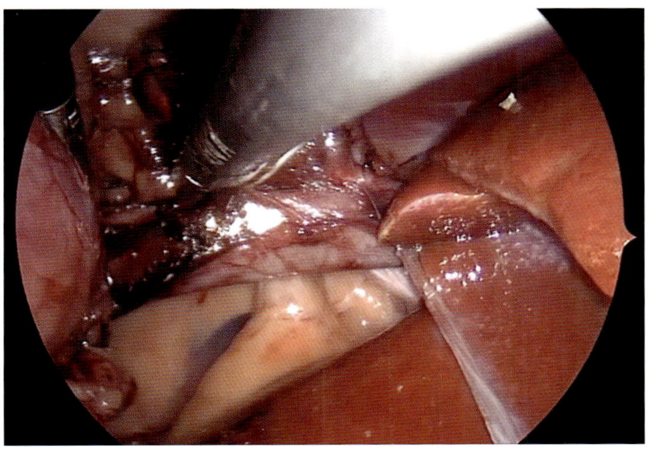

FIGURE 10. The ventral side, including the vena cava.

B ADRENALECTOMY IN LATERAL RECUMBENCY

PATIENT PREPARATION AND POSITIONING

The caudal aspect of the hemithorax and the lateral abdomen on the affected side are clipped and prepared for aseptic surgery. The patient is placed in lateral recumbency on the unaffected side. A cushion is placed under the erector spinae muscle group to raise the spine toward the surgeon.

OPERATING ROOM LAYOUT

The surgeon and the assistant stand facing the patient's ventral side. The video monitor is placed in front of them, on the dorsal side of the patient (**Fig. 11**).

Instruments

- Irrigation/suction unit (Surgiwand II, Tyco Healthcare, Elancourt, France)
- Self-retaining retractor (Endo Retract II, Tyco Healthcare)
- Bipolar forceps (Bipolar-Zangen 5 mm, Karl Storz Endoscope, Reims, France)
- Grasping forceps (Endo Grasp, Tyco Healthcare)
- Scissors (Endo Shears, Tyco Healthcare)
- Dissectors (Endo Dissect, Tyco Healthcare) connected to an electrosurgical unit
- Endoclips (Endo Clip II ML, Tyco Healthcare)
- LigaSure device (LigaSuret Lap, LigaSure Atlast, Valley ab, Tyco Healthcare, Brunn Gebirge, Austria)
- Feedback-controlled, bipolar vessel-sealing system used to achieve hemostasis

PORT PLACEMENT (FIG. 12)

- T1, 2–5 cm lateral to the umbilicus
- T2, 5–8 cm lateral to the subumbilical port in the lower left quadrant
- T3, 5–10 cm cranial to umbilicus on the left side

PROCEDURE

- After draping, a Veress needle is inserted just caudal to the 13th rib in the paralumbar fossa ipsilateral to the affected side. The abdomen is inflated with CO_2 until an intra-abdominal pressure of 8–10 mmHg is achieved. Inflation is adjusted according to the patient's size and physiologic variables.

Tips

It is important that T3 remains caudal to the last rib to avoid inadvertent penetration into the thoracic cavity.

- Laparoscopic examination of the tissues surrounding the affected adrenal gland and partial examination of the liver (incomplete because of the lateral position) is performed.
- Absence of liver macrometastases and macroscopic vascular invasion into the caudal vena cava should be confirmed in all patients.

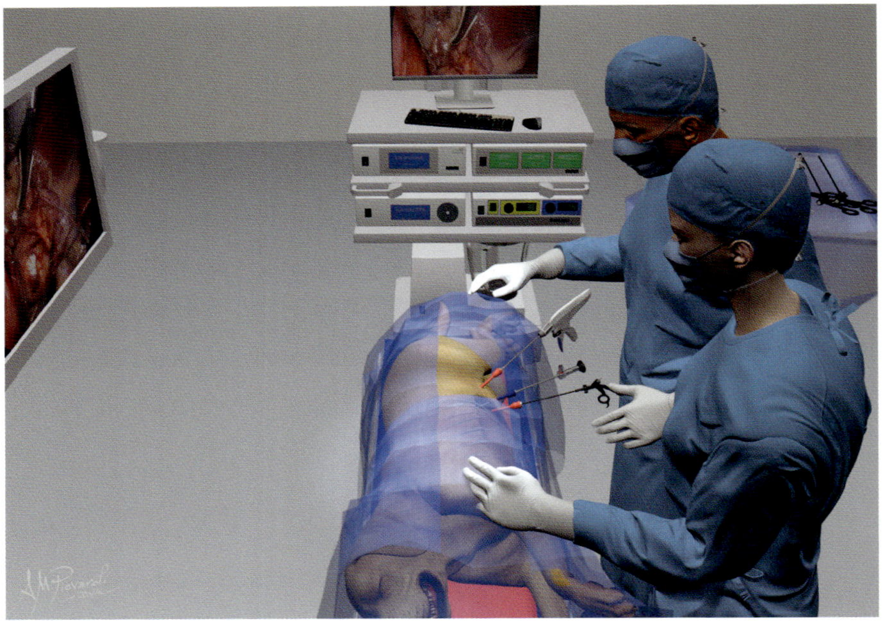

FIGURE 11. Operating room layout for laparoscopic adrenalectomy in lateral recumbency.

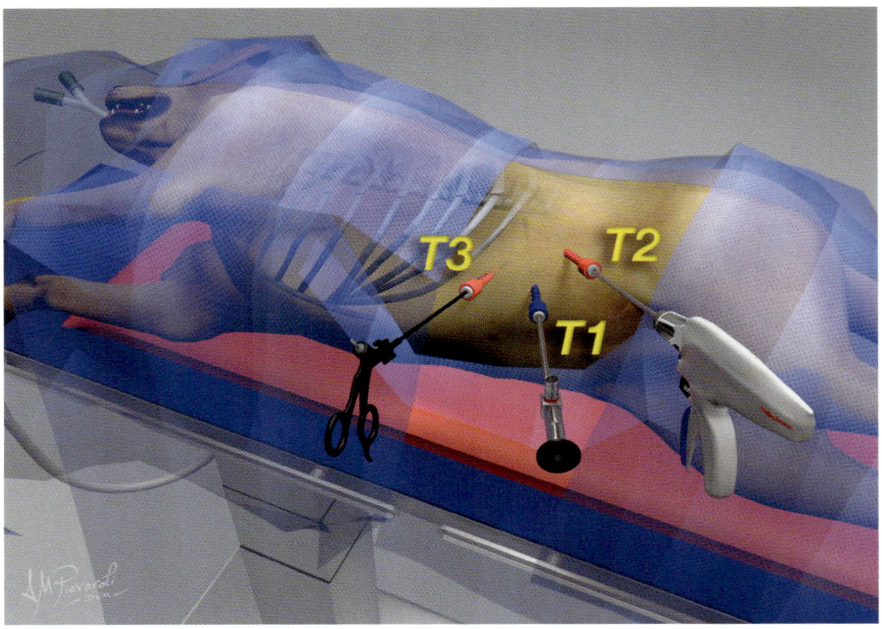

FIGURE 12. Port placement for laparoscopic adrenalectomy in lateral recumbency.

- Exposure and dissection of the adrenal glands are performed differently on the right and left sides because of anatomic differences.
- To achieve broad exposure of the right adrenal gland, the right lateral hepatic lobe is retracted cranially while the kidney is retracted dorsally. Because the patient is positioned in lateral recumbency with a cushion under the erector spinae muscle group, the descending duodenum or other organs are displaced by gravity. Dissection between the right adrenal gland and the caudal vena cava is carefully performed using an endoscopic dissector (**Fig. 13**).
- For exposure of the left adrenal gland, the descending colon is reflected medially, the left kidney dorsally, and the spleen ventrally.
- To minimize manipulation of the adrenal gland, the peritoneum is incised lateral to the adrenal gland.
- Care should be taken not to grasp the tumor directly but to use the periadrenal fat as a handle for grasping or simply to push the tumor in different directions using a blunt probe or the shaft of laparoscopic instruments to assist any manipulation.
- The phrenicoabdominal vein and artery are sealed with a vessel-sealing device, but laparoscopic hemoclips may be used in addition to the vessel-sealing device.
- When the gland is friable and under tension, or in the case of spontaneous rupture, a small window in the capsule is used to aspirate the necrotic semiliquid content at the center of the gland by using an irrigation/suction unit.
- After careful dissection, the remaining glandular tissue is progressively entirely removed in small pieces through the 12 mm protected trocar to prevent abdominal wall contamination.
- The abdomen is inspected for hemorrhage, and the adrenalectomy site is locally rinsed with small volumes of warmed lactated Ringer solution and concurrent use of close suction to avoid abdominal contamination with neoplastic cells (**Fig. 14**).
- After abdominal deflation, the laparoscopic ports are closed.
- The excised adrenal tissue is submitted for pathologic examination.

Key points

- The periadrenal tissue should be grasped as little as possible to minimize the risk of capsular rupture.
- The quality of the supportive care available for the postoperative period.

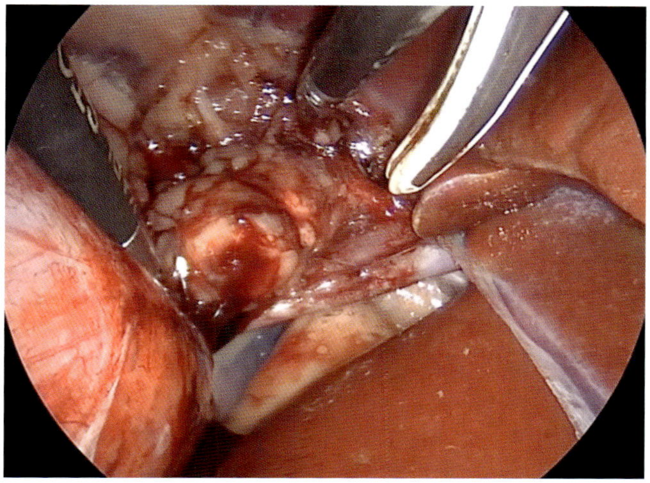

FIGURE 13. Dissection between the right adrenal gland and the caudal vena cava.

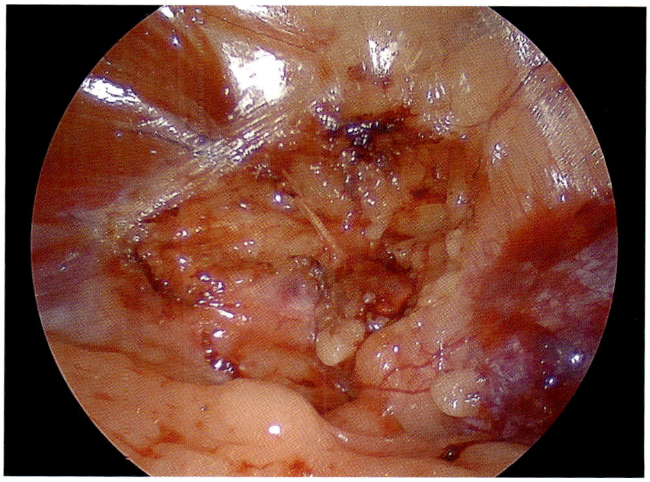

FIGURE 14. The adrenalectomy site is locally rinsed with small volumes of warmed lactated Ringer solution and the concurrent use of close suction to avoid abdominal contamination with neoplastic cells.

POSTOPERATIVE MANAGEMENT

- In dogs with functional adrenocortical tumors, monitoring for postoperative hypoadrenocorticism is necessary. Ongoing therapy with corticosteroids should be continued for 2–3 weeks postoperatively until the results of ACTH stimulation tests confirm normal corticosteroid production from the contralateral adrenal gland.
- Postoperative complications occur with high incidence following adrenalectomy (30%, according to Lang et al., 2011).
- Close monitoring in ICU settings.
- Hypo- or hypertension.
- Arrhythmias.
- Vomiting.
- Esophagitis.
- Seizures.
- Pancreatitis.
- Acute renal failure.
- Hemoperitoneum.
- Hyperthermia.
- Hypokalemia.
- Tachypnea and cardiopulmonary arrest.

Complications of laparoscopic adrenalectomy in sternal or lateral recumbency

- Dissection close to major vascular structures makes profuse hemorrhage possible. If significant hemorrhage occurs in laparoscopic cases, immediate conversion to an open approach should be performed.
- The most significant arterial bleeding the author has encountered came from the cranial abdominal branch of the phrenicoabdominal artery as it dives dorsal to the kidney. If it is possible to suction enough blood to visualize the bleeding vessels, clamping or clip application can be performed laparoscopically.
- The most common problem is “nuisance” hemorrhage that is not hemodynamically significant but prevents visualization of the surgical field and prolongs surgical time.
- Thromboembolism is a potentially fatal complication seen after both open and laparoscopic adrenalectomy in dogs and necessitates careful monitoring.
- Other important postadrenalectomy complications that can be fatal include pancreatitis and renal failure.

C RETROPERITONEAL ADRENALECTOMY

When laparoscopic adrenalectomy was performed in lateral recumbency, as described by Jiménez Peláez et al., the surgery was feasible and without intraoperative complications. Laparoscopic adrenalectomy performed with the patient in sternal recumbency has the advantages of allowing gravitational displacement of the abdominal organs, better visualization of the adrenal gland, and a shorter surgical time than conventional laparoscopy or open adrenalectomy. The mean surgical time was reported to be 78.7 minutes. However, both methods require retraction of the abdominal organs.

In human medicine, operative times for laparoscopic adrenalectomy have not shortened since the procedure was first performed in 1992. Retroperitoneoscopic adrenalectomy was devised in 1994 to address this issue. After standardization of the procedure, it has been reported that retroperitoneoscopic adrenalectomy had the advantages of a shorter operative time, less blood loss, and less pain compared with transperitoneal laparoscopic adrenalectomy. It has been suggested that these advantages are due to minimal organ retraction allowing direct access to the adrenal gland. Recently, surgical procedures performed through a single port have become popular in human medicine because they afford better patient comfort, superior cosmetic results, less pain, and faster functional recovery.

In dogs, right adrenalectomy is a challenging and time-consuming surgery compared to the left one. It is particularly hard to have good visualization and separation. The laparoscopic transperitoneal approach is completely suitable for left adrenalectomy, but in right adrenal tumors, extra separation and caution are usually needed to avoid bipolar-related organic lesions or vascular lesions during dissection of the caval margin of the gland that could cause massive and possibly fatal hemorrhages.

> Single-port retroperitoneoscopic adrenalectomy is a minimally invasive surgery with the additional advantages of using a single-port access and the ability to use a retroperitoneal approach.

Jeong et al. proved in 2016 the feasibility of pneumoretroperitoneum in dogs. One year later, the same Korean group published an article about single-port retroperitoneal adrenalectomy in healthy Beagle dogs. Clinical cases were successfully performed in selected patients with noninvasive middle-sized adrenal masses.

PATIENT PREPARATION AND POSITIONING

The patient is placed in lateral recumbency with lumbar elevation using a cushion and secured with self-adhesive tape. The dorsal and lateral aspects of the hemithorax and hemiabdomen are clipped from the 11th thoracic vertebra to the 7th lumbar vertebra for aseptic surgery. It is necessary to transect the skin and fascia and to separate muscular layers to access the retroperitoneal space.

OPERATING ROOM LAYOUT

The video monitor is placed in front of the surgeons on the patient's dorsal side (**Fig. 15**).

PORT PLACEMENT (FIGS. 16 AND 17)

- SILS port (T1, T2, T3), in the flank of the affected adrenal gland

Instruments

- SILS port (Covidien, New Haven, CT)
- Three 5 mm cannulas
- Telescope 5 mm – 0° (Karl Storz, Tuttlingen, Germany)
- Ultrasonic scalpel (Harmonic or Sonicision)
- Vascular dissection and sealing
- Advanced bipolar sealers

PROCEDURE

- After draping, a Veress needle is inserted caudal to the 13th rib in the paralumbar fossa ipsilateral to the affected side.
- A 3 cm skin incision is made immediately lateral to the epaxial muscles and 10 cm caudal to the last rib.
- An electrocautery is used for hemostasis to prevent hemorrhage after the skin incision is made with a scalpel.
- Blunt dissection with Metzenbaum scissors, with the index finger positioned below the epaxial muscle, is used to access the retroperitoneal space through the muscle structures (external oblique, internal oblique, and transverse abdominis).
- The ability to palpate the dorsal aspect of the kidney indicates successful entry into the retroperitoneal space after dissection of the thoracolumbar fascia.

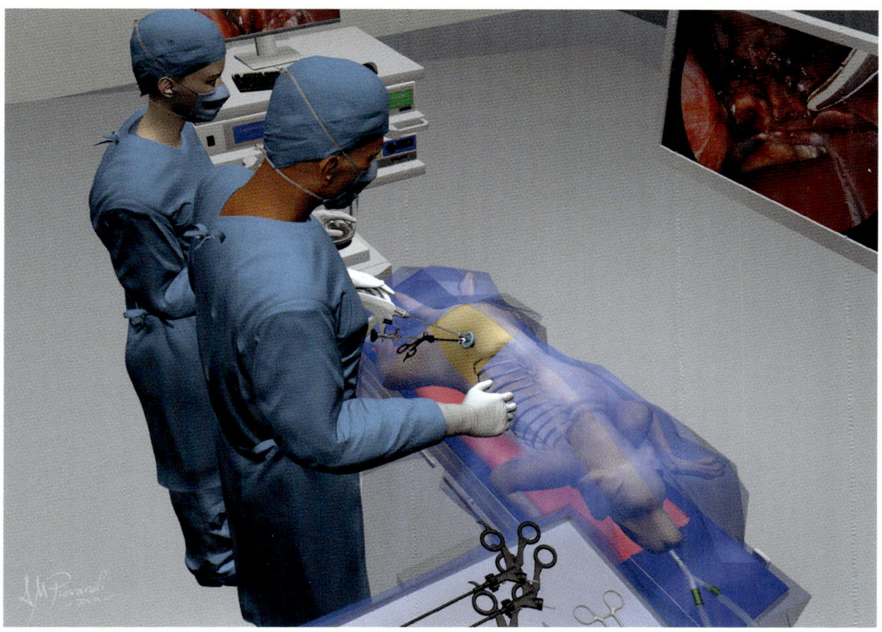

FIGURE 15. Operating room layout for laparoscopic retroperitoneal adrenalectomy.

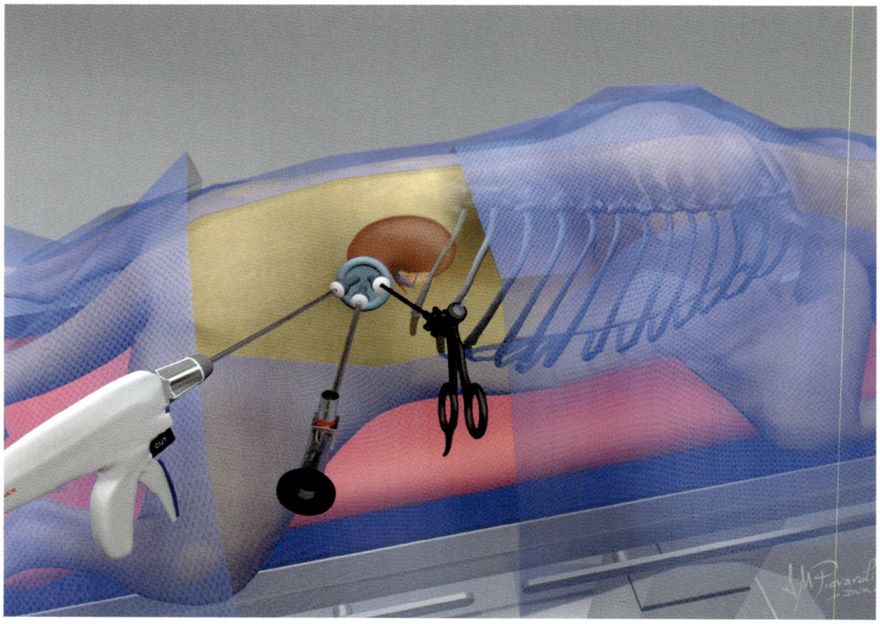

FIGURE 16. Port placement for retroperitoneal adrenalectomy.

- This maneuver can be assisted with transperitoneal laparoscopic visualization using a sublumbar laparoscopic port.
- When the pneumoretroperitoneum is established, the pneumoperitoneum must be extracted, and this optical port can be closed or reserved in case conversion from a retroperitoneoscopic to a laparoscopic approach.
- The SILS port is implanted, placing a stay suture for retraction of the skin and muscles.

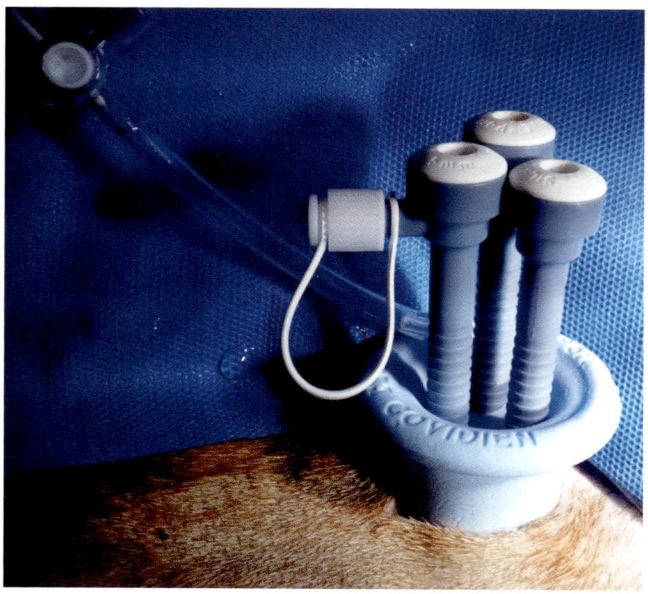

FIGURE 17. Intraoperative image of port placement.

- After placing the three 5 mm cannulas through the SILS port to triangulate the laparoscopic instruments, the retroperitoneal space is investigated using the telescope (**Fig. 18**).
- When the retroperitoneal space is visualized, pneumoretroperitoneum is induced using an insufflator (Karl Storz) at a pressure of 5 mmHg (**Figs. 19 and 20**).
- An ultrasonic scalpel is recommended to accomplish the vascular dissection and sealing. Other devices, such as advanced bipolar sealers, can also be used.
- Separation and/or excision of the perirenal fat pad is made. The surgical plane between the fat pad and the lateral aspect

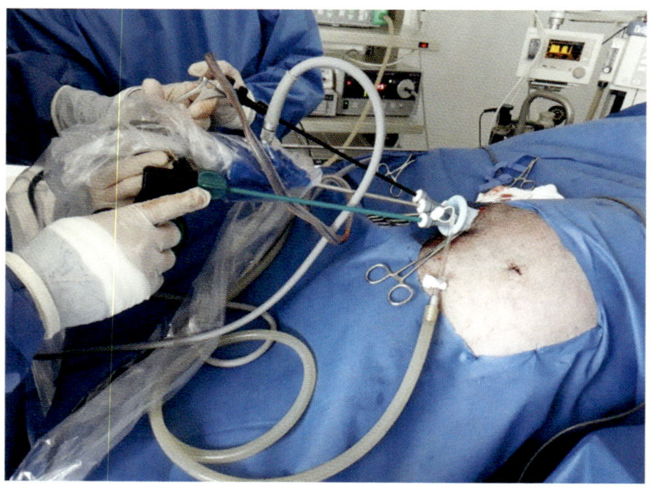

FIGURE 18. Three 5 mm cannulas are inserted through the SILS port for triangulation of the laparoscopic instruments.

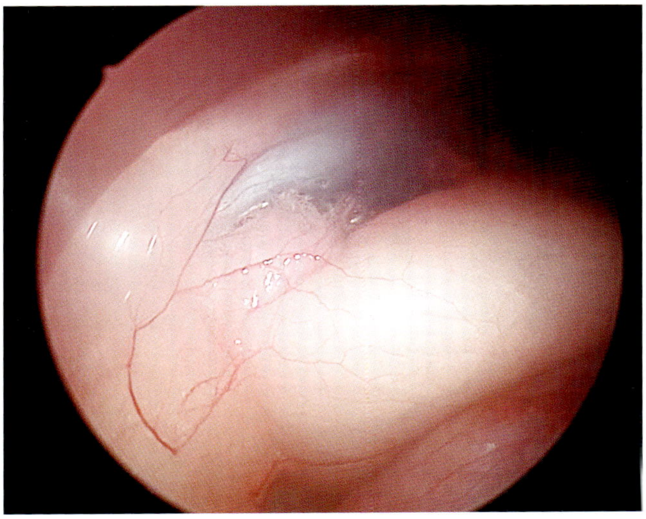

FIGURE 19. Retropneumoperitoneum creation and SILS port installation.

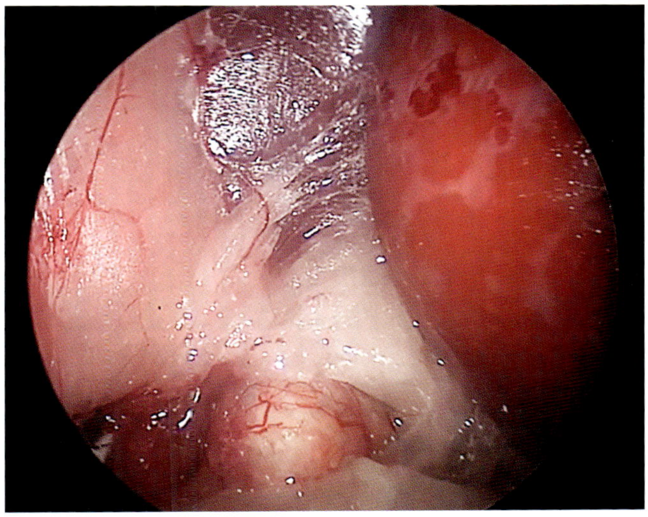

FIGURE 20. Pneumoretroperitoneum.

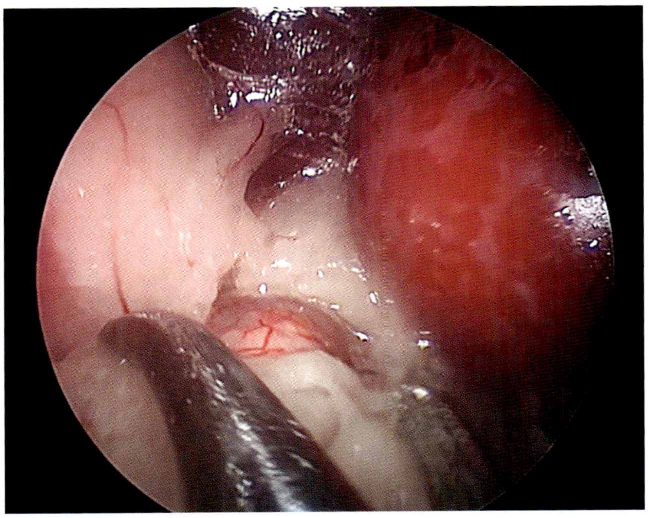

FIGURE 21. The fat pad and the lateral aspect of the kidney to gain access to the adrenal gland.

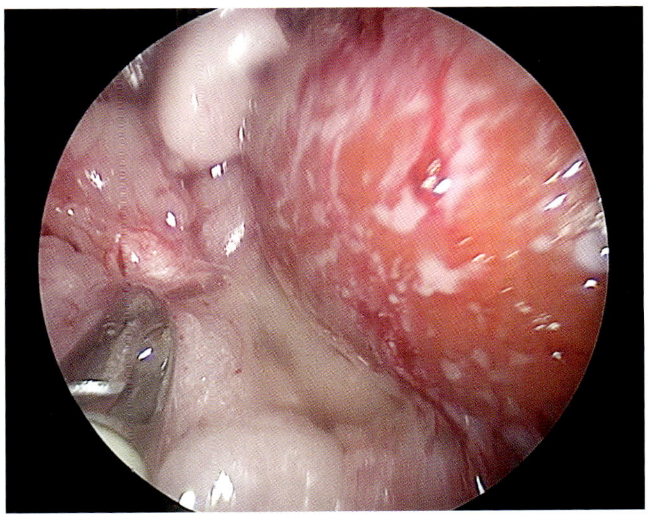

FIGURE 22. Absence of liver macrometastases and macroscopic vascular invasion.

of the kidney is dissected to gain access to the adrenal gland (**Fig. 21**).

- Retroperitoneoscopic examination of the kidney and its pedicle, adrenal gland, vena cava, and integrity of the peritoneum is performed.
- Absence of liver macrometastases and macroscopic vascular invasion into the caudal vena cava should be confirmed in all patients (**Fig. 22**).
- The distal segment of the phrenicoabdominal vein is identified, sealed, and transected.
- Exposure and dissection of the adrenal glands are performed from caudal to cranial (close to far from the camera) (**Fig. 23**).
- To achieve the dissection of the adrenal-cava plane, the gland must be elevated from the caudal pole, grasping the gland from a sealed and transected small pedicle.
- At about half of the adrenal-cava dissection plane, it is possible to identify the proximal segment of the phrenicoabdominal vein. This vessel must be sealed and transected as close to the gland as possible.

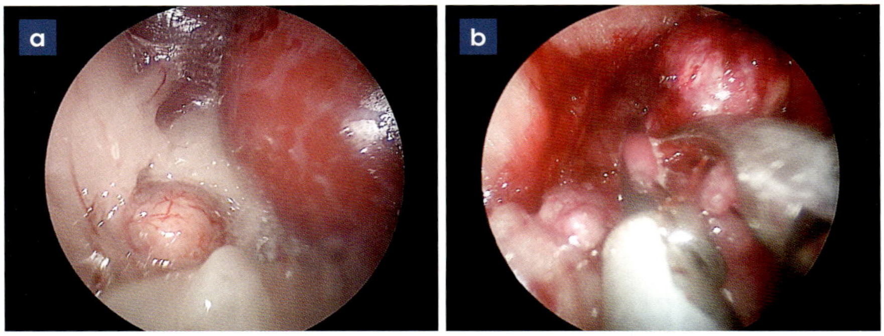

FIGURE 23. Dissection of the adrenal glands performed from caudal to cranial.

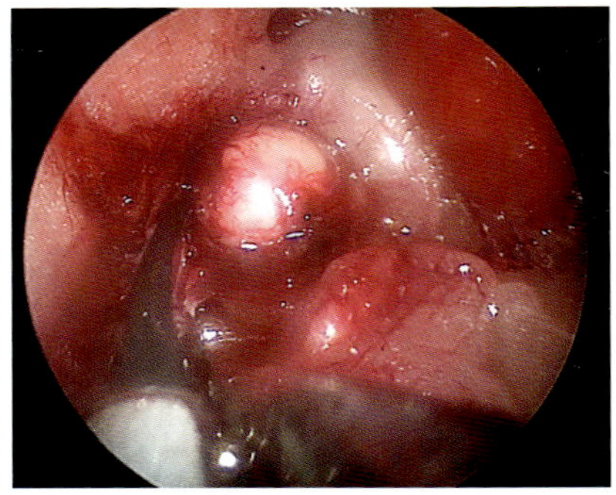

FIGURE 24. Periadrenal fat.

- Care must be taken not to grasp the tumor directly but to use the periadrenal fat as a handle for grasping or simply to push the tumor in different directions using a blunt probe or the shaft of laparoscopic instruments to assist any manipulation (**Fig. 24**).
- When the gland is friable and under tension, or in case of spontaneous rupture, a small window in the capsule is used to aspirate the necrotic semiliquid content at the center of the gland by using an irrigation/suction unit.
- After careful dissection, the remaining glandular tissue is progressively entirely removed along with the SILS port to prevent abdominal wall contamination.
- The retroperitoneal space is inspected for hemorrhage, and the adrenalectomy site is locally rinsed with small volumes of warmed lactated Ringer solution and concurrent use of close suction to avoid abdominal contamination with neoplastic cells. All remaining gas must be aspirated to avoid postsurgical pain.
- After total gas elimination, the incision is closed.
- The excised adrenal tissue is submitted for histopathological examination.

Complications of laparoscopic retroperitoneal adrenalectomy

- Subcutaneous emphysema.
- Hematoma.
- Hernia.
- Dehiscence.
- Hemorrhage.
- Substantial hemorrhage, which is a possible complication during surgery, will not occur if the renal vessels, aorta, and caudal vena cava are securely separated in the approach and during the resection of the adrenal gland.
- If severe bleeding occurs, conversion to open surgery would be required, but this should not affect the outcome for the patient.

SUGGESTED READINGS

CLINICAL CASES

40.1 RIGHT LAPAROSCOPIC ADRENALECTOMY

William T. N. Culp

CASE DESCRIPTION

A 10-year-old spayed female Samoyed was evaluated for treating a right-sided adrenal tumor (adrenocortical adenoma). The adrenal mass was found incidentally during abdominal ultrasonography performed for staging of a mammary mass. A CT-angiography scan revealed a noninvasive right-sided adrenal gland mass that was 2×2×2.3 cm. A three-port laparoscopic approach was used.

Key points

- A CT angiography scan is very useful preoperatively to determine if vascular invasion has occurred.
- It is crucial to be sure of the location of the vena cava during the entire procedure, especially during dissection of right-sided masses.

PORT PLACEMENT

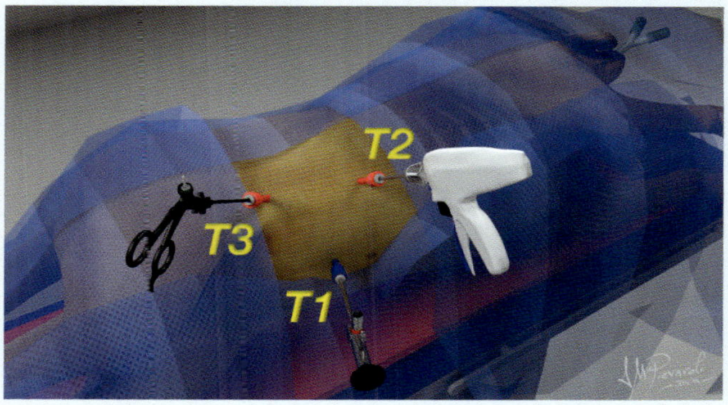

The patient was placed in lateral recumbency. A 1 cm incision was made approximately 3 cm caudal to the umbilicus and 1 cm to the right of the midline. A modified Hasson technique was used to create a camera port, and the tip of a 6 mm Endotip trocarless cannula (Ternamian Endotip Cannula, Karl Storz) was introduced into the peritoneal cavity. A 5 mm 30° telescope (T1) (Hopkins Forward-Oblique Telescope, Karl Storz) was introduced and used to help place two instrument cannulas. One instrument port was created a few centimeters caudal to the 13th rib (T2), with the second instrument port (T3) created several centimeters caudal to T2 in a triangulated pattern. During part of the procedure, the operating table may be tilted, dropping the ventral aspect of the patient.

PROCEDURE

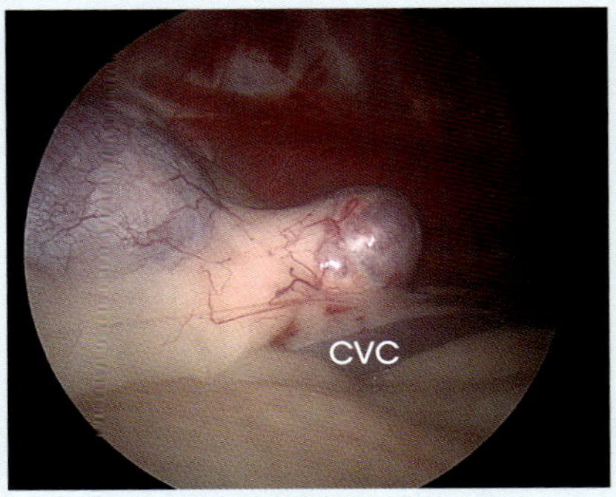

FIGURE 1. Laparoscopic image of a right-sided adrenal mass prior to dissection. The cranial vena cava (CVC) can be seen in close proximity to the mass.

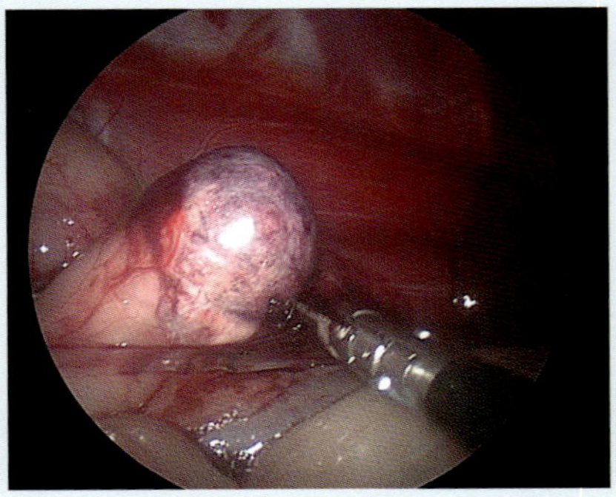

FIGURE 2. Blunt dissection of the adrenal gland mass from the surrounding retroperitoneal attachments and the vena cava starts at the cranial aspect of the mass using a right-angle forceps.

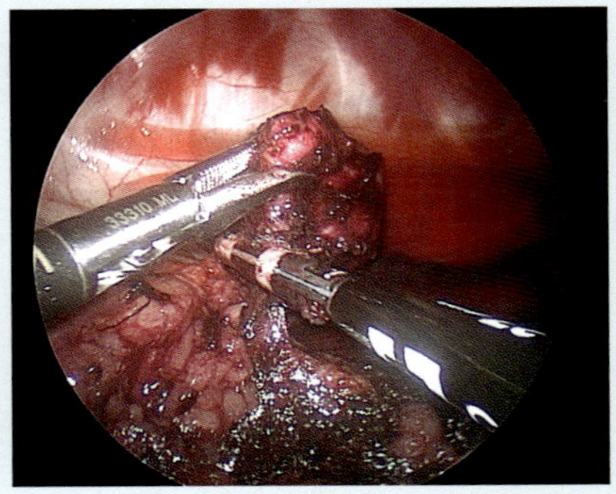

FIGURE 3. A combination of dissection is performed with a right-angle forceps and a vessel-sealing device.

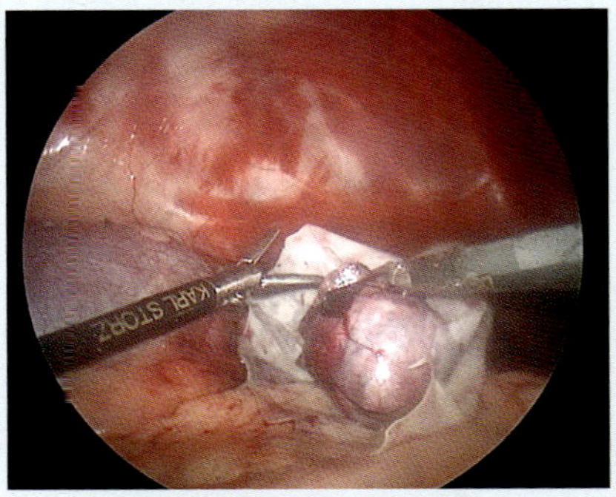

FIGURE 4. Once the adrenal gland mass has been completely freed from attachments and vascular supply, the gland is placed into the cut thumb of a sterile surgical glove for extraction.

Tips and tricks

- ✓ Try to maintain some noncapsular tissue attached to the mass so that this tissue can be grasped during dissection and allow for improved visualization of new dissection planes.
- ✓ For dissection of the caudal pole of the adrenal gland, a probe can be inserted through the caudal cannula to apply caudal traction on the kidney to improve visualization.

40.2 LAPAROSCOPIC RIGHT ADRENALECTOMY FOR ADRENAL ADENOCARCINOMA IN A DOG

Hiroo Kanai

CASE DESCRIPTION

A 12-year-old intact female 6.1 kg toy Poodle presented for polyuria and polydipsia. An adrenal tumor was suspected based on hormone measurement and echography results. After adrenalectomy, histopathological examination of the gland showed adrenal adenocarcinoma, and no damage to the adrenal gland capsule was observed histopathologically. Six months after the operation, this dog had not experienced recurrence and was in good general health.

Key points

- Ultrasound examination revealed a major axis of the right adrenal gland of 1.8 cm, with an irregular surface.
- After CT (**Fig. 1**), it was confirmed that the blood vessels ran around the adrenal gland, so the right adrenal gland was removed laparoscopically.
- Finally, the cranial abdominal vein, which flows into the cranial vena cava, was transected.

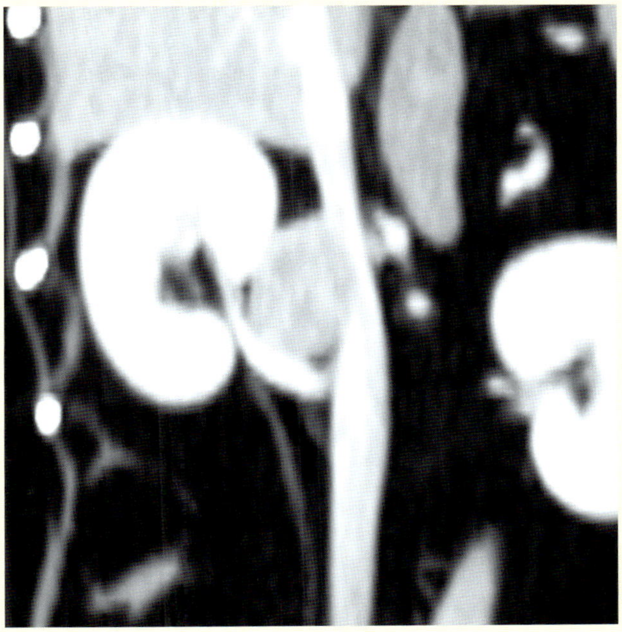

FIGURE 1. CT image showing enlargement of the right adrenal gland (1.8 cm in diameter). Note that the adrenal glands are close to the renal vein.

PORT PLACEMENT

The patient was placed in left lateral recumbency. Three ports were placed in a triangulating fashion around the site of the adrenal gland. A 10 mm trocar was placed for a camera port (T1). In the right flank on the center of the area, T2 and T3 were placed cranial and caudal to T1, respectively, to achieve triangulation.

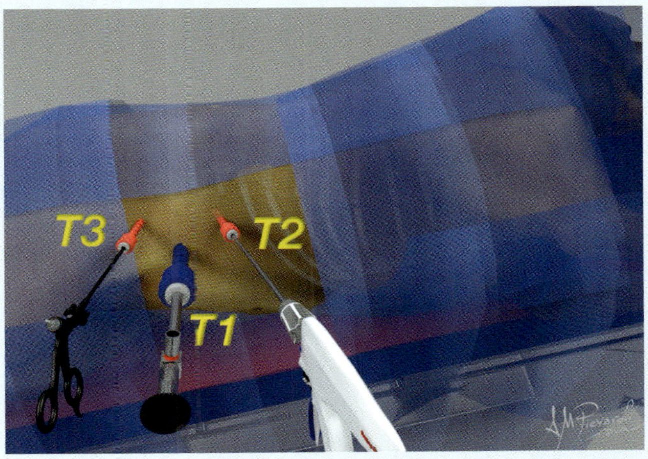

PROCEDURE

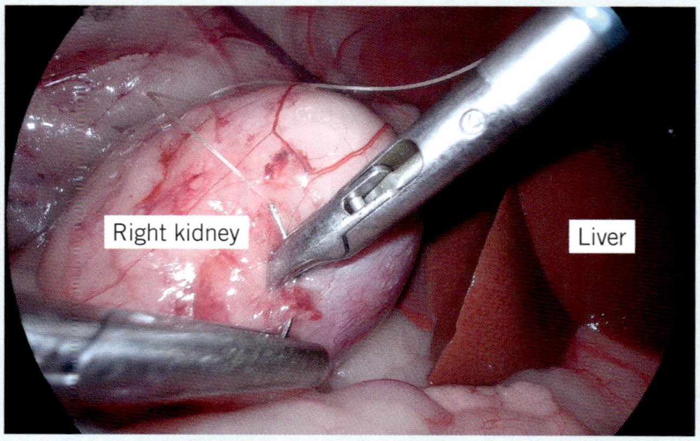

FIGURE 2. The adrenal gland is dissected firstly from the caudal side using the marionette method to pull the right kidney caudally. A one-needle suture is ligated on the renal serosa, and the end of the thread is pulled out of the abdominal cavity and clamped with forceps.

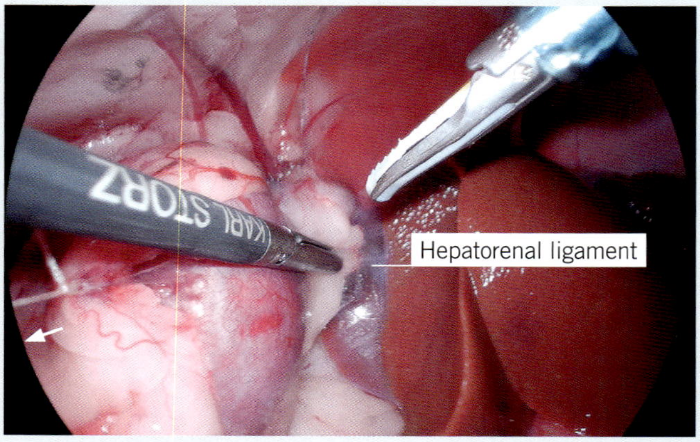

FIGURE 3. Pulling the kidney caudally with the marionette method (arrow) makes it easier to approach the right adrenal gland. The hepatorenal ligament is dissected with an ultrasonic coagulation and incision device.

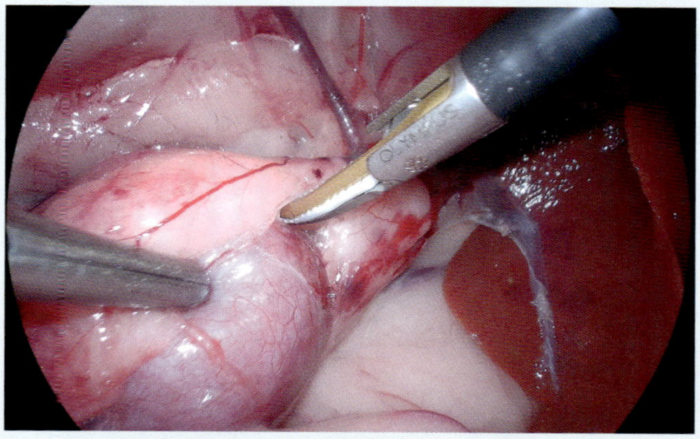

FIGURE 4. The adrenal gland is dissected from the back, exposing the major psoas muscle. The fat layer in contact with the kidney is peeled so the kidney can be pulled further caudally.

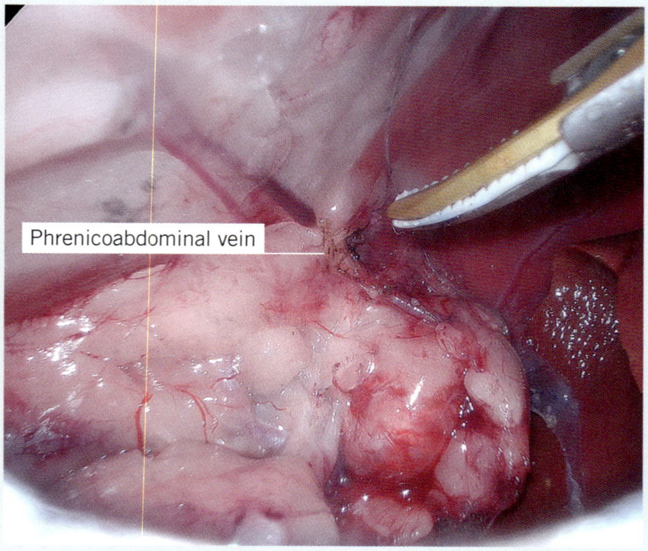

FIGURE 5. The phrenicoabdominal artery and vein flowing into the adrenal glands are dissected with an ultrasonic coagulation and incision device.

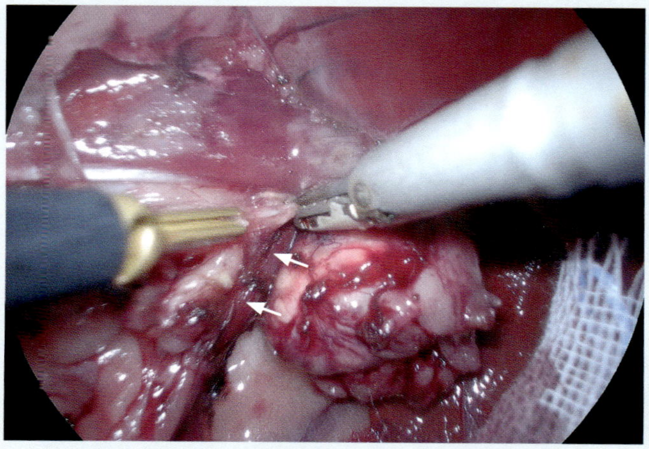

FIGURE 6. The adrenal artery is coagulated with a bipolar electrosurgical knife. Care should be taken not to damage the renal veins (arrows) that run nearby.

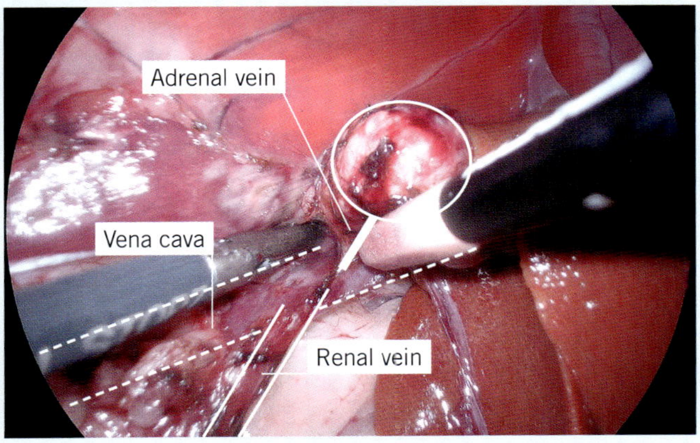

FIGURE 7. Local anatomical photograph before ligating the adrenal vein. Because the kidney is pulled caudally, proper dissection can be performed, even though the renal vein and adrenal vein are very close to each other.

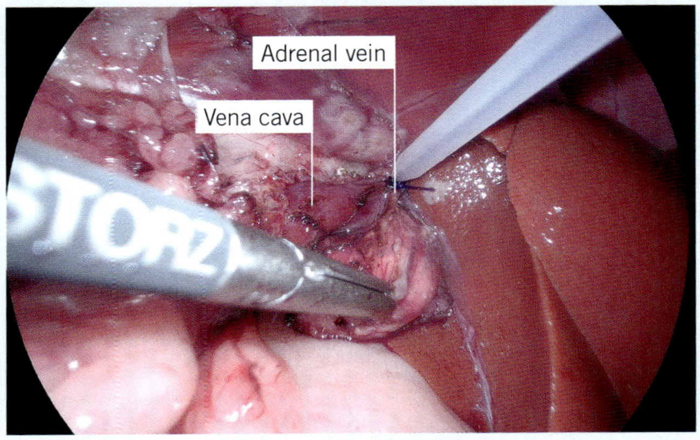

FIGURE 8. The adrenal vein is ligated with an Endoloop Ligature (J&J Medical Devices). Adjusting the ligation position by applying appropriate traction with left-hand forceps is important.

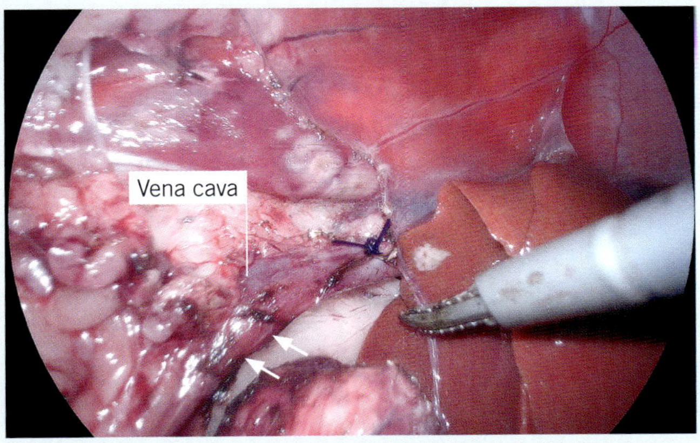

FIGURE 9. Local anatomical photograph after left adrenal resection. The renal veins are protected (arrows), and the adrenal glands are properly resected.

Tips and tricks

- ✓ Placing a small thin towel beneath the patient's lumbar area will alter the patient's position from standard lateral recumbency to a slightly more dorsal recumbency and may improve visibility by shifting the intestinal tract away from the adrenal glands.
- ✓ The operating table may be moved during surgery but should be kept flat to avoid accidents such as falling of instruments.
- ✓ The patient was placed in left lateral recumbency but can be tilted slightly towards ventral recumbency if the view becomes obstructed by bowels. Three ports were placed on the right flank.

40.3 RIGHT ADRENALECTOMY IN A YORKSHIRE TERRIER DOG

David García Rubio

CASE DESCRIPTION

A 12-year-old Yorkshire Terrier with an incidental ultrasound finding of an increase in the size of the right adrenal gland, although it has not lost its shape, was presented. The CT scan findings did not show encroachment into the caudal vena cava and raised suspicions about the neoplastic origin of the mass.

Key points

- The necessary tests should be carried out to discern whether it is a functional tumor with a view to prior medical stabilization of the patient.
- The adrenal gland receives arterial flow from small vessels stemming from the aorta, the renal artery, and the phrenicoabdominal trunk, and it is superficially crossed by a single phrenicoabdominal vein.
- The right adrenal gland is closely associated with the caudal vena cava, sharing the adventitia layer.

PORT PLACEMENT

The patient was placed in sternal recumbency and approached from the right abdomen. Three trocars triangulated the adrenal area, positioning the most cranial behind the last rib (T2). The central trocar was used for the telescope (T1), and the two lateral trocars were used for instrumentation (T2, T3). Inserting a fourth trocar for the use of a separator (T4) may be useful.

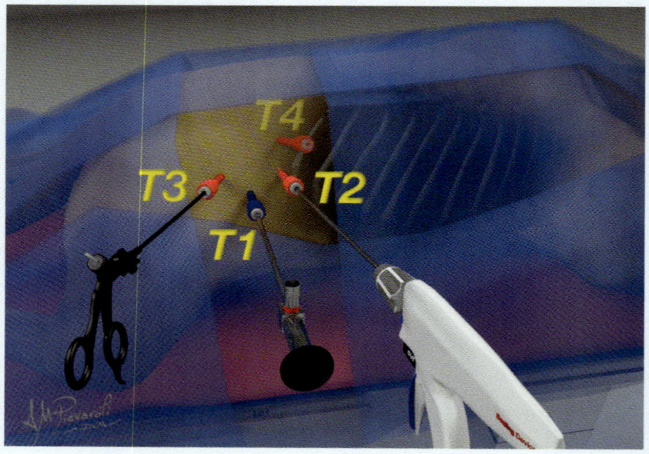

PROCEDURE

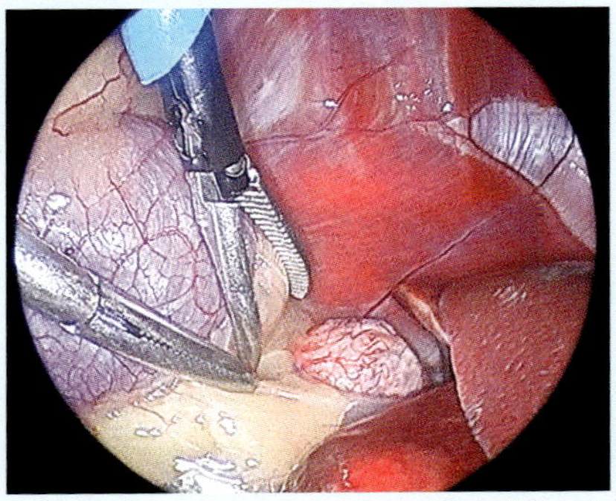

FIGURE 1. First view of the cranial abdomen. Cranial is to the right of the image. The image shows the right kidney in a caudal direction, the right adrenal gland, and the right lateral and caudate lobes of the liver in the cranial area.

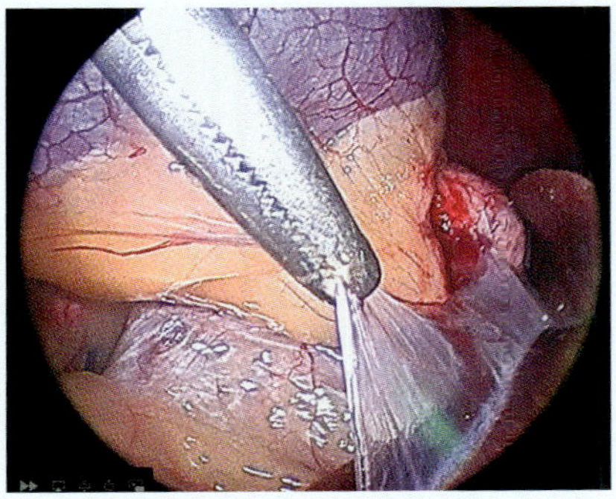

FIGURE 2. The hepatorenal ligament that joins the right kidney with the caudate process of the caudate lobe can be sectioned to improve visualization of the area.

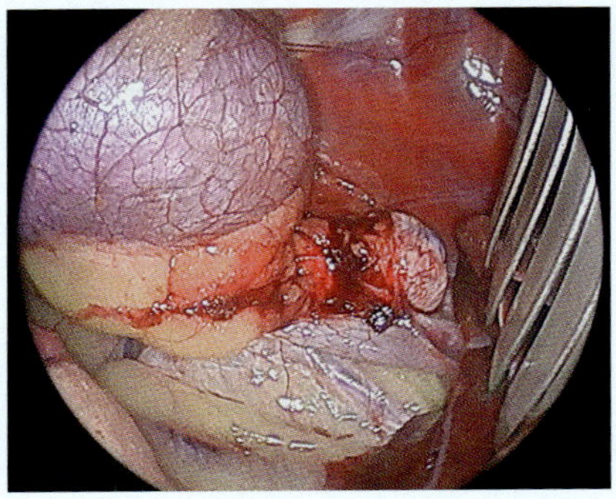

FIGURE 3. Detailed view of an articulating fan retractor to separate the hepatic lobes.

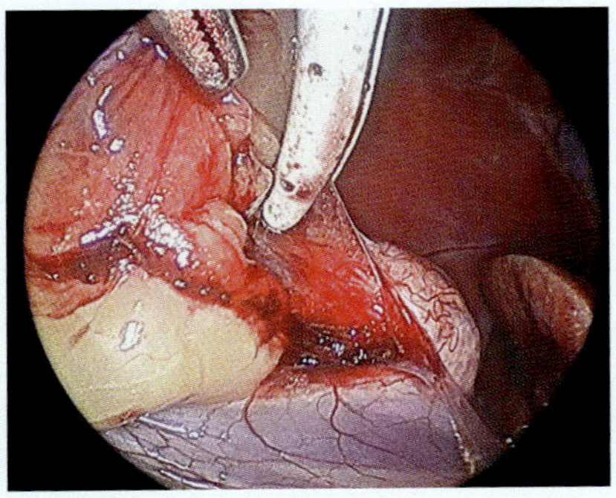

FIGURE 4. Dissection of the lateral part of the gland via cauterization of the arterial branches using a bipolar LigaSure system (Medtronic, Minneapolis, MN).

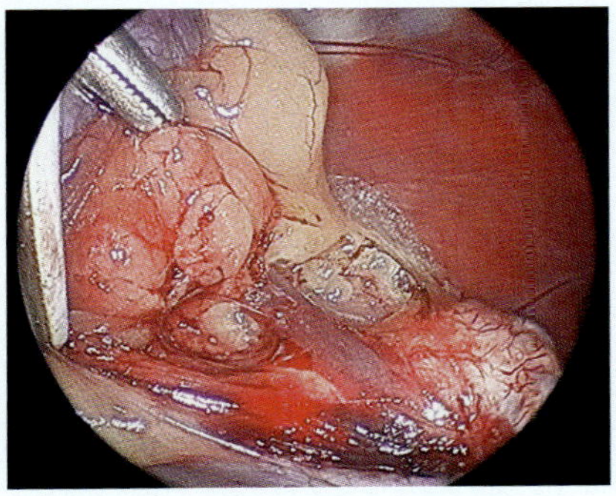

FIGURE 5. Detailed view of the phrenicoabdominal vein. This should be bound or cauterized at its medial and lateral aspects.

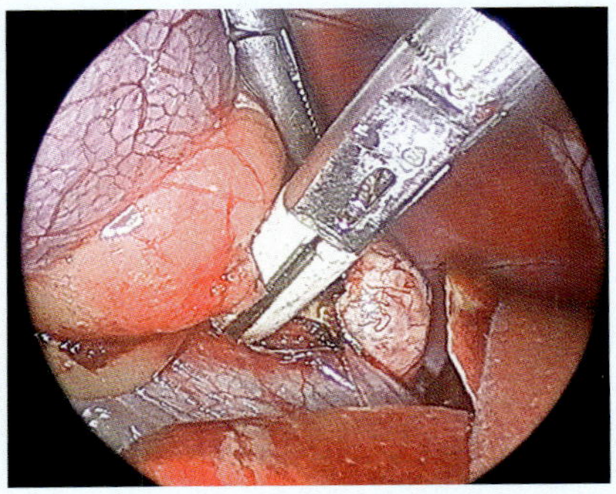

FIGURE 6. Careful dissection of the gland at its medial aspect. Exercise great caution to ensure the vena cava and right renal vein are not lacerated.

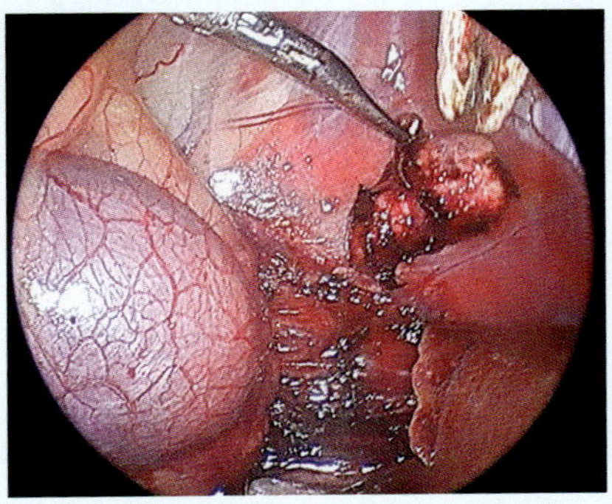

FIGURE 7. Full separation of the gland for its extraction via collection bag.

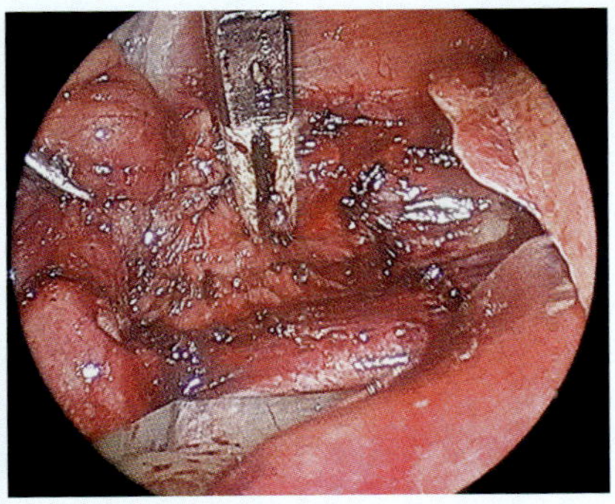

FIGURE 8. Final appearance of the surgical area and check for absence of bleeding.

Tips and tricks

- ✓ Be extremely careful when handling the gland. Never hold it directly, but rather grasp the peripheral tissue or stump of the phrenicoabdominal vein once it has been sectioned.
- ✓ The use of advanced coagulation systems is highly useful, but they are not recommended for use in areas near the vena cava to prevent the risk of subsequent sores.
- ✓ In secreting adrenal tumors, Cushing syndrome may generate hepatomegaly, and the lobes may block the view of the gland, so a separator may be useful.

40.4 LEFT ADRENALECTOMY IN A DOG

Ikuya Ehara

CASE DESCRIPTION

A 12-year-old female Shih Tzu (body weight 8.2 kg) was presented with an enlarged left adrenal gland that was noted during an annual examination.

Key points

- Placing a small thin towel beneath the patient's lumbar area will alter the patient's position from standard lateral recumbency to a slightly more dorsal recumbency and may improve visibility by shifting the intestinal tract away from the adrenals.
- The operating table may be moved during surgery but should be kept flat to avoid accidents such as falling of instruments.

PORT PLACEMENT

Three ports were placed in the right flank in a triangulating fashion: T1 on the center of the area, T2 cranial to T1, and T3 caudal to T1.

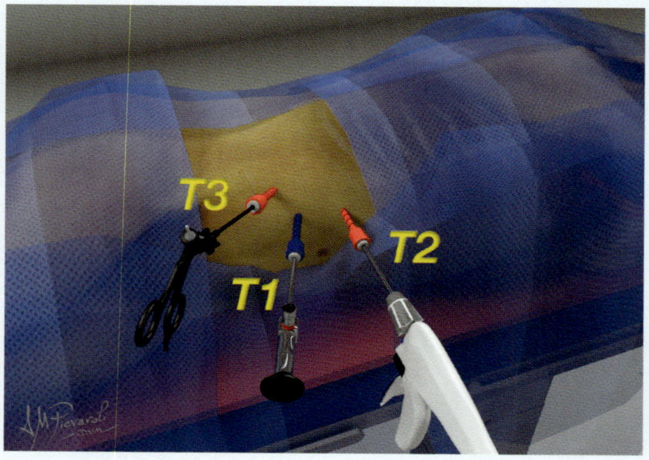

PROCEDURE

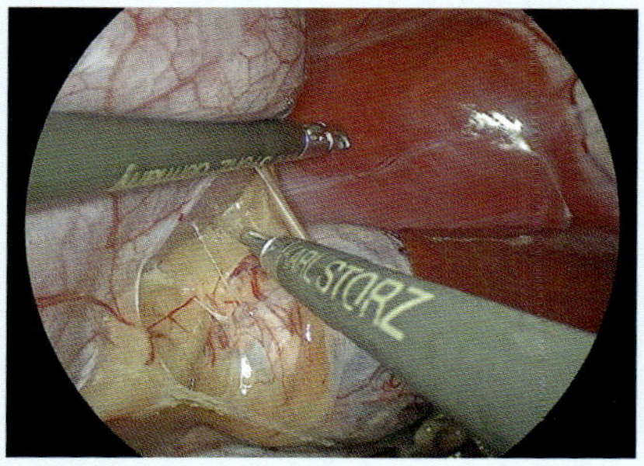

FIGURE 1. First, the adipose tissue between the adrenal gland and the kidney, and the adrenal gland and the liver are dissected with an ultrasonic coagulation and a cutting device.

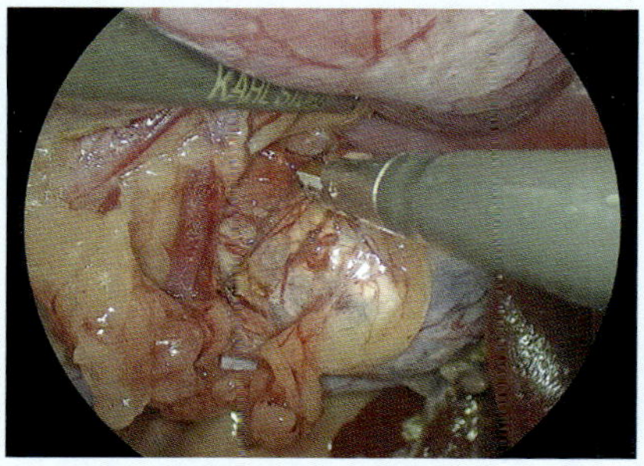

FIGURE 2. After dissection of the surrounding tissue to the renal vein region, gradual dorsal dissection reveals newly formed vessels in the adrenal gland.

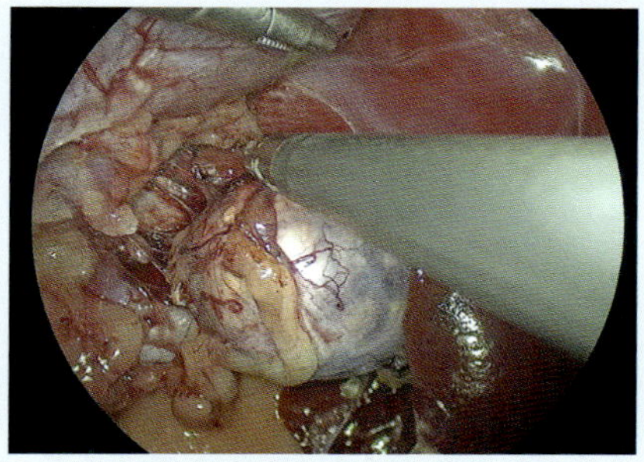

FIGURE 3. The neovasculature to the adrenal gland is sealed close with an ultrasonic coagulation and cutting device.

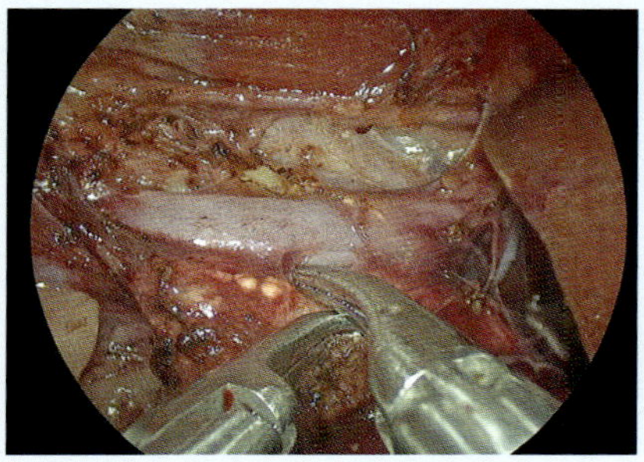

FIGURE 4. After dissection of the dorsal aspect, the adrenal gland is reflected ventrally to dissect the connective tissue between the gland and the caudal vena cava with Maryland forceps.

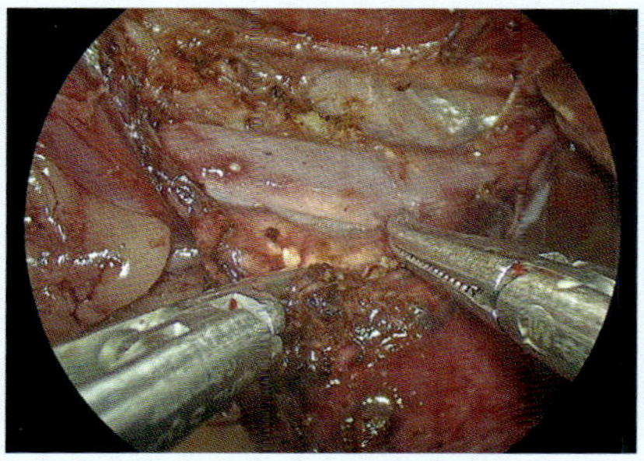

FIGURE 5. Dissection of connective tissue between adrenal gland and caudal vena cava, caudal to the phrenicoabdominal vein.

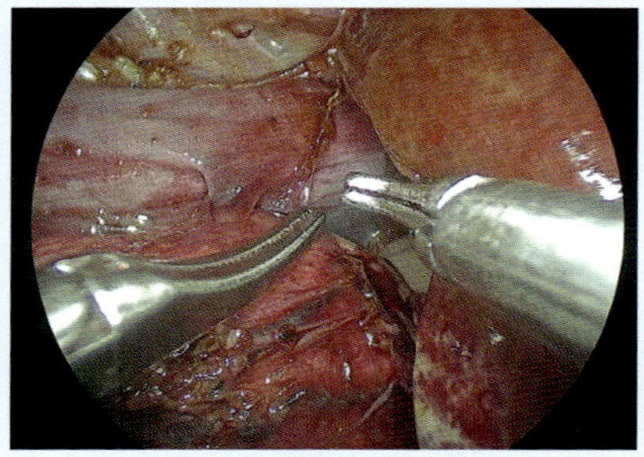

FIGURE 6. Dissection of connective tissue between the adrenal gland and the caudal vena cava.

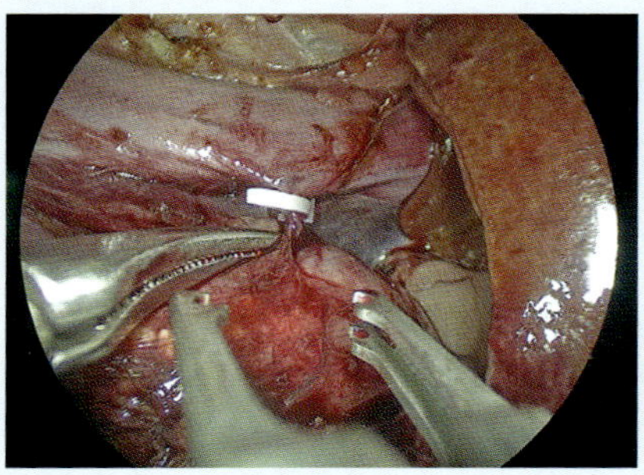

FIGURE 7. The phrenicoabdominal vein is closed with a hemoclip (5 mm Hem-o-lok, ML).

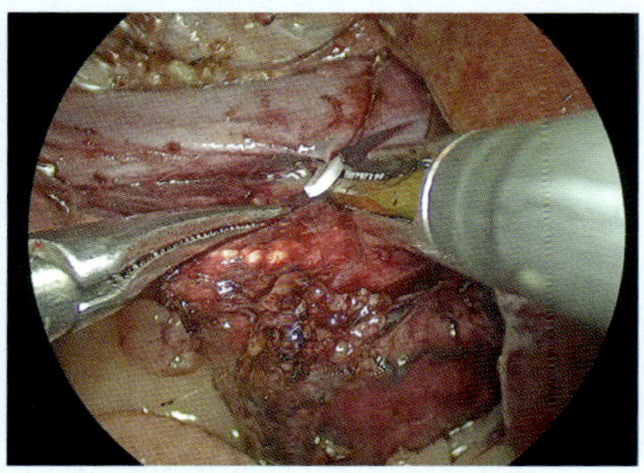

FIGURE 8. The phrenicoabdominal vein is transected after creating an entry point for the blade of the ultrasonic coagulation and cutting device in the connective tissue on the adrenal aspect of the vein to avoid traumatizing the gland.

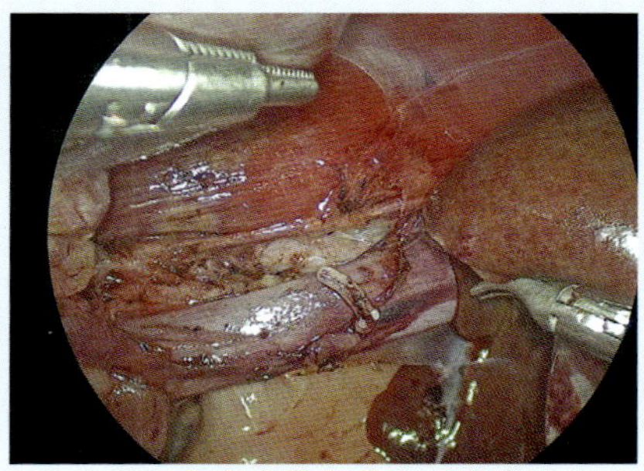

FIGURE 9. Completed adrenalectomy.

Tips and tricks

- ✓ Approach under lateral recumbency.
- ✓ Take care to avoid traumatizing the renal vein and the caudal vena cava.
- ✓ Take care to avoid traumatizing the adrenal capsule.

40.5 LAPAROSCOPIC RIGHT ADRENALECTOMY

Przemysław Prządka, Stanisław Dzimira, Agnieszka Antończyk, Łukasz Juźwiak, Bartłomiej Liszka

CASE DESCRIPTION

A 9.5-year-old male American Staffordshire Terrier (weight 24 kg) was evaluated for the treatment of a right-sided adrenal tumor (adrenocortical adenoma). The tumor was 3.6×1.73×1.63 cm in size. After ultrasound examination and contrast tomography, the patient was qualified for laparoscopic adrenalectomy. The procedure was performed with a four-trocar access.

Key points

- Qualifying a patient for laparoscopic adrenalectomy requires proper imaging diagnostics and blood tests.
- Adequate hemostasis is essential during adrenal gland removal—this ensures adequate visibility during laparoscopy.

PORT PLACEMENT

The patient was placed in left lateral recumbency and a foam wedge was placed under the patient's back to elevate the spine. The Hasson technique was used to introduce an optical trocar (T1) into the peritoneal cavity 3 cm lateral to the umbilicus on the right side. After obtaining a pneumoperitoneum and visualizing the viscera and abdominal wall, three trocars for instruments were placed. Two trocars on both sides of the optical trocar (T2, T3) and one caudodorsally in a triangulating fashion (T4).

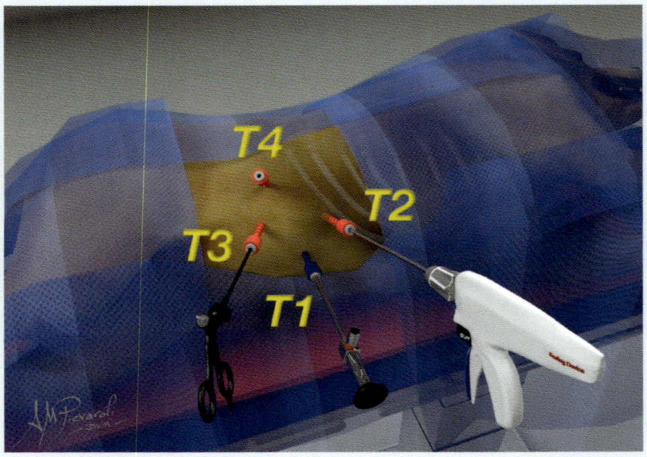

PROCEDURE

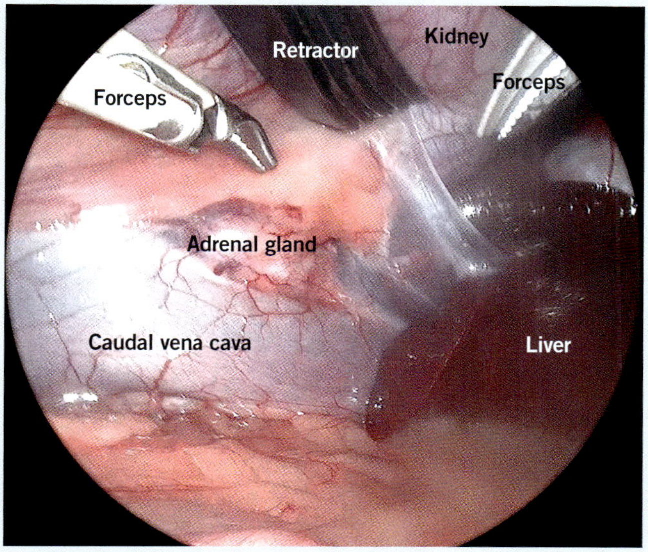

FIGURE 1. Intraoperative view of a right-sided adrenal mass prior to dissection during laparoscopy.

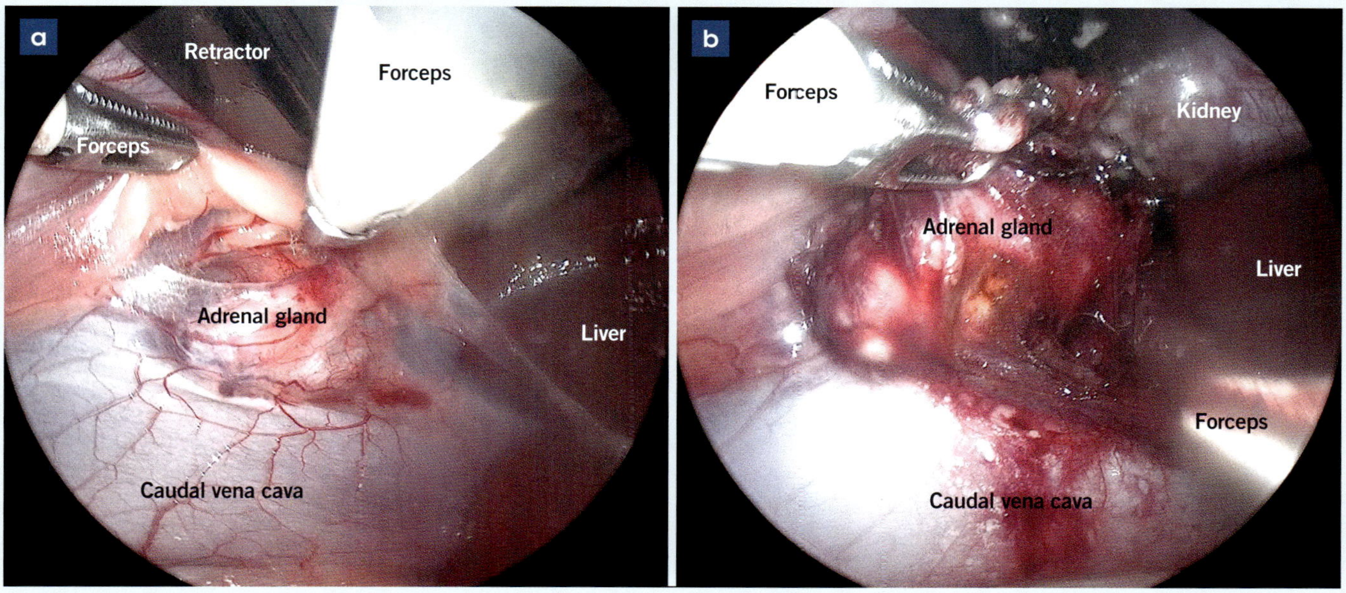

FIGURE 2. Blunt dissection of the right-sided adrenal mass from the surrounding retroperitoneal attachments and the vena cava using a forceps and a vessel-sealing device.

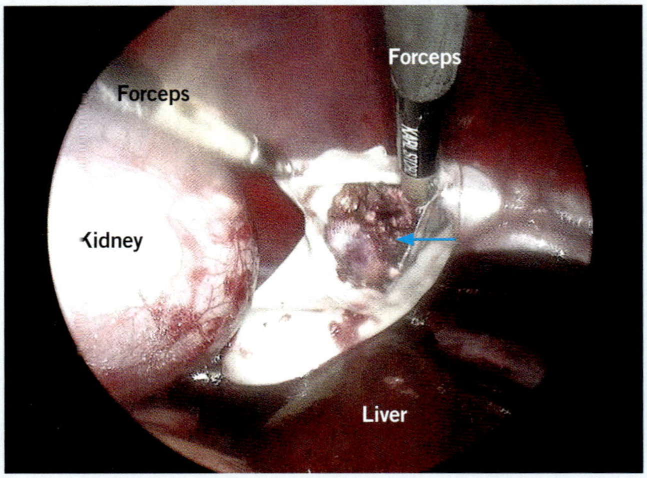

FIGURE 3. Image of a completely dissected right-sided adrenal mass placed in the thumb of a sterile surgical glove before removal from the abdominal cavity through the caudal port. The arrow indicates the resected adrenal gland tumor.

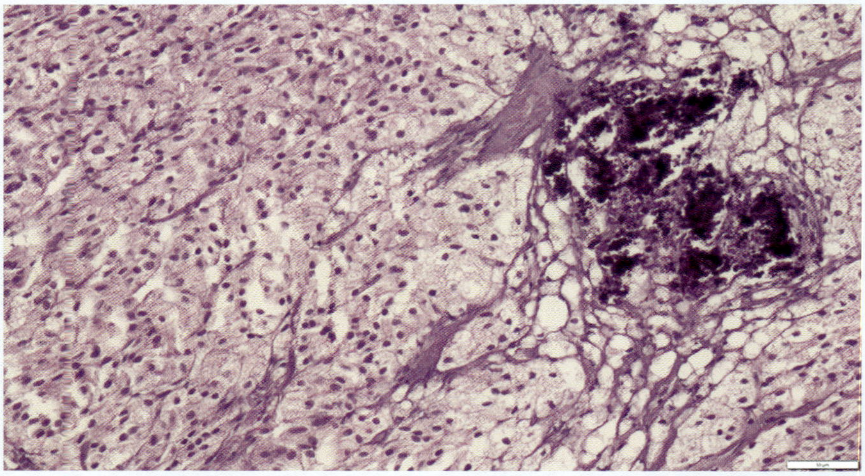

FIGURE 4. The microscopic view shows the adrenocortical adenoma with a focus of calcification (HE, ×200).

Tips and tricks

- ✓ The retractor inserted through the additional trocar allows the kidney to be moved—this improves visibility and increases the operating space.
- ✓ Grasping a thin adrenal capsule with laparoscopic forceps carries the risk of capsular rupture.

41 LAPAROSCOPIC DIAPHRAGMATIC HERNIORRHAPHY

J. Brad Case, Maurício Veloso Brun

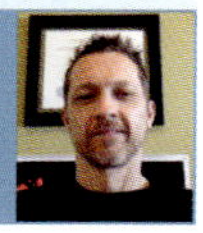

Indications

- Diaphragmatic herniation in cardiovascularly stable dogs
- Dogs with diaphragmatic hernia with mid-to-ventral diaphragm tears
- Dogs with diaphragmatic hernia with reducible visceral herniation into the thorax

Contraindications

- Dogs that are unstable or do not stabilize well
- Patients with an anatomical size or conformation that impose an important limit on the execution of intracorporeal suturing
- Surgeon inexperience with laparoscopic suturing and knot tying

Diaphragmatic hernias are relatively common in dogs and are typically the result of previous blunt trauma, such as being hit by a car, although congenital diaphragmatic hernias have been reported. In some cases, the diaphragmatic rupture may go unnoticed if the dog does not demonstrate significant clinical signs acutely or if thoracic radiography is not performed. The typical clinical sign is dyspnea relating to abdominal viscera retained within the thorax, restricting the expansion of the lungs during inspiration. Pain from trauma can further exacerbate this sign. Additionally, a physical examination may reveal tachycardia, prolonged capillary refill time, and hypotension, indicating shock.

In the case of a traumatic diaphragmatic hernia in which the dog is clinically ill and/or unstable, immediate consideration is given to stabilization before any surgical procedure is performed. Controversy regarding the timing of surgery exists, but most recent studies have demonstrated that early surgical intervention is not associated with poor clinical outcome. Unfortunately, similar data with laparoscopic diaphragmatic herniorrhaphy does not exist. Still, given the authors' experience, caution should be exercised during case selection if considering laparoscopy with pneumoperitoneum, as significant complications can arise.

Once the dog is considered stable and the whole patient has been evaluated, a minimally invasive approach to diaphragmatic hernia may be considered. An open abdominal approach is strongly recommended if the dog remains unstable or cannot be stabilized without surgery. Conversely, a minimally invasive approach may be reasonable if the dog is stable and has been completely evaluated. Diaphragmatic herniorrhaphy in small animals can be treated by conventional laparoscopy, thoracoscopy, video-assisted thoracic surgery (VATS), video-assisted abdominal surgery, or by laparoscopy without capnopneumoperitoneum (gasless surgery).

In the case of "conventional" laparoscopic access, CO_2 insufflation will cause hypertensive pneumothorax due to communication between the cavities. Thus, for conventional laparoscopic access, the use of pneumoperitoneum at a pressure of 3–5 mmHg is indicated, and in cats, it is indicated to use 3 mmHg, considering the associated cardiorespiratory changes. Access via total thoracoscopy may be more suitable for unilateral hernias, impractical in small dogs and cats, and usually requires one-lung ventilation or pneumothorax with CO_2 at low-pressure capnoperitoneum.

Access via VATS can be an excellent choice in large animals with adhesions from the liver to the pericardium and diaphragm. Gasless access is based on the traction of the abdominal wall, creating a workspace in the cranial abdomen without using CO_2. This approach produces isobaric pneumothorax with fewer physiological repercussions for the patient. A considerable number of patients treated have extensive, chronic diaphragmatic hernias involving both hemithoraces. Therefore, conventional laparoscopic surgery with reduced pneumoperitoneum or a gasless laparoscopic approach is preferred in most cases.

> In the authors' experience, diaphragmatic herniation is a technically challenging and potentially risky disease to treat with endoscopy, so caution is highly recommended.

DESCRIBED SURGICAL PROCEDURES

A three-port technique is adequate in most cases and has been previously described. This minimally invasive approach allows extensive cavity exploration and hernia reduction by applying intracorporeal sutures, surgical meshes, or a combination of both. This technique facilitates using a 30° laparoscope and two instrument cannulas. Dual-instrument cannulas will be needed to manipulate organs and to suture the diaphragmatic defect.

The authors consider diaphragmatic herniorrhaphy an advanced procedure for two reasons. First, the safe reduction of abdominal viscera from the chest to the abdomen can be challenging. Secondly, laparoscopic diaphragmatic herniorrhaphy requires the surgeon to possess intracorporeal suturing competency. Finally, the use of positive pressure insufflation is controversial.

Some dogs will not tolerate even low-pressure (<3 mmHg) pneumoperitoneum, and acute decompensation may occur at the initialization of the pneumoperitoneum. Pneumoperitoneum should be started at a low insufflation pressure and flow rate. The authors generally begin at a maximum pressure of 1–3 mmHg and a gas flow rate of 0.5–1.0 L/minute. If pneumoperitoneum causes instability, it is highly advised to be ready to convert immediately or to have a chest tube placed preemptively in case of complications. Converting to an open abdomen approach can be done safely in seconds if necessary. Alternatively, a gasless or lift laparoscopic approach can also be utilized.

The following procedures are described below:

A. Three-port laparoscopic diaphragmatic herniorrhaphy

B. Three-port gasless laparoscopic diaphragmatic herniorrhaphy

A THREE-PORT LAPAROSCOPIC DIAPHRAGMATIC HERNIORRHAPHY

PATIENT PREPARATION AND POSITIONING

A physical examination, blood work (CBC and serum biochemistry), and thoracic and abdominal radiography are completed prior to laparoscopic diaphragmatic herniorrhaphy. Most dogs with diaphragmatic hernias will have a recent traumatic history, so careful attention to physical assessment and resuscitation is critical.

Dogs with diaphragmatic herniation should be fasted for at least 12 hours before anesthesia and have an IV catheter placed for fluid and medication therapy during the procedure. The urinary bladder should be expressed or drained with a urinary catheter at the time of anesthesia induction. Premedications that result in splenic enlargement, such as acepromazine, should be avoided. Perioperative analgesia may include opioid and/or nonsteroidal medications. Local anesthesia with bupivacaine is recommended at individual port sites prior to incision.

The patient is placed in dorsal recumbency and clipped from the cranial thorax to the pubis and dorsally to the level of the epaxial musculature. If a hydraulic float table is available, the patient may be positioned directly on the operating table in dorsal recumbency (**Fig. 1**). In contrast, if a standard

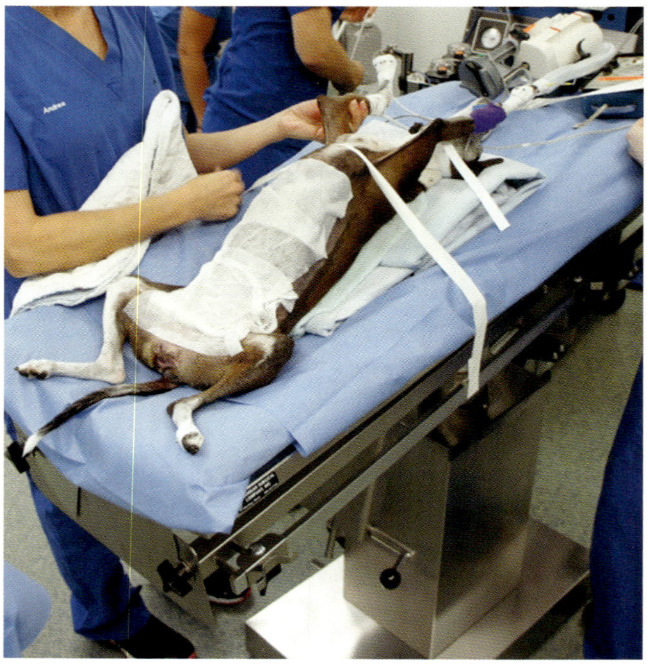

FIGURE 1. Position of the patient on the operating table for laparoscopic diaphragmatic herniorrhaphy.

operating table is used, ensure that the table can be tilted to allow reverse-Trendelenburg patient positioning (about 20°). Lateral tilting of the table may also be necessary depending on the location of the diaphragmatic rupture.

The laparoscopic approach allows extensive evaluation of the pars muscularis (subdivided into pars sternalis, pars costalis, and pars lumbalis) and central tendon (triangular). The triangular ligament attaches the liver to the diaphragm and surrounds the vena cava. In cases of hiatal hernia, it is necessary to explore the diaphragmatic pillars, the esophageal hiatus, and the pars lumbalis. The falciform ligament can be partially detached from the ventral midline if necessary. In the authors' routine, most hernias are composed, having a circumferential lesion in the pars muscularis associated with a radial lesion close to the vena cava (which enters the abdomen through the caval foramen).

OPERATING ROOM LAYOUT

The surgeon and the assistant stand at the foot of the table, so the patient is positioned with the pelvic limbs at the end of the table. The anesthesia staff and laparoscopic tower should be positioned near the front of the table to facilitate room for the surgical team to work. The instrument table is best positioned over the operating table or off to one side of the patient (**Fig. 2**). There must be enough room for the surgeon and the assistant to maneuver near the end of the table with the abdomen unobstructed.

Triangulation between the laparoscope, instruments, and diaphragmatic defect is critically important, especially when performing intracorporeal suturing. Suturing for laparoscopic diaphragmatic herniorrhaphy is even more challenging, as interrupted sutures may need to be placed to support attachment points, such as the costal arch, and to approximate the central point of the hernia in cases of chronic hernias. Interrupted sutures require proficiency with intracorporeal knots using large monofilament suture that can be challenging.

PORT PLACEMENT

Configuration 1 (**Fig. 3**):

- T1, on the midline, 1–2 cm caudal to the umbilicus
- T2 (T3), on the midline, 6–8 cm cranial to T1
- T3 (T2), left or right abdomen (depending on the side of the defect), 4–6 cm lateral to the midline at the level of the umbilicus

Configuration 2 (**Fig. 4**):

- T1, on the midline, caudal to the umbilicus (in the middle or cranial third of the distance between the umbilicus and the edge of the pubis)
- T2, on the left abdomen, cranial to T1, in triangulation considering T3
- T3, on the right abdomen

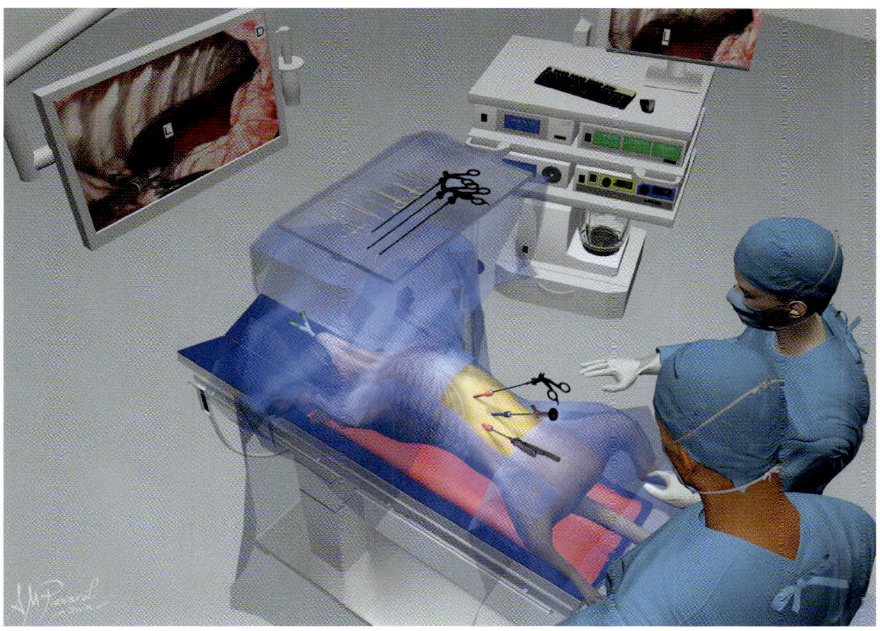

FIGURE 2. Operating room layout for laparoscopic diaphragmatic herniorrhaphy.

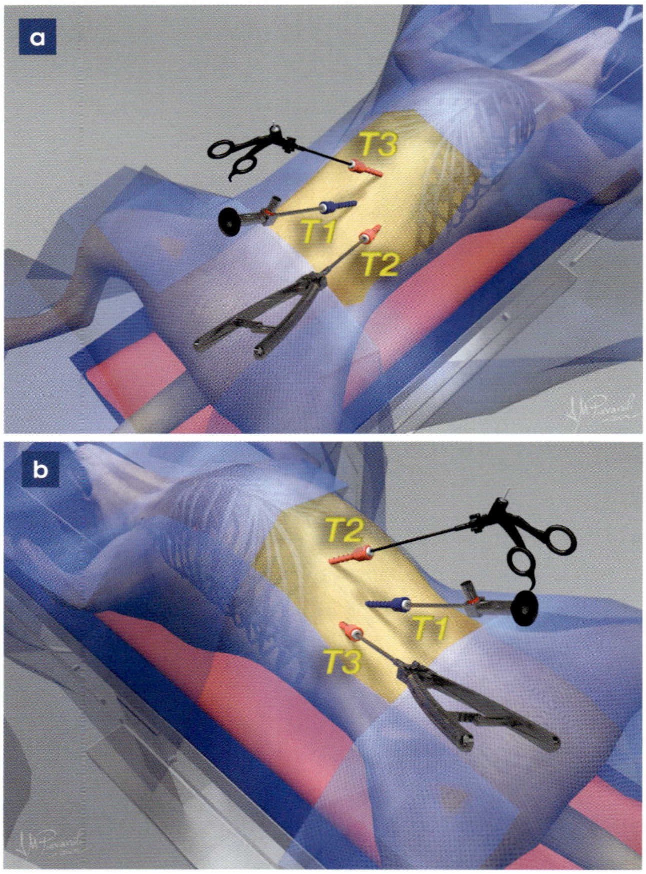

FIGURE 3 Port placement for laparoscopic diaphragmatic herniorrhaphy. a) Defect on the left side. b) Defect on the right side.

Instruments

On the table:

- Standard abdominal surgical pack
- Thoracic drains of different sizes
- High-definition video camera
- Telescope 5 or 10 mm – 30°
- Three 5 mm cannulas (or two 10 mm cannulas + one 5 mm cannula)
- Straight laparoscopic DeBakey forceps, 5 mm
- Straight laparoscopic Kelly/Maryland forceps, 5 mm
- Laparoscopic needle drivers, 5 mm
- Laparoscopic Metzenbaum scissors
- L- or J-hook style monopolar probes
- Different sizes of suture with needle stamped (including 12 cm barbed suture)
- Vessel-sealing device

Ready to use:

- Endoscopic cannula for aspiration/irrigation
- Hemostatic materials (in case of superficial hepatic laceration)
- Surgical mesh

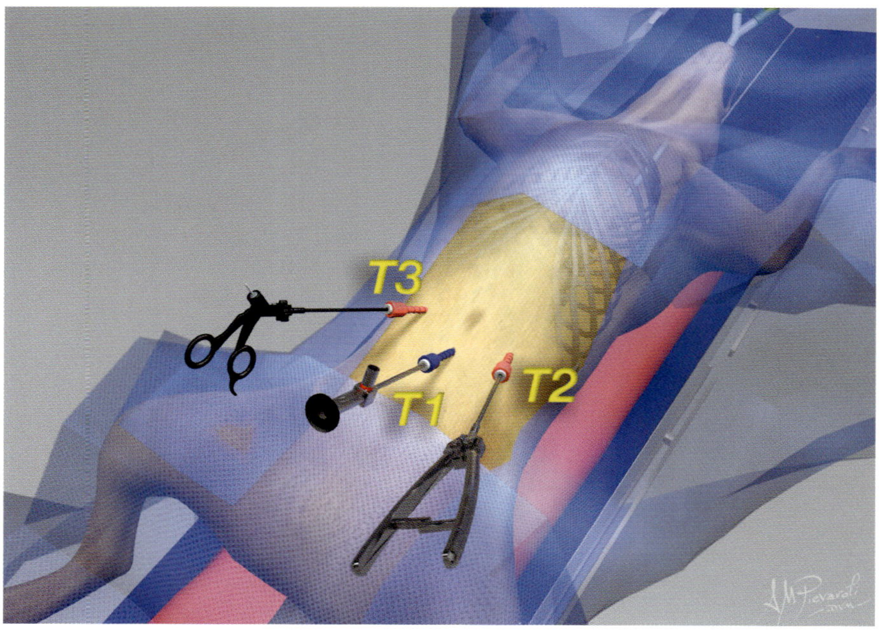

FIGURE 4. Alternative port placement for laparoscopic diaphragmatic herniorrhaphy.

PROCEDURE

- After all the ports have been placed and pneumoperitoneum of 1–3 mmHg (at maximum 5 mmHg in dogs if they do not show decompensation) has been achieved, an initial exploration of the abdomen, diaphragm, and thorax is completed. Special attention should be paid to the size and location of the diaphragmatic defect and the herniated viscera (**Fig. 5**).
- If abdominal viscera can be reduced safely and effectively and the defect is amenable to laparoscopic reconstruction, continuation to herniorrhaphy can be performed (**Fig. 6**). Alteration of patient position to best access the defect may be needed before herniorrhaphy. Slight lateral tilting to the left was utilized for the dog in **Figure 1** to facilitate access to the right diaphragmatic crus.
- Once the abdominal content has been reduced, laparoscopic Metzenbaum scissors or J-monopolar electrosurgical devices can be used to scarify the edges of the ruptured diaphragmatic muscles in cases of chronic herniation. This will encourage mature adhesion formation as the repaired tissues heal.
- Prior to suturing the defect, the authors prefer and encourage the placement of a small (e.g., 14-gauge) chest drain to create negative intrathoracic pressure once the hernia is repaired. The percutaneous drain can be placed under thoracoscopic visualization by advancing the laparoscope through the diaphragmatic defect into the thorax.
- Once the chest drain has been placed and the crus muscles scarified, laparoscopic suturing is performed (**Fig. 7**).
- Barbed suture (e.g., V-Loc 180 12 cm, Medtronic; or Stratafix 12 cm, Ethicon, J&J) is most commonly used in acute hernias. An initial bite is placed at the most dorsal aspect of the defect, ensuring a wide, full-thickness bite of the crus. A continuous suture pattern is started from dorsal and is continued ventrally to the termination of the diaphragmatic defect. Making at least two backstitch bites is important before terminating the continuous suture line. Backstitch bites are created by orienting the suture pattern in the opposite direction of the original pattern. The easiest way to do this is to reverse the orientation of the needle in the needle drivers so that each backstitch bite is 180° to the original pattern. The backstitch locks the barbed suture strand in place to prevent backing out of the suture.
- In some cases, the defect includes a muscular attachment to the costal arch. In these cases, the authors advise placing deep bites, including the perichondrium, and/or using interrupted sutures to strengthen the repair.
- In cases of chronic and large hernias, isolated tension sutures (as a cruciate or horizontal mattress) allow better apposition of the wound's edges. Placing the first suture at

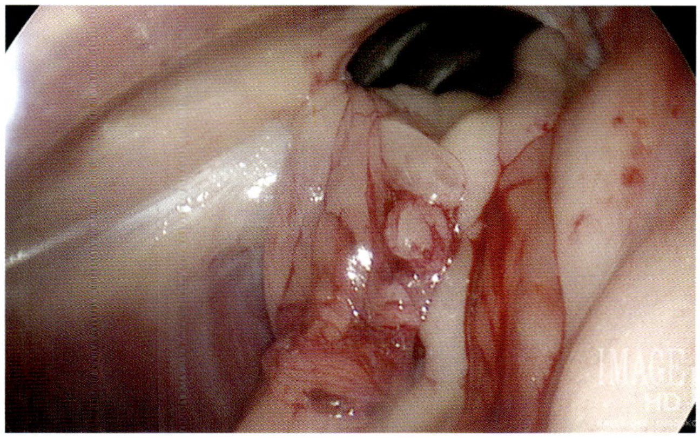

FIGURE 5. Chronic diaphragmatic hernia with herniation of the omentum to the thorax approached by laparoscopy.

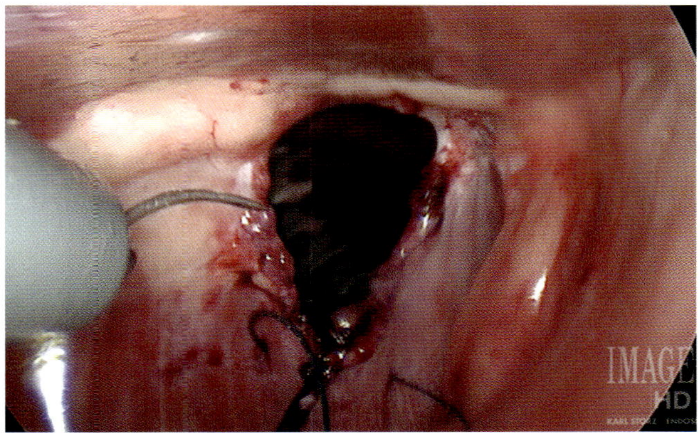

FIGURE 6. Laparoscopic diaphragmatic herniorrhaphy with intracorporeal suture using barbed thread.

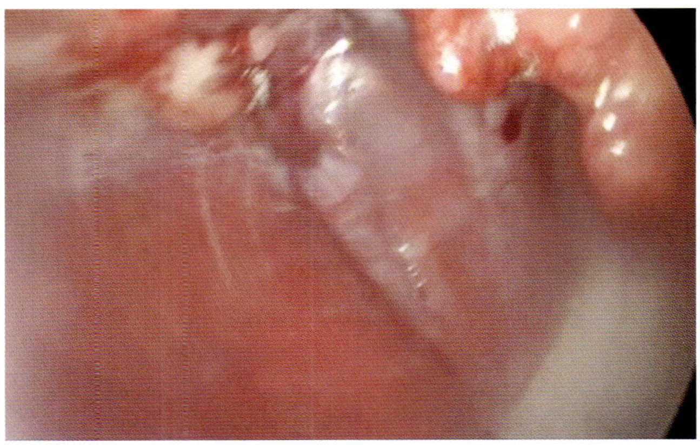

FIGURE 7. Postoperative result of the laparoscopic herniorrhaphy with intracorporeal suture.

the central point of the defect facilitates the application of the remaining sutures, even if the edges cannot be completely apositioned. The authors recommend occluding the triple half knot suture for chronic hernias, overlaid by a double half knot, and adding three other simple half knots (configuration 3=2=1=1=1).

- In some cases, the defect is extensive and irreducible with intracorporeal sutures, requiring mesh application over the sutures. The mesh should be covered with the omentum to reduce intra-abdominal adhesions.
- Once the herniorrhaphy has been performed and the chest has negative pressure, the repair is assessed. The diaphragm should regain its concave appearance, and the chest drain should be negative. The authors are generally slow in their approach to recreate a normal negative thoracic pressure, as some concern for reexpansion pulmonary edema exists, especially in more chronic cases. The authors also advise limiting the degree of positive pressure the anesthesia team applies during the procedure and recovery for the same reasons.
- Capnoperitoneum is discontinued, and all ports are removed. Individual port sites are closed routinely. Typically, only a two-layer (subcutaneous and skin) closure is required when closing port sites <5 mm. Port sites of 5 mm or 10 mm require muscular occlusion.

B THREE-PORT GASLESS LAPAROSCOPIC DIAPHRAGMATIC HERNIORRHAPHY

PROCEDURE

- The gasless technique follows the principles of the laparoscopic "conventional" technique with capnoperitoneum. However, abdominal distention is achieved by pulling the muscle wall without using CO_2. Thus, the defects that communicate the thoracic and abdominal cavities with loss of the peritoneal and pleural barrier (most cases seen) allow the formation of isobaric pneumothorax, which causes less hemodynamic and cardiorespiratory repercussions than the hypertensive pneumothorax originating from the capnoperitoneum.
- A recent study on dog cadavers demonstrates that diaphragmatic herniorrhaphy performed with a new device for gasless surgery allows adequate creation of workspace and effective diaphragm reconstruction. This condition has also been verified in clinical cases (**Figs. 8–13**).
- Diaphragmatic reconstruction can be obtained with barbed intracorporeal sutures, interrupted tension sutures, or from an intracorporeal suture at the central point of the defect associated with the polypropylene mesh fixed with hernia clips and/or suture. The defect conditions define which technique should be used.

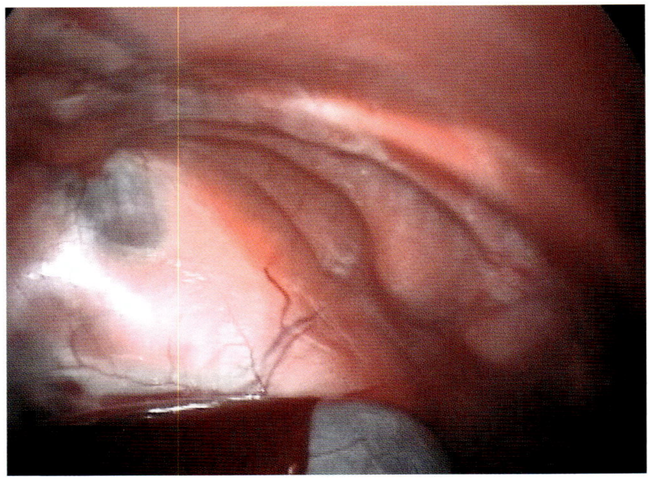

FIGURE 8. Laparoscopic observation of the diaphragm (pars muscularis and central tendon) using the gasless approach in a dog with hiatal hernia. There is adequate exposure of the working area for herniorrhaphy without the need for hypertensive capnoperitoneum.

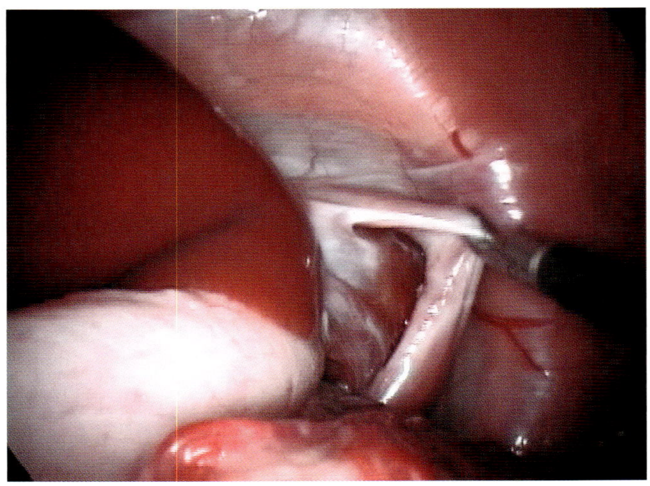

FIGURE 9. Gasless laparoscopy in a dog with hiatal hernia and extensive intrathoracic adhesion between the liver and the diaphragm. Due to the great difficulty of adhesiolysis, the authors chose to convert to celiotomy with reduced access in the ventral midline.

- The first port can be placed in the umbilicus or caudally to it by the open technique (modified Hasson), being triangulated with two other lateral ports, one in each hemiabdomen. If necessary, a fourth port can be used to expose the defect better and pull the stomach in cases of hiatal hernia.
- Permanent cannulas can be disassembled from their valves after they have been positioned, making it easier to move instruments and place and remove materials from the abdomen.

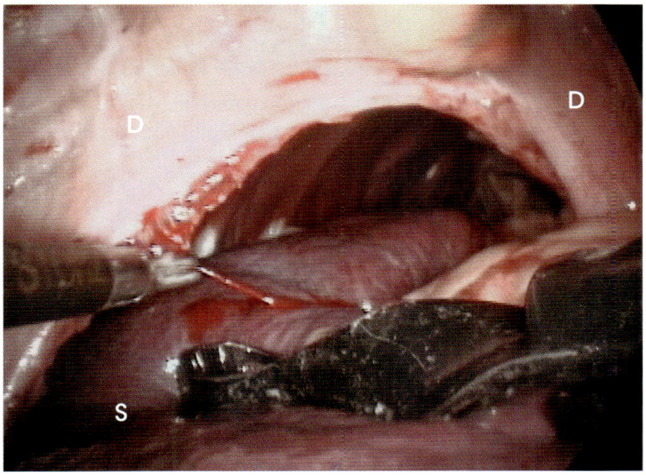

FIGURE 10. Patient with an extensive and chronic traumatic diaphragmatic hernia submitted to a laparoscopic gasless approach (A). The liver presented extensive intrathoracic adhesions that made it impossible to reduce the hernia by minimally invasive surgery (A). The surgery was converted to celiotomy with reduced access. D, diaphragm; S, spleen; L, liver.

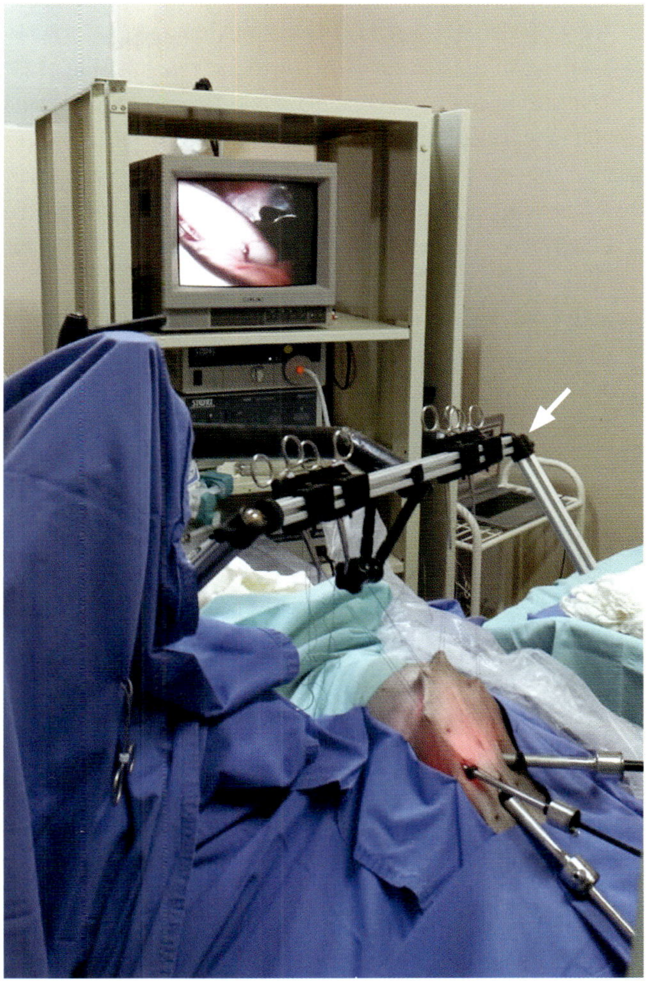

FIGURE 11. Multidirectional traction device (arrow) being used in diaphragmatic herniorrhaphy in a dog with hiatal hernia.

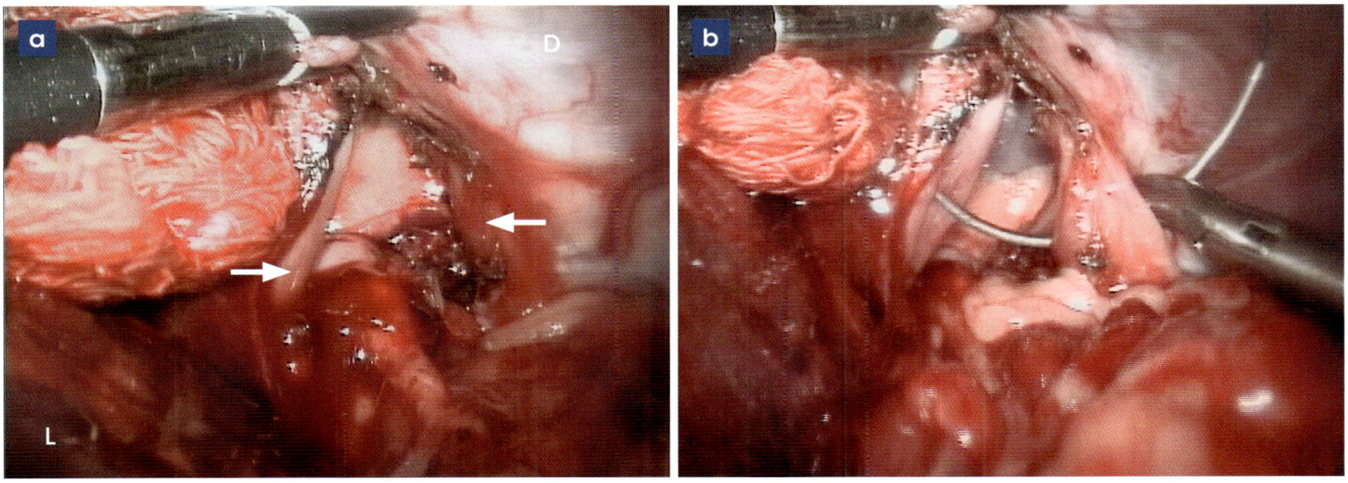

FIGURE 12. Hiatal hernia reconstructed by gasless laparoscopy using intracorporeal suture. a) The dissected diaphragmatic pillars (arrows) are observed. b) The application of the barbed suture in the occlusion of the diaphragmatic pillars is observed. D, diaphragm; L, liver.

- The abdominal wall is suspended with four external sutures attached to the subcutaneous or muscle fascia (**Fig. 11**). The sutures are applied cranially and laterally to the optical port (first one) and parallel to the costal margin.
- Four traction sutures are fixed by hemostatic forceps, which are accommodated to the multidirectional traction device in specific case building. All sutures are pulled, lifting the abdominal wall. The configurations of this device allow abdominal traction in different directions and manual adjustment of the traction force.

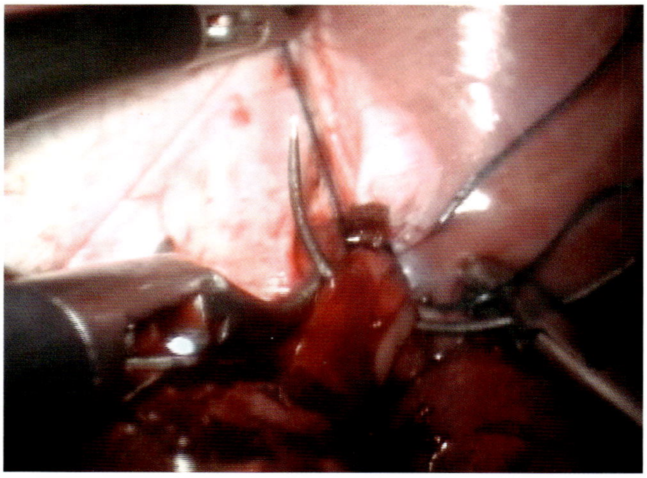

FIGURE 13. Simple continuous intracorporeal suture with a barbed thread applied in the reconstruction of diaphragmatic hernia via gasless laparoscopy.

POSTOPERATIVE MANAGEMENT

- Respiratory rate and effort monitoring are continued for at least 48 hours after surgery. The chest tube can be removed after 12–24 hours as long as it is not productive.
- Analgesic requirements for dogs undergoing laparoscopic diaphragmatic herniorrhaphy appear to be minimal but may be complicated by concurrent injuries.
- Intraoperative infiltration of all port sites with local anesthetic affords 4–6 hours of analgesia postoperatively and, when coupled with nonsteroidal anti-inflammatory medication (2–3 days), is generally effective for uncomplicated laparoscopic surgery.
- If further analgesia is indicated, the addition of opioid medications can be included postoperatively, but opioids are rarely needed beyond 48–72 hours following uncomplicated laparoscopic herniorrhaphy.

Complications of laparoscopic diaphragmatic herniorrhaphy

- Complications are not well established, given the paucity of literature on the subject. However, general complications such as injury to the viscera (e.g., spleen or bowel) or hemorrhage are possible.
- Pneumothorax created by the pneumoperitoneum or due to adhesiolysis between abdominal viscera and lung is perhaps the most concerning issue, as acute decompensation can occur even at low insufflation pressures. Desaturation and bradycardia, as well as increased respiratory resistance and a decrease in blood pressure, are signs that conversion should be performed immediately. Awareness of this complication and careful patient management should be practiced for any surgeon considering or performing laparoscopic diaphragmatic herniorrhaphy.
- Herniorrhaphy failure may also occur consequent to poor surgical technique or over-physical activity in the healing period.
- Postoperative complications such as aspiration pneumonia or port-site infection are also possible and should be monitored for and addressed as needed.

Clinical outcome

- The outcome for laparoscopic diaphragmatic herniorrhaphy should be good as long as a careful and technically sound approach is utilized. However, no clinical reports characterizing results in a significant number of dogs exist to date.
- Be very careful: future performance of pneumoperitoneum in an animal previously submitted to laparoscopic herniorrhaphy may present with gradual tension pneumothorax.

Key points

- Laparoscopic diaphragmatic herniorrhaphy is minimally invasive and can be associated with good clinical outcomes in certain cases.
- Laparoscopic diaphragmatic herniorrhaphy is both technically challenging and potentially risky from an anesthesia perspective due to discontinuity between the abdomen and thorax.
- To reposition the liver in the abdomen, a delicate apprehension of the apex of the gallbladder can be performed with Babcock or DeBakey forceps. Another way is to use forceps to support and relocate the hepatic lobules (do not pinch, because the liver tears easily).
- The use of an intracorporeal tension suture (cruciate or horizontal mattress) at the central point of the hernia facilitates the other sutures and may create a support base for mesh implantation.
- In case of interrupted sutures, perform the first one at the midpoint of the hernia. Occlude the suture without exaggerating the tension, even if it does not completely bring the edges of the defect together.
- Careful case selection and management are critical to ensure a successful outcome.

SUGGESTED READINGS

CLINICAL CASES

41.1 DIAPHRAGMATIC HERNIA IN A CAT

David García Rubio

CASE DESCRIPTION

A 2-year-old European Shorthair cat with acute respiratory distress was rescued from the street. Radiographies and a transthoracic ultrasound scan confirmed the presence of a diaphragmatic hernia with partial presence of liver tissue in the thorax.

Key points

- The patient must be stabilized prior to any surgical intervention.
- Not all diaphragmatic hernias may be operated on via laparoscopy. Its size and location must be assessed, along with its herniated content and any possible adhesions formed.
- It is essential that CO_2 pressures as low as possible are used, as they will significantly impact the patient's ventilatory capacity. In this case, pressures of 5 mmHg were used.

PORT PLACEMENT

The patient was placed in dorsal recumbency and anti-Trendelenburg position at an angle of 10°–15°. Three 5 mm trocars were used. The optical trocar (T1) was inserted using the open entry technique in an infraumbilical position through which pneumoperitoneum was established at 5 mmHg. The two lateral ports (T2, T3) were positioned slightly more cranial to both sides of the first.

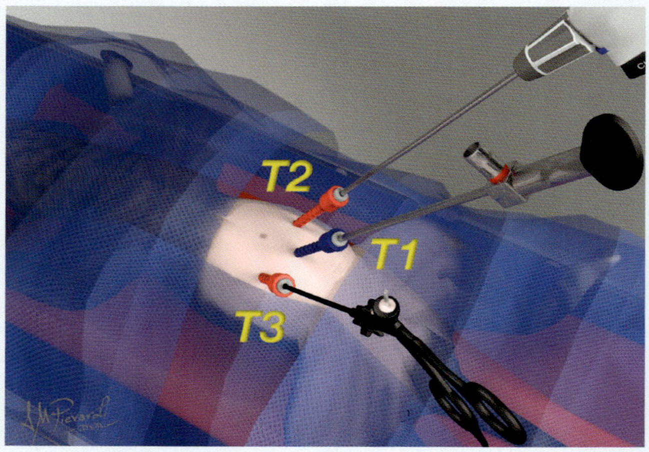

PROCEDURE

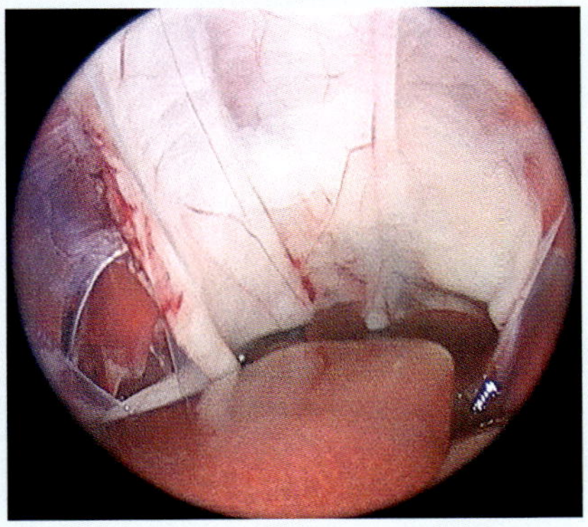

FIGURE 1. Initial view following entry into the abdomen where an absence of continuity in the diaphragm is noted along with displacement of the liver in a cranial direction.

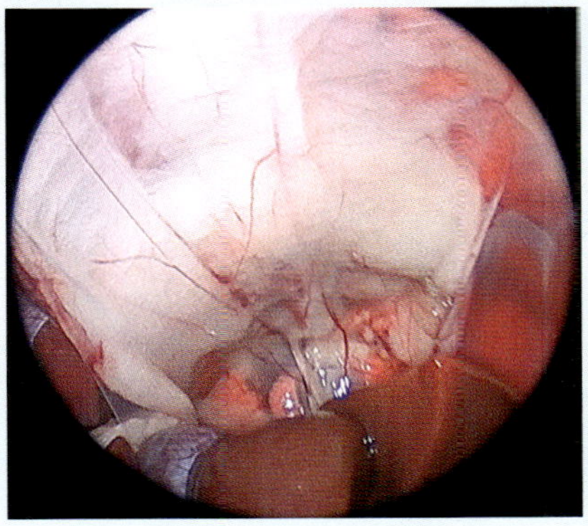

FIGURE 2. After lowering the herniated liver, a direct view of the pulmonary caudate lobes is obtained.

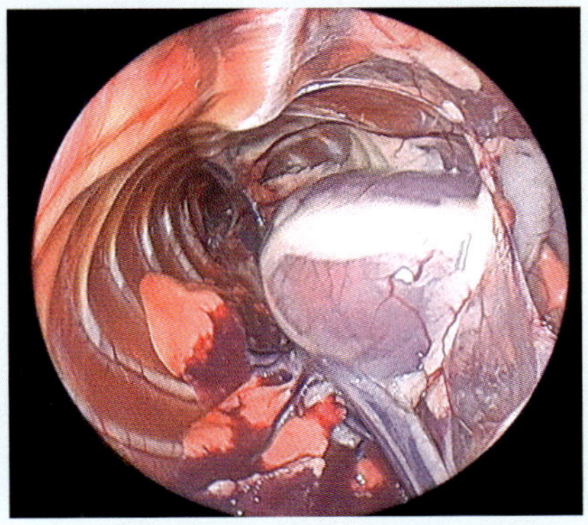

FIGURE 3. View of the thorax (after crossing the diaphragmatic defect), heart, and partially collapsed lungs.

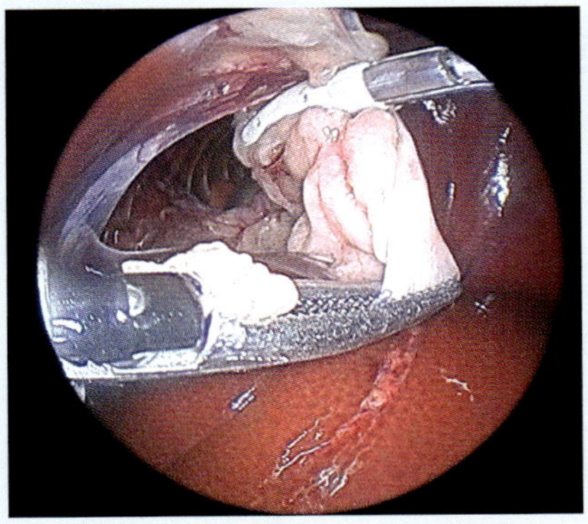

FIGURE 4. The first surgical step is to clean any adhesions to be then able to reconstruct the diaphragmatic cupola suitably. In the image, the falciform ligament is being dissected using bipolar LigaSure forceps (Medtronic, Minneapolis, MN).

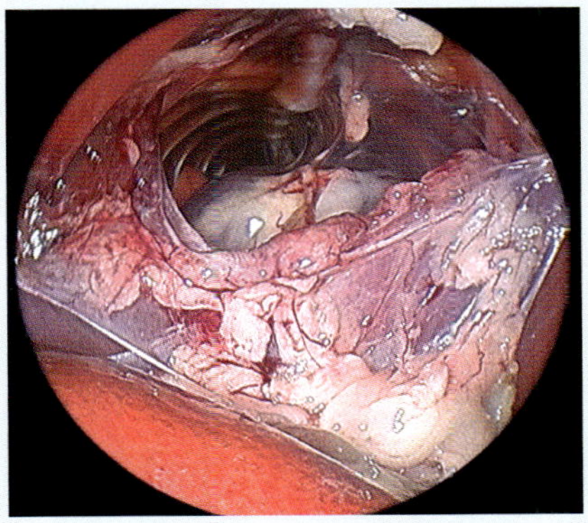

FIGURE 5. Assessment of the diaphragmatic defect after cleaning and dissecting the adhesions. In this case, circumferential tugging of the muscular part of the same from its costal fixing has occurred.

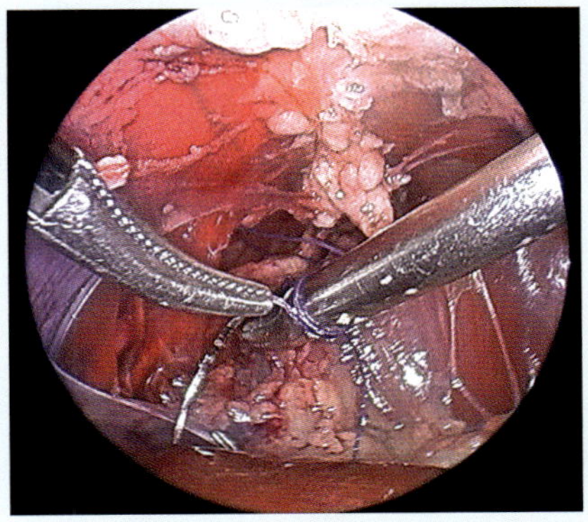

FIGURE 6. First intracorporeal stitch using long-lasting absorbable multifilament material.

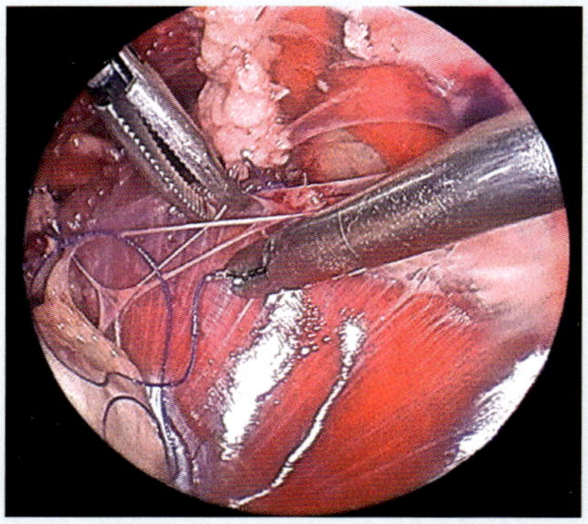

FIGURE 7. Single sutures are placed until the defect is completely closed.

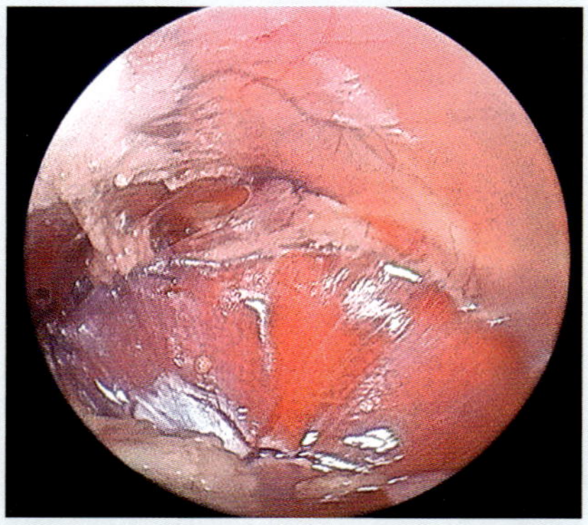

FIGURE 8. Final appearance after closing the defect. Five single stitches were required.

Tips and tricks

✓ Observe whether the diaphragm regains its concave shape to assess if the seal has been completed correctly.

✓ Sealing of the diaphragm can be carried out using absorbable or nonabsorbable, multifilament or monofilament material. The author prefers using multifilament over monofilament material because it is easier to handle.

✓ Occasionally, such as in this case, the herniated content may be reduced atraumatically by the anesthetist performing manually forced inspiration.

42 LAPAROSCOPIC HIATAL HERNIORRHAPHY

J. Brad Case

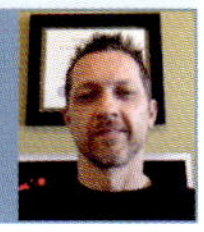

Indications	Contraindications
▪ Regurgitation, discomfort, and aspiration pneumonia in dogs with sliding hiatal hernia ▪ Dogs with hiatal hernia when medical management fails to control clinical signs	▪ Dogs with diaphragmatic compromise that may cause pneumothorax ▪ Dogs with cardiopulmonary disease that will not tolerate peritoneal insufflation ▪ Surgeon inexperience with laparoscopic suturing and knot tying

Hiatal hernias are rare in dogs but commonly seen in certain breeds. For example, French Bulldogs are reported to have a risk of up to 40%. Hiatal hernias vary based on the anatomic regions that displace into the thorax, but type 1, or sliding hiatal type, is most common in dogs. Sliding hiatal hernias result from the weakening of the diaphragmatic muscles and enlargement of the esophageal hiatus, allowing the gastroesophageal junction to move in and out of the thoracic cavity. This disruption results in gastroesophageal reflux, regurgitation, esophagitis, discomfort, and aspiration pneumonia. Although some nonbrachycephalic breeds (e.g., Shar Peis) are reported to have a congenital form of sliding hiatal hernia, most cases are associated with upper airway obstruction. In some situations, clinical signs are mild, and correction of upper airway abnormalities such as elongated soft palate or stenotic nares may improve regurgitation. However, in more severe cases, correction of upper airway obstruction may be inadequate. Surgical treatment is aimed at hiatal plication, esophagopexy, and fundopexy. Laparoscopic treatment of hiatal hernia is a standard of care in humans and has recently been reported in dogs. Results demonstrate improvement in clinical signs in most dogs and are similar to those reported via laparotomy.

DESCRIBED SURGICAL PROCEDURES

A three-port laparoscopic phrenoplasty, esophagopexy, and gastric fundopexy technique has recently been described and is preferred. However, no reports using single-port technology have been published. Because phrenoplasty and esophagopexy require laparoscopic intracorporeal suturing, at least three correctly triangulated ports are necessary for this procedure. For gastric fundopexy (left-sided gastropexy), an intracorporeal or extracorporeal (laparoscopic-assisted) approach can be used. The intracorporeal approach is preferred and does not add significant time to the operation. However, laparoscopic hiatal hernia repair requires the surgeon to possess intracorporeal suturing competency.

PATIENT PREPARATION AND POSITIONING

A physical examination and basic blood work (packed red blood cell volume, total solids, blood glucose, and blood urea nitrogen) are completed prior to elective laparoscopic hiatal herniorrhaphy. Most dogs with sliding hiatal hernias will be brachycephalic and thus have some degree of upper airway obstruction. Antacid medications should be continued or initiated before surgery. Many dogs will require these medications lifelong despite clinical improvement following surgery. Both histamine-2 blocker (H2B) and proton-pump inhibitor (PPI) medications are appropriate, although the latter is typically more potent. Cisapride, a 5HT receptor agonist, appears to be effective at improving gastric emptying and increasing lower esophageal sphincter tone and is considered routine in the author's management of hiatal hernia patients.

In general, dogs with hiatal herniation should be fasted for at least 12 hours (if not longer) prior to anesthesia and have an IV catheter placed for fluid and medication therapy during the procedure. The urinary bladder should be expressed or drained with a urinary catheter at the time of anesthesia induction. Premedications that result in splenic enlargement, such as acepromazine, should be avoided. Perioperative analgesia may include opioid and/or nonsteroidal medications. Local anesthesia with bupivacaine is recommended at individual port sites prior to incision. The patient is positioned in dorsal recumbency and clipped from the caudal third of the thorax to the pubis and dorsally to the level of the hypaxial musculature. If a hydraulic float table is available, the patient may be positioned directly on the operating table in dorsal recumbency. In contrast, if a standard operating table is being used, a sandbag can be placed to the right of the patient to allow for right-lateral oblique patient positioning.

OPERATING ROOM LAYOUT

The operating surgeon and surgeon assistant will stand at the foot of the table, so it is important that the dog is positioned with the pelvic limbs at the end of the table. The anesthesia team and laparoscopic tower should be positioned near the front of the table to facilitate room for the surgical team to work. The instrument table is best positioned over the operating table but cranial to the dog's abdomen (**Fig. 1**).

Triangulation between the laparoscope, instruments, and surgical target is critically important, especially when performing intracorporeal suturing. Suturing for laparoscopic hiatal herniorrhaphy is even more challenging as interrupted sutures must be used during phrenoplasty, and these will require intracorporeal knots.

Instruments

On the table:

- Standard abdominal surgical pack
- High-definition video camera
- Telescope 5 mm – 30°
- Three 5 mm cannulas
- Laparoscopic DeBakey forceps, 5 mm straight
- Laparoscopic needle drivers, 5 mm
- Laparoscopic Metzenbaum scissors
- L- or J- hook style monopolar probes
- 12 cm barbed suture
- DeBakey forceps
- Needle driver

PORT PLACEMENT (FIG. 2)

- T1, on the midline, 2 cm caudad to the umbilicus
- T2, left abdomen, 4 cm lateral to the midline at the level of T1
- T3, on the midline, 6–8 cm cranial to T1

PROCEDURE

- After all ports are placed, and pneumoperitoneum of 8 mmHg has been achieved, an initial exploration of the abdomen and diaphragm is completed.
- If the dog was not positioned in right lateral oblique recumbency, rotation into this position is performed. This will cause the liver lobes to displace to the right and expose the triangular ligament (**Fig. 3**).
- Once the triangular ligament of the left lateral liver lobe is observed, it is sectioned using Metzenbaum scissors or J-monopolar electrosurgical devices (**Fig. 4**). This will expose the esophageal hiatus.
- The crural margins are usually easy to identify as the defect in the hiatus. DeBakey forceps are used to grasp the fundus of the stomach and to maneuver it in and out of the hiatus gently. This gross assessment will help to guide the degree of hiatal plication (i.e., number of sutures to be placed).
- Once gross assessment of the hiatus is made, scarification of the crural margins (tissue intended for suture placement) using the J-hook monopolar electrosurgery is performed.

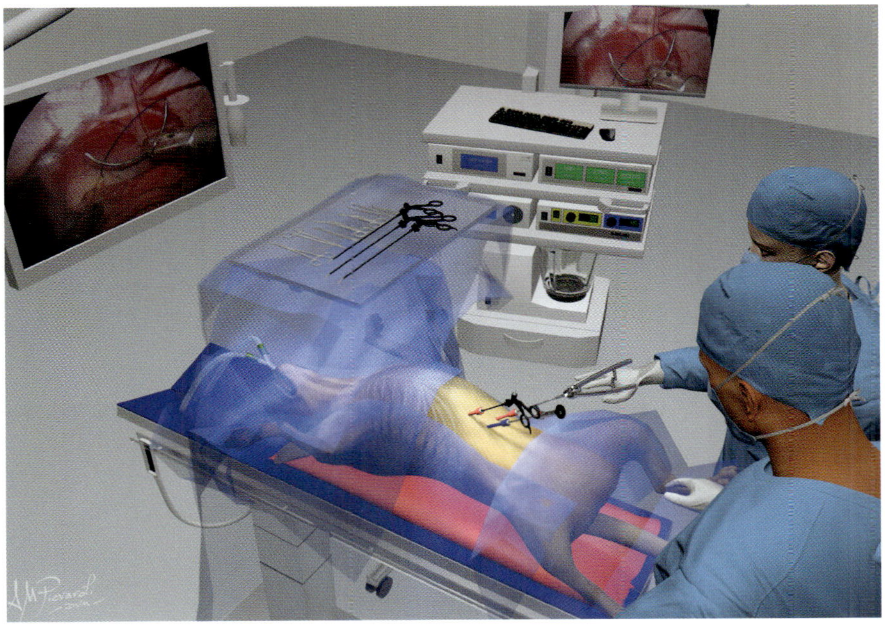

FIGURE 1. Operating room layout for intracorporeal hiatal herniorrhaphy.

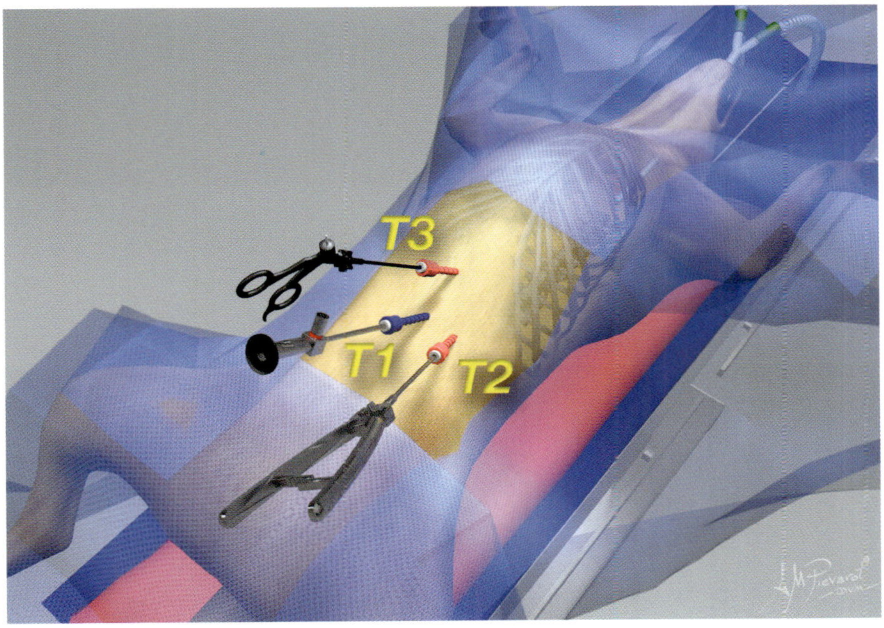

FIGURE 2. Port placement for intracorporeal hiatal herniorrhaphy.

This will help encourage mature fibrous adhesion following healing of the phrenoplasty.

- An initial interrupted stitch (using 2-0 Prolene) is placed at the most ventral aspect of the hiatus, followed by repeated assessment of the hiatal defect (**Fig. 5**). If significant cranial movement of the fundus into the thorax is present, then additional sutures are placed. In most cases, 2–3 interrupted sutures will be required (**Fig. 6**). Caution should be exercised not to narrow the hiatus too much. While there is no validated or objective method to assess this in veterinary medicine, special devices (EndoFLIP, Medtronic) are being investigated and may help in the future.
- Following completion of the phrenoplasty, an esophagopexy is performed. The most commonly used is a barbed suture (V-Loc 180, 12 cm, Medtronic). An initial bite is placed at the most ventral aspect of the left crus (**Fig. 7**). A continuous

suture pattern engaging the left crus and the distal esophagus is continued approximately to the level of the cardia. In most cases, between 4–5 bites will be placed. It is important to reverse the orientation of the needle (so-called back stitch) for the last suture pass to lock the barbed suture strand in place.

- The third and last procedure is the fundopexy to the left side of the abdomen (**Fig. 8**). The procedure is performed similarly to the traditional prophylactic gastropexy (see Chapter 30) but involves the gastric fundus (instead of the antrum) and is sutured to the left transversus muscle instead of the right. The objective of gastropexy is to prevent cranial displacement of the stomach through the hiatus.
- Once phrenoplasty, esophagopexy, and gastropexy have been performed (**Fig. 9**), capnoperitoneum is discontinued, and all ports are removed. Individual port sites are closed routinely. Typically, only a two-layer (subcutaneous and skin) closure is required when closing port sites <5 mm.

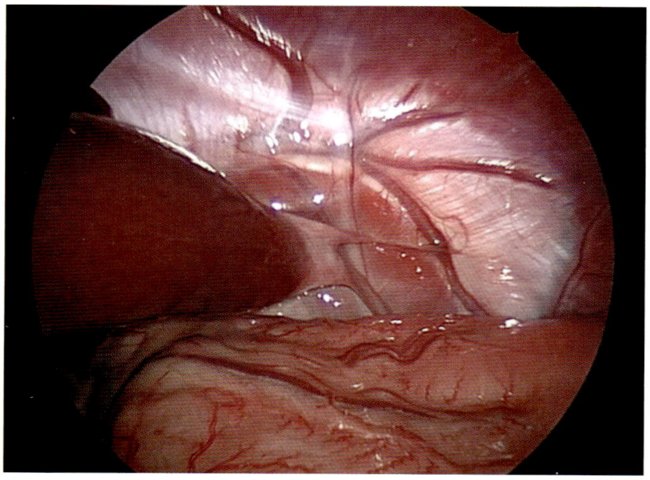

FIGURE 3. Intraoperative, laparoscopic image of the cranial abdomen. The left lateral liver lobe and associated triangular ligaments are present.

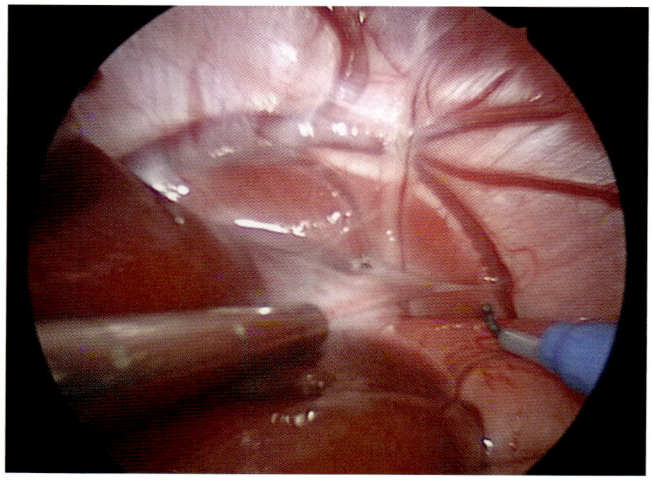

FIGURE 4. Intraoperative, laparoscopic image during dissection of the triangular ligaments using laparoscopic DeBakey forceps and an electrosurgical L-hook dissector.

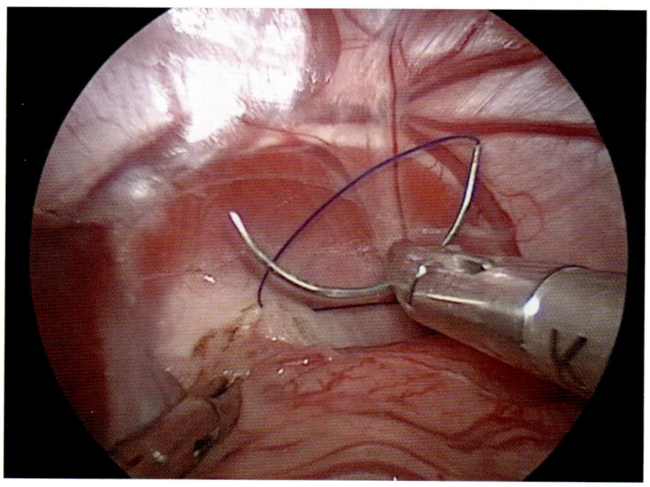

FIGURE 5. Intraoperative, laparoscopic image of the cranial abdomen following scarification of the hiatus and reduction of the cardia into the abdomen. In this image, the first of three interrupted sutures is being placed using 2-0 Prolene.

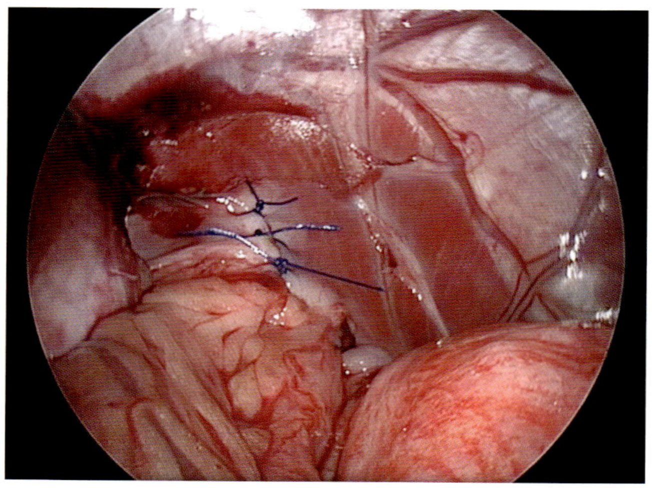

FIGURE 6. Intraoperative image following placement of three simple interrupted sutures for herniorrhaphy (phrenoplasty).

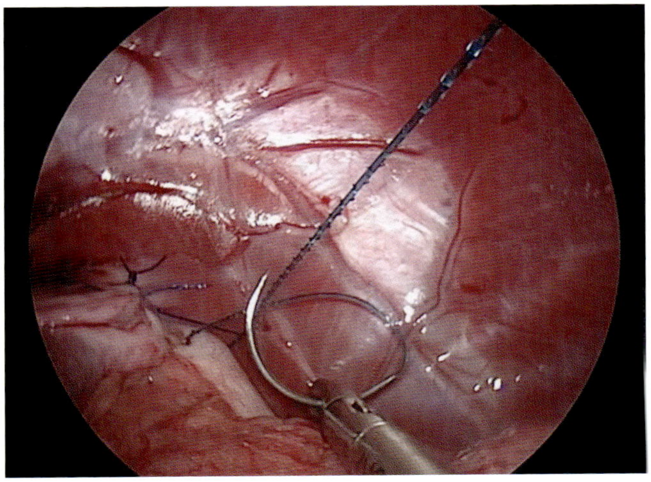

FIGURE 7. Laparoscopic image of the initiation of the esophagopexy using 3-0 barbed suture.

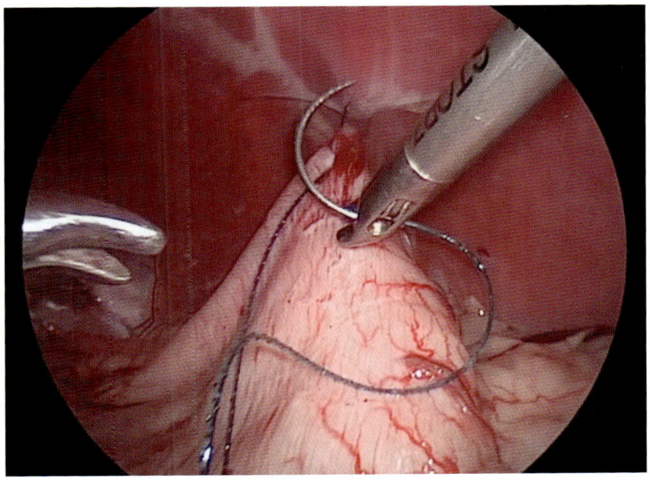

FIGURE 8. Intraoperative, laparoscopic image of the intracorporeal gastric fundopexy being performed. Again, barbed suture using a continuous pattern is preferred.

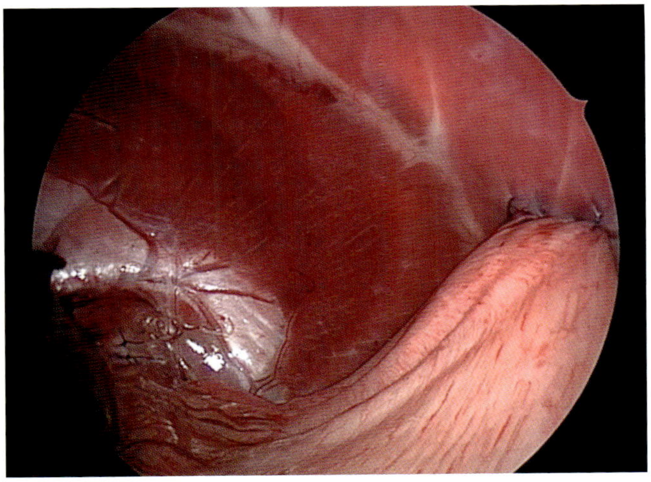

FIGURE 9. Final laparoscopic image following phrenoplasty, esophagopexy, and left-sided gastric fundopexy.

POSTOPERATIVE MANAGEMENT

- Because many dogs undergoing laparoscopic hiatal herniorrhaphy are brachycephalic, more intensive monitoring and postoperative care may be required. In general, maintaining a patent, unobstructed airway is critical. Evaluation and removal of any regurgitant fluid from the oropharynx before extubation should be performed.
- Continuation of antacid, prokinetic and antinausea medications (see above) is recommended during the postoperative period and may be necessary long-term.
- Analgesic requirements for dogs undergoing laparoscopic hiatal herniorrhaphy appear to be minimal.
- Intraoperative infiltration of all port sites with local anesthetic provides 4–6 hours of analgesia postoperatively and, when coupled with nonsteroidal anti-inflammatory medication (2–3 days), is generally effective for uncomplicated laparoscopic surgery in general.
- If further analgesia is indicated, the addition of opioid medications can be included postoperatively, but it is rare to require opioids beyond 48–72 hours following uncomplicated laparoscopic herniorrhaphy.

Complications of laparoscopic hiatal herniorrhaphy

- Complications of laparoscopic hiatal herniorrhaphy are not well established, given the paucity of literature on the subject. However, general complications such as injury to the viscera (e.g., spleen or bowel) or hemorrhage are certainly possible.
- Perhaps the most concerning operative complication is acute pneumothorax, which has been reported in humans and in a dog in a previous report. Pneumothorax appears to result from communication between the abdomen and thorax either by dissection through the pleura or by a preexisting defect. In either scenario, positive pressure insufflation creates a significant pneumothorax that may require emergent thoracocentesis and conversion to an open abdominal surgical approach. Awareness of this complication and careful assessment/dissection of the hiatus should be practiced for any surgeon considering or performing laparoscopic hiatal herniorrhaphy.
- Postoperative complications such as aspiration pneumonia or port-site infection are also possible and should be monitored for and addressed as needed (**Fig. 10**).

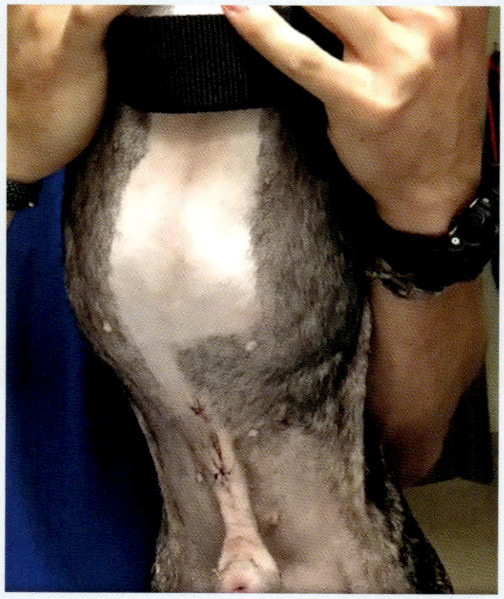

FIGURE 10. Image of the three abdominal port sites at the time of suture removal 14 days after surgery.

Clinical outcome

Although most dogs with type 1 hiatal hernias will improve following laparoscopic surgery, many will have persistent clinical signs. Ongoing medical management for gastroesophageal reflux should be anticipated, and the owners should be made aware prior to surgery. In some cases, the owner will report the resolution of clinical signs. However, given the subtle nature of silent regurgitation and esophagitis in some cases, a thorough interrogation and assessment may uncover ongoing gastroesophageal reflux.

Key points

- Laparoscopic hiatal herniorrhaphy is minimally invasive and associated with equivalent to improved outcomes compared to the open abdominal approach.
- Most dogs will improve following surgery, but clinical signs may still be present in a fair number of cases.
- Ongoing medical management is expected in most dogs despite surgical improvement.

SUGGESTED READINGS

43 LAPAROSCOPIC INGUINAL HERNIORRHAPHY

Alexander Chernov

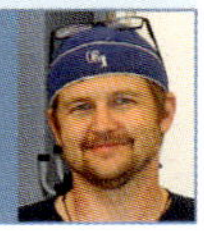

Indications

- Unilateral or bilateral inguinal hernia
- Availability of equipment, a trained specialist, and conditions to perform the laparoscopic hernioplasty
- The procedure is technically feasible for animals of any size

Contraindications

- Constricted inguinal hernia
- Severe general conditions
- Operating room not prepared for specialized care and lack of specialist experience

The open and closed (laparoscopic) techniques for treating inguinal hernias have some fundamental differences. For laparoscopic hernioplasty, instruments and devices (i.e., manual and automatic sutures, stapler technology, mesh) are specific and used to reconstruct and repair anatomical structures, eliminating certain defects.

It is recommended to use biocompatible material adapted to laparoscopic operations. An important role is played by the ability to use implantation materials customized in size and shape for each specific operation.

Tips

The quality of surgical hemostasis and controlled bloodless dissection play an important role and depend on the accuracy without excessive tissue injury.

DESCRIBED SURGICAL PROCEDURES

As in open hernioplasty, the access is in the subcutaneous protrusion area. With the laparoscopic technique, it should be outside of the hernia and the hernial gate site. Thus, the approach is the first important principle of laparoscopic hernioplasty.

The size of the surgical approach (port) is critical, determining the traumatic nature of hernioplasty. Closure of the hernia defect is carried out directly inside the abdominal cavity.

PATIENT PREPARATION AND POSITIONING

The bladder and colon should be emptied. The abdomen is clipped, including both sides of the inguinal area up to the medial femoral area. The patient is placed in dorsal recumbency, with the possibility of tilting the table 45° to the left or to the right (depending on the side of the hernia).

After a diagnostic examination of the abdominal cavity, the animal is turned to the contralateral side of the hernial protrusion. If the hernia is bilateral, then symmetrical actions are performed on the other side, and the surgeon moves to the opposite side of the operating table (**Fig. 1**).

The endoscopic anatomy of an inguinal hernia demonstrates that the hernial gate (regardless of size) extends from the cranial to the caudal direction, following the inguinal canal, ending at the junction of the aponeurosis with the pubic bone (left and right). The appearance of the defect in the abdominal cavity often resembles a drop, with the rounded part directed cranially. Thus, very often, one of the sutures in the caudal zone of the defect is superimposed with a gripper on the epigastrica caudalis artery and vein.

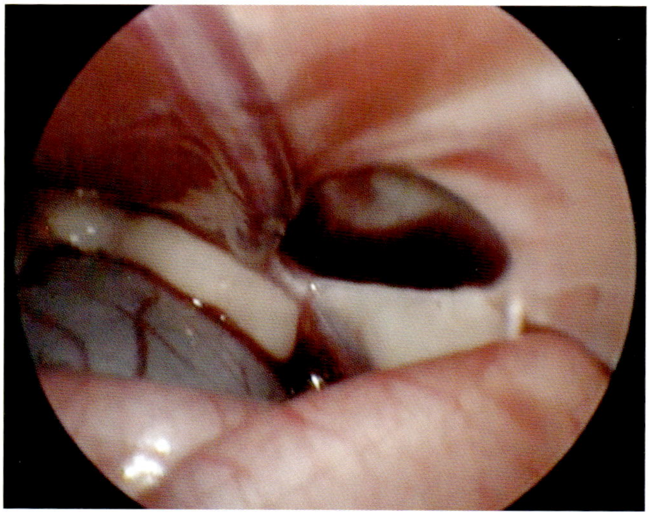

FIGURE 1. Endoscopic view of a unilateral inguinal hernia. The inguinal ring is on the right side. The hernial gate, immediately identified during the initial laparoscopy, lacks adhesions to the surrounding tissues and organs.

It is necessary to remember that:

- The tension of the musculoaponeurotic tissues by single or some barbed sutures is very high (especially with huge hernias and/or in addition to hernias), and it is not considered a good treatment.
- The laparoscopic application of caudal nodal sutures in the defect area (in all dog sizes) is accompanied by ligation of the epigastrica caudalis artery and vein.

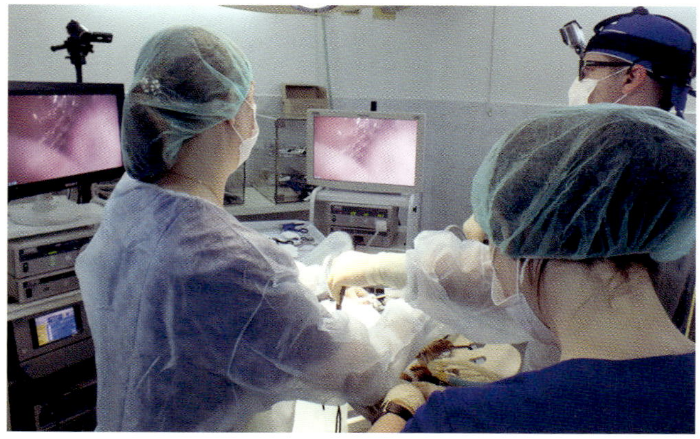

FIGURE 2. Arrangement of the operating team and equipment for the laparoscopic approach to an inguinal hernia.

OPERATING ROOM LAYOUT

The technological features of endoscopic operations require a higher level of visualization of the endoscopic image. Therefore, the video equipment should improve visual–tactile interaction and image transmission from the object to the surgeon. The 3D visual effects can provide higher precision during laparoscopic hernioplasty (**Fig. 2**).

The surgeon and the assistant stand on each side of the patient. The monitor is placed at the caudal end of the operating table (**Fig. 3**).

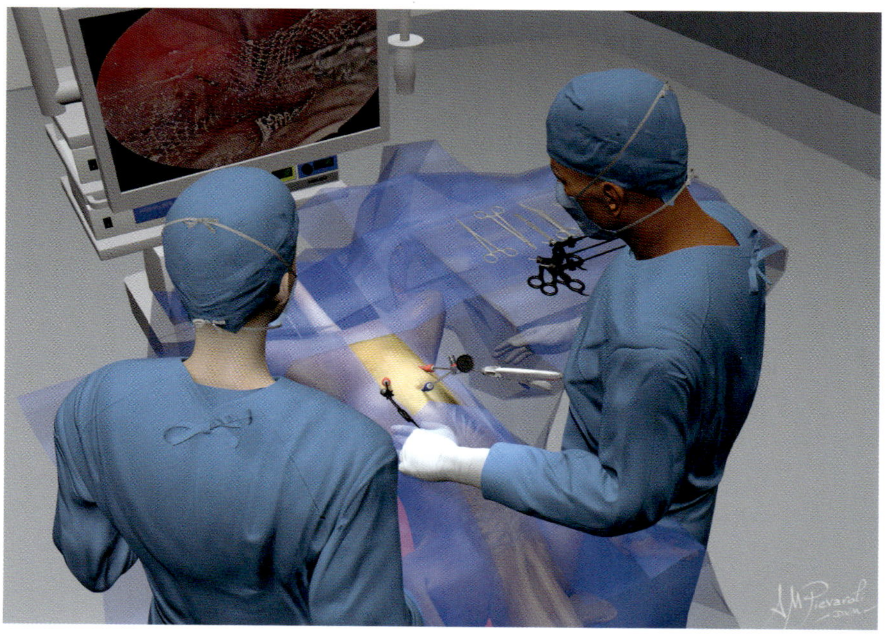

FIGURE 3. Operating room layout for laparoscopic inguinal herniorrhaphy.

Instruments (Fig. 4)

On the table:

- Telescope 5 mm – 30°
- Two or three 5 mm diameter cannulas
- 10–12 mm diameter cannulas for laparoscopic clamp
- Needle holders to apply percutaneous sutures with the help of a gripping thread loop

Ready to use:

- Endoscopic aspiration/irrigation device
- Laparoscopic retractor (palpation probe)
- General surgery set

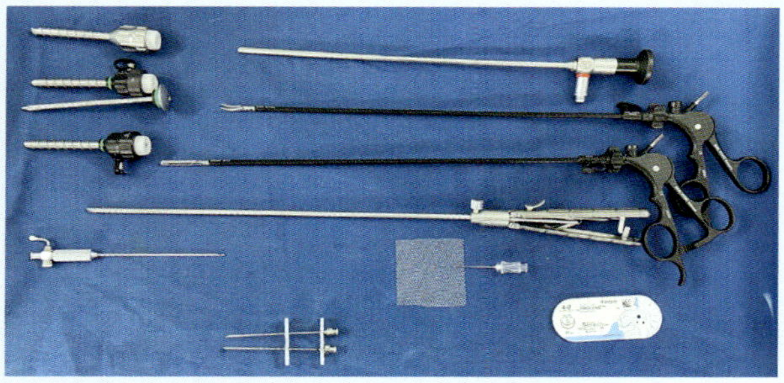

FIGURE 4. Standard laparoscopic set.

PORT PLACEMENT (FIG. 5)

- T1 (telescope port), on the midline, 1–2 cm cranial to the umbilicus
- T2, on the right mammillary line (between cranial and caudal nipples)
- T3, on the left mammillary line (between cranial and caudal nipples)

PROCEDURE

- The choice of endoscopic ports depends on the location of the hernial defect.
- The endoscope is introduced for laparoscopic examination. A preliminary search for endoscopic landmarks of the hernial orifice and hernial contents is made, simultaneously checking the whole abdominal cavity (**Fig. 6**).
- A direct examination of the hernial sac and hernial gate is performed (**Fig. 7**).
- The release of the hernial sac depends on its content. If there are no signs of constriction and adhesions, hernia reduction can be easier, especially with bimanual pushing from the outside, with mobilization or isolation of the hernial sac (if possible).
- The goal of the previous stages is a clear visualization of the hernial gate.

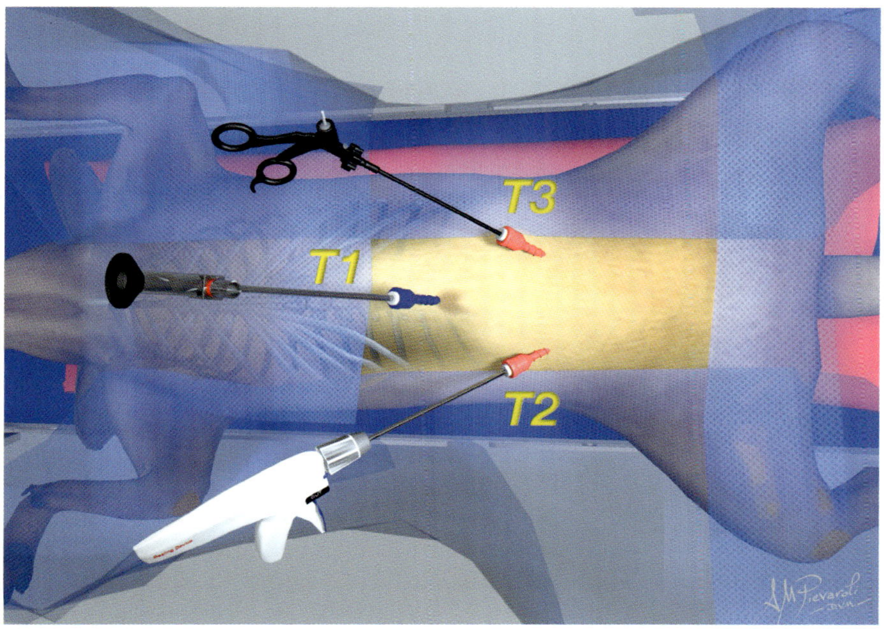

FIGURE 5. Port placement for laparoscopic inguinal herniorrhaphy.

- The musculofascial structures that form the hernial gate are additionally dissected if needed. Hemostasis and internal anatomy are rechecked.
- Then, the question of what to do with a herniated sac that remains in the soft tissues must be solved. It is important to clearly mark, select and close the hernia gate (**Fig. 8**).
- The method of hernia gate suturing (manual suture, pouch suture, nonabsorbable material, hardware suture, paper clip suture, plug-in, gel) is selected. Occasionally, it is necessary to create an additional port for grasping or retraction (3 or 5 mm port). The recommended method for hernia suturing is manual (barbed suture or/without a duplicate), with an additional autoplasty or alloplasty (with mesh) implant. Mesh materials and structures can be used to strengthen the operation area (in addition to any method) (**Fig. 9**). Attention must be paid to the mesh shape. Ideally, its size should correspond to the size of the hernial defect.
- In the case of recurrent hernias, an alloplastic method with mesh is preferred. Omentalization of the implantation area is essential. If postoperative hernia recurrence occurs, more delicacy for the laparoscopic hernial examination must be used.
- Be ready for traditional hernioplasty if necessary.

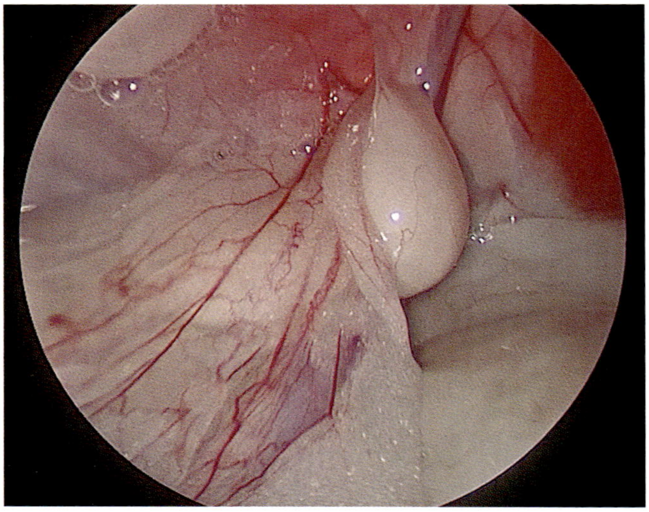

FIGURE 6. Left inguinal ring zone. During preliminary laparoscopy, the hernial gate is not visually identified. Adhesions and the peritoneal fat are visualized.

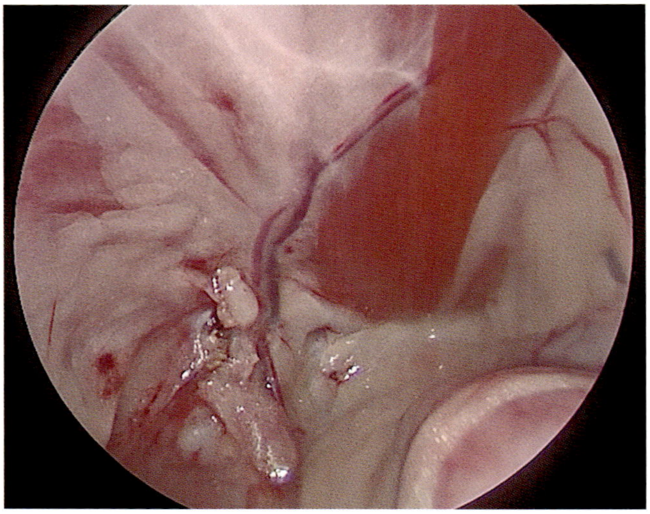

FIGURE 7. Hernial gate after tissue dissection.

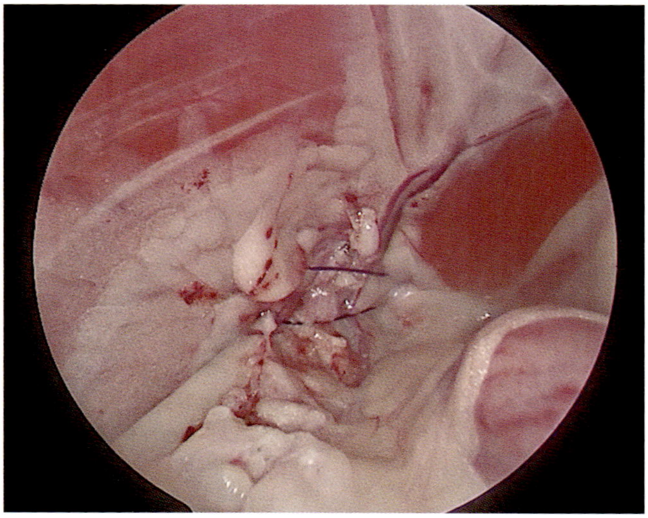

FIGURE 8. Two single external ligatures are placed on the hernial gate under endoscopic-assisted control.

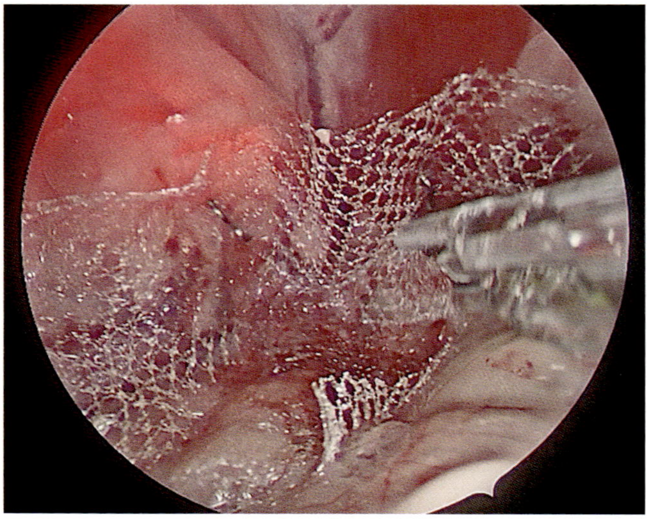

FIGURE 9. Duplication of the single sutures using a mesh.

POSTOPERATIVE MANAGEMENT

- Rest and reduction of irritating factors that can provoke the animal's barking and aggression.
- Control of bladder emptying and bowel peristalsis.
- Treatment of underlying diseases and conditions that are important in increasing intra-abdominal pressure.
- Analgesia.
- Monitoring the state of soft tissues in the port sites and other postoperative wounds (**Figs. 10 and 11**).
- Control of changes in local and regional sensitivity (hyper-esthesia, paresthesia, insensitivity).

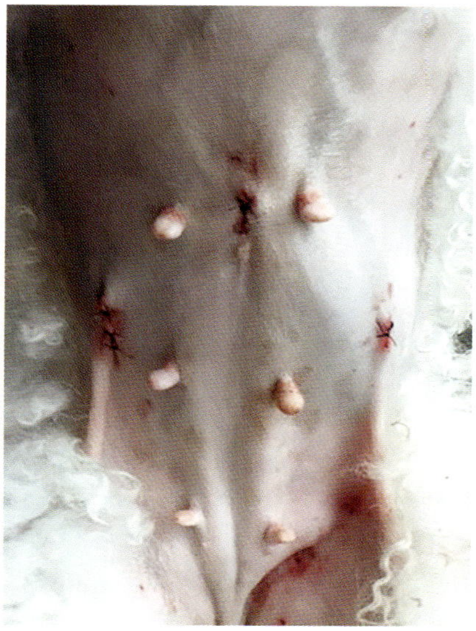

FIGURE 10. View of postoperative wounds in a dog after laparoscopic unilateral inguinal hernioplasty. Three small skin wounds are seen away from the inguinal hernial defect.

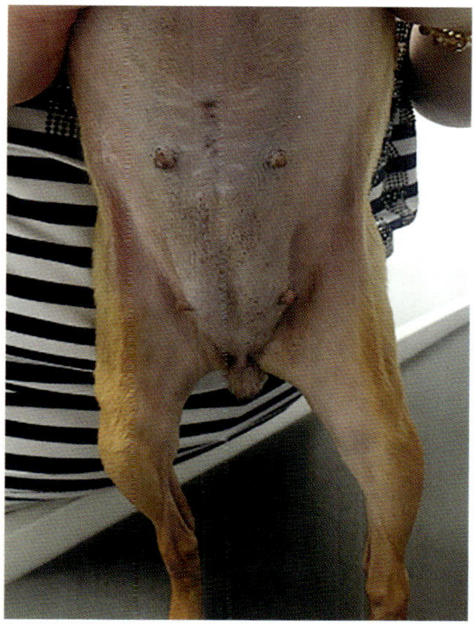

FIGURE 11. A patient 1.5 months after the surgery.

Complications of laparoscopic inguinal herniorrhaphy

Immediate (2–3 hours)

- Heart, renal, and respiratory failure.
- Bleeding.

Early (5–7 days)

- Heart, renal, respiratory, liver failure, allergy.
- Pain syndrome.
- Urinary incontinence and retention.
- Coprostasis, diarrhea.
- Intraoperative damage resulting from endosurgery (e.g., hemoperitoneum, peritonitis, foreign body).
- Changes in port soft tissue wounds (e.g., pus, hematoma, seroma, burn, allergy).

Late (after 2 weeks)

- Recurrence. The hernial gate is not anatomically distinguished, and suturing occurs without observing the interposition of tissues. A large tension of musculoaponeurotic tissues is produced.
- Suture dehiscence.
- Abdominal adhesions (**Fig. 12**).

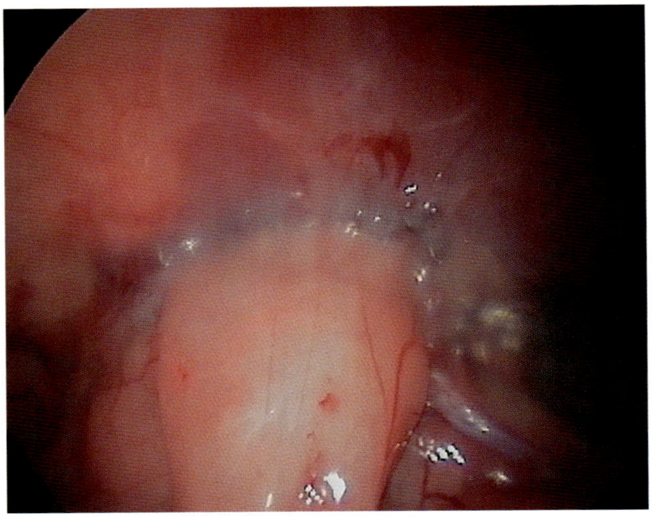

FIGURE 12. Laparoscopic control 3 months after laparoscopic tension-free mesh implant surgery. There are some adhesions with the great omentum.

Key points

- The general principle of laparoscopic hernioplasty is obtained with nonabsorbable suture materials, so it is possible to tighten the hernial gate and close it with the development of fibrosis. Obviously, this principle of hernia surgery is somewhat different from the classical canons of hernia repair in several aspects (e.g., isolation of the hernial sac). However, as many years of practice show, this method is not worse than the classical open principles when used with knowledge of the details.
- It should be clear that both total laparoscopic (suturing of the hernia gate in the abdominal cavity) and laparoscopic-assisted ligatures from the abdominal wall under laparoscopic control are possible. For small-sized hernial defects in young animals, sometimes single sutures on the aponeurotic defect without isolating the hernial sac—as well as assisted annular suture on the inguinal opening— are acceptable with the help of needles (ligature guides), together with the simple use of single contraction sutures applied using laparoscopic needle holders.
- In large hernial protrusion, the laparoscopic approach should be considered an exception because the risk of recurrence is very high. In some cases, as a rule, it should be applied, according to the author, a method of combining tension and non-tension techniques using a mesh structure.

SUGGESTED READINGS

CLINICAL CASES

43.1 LAPAROSCOPIC-ASSISTED PERCUTANEOUS HERNIORRHAPHY IN DOGS USING THE PIRS TECHNIQUE AND LAPAROSCOPIC OVARIECTOMY

Przemysław Prządka, Bartłomiej Liszka, Agnieszka Antończyk, Zdzisław Kiełbowicz, Dariusz Patkowski

CASE DESCRIPTION

A 1-year-old intact female Dachshund was evaluated for treating a right-sided inguinal hernia and bilateral ovariectomy. The inguinal hernia was treated with the PIRS technique. The technique described in dogs was modified in this case by introducing two additional trocars for ovariectomy instruments during the same operation.

The hernia contents were moved back to the abdominal cavity with the aid of both manual pressure on the hernia sac and laparoscopic forceps. The PIRS procedure was performed under camera control to close the internal inguinal ring with 2-0 nonabsorbable multifilament suture material.

Ovariectomy was performed through a three-trocar access. A vessel-sealing device was used to dissect the ovaries. The ovaries were removed from the abdominal cavity in the thumb of a sterile glove through the widened cut in the midline for the optical trocar.

Key points

- In the PIRS technique, it is important to correctly determine the point of insertion of the needle above the level of the internal ring. This will allow the needle tip to pass through the edges of the inguinal ring.
- Good visualization of the inguinal ring while passing the needle is necessary
- While closing the internal ring, both needle insertions should be done through the same puncture point on the skin to place the suture under the skin.

PORT PLACEMENT

The Hasson technique was used to introduce an optical trocar into the peritoneal cavity through the umbilicus. After obtaining a pneumoperitoneum and visualization of the viscera and abdominal wall, two trocars for instruments were placed on both sides of the optical trocar in a triangular fashion.

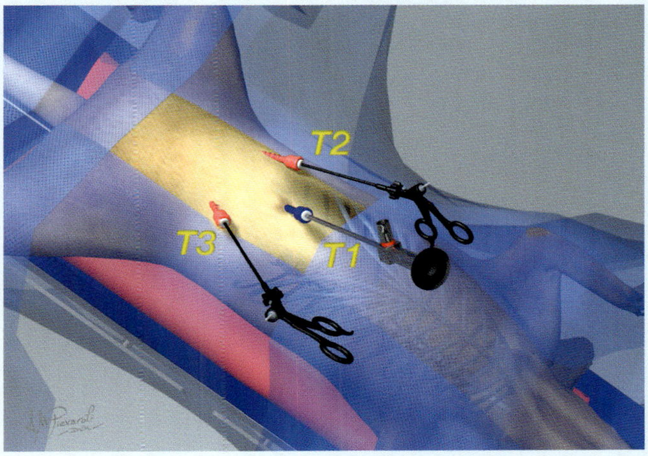

PROCEDURE

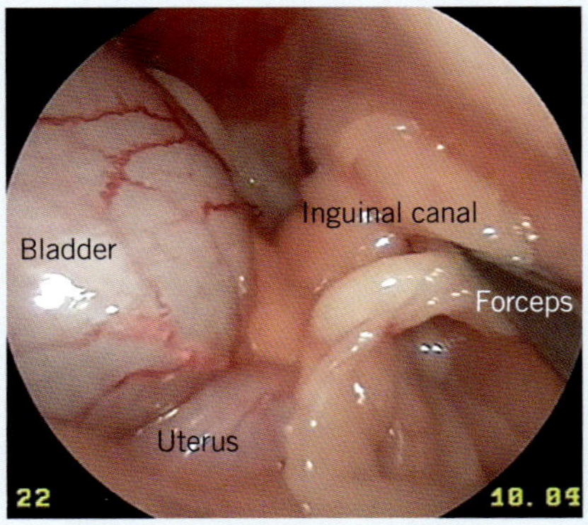

FIGURE 1. Laparoscopic view of the right inguinal hernia. Reduction of hernia content.

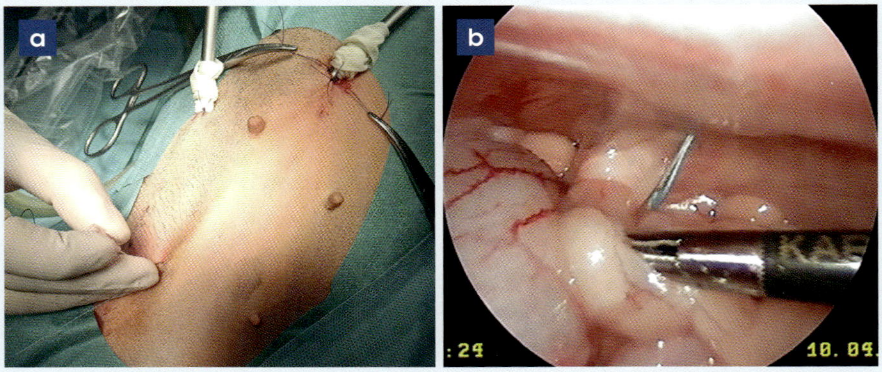

FIGURE 2. Insertion of the needle into the previously designated place and its passage through the outer half of the internal inguinal canal ring. a) External view. b) Laparoscopic view of the abdominal cavity.

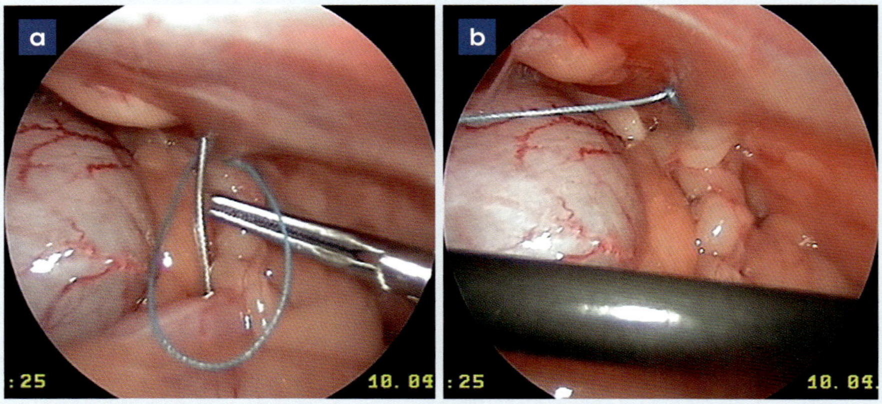

FIGURE 3. Stages of a needle passing through the medial part of the internal inguinal ring and introduction of the polyester suture through the needle into the previously formed loop.

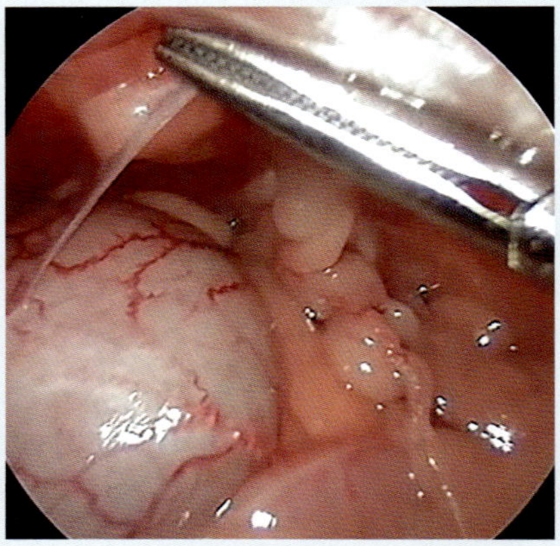

FIGURE 4. Laparoscopic view of the closed inguinal canal.

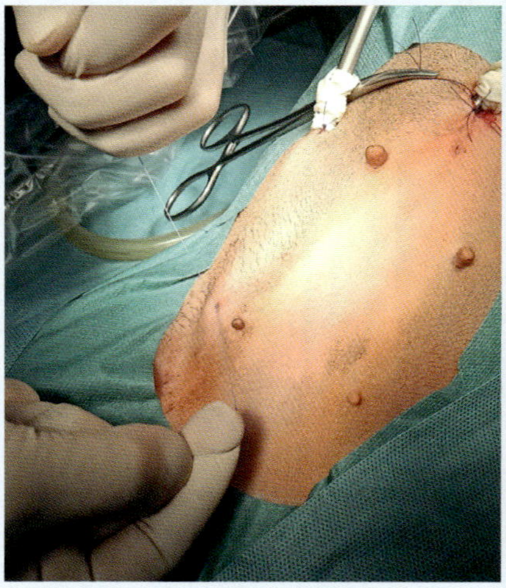

FIGURE 5. Knotting a polyester suture that closes the internal ring of the inguinal canal.

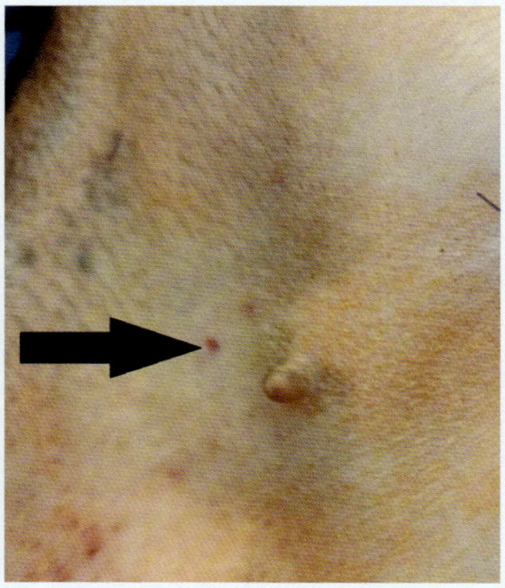

FIGURE 6. View of postoperative wounds. The arrow indicates the site of needle insertion above the inguinal canal.

Tips and tricks

✓ The use of an additional laparoscopic instrument during laparoscopic-assisted percutaneous herniorrhaphy may help reduce the inguinal hernia content in female dogs.
✓ The PIRS technique can be used regardless of trocar placement for ovariectomy.

43.2 LAPAROSCOPIC-ASSISTED PERCUTANEOUS INGUINAL HERNIORRHAPHY

F. Martínez Gomariz, C. Sánchez, J. D. Carrillo

CASE DESCRIPTION

An 8-year-old, intact dog was presented with evidence of bulging in the left inguinal region that could be reduced by pressure. An ultrasound was performed, observing the presence of content inside, leading to the diagnosis of a left inguinal hernia. Laparoscopic-assisted surgical treatment was recommended for its resolution. An analytical study was carried out that consisted of hematology and blood biochemistry as preparatory treatment.

Key points

- The hernial content, composed of epiploic fat, was emptied with the help of grasping forceps using traction.
- After this maneuver under direct laparoscopic visualization and using an 18-gauge needle threaded with a 2-0 nonabsorbable monofilament suture in a loop, it was introduced through the lateral edge of the hernial defect.
- The hernial defect was closed using 2-0 nonabsorbable monofilament suture. The suture was introduced through the previously created loop to finally retract the loop, achieving passage of the suture between both edges of the defect, knotting extracorporeally and leaving it included in the subcutaneous plane.
- Finally, the two port incisions were closed with simple stitches after removing the pneumoperitoneum with light abdominal pressure.

PORT PLACEMENT

The 6 mm trocars were implanted with the patient in supine recumbency. A ventral midline incision was made approximately 5 mm caudal to the umbilicus (T1) using the modified Hasson technique to open a subumbilical chamber port. Pneumoperitoneum was created at an intra-abdominal pressure of 9 mmHg. The second (T2) trocar was implanted in midway between the first port and the prepubic area. After observing both inguinal rings, the defect was located on the left side, so the patient was lateralized in right lateral decubitus, performing the Trendelenburg maneuver with a 15° inclination angle.

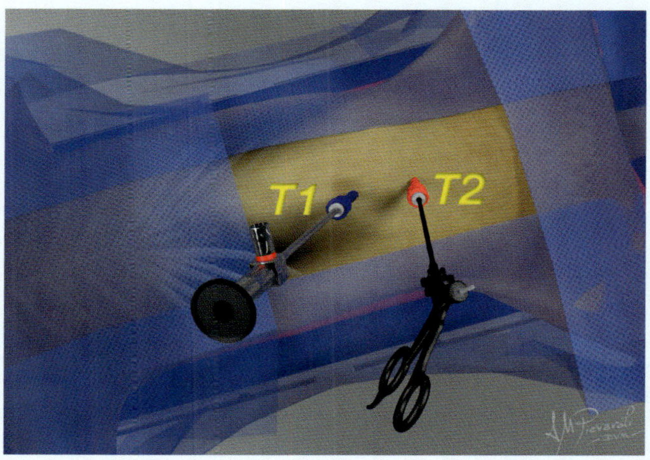

PROCEDURE

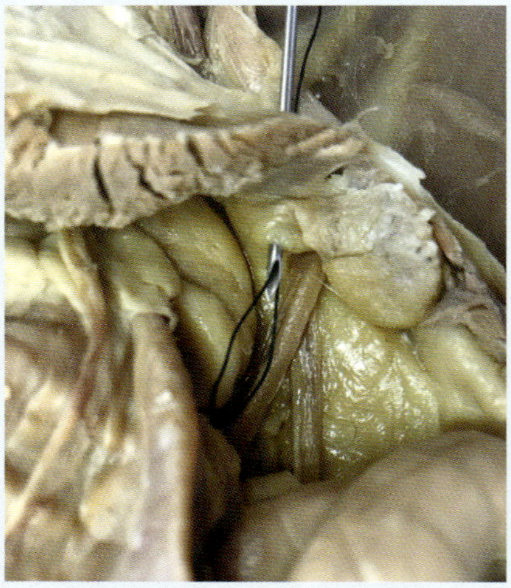

FIGURE 1. Suture passage in a cadaver model. Insertion of the medial edge threaded needle for the creation of a loop.

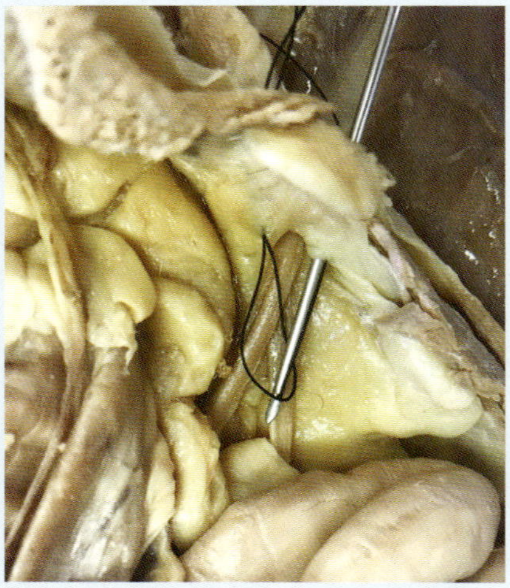

FIGURE 2. Needle insertion at the lateral edge in a cadaver model.

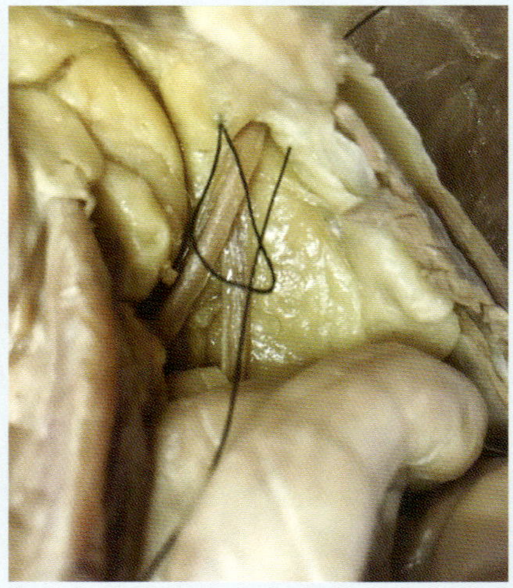

FIGURE 3. Appearance of the suture trapped in the loop.

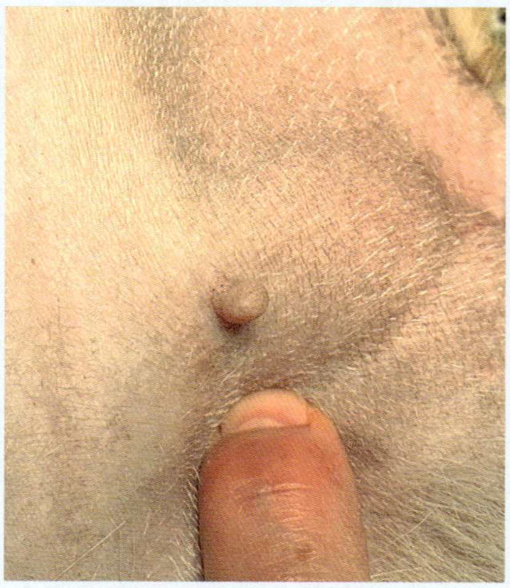

FIGURE 4. Laparoscopic-assisted procedure. External appearance of the left inguinal hernia.

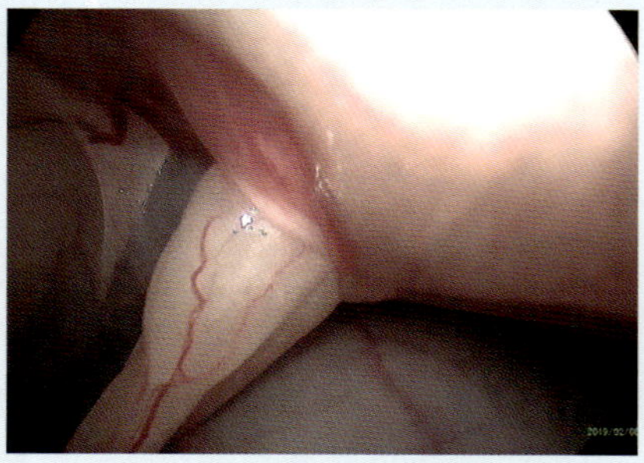

FIGURE 5. Laparoscopic appearance of the hernial defect and its content.

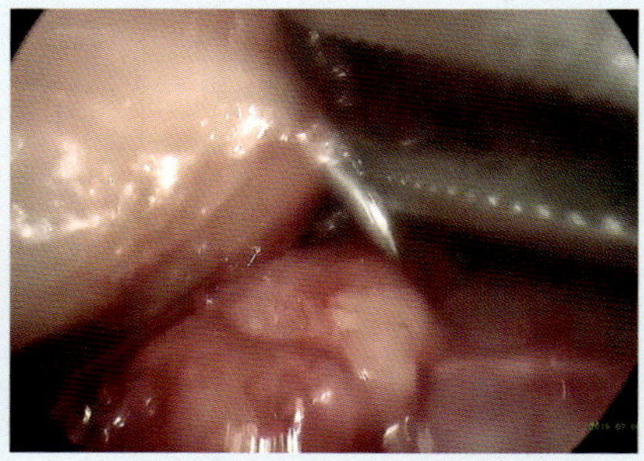

FIGURE 6. Introduction of an 18-gauge needle threaded in a 2-0 nonabsorbable monofilament suture.

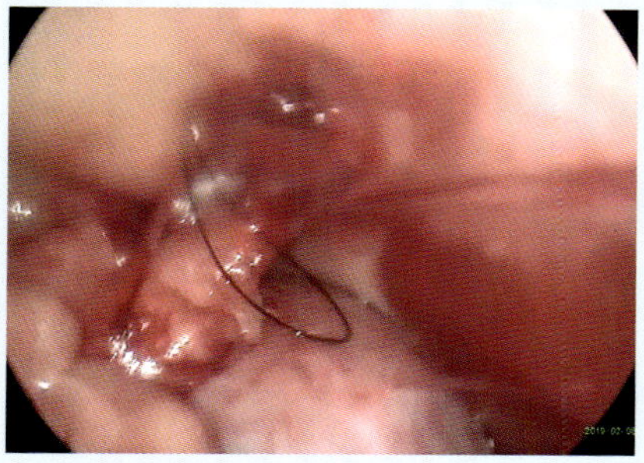

FIGURE 7. Appearance of the created loop.

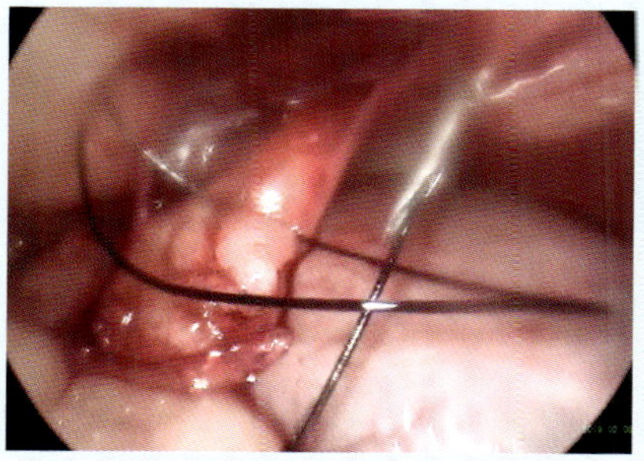

FIGURE 8. Insertion of the 18-gauge needle threaded and caught in the loop.

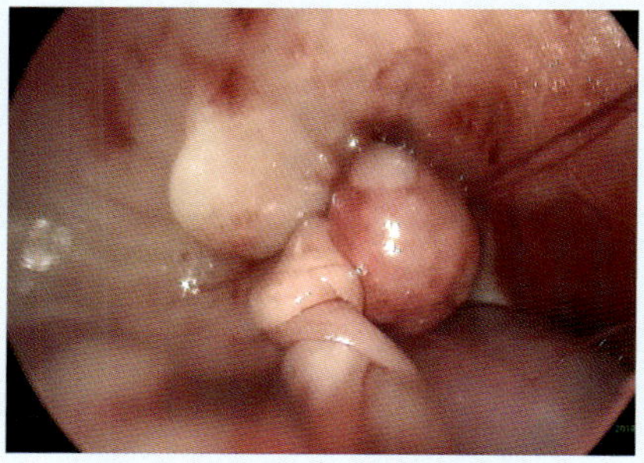

FIGURE 9. Final appearance after suturing.

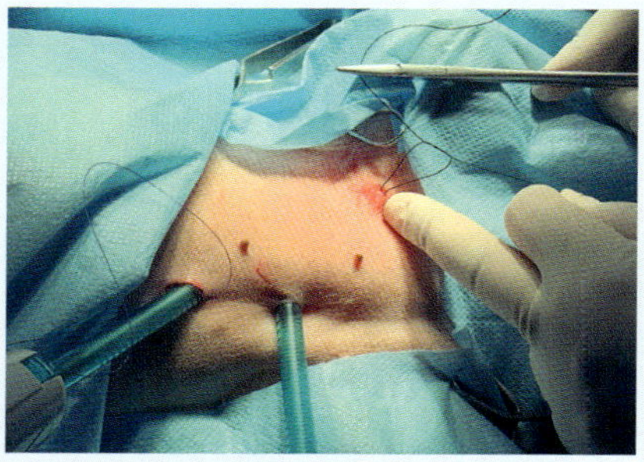

FIGURE 10. Tying the extracorporeal knot.

Tips and tricks

- ✓ The use of the end of a laparoscopic dissector applying pressure to each edge of the defect will allow to identify the point where the needle should be inserted extracorporeally from the outside.
- ✓ The 15° Trendelenburg position facilitates all maneuvers for the laparoscopic-assisted resolution of the inguinal hernia.
- ✓ It is important to carry out a previous ultrasound study to have proof of the hernial content.
- ✓ It is also advisable to empty the bladder of urine, allowing higher space for maneuver in the abdominal cavity.
- ✓ It is crucial not to injure the caudal epigastric vessels with the introduction of the 18-gauge needle, since bleeding can hinder the surgical procedure.

44 LAPAROSCOPIC PERINEAL HERNIORRHAPHY

Alexander Chernov

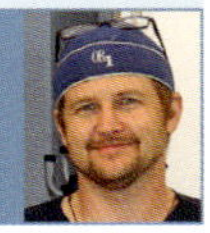

Indications

- Perineal hernia (unilateral or bilateral) (**Fig. 1**)
- Availability of equipment, a trained specialist, and conditions for performing a laparoscopic hernioplasty
- The procedure is technically feasible for animals of any size

Contraindications

- Constricted perineal hernia
- Severe general condition
- Operating room not prepared for specialized care and lack of specialist experience

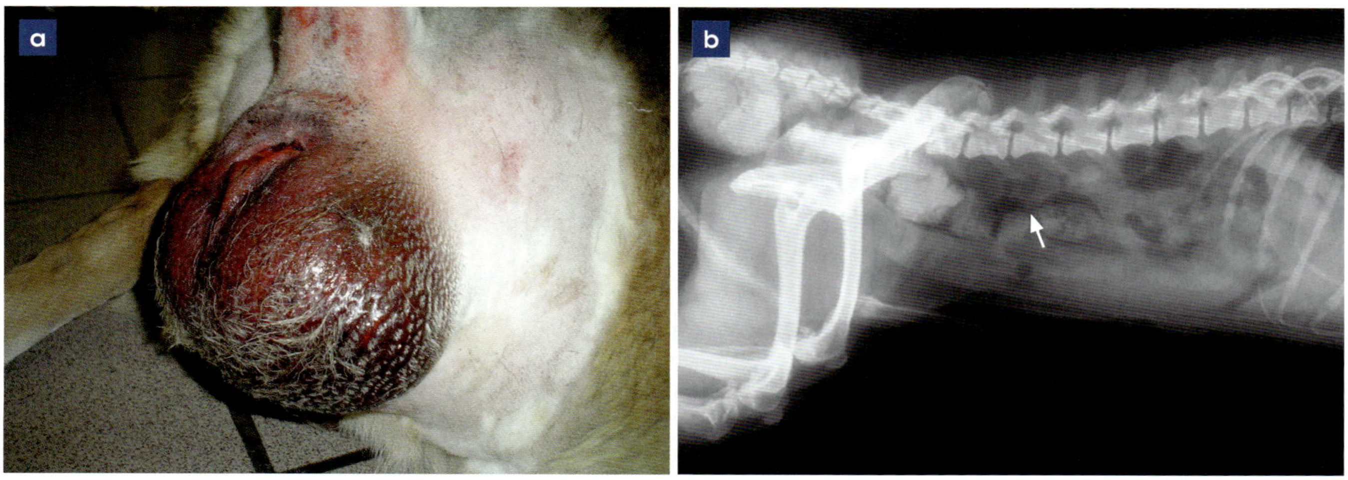

FIGURE 1. Perineal hernia in a dog. a) General view after clipping. b) X-ray image.

The minimum injury rate and compliance with the necessary asepsis in open (classic) surgery to possible infection remain relevant. For this reason, the intra-abdominal laparoscopic approach and further developments in hernioplasty for perineal hernia deserve attention.

The reliability of hernioplasty for perineal hernia is closely related to the problem of accessibility of the hernial gate and the possibility of eliminating the musculoaponeurotic defect.

The existing traditional methods for open perineal hernioplasty do not lack failures. They are obviously associated with an intervention in a slightly infected area. With classical methods, the boundaries of the hernial defect are difficult to reach; they are traumatic, and open hernioplasty does not solve another problem with perineal hernias. With this method, eliminating certain factors contributing to hernia recurrence is practically unattainable.

It is worth choosing the best option for hernioplasty to prevent the described complications of the surgical treatment of "classic" perineal hernia surgery. These include:

- Wound infection (6%–62%)
- Postoperative hernial protrusion on the operated or contralateral side (5%–60%)
- Infringement of protruding organs in the hernial protrusion of the contralateral side (10%–27%)

- Tenesmus (10%–25%)
- Fecal incontinence (10%–15%)
- Perineal fistula (7%)
- Paralysis of the sciatic and rectal s caudalis nerves (1%–3%)
- Complications after associated colopexy and cystopexy (dysuria, ischemia, obstruction, bleeding, stricture)

The diagnosis of a perineal hernia consists of identifying a characteristic protrusion dorsolaterally to the anus (right or left, but it can also be on both sides). When probing in the hernial gate, the colon, bladder, large omentum, intestinal loops, uterine horn, ovary, and/or spleen can be felt. Differential diagnosis is performed with tumor diseases in this area, such as lipoma, hemangioma, and so on. Perineal hernias are most often observed on the right side in males, but there are also bilateral hernias (less often in females).

There is the theory of degenerative changes in the soft tissues of the pelvis and perineum diaphragm (myopathy, neurogenic atrophy, prostate disease, increased intra-abdominal pressure).

The search for perineal hernioplasty methods is based on two classical approaches: suturing the hernial gate (by tension or unreliable method) and mostly plus performing colopexy and/or cystopexy.

The first description of a perineal hernia in the dog was made by C. F. Burrows and C. E. Harvey in 1973.

PATIENT PREPARATION AND POSITIONING

The bladder and colon are emptied. The abdominal wall is clipped (including the inguinal area from the medial femur to the perianal area). The legs are pulled as much as possible to the head (frog position) (**Fig. 2**).

Depending on the side of the hernia, the dog is placed in dorsal recumbency inclined 45° to the left or right laterally. After a diagnostic examination of the abdominal cavity, the animal is turned to the contralateral side of the hernial protrusion (if the hernia is bilateral symmetrical actions are performed on the other side, with the surgeon moving to the opposite side of the operating table).

The principle of visualization of the tissues that form the hernial orifice of the perineum (muscular aponeurotic tissues) is important. Laparoscopic examination is performed from the contralateral to the side of the hernial protrusion (**Fig. 3**).

Endoscopic description of the perineal hernia is complicated by the abundance of organs inside the hernial sac. For examination during laparoscopy, removal of the elements of hernial protrusion inside the abdominal cavity is required (e.g., intestines, bladder, large omentum).

The endoscopic picture of a perineal protrusion from the abdominal cavity is characterized by a close fit of the rectum (sometimes urinary bladder) to the defect zone. The pelvic bones significantly limit the range of all movements.

For small animals (weight <3 kg), the endoscopic hernia gate is difficult to visualize with a direct laparoscopic examination due to the size of the pelvis and organs (rectum, urinary bladder).

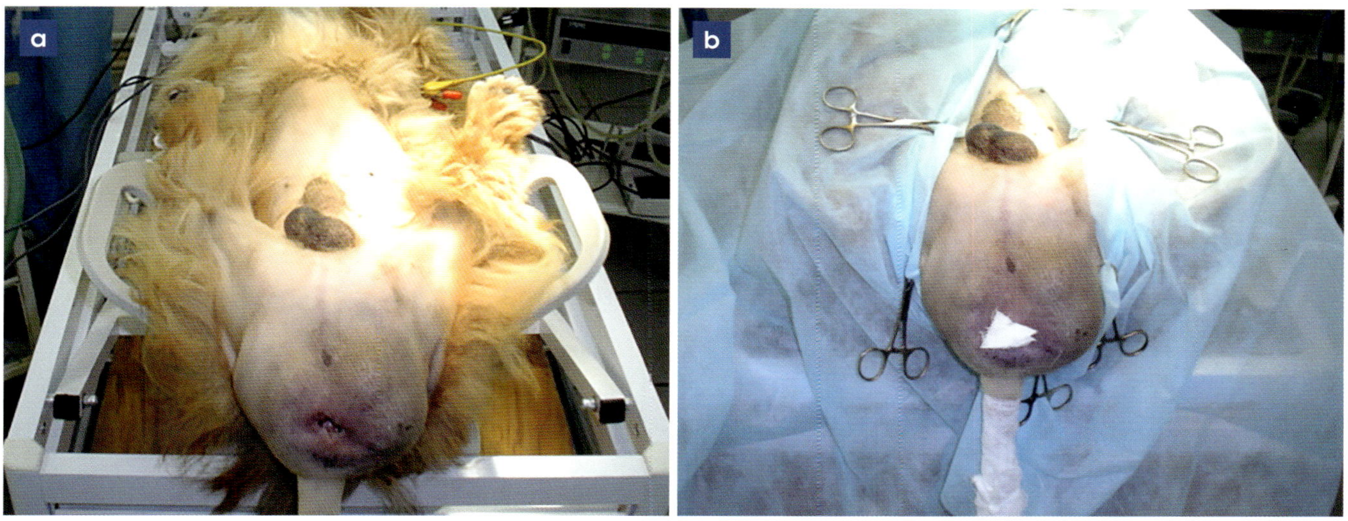

FIGURE 2. Dog with a bilateral perineal hernia in dorsal recumbency ("frog position"), a) before and b) after aseptic preparation.

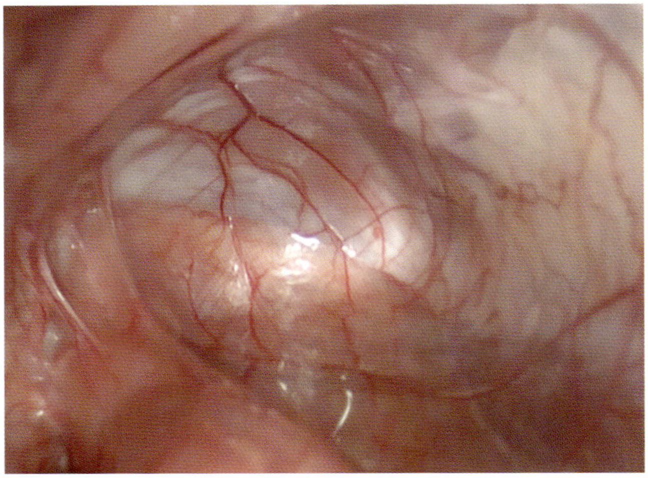

FIGURE 3. Endoscopic view of the right-side perineal hernial sac protrusion after suitable cystopexy and colopexy.

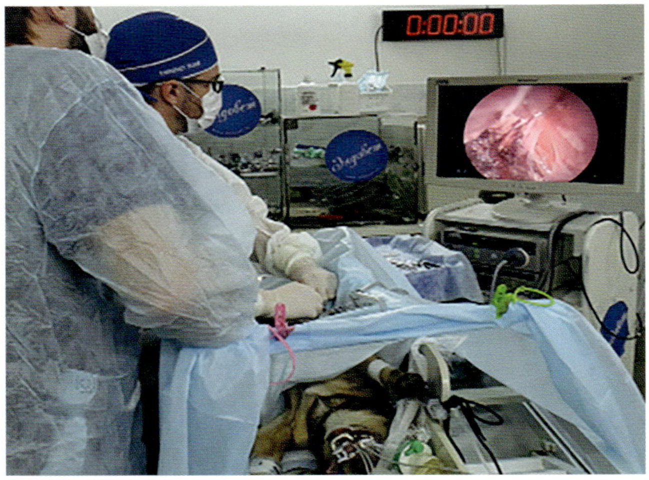

FIGURE 4. Location of the operating team and equipment for a right-sided perineal hernia.

OPERATING ROOM LAYOUT (FIG. 4)

The tasks necessary for the development of the laparoscopic perineal hernioplasty technique during endosurgery are the following:

- Selecting the access method (it should be adapted to the location and shape of the abdominal wall hernia defect and provide visualization of the intervention area).
- Choosing high-quality endoscopes and instruments.
- Additional tools can be placed on another operating table.
- The surgeon and the assistant stand on the same side of the operating table, and the monitor is placed at the caudal end of the table (**Fig. 5**).

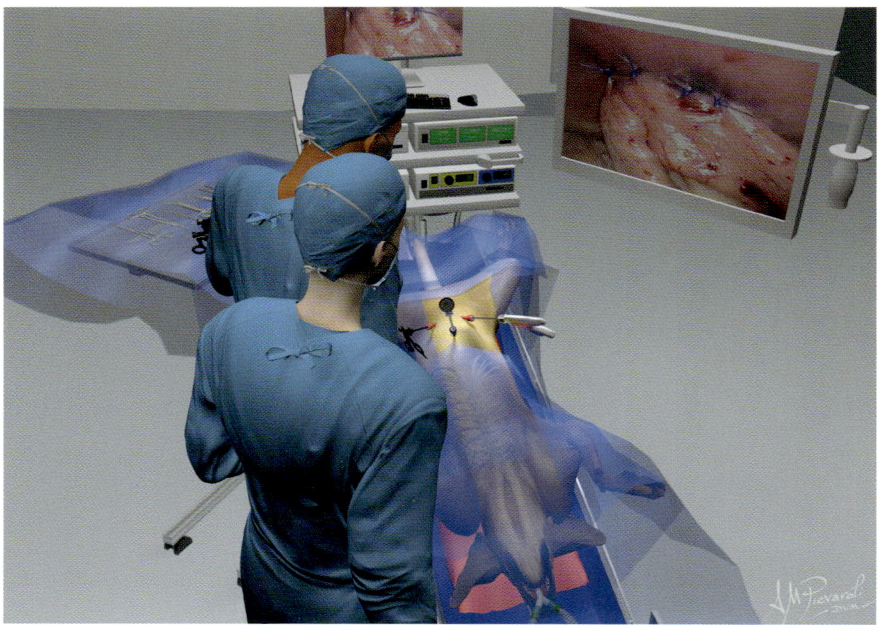

FIGURE 5. Operating room layout for laparoscopic perineal hernia repair.

Instruments (Fig. 6)

On the table:

- Telescope 5 mm – 30°
- Two or three 5 mm cannulas
- 10–12 mm cannulas for laparoscopic clamping
- Elongated needles for performing percutaneous sutures with the help of a gripping thread-loop
- Mesh (polypropylene is recommended)
- Devices and methods for temporary or permanent pexy of organs can also be used for this purpose (EndoGrab, extra- and/or intra-abdominal sutures)

Ready to use:

- Endoscopic cannula and aspiration/irrigation device
- Laparoscopic retractor (palpation probe)
- Set for general surgery

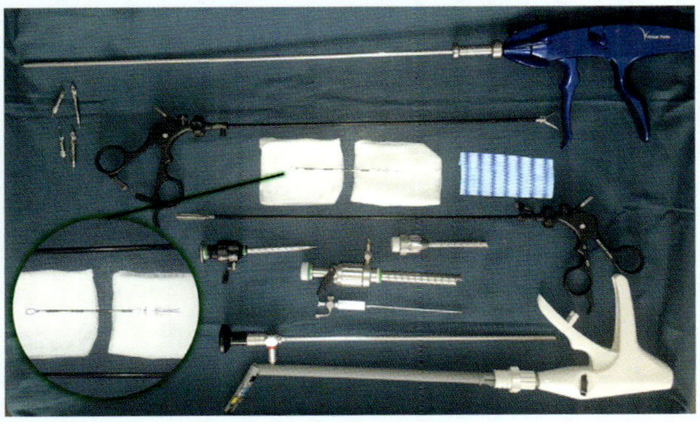

FIGURE 6. Standard laparoscopic set.

PORT PLACEMENT (FIG. 7)

- T1 (telescope port), on the midline, 1–2 cm cranial to the umbilicus
- T2, on the right mammary line (between the cranial and caudal mammary nipples)
- T3, on the left mammary line (between the cranial and caudal mammary nipples)

PROCEDURE

- During laparoscopy, the internal organs of the pelvis (bladder, prostate, rectum) are differentiated.
- Through the trocar ports (2–3 in total), instrumental control is provided (scope, palpation probe, intestine grasper). Laparoscopy significantly facilitates control of the perineal hernia contents.
- The detection of a hernia defect is mutually complemented by visual laparoscopic control and bimanual palpation (instrumental and external palpation towards each other) (**Fig. 8**).
- A suitable/constant colopexy/cystopexy is performed to appose the hernia sides (**Fig. 9**).
- A polypropylene patch 1–2 cm larger than the hernial defect is prepared and introduced into the abdomen through a port (**Fig. 10**).
- The implant is fixed to the peritoneum, muscle, and fascial tissues of the pelvic floor with nonabsorbable sutures or

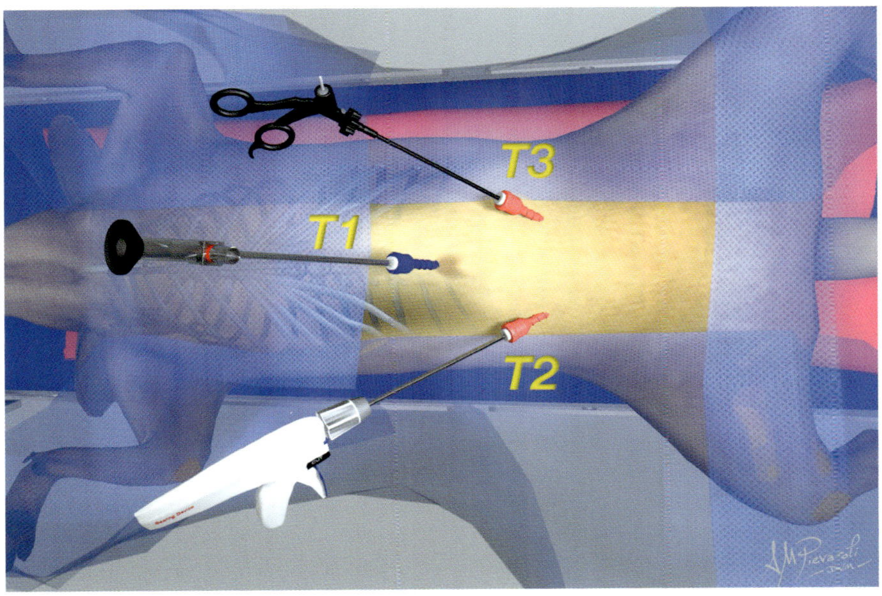

FIGURE 7. Port placement for laparoscopic perineal hernia repair.

staplers around the defect. A more useful endoscopically assisted suturing when inserting the wire into the abdomen through the system consists of two needles catching the wire out (the knot is tied outside and pulled under the skin) (**Fig. 11**).

- These sutures (5–10 ligatures) can be fixed to the mesh across the triangle or rhombus that connects the external sphincter ani and the gluteus superficialis muscles, and the tuber ischiaticum). All sutures fix the mesh to the abdominal wall (**Fig. 12**).
- If possible, additional endoscopic staplers can be used to clip the mesh from the abdominal cavity.
- Laparoscopic colopexy and cystopexy are performed as needed in a final step (if this has not been done before) (**Fig. 13**).
- The operation is completed by monitoring the hemostasis and pelvic organ integrity. Be ready to make a traditional open hernioplasty if anything goes wrong.

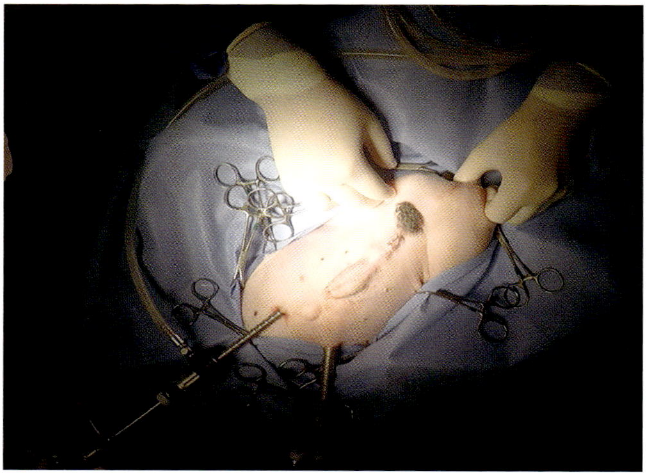

FIGURE 8. Determination of the perineal hernia orifice by external digital pressure under endoscopic control.

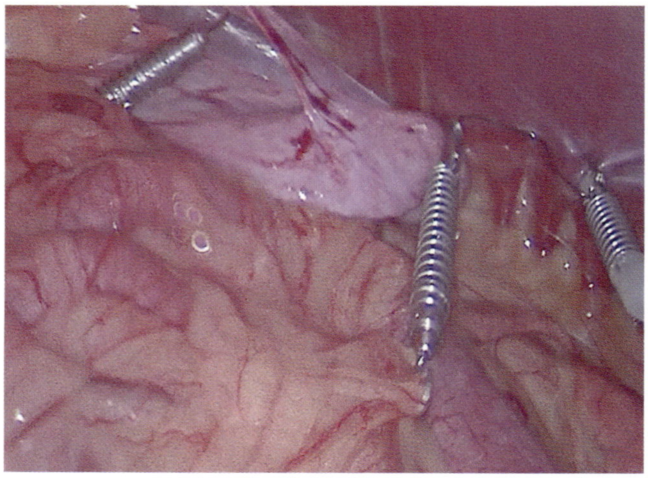

FIGURE 9. Stages of laparoscopic hernioplasty for perineal hernia: suitable cystopexy and colopexy with EndoGrab.

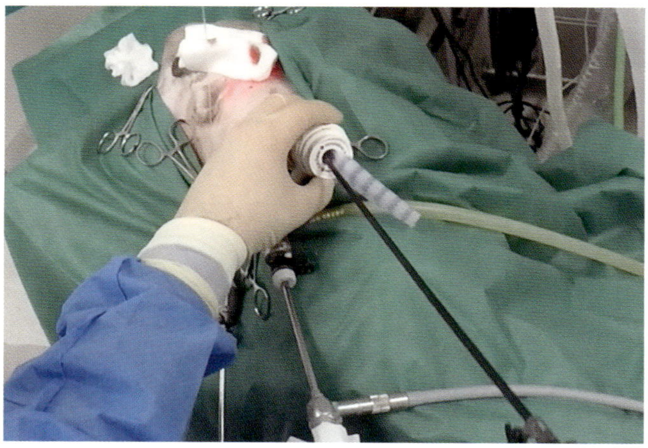

FIGURE 10. Passing the polypropylene mesh of the desired size into the abdominal cavity through a 10 mm trocar.

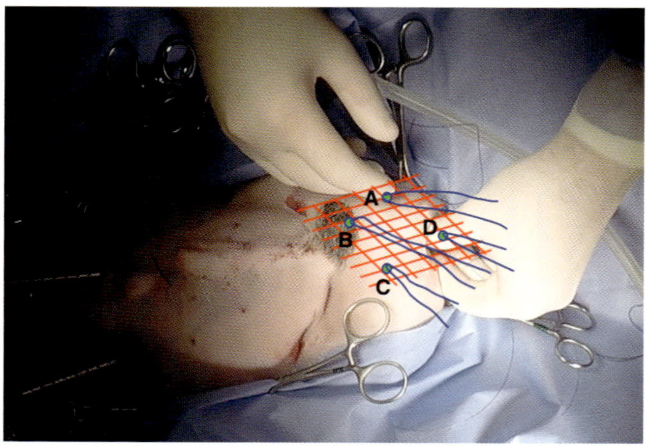

FIGURE 11. External scheme.

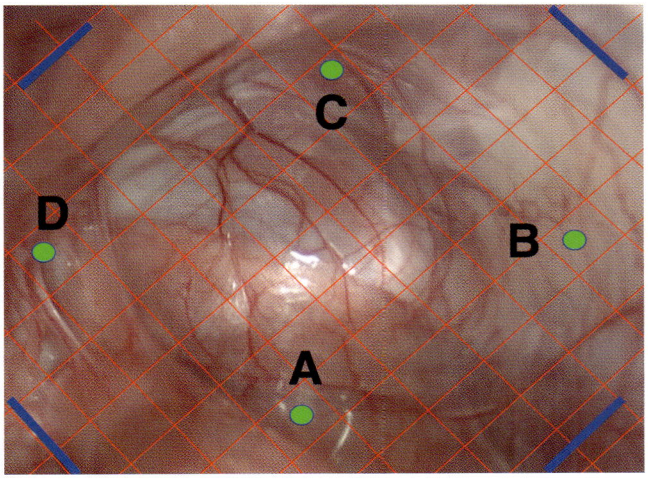

FIGURE 12. Endoscopic view and scheme of a mesh placement into the perineal hernia. Red: mesh; green: sutures; blue; endoclips; A: ligature passed through the mesh and the levator ani, and the sphincter ani muscles; B, C: ligature passed through the mesh and periosteum of the tuber ischiaticum; D: ligature passed through the mesh and the coccygeus lateralis muscle, the sacrotuberous ligament, and the levator ani muscle.

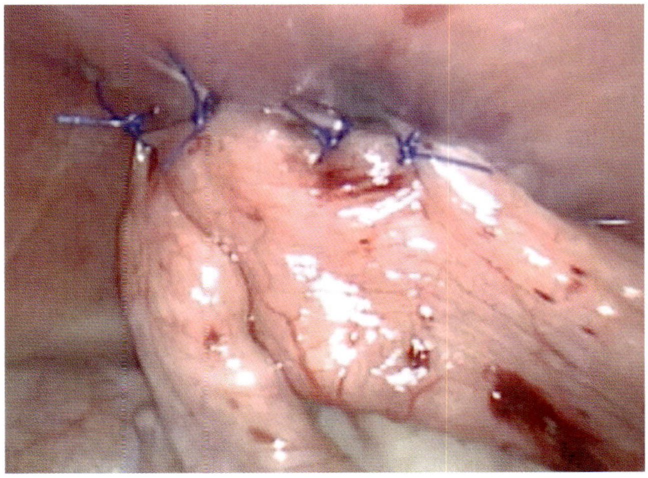

FIGURE 13. Total laparoscopic colopexy performed.

POSTOPERATIVE MANAGEMENT

- In the early postoperative period, factors that predispose to increased intra-abdominal pressure must be excluded (cough, excessive delay in restoration of physiological functions, constipation, aggressive behavior). Therefore, the use of sedatives, laxatives and other symptomatic drugs is recommended.
- It should be noted that in the early postoperative period there may not be a significant decrease in the external protrusion of the skin in the area of the former hernia. Within 3–4 months, this skin protrusion progressively decreases due to the closure of the mesh structure by connective tissue and the obliteration and fibrosis of the cavity of the former hernial sac.

Complications of laparoscopic perineal herniorrhaphy

Direct (2–3 hours):

- Heart, renal, and respiratory failure.
- Bleeding.

Early (5–7 days):

- Heart, renal, respiratory, and liver failure; allergy.
- Pain syndrome.
- Urinary incontinence and retention.
- Coprostasis, diarrhea.
- Intraoperative damage and consequences of endosurgery (e.g., hemoperitoneum, peritonitis, foreign body).
- Changes in soft tissue wounds of the ports (e.g., purulence, hematoma, seroma, burn, allergy).

Late (after 2 weeks):

- Recurrence.
- Suture fistula.
- Abdominal adhesions.

Excessive long-term exposure to friction or sprouting of polypropylene mesh in contact with the rectum and urethra should be studied (until now, the author has not encountered such complications).

Key points

- With unilateral perineal hernia, the laparoscopic examination is performed on the contralateral side of the hernial protrusion in the dog.
- The parietal peritoneum lines the inner surface of the hernial protrusion, which protrudes aside to the defect, forming a hernial sac (while determining the exact size of the herniated sac in a perineal hernia from the abdominal cavity endoscopically is not easy).
- It is convenient to use the bimanual finger method to manage organs and tissues that have fallen into a hernia (from the outside, pressing a finger on the center of the hernia). In females, it is recommended to use a vaginal retractor.
- Laparoscopic hernioplasty of a perineal hernia is performed with the simplest method of closing the hernial defect without isolating the hernial sac. However, the dissection of adhesions between the hernial sac and adjacent internal organs is sometimes required.
- One of the most important management stages of the operation, in terms of the possibility of performing hernioplasty, is the creation of a temporary or permanent colopexy.
- During the mesh fixation to the pelvic floor, the most important part is placing 5–10 sutures along the perimeter of the implant, passing through the fixation points.
- Each suture should securely capture both the mesh and the muscle-fascial elements.
- When through-sutures are applied through the peritoneum under laparoscopic control, the knots tied from the outside are tightened and sunk under the skin.
- It is important to assess the primary intraoperative effect if the hernial protrusion during the pneumoperitoneum creation increases from the outside. In this case, a few more fixing stitches are applied.

SUGGESTED READINGS

45 LAPAROSCOPIC PERITONEOPERICARDIAL HERNIORRHAPHY

Valery F. Scharf

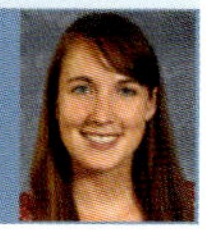

Indications

- Elimination of clinical signs secondary to peritoneopericardial hernias
- Prevention of sequelae from peritoneopericardial hernias

Contraindications

- Substantial adhesions
- Large peritoneopericardial hernias
- Emergent gastrointestinal entrapment or strangulation
- Cats: laparoscopic repair should be approached with caution

Peritoneopericardial hernias (PPDHs) are an uncommon congenital anomaly in cats and dogs in which separation of the peritoneal and pericardial cavities is incomplete. This defect allows abdominal organs, most commonly the liver, gallbladder, and small intestines, to herniate into the pericardial space. Clinical signs are usually gastrointestinal and/or respiratory in nature, although it is not uncommon for PPDHs to be diagnosed incidentally. Radiographic evidence of a PPDH includes an enlarged cardiac silhouette, with inability to distinguish normal diaphragmatic borders. If the gastrointestinal tract is herniated, gas-filled viscera may also be visible within the pericardium on radiographs.

Repair of PPDHs in cats and dogs remains controversial due to the incidental nature of many of these hernias when diagnosed. Surgical repair is generally recommended when clinical signs are present, or to prevent the development of clinical signs or life-threatening sequelae in the future (i.e., gastrointestinal entrapment). A recent large retrospective study evaluating dogs with surgical repair versus conservative management of PPDHs found low operative mortality rates and good long-term survival for dogs following surgical repair.

Experience with laparoscopic repair of PPDHs in both people and small animals is limited. A case series of three dogs and three cats pending publication suggests that laparoscopic herniorrhaphy is feasible in dogs but should be approached with caution in cats due to a high risk of complications, including cardiovascular arrest. Although rare, intrapericardial cystic lesions may also be associated with PPDHs and may be addressed thoracoscopically concurrently with laparoscopic PPDH repair.

> The first report of laparoscopic repair of peritoneopericardial hernias in two dogs was presented by Scharf at the 2021 World Veterinary Endoscopy and Minimally Invasive Surgery meeting.

PATIENT PREPARATION AND POSITIONING

The patient should be clipped to be prepared for potential conversion to open celiotomy and/or median sternotomy. Thus, the entire ventral abdomen and thorax should be clipped and draped into the surgical field with enough distance laterally to place paramedian ports as needed for triangulation (**Fig. 1**). It is recommended to drape from the manubrium cranially to the pubis caudally to allow for placement of thoracic ports in the case that a thoracoscopic approach can aid in the dissection of adhesions.

Reverse Trendelenburg positioning is critical to successful laparoscopic reduction of a PPDH (**Fig. 2**). Steep (>15°) reverse Trendelenburg may impair venous return to the heart and contribute to systemic hypotension.

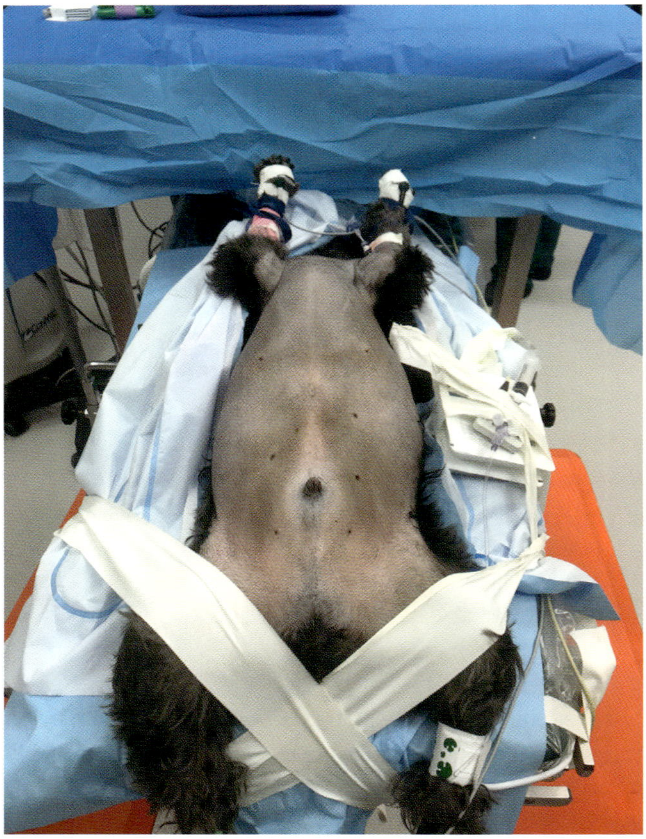

FIGURE 1. Patient preparation should include the entire ventral thorax and abdomen to allow for conversion to open celiotomy and/or median sternotomy. The clipped area should extend laterally to facilitate lateral port placement for articulation of needle drivers.

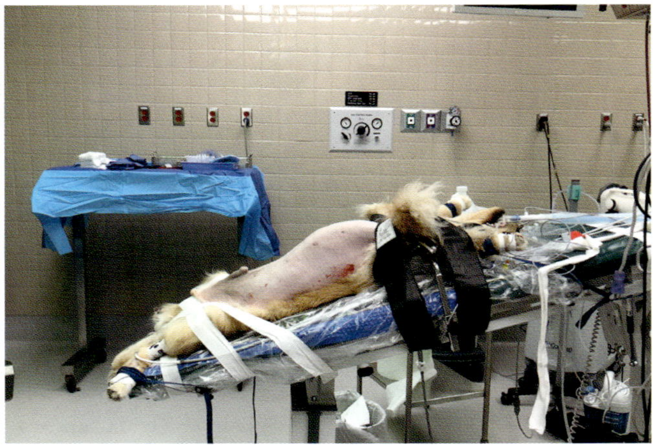

FIGURE 2. Reverse Trendelenburg positioning can greatly assist with the reduction of herniated organs.

OPERATING ROOM LAYOUT

The patient should be placed in dorsal recumbency with the hind end positioned at the caudal edge of the table. The surgeon stands at the caudal edge of the table with the assistant to the side. The monitor is positioned directly over the head of the patient, and the instrument table is positioned over the head, making sure there is enough room for reverse Trendelenburg positioning (**Fig. 3**). Alternatively, the instrument table may be positioned alongside the patient or adjacent to the surgeon and assistant at the caudal edge of the table.

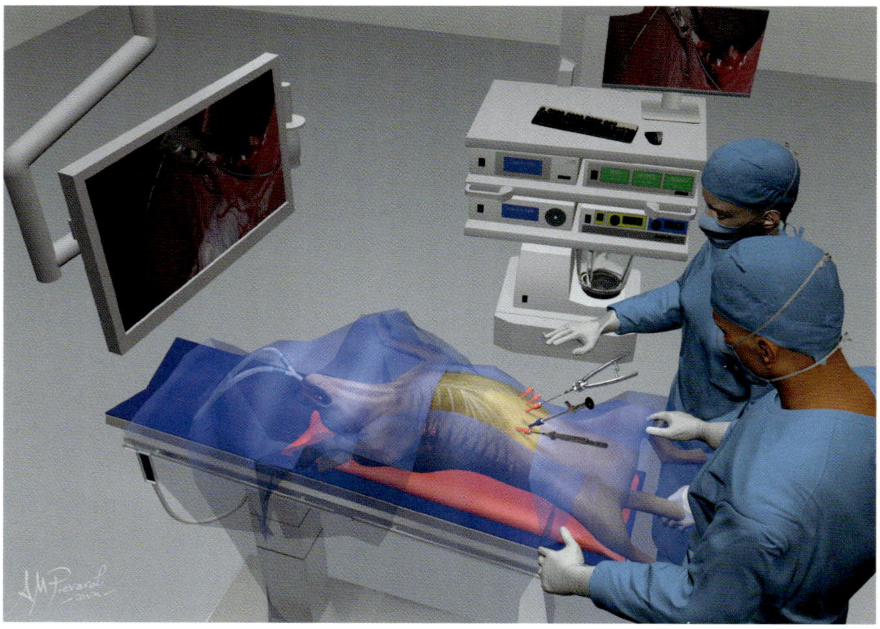

FIGURE 3. Operating room layout for laparoscopic peritoneopericardial herniorrhaphy.

Instruments

On the table:

- Laparoscope 5 or 10 mm – 30°
- Two 4–5 mm cannulas
- Endoscopic atraumatic grasping forceps
- Endoscopic Metzenbaum scissors
- Blunt probe
- Fan retractor
- Vessel-sealing device
- Endoscopic needle drivers or suture-assisting device
- Barbed suture with large needle
- 3 Fr red rubber catheter or pericardiocentesis catheter

Ready to use:

- Additional cannulas as needed for additional retraction
- A 10 mm cannula may be needed for introduction of a suture-assisting device or specimen retrieval bag

PORT PLACEMENT (FIG. 4)

- T1, on the midline, 1–2 cm caudal to the umbilicus, to facilitate initial endoscope placement
- T2, left paramedian, 4–6 cm cranial to T1
- T3, right paramedian, 4–6 cm cranial to T1
- Additional paramedian ports (T4, T5) may be placed as needed to aid in the retraction of falciform fat to improve visualization and to place a catheter to evacuate the pericardial space

Paramedian placement of T2 and T3 accommodate graspers for reduction and needle drivers for herniorrhaphy.

In large dogs, T1–T3 may be shifted 2–6 cm cranially to ensure instruments can reach the diaphragm.

Changing the endoscope to T2 or T3 may aid in visualization of the hernia for suturing if falciform fat obscures visualization.

PROCEDURE

- Following T1 placement, initial insufflation should be started at approximately 5 mmHg, and hemodynamic parameters (blood pressure, heart rate, oxygenation) should be monitored carefully for severe hypotension. T2 and T3 are then placed under laparoscopic guidance.
- The PPDH is visualized cranially; the extent of adhesions and herniated organs is assessed (**Fig. 5**). Atraumatic grasping forceps are used to reduce herniated falciform, omental fat, and stomach (**Fig. 6**).
- A blunt probe or fan retractor is used to gently sweep herniated liver lobes, gallbladder, and intestines through the PPDH back into the peritoneal cavity (**Fig. 7**). Reverse Trendelenburg positioning can be temporarily increased to facilitate organ reduction.

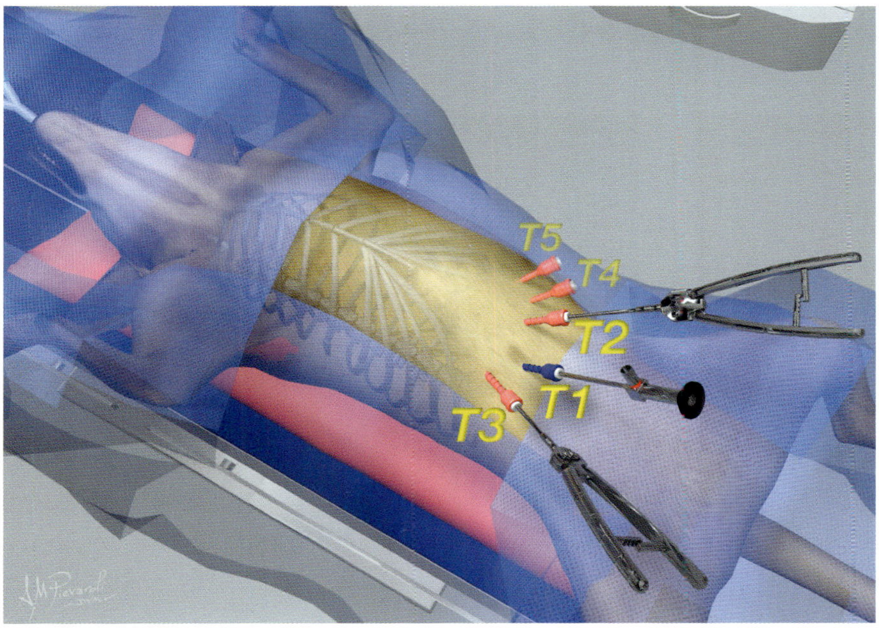

FIGURE 4. Port placement for laparoscopic peritoneopericardial herniorrhaphy.

- If a large amount of falciform or omental fat is herniated, additional retractors may be needed once the fat is reduced to improve visualization of the hernia. Alternatively, a vessel-sealing device can be used to resect falciform fat, although extraction of extensive falciform likely necessitates a single-incision laparoscopic surgery port to facilitate removal without extension of a port site.
- A vessel-sealing device is used to transect adhesions between organs and the hernial ring (**Fig. 8**). Caution should be taken when using a bipolar vessel-sealing device near the epicardium to avoid inducing fatal arrhythmias.
- The endoscope is then advanced into the pericardial space to confirm the reduction of all herniated contents.
- A 3 Fr red rubber or pericardiocentesis catheter is then introduced through a separate paramedian cannula into the pericardial space (**Figs. 9 and 10**).
- Large (0 or 2-0) suture is used to close the diaphragmatic defect in a simple continuous or interrupted pattern (**Fig. 11**). Barbed suture allows for easier maintenance of tension along the suture line when using a simple continuous pattern.
- Triangulation of the needle drivers to the ventral aspect of the hernia is challenging; for this reason, the use of a suture-assisting device is recommended to improve the ease of suturing the diaphragmatic defect (**Fig. 12**).
- Following closure of the diaphragmatic defect around the pericardial catheter, negative suction is applied to the catheter to evacuate air from the pericardial space. The pericardial catheter is then withdrawn from the pericardial space and the abdomen.
- Pneumoperitoneum is evacuated, and the port sites are closed routinely.

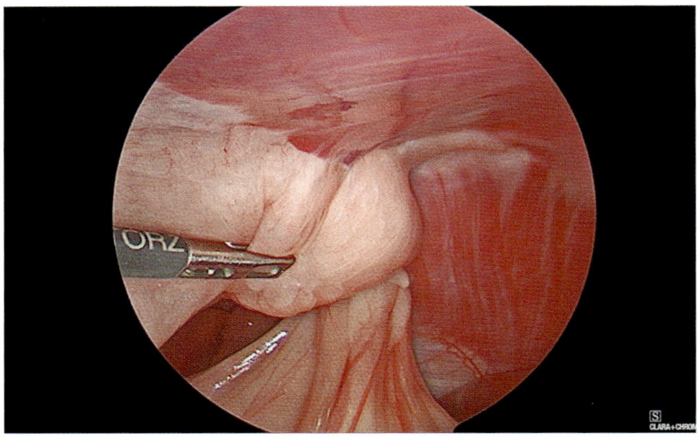

FIGURE 5. Initial view of a PPDH with herniated falciform and omental fat.

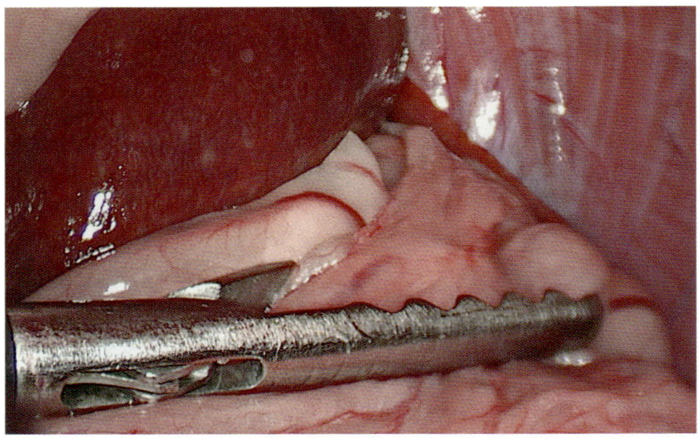

FIGURE 6. Reduction of herniated omental fat using atraumatic grasping forceps.

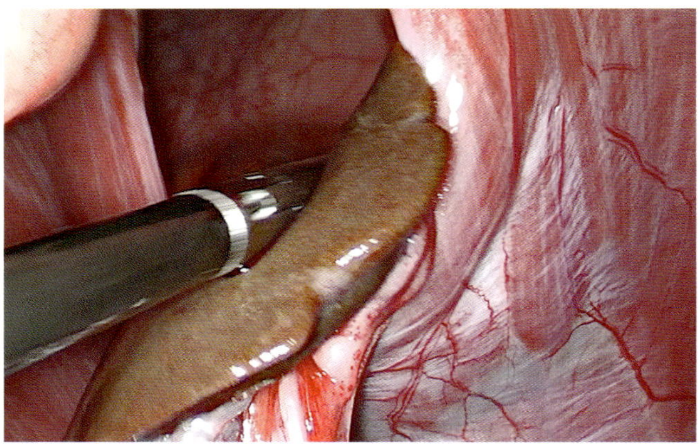

FIGURE 7. Reduction of herniated liver lobe and gallbladder using a sweeping motion with a blunt instrument. Gentle reduction is assisted by gravity by using reverse Trendelenburg positioning.

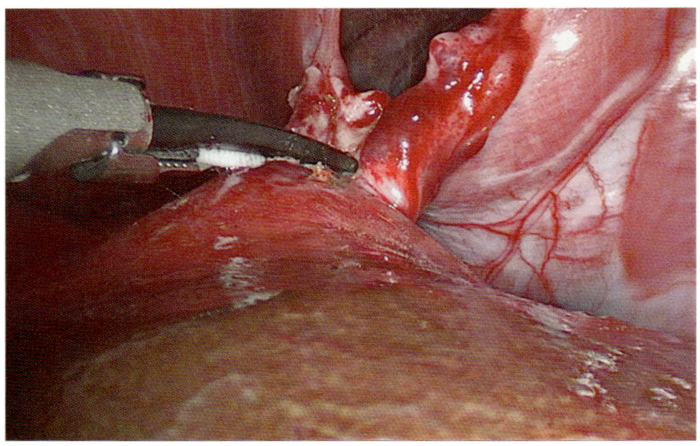

FIGURE 8. An ultrasonic vessel-sealing device is used to dissect adhesions between the liver and the hernia ring.

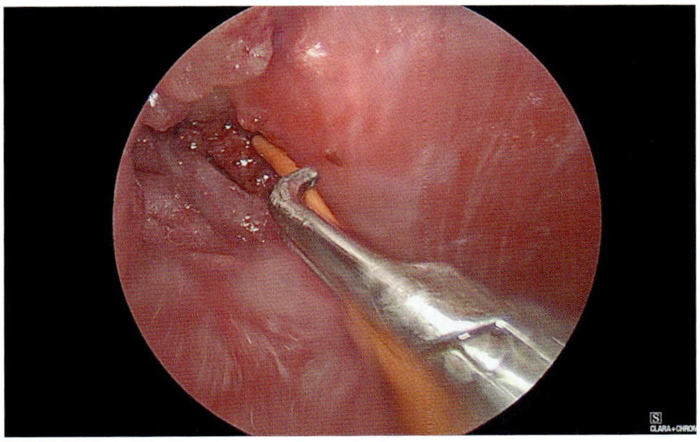

FIGURE 9. Placement of a 3 Fr red rubber catheter into the pericardial space prior to closure of the hernia. The catheter may be placed percutaneously or through an instrument cannula.

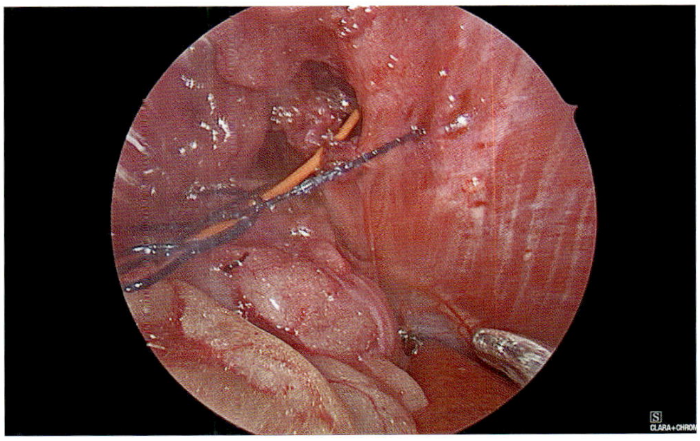

FIGURE 10. Positioning of the red rubber catheter exiting the pericardial space while the hernia is sutured closed.

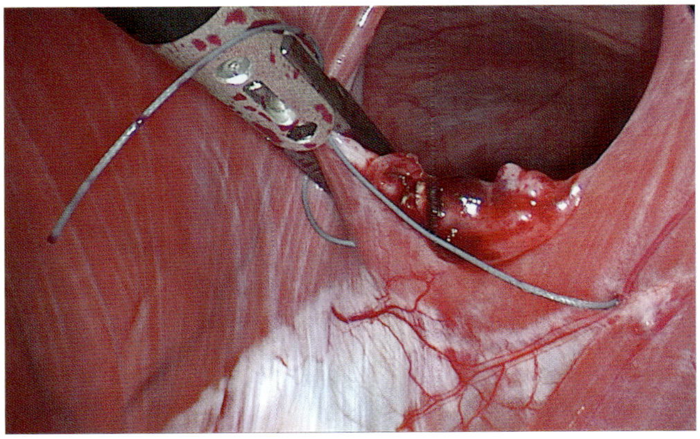

FIGURE 11. Initial suture placement to close the hernia starting at the dorsal aspect of the defect.

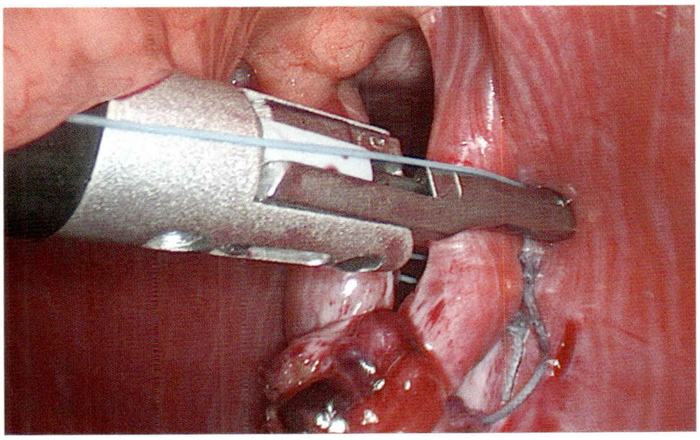

FIGURE 12. The use of a suture-assisting device facilitates the placement of suture through the edges of the hernia ring; triangulation of traditional needle drivers for hernia closure can present an additional challenge.

POSTOPERATIVE MANAGEMENT

- Patients should be monitored postoperatively for any evidence of tachycardia, hypotension, or hypoxemia. If the pleural space was breached and a thoracostomy tube was placed, the pleural space should be evacuated every hour for 4 hours and then every 6 hours; the thoracostomy tube may be removed within 12 hours if the air is evacuated and fluid is minimal.
- Postoperative analgesia is provided intravenously initially and may be supplemented with pre- or intraoperative local blocks.
- Patients may be discharged as soon as comfortable on oral analgesics, often within 24 hours.

Complications of laparoscopic peritoneopericardial herniorrhaphy

- Severe systemic hypotension may result from insufflation of the pericardium and compression of the right side of the heart. For this reason, insufflation pressures should be maintained at the lowest pressure possible, allowing for adequate visualization. The author recommends using an initial insufflation pressure of 5 mmHg and decreasing it to 2–3 mmHg as needed. Prior to reducing herniated contents, peritoneal pressures of up to 8 mmHg may be tolerated. If hypotension is noted, insufflation should be reduced until pressures improve and then cautiously restarted at low (2–3 mmHg) pressures. Alternatively, lift laparoscopy may be utilized to assist exposure. The author has temporarily placed a large percutaneous suture through the cranial body wall and falciform fat to aid in the retraction of the ventral body wall and falciform fat (**Fig. 13**).
- Pneumothorax may occur if the pleural space is breached during dissection of adhesions or suturing of the diaphragm; ventilation and oxygenation should be carefully monitored as the creation of pneumothorax may not be recognized by the surgeon. If pneumothorax occurs, the pleural space may be evacuated through the diaphragm in a similar manner to that previously described for the pericardium, or a thoracostomy tube may be placed. If tension pneumothorax is suspected, a thoracic cannula may be rapidly placed to allow rapid evacuation of the pleural space and mitigate any pleural insufflation that may occur as the result of the pneumoperitoneum.
- Reduction of herniated organs may prove challenging due to extensive adhesions. Careful case selection is important: the author recommends that traditional open PPDH repair be considered for older dogs or those with more than 1–2 liver lobes herniated due to potentially increased likelihood of substantial adhesions between the liver and the pericardium. Similarly, laparoscopic repair of PPDHs in cats should only be pursued with extreme caution and minimal abdominal insufflation due to anecdotal evidence that cats may be more susceptible to cardiovascular arrest during laparoscopic PPDH repair.
- Hemorrhage may occur during dissection of adhesions and reduction of liver lobes. Careful case selection, gentle use of a blunt instrument for liver reduction, use of a vessel-sealing device to dissect adhesions, and increased reverse Trendelenburg position are recommended to facilitate challenging reduction and decrease the risk of significant hemorrhage.

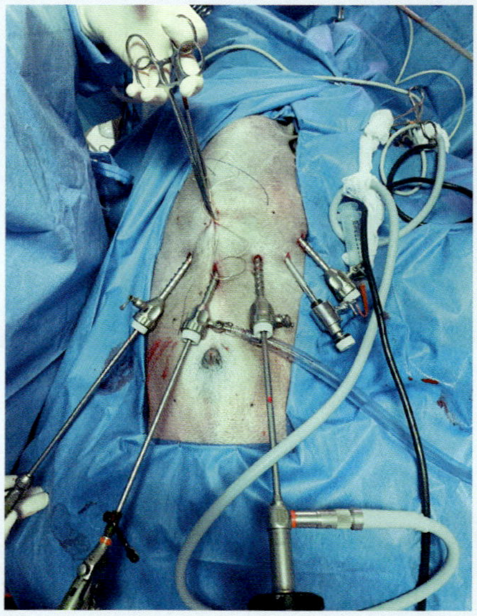

FIGURE 13. A large-gauge percutaneous stay suture was placed approximately 3 cm caudal to the xiphoid to facilitate retraction of the falciform fat and lift laparoscopy to allow for lower peritoneal (and pericardial) insufflation pressures while improving visualization during suturing of the hernia.

Key points

- Case selection is critical for successful laparoscopic PPDH repair: laparoscopic repair of chronic PPDHs with extensive liver lobe herniation and PPDHs in cats is contraindicated based on currently available clinical data.
- Patients undergoing laparoscopic repair of PPDHs should be monitored closely for severe hypotension, which may be addressed by decreasing or discontinuing abdominal insufflation.
- Abdominal insufflation should be initiated at 5 mmHg or less and should be monitored carefully in conjunction with the patient's blood pressure during laparoscopic PPDH repair.
- Tension pneumothorax may occur and should be addressed by discontinuing abdominal insufflation and/or rapidly placing a thoracic (intercostal) port.

SUGGESTED READINGS

CLINICAL CASES

45.1 LAPAROSCOPIC TREATMENT OF PERITONEAL-PERICARDIAL DIAPHRAGMATIC HERNIA IN A PUPPY DOG

Andrea M. Pievaroli

CASE DESCRIPTION

A 3-month-old male Weimaraner dog was referred to undergo surgery for a congenital PPDH. The defect was diagnosed as an incidental finding following an echocardiographic examination for the presence of a mild heart murmur. The patient was asymptomatic. Despite the absence of clinical signs, it was decided to perform surgery to reposition the herniated organs early, close the defect, and prevent future complications. To reduce invasiveness, the surgery was performed under laparoscopy, although the author's case history is small and there are, to date, few reports of the laparoscopic treatment of PPDHs in dogs and cats. Through the diaphragmatic defect, part of the liver, gallbladder, and small intestines were herniated in the pericardial space. The hernia was closed using a barbed suture. The patient recovered quickly after surgery and had no complications in the following months.

Key points

- Early treatment in young patients has a greater chance of success in repositioning herniated organs.
- Set low abdominal insufflation pressures (3–4 mmHg) to reduce the risk of cardiac complications. Careful anesthetic monitoring is essential.
- Be careful not to interfere with the heart during the procedure.
- Be careful not to create iatrogenic pneumothorax.

PORT PLACEMENT

- Patient in dorsal recumbency
- T1, 1 cm cranial to the umbilicus
- T2, on a left paramedian position, 2–3 cm cranial to T1
- T3, on a right paramedian position, 2–3 cm cranial to T1

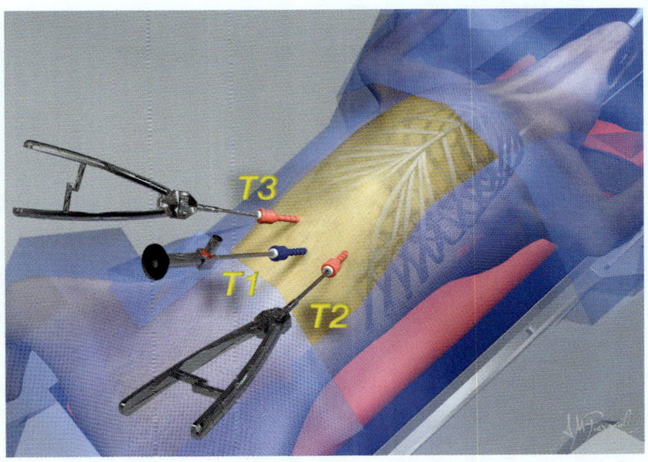

PROCEDURE

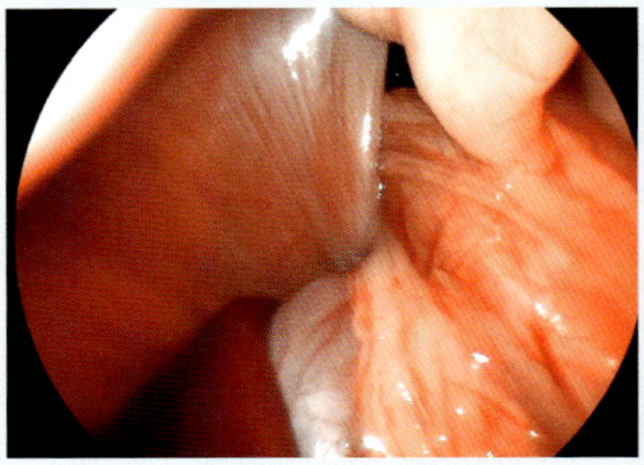

FIGURE 1. Initial endoscopic appearance of the PPDH. Some abdominal organs are seen herniated in the pericardial sac.

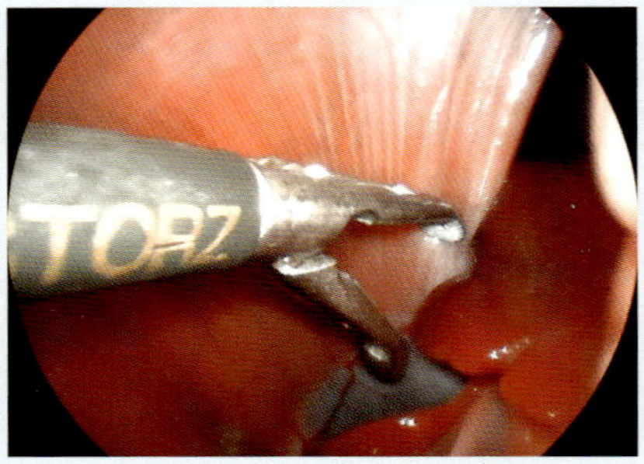

FIGURE 2. A blunt probe or atraumatic forceps is used to gently sweep the herniated intestine, stomach, liver lobes, and gallbladder back into the peritoneal cavity.

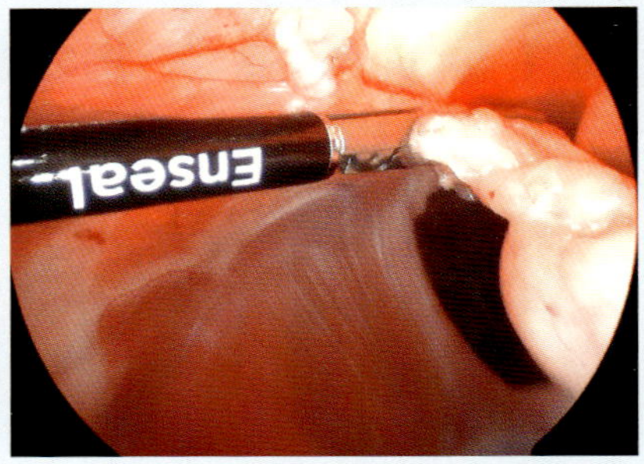

FIGURE 3. Use a sealing device to resect the falciform fat. It is mandatory to have a clear view of the surgical field before starting the intracorporeal suture.

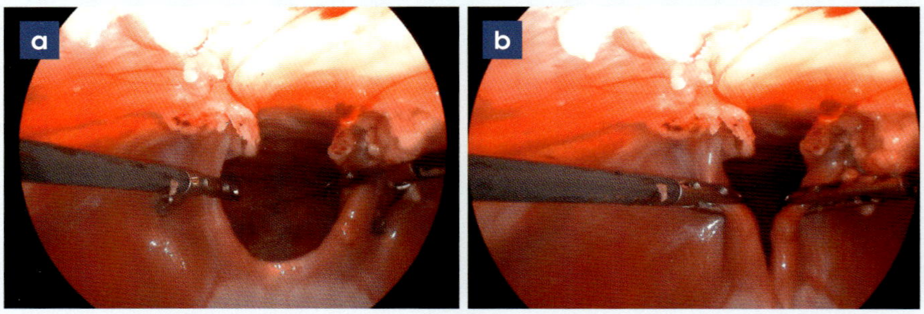

FIGURE 4. A test can be done, using two atraumatic forceps, to bring the margins closer and evaluate the tension.

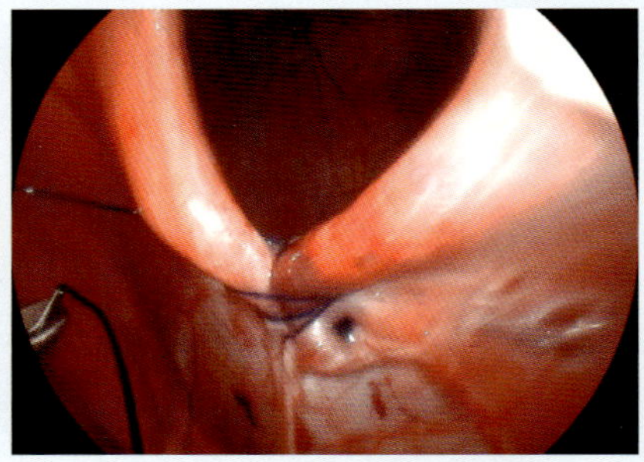

FIGURE 5. Herniorrhaphy is performed with two needle holders, in a continuous suture pattern suture, starting from the lower margin. For an optimal result, it is necessary to use a barbed suture.

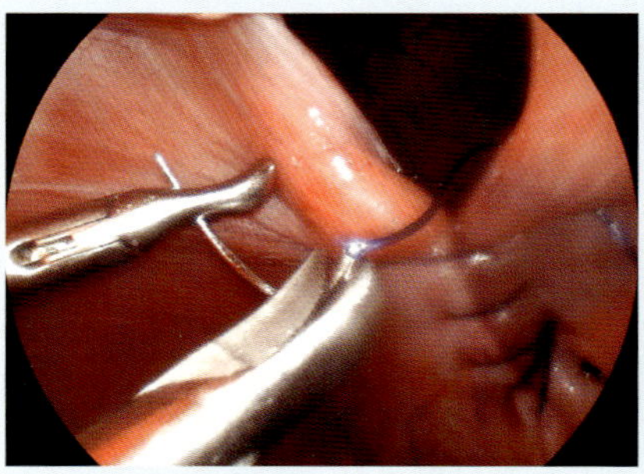

FIGURE 6. When performing intracorporeal suturing, the optimal arrangement of the needle holders must be found. In this case, the telescope (T1) is temporarily inserted in the right-hand port (T2) and the needle holder in the central port ("off-axis viewing").

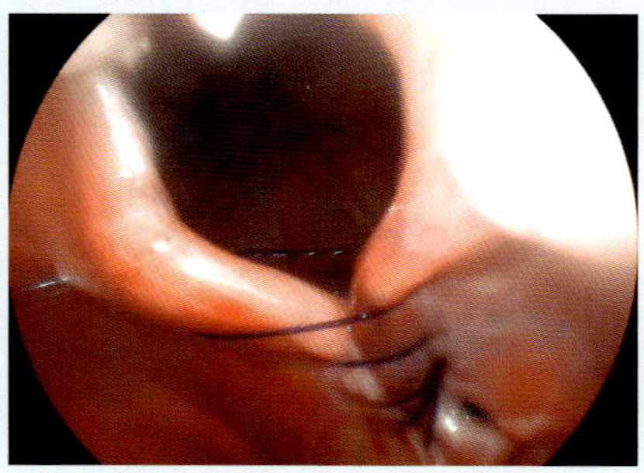

FIGURE 7. As the hernia edges get closer, the tension is reduced. The technical features of the barbed suture prevent the suture from loosening.

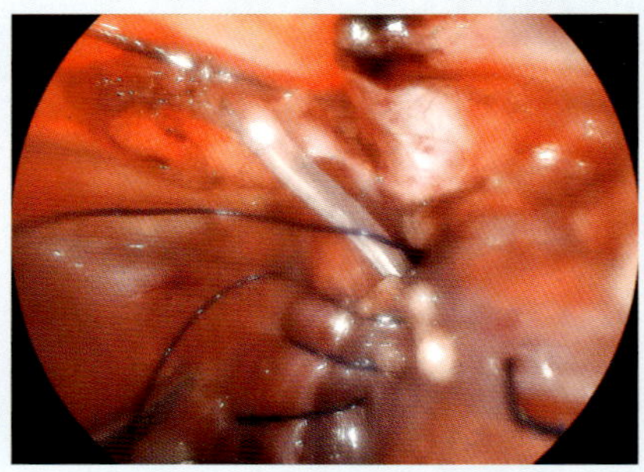

FIGURE 8. Before tying the last knot to close the defect, a silicone foley catheter is placed into the pericardial sac, and the balloon is inflated. This device is helpful at the end of the surgery to remove the trapped gas, and the presence of any effusion is checked.

Tips and tricks

- ✓ Tilt the table in reverse Trendelenburg position to facilitate the displacement of herniated organs.
- ✓ Use a barbed absorbable suture.
- ✓ Place a temporary foley catheter in the pericardial sac to drain gas and fluid.

45.2 LAPAROSCOPIC REPAIR OF PERICARDIAL DIAPHRAGMATIC HERNIA IN A DOG

Hiroo Kanai

CASE DESCRIPTION

A 4-year-old intact female Papillon (body weight 4.2 kg) was brought to the hospital for a laparoscopic ovarian hysterectomy. A defect was found in the diaphragmatic part intraoperatively. At this time, the surgeon removed the ovaries and uterus, then closed the abdomen as usual. On discharge, the patient's owner was informed of this situation. As a result, surgery was later performed to close the defect in the diaphragm. In this case, even if pneumoperitoneum was performed intraperitoneally, no abnormalities were observed in lung ventilation or hemodynamics, so the hernial orifice could be closed under laparoscopic surgery. At the final stage of closure with sutures, CO_2 in the pneumoperitoneum invaded the pericardial cavity, resulting in ventilatory insufficiency. This was improved by removing CO_2 from the pericardial cavity by catheterization. The operation was completed by normal laparoscopic surgery, but in some cases, anesthesia may be difficult to maintain due to CO_2 entering the pericardial or thoracic cavity. In such cases, a gasless laparoscopic surgery may be effective. In addition, suturing may be facilitated with the use of sutures such as V-Loc. Further studies on the surgical procedure are needed in the future.

Key points

- Laparoscopic surgery for pericardial diaphragmatic hernia.
- Slipknot method in hernia closure.
- Respiratory and circulatory dynamics are carefully monitored as CO_2 flows into the pericardial cavity.
- CO_2 is removed from the pericardial cavity with a catheter before completely closing the hernial orifice.

PORT PLACEMENT

A 5 mm trocar was placed 1 cm to the caudal side of the umbilicus for a camera port (T1). Two further ports (T2, T3) were placed in a triangulating pattern around the anticipated location of the diaphragmatic hernia.

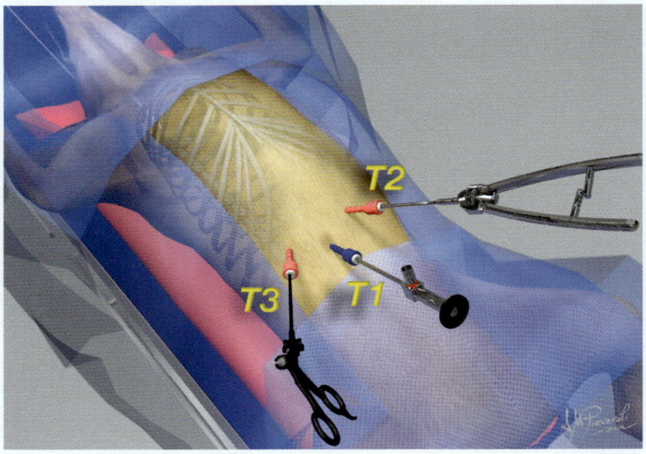

PROCEDURE

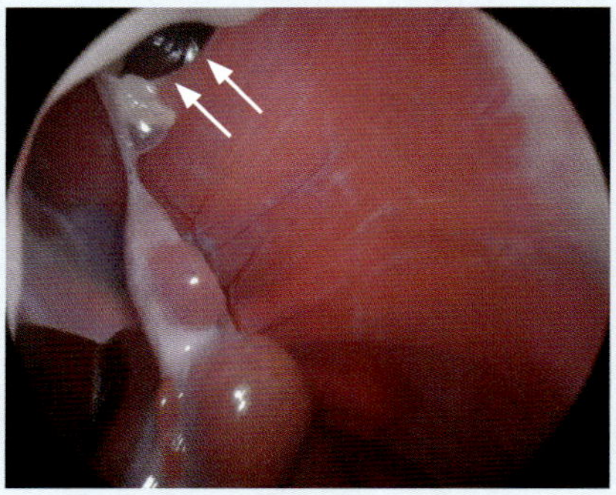

FIGURE 1. Diaphragmatic defect found incidentally during laparoscopic ovarian hysterectomy. The defect is evident in the ventral center of the diaphragm, with the entry of some of the fat in the hepatic falciform ligament (arrows). However, no intrusion of the liver or gastrointestinal tract is seen, and the finding is considered incidental with no clinical signs.

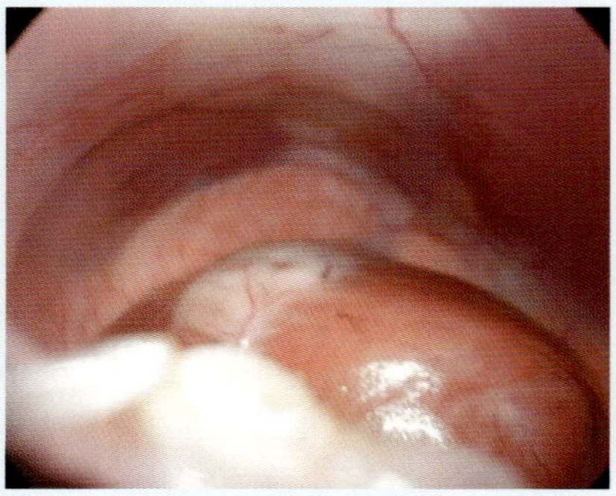

FIGURE 2. Image from a rigid endoscope inserted through the diaphragmatic defect. The inside of the thoracic cavity is observed. The heart is seen inside the pericardium. Laparoscopic surgery is continued because no changes are seen in respiratory or circulatory dynamics even after continuing pneumoperitoneum from the abdominal cavity.

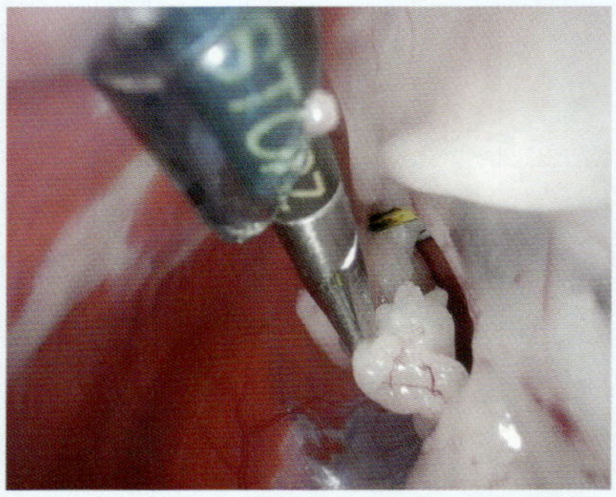

FIGURE 3. Fat removal from the hepatic falciform ligament inserted into the hernial orifice. Since the fat of the hepatic falciform ligament has protruded into the pericardium, excision is achieved using an ultrasonic coagulation and incision device. This allows the hernial orifice to be clearly observed.

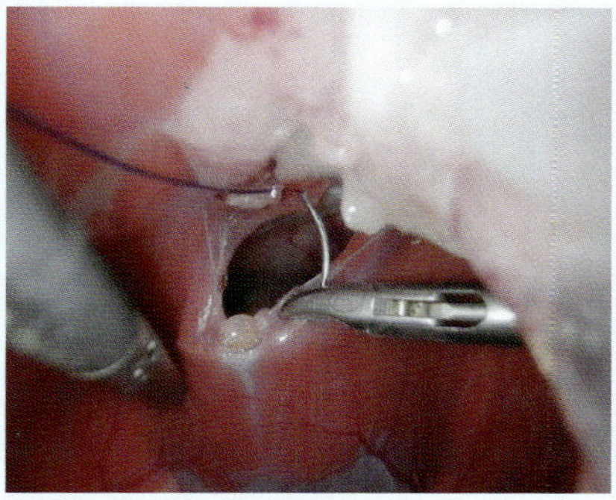

FIGURE 4. Closure of the hernial orifice. The diaphragmatic defect is ligated using simple ligature suture with PDS2 4-0. Suturing is technically difficult because the angle of forceps insertion is higher than in other surgeries. In addition, when suturing from the lower side to the upper side, hand movement tends to become more difficult as the sutures progress.

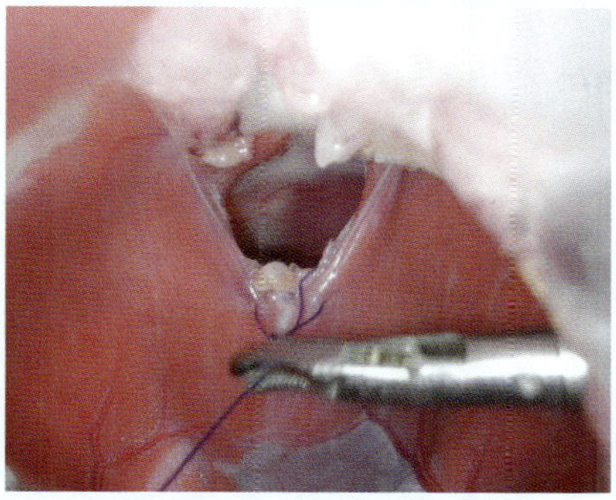

FIGURE 5. Closure of the hernial orifice using the slipknot method. The defect is sutured using the slipknot method so that sutures do not loosen. To firmly ligate the muscular part of the diaphragm, the slipknot method is used to tighten the knot.

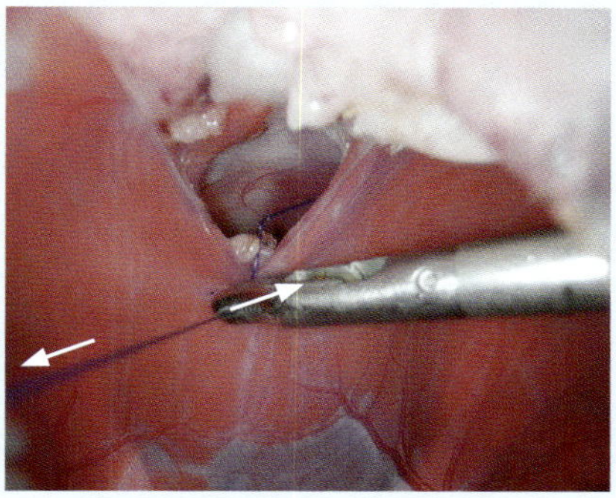

FIGURE 6. Fastening sutures using the slipknot method. The knot is pushed with a needle to complete firm ligation. The arrows indicate the direction of tension from the left and right forceps.

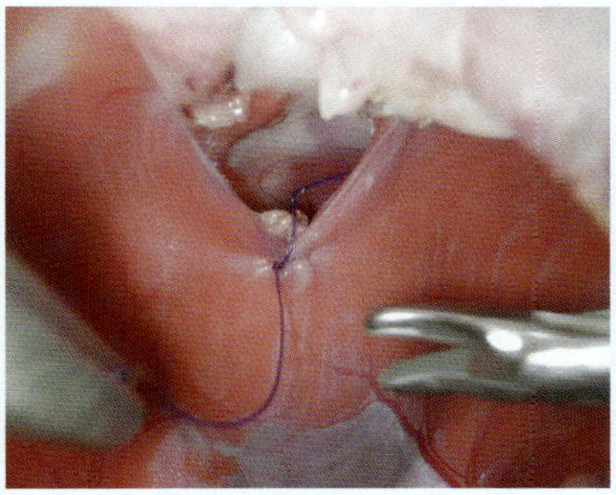

FIGURE 7. Completed slipknot. The ligation is completed without any loss of tension.

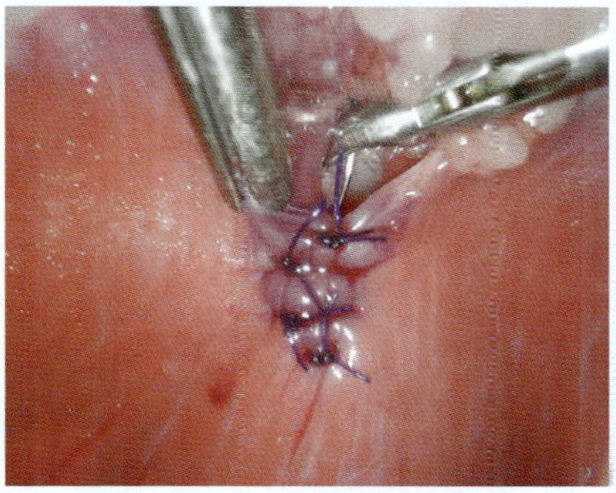

FIGURE 8. Several completed suture ligations. The ligation is completed without any loss of tension. Simple ligation and suture are continued. This procedure becomes more difficult with progression to the ventral side.

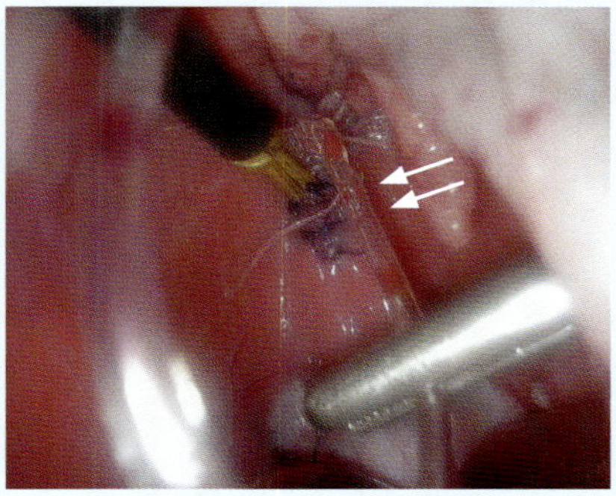

FIGURE 9. Catheter insertion and deaeration of the pericardial cavity. Prior to the final closure of the hernial orifice, a catheter is inserted into the pericardium to remove the CO_2 that entered the pericardium (arrows).

Section III

THORACOSCOPY

LEARNING FROM THE PAST

Without doubt, the predominant value of endoscopy centers around the examination of the pleural cavities, the so-called thoracoscopy.

H. C. Jacobaeus (1910)

46 ANESTHESIA IN THORACOSCOPY

Elisa Bortolami

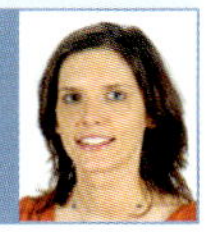

Minimally invasive surgery is becoming more and more popular in veterinary medicine thanks to the advances in both theoretical knowledge and practical skills. Thoracoscopy, in particular, may be useful to perform diagnostic procedures and esophageal, mediastinal, vascular, or cardiothoracic surgery.

Video-assisted thoracoscopic surgery (VATS) is less invasive in comparison to lateral thoracotomy or sternotomy requiring relatively large incisions; indeed, 1–4 incisions a few centimeters long are generally carried out in order to introduce the camera and the surgical instruments. For this reason, in the medical field, thoracoscopic procedures have been associated with less pain and quicker recoveries. This has also been proven for some veterinary procedures, such as pericardiectomy and correction of persistent right aortic arch.

Although there are potential benefits to thoracoscopic procedures, the relative disadvantages have to be considered as well. As clearly described in a review paper, "the anesthetist and surgeon are very much rivals for the same anatomy"; indeed, although lung inflation is necessary for oxygenation, the expansion of the lungs interferes with the surgical maneuvers and visualization. This is the most important challenge that the anesthetist has to deal with during this kind of procedures.

As in human medicine, a multidisciplinary team approach to the veterinary patient is paramount, with the involvement of surgeons, anesthesiologists, and intensive care specialists.

INDICATIONS FOR THORACOSCOPIC PROCEDURES

VATS is described in veterinary medicine for several procedures, including various diagnostic procedures, persistent aortic arch ligation, patent ductus arteriosus ligation, pericardiectomy, lung lobectomy, management of pyothorax, treatment of spontaneous pneumothorax and pulmonary bullae, thoracic duct ligation, and removal of cranial mediastinal masses, just to cite a few.

PATIENT SELECTION

The patient should be carefully assessed, and a discussion with the owner should precede the procedure. The potential risks and complications must be discussed, especially the possibility of conversion to an open thoracic procedure due to intraoperative complications, such as bleeding or poor visualization. There are data in the literature on the outcomes of dogs undergoing thoracic surgery, but to date there are no reviews regarding thoracoscopic procedures. However, there are studies evaluating the outcome of specific procedures, and the results seem promising.

PREOPERATIVE WORK-UP

Before performing a thoracoscopic procedure, it is important to conduct a full clinical examination. The preanesthetic work-up should include complete blood work (hematology, biochemistry, coagulation, blood gas analysis), a urinalysis, and, according to the reason why the procedure should be performed, diagnostic imaging. Due to the risks of bleeding, blood typing should be performed, and blood products should be available in case they are needed. The status of the cardiovascular and the respiratory systems should be assessed because, as selective ventilation or insufflation of carbon dioxide may be necessary, the effects on the cardiorespiratory system may worsen a preexisting clinical situation. Blood gas analysis is useful to assess the efficiency of oxygenation and ventilation. Echocardiography, chest X-rays, or advanced imaging exams may also be recommended. A CT or MRI scan can be useful not only to assess the clinical condition of the patient but also to decide which airway device should be used and its size. In some situations, airway endoscopy and a bronchoalveolar lavage may be necessary. Accurate preoperative evaluation is mandatory to identify patients that are more likely to incur perioperative complications, such as patients with cardiorespiratory problems or other comorbidities.

PATIENT STABILIZATION

Patients might need to be stabilized before performing anesthesia for thoracoscopy. For example, in some cases, fluid therapy may be necessary to reach euvolemia and decrease the impact of anesthetic drugs and thoracoscopic procedures on the cardiorespiratory system. In other cases, a thoracocentesis may be necessary to improve the patient's cardiorespiratory performance during anesthesia.

PATIENT PREPARATION AND POSITIONING

During VATS, the patient is usually placed in lateral recumbency, with the hemithorax to be investigated being the nondependent side. If examination of both hemithoraces is necessary, the animal is placed in sternal or dorsal recumbency. Wide clipping and prepping of the thorax must be performed, should it be necessary to convert the VATS to an open thoracotomy. If selective one-lung ventilation (OLV) is used, a fiberoptic bronchoscope (FOB) should be available to confirm correct placement of the respiratory device utilized.

ANESTHESIA

During anesthesia for thoracoscopic procedures, challenges may arise due to the compression or deflation of the operative lung caused by the creation of the pneumothorax, inflation of the thorax with carbon dioxide, or selective lung ventilation with consequent impairment of oxygenation and hemodynamics. Focus should be set on protective lung ventilation strategies, optimization of cardiac output, analgesia, and fluid management in order to achieve better recoveries and avoid postoperative complications. Good knowledge of respiratory pathophysiology is required, especially when selective lung ventilation is used.

The anesthetic protocol should achieve cardiovascular stability, optimization of respiratory function, and analgesia. This may be particularly challenging when OLV is required. In order to facilitate surgical maneuvers and decrease the likelihood of displacement of the endotracheal device, the use of neuromuscular blocking agents may be useful.

PREMEDICATION

According to the author's experience, premedication may consist of a full mu-opioid agonist, such as methadone (0.1–0.3 mg/kg IV or IM), associated with a low dose of dexmedetomidine (0.5–1.0 µg/kg IV or IM) if the patient is cardiovascularly stable. A low dose of acepromazine (0.005–0.01 mg/kg IV or IM) may be used in euvolemic patients, but hypotension, especially if caused by hemorrhage, may be more challenging to treat. Blood pressure should be monitored closely to promptly detect the occurrence of hypotension.

INDUCTION OF ANESTHESIA

Preoxygenation for about 5 minutes is recommended, especially in patients suffering from cardiorespiratory disease, as this will increase the oxygen reserve in the lungs.

Anesthesia can be induced with either propofol or alfaxalone titrated to effect. If only an opioid is used as premedication, coinduction with midazolam (0.1–0.2 mg/kg IV) can be helpful in decreasing the amount of induction agent required.

MAINTENANCE OF ANESTHESIA

Anesthesia can be maintained with inhalants, such as isoflurane or sevoflurane, or intravenous agents, such as propofol or alfaxalone. Whether to maintain anesthesia with inhalation or intravenous agents is still controversial in people undergoing OLV and depends on the anesthetist's preference. On the one hand, the use of injectable agents seems to maintain the pulmonary vasoconstriction reflex and may reduce intraoperative shunt and hypoxemia; on the other hand, when modern inhalation agents are used at values equal or lower than 1 minimal alveolar concentration (MAC), alveolar inflammation, and thus postoperative acute lung injury, seems to be lower. Nevertheless, the effects of inhalants or intravenous agents on postoperative outcomes are still being studied. In veterinary medicine, maintaining anesthesia with either isoflurane or propofol does not seem to result in a different outcome of pulmonary hemodynamics and oxygenation during canine OLV.

Propofol (0.1–0.3 mg/kg/h) or alfaxalone (0.1 mg/kg/min) can be started via intravenous infusion, with the infusion rate titrated to effect according to vital parameters. If inhalation agents such as isoflurane or sevoflurane are used, they should be administered at 1 MAC or less so that hypoxic pulmonary vasoconstriction is not completely abolished. Consequently, a balanced anesthetic protocol should be used.

NEUROMUSCULAR BLOCKING AGENTS

The use of neuromuscular blocking agents may be beneficial in facilitating controlled ventilation and decreasing the likelihood of displacement of selective ventilation devices. Atracurium (0.25–0.5 mg/kg, or 0.25 mg/kg bolus followed by 0.4–0.5 mg/kg/h IV infusion) or rocuronium (0.5–0.6 mg/kg followed by 0.2 mg/kg/h IV infusion), to cite a few, can be administered. Whenever neuromuscular blocking agents are used, the degree of muscle relaxation should be monitored. For this, most commonly a nerve stimulator is used on the ulnar or peroneal nerve, and the response to electrical stimulation is noted. The train of four (TOF) is a pattern of stimulation that can be used for neuromuscular monitoring. If necessary, neuromuscular blocking agents can be antagonized at the end of the procedure by the use of anticholinesterases together with antimuscarinic agents (neostigmine 0.01–0.05 mg/kg + glycopyrronium 0.01–0.02 mg/kg or edrophonium 0.1–0.5 mg/kg + atropine 0.04 mg/kg) or sugammadex (8 mg/kg), a modified cyclodextrin, in order to avoid muscle weakness and respiratory impairment in the recovery phase. It is imperative to ensure that the neuromuscular function is completely restored before discontinuing the anesthetics. When using TOF stimulation, the T1:T4 ratio should be equal to 1 to ensure the patient has adequate ventilatory and laryngeal function.

ANALGESIA

According to the medical literature, persistent pain is very common after thoracic surgery, and a multimodal analgesia approach, including regional anesthesia, is recommended. Although the expected level of pain may be lower for thoracoscopic procedures than for thoracotomies or sternotomies, the same principles can be translated to the former, aiming at a multimodal approach, especially when VATS associated with minithoracotomy is performed. Different analgesic techniques can be used and are described below.

INFUSION OF SYSTEMIC DRUGS

- Fentanyl infusion (1–10 μg/kg/min) can be used in cats and dogs.
- Ketamine infusion (0.5mg/kg bolus and 0.6–1.2 mg/kg/h infusion) can also be used to decrease the amount of maintenance agent, increase cardiovascular stability, and provide antihyperalgesic effects.
- Lidocaine infusion (1 mg/kg bolus and 10–50 μg/kg/min infusion) provides maintenance agent sparing effects and analgesia. Since lidocaine decreases the cardiac index and thus the blood pressure, its use is not recommended in cats.

Therefore, although the evidence in veterinary medicine is unclear, the use of ketamine and lidocaine may be useful not only to decrease the amount of the anesthesia maintenance agent but also to prevent hyperalgesia and central sensitization and possibly the occurrence of chronic postoperative pain.

LOCOREGIONAL TECHNIQUES

Perioperative regional anesthesia is one of the most important aspects of multimodal analgesia, as local anesthetics block the activation and sensitization of both the peripheral and central nervous systems and may be effective in preventing chronic postoperative pain. Moreover, the use of regional anesthesia is correlated with better respiratory function after thoracotomy in dogs, and this conclusion can be transposed to VATS.

Several locoregional techniques can be used. Some of them are performed blindly, others under nerve stimulator or guided by ultrasound. Nerve location techniques are important to reduce potential complications, including intravascular injection, hematoma formation, and nerve damage. Ultrasound-guided techniques have the advantages of less amount of drug needed and potentially fewer side effects due to the anatomically targeted spread of the local anesthetic around the peripheral nerve. The technique chosen depends on practical skills and availability of instrumentation. The most common locoregional techniques are as follows:

- Thoracic epidural anesthesia (TEA). It provides excellent somatic and visceral analgesia of the thorax, but side effects including urinary retention (when an opioid such as morphine is used), hypotension, and pulmonary complications have been reported in people. It requires advanced technical skills. A technically easier technique is lumbosacral epidural analgesia, which has been proven effective in early studies evaluating analgesia options in dogs undergoing lateral thoracotomy.
- Thoracic paravertebral block (TPVB). In people, TPVB provides similar analgesia to TEA but has fewer side effects. TPVB was used to provide analgesia during thoracotomy in dogs and seems very promising for VATS as well. This

technique is relatively easy to perform, either with the aid of a neurostimulator or guided by ultrasound, and provides somatic and visceral analgesia of the thorax. Possible complications include epidural spread and pneumothorax.

- Intercostal nerve block (ICNB). It is easy to perform, either blindly or with a neurostimulator or ultrasound machine. This technique provides analgesia only to the ventrolateral aspect of the thoracic wall; therefore, visceral analgesia is not guaranteed. Nevertheless, in dogs undergoing lateral thoracotomy, ICNB provided comparable analgesia to epidural and systemic opioid administration. Complications may include pneumothorax, intravascular administration, nerve injury, and local anesthetic toxicity.
- Transversus thoracis plane block. It is an ultrasound-guided technique recently described in canine cadavers. This technique is used to provide effective analgesia in people undergoing median sternotomy, and it may find a role in some VATS procedures too, depending on where the surgical access is performed.
- Serratus plane block. It has been used as an adjunct to systemic analgesia in dogs undergoing thoracotomy. As the lateral cutaneous branches of the intercostal nerves between the serratus muscle are blocked, it may also be useful for VATS.
- Intrapleural administration of local anesthetics. It is an easy way to provide postoperative analgesia, especially when a chest drain is used. Care should be taken not to reach toxic doses, especially when repeated administration is necessary.

The local anesthetic agents most commonly used are lidocaine, bupivacaine, and ropivacaine. Doses and volumes depend on the specific drug and anesthetic techniques. It must be remembered that the toxic doses of lidocaine, bupivacaine, and ropivacaine are in the order of 4–6 mg/kg, 1–4 mg/kg, and 5 mg/kg, respectively, with cats being more sensitive than dogs. In order not to exceed the maximum recommended doses, especially if large drug volumes are needed, the concentration may be decreased without affecting sensory blockade.

POSTOPERATIVE ANALGESIA

Postoperatively, pain should be regularly assessed using validated pain scales and analgesia tailored to the patient's requirements. At the end of the procedure, the administration of a nonsteroidal anti-inflammatory drug is advisable, whenever the clinical conditions allow it. The use of opioids may also be necessary postoperatively.

VISUALIZATION OF THE SURGICAL FIELD AND LUNG SEPARATION

To facilitate the surgical procedure, several techniques may be used, including:

- Endotracheal intubation with a single-lumen tube (SLT) and collapse of the operative lung caused by the introduction of the thoracoscopic instruments. When pleural pressure is not negative anymore, the lung's intrinsic elasticity favors its retraction toward the hilum (**Fig. 1**).
- Endotracheal intubation with an SLT and collapse of the lung caused by the insufflation of the thorax with carbon dioxide. It is important to perform a low-pressure carbon dioxide insufflation (intrathoracic pressure of 2–3 mmHg). If the insufflation pressure is excessive, a tension capnothorax may occur and cause a dramatic decrease in cardiac output. This technique is not commonly performed due to its deep impact on hemodynamics. It has mainly been described in cats, in which it is more difficult to achieve selective ventilation due to the lack of respiratory devices suitable for small-sized animals.

If lung separation can be achieved, different methods have been described:

- Selective endobronchial intubation using an SLT.
- Bronchial blockers (BBs).
- Double-lumen tubes (DLTs).

All these methods have been described in veterinary medicine and each has advantages and disadvantages. When DLTs or BBs are used, the establishment of OLV has to be

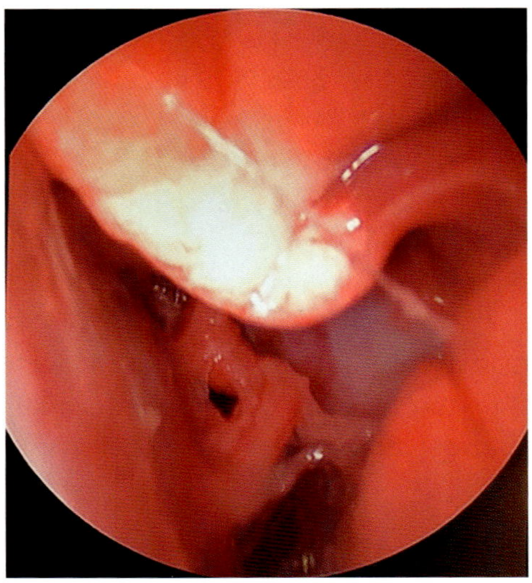

FIGURE 1. Lung deflation caused by VATS-induced pneumothorax.

bronchoscopically assisted. The correct position of the respiratory device must be confirmed endoscopically any time there is a change in the patient's recumbency.

SELECTIVE ENDOBRONCHIAL INTUBATION

Selective bronchial intubation using an SLT, which is advanced into one of the main bronchi, is a less refined way to perform selective lung intubation and can be useful in situations when other respiratory devices are too big for the animal's anatomy.

BRONCHIAL BLOCKERS (FIGS. 2–4)

BBs are introduced inside a standard endotracheal tube, and the cuff should be positioned inside the main bronchus or a smaller bronchus if lobar isolation is required. The correct position of the BB must be confirmed with an endoscope. When BBs are used, it takes more time for the lung to collapse due to their narrower diameter. Placement of a BB is performed as follows:

- Before starting the procedure, make sure that the chosen BB is the correct size for the patient and that the cuff inflates properly and symmetrically. Make also sure that the FOB fits into the endotracheal tube.
- Perform endotracheal intubation using an SLT and inflate the cuff.
- Connect the patient to the breathing system.
- Place the patient in the correct position for the procedure.
- Insert the FOB into the endotracheal tube.
- Insert the BB inside the endotracheal tube and, with the assistance of the FOB, place it in the desired position.
- Inflate the cuff and check its position using the FOB.
- Make sure that the cuff of the BB is inflated and start OLV just before commencing the procedure in order to decrease the duration of OLV.

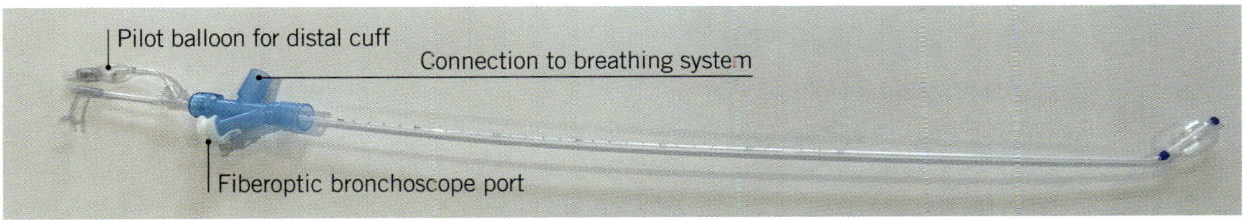

FIGURE 2. Example of an angled bronchial blocker with its connector.

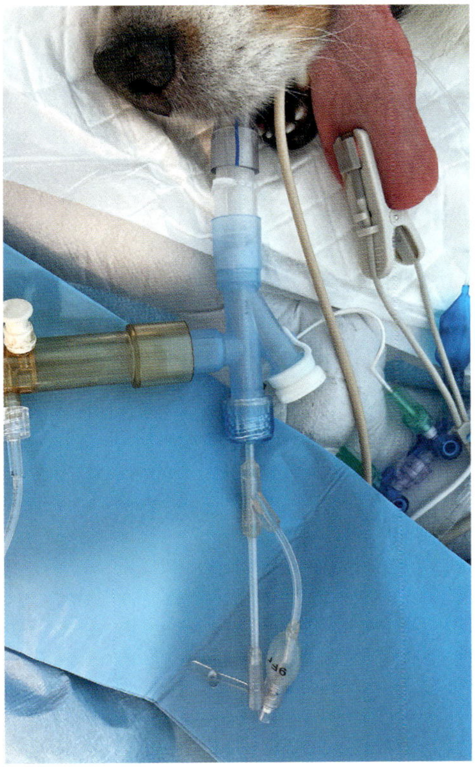

FIGURE 3. Intra-operative setup of a bronchial blocker. The bronchial blocker was inserted into the endotracheal tube and positioned with the aid of a fiberoptic bronchoscope. The bronchoscope port cap is on to provide a seal.

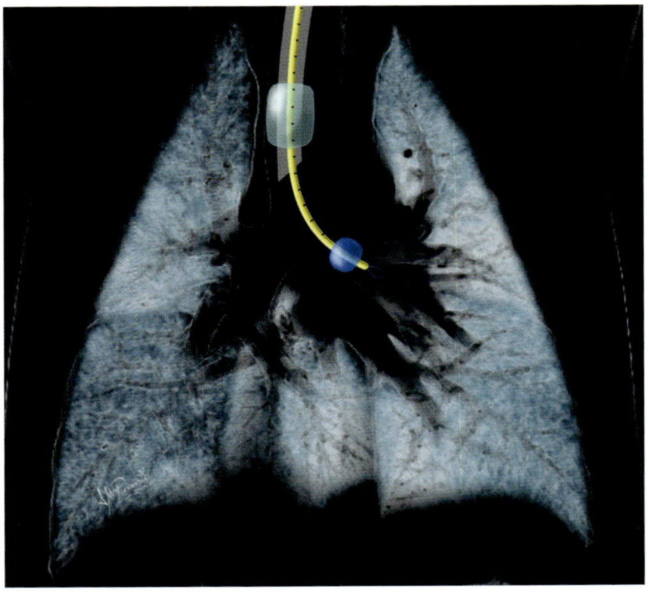

FIGURE 4. Three-dimensional volume-rendered CT image of a canine trachea and bronchi with graphic superimposition of a bronchial blocker inserted inside an endotracheal tube. Ventilation to the side where the bronchial blocker is placed is occluded. CT image courtesy of Dr. Giovanna Bertolin, Diagnostic and Interventional Radiology Division, San Marco Veterinary Clinic and Laboratory, Veggiano, Italy.

DOUBLE-LUMEN TUBES (FIGS. 5–8)

DLTs are composed of two endotracheal tubes of unequal length connected longitudinally, both provided with cuffs. The end of the shorter tube is placed in the trachea, while the end of the longer tube is placed in one of the mainstem bronchi. This conformation allows selective lung ventilation. DLTs have the advantage of permitting alternate ventilation of the two lungs without the need to reposition the tube. These devices are designed for human medicine, and it must be remembered that the canine trachea is proportionally longer and the mainstem bronchi shorter in comparison to those of humans. This is why a preanesthetic evaluation of the patient's upper respiratory tract anatomy is advisable, ideally via a chest X-ray or a CT or MRI scan. Moreover, different designs of left- and right-sided DLTs are available for use in human patients to best fit the different anatomy of the right and left airways and consequently to optimize tube positioning. In veterinary medicine, left-sided DLTs are usually utilized for selective ventilation of either the right or left lung. There are different types and sizes of commercially available DLTs. If the tube is too small, there is a risk of cuff hyperinflation, with consequent trauma and ischemia to the airways, and distal migration. If the tube is too large, positioning may cause airway trauma. Similar to an endotracheal tube, a properly fitted DLT should be able to be smoothly inserted into the airways without encountering excessive resistance.

Placemen of a DLT is as follows:

- Before placement of the DLT, check its integrity and that the cuffs inflate properly and symmetrically.
- Insert the stylet in the bronchial side and make sure it does not protrude beyond the end of the tube.
- Make sure that a FOB which will fit inside the DLT and the DLT connector is available.
- Make sure the size of the DLT is appropriate. Usually, left-sided DLTs are used in veterinary medicine due to the shape of the bronchial cuff. The endobronchial part of the DLT can be placed in the left or right bronchus depending on the procedure to be performed.
- Place the patient in the correct position for the procedure.
- Perform bronchoscopic intubation: pass the FOB into the bronchial lumen and guide the DLT over the FOB, introducing the bronchial port in the right or left bronchus.
- Move the FOB from the bronchial tube lumen to the tracheal tube lumen and check the correct position of the bronchial tube. Make sure that the DLT is not too far in (bronchial cuff occluding the lobar bronchi) or too proximal (bronchial cuff occluding the trachea).
- Inflate the bronchial cuff and check with the FOB.
- Connect the Y connector to the DLT and the breathing system. The Y connector will allow either one-lung or two-lung ventilation.
- Inflate the tracheal cuff and make sure that bilateral ventilation occurs by visualizing bilateral chest movements and auscultating bilateral air flow into the lungs.
- Make sure that the bronchial cuff is in the correct position: deflate the tracheal cuff, inflate the bronchial cuff gradually, clamp the connector for tracheal ventilation, and check for unilateral ventilation.
- Occlude either the tracheal or the bronchial port depending on which lung has to be ventilated. For example, with the dog in left lateral recumbency, if a left-sided DLT was placed with the bronchial port on the left mainstem bronchus, the tracheal port has to be clamped to ventilate the dependent nonsurgical left lung.
- The lung that is not ventilated passively deflates or is displaced by the surgeon.
- Continuous positive airway pressure (CPAP) can be applied to the surgical lung to decrease the shunt fraction, but this may impair visualization of the surgical field.
- Any time the recumbency or position of the patient is changed, the correct position of the DLT should be endoscopically checked.

Key points

- Thoracoscopic procedures can be performed using OLV, which can be achieved via different methods.
- In human medicine, BBs and DLTs are used, depending on the anesthetist's preference.
- Whenever OLV is established, its duration should be minimized. In people, it has been shown that the longer the OLV, the higher the risk of postoperative pulmonary complications.

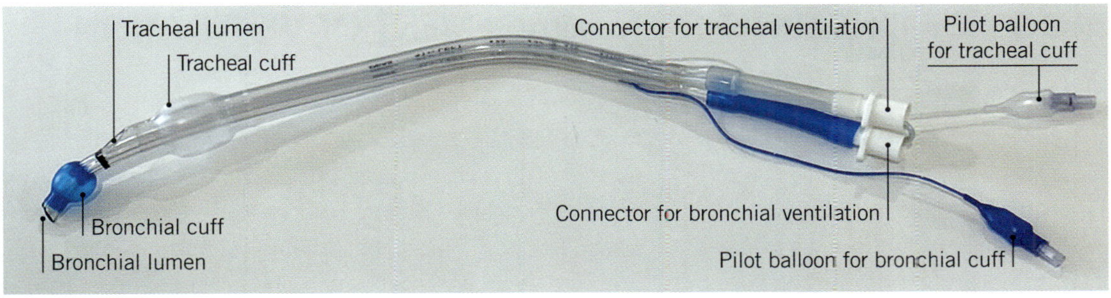

FIGURE 5. Left-sided double-lumen tube with color-coded tracheal and bronchial cuffs.

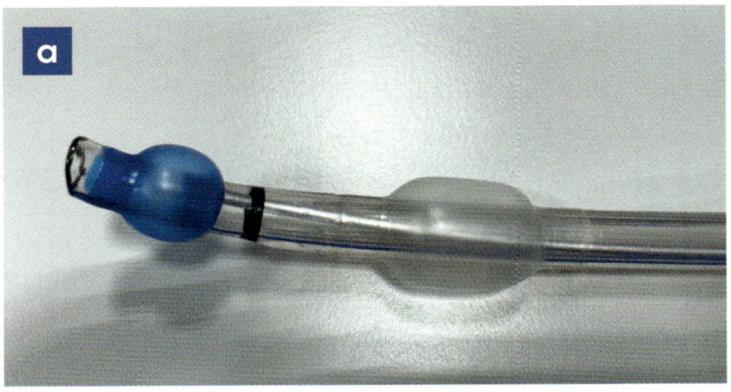

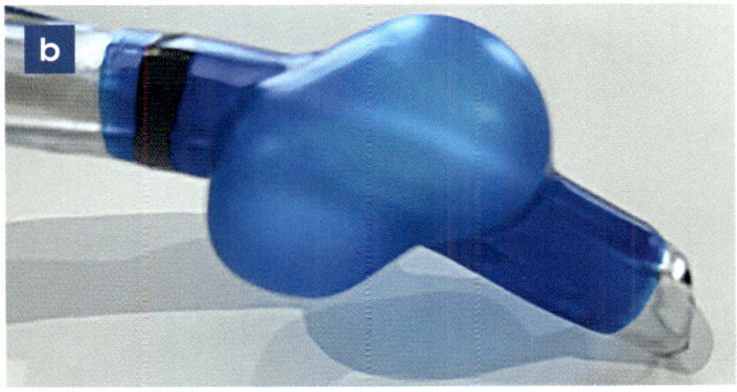

FIGURE 6. a) Left-sided and b) right-sided double-lumen tube cuffs. Note the different shape of the cuffs to better fit the different human tracheal and bronchial anatomy. In veterinary medicine, left-sided double-lumen tubes are typically used.

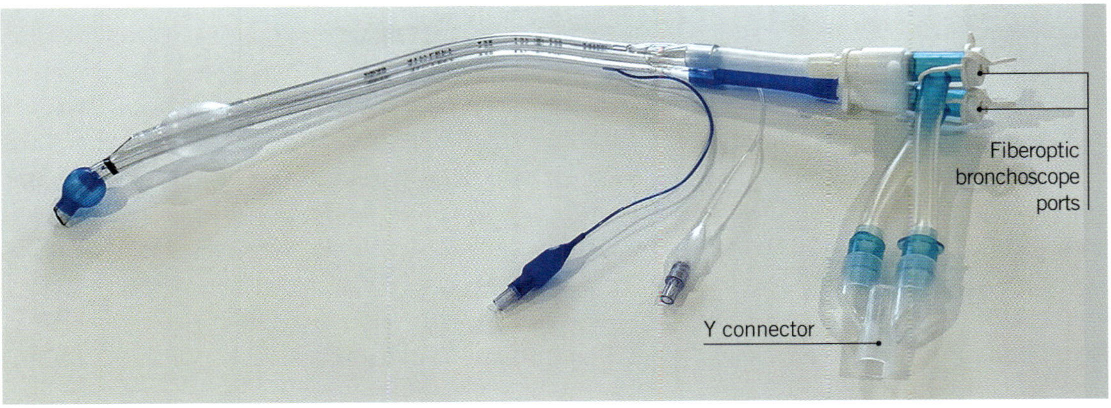

FIGURE 7. Double-lumen tube with ports for the fiberoptic bronchoscope and Y connector to allow two-lung ventilation.

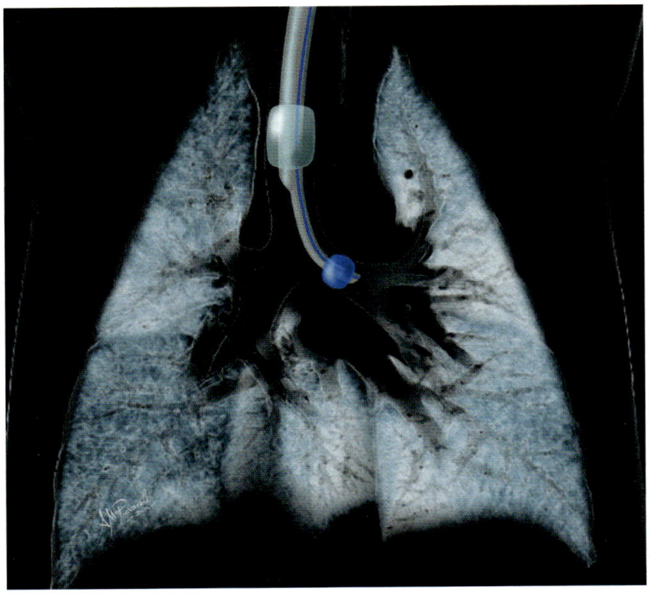

FIGURE 8. Three-dimensional volume-rendered CT image of a canine trachea and bronchi with graphic superimposition of a left-sided double-lumen tube. Selective ventilation can be provided with either the tracheal or bronchial lumen. CT image courtesy of Dr. Giovanna Bertolini, Diagnostic and Interventional Radiology Division, San Marco Veterinary Clinic and Laboratory, Veggiano, Italy.

PATHOPHYSIOLOGY OF ONE-LUNG VENTILATION

The lung is not a homogeneous organ, as different regions have different degrees of ventilation and perfusion. The ratio of ventilation to perfusion (V/Q) is used to measure collective changes in lung ventilation and perfusion. Normally, these parameters are anatomically matched, as perfusion and ventilation are greater in the dependent regions of the lung than in the nondependent regions due to the gravity force and gravitational effects of lung compliance, respectively.

Whenever OLV is instituted, due to the collapse of the operative lung, an area which is perfused but not ventilated is created, that is, a right-to-left "shunt" area. The degree of the shunt is greater when the right lung is not ventilated because of its larger size compared to the left lung. This change in the V/Q ratio can impair gas exchange and cause or worsen hypoxemia, especially if the lung is diseased. Hypoxemia is one of the most common complications encountered during OLV anesthesia.

A physiological mechanism to decrease V/Q mismatch is provided by hypoxic pulmonary vasoconstriction. Different species have different degrees of hypoxic pulmonary vasoconstriction (e.g., it is well developed in humans and horses). Thanks to the contraction of pulmonary vascular smooth muscles in areas of low oxygen partial pressure, the blood is diverted from nonventilated to ventilated areas of the lung to reestablish V/Q matching and improve oxygenation. Several factors influence hypoxic pulmonary vasoconstriction, including temperature, pH, carbon dioxide partial pressure, age, and anesthetic drugs. In veterinary experimental and clinical studies, maintenance of anesthesia with either inhalants or intravenous agents was correlated with good clinical parameters. In healthy dogs with an open thoracic cavity, OLV caused a decrease in the partial pressure of oxygen, arterial oxygen saturation, and alveolar–arterial oxygen difference and an increase in the physiological dead space and arterial partial pressure of carbon dioxide, with hemodynamics not being clinically affected. Similarly, OLV increased the shunt fraction, with a consequent decrease in arterial oxygen saturation and arterial oxygen content in anesthetized dogs with a closed thoracic cavity. During OLV, in healthy anesthetized dogs, the use of positive end-expiratory pressure (PEEP) has been proven beneficial for oxygenation without significantly affecting cardiac output. Although these promising results in healthy experimental animals may not be as good in patients with cardiorespiratory compromise, there are a several clinical studies and case reports showing good outcomes.

MANAGEMENT OF VENTILATION

The most challenging aspect of anesthesia is the management of ventilation, especially if OLV is performed (it should be noted that some procedures can be carried out without OLV). Whether or not OLV is performed, controlled mechanical ventilation should be instituted. Volume-controlled ventilation or pressure-controlled ventilation can be used, and each has advantages and disadvantages, but there is no zero-risk ventilatory mode. Avoiding lung damage in the form of volutrauma, atelectotrauma, barotrauma, or biotrauma is crucial, especially if the lung is diseased. In this case, it is even more important to use lung-protective ventilation with low tidal volumes, higher respiratory rate, moderate PEEP, low peak and plateau pressures, and inspired oxygen fraction (FiO_2) as low as possible in order to maintain oxygen saturation (SpO_2) greater than 90%. The principles of protective lung ventilation should also be applied when OLV is performed. Although the ranges for protective ventilatory settings are well recognized in human medicine, they are still to be validated in veterinary medicine. Nevertheless, considering that it has been shown that a tidal volume of 15 mL/mg with a PEEP of 5 cmH_2O provides good oxygenation and lung compliance in mechanically ventilated healthy dogs, when switching from two-lung to one-lung ventilation the tidal volume in cats and dogs should be decreased to 6–10 mL/kg. According to the author, when choosing the ventilatory settings, a respiratory rate of 10–18 breaths per minute and a PEEP of 2–5 cmH_2O seem to be reasonable values, with a FiO_2 of 0.5% that can be increased to maintain a SpO_2 greater than 90% (**Table 1**). These values have also been described in veterinary case reports and studies, but, obviously, they should only be considered as a guide and have to be tailored according to the patients' status and disease, the surgical procedure, and which lung is ventilated, considering that the right lung is larger than the left one.

As mentioned before, damage to the lung should be avoided. When ventilating the patient, plateau pressure, which indicates the pressure at the level of the alveoli and is more relevant than peak inspiratory pressure, should be carefully monitored.

When using lung-protective strategies, the use of PEEP is useful in preventing alveolar derecruitment and consequently desaturation. When utilizing PEEP, careful assessment of hemodynamics is necessary, and target use of fluids and vasoactive drugs may be necessary to optimize cardiovascular function. The use of high respiratory rates is necessary to compensate for low tidal volumes. This may cause air trapping; therefore, higher carbon dioxide partial pressures are usually tolerated (permissive hypercapnia, maximum 60 mmHg). Accurate monitoring should be performed in patients with cardiopulmonary disease, as they may not tolerate excessive hypercapnia.

A high FiO_2 has been associated with absorption atelectasis, even in healthy lungs, and with the production of reactive oxygen species and pro-inflammatory cytokines. Ischemia-reperfusion injuries induced by these mediators may happen during lung re-expansion after OLV. These cellular mechanisms are reflected clinically as acute lung injury. This is another reason why OLV time should be minimized as much as possible.

Moreover, in order to prevent atelectasis in the nonoperative lung, periodic alveolar recruitment maneuvers may be necessary, the duration and pressures of which are still debated. There is a negative correlation between acute lung injury in the operative lung and slow, gradual re-expansion of the lung with low FiO_2. Ideally, unilateral re-expansion should be performed, if possible.

TABLE 1. Ventilatory parameters during one-lung ventilation*

Mode of ventilation	Volume-controlled ventilation Pressure-controlled ventilation
Tidal volume	6–10 mL/kg
Respiratory rate	10–18 breaths per minute
PEEP	0–5 cmH_2O
FiO_2	50% or as low as possible to maintain SpO_2 >90%
End-tidal carbon dioxide tension	35–60 mmHg
Inspiratory:expiratory ratio	1:2–1:3

*Values depend on the patients, their clinical status, and the procedures to be performed.

COMPLICATIONS DURING ONE-LUNG VENTILATION

Common complications during OLV include:

- hypoxemia
- overdistention of the lung
- barotrauma
- iatrogenic airway rupture

Whenever hypoxemia occurs during OLV, the following actions should be taken:

- Check the correct positioning of the respiratory device with the FOB. DLTs and BBs can displaced and impair the ventilation to other parts of the lung which were intended to be ventilated.
- Aspirate tracheobronchial secretions, if present.
- Rule out pneumothorax in the ventilated lung.
- Gradually increase FiO_2.
- Apply or increase PEEP to the ventilated lung, making sure this does not impair hemodynamics.
- Insufflate oxygen or apply CPAP to the nonventilated lung (although this may impair visualization of the surgical field). CPAP can be provided using commercial devices or using a nonrebreathing breathing system.
- Perform recruitment maneuvers. In veterinary medicine, a few strategies have been described, including the provision of three manual breaths of 30 cmH_2O for 10 seconds, or provision of an airway pressure of 30 cmH_2O for 30 seconds.
- Use intermittent two-lung ventilation.
- Improve oxygen delivery through optimization of hemoglobin and cardiac output.

MONITORING

Advanced constant monitoring is suggested during thoracoscopy, including:

- pulse oximetry
- capnography
- arterial blood pressure (preferably invasive) to monitor hemodynamics
- electrocardiography to monitor heart rhythm
- Temperature
- spirometry to assess respiratory system mechanics
- blood gases analysis to assess oxygenation and ventilation.

POSTOPERATIVE COMPLICATIONS

Postoperative complications may include:

- pneumothorax
- bleeding
- residual neuromuscular blockade
- hypoxemia due to incomplete re-expansion of the lungs
- postoperative pulmonary complications.

Noncardiogenic pulmonary edema is caused by dynamic hyperinflation, prolonged surgical handling, or patient's predisposition. Intraoperative ventilator settings play a major role; however, evidence for optimal ventilator settings is still lacking. Together with low tidal volumes, optimization of PEEP and compliance (tidal volume/driving pressure) are important factors to consider during OLV.

POSTOPERATIVE MANAGEMENT

At the end of the thoracoscopic procedure, the following should be performed:

- Chest X-rays to exclude pneumothorax.
- Blood gases analysis to assess ventilation and oxygenation.
- Admission to the ICU department for postoperative monitoring, oxygen therapy if necessary, analgesia, and fluid therapy.

Disclaimer. Not all drugs mentioned in this chapter are licensed for use in veterinary patients, and marketing authorizations vary between different countries.

Key points

- Nowadays, many thoracoscopic procedures are performed in veterinary patients.
- The anesthetist should implement anesthetic management (anesthetic and analgesic protocol, ventilation, hemodynamics, and fluid therapy) based on the expected challenges.
- The anesthetist should be ready to respond promptly to possible complications.

SUGGESTED READINGS

47 PATIENT POSITIONING, ACCESS, AND PORT PLACEMENT IN THORACOSCOPY

Roberto Properzi

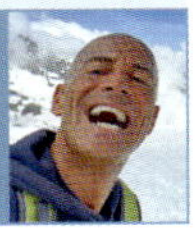

Human thoracoscopy was invented in 1910 by the Swedish urologist Jacobeus, using a cystoscope.

PATIENT POSITIONING

Correct patient positioning is pivotal for the success of thoracoscopic surgery. The patient can be positioned in lateral, dorsal, or sternal recumbency. As a general rule, lateral recumbency is preferred in those procedures that are performed using the same lateral approach in thoracotomy, while the patient is placed in dorsal recumbency in those procedures in which a median sternotomy approach is used in open surgery (**Fig. 1**). Sternal recumbency, sometimes with a slightly oblique tilt, has only been described in a few procedures, such as thoracic duct ligation. After positioning, it is very important to secure the patient properly to the operating table to prevent them from falling during table tilting.

THORACOSCOPIC ACCESS AND PORT PLACEMENT

As for laparoscopic procedures, several techniques can be used for thoracoscopic access. The choice of technique is based on the surgeon's experience and equipment available. During the access procedure, care must be taken to avoid lesions to thoracic structures and organs; for this, a blunt-tipped trocar or a trocarless cannula can be used (**Fig. 2**).

Whatever access, intercostal or subxiphoid, is chosen for placement of the first port, the author prefers to use an open technique similar to the Hasson technique used for laparoscopy. Before the skin incision is created, the end of the cannula is used to make an impression on the skin in order to establish the correct length of the incision (**Fig. 3**). A number 15 scalpel blade is typically used to cut the skin and subcutaneous tissue (**Fig. 4**). Then, the deeper layers are bluntly dissected with a curved Crile mosquito forceps (**Fig. 5**).

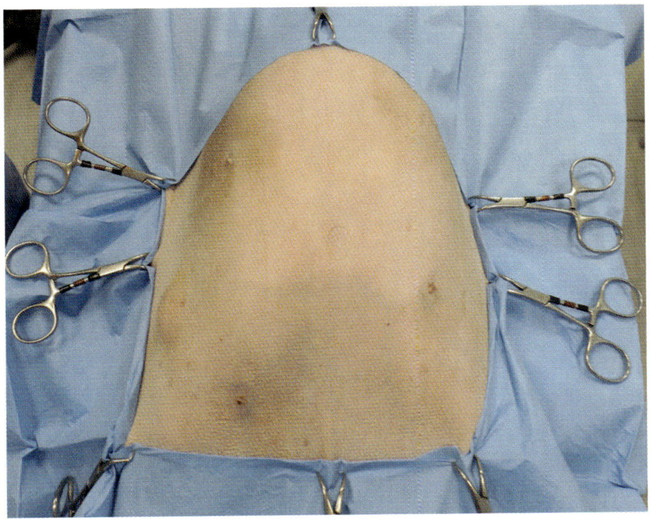

FIGURE 1. Patient positioned in dorsal recumbency.

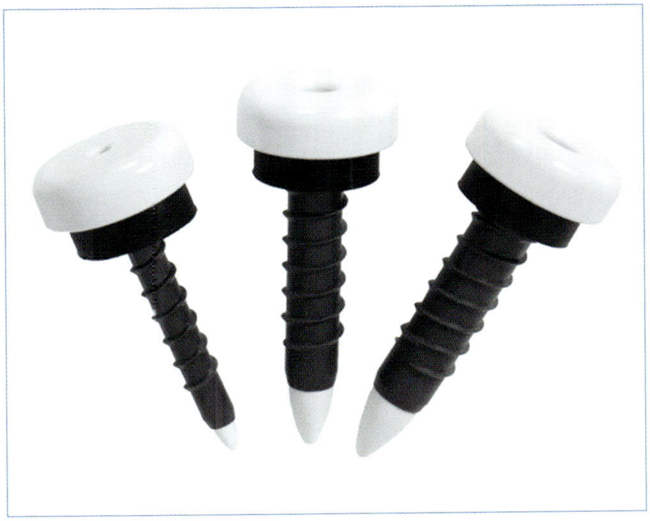

FIGURE 2. Different sizes of plastic thoracoscopic cannulas and trocars.

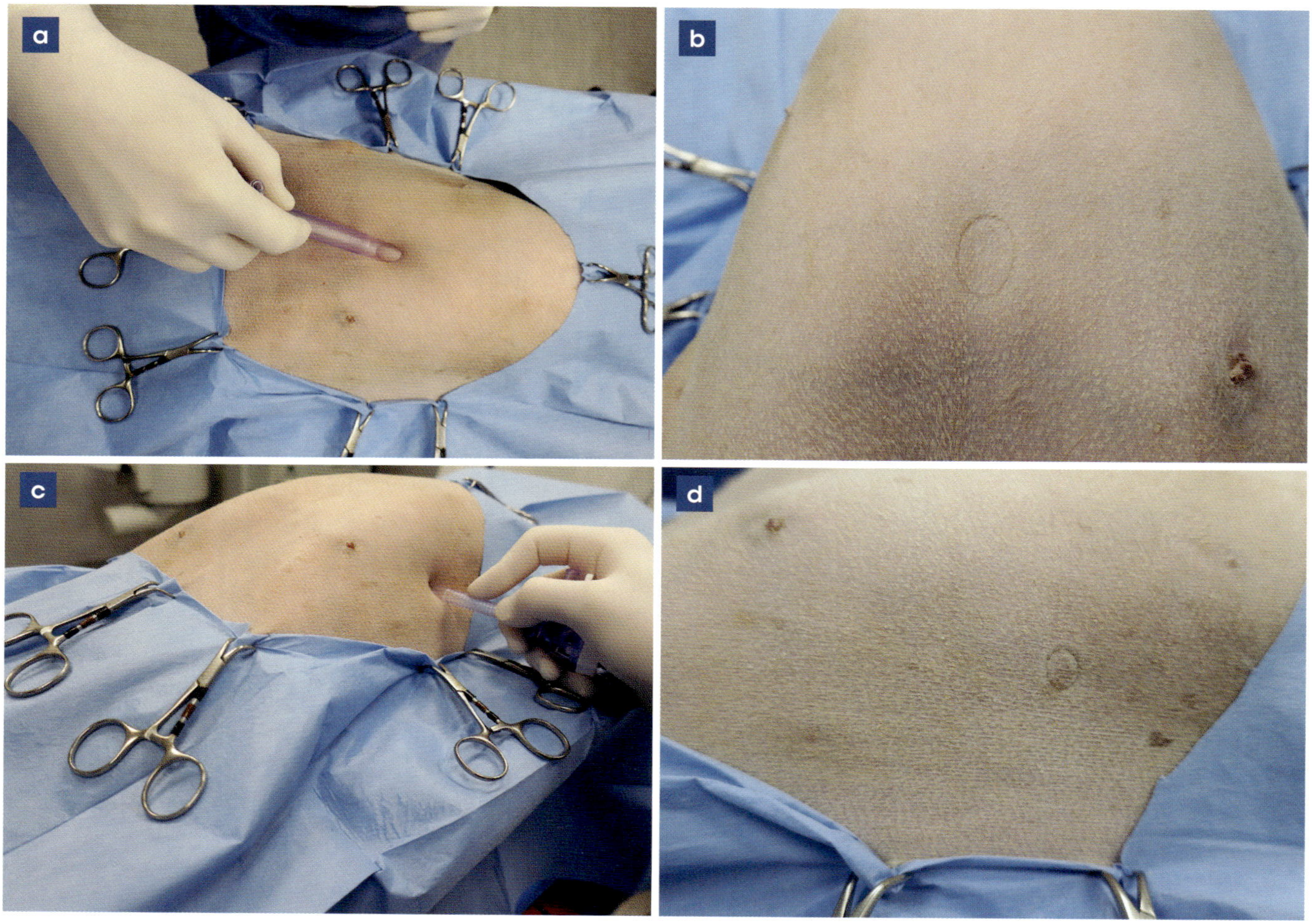

FIGURE 3. An impression is made on the skin using the cannula to determine the length of the incision. a,b) Subxiphoid access. c,d) Intercostal access.

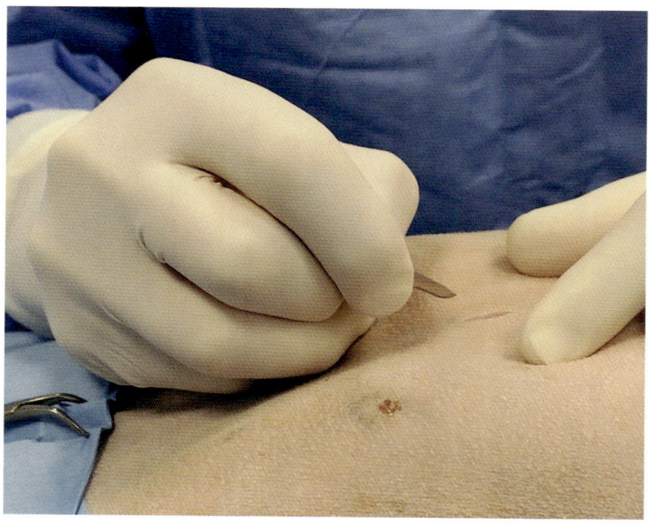
FIGURE 4. Incision of the skin and subcutaneous tissue using a number 15 scalpel blade.

In the subxiphoid port placement, after blunt dissection of the deeper layers, the author uses a cannula with a blunt-tipped trocar (or a trocarless cannula, such as Endotip) inclined at an angle of 45° with respect to the sagittal plane and oriented slightly laterally towards the left or right side depending on the hemithorax of interest (**Fig. 6**). A fair amount of strength is needed to perforate the diaphragmatic muscle with the cannula. Cannulas 6.5 cm in length are the most frequently used; however, in large-sized dogs with a deep chest, a longer cannula should be selected to ensure adequate penetration through the diaphragm.

Pitfalls of this access include absence of diaphragmatic muscle perforation and penetration of the mediastinal attachment to the sternum. In the former, the cannula is inserted into the abdomen between the diaphragm and the liver lobes; in the latter, the cannula drags the mediastinal tissue. In both cases, the thorax cannot be explored.

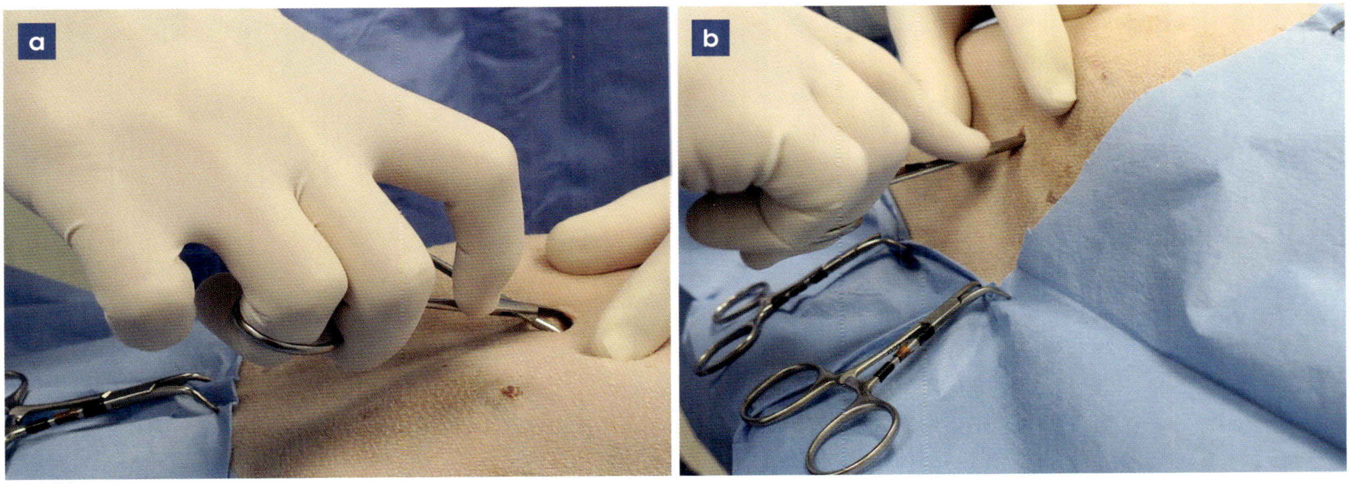

FIGURE 5. Blunt dissection of the deeper layers with a curved Crile mosquito forceps. a) Subxiphoid access. b) Intercostal access.

For the intercostal approach (**Video 1**), the choice of intercostal space depends on the surgical procedure to be performed. After incising the skin and subcutaneous tissue, blunt dissection of the deeper layers is quite easy because the intercostal muscles are very thin. For the same reason, it is not necessary to apply great pressure to introduce the cannula into the thorax (**Fig. 7**). It is advisable to use the smallest possible cannula diameter to allow for maximal cannula angulation. Care must be taken to avoid the intercostal neurovascular bundle that lies in the intercostal space, at the caudal border of each rib. The parietal pleura is pierced using a blunt-tipped trocar or a trocarless cannula to avoid an excessively deep positioning.

Once the first port has been placed and the telescope has been inserted in the thorax, the other ports are placed under thoracoscopic visualization depending on the surgical procedure to be performed (**Fig. 8**).

VIDEO 1. Placement of the first port for intercostal thoracoscopy.

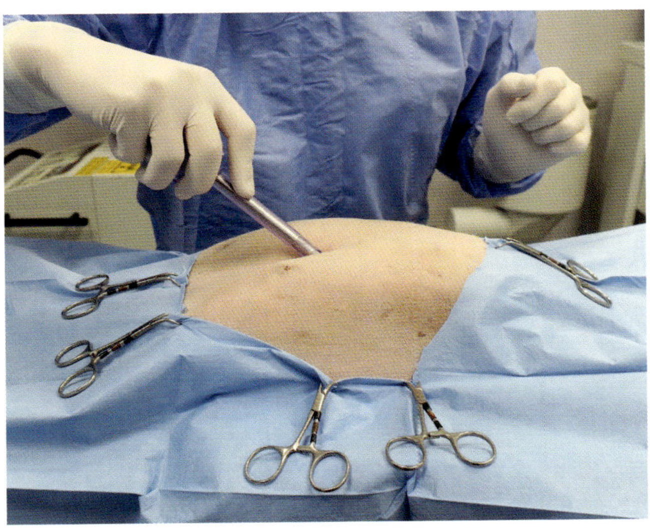

FIGURE 6. Insertion of the cannula and trocar in the subxiphoid access.

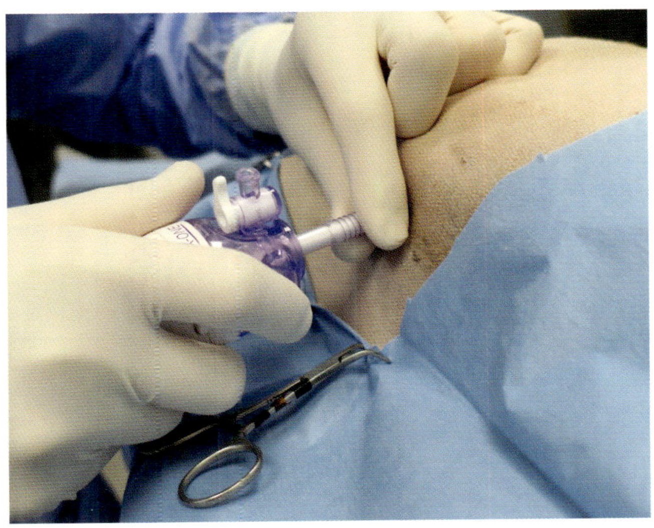

FIGURE 7. Insertion of the cannula and trocar in the intercostal access.

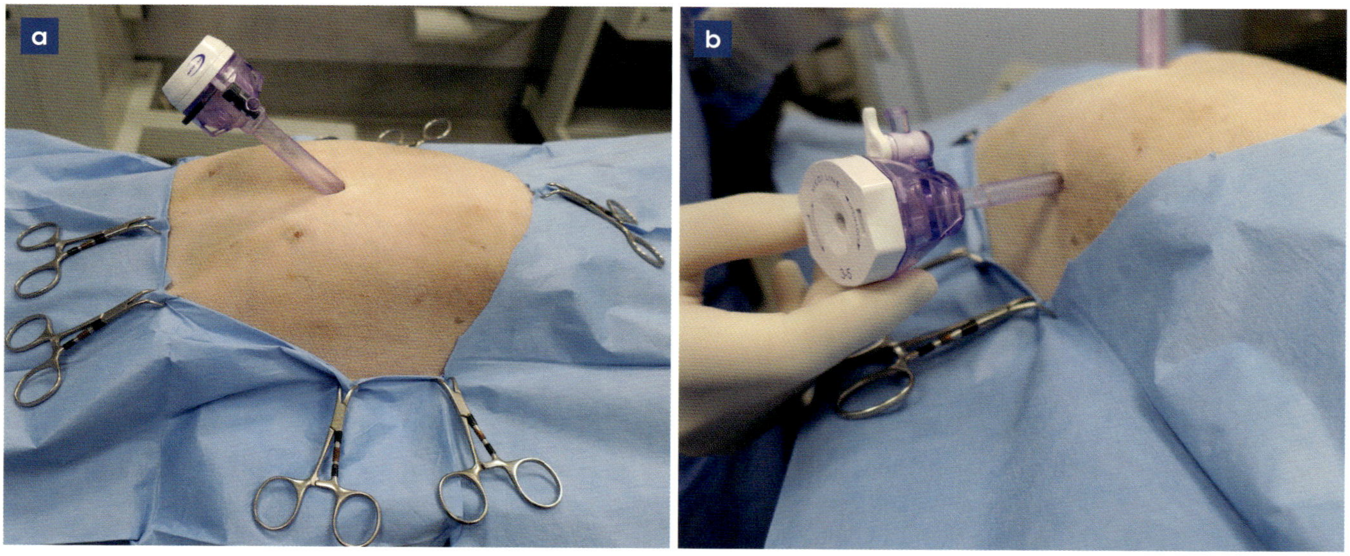

FIGURE 8. Inserted cannula. a) Subxiphoid access. b) Intercostal access.

Tips and tricks

- ✓ Attention must be paid not to damage the lung lobes during port placement, especially in small-sized animals, in which the working space is very limited.
- ✓ Sometimes it is necessary to cut the mediastinum to inspect both hemithoraces.
- ✓ One-lung ventilation can help to avoid iatrogenic injury during port placement, as it increases the working space.
- ✓ Both the right and left hemithorax should be clipped from the sternum to the dorsal third of the rib cage, and the clip should extend to the cranial abdomen.
- ✓ Insufflation of CO_2 is rarely required during thoracoscopic surgical procedures; if indicated, it can be used at 1–2 mmHg.

SUGGESTED READINGS

48 CONTRAINDICATIONS AND COMPLICATIONS IN THORACOSCOPY

J. Brad Case

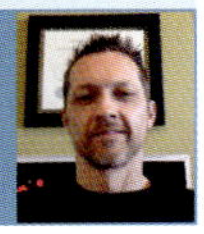

Contraindications

- Dogs with conditions not amenable to effective and safe treatment via thoracoscopy
- Dogs with cardiopulmonary disease that will not tolerate one-lung ventilation
- Dogs with significant pleural–pulmonary adhesions
- Dogs with invasive neoplasms (e.g., thymoma)
- Surgeon or surgical support team inexperience

The indications and, consequently, contraindications for thoracoscopy in veterinary surgery are numerous and constantly evolving as new procedures are developed and experience is gained. In human surgery, thoracoscopy has numerous accepted indications; however, a number of explicit contraindications also exist, including diffuse body wall neoplasia, diffuse pleural adhesions, and lack of cardiopulmonary reserve to tolerate lung collapse. Currently, veterinary patients are considered candidates for thoracoscopy if they are hemodynamically stable and have a disease that can be treated effectively and safely with a thoracoscopic approach. Obviously, subjectivity exists when determining a patient to be suitable for a particular thoracoscopic procedure, partially because guidelines in veterinary medicine are limited. The experience and training of the surgeon and surgery team, the facilities and equipment, and the capabilities for intraoperative as well as postoperative support further complicate the decision-making process.

> Thoracoscopy was first described for diagnosing and treating humans with pulmonary adhesions secondary to tuberculosis by H. C. Jacobaeus in 1910.

STRATEGIC AVOIDANCE OF COMPLICATIONS

INITIAL ASSESSMENT

Preoperative evaluation, including a complete physical and neurologic examination, complete blood count, serum biochemistry, urinalysis, and thoracic imaging, are encouraged prior to thoracoscopic surgery. Fluid, electrolyte, and acid–base alterations should be corrected prior to anesthesia. Anemic dogs should be transfused with packed red blood cells or whole blood to replenish oxygen-carrying capacity before surgery. Acute hemorrhage or preexisting anemia can compromise the patient during thoracoscopy. Because oxygen delivery to the tissues is dependent on the oxygen content of the blood, most significantly hemoglobin, patients undergoing thoracoscopy should have a minimum preoperative hematocrit of 30%. A crossmatch should be performed ahead of surgery, and donor blood should be readily available. Rupture of a large thoracic vessel may result in the near-immediate death of the patient if not addressed rapidly. Immediate surgical control of significant hemorrhage and rapid administration of blood products may be crucial. Additionally, the surgeon must avoid this complication by judicious preparation, attention to technique, and by converting to thoracotomy when the thoracoscopic procedure cannot be completed safely.

Preoperative imaging and surgical planning are important for thoracoscopic surgery. The specific pathological disease may be imaged using thoracic radiography, echocardiography, contrast-enhanced CT, or MRI. Typically, dogs with pericardial disease should undergo echocardiography in addition to survey radiography and electrocardiography before video-assisted thoracic surgery (VATS) pericardiectomy and pericardioscopy. If diastolic function is compromised by cardiac tamponade, pericardiocentesis should be performed before surgery. Echocardiography is more sensitive in detecting epicardial masses if pericardial fluid is present. In dogs with a pronounced pneumothorax or pleural effusion, preoperative thoracocentesis or thoracostomy drain placement should be considered. Pulmonary neoplasia typically requires CT for staging and preoperative determination of suitability for thoracoscopic lung lobectomy. Large lung tumors, those near the hilus, and/or in smaller dogs are typically nonideal candidates for thoracoscopic lung lobectomy. Thorough preoperative assessment facilitates patient selection for a VATS approach and therefore reduces the risk for conversion to thoracotomy and allows for more accurate surgical planning.

PATIENT PREPARATION

Preparation of cats and dogs undergoing thoracoscopic surgery is similar to that of patients undergoing thoracotomy, including a wide presurgical clipping of most, if not all, of the fur over the hemithorax involved in the approach (**Fig. 1**). This is in part because basic surgical principles apply to both open and thoracoscopic operations, and because elective or emergent conversion may be necessary. Consequently, a site prepared for open conversion should be available in all thoracoscopic procedures. Typically, conversion is performed via intercostal thoracotomy or sternotomy. Instrumentation such as Finocietto retractors, oscillating saws, electrosurgical devices, vascular forceps, and staplers normally used for open thoracic surgery should be readily available in the operating room. Thoracic surgical site infections can be morbid and have the potential to progress to pyothorax if not managed early. Careful attention to surgical asepsis and patient preparation is important despite the minimally invasive nature of thoracoscopy.

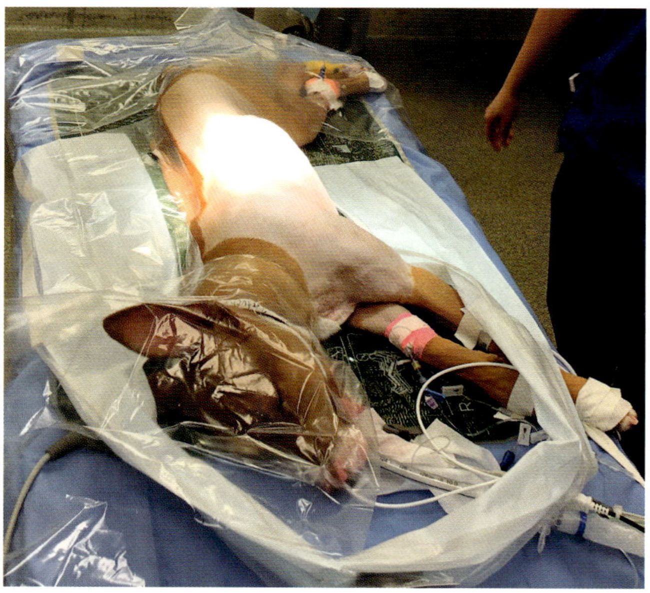

FIGURE 1. Patient being prepared for thoracoscopic persistent right aortic arch surgery. Note the wide clipping that extends below the sternum and beyond the epaxial musculature.

WORKING SPACE

Thoracoscopic surgery requires an active pneumothorax to facilitate exposure of pleural space structures. Pneumothorax causes reduction of lung volume, retraction of lungs, and expansion of the thoracic wall which create some degree of working space in the closed thorax. However, in some cases, these expected processes may be inadequate to facilitate safe thoracoscopic surgery. Thus, increasing the amount of working space beyond that created by the initial pneumothorax may be necessary in some clinical scenarios. Numerous factors play a role in limiting the actual amount of operable space during thoracoscopy, including small patient size, thoracic morphology, positioning, instrumentation, and attributes of the patient's underlying disease (e.g., adhesions, effusion, tumor size). Various techniques have been used to circumvent some of these limitations, including patient tilting or positioning (**Fig. 2**), organ retraction, intermittent ventilation, pleural space CO_2 insufflation, and one-lung ventilation. Pleural space insufflation and one-lung ventilation are covered in Chapters 46 and 53.

One of the simplest and safest methods for increasing working space in the thoracic cavity is by specific positioning or tilting of the patient. Trendelenburg principles also apply to the thoracic cavity during thoracoscopy. Using a mechanical tilt or hydraulic table, patients can be readily positioned into lateral-oblique, Trendelenburg, or reverse Trendelenburg recumbency during the operation. Slight lateral tilting of the patient while in dorsal recumbency is often helpful in shifting the heart and lungs to provide increased exposure in the thoracic cavity. Thoracoscopic instruments such as blunt probes and fan-style retractors can be used to atraumatically manipulate tissues (e.g., lung) away from the surgical site. Alternatively, the shaft of the dissection instrument can be used to

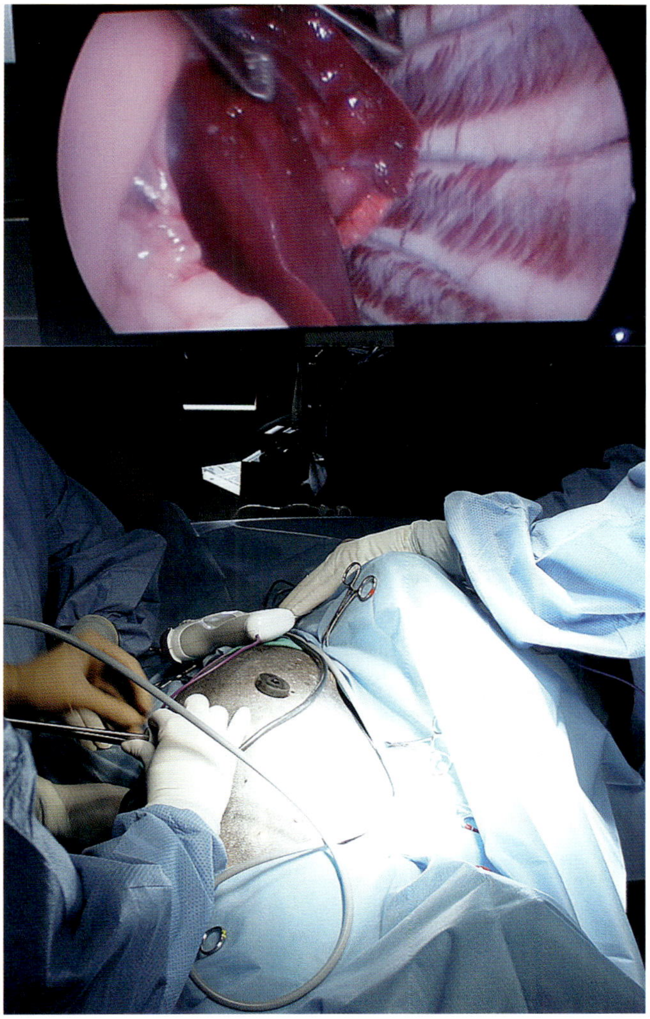

FIGURE 2. Patient positioned in dorsal-oblique recumbency to improve exposure of the left lung. In this dog, pulmonary exclusion was also performed and the right middle lung lobe was removed.

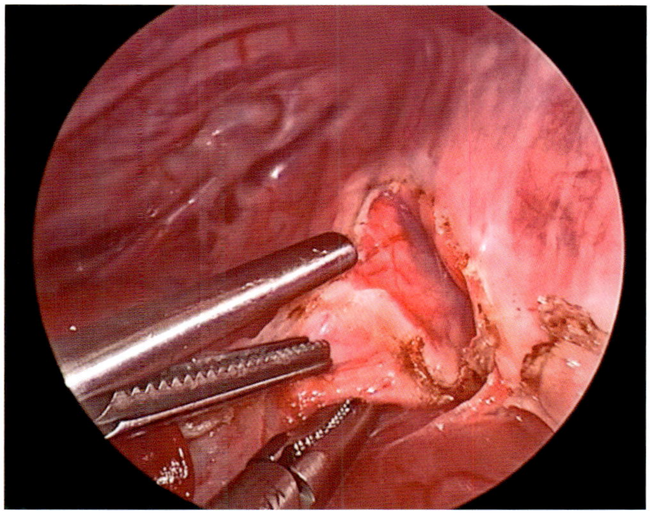

FIGURE 3. Intraoperative image of a young dog undergoing persistent right aortic arch surgery. Due to the small size and delicate nature of the tissues, pediatric instrumentation is used. In the image, 3.9 mm DeBakey and curved dissecting forceps are being utilized for dissection of the ligamentum arteriosum.

indirectly maintain retraction of tissues such as the lung. In small dogs or puppies undergoing thoracoscopy (e.g., vascular ring ligation), the use of pediatric instrumentation is extremely useful to improve the working space (**Fig. 3**). The smaller size of the instruments not only increases the accuracy of the dissection but also dramatically improves working space and visualization during procedures such as vascular ring division. Finally, intermittent ventilation or reduction in inspiratory pressure may also improve working space. Creating and maintaining adequate working space is mandatory for performing any thoracoscopic procedure. If a safe working space is not available or cannot be acquired, conversion to an open approach should be applied.

MOST FREQUENT COMPLICATIONS

PERICARDIAL COMPLICATIONS

Perhaps the most commonly performed thoracoscopic procedure in dogs is pericardiectomy. The pericardium can become thickened and opaque in cases of chronic effusion, while some dogs may have excessive pericardial fat. These factors increase the risk of inadvertent transection of the phrenic nerves, which pass through the pericardium at the level of the dorsal third of the heart, and may predispose some dogs to elective conversion. Another potential complication during pericardiectomy is accidental laceration of epicardial structures such as the auricles or myocardium. The auricle tips aim ventrally, which places them at risk for laceration during pericardiectomy. Careful pericardioscopic visualization during pericardiectomy to ensure that the auricles are not entrapped within the bipolar or scissor device is critical to avoid this complication. Similarly, the myocardium must also be protected during pericardiectomy. Excitation of the myocardium by contact from a bipolar vessel-sealing device or monopolar scissor may induce fatal ventricular arrhythmias.

VASCULAR COMPLICATIONS

The heart base, aortic root, and cranial vena cava are typically exposed during pericardiectomy. These are common locations for small nodules or masses and can be biopsied in some instances. Given the adjacency to large vascular structures, hemorrhage is certainly possible. Attention to preoperative imaging and caution during thoracoscopy can limit this risk. The right auricle is also visible in a similar region and may be intimately involved with the right atrium in the case of a large auricular mass. In some instances, the mass may be friable and prone to significant hemorrhage if it is injured during thoracoscopy (**Fig. 4**). In dogs with small apically located masses, the auricle can usually be displaced away from the epicardium for evaluation and possible resection. Endoscopic staplers are required for thoracoscopic auriculectomy, but severe hemorrhage is a risk if auriculectomy is performed in an unsafe manner.

Hemorrhage is also a concern in dogs with vascular ring anomalies undergoing ligamentum arteriosum transection with or without aberrant left subclavian ligation/division. Pediatric small dogs are a significant challenge as a result of a small thoracic volume which limits the working space, but also because of the greater risk for hemorrhage. Careful attention to preoperative imaging (e.g., CT angiography) to rule out patency of a persistent right aortic arch or aberrant subclavian artery and to plan safe ligation is critical.

VATS thymectomy is another procedure that involves substantial risk for hemorrhage, and preoperative CT angiography is a requirement in patient selection and preoperative planning. Thymomas are usually located in the cranial mediastinum and may be associated with structures like the cranial vena cava, brachiocephalic artery, and internal thoracic arteries, which require cautious dissection during thoracoscopic thymectomy.

The thoracic duct in dogs is typically situated in the dorsolateral right side of the aorta in the caudal thorax. Ligation requires dissection among the thoracic aorta and azygos vein, which can be technically challenging. Proper identification of the thoracic duct and its surrounding structures is vital to reduce the chances of damaging the adjacent vasculature (**Fig. 5**).

Intercostal ports run the risk of lacerating the intercostal vessels, which, if unaddressed, can lead to severe hemorrhage and the need for emergent conversion or reoperation. Careful thoracoscopic observation of all port sites as the ports are removed is considered mandatory. If significant hemorrhage is observed, digital pressure or reinsertion of the port can be performed to temporarily halt bleeding (**Fig. 6**). Passage of an extracorporeal suture around the vessel, via the port incision, is typically adequate but can be challenging in some dogs.

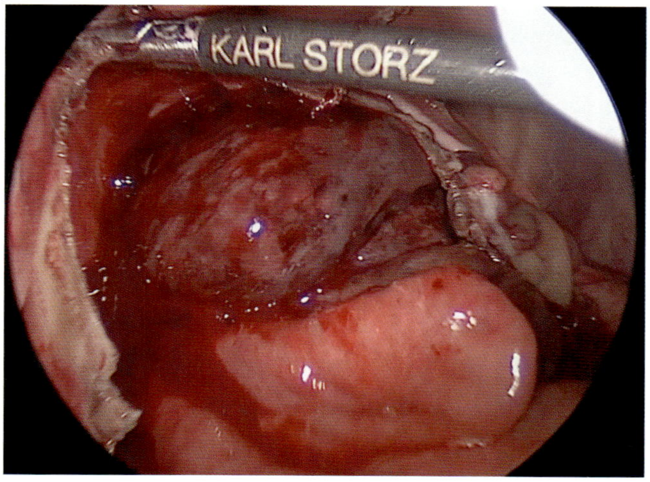

FIGURE 4. Thoracoscopic image of a patient following pericardiectomy due to pericardial tamponade from a bleeding right auricular mass. The mass was not resectable due to its large size and broad attachment to the right atrium.

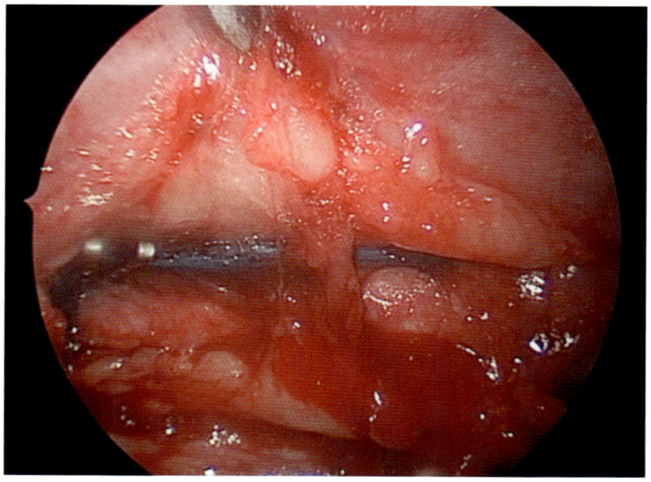

FIGURE 5. Vertebral artery hemorrhage that occurred during thoracoscopic dissection of the thoracic duct in a dog with idiopathic chylothorax. The hemorrhage was ultimately controlled with a bipolar sealing device.

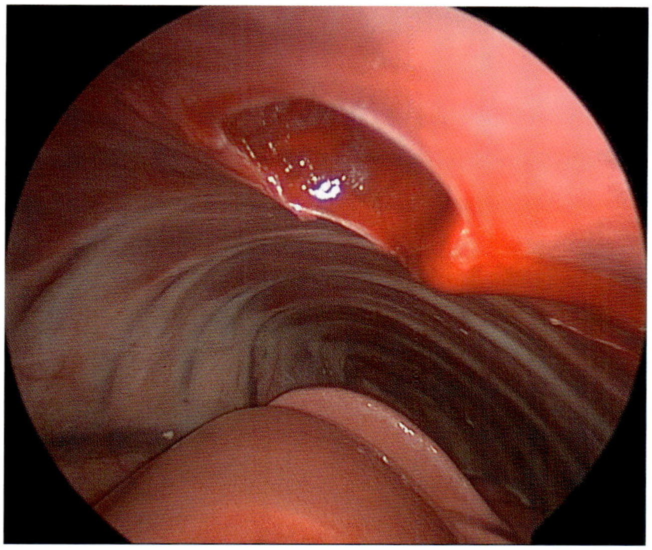

FIGURE 6. Intercostal artery bleed seen at the time of port removal. In this case, an interrupted suture was placed around the vessel to arrest the bleeding.

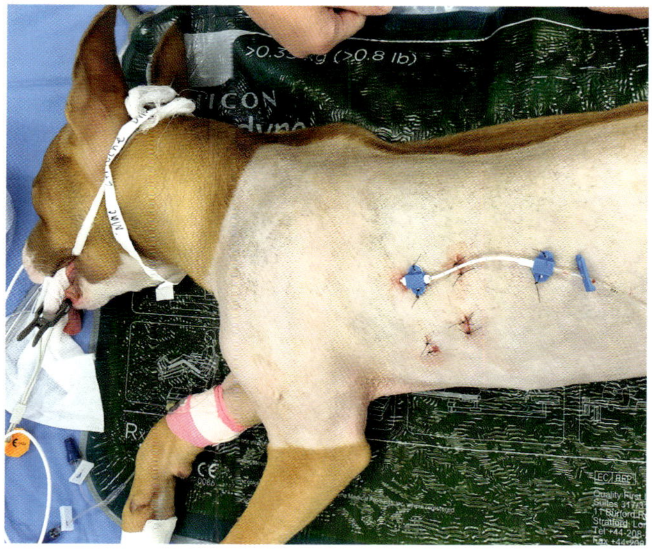

FIGURE 7. Postoperative image of a puppy following thoracoscopic persistent right aortic arch surgery. An appropriately placed 14-gauge chest drain is seen.

MONITORING FOR COMPLICATIONS

All patients undergoing thoracoscopy should be supported and monitored postoperatively as if they had undergone intercostal thoracotomy or median sternotomy. Patients should have a thoracostomy tube placed (**Fig. 7**), anchored with at least a 2-0 suture at the base of the incision and secured using a finger trap pattern including at least four throws. Thoracostomy tubes should be monitored hourly for the first few hours, and quantification and characterization of the fluid/air produced should be documented in the medical record and assessed for trends. In the event of large or increasing volumes of hemorrhage, consideration for reoperation should be made based on the patient's status and the severity of the hemorrhage. Increasing volumes of or nonresolving air accumulation after a thoracoscopic procedure may be the result of pulmonary leakage or transthoracic air movement, usually because of an inappropriately placed thoracostomy tube. As such, the housing and insertion site of the tube should be assessed for compromise. If the thoracostomy tube device is not compromised but significant air accumulation persists, continuous evacuation from the pleural space may be indicated. If the pneumothorax fails to resolve after 2 or 3 days with continuous pleural drainage, the patient may require reexploration.

SUGGESTED READINGS

49 EXPLORATORY AND DIAGNOSTIC THORACOSCOPY

Francisco Miguel Sánchez-Margallo, Isabel López-Agudelo, Manuel Ramón González-Portillo, David Durán-Rey

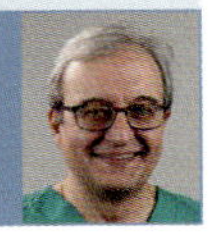

Indications

- Lung biopsy and lung lobectomy
- Pericardial window and subtotal pericardiectomy
- Placement of epicardial pacemakers
- Right auricular mass resection
- Chylothorax
- Treatment of vascular ring anomalies
- Mediastinal mass resection
- Cancer staging

Contraindications

- Intracranial disease
- Adhesions from previous surgery
- Coagulopathy

Surgery on the chest by means of a thoracoscope is usually called video-assisted thoracoscopic surgery (VATS). In veterinary surgery, VATS uses specialized ports to access the thoracic space and specialized instruments to perform the surgery. This approach has been used to collect biopsy samples from different organs, explore the pleural space, and perform advanced surgical procedures in cats and dogs.

The following procedures are described below:

A. Thoracoscopic exploration

B. Thoracic biopsy:

- Lung biopsy using a loop or biopsy forceps
- Lung lobectomy
- Mediastinal mass biopsy
- Pericardial effusion biopsy

A THORACOSCOPIC EXPLORATION

VATS is more suitable for adjuvant treatment than conventional surgery because it has fewer complications, less postoperative pain, and shorter hospital stays. However, the working space for VATS is limited, and the surgeon cannot directly observe lesions that are not detected by imaging examination.

PATIENT PREPARATION AND POSITIONING

The animal is placed in dorsal or lateral recumbency, and the entire ventral and lateral thorax is aseptically prepared. The intercostal approach provides good visualization of a limited region of the thorax, while the transdiaphragmatic subxiphoid approach offers complete exploration of the thoracic cavity and provides access to both hemithoraces. Transdiaphragmatic entry of the first trocar into the thoracic cavity can lead to lung injury and lacerations.

OPERATING ROOM LAYOUT

Thoracoscopic exploration is performed with the patient's hind end positioned at the caudal edge of the table. The operating surgeon and the assistant stand side by side at the end of the operating table. The monitor is placed in front of the surgeons, towards the patient's head. The anesthesia machine and staff are placed at the head of the operating table, while the instrument table may be positioned alongside the patient or adjacent to the surgeons at the caudal edge of the table (**Fig. 1**).

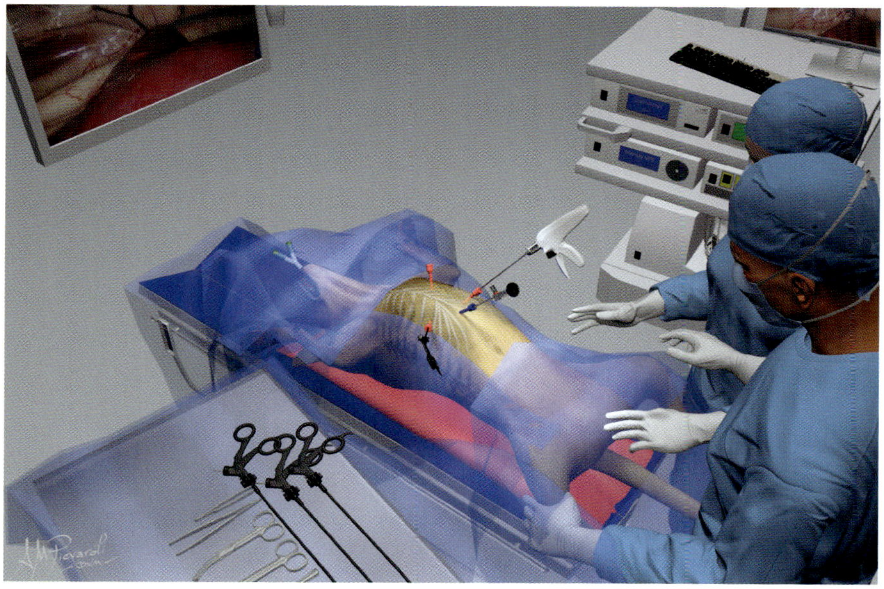

FIGURE 1. Operating room layout for thoracoscopic exploration.

Instruments

On the table:

- Standard surgery set
- Telescope 10 mm – 30°
- Two 5 mm cannulas (or one 5 mm cannula + one 10 mm cannula)
- Grasping forceps
- Vessel-sealing device

Ready to use:

- Endoscopic cannula for aspiration/irrigation
- Third cannula to switch to the three-port technique

PORT PLACEMENT

The creation of a pneumoperitoneum is not needed for thoracoscopic exploration because the ribs provide an adequate working space due to their rigidity. The ports for the instruments and for the endoscopic camera are placed in a triangular configuration around the organ to be visualized. The endoscopic camera should be placed away from the surgical field to allow adjustment of the field of view magnification if necessary.

For the transdiaphragmatic subxiphoid approach, port placement may vary depending on the patient's size and the structures of interest. The following is an example (**Fig. 2**):

- T1, subxiphoid position
- T2, on the midline, in the 9th intercostal space
- T3, on the midline, in the 7th intercostal space
- T4, on the midline, in the 5th intercostal space

PROCEDURE

- If pleural effusion is present, it should be drained before starting the examination.
- Thoracic examination begins at the cranial part of the right hemithorax, and the right cranial, middle, and caudal lung lobes are assessed (**Figs. 3a–3c**).
- Similarly, from cranial to caudal, the left hemithorax is evaluated. The cranial and caudal subsegments of the left cranial lobe lobe are assessed, followed by the left caudal lobe (**Figs. 3d and 3e**).
- After making a window in the vena cava fold and the left caudal mediastinal pleura on the left, the accessory lobe is visualized (**Fig. 3f**).
- The use of forceps may be necessary for retraction of the vena cava and mediastinal pleura.
- In cases of mediastinal swelling, the mediastinum should be fenestrated using laparoscopic scissors or a vessel-sealing device, the latter instrument being useful to improve visualization and minimize bleeding.

Tips

To ensure that the evaluation is complete, examination of the thoracic cavity should be performed systematically.

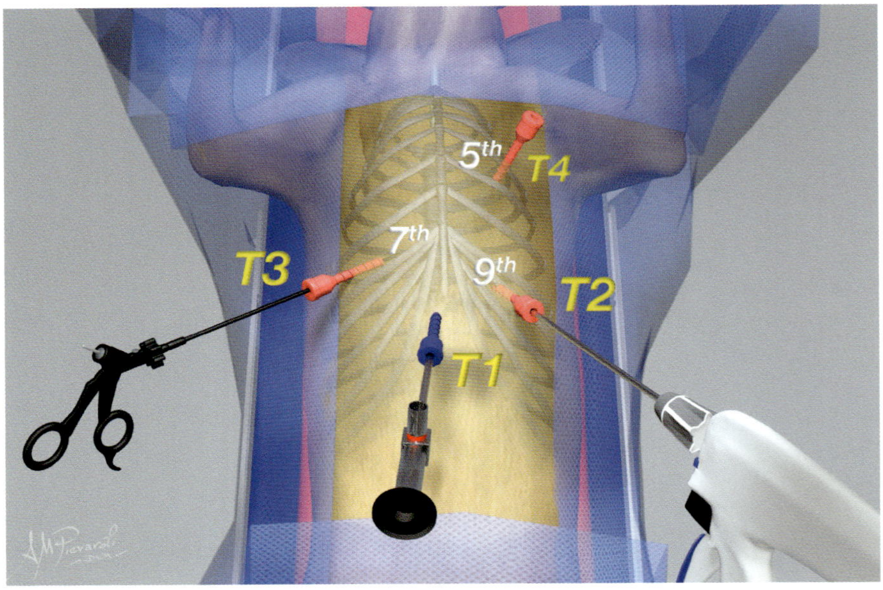

FIGURE 2. Port placement for thoracoscopic exploration. Transdiaphragmatic subxiphoid approach.

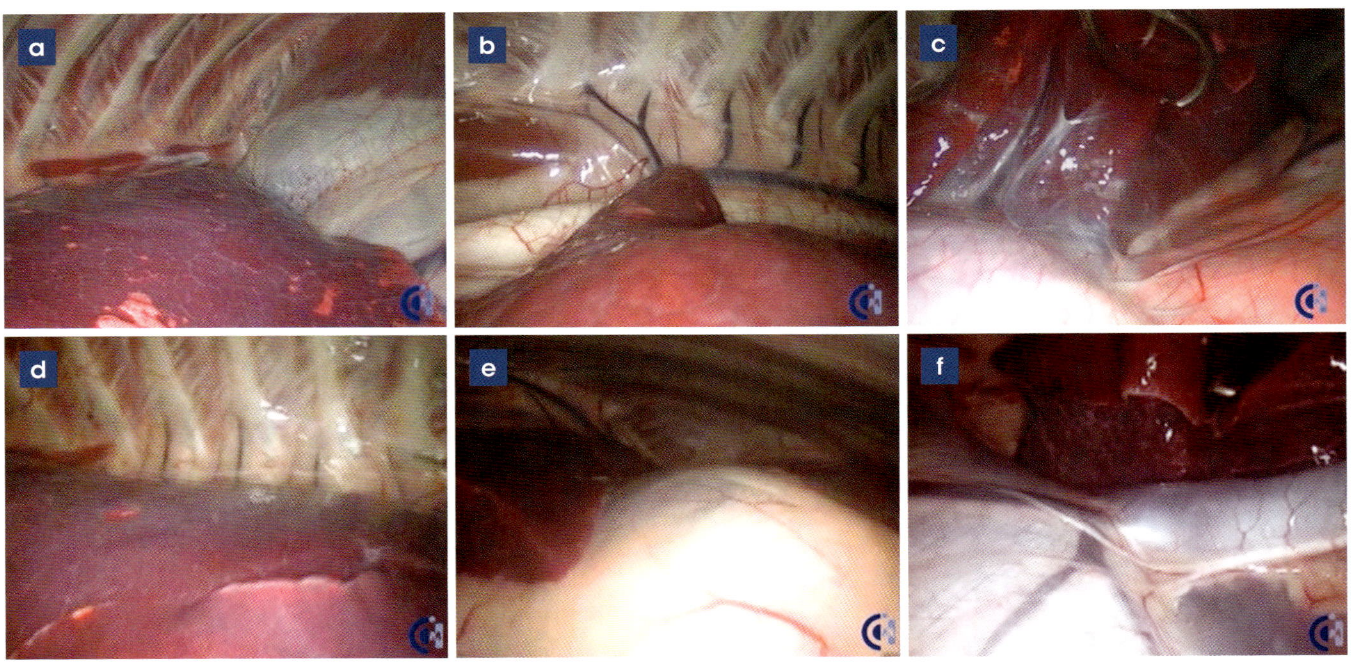

FIGURE 3. Intraoperative exploration of the thorax. a) Left cranial view. b) Left middle view. c) Left caudal view. d) Right cranial view. e) Right middle view. f) Right caudal view.

Key points

- Thoracoscopic examination allows localization and confirmation of thoracic pathologies and facilitates the treatment of intrathoracic diseases.
- Diagnostic thoracoscopy aids in patient preparation and selection.
- Thoracoscopic surgery is associated with higher morbidity than laparoscopic surgery. Exploration should be performed with care due to the presence of vital organs in the thorax.

B THORACIC BIOPSY

Minimally invasive exploration of the thoracic space allows biopsy of pleural surfaces, lymph nodes, pericardium, and lungs. In cases of pericardial effusion, thoracoscopy can be used as a diagnostic and therapeutic tool. Pericardiectomy provides the opportunity for reduction of pericardial tamponade and the capacity to obtain diagnostic samples, as well as inspection for cardiac masses. Exploratory thoracoscopy and biopsy procedures are well tolerated, with just a few complications. However, cases of port-site metastasis after thoracoscopy have been described.

Evaluating lymph node metastasis in cancer patients is important staging information for several tumor types. VATS has the benefits of direct visualization, potentially minimizing damage to surrounding tissue, and the obtainment of larger tissue samples for histopathology. Intraoperative imaging such as lymphoscintigraphy, blue dye techniques, and near-infrared imaging dyes are very useful to the surgeon, especially when dissecting lymph nodes. Within seconds to minutes after injecting a small amount of dye peritumorally, uptake should be visualized in the lymphatics and finally in the sentinel lymph node.

PATIENT PREPARATION AND POSITIONING

For thoracic biopsy, the transdiaphragmatic subxiphoid approach is the best option. Sternal and mediastinal lymph nodes will be easily accessible for biopsy, but hilar lymph nodes will not be seen. If the pathology is unilateral, an intercostal approach would be more appropriate, and the hilar lymph nodes would be visible. Additionally, lateral recumbency with intercostal port placement is the preferred technique for complete lung lobectomy.

OPERATING ROOM LAYOUT

The surgeon and the assistant are positioned on the patient's side, facing the dog's thorax. The endoscopic tower is placed on the contralateral side of the patient (**Fig. 4**).

PORT PLACEMENT

For the transdiaphragmatic subxiphoid approach, port placement may vary depending on the patient's size and the structures of interest. The following is an example (**Fig. 2**):

- T1, subxiphoid position

Instruments

On the table:

- Standard surgery set
- Telescope 10 mm – 30°
- Three 5 mm cannulas
- 10 mm cannula
- Grasping forceps
- Vessel-sealing device
- Biopsy forceps
- Biopsy loop
- Linear stapler
- Suction device

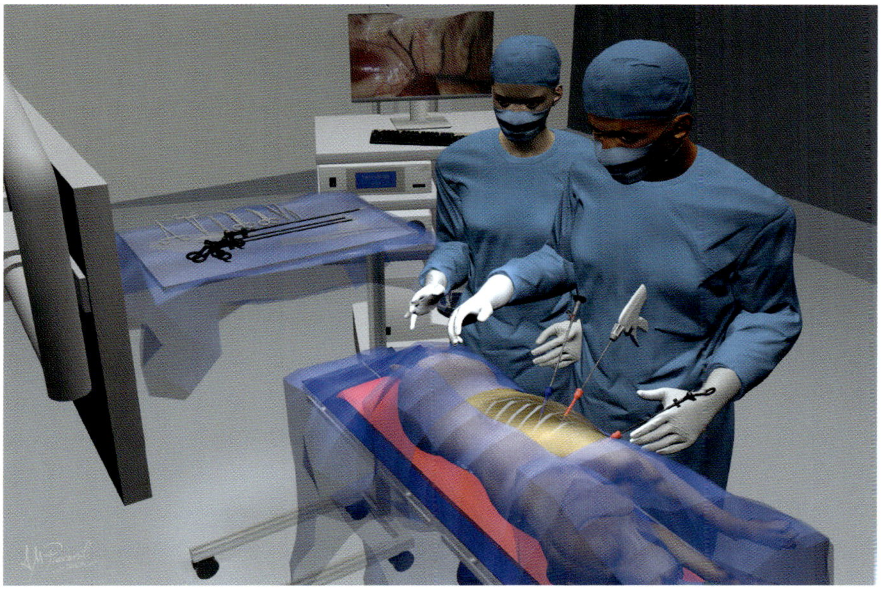

FIGURE 4. Operating room layout for thoracic biopsy.

- T2, on the midline, in the 9th intercostal space
- T3, on the midline, in the 7th intercostal space
- T4, on the midline, in the 5th intercostal space

If the patient is in lateral recumbency, the ports are placed as follows (**Fig. 5**):

- T1, on the midline, in the 9th intercostal space
- T2, under the tip of the scapula, in the 7th intercostal space
- T3, on the midline, in the 3rd or 4th intercostal space

PROCEDURE

Lung biopsy using a loop or biopsy forceps

- When using a loop ligature, the device is introduced through one of the ports, and the grasping forceps are then passed through the loop.
- The tip of a lung lobe is grasped and pulled into the loop.
- The distal tip of the loop ligature is broken and the slip knot tightened around the lung parenchyma.
- The knot pusher is used to conduct the suture where it should be positioned for the biopsy.
- The lung biopsy is then cut, making sure that 0.5 cm of tissue extends passed the ligature.
- If a leak is observed on the incision, a second loop ligature can be applied.
- If a solid mass is present in the center of a lung lobe, biopsy forceps can be used to biopsy the center of the mass.
- A palpation probe or hemostatic absorbable foam can be used to help control bleeding.

Lung lobectomy

- Lung lobectomy via VATS is most appropriate for smaller masses that are located at the periphery of the lung lobe. The accessory lung lobe is more difficult to access.
- Successful thoracoscopy requires various ports and placement of bronchial blockers for one-lung ventilation.
- The linear stapler is the preferred device (**Fig. 6**). It is important to place it as perpendicular as possible to the hilus of the lung, optimizing the length of the cartridge of staples. Hence, the port for the stapling device should be placed last, after visualization of the hilus of the lung. The linear stapler is articulated, so its position can be adjusted even if the port is not in a perfect position.
- Before releasing the staples, it is important to make sure that no other structures are caught.
- After releasing the staples, the resected lung lobe is placed in a sterile bag to prevent seeding of tumor cells.
- A port site is enlarged to allow exteriorization of the lung lobe in the retrieval bag.
- Enlarged hilar lymph nodes should be biopsied or removed as well (**Fig. 7**).
- For hemostasis, electrosurgical assistance and clip application can be used.
- Before removing the optic, the hilus is observed for air outflow or bleeding.

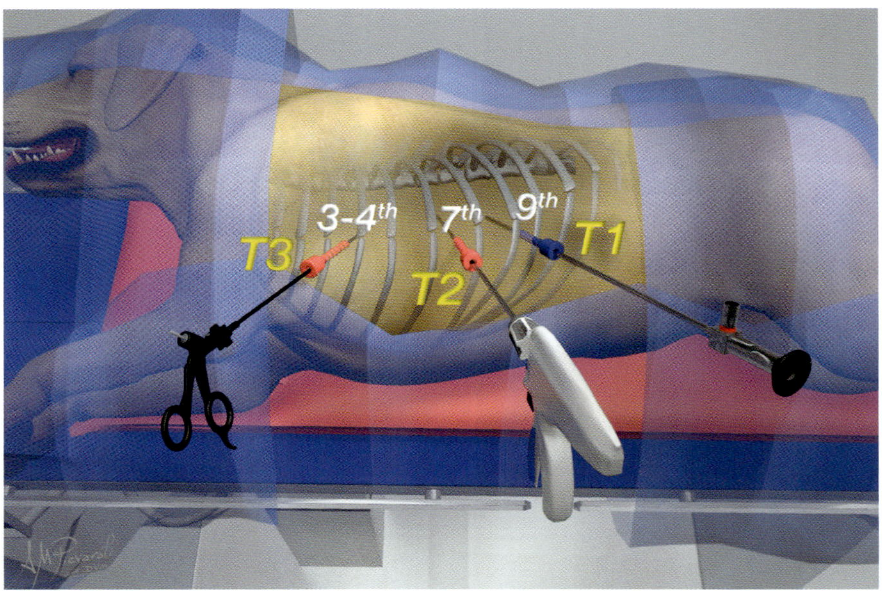

FIGURE 5. Port placement for thoracic biopsy. Patient in lateral recumbency.

Mediastinal mass biopsy

- Thoracoscopic removal of mediastinal masses has been reported in cats and dogs. For this purpose, the transdiaphragmatic subxiphoid approach should be used.
- A vessel-sealing device used as a dissection tool significantly reduces surgical time.
- Monopolar hook electrosurgery can also be helpful in the dissection of tissue planes, particularly when close to vital structures.
- After identifying the mass, the optic should be inserted deeper enough for localization of the phrenic nerves.
- The mass is then carefully dissected from the surrounding mediastinum and pericardium while trying to not damage the phrenic nerves.
- Usually, an attempt is made to remove one or more sternal lymph nodes.

Pericardial effusion biopsy

- In pericardial effusion, thoracoscopy can be used as a diagnostic and a therapeutic tool.
- VATS pericardiectomy provides the opportunity for alleviation of pericardial tamponade and the ability to obtain diagnostic samples, as well as inspection for possible cardiac masses.
- Resected portions of pericardium should be submitted for histopathology.
- After moderate collapse of the lungs, the optic is inserted and a small window in the ventral mediastinum is made.
- The second port is then placed on the contralateral side.

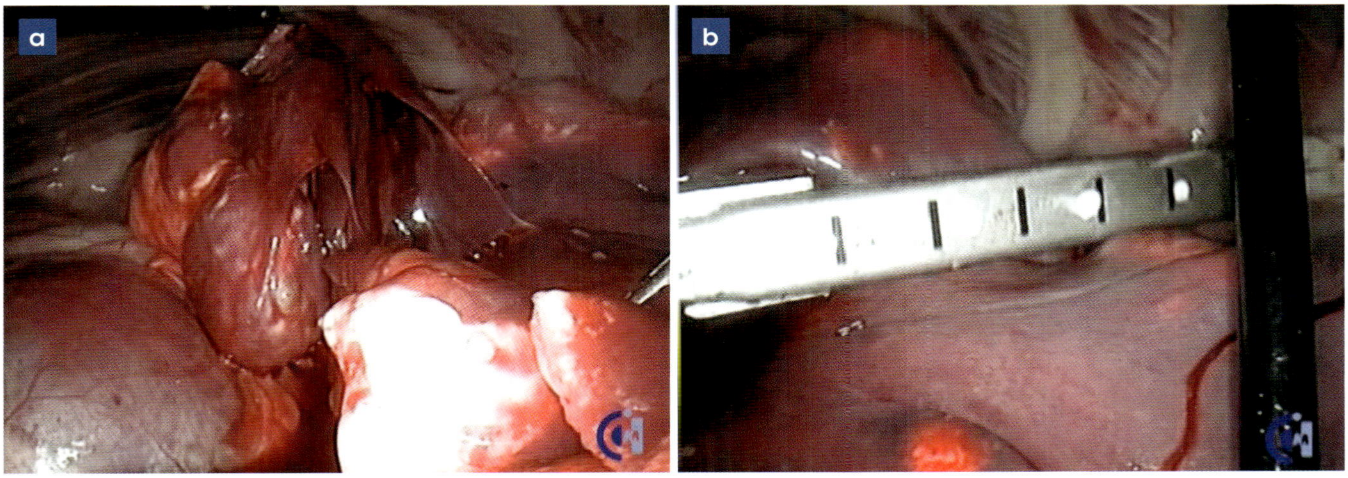

FIGURE 6. Intraoperative view of lobectomy. a) Dissection of the cranial lobe. b) Application of the linear stapler.

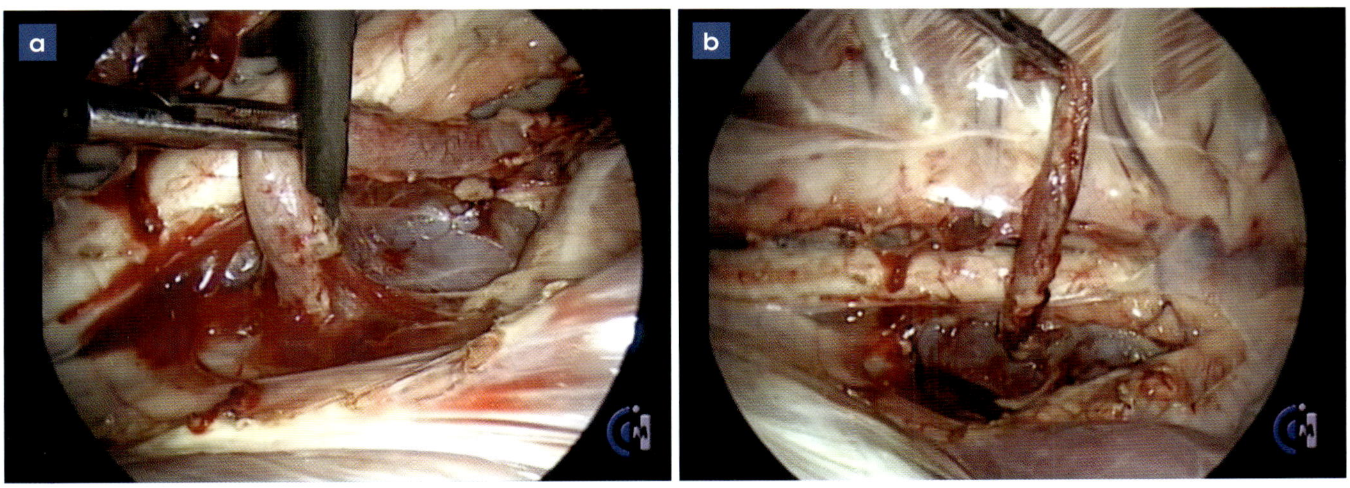

FIGURE 7. Intraoperative view of a) caudal and b) para-aortic lymphadenectomy.

- An additional 5 mm port can be placed for the irrigation unit.
- To allow for 360° visualization, the ventral mediastinum is dissected from its sternal fixation, preferably using a bipolar electrocoagulation or vessel-sealing device.
- The pericardial sac is held with the grasping forceps and opened with scissors. Its contents are evacuated with the endoscopic suction unit.
- For a right-handed surgeon, standing on the patient's right side with the vessel-sealing device in the subxiphoid port and the grasping forceps in the right intercostal port will facilitate the pericardiectomy. The assistant, with the camera, should stand on the patient's left side.
- After excision, the pericardium is placed in a bag to prevent seeding of tumor cells if malignancy is a possibility and retrieved from the thorax through the subxiphoid port (**Fig. 8**).
- Pericardial specimens are submitted for histological examination.

POSTOPERATIVE MANAGEMENT

- Analgesia with low-dose opioids.
- Nonsteroidal anti-inflammatory drugs if not contraindicated in the patient.
- Thoracic drainage if necessary.
- Empirical antimicrobial therapy.

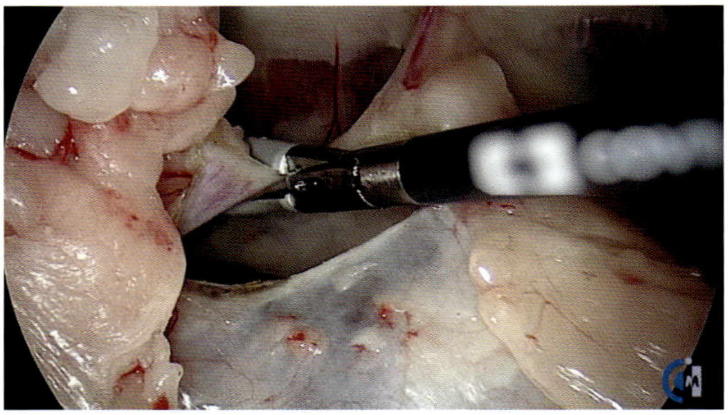

FIGURE 8. Intraoperative view of pericardiectomy.

Key points

- The use of electrosurgery or vessel-sealing devices is very helpful.
- Minimize sample handling by grasping the tissues adjacent to the desired biopsy site to avoid damage to the specimen.
- Protected specimen removal should be used to minimize the risks of port-site metastasis.

Complications of exploratory and diagnostic thoracoscopy

- Inappropriate port placement
- Perforation of intercostal vessels at port placement
- Transection of phrenic nerves
- Hemorrhage
- Pulmonary injury
- Pneumothorax
- Port-site metastasis

SUGGESTED READINGS

CLINICAL CASES

49.1 THORACOSCOPY IN COMBINATION WITH DIGESTIVE ENDOSCOPY FOR THE DIAGNOSIS OF INTRATHORACIC NEOFORMATIONS

Francesca Molinari, Enrico Sponza, Giacomo Federici

CASE DESCRIPTION

Chest X-ray examination of a 10-year-old sterilized female German Shepherd Dog showed the presence of moderate pleural effusion. After draining the effusion, an intrathoracic neoformation was suspected (no cancer cells from the effusion cytology). CT examination confirmed the presence of a mass in the right caudal paraesophageal mediastinum and showed multifocal pleural thickening without lymph node enlargement. Thoracoscopy was performed with simultaneous digestive endoscopy to highlight, in transillumination, the position and appearance of the neoformation. The mass had a homogeneous consistency, and it was decided to perform biopsy. Histological examination was compatible with poorly differentiated epithelial neoplasia, which, following immunohistochemical staining with cytokeratin and vimentin, was typified as epithelioid mesothelioma.

Key points

- Place the three ports according to the guidelines below.
- Place the patient in dorsal recumbency and prepare a wide surgical field (from the 3rd intercostal space to the mid-abdomen).
- Always perform multiple biopsies to increase diagnostic sensitivity.
- It is imperative to have the correct equipment and be prepared to handle any complications.

PORT PLACEMENT

- T1, telescope port, in the 8th right intercostal space
- T2, right-hand port, in the 10th right intercostal space
- T3, left-hand port, in the 6th right intercostal space

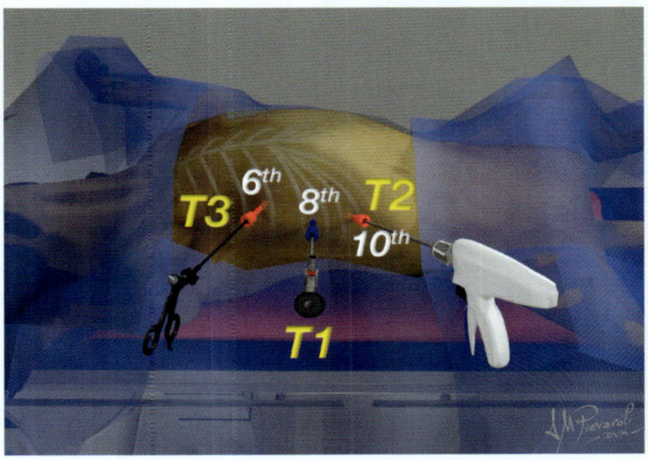

PROCEDURE

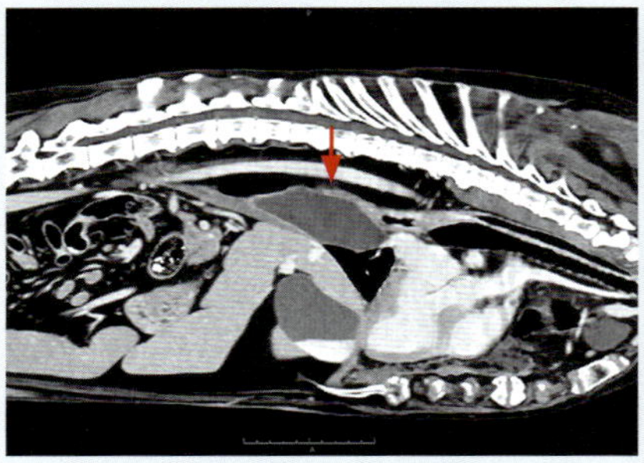

FIGURE 1. CT image showing the neoformation (arrow), caudal to the heart.

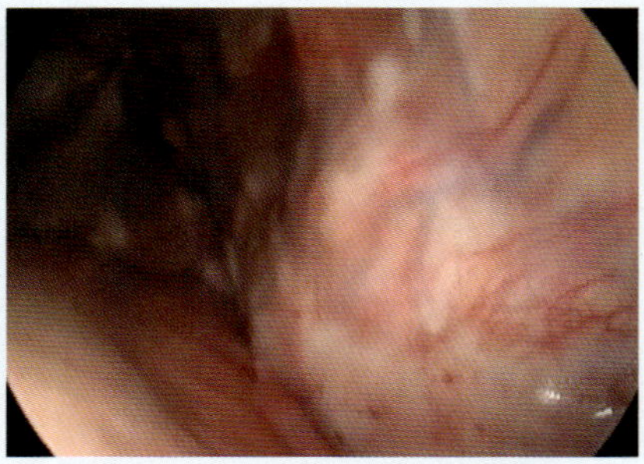

FIGURE 2. Thoracoscopic appearance of the pleura.

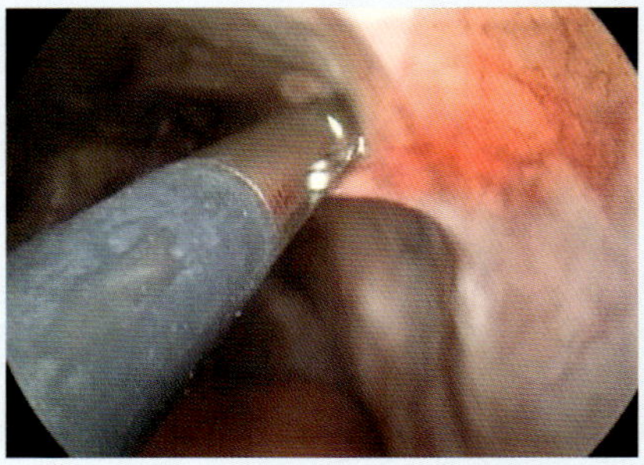

FIGURE 3. Biopsy of the pleural lesion.

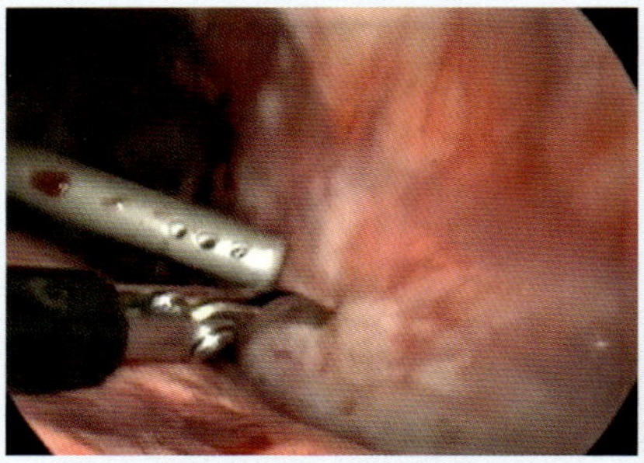

FIGURE 4. First approach to the neoformation.

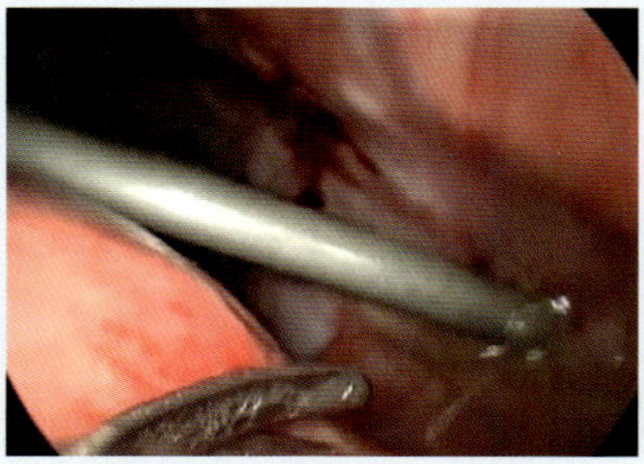

FIGURE 5. Effusion after cutting the neoformation.

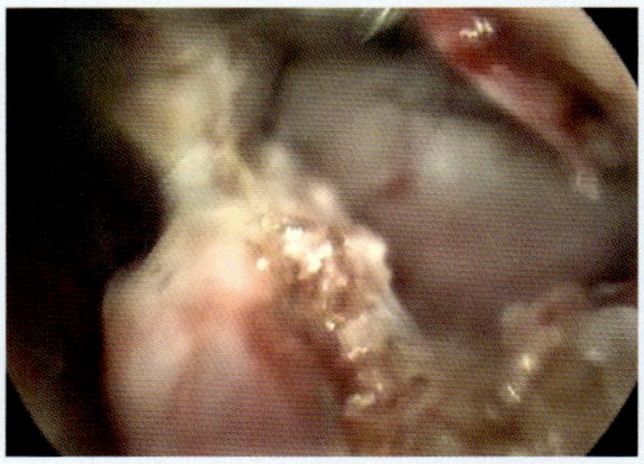

FIGURE 6. Internal appearance of the neoformation.

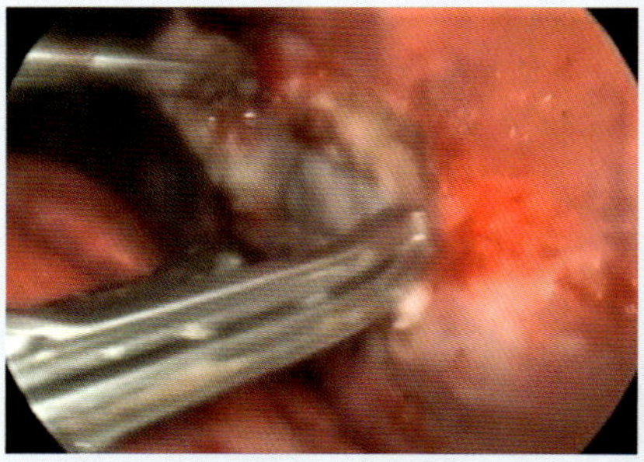

FIGURE 7. First biopsy of the mass.

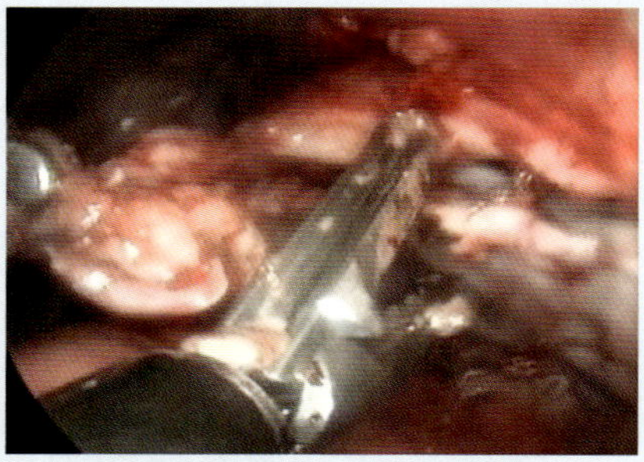

FIGURE 8. Second biopsy of the mass.

Tips and tricks

✓ Based on the localization of the lesion, consider the use of digestive endoscopy to better identify the biopsy site.

49.2 GUNSHOT WOUND TO THE CHEST CAVITY IN A DOG

P.V. Osichkin, P.A. Kuznetsov

CASE DESCRIPTION

A 5-year-old Belgian Shepherd police dog was presented with a chest traumatic gunshot wound that happened 2 days prior. A passive subcutaneous drain was immediately installed in the inlet of the rubber bullet. X-ray confirmed the presence of a foreign body in the chest cavity. Other concomitant pathologies, such as pneumothorax and hydrothorax, were excluded. Thoracoscopy was performed to rule out lung damage and to remove the foreign body.

Key points

- X-ray diagnosis before surgery is useful for initial assessment of the extent of the injury, detection of a foreign body, and evaluation of signs of lung damage, hydrothorax, and pneumothorax.
- The contused lung was tested for leaks with a submersion test. There were no signs of air leaks.

PORT PLACEMENT

The patient was placed in dorsal recumbency. The first optical port (T1) was placed paraxiphoidally. Two working ports were placed laterally on both sides at the level of the 7th (T2) and 8th (T3) intercostal spaces under thoracoscopic visualization.

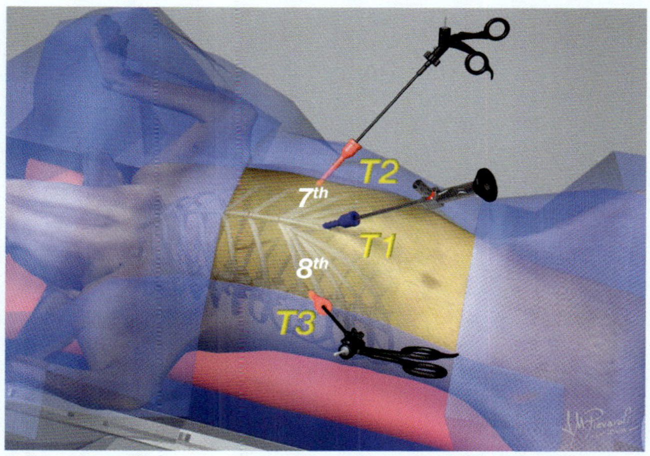

PROCEDURE

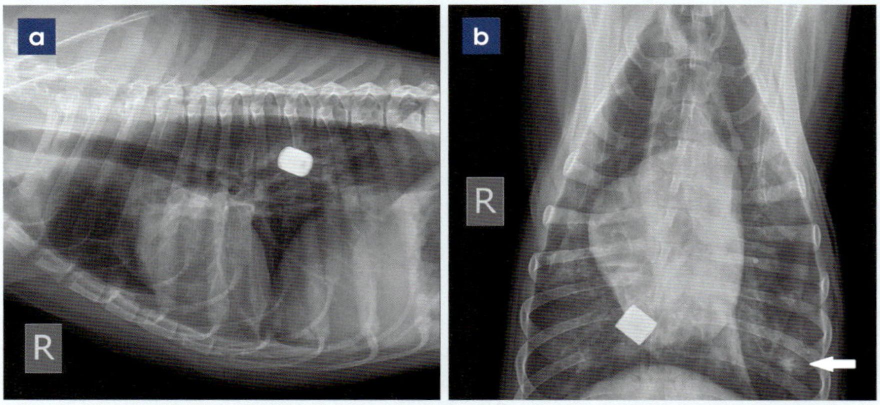

FIGURE 1. a) Lateral and b) ventrodorsal chest X-rays showing a high-density foreign body (rubber bullet) in the thoracic cavity. The arrow points to an area of increased contrast in the caudal lobe of the left lung, indicating an area of interstitial lung damage due to contusion.

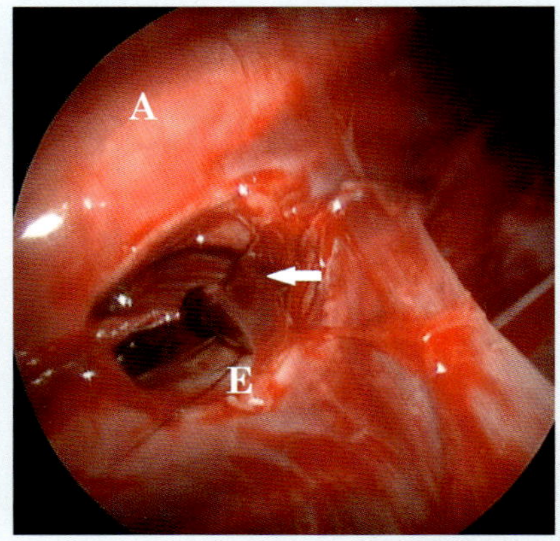

FIGURE 2. With the patient in right lateral recumbency, a thoracoscopic exploration was performed. The image shows the area of injury caused by the bullet (arrow) between the aorta (A) and the esophagus (E). The aorta and esophagus were intact.

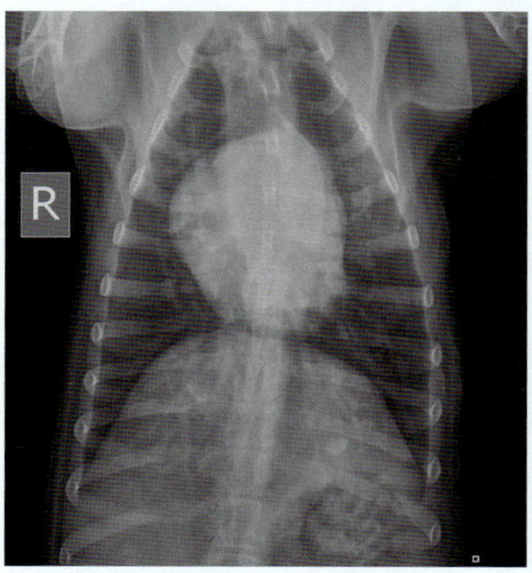

FIGURE 3. Ventrodorsal chest X-ray 2 weeks after surgery.

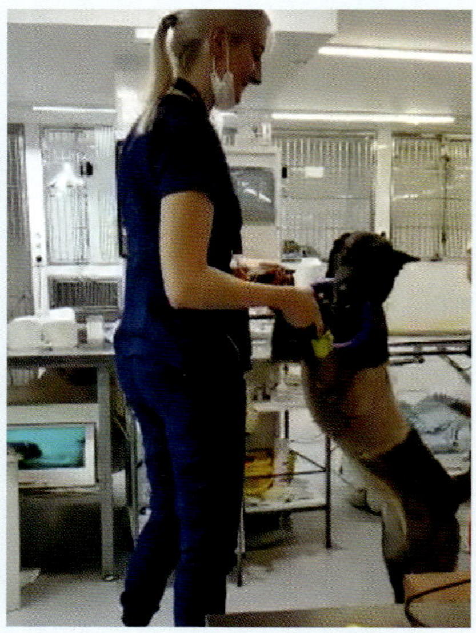

FIGURE 4. The patient 1 day after surgery.

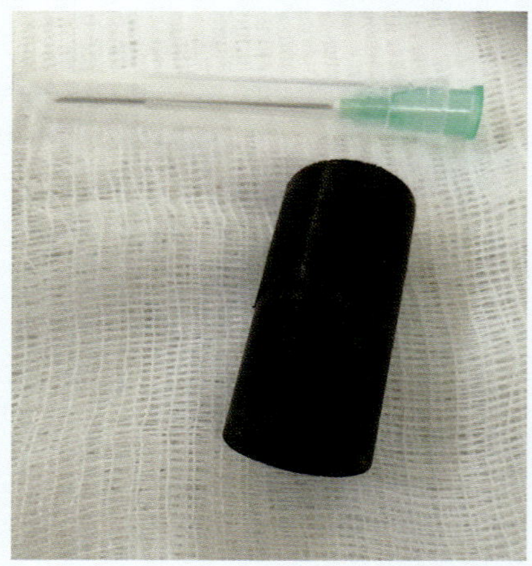

FIGURE 5. The rubber bullet extracted from the chest cavity.

Tips and tricks

- ✓ The bullet was deep in the soft tissue of the dorsal mediastinum, between the aorta and the esophagus. After constantly changing the position of the patient, the bullet moved into the pleural cavity. The constant hemorrhage, and the lung movement when breathing, created difficulty finding and visualizing the foreign body.
- ✓ Blunt trauma to the caudal lobe of the left lung resulted in pulmonary hemorrhage and swelling, which prevented air leakage. Constant bleeding acted as autohemopleurodesis; therefore, there was no leak of air or blood. Thoracic X-rays 14 days after bullet removal showed no abnormalities.

50 THORACOSCOPIC PERICARDIECTOMY

Roberto Bussadori, Andrea Pievaroli, Roberto Properzi, Deborah De Bastiani

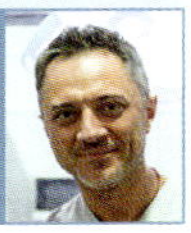

Indications

- Pericardial effusion (idiopathic, neoplastic)
- Constrictive pericarditis
- Idiopathic chylothorax

Contraindications

- Hemodynamically unstable patients
- Dogs with large or invasive tumors
- Surgeon or surgical support team inexperience

Pericardiectomy is the treatment of choice for the management of cardiac and pericardial diseases such as pericardial effusions, constrictive pericarditis, and cardiac and pericardial tumors. It is considered curative for idiopathic pericardial effusion but palliative in cases of malignant effusion. Pericardiectomy is also considered the surgical procedure of choice for the management of idiopathic chylothorax.

Pericardiectomy can be performed with a thoracoscopic approach, reducing perioperative morbidity and pain and hospitalization time compared to the thoracotomy approach. It can be subphrenic (subtotal) or partial (pericardial window). Subphrenic pericardiectomy is the removal of the pericardium ventral to the phrenic nerves, while the pericardial window allows the removal of a portion of pericardium. Recently, some studies have described the advantages of a novel technique using a pericardial window associated with vertical pericardial fillets to improve the exposure of the epicardium compared to standard pericardial window. Thoracoscopy also allows the execution of pericardioscopy, a procedure that must always be performed to improve diagnostic accuracy and which permits the detection of lesions (e.g., nodules, masses, adhesions) that could influence the prognosis of the patient (**Figs. 1 and 2**).

Currently, great debate exists about the ideal amount of pericardium to be removed in cases of idiopathic pericardial effusion. The authors' recommendation is to remove as much pericardial tissue as possible. Subphrenic pericardiectomy allows a greater portion of pericardium to be submitted for histopathology, increasing diagnostic accuracy, and it remains the treatment of choice in case of constrictive pericarditis. A pericardial window can be used in cases of malignant pericardial effusion.

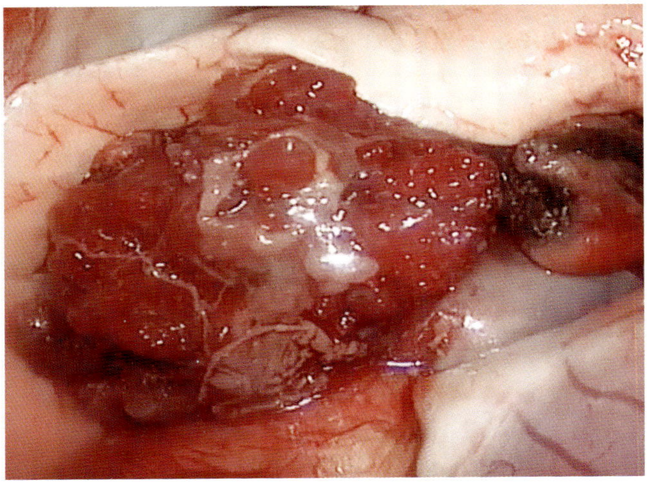

FIGURE 1. Pericardioscopy. Visualization of a mass in the right atrium.

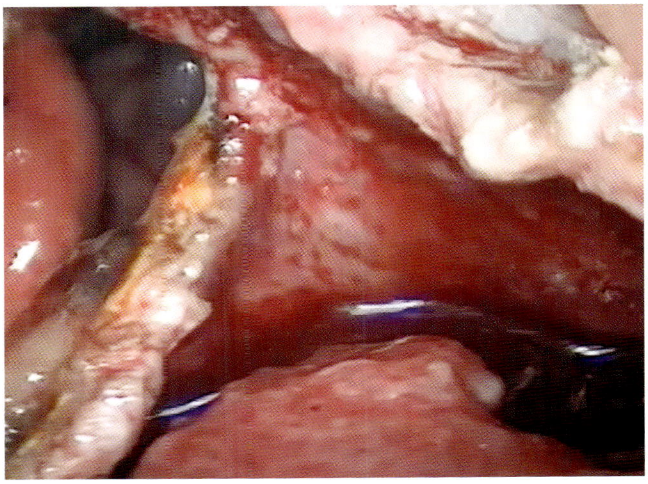

FIGURE 2. Evaluation of the inside of the pericardium using the optic.

The creation of a working space during thoracoscopic pericardiectomy can be achieved in different ways. Usually, for procedures performed with the patient in dorsal recumbency, the open pneumothorax is enough for adequate visualization. In other patient positions, pulmonary exclusion and one-lung ventilation may be necessary. The use of selective intubation or bronchial blockers has been described.

The first partial thoracoscopic pericardiectomy was described in 1999 by Jackson et al. in 13 dogs.

Instruments

On the table:

- Standard surgery set
- Telescope 5 mm – 30°
- Three 5 mm cannulas (or two 5 mm cannulas + one 10 mm cannula)
- Grasping forceps
- Endoscissors
- Vessel-sealing device or harmonic scalpel device

Ready to use:

- Endoscopic cannula for aspiration/irrigation
- Retrieval bag
- Probe

Pericardial window

A pericardial window allows a portion of 3–5×3–5 cm of pericardium to be removed. It is indicated in cases of neoplastic or idiopathic pericardial effusions. It is considered easier to perform compared to subphrenic pericardiectomy because there is a decreased risk of phrenic nerve damage. Some studies suggest that the portion of pericardium removed could be insufficient to resolve the clinical signs associated with cardiac tamponade in cases of idiopathic pericardial effusion. Moreover, this technique allows for a smaller specimen of pericardium to be collected for histopathology and does not permit a thorough epicardial exploration compared to subphrenic pericardiectomy. Pericardial window can be performed with the patient in either dorsal or lateral recumbency; dorsal recumbency is preferred.

The following procedures are described below:

A. Pericardial window in dorsal recumbency
B. Pericardial window in lateral recumbency
C. Subtotal pericardiectomy

A PERICARDIAL WINDOW IN DORSAL RECUMBENCY

PATIENT PREPARATION AND POSITIONING

Pericardial window in dorsal recumbency can be performed using ports on either the left or right side of the patient. Alternatively, single right-side port placement has also been described.

The patient is placed in dorsal recumbency. Both hemithoraces are clipped from the sternum to the dorsal third of the rib cage. Clipping should extend to the cranial abdomen.

OPERATING ROOM LAYOUT

Thoracoscopic pericardial window is performed with the patient's hind end positioned at the caudal edge of the table. The surgeon and the assistant stand side by side at the end of the operating table. The monitor is placed in front of the surgeons, towards the dog's head. The anesthesia circuit and staff are positioned at the head of the operating table. The instrument table may be placed alongside the patient or adjacent to the surgeons at the caudal edge of the table (**Fig. 3**).

PORT PLACEMENT

Left- and right-side approach, paraxiphoid or subxiphoid telescope location (**Fig. 4**):

- T1, subxiphoid (caudal and dorsal to the xiphoid process) or paraxiphoid position (between the xiphoid process and the last sternocostal junction)
- T2, in the ventral third of the 6th–9th left intercostal space
- T3, in the ventral third of the 6th–9th right intercostal space
- T4 (optional), in the ventral third of the 6th–5th left/right intercostal space (for irrigation/aspiration unit)

Right-side approach, paraxiphoid or subxiphoid telescope location (**Fig. 5**):

- T1, subxiphoid position or paraxiphoid position
- T2, in the ventral third of the 8th–10th right intercostal space
- T3, in the ventral third of the 4th–6th right intercostal space

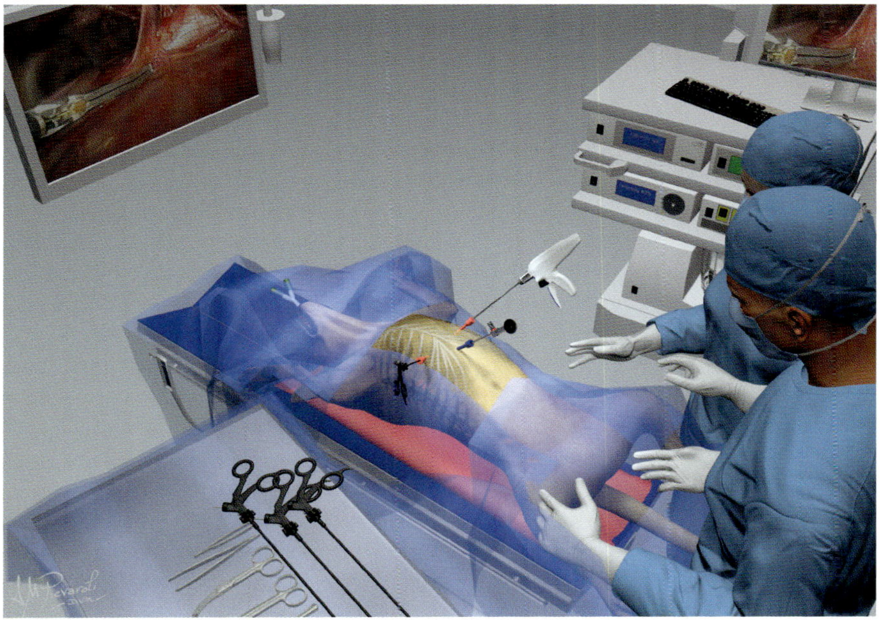

FIGURE 3. Operating room layout for pericardial window in dorsal recumbency.

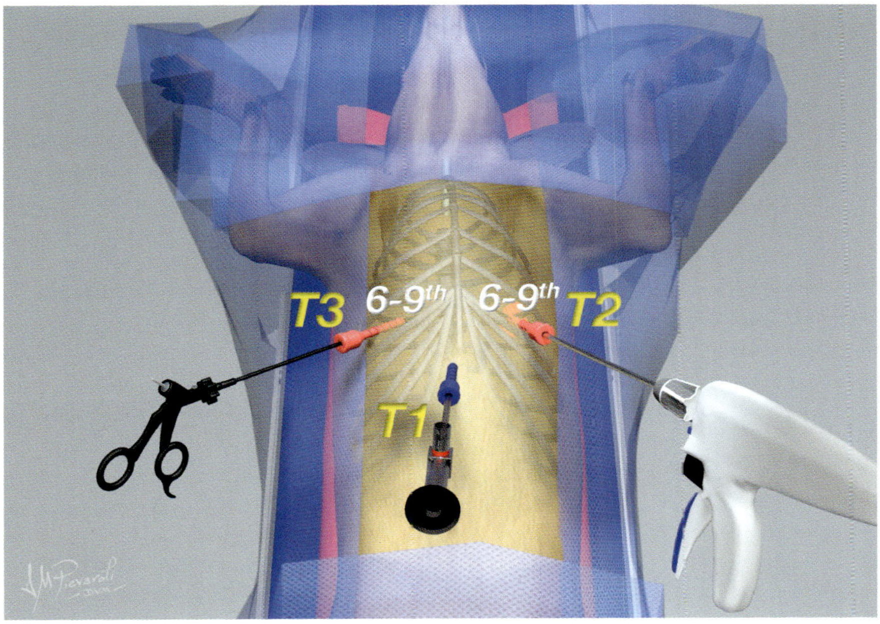

FIGURE 4. Port placement for left- and right-side approach, paraxiphoid or subxiphoid telescope location.

PROCEDURE (VIDEO 1)

- A 0.5–1 cm incision is made in a paraxiphoid or subxiphoid position for the insertion of a 5 mm cannula (T1). The 5 mm telescope is then inserted and a first exploration of the thorax is performed (**Fig. 6**).
- Under direct visualization, the second port is placed (T3 or T2) (**Fig. 7**).

VIDEO 1. Thoracoscopy for pericardial fenestration. Paraxiphoid access for the insertion of the camera and placement of two ports on the right hemithorax for the insertion of surgical instruments.

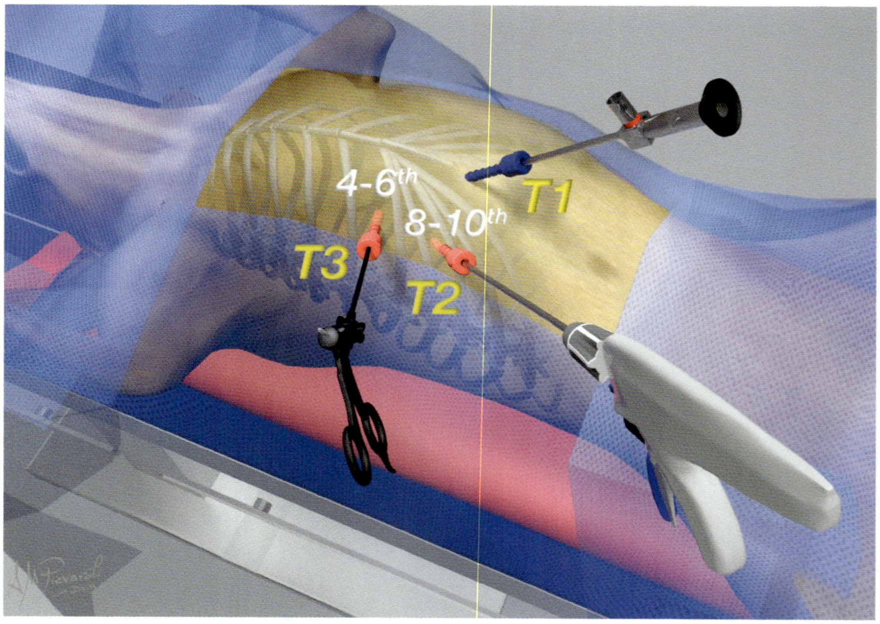

FIGURE 5. Port placement for right-side approach, paraxiphoid or subxiphoid telescope location.

- The ventral mediastinum is dissected free to improve visualization. The use of a vessel-sealing device is recommended to reduce bleeding (**Fig. 8**).
- The third port is placed (T3 or T2) (**Fig. 9**).
- Before starting the pericardiectomy, a thorough exploration of the thoracic cavity is performed to check for lesions (**Fig. 10**).
- Using grasping forceps, the pericardium over the cardiac apex is grasped and an incision is made using scissors (**Fig. 11**). If a lot of effusion is present, it may be difficult to grasp the pericardium due to excessive distension. In this case, a pericardiocentesis can be performed under direct visualization. The first pericardial incision can also be made using a vessel-sealing device, but a fold must be lifted to avoid touching the epicardium while the device is being operated.
- A variable amount of pericardial fluid will exit from the incision. To optimize visualization, an aspiration device can be inserted in T4 for the removal of the fluid (**Fig. 12**).
- While tension is exerted with the grasping forceps, a portion of at least 3–5×3–5 cm of pericardium over the cardiac apex is dissected using scissors or a vessel-sealing device (thus reducing hemorrhage) (**Fig. 13**).
- The authors recommend removing as much pericardial tissue as possible (**Fig. 14**).
- Small fragments of the pericardium can be extracted directly through the port cannulas. For the extraction of larger pieces of tissue, especially if the effusion is of neoplastic origin, the pericardium is retrieved from the thorax using a retrieval bag to minimize the risk of port-site metastasis.
- After performing the pericardial window, it is recommended to explore the pericardial sac (pericardioscopy). This is useful for visualizing lesions not always identifiable with preoperative investigations (**Fig. 15**).
- A chest drain is inserted and port incisions are closed in a routine manner (**Fig. 16**).

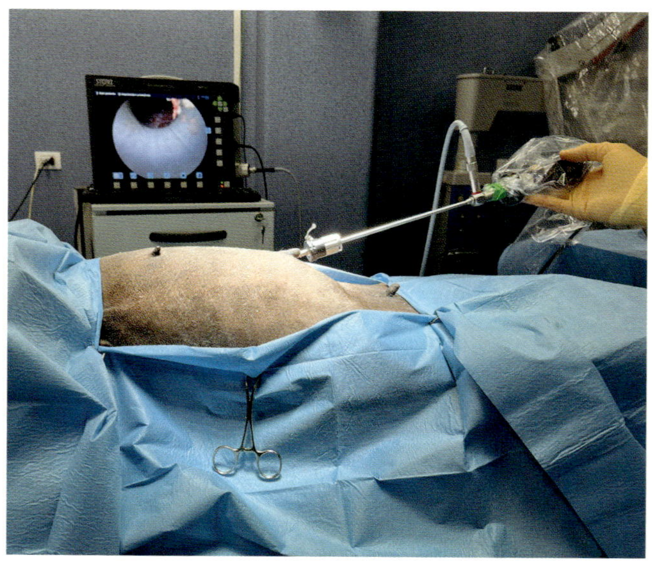

FIGURE 6. Placement of the first port, for the optic.

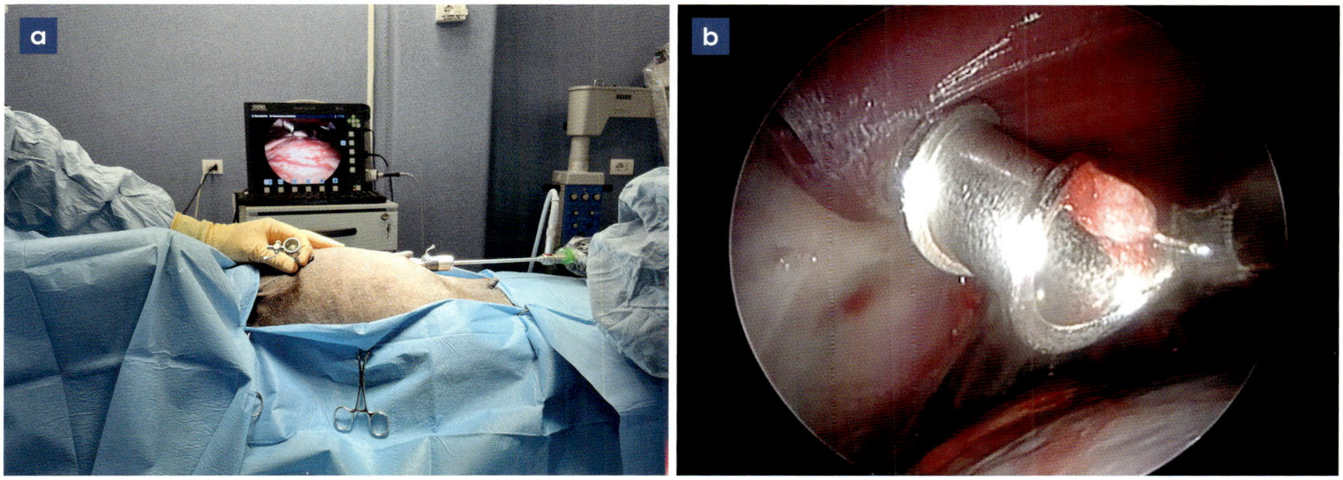

FIGURE 7. Placement of the second port under direct vision. a) From the outside. b) From the inside.

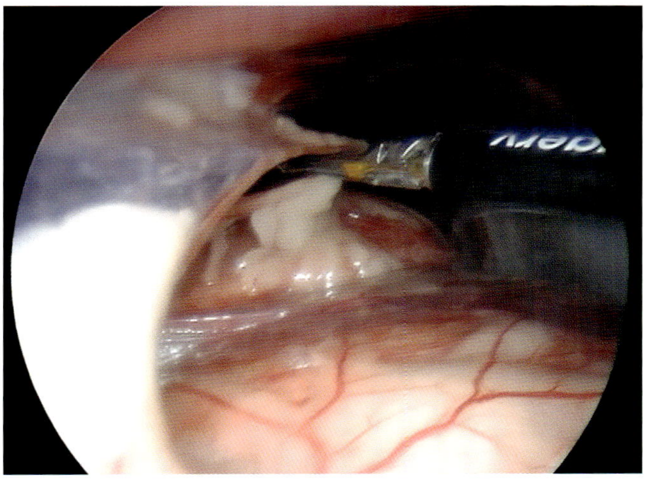

FIGURE 8. Mediastinum dissection with a vessel-sealing device.

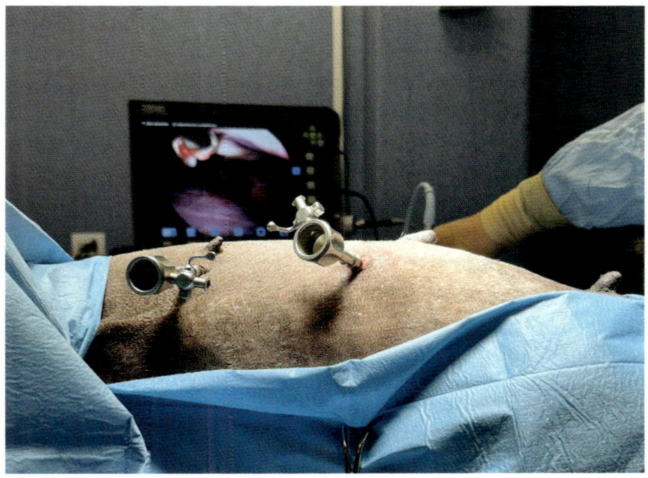

FIGURE 9. Placement of the third port.

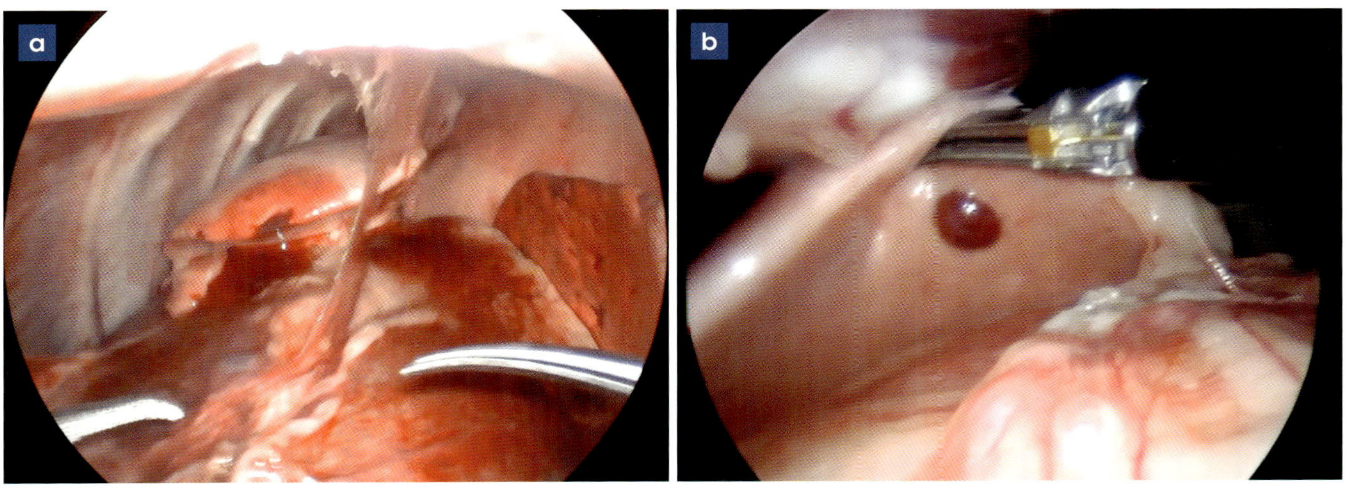

FIGURE 10. Initial exploration of the thorax. a) After dissection of the ventral mediastinum, both sides of the thoracic cavity are explored. This inspection is not always feasible in some flat-chested dogs. b) During the inspection, a lung lesion is detected after lifting a lobe.

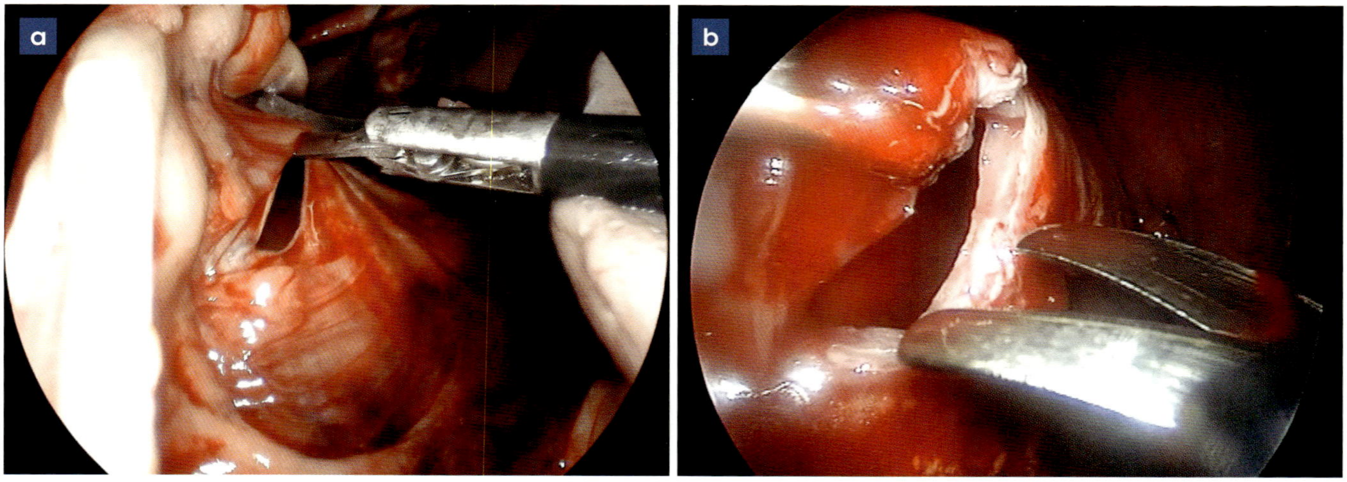

FIGURE 11. a) The cardiac apex is grasped and an incision is made using scissors. b) In chronic inflammatory diseases, thickening of the pericardium is evident.

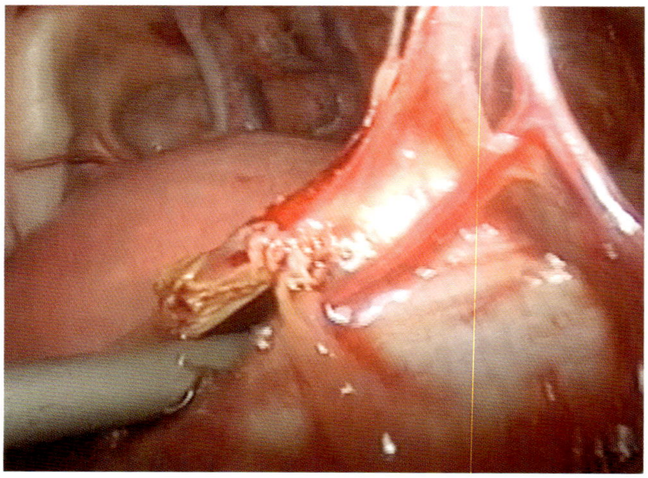

FIGURE 12. Pericardial fluid removal with an aspiration device.

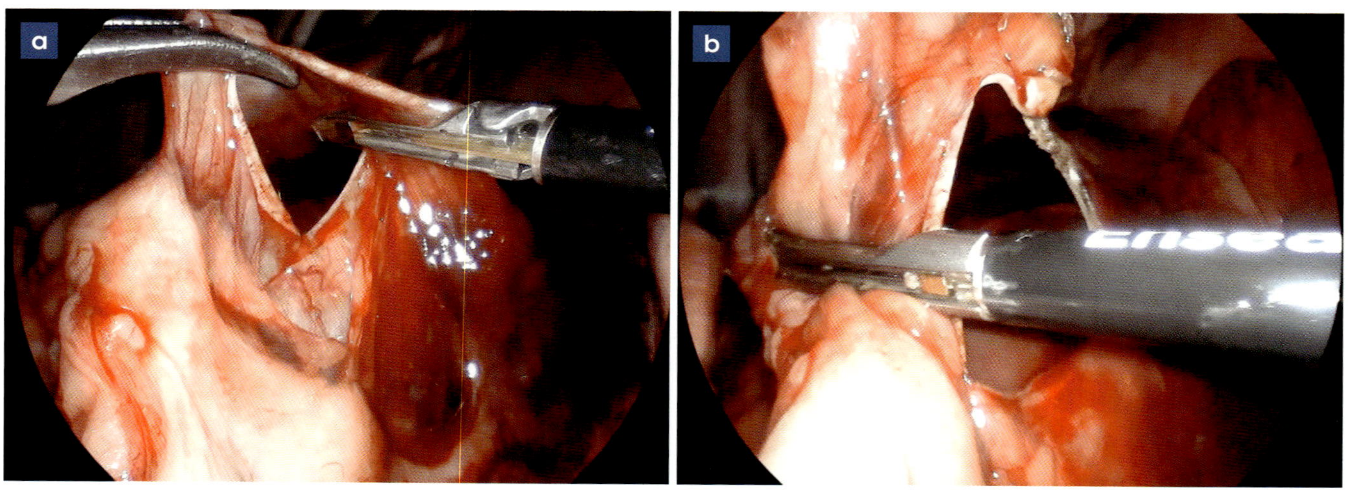

FIGURE 13. Pericardium dissection using a vessel-sealing device. This is useful, especially in cases of chronic disease with significant vascularization, to reduce bleeding.

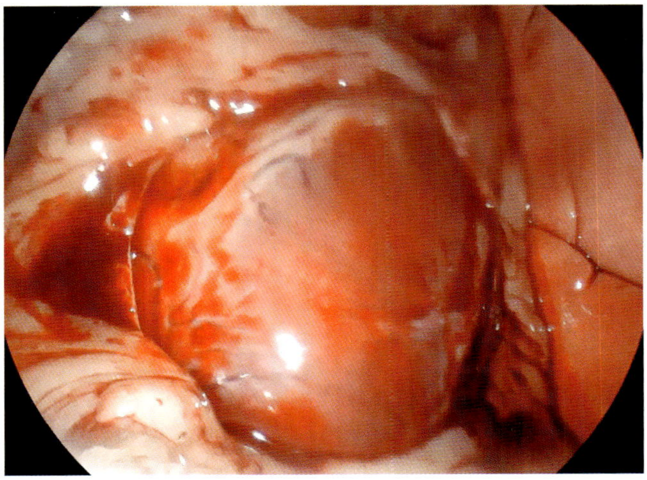

FIGURE 14. Image of the pericardial window.

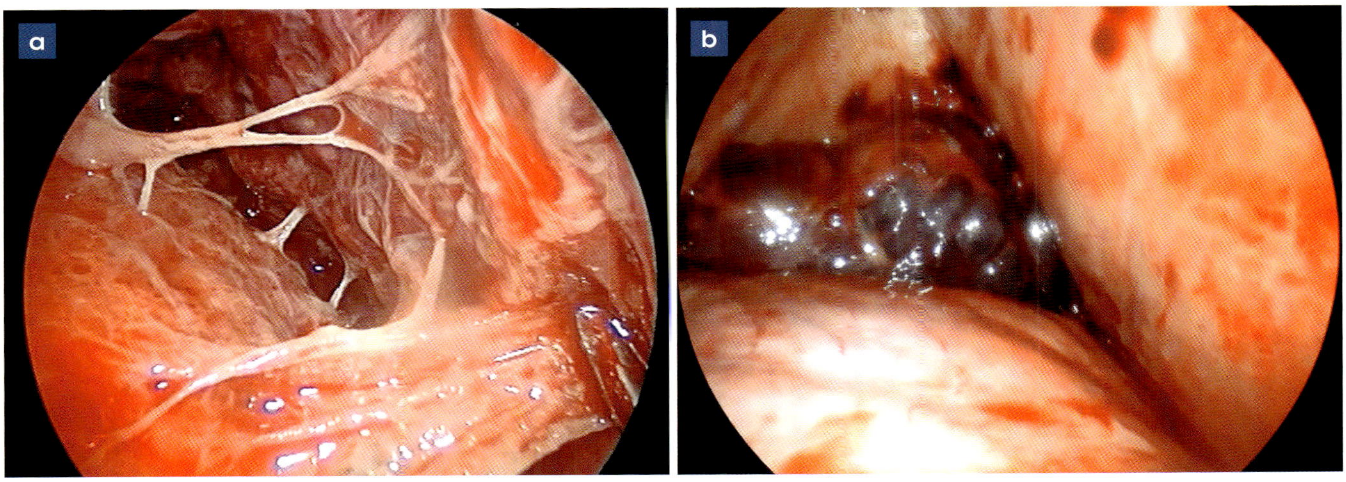

FIGURE 15. Pericardioscopy is useful for visualizing lesions not always identifiable with preoperative investigations. a) Adhesions in idiopathic pericarditis. b) Mass arising from the left atrium.

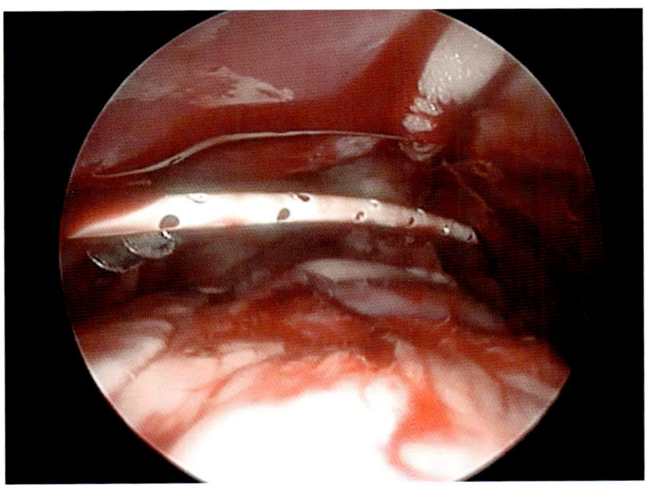

FIGURE 16. Insertion of a chest drain.

B PERICARDIAL WINDOW IN LATERAL RECUMBENCY

PATIENT PREPARATION AND POSITIONING

The patient is placed in right or left lateral recumbency. The entire hemithorax is clipped, from the scapular spine to the cranial abdomen and from the dorsal spine to the sternum. Right lateral recumbency allows better visualization of the heart base and right atrium.

OPERATING ROOM LAYOUT

The surgeon and the assistant position themselves on the patient's side, facing the dog's thorax. The endoscopic tower is placed on the patient's contralateral side (**Fig. 17**).

PORT PLACEMENT (FIG. 18)

- T1, in the ventral third of 5th–7th intercostal space (alternatively, 10th intercostal space)
- T2, in the mid to dorsal third of the 8th–10th intercostal space (alternatively, 8th intercostal space)
- T3, in the mid to dorsal third of the 3rd–7th intercostal space (alternatively, 6th intercostal space)

PROCEDURE

- The procedure is similar to that described for the pericardial window in dorsal recumbency.
- After placing the ports, the pericardium is grasped ventral to the phrenic nerve and a lateral incision is made with scissors, avoiding damage to the ipsilateral lung. Exerting traction on the pericardium, the dissection is continued using a vessel-sealing device as previously described.

C SUBTOTAL PERICARDIECTOMY

The right and left phrenic nerves run in a narrow plica of pleura near the base of the heart and spread out on their respective half of the diaphragm (**Fig. 19**). Subtotal pericardiectomy allows the removal of the entire pericardium 1–2 cm ventral to the phrenic nerves. It is indicated in cases of idiopathic or neoplastic pericardial effusion and infections and is considered the treatment of choice for constrictive pericarditis.

The procedure is more challenging than creating a pericardial window due to the increased risk of phrenic nerve damage. However, it allows a larger portion of pericardium to be submitted for histopathology, improving diagnostic accuracy. It also permits a thorough exploration of the epicardium and part of right and left atria and auricles, aortic root and pulmonary artery.

Subtotal pericardiectomy can be performed with the patient in dorsal or lateral recumbency. When the patient is placed in dorsal recumbency, subtotal pericardiectomy can be performed using a right–left approach or a right approach.

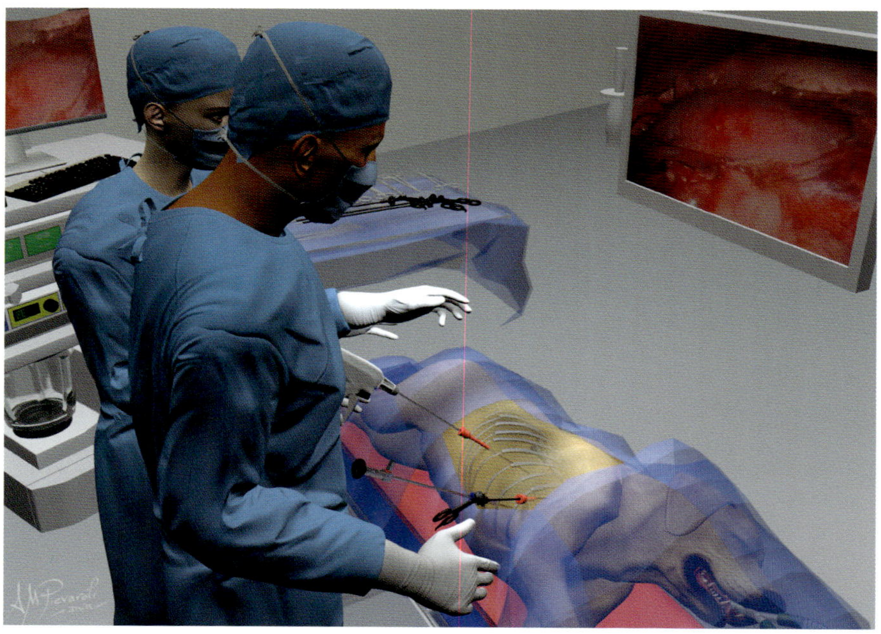

FIGURE 17. Operating room layout for pericardial window in lateral recumbency.

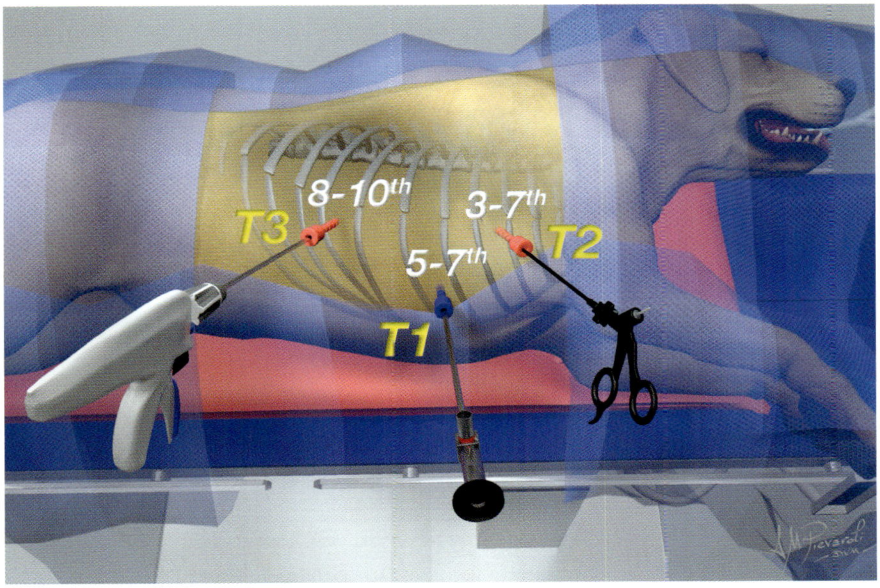

FIGURE 18. Port placement for pericardial window in lateral recumbency.

PROCEDURE

- Port placement for subtotal pericardiectomy is the same as described for pericardial window, with the patient either in dorsal or in lateral recumbency (see procedures A and B above).
- The ventral mediastinum is dissected free to improve visualization. The use of a vessel-sealing device is recommended to reduce bleeding.
- Using grasping forceps, the pericardium over the cardiac apex is grasped and an incision is made using scissors.

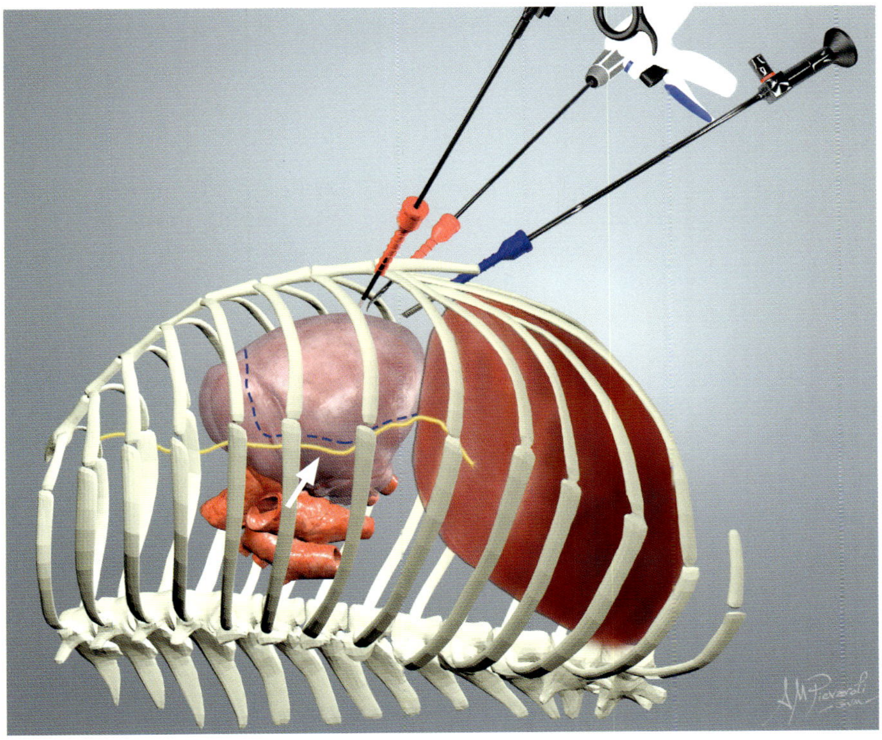

FIGURE 19. Illustration showing the course of the right phrenic nerve (arrow). It runs in a narrow plica of pleura near the base of the heart and spreads out on the right half of the diaphragm. The dotted line indicates the ideal safety margin to avoid damaging the phrenic nerves.

- A variable amount of pericardial fluid will exit from the incision. To optimize visualization, an aspiration device can be inserted in T4 for the removal of the fluid.
- Pericardiectomy is started caudolaterally from the initial rent, toward the diaphragm and up to 1–2 cm to the right phrenic nerve. It is then directed cranially while placing caudoventral tension on the pericardium to help the maneuver.
- A similar procedure is performed on the left side of the pericardium until the lines of dissection join (**Fig. 20**).
- The pericardium is retrieved from the thorax using a retrieval bag to minimize the risk of port-site metastasis.
- A chest drain is inserted and port incisions are closed in a routine manner.

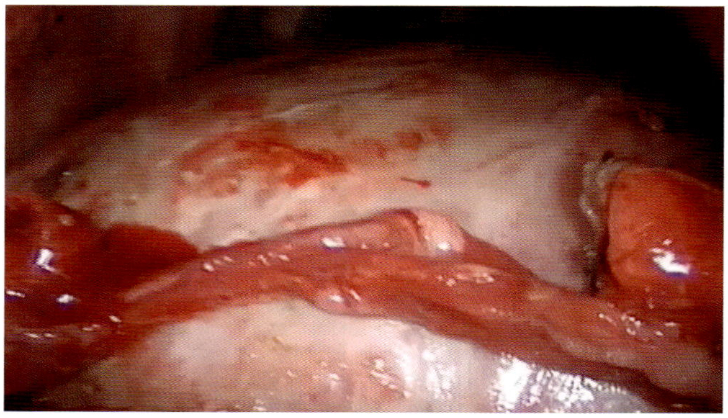

FIGURE 20. Completed subtotal pericardiectomy.

POSTOPERATIVE MANAGEMENT

- Postoperative X-rays are essential to rule out the presence of residual air or fluid and to evaluate the correct placement of thoracostomy tube.
- In the postoperative period, aspiration from the chest drain can be performed every 12–24 hours. The chest drain is left in place until small quantities of air or fluid are collected in a day.
- Even though thoracoscopy is associated with less pain than thoracotomy, analgesia is warranted to control pain that can cause hypoventilation and hypoxia. Local anesthetics, intrapleural application of anesthetics, systemic analgesia, and the use of flexible ports contribute to pain control.

Complications of thoracoscopic pericardiectomy

- Bleeding from lesions to intercostal vessels during port placement or pleural biopsy, thoracic structures (mediastinum, lymph nodes, lungs, heart), and masses/tumors.
- Pneumothorax due to inadvertent lung injury.
- Difficulty in visualization caused by adhesions, excessive bleeding, inadequate working space, or patient's anatomy. This may warrant conversion to an open approach.
- To the authors' knowledge, there are no reports of port-site metastasis following pericardiectomy, as there are in a case of mesothelioma and of a mediastinal mass. The use of a retrieval bag is helpful to reduce the risk of port-site metastasis.

Key points

- In cases of cardiac tamponade, perform pericardiocentesis before thoracoscopy to reduce the risk associated with anesthesia.
- Rolling the pericardium around the grasping forceps helps maintain adequate tension during pericardiectomy.
- Pericardioscopy is warranted to rule out the presence of masses or nodules not detected with ultrasonography.
- If the pericardium is very thick and inflamed, great care must be taken during dissection to reduce the risk of phrenic nerve injury.
- Be careful not to touch the myocardium with electric devices because arrhythmias, even severe, can occur.

SUGGESTED READINGS

CLINICAL CASES

50.1 TWO-PORT THORACOSCOPIC PERICARDIECTOMY AS A NOVEL TECHNIQUE IN FLAT-CHESTED DOGS WITH REDUCED THORACIC WORKING SPACES

Andrea M. Pievaroli

CASE DESCRIPTION

An English Bulldog with pericardial effusion, pleural effusion, and ascites due to a neoplastic lesion at the base of the heart was referred for thoracoscopic pericardiectomy. X-rays also showed an increased cardiac silhouette that occupied a large part of the chest cavity, close to the diaphragm and thoracic walls. Before surgery, the patient was sedated to perform a pericardiocentesis to reduce the pressure over the cardiac muscle and to reduce anesthesiological risks. Fluid was also aspirated from the abdominal cavity to reduce the compression of the diaphragm during surgery.

As expected, the conformation of the patient's chest made the thoracoscopic procedure very difficult to perform. There was no working space after inserting the first lateral intercostal instrument. In addition, the view from the telescope at the central paraxiphoid port was very limited. After 30 minutes without success, it was decided to approach the pericardium exclusively via the central access, the only port that allowed a minimum view of the apex of heart. A second paraxiphoid port was placed parallel to the first one, through which an arthroscopic hook knife was inserted to make a longitudinal cut in the pericardium, carefully under telescope view. Then, with endoscopic scissors and the hook knife, more incisions were made in different directions to release the pericardium as if peeling a banana. Fluid was aspirated, and a drainage was placed to continue suction in the following hours. This technique was later repeated with success in other dogs with a reduced thoracic working space.

Key points

- Safe procedure that avoids conversion, but more challenging to perform than three-port pericardiectomy.
- Pericardiocentesis should be performed before surgery.

PORT PLACEMENT

- Patient in dorsal recumbency
- T1, right paraxiphoid access for the telescope
- T2, left paraxiphoid access for the instruments

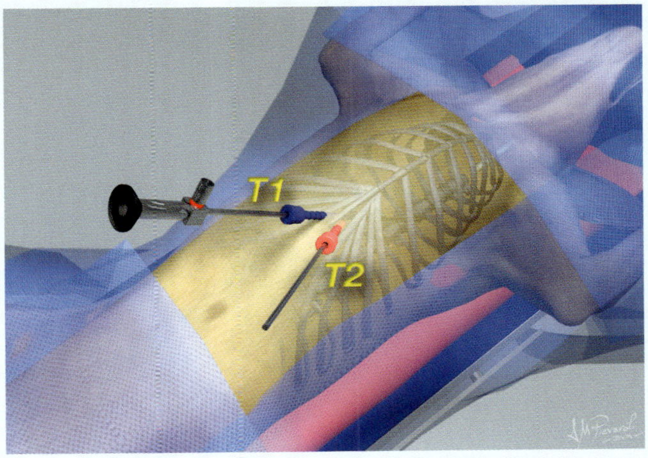

PROCEDURE

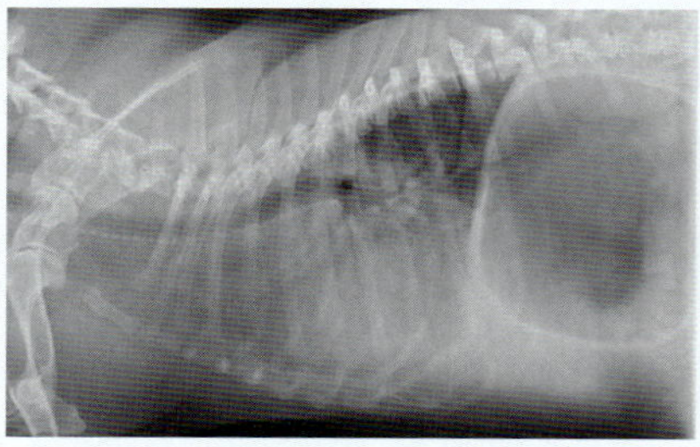

FIGURE 1. Preoperative X-ray showing a large cardiac silhouette that extends near the diaphragm.

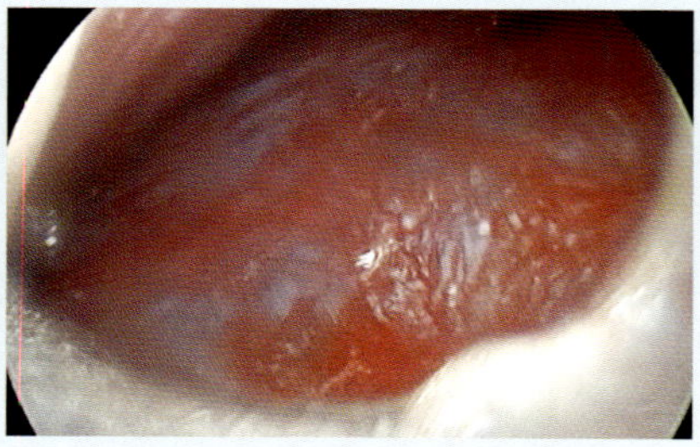

FIGURE 2. Thoracoscopic view from paraxiphoid access (T1). The pericardial sac is adjacent to the diaphragm and the working space is extremely limited.

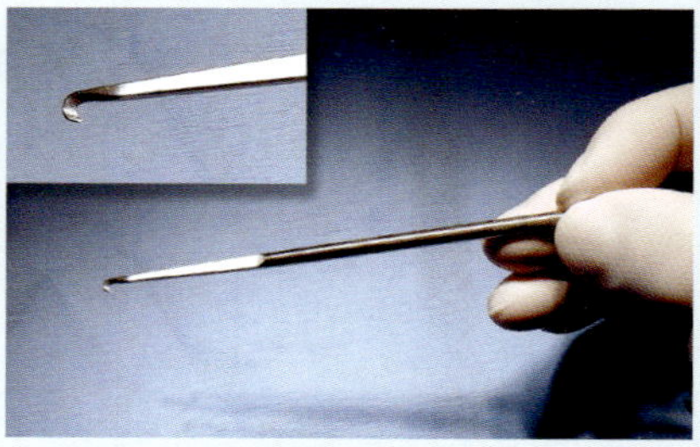

FIGURE 3. Arthroscopy hook knife used to make the incision in the pericardium.

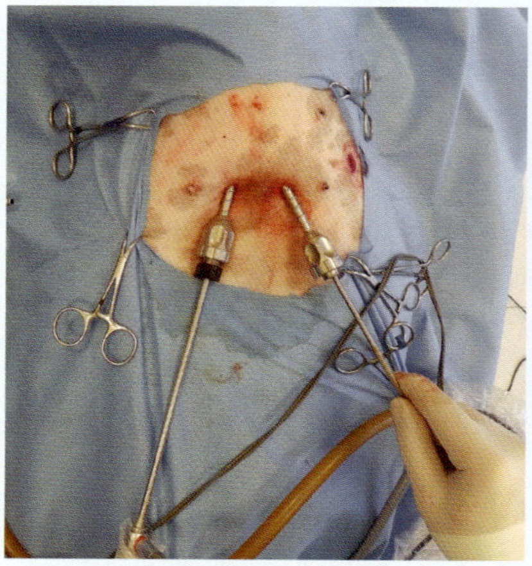

FIGURE 4. Image of the operative field for the two-port technique.

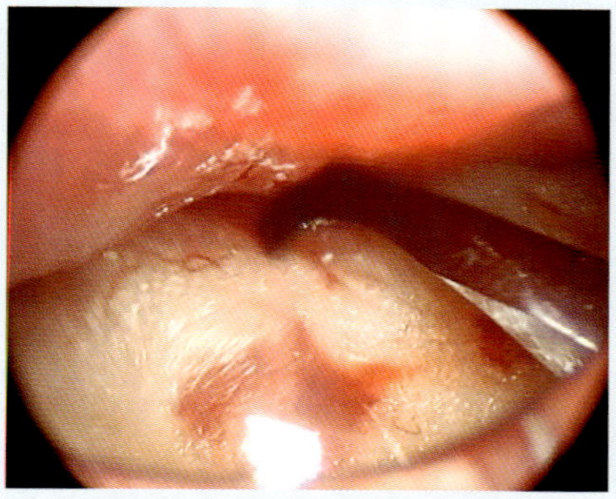

FIGURE 5. The hook knife is inserted in T2.

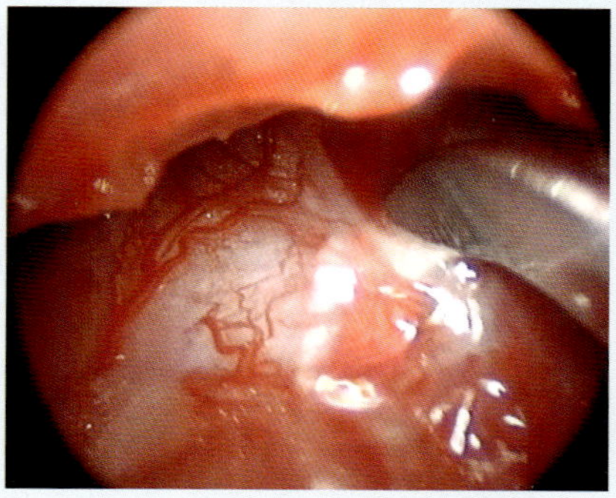

FIGURE 6. The tip of the hook has just started to make the incision in the pericardium.

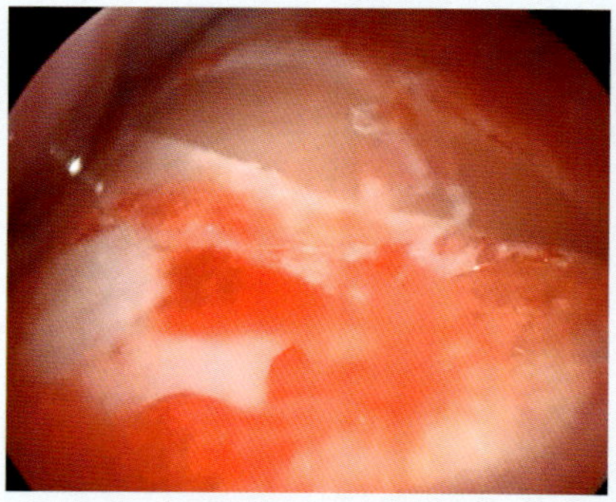

FIGURE 7. View of the longitudinal incision.

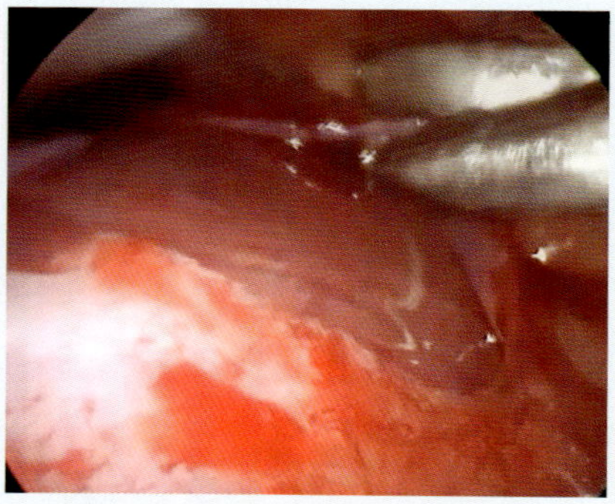

FIGURE 8. After draining the pericardium, more working space is available. Endoscopic scissors are used to make radial incisions.

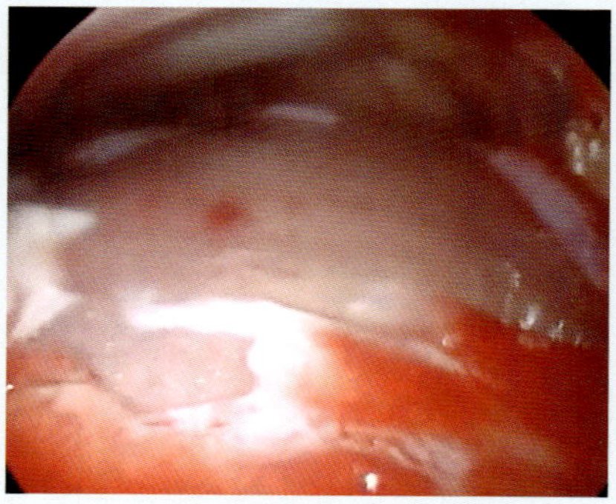

FIGURE 9. Finally, a large pericardial window is obtained.

Tips and tricks

✓ The cutting edge of the hook must be sharp.

✓ If there is little pericardial effusion, be careful not to damage the myocardium.

50.2 THORACOSCOPIC SUBPHRENIC (SUBTOTAL) PERICARDIECTOMY

Giovanni Allevi

CASE DESCRIPTION

An 8-year-old spayed female German Shepherd Dog was referred for surgical treatment of recurrent pericardial effusion. Ultrasound and CT scans led to the diagnosis of idiopathic pericarditis. A three-port thoracoscopic subphrenic pericardiectomy was performed (trocar 5 mm) (VersaPort, Covidien, Medtronic, Milano, Italy) using a vessel-sealing device (LigaSure, Medtronic).

Key points

- Incising the pericardium is the most challenging part of the procedure. It is important to lift the pericardium away from the myocardium to avoid thermal and electrical injury.
- Care should be taken not to damage the phrenic nerve.

PORT PLACEMENT

The patient was placed in dorsal recumbency and prepared for surgery. A 0.5 cm incision was made at the level of the 6th right intercostal space and the first trocar was inserted. The subxiphoid port was then placed and a 5 mm 30° telescope (Karl Storz Veterinary Endoscopy) was introduced. Finally, the third port was placed at the level of 6th left intercostal space.

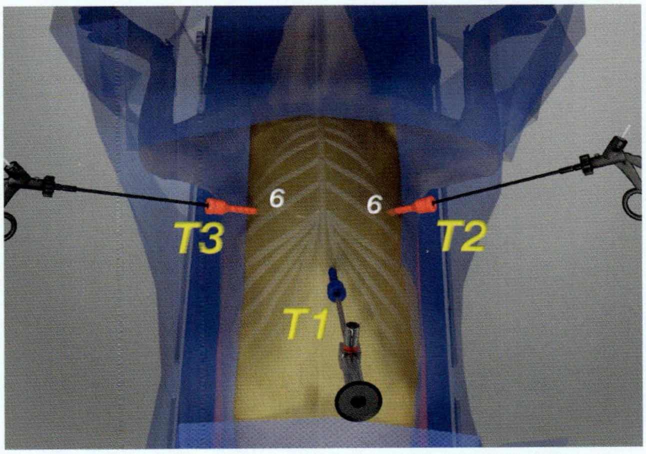

PROCEDURE

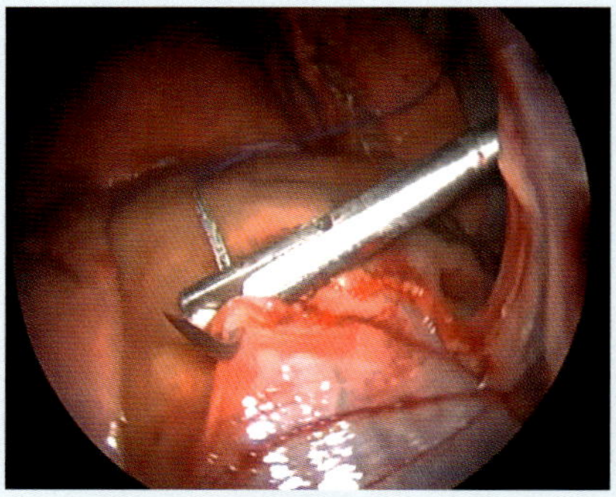

FIGURE 1. A stay suture is placed in the pericardium to lift it and cut it without damaging the myocardium.

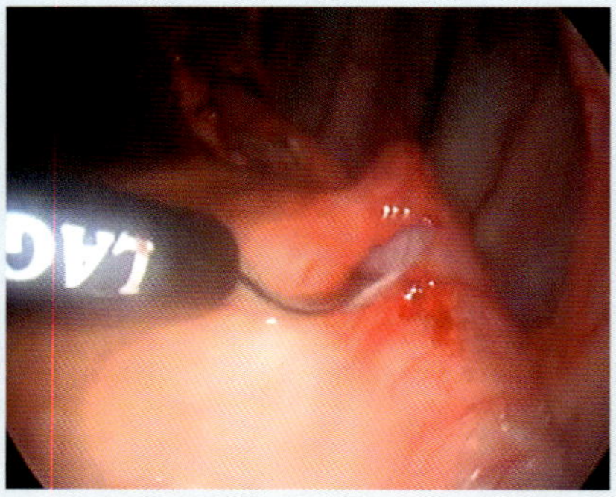

FIGURE 2. The pericardium is incised with laparoscopic scissors.

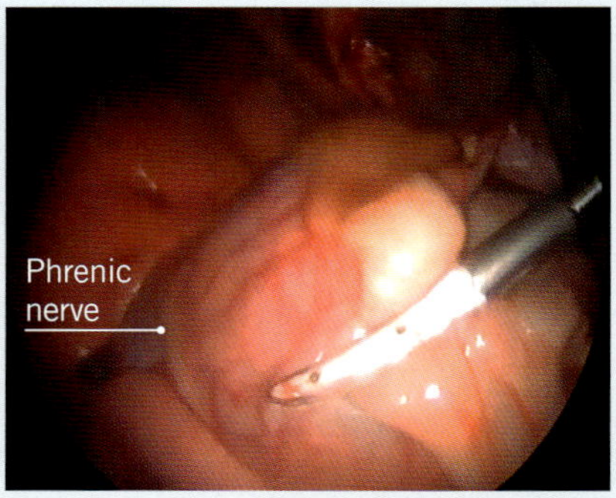

FIGURE 3. A 4×4 cm portion of pericardium was removed and a subphrenic pericardiectomy was performed with a vessel-sealing device. During pericardiectomy, attention must be paid not to damage the phrenic nerve.

Tips and tricks

✓ It is easier to insert one trocar into the intercostal space first and then place the subxiphoid port under endoscopic vision.

✓ The author recommends stretching the pericardium with a stay suture before cutting it, especially if a small amount of pericardial effusion is present.

51 THORACOSCOPIC THORACIC DUCT LIGATION FOR TREATMENT OF CHYLOTHORAX

J. Brad Case

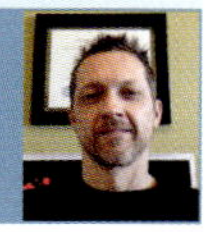

Indications

- Treatment of idiopathic chylothorax
- Thoracic duct anatomy amenable to ligation via thoracoscopy

Contraindications

- No explicit contraindications for thoracoscopic thoracic duct ligation have been identified
- Unstable dogs with cardiopulmonary disease
- Inexperience with thoracoscopic surgery

Chylothorax is the pathological accumulation of chyle within the thoracic cavity. Although it is rare in dogs and cats, it is associated with significant morbidity and mortality. The potential causes include traumatic thoracic duct rupture, neoplasia, cardiomyopathy, heartworm disease, restrictive pericarditis, and lung lobe torsion. However, most cases in dogs are idiopathic. Chronic idiopathic chylothorax will result in restrictive pleural fibrosis and is labor-intensive to manage medically in many cases. Consequently, early surgical treatment is indicated to minimize the risk of pleural fibrosis. Clinical signs such as restrictive dyspnea, tachycardia, lethargy, and hyporexia are commonly reported. Reduced or absent bronchovesicular sounds on thoracic auscultation is a typical finding. Afghan Hounds, Shetland Sheepdogs, and Shiba Inus are overrepresented. The definitive diagnosis of chylothorax is made by measuring fluid triglyceride levels and comparing them with serum triglyceride levels. Dogs with true chylous effusion will have fluid triglyceride levels significantly higher than serum levels.

Chest X-rays demonstrate increased radiopacity in the pleural space, with concomitant dorsal elevation and scalloping of the lung lobes on the lateral view. CT lymphangiography is the procedure of choice for imaging of the thoracic duct and cisterna chyli. It is an important diagnostic test in the presurgical evaluation of patients with chylothorax.

Thoracic duct ligation (TDL) is the most common surgical treatment for dogs with chylothorax, and it can readily be performed via thoracoscopy. It is routinely combined with thoracoscopic pericardiectomy, although cisterna chyli ablation or lymphatic embolization have also recently been described.

> The first clinical report of thoracoscopic thoracic duct ligation in dogs was published in 2010 by Allman D. A. et al.

DESCRIBED SURGICAL PROCEDURES

A three-port thoracoscopic technique with or without a flank minilaparotomy has been described. If the flank minilaparotomy is not used, access to a popliteal lymph node is necessary. Advantages of the minilaparotomy are improved access to mesenteric lymph nodes and lymphatic channels and improved opacification of the thoracic duct with dyeing agents. The main advantage of the popliteal approach is less tissue trauma.

PATIENT PREPARATION AND POSITIONING

A physical examination, complete blood count, serum biochemistry, heartworm test, and pleural fluid analysis including triglycerides should be performed prior to surgery. Diagnostic imaging including thoracic radiography, echocardiography, and CT lymphangiography are also essential. In general, the patient should be fasted for at least 8 hours prior to anesthesia and have an IV catheter placed for fluid and medication therapy during the procedure. Cream can be administered orally the evening prior to surgery to improve visualization of the lymphatics. Perioperative analgesia may include opioid and/or nonsteroidal medications. Local anesthesia with bupivacaine is recommended at individual port sites prior to incision.

Following a 360° clip including the chest and abdomen, the patient is aseptically prepared according to standard techniques. Both sternal and semilateral patient positioning have been described, but the author prefers to place the patient in sternal recumbency, as disruption of the operative field by lung motion and pleural fluid is eliminated due to gravity. Sternal recumbency is facilitated by placing rolled towels under the patient's axillary and inguinal regions (**Fig. 1**).

OPERATING ROOM LAYOUT

Thoracoscopic TDL is typically performed with the operating surgeon and the assistant standing on the patient's right side. The monitors should be placed on the patient's left side to facilitate appropriate triangulation. The anesthesia circuit and staff are placed at the head of the operating table. The instrument table is placed near the patient's head (**Fig. 2**). If thoracoscopic pericardiectomy is also performed, repositioning of the patient into dorsal recumbency is typically required. See Chapter 50 for details on the operating room layout for pericardiectomy.

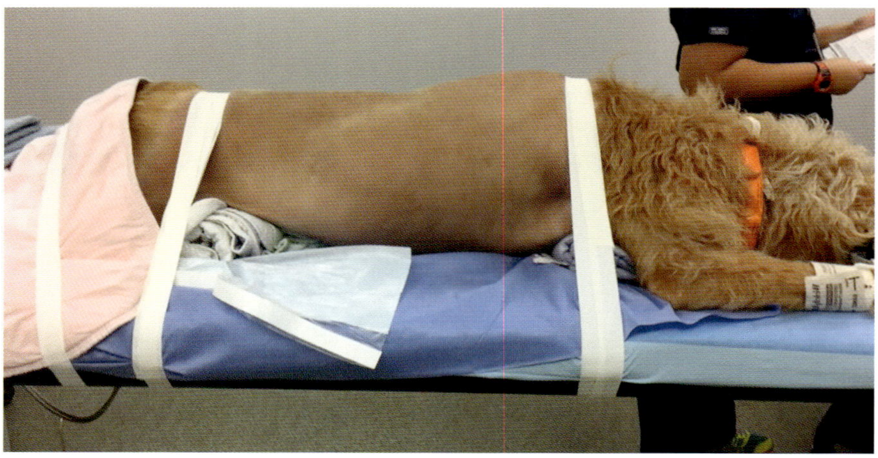

FIGURE 1. Preoperative patient positioning in sternal recumbency for thoracoscopic thoracic duct ligation. Note the rolled towels under the inguinal and axillary regions to help stabilize the patient during the procedure.

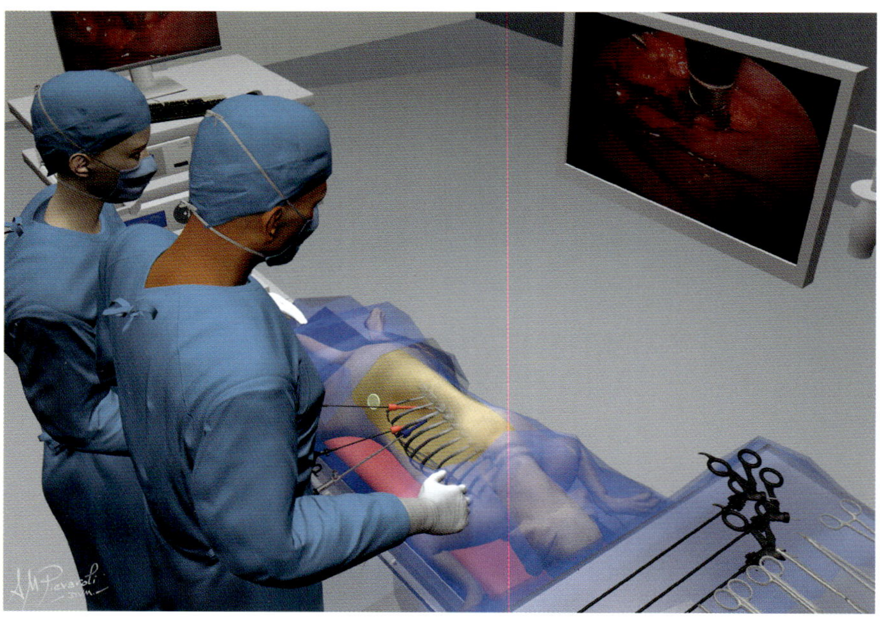

FIGURE 2. Operating room layout for thoracoscopic thoracic duct ligation.

Instruments

On the table:

- Standard surgical pack
- High-definition video camera
- Telescope 5 mm – 30°
- Two 5 mm threaded cannulas + one 12 mm threaded cannula
- Laparoscopic Babcock, Kelley, right-angle forceps, 5 mm
- Laparoscopic cotton-tip (endopeanuts), blunt dissection probes, 5 mm
- L- or J-hook monopolar electrosurgical tip, 5 mm
- 10 mm titanium endoscopic clips (endoclips)
- Pharmaceutical grade methylene blue
- 3–5 cm wound retractor

PORT PLACEMENT (FIGS. 3 AND 4)

- T1, in the middle third of the 10th intercostal space, thoracoscope port
- T2, in the dorsal third of the 11th intercostal space, dissection instrument port
- T3, in the dorsal third of the 12th intercostal space, dissection instrument port
- Wound retractor, in the caudoventral region of the right flank

PROCEDURE

- After all the ports have been placed, suction of the remaining chylous effusion in the right hemithorax is advised to improve the working space and visualization of the caudal mediastinum.
- A mesenteric lymph node is then isolated (**Fig. 5**). Typically, 1–2 mL of a 1:1 mixture of methylene blue and sterile saline is injected slowly at the ileocecocolic junction using a 25-gauge needle. This will opacify the thoracic duct within 2–3 minutes.

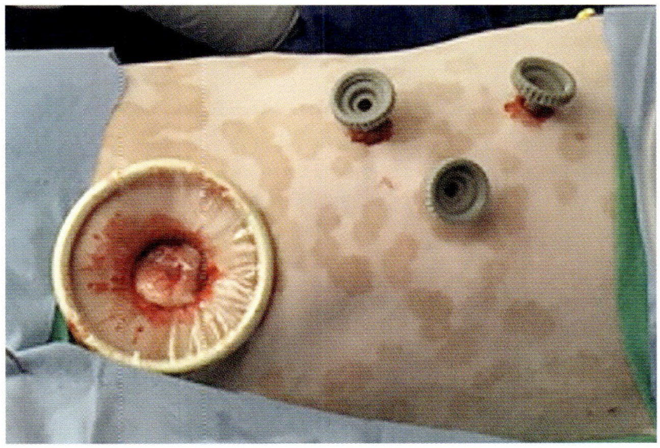

FIGURE 4. Port placement for thoracoscopic thoracic duct ligation, with the patient in sternal recumbency. Note the caudal thoracic thoracoscopy ports and the wound retractor placed in the flank minilaparotomy for lymph node access.

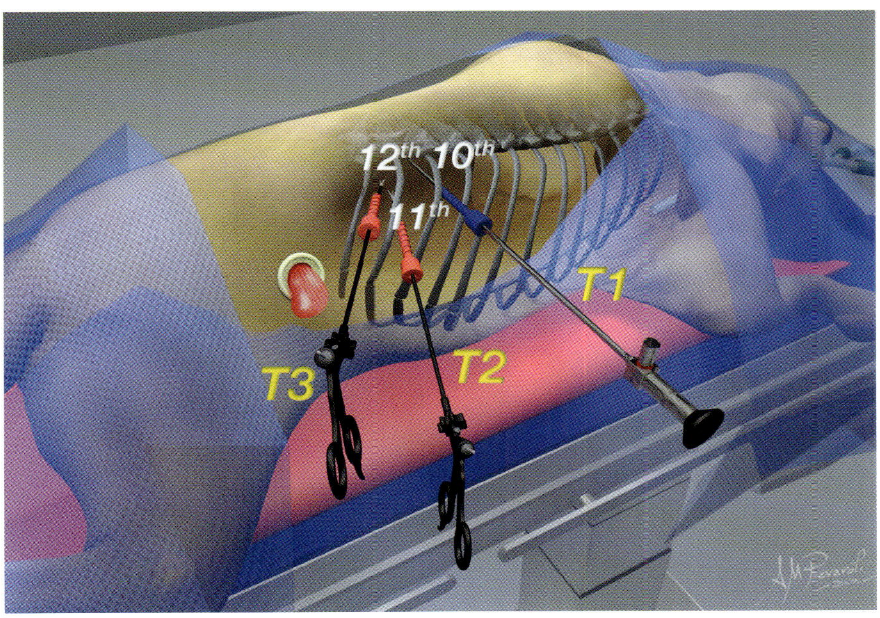

FIGURE 3. Port placement for thoracoscopic thoracic duct ligation.

- Dissection of the mediastinum is initiated after thoracic duct branches have been dye opacified to reduce the risk of inadvertent laceration (**Fig. 6**). Dissection begins in a region in the right caudal hemithorax near the lateral aorta and is extended as dorsal as is necessary but below the sympathetic trunk. Further dissection dorsal and medial to the aorta may be needed to access all the thoracic duct branches. Individual branches are isolated, undermined with dissection forceps, and clipped with an endoscopic clip applier. It is important to place at least two clips per branch and to make sure that the clips are placed across the entire width of the branch.

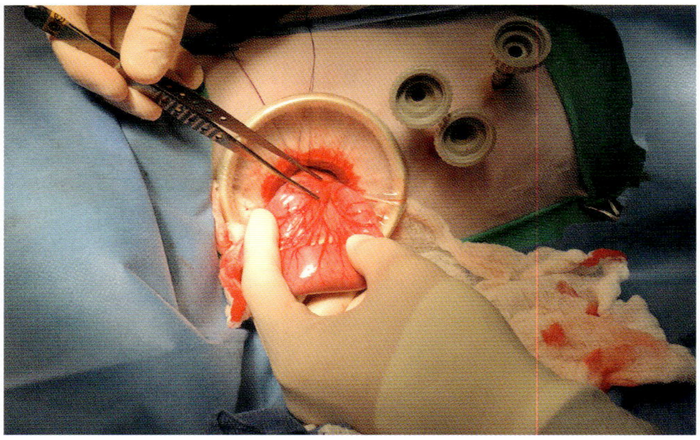

FIGURE 5. Isolation of a mesenteric lymph node for lymphangiography. Note the caudal thoracic intercostal ports between the 9th and 11th intercostal spaces and the 3–5 cm wound retractor.

- All the thoracic duct branches observed on preoperative CT lymphangiography should be accounted for (**Fig. 7**). In some cases, up to five individual branches may be present. Caution and careful dissection are critical to avoid damage to the regional vasculature (aorta, azygous vein, vertebral vessels).
- Following ligation of the branches, a thoracostomy tube is placed. The author prefers to use a small-gauge drain (e.g., Mila 14 Fr) for postoperative monitoring.
- Thoracoscopic ports are removed under endoscopic visualization to ensure that no hemorrhage from the intercostal

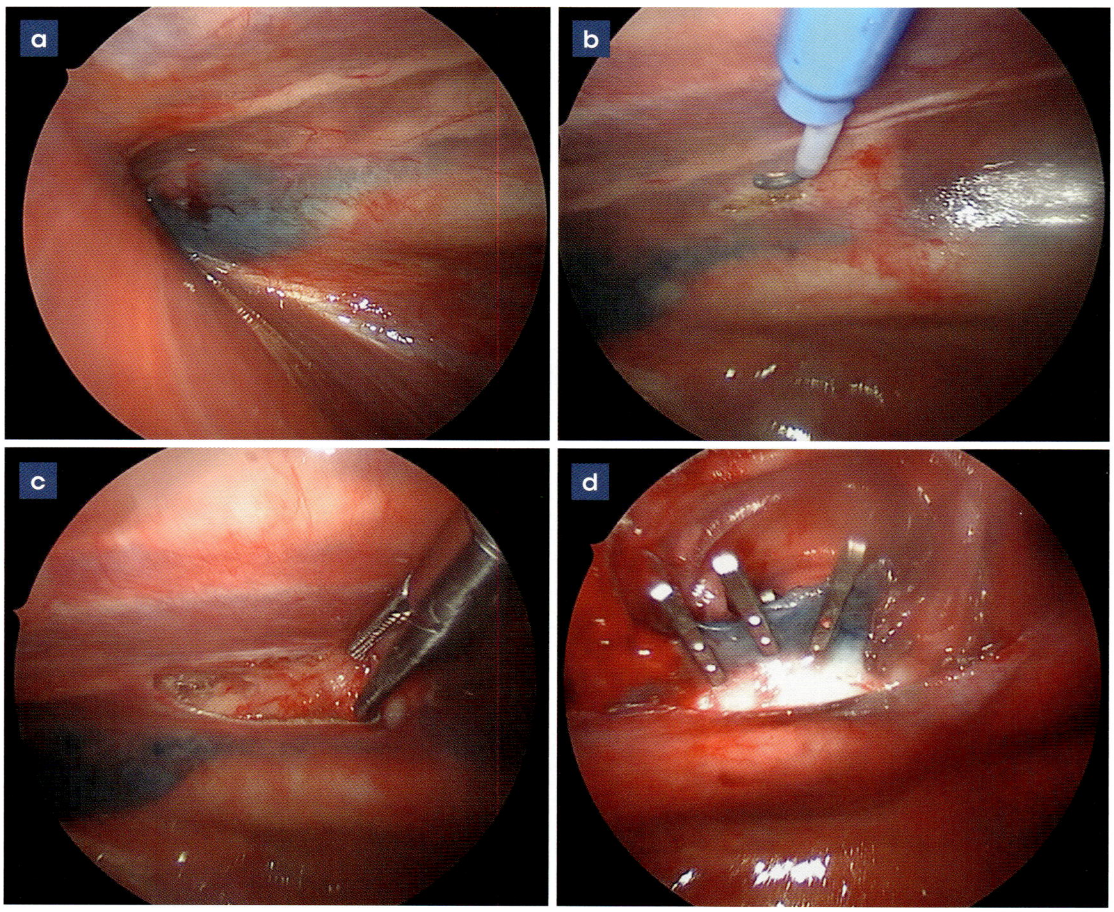

FIGURE 6. Thoracoscopic series of images showing dissection of the cisterna chyli and caudal thoracic duct. Electrosurgical and blunt dissection are performed prior to ligation of all the thoracic duct branches.

vessels is present. Port incisions are typically closed in two layers.

- The flank minilaparotomy is closed routinely, being sure to close all abdominal muscle layers individually followed by the subcutaneous tissue and skin.
- If pericardiectomy is performed, the patient needs to be repositioned into dorsal recumbency and standard subxiphoid ports are placed. See Chapter 50 for further details on the pericardiectomy procedure

POSTOPERATIVE MANAGEMENT

- Intraoperative infiltration of the port sites with local anesthetic affords 4–6 hours of analgesia postoperatively.
- The combination of nonsteroidal anti-inflammatory medication (3–5 days) and systemic opioids (12–36 hours) is generally effective for uncomplicated thoracoscopic surgery.
- Monitoring of pleural fluid production via the chest drain is recommended for 2–3 days postoperatively.
- Recheck examination with chest X-rays at 2 and 6 weeks is recommended.

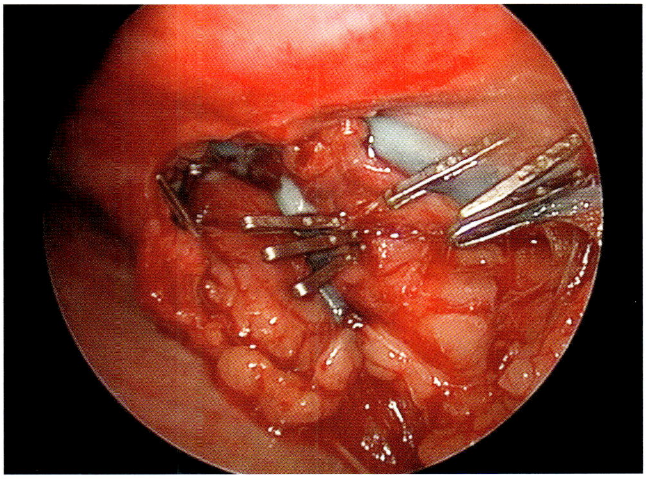

FIGURE 7. Thoracoscopic image after isolation and ligation of three thoracic duct branches.

- If continued pleural fluid accumulation is seen, the triglyceride content of the effusion is measured. If consistent with chylothorax, repeat CT lymphangiography is indicated for detection of missed thoracic duct branches or collateral vessel formation.

Complications of thoracoscopic thoracic duct ligation

- Port-site hemorrhage can occur after removal of intercostal ports. In some cases, bleeding from intercostal arteries may necessitate reoperation to locate and ligate the affected intercostal vessel. It is recommended that all ports sites are monitored endoscopically during port removal.
- Significant intercostal vessel hemorrhage may occur during dissection of the thoracic duct branches. It is important to have bipolar energy or vascular clips available to ligate the ruptured vessel.
- Thoracic duct laceration is also a risk during dissection. Placement of endoclips on both sides of the affected branch is necessary if this occurs. Thoracic duct branches can be adhered to the aorta or free in the dorsal mediastinum and tend to be relatively friable. Thus, caution should be exercised when manipulating and dissecting thoracic duct branches.

Key points

- Preoperative CT lymphangiography and intraoperative dye opacification of the thoracic duct is necessary to ensure that all the thoracic duct branches are ligated.
- Thoracoscopic TDL and pericardiectomy is associated with an 86% long-term success rate for the treatment of idiopathic chylothorax in dogs.

SUGGESTED READINGS

CLINICAL CASES

51.1 BILATERAL EN BLOC THORACIC DUCT LIGATION IN COMBINATION WITH PERICARDIECTOMY BY VIDEO-ASSISTED THORACOSCOPIC SURGERY FOR IDIOPATHIC CHYLOTHORAX IN A DOG

Hiroo Kanai

CASE DESCRIPTION

A 4-year-old neutered female Shiba Inu weighing 12.4 kg was referred by another veterinary hospital with a diagnosis of idiopathic chylothorax. The dog was treated with thoracentesis and medications to resolve the pleural effusion but experienced recurrence that was difficult to control. Initial CT lymphangiography was performed before video-assisted thoracoscopic surgery, and thoracic ducts were identified on the right side cranial to the diaphragm.

Key points

- Video-assisted thoracoscopic surgery for idiopathic chylothorax: pericardiectomy and en bloc TDL.
- The author's hypothesis is that there might be fine ducts that are collapsed and do not contain lymphatic fluid, so they are not visible on preoperative CT lymphangiography. These "dormant" thoracic ducts could affect the efficacy of surgery and influence the recurrence of canine idiopathic chylothorax. Therefore, it is important to ligate the thoracic ducts on both sides.
- All the tissues on both sides of the aorta are ligated using 3-0 Vicryl to complete the bilateral en bloc TDL.
- In this case, pleural effusion disappeared several days after surgery, and no recurrence was observed after 1 year of follow-up.

PORT PLACEMENT

The patient was placed in dorsal recumbency, and the first trocar (T1) was inserted from the right side of the xiphoid process using the optical view. Two 5 mm trocars (T2, T3) were inserted bilaterally at the 8th intercostal space for subtotal pericardiectomy. After pericardiectomy, the dog was placed in left lateral recumbency for TDL. A stereoscopic camera port (T1) was placed at the 10th intercostal space, a right-hand instrument port (T2) was set at the 8th or 9th intercostal space, and a left-hand instrument port (T3) was placed at the 11th intercostal space.

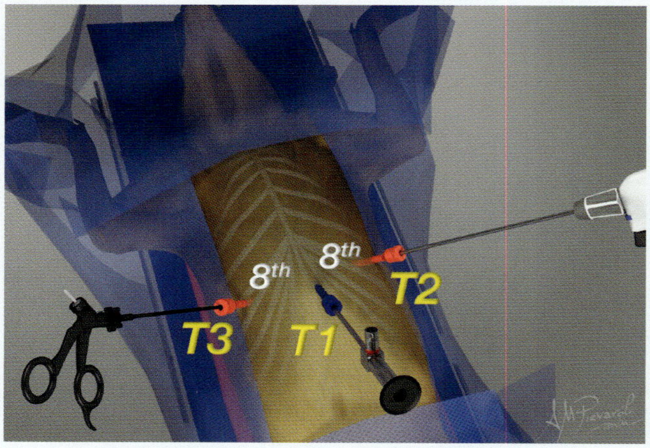

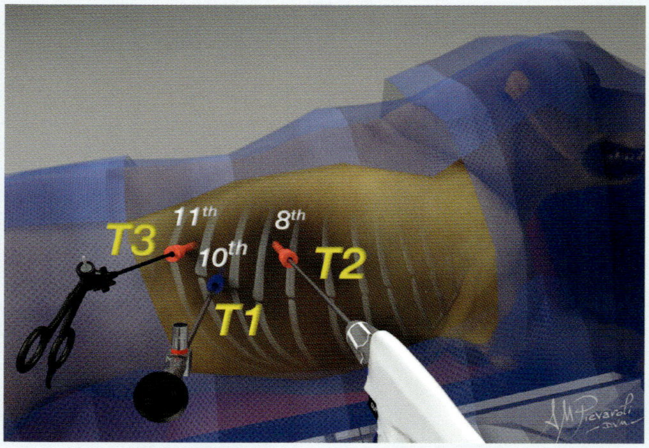

PROCEDURE

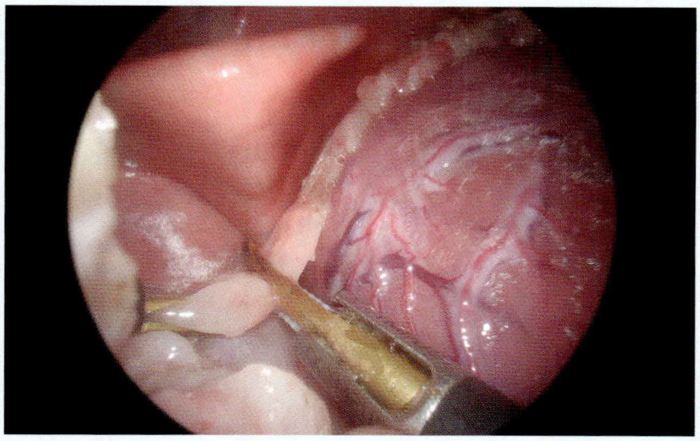

FIGURE 1. Subtotal pericardiectomy by video-assisted thoracoscopic surgery. The pericardium is grasped with forceps and a small incision is made with scissors. The pericardium ventral to the phrenic nerve is removed piece by piece, starting from the initial small incision.

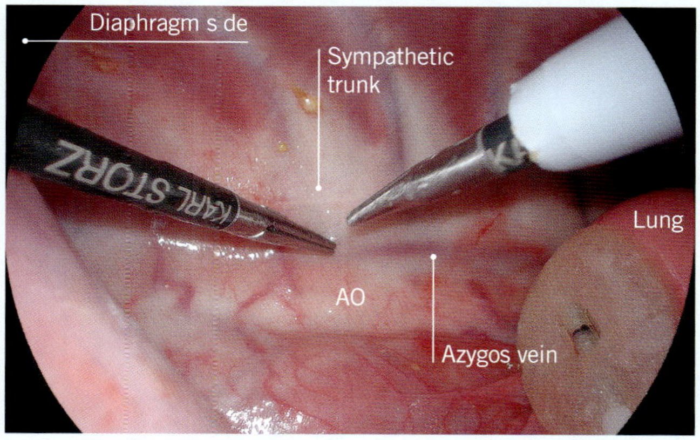

FIGURE 2. After pericardiectomy, bilateral en bloc thoracic duct ligation is performed by video-assisted thoracoscopic surgery. The image shows the anatomy of the sympathetic trunk, aorta (AO), azygos vein and diaphragm.

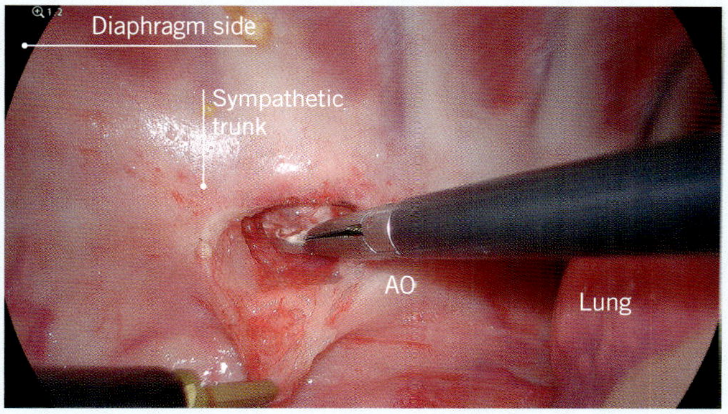

FIGURE 3. The thickened pleura is dissected on the ventral side of the sympathetic trunk. The dissection is continued to vertebral body level using Maryland forceps.

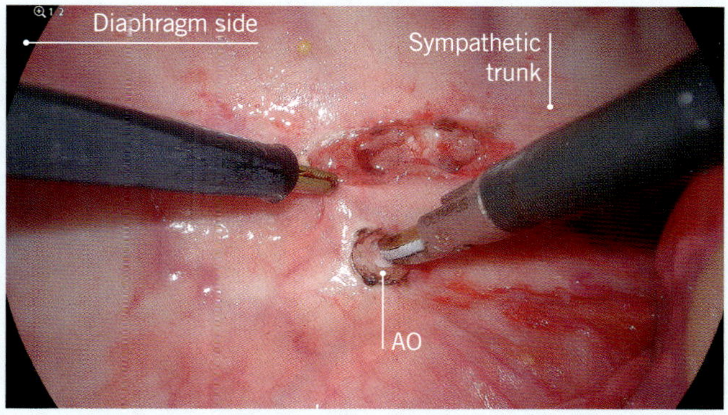

FIGURE 4. After making a deep dissection, a tunnel is created between the dissection site and the dorsal aspect of the aorta.

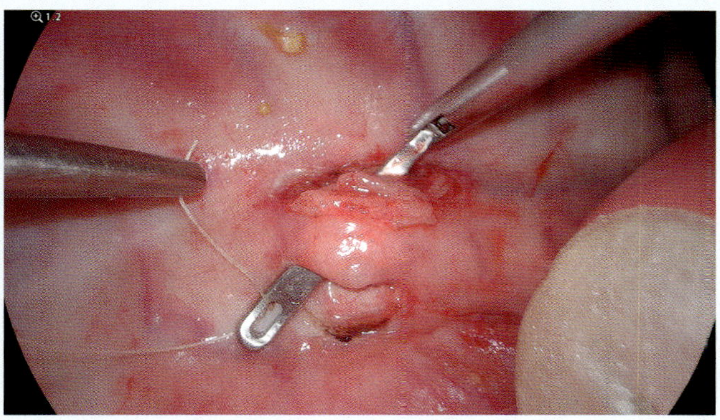

FIGURE 5. The maneuver of threading the suture through the tunnel is performed safely using atraumatic instruments. Then, ligation is performed using 3-0 Vicryl

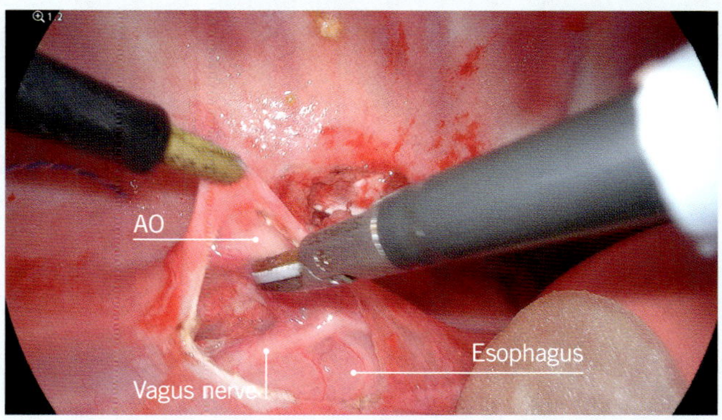

FIGURE 6. The tissue surrounding the aorta is peeled. The aorta is pulled upward using forceps. Next, the tissues on both sides of the aorta are collectively ligated to achieve bilateral en bloc thoracic duct ligation. In the image, the esophagus and vagus nerve can be observed in the left thoracic cavity; care must be taken not to damage them.

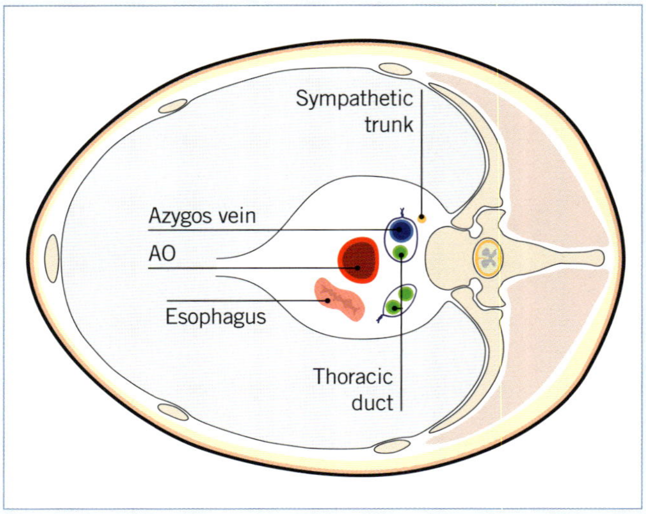

FIGURE 7. Schematic representation of the anatomy of the mediastinum after bilateral en bloc thoracic duct ligation.

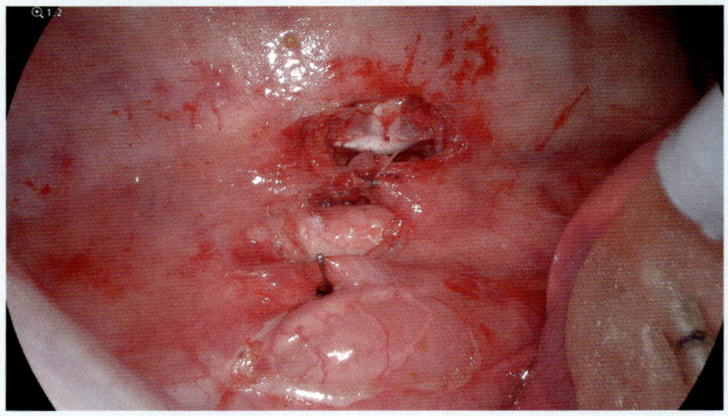

FIGURE 8. A metal clip is applied in the ligature position so that it can be confirmed by postoperative CT examination. The image shows the surgical site where bilateral ligation has been completed.

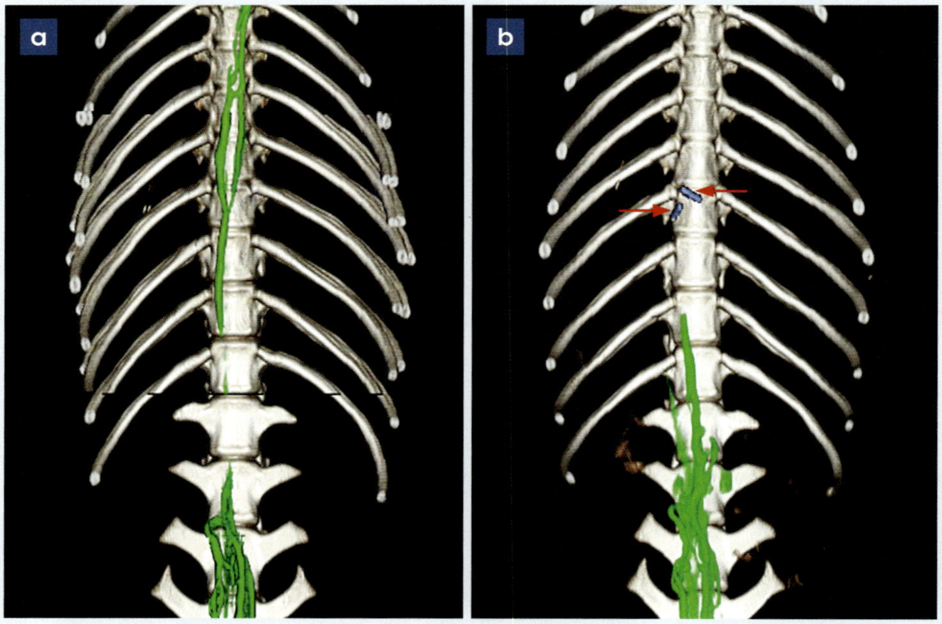

FIGURE 9. Three-dimensional volume rendered images of the thoracic duct. a) Preoperative CT lymphangiography. Multiple thoracic ducts branches are observed in the thoracic cavity. b) Postoperative CT lymphangiography performed 7 days after surgery. Lymph flow is interrupted at the ligation site (arrows).

Tips and tricks

- ✓ Pass the suture through the tunnel dorsal to the aorta.
- ✓ Ligate the thoracic duct branches using 3-0 Vicryl.
- ✓ Place a metal clip at the ligature position for confirmation by postoperative CT examination.

51.2 THORACOSCOPIC THORACIC DUCT LIGATION FOR IDIOPATHIC CHYLOTHORAX

F. J. Pérez Duarte, J. Gutiérrez del Sol, M. A. Sánchez Hurtado

CASE DESCRIPTION

A 5-year-old 26 kg Labrador Retriever dog was presented with dyspnea and lethargy. Radiographs showed bilateral pleural effusion. Fluid analysis confirmed a diagnosis of chylothorax. Echocardiography and CT did not reveal any underlying pathology that could explain the chylothorax. Thoracoscopic TDL and pericardiectomy were performed as surgical treatment. No complications were noted during the procedure. The patient had minimal postoperative morbidity, and the chylothorax resolved.

Key points

- If there is a primary condition that is causing the chylous effusion, it must be treated first; otherwise, surgical treatment will have very poor results.
- The surgical approach is different between dogs and cats, as the anatomy of the thoracic duct varies between species.
- If medical treatment has failed after 2 weeks, surgical treatment should be considered, since chyle is irritant and causes pleuritis.
- The thoracic duct usually has several branches. If the duct has not been colored (with methylene blue or indocyanine green), it is recommended that all structures be ligated between the aorta and the sympathetic trunk.

PORT PLACEMENT

The first 5 mm trocar (T1) was placed in the 10th intercostal space, in the middle area of the right hemithorax. Under direct vision, two other 5 mm trocars were placed in the 11th (T3) and 9th (T2) intercostal spaces, slightly dorsal to the first trocar, thus achieving triangulation between instruments and optics. Two other trocars (5 and 3 mm) were placed in the left hemithorax to simultaneously guide the dissection maneuvers from the other side.

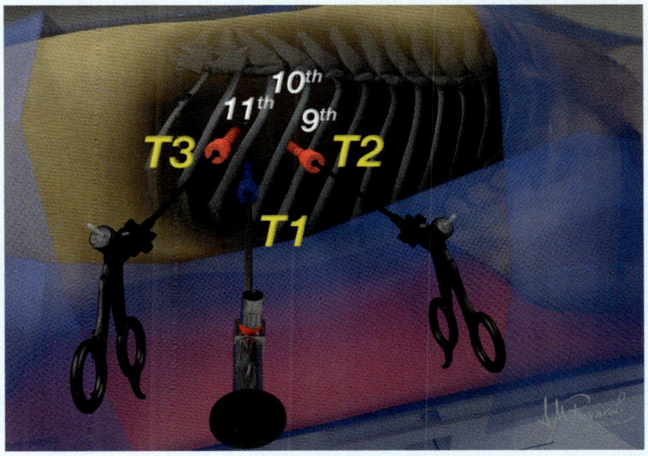

PROCEDURE

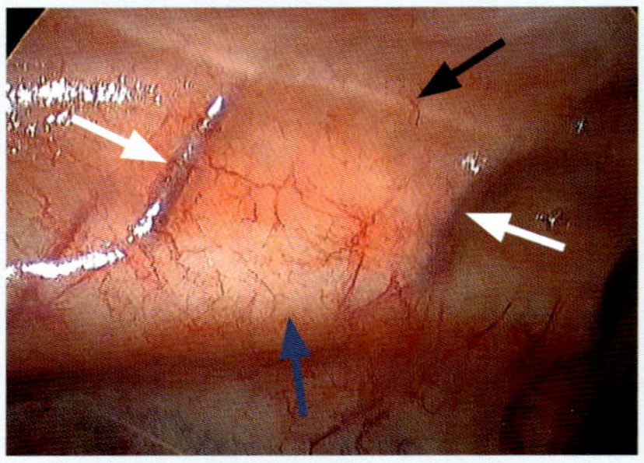

FIGURE 1. The first step of the procedure involves the identification of the anatomical structures cranial to the lumbodiaphragmatic recess: aorta (blue arrow), intercostal vessels (white arrows), and sympathetic nerve (black arrow).

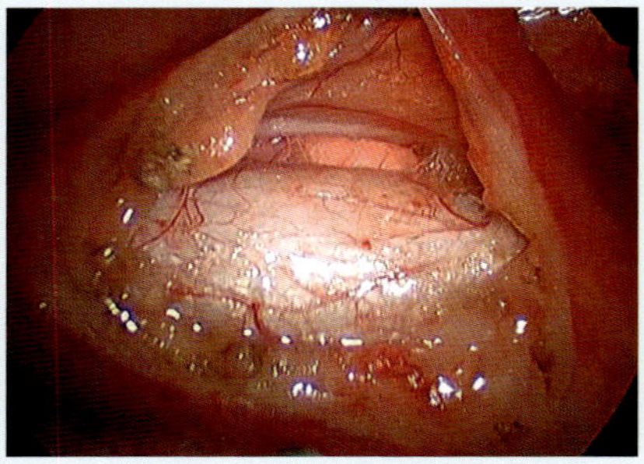

FIGURE 2. The mediastinal pleura is incised in the middle area of the aorta, dissecting this vessel until its dorsal area is exposed.

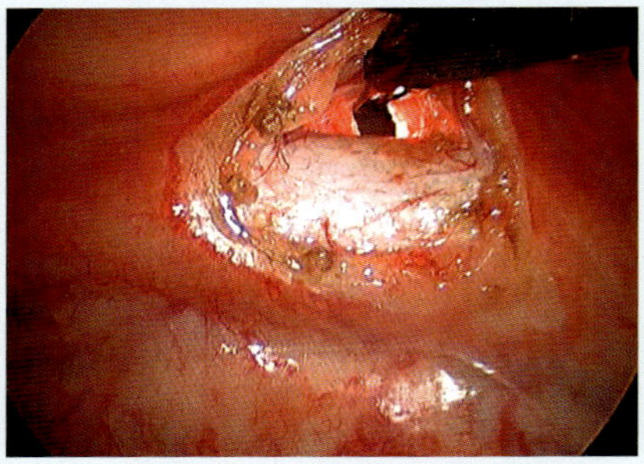

FIGURE 3. Dorsal to the aorta, the entire thickness of the mediastinum is dissected up to the contralateral hemithorax, controlling this maneuver from the other hemithorax.

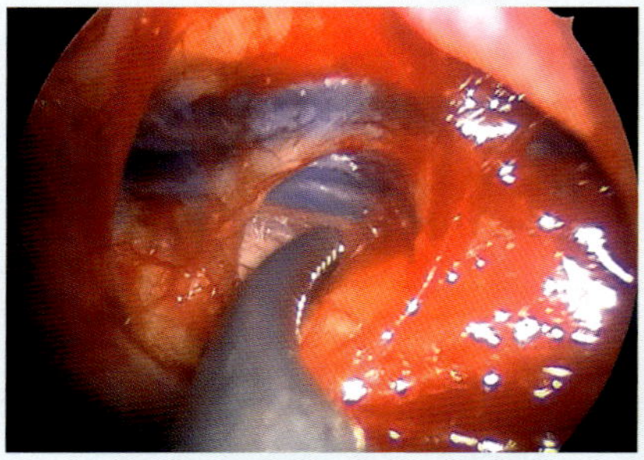

FIGURE 4. If methylene blue has been injected in a lymph node, the thoracic duct and its branches will be easily identifiable.

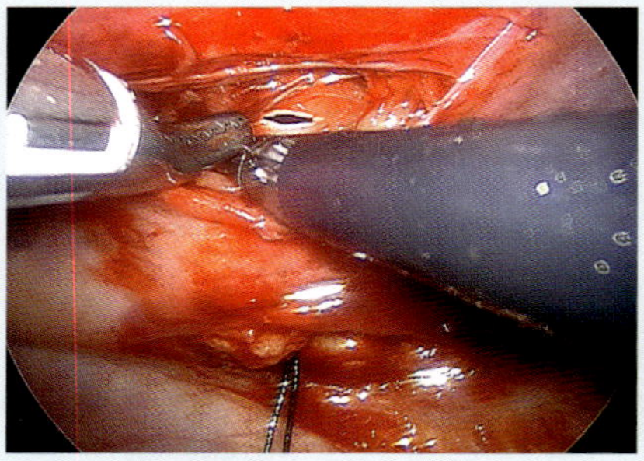

FIGURE 5. The thickness of the mediastinum is dissected in the same way, ventral to the sympathetic nerve, accessing the contralateral hemithorax.

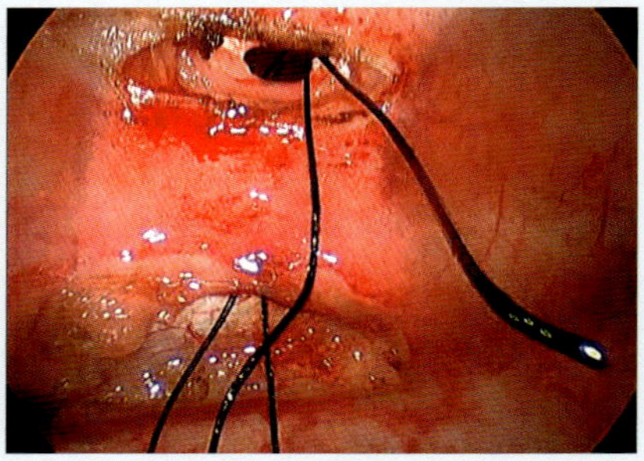

FIGURE 6. A double ligature of nonabsorbable surgical material (2/0 or 3/0) is passed through both dissections, thus including all the structures between the aorta and the sympathetic trunk.

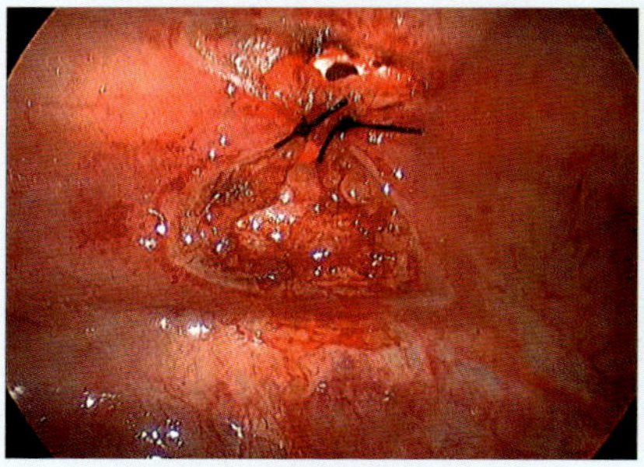

FIGURE 7. The ligatures are knotted intracorporeally, and a vascular clip is placed between the two ligatures.

Tips and tricks

- ✓ The patient should be placed in sternal recumbency with a pendulous abdomen in order to increase the working space in the caudal area of the thorax.
- ✓ Since the thoracic duct is a semitransparent structure, methylene blue or indocyanine green can be injected in a mesenteric or popliteal lymph node to facilitate identification.
- ✓ Simultaneously approaching both hemithoraces facilitates the identification of thoracic duct branches that could run through the contralateral hemithorax.
- ✓ Dissection of the mediastinum should be performed in a perpendicular way to reduce the risk of injuring the contralateral intercostal artery.

51.3 THORACIC DUCT LIGATION AND PERICARDIECTOMY IN A CAT WITH CHYLOTHORAX

Antoine Adam

CASE DESCRIPTION

A cat was presented with the typical clinical signs of chronic thoracic disease and effusion. A complete workup including blood tests and CT lymphangiography was done preoperatively. The thorax was accessed several times before surgery for fluid removal.

After surgery, cats should be hospitalized for 4 days to 1 week. An esophageal tube can be placed to help for a quicker recovery. The thorax is drained 2–3 times a day until there is no fluid production. Before discharge, CT lymphangiography should be performed to assess the thoracic duct and to search for any leakage. Clinical recheck is recommended at 1 week, 2 weeks, and 1 month postoperatively.

Key points

- The cat is positioned at the border of the operating table.
- The patient must always be ventilated with positive pressure (volume-controlled).
- The thorax is accessed from the left side.
- The working space involves the dorsal thorax.
- Specimens retrieved should be sent for histopathology.

PORT PLACEMENT

- T1, 3 mm camera port, in the 8th–9th intercostal space, two-thirds dorsal
- T2, 3 mm port for instrument, approximately in the 6th–8th intercostal space
- T3, 5 mm port for instrument and vessel-sealing device or stapler

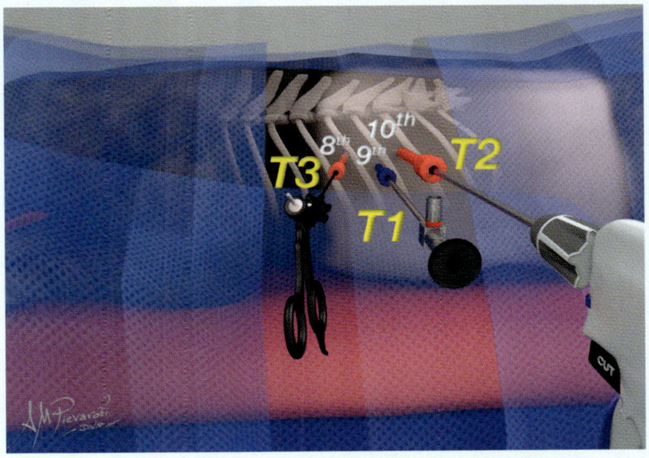

PROCEDURE

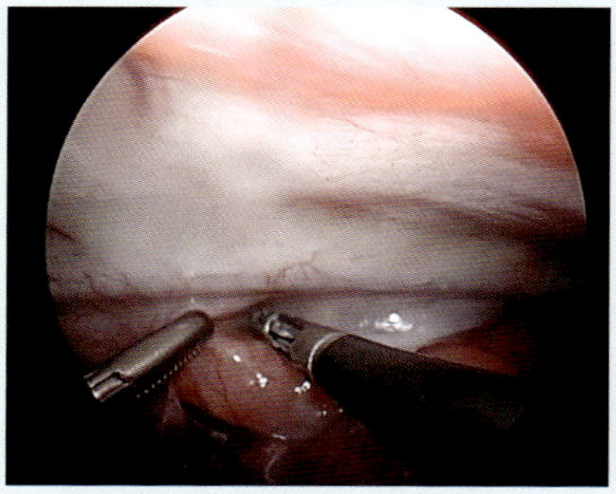

FIGURE 1. Dissection of the thoracic duct dorsal to the aorta is started. Intrathoracic insufflation may be used (up to 4 mmHg).

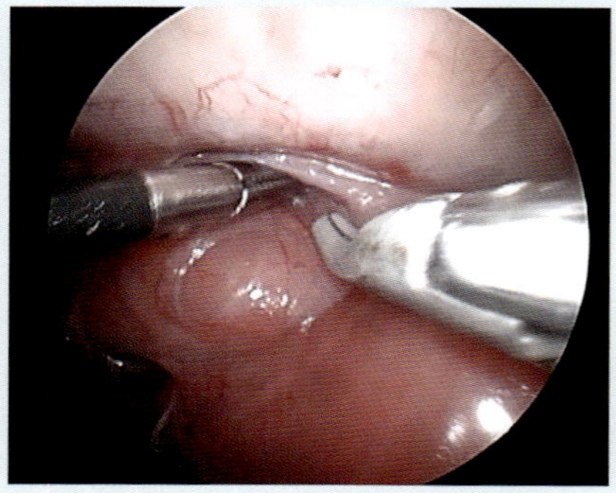

FIGURE 2. A suction device is used to remove the remaining chyle and thoracic fluid. Maryland forceps helps find the plane between the thoracic duct and the aorta.

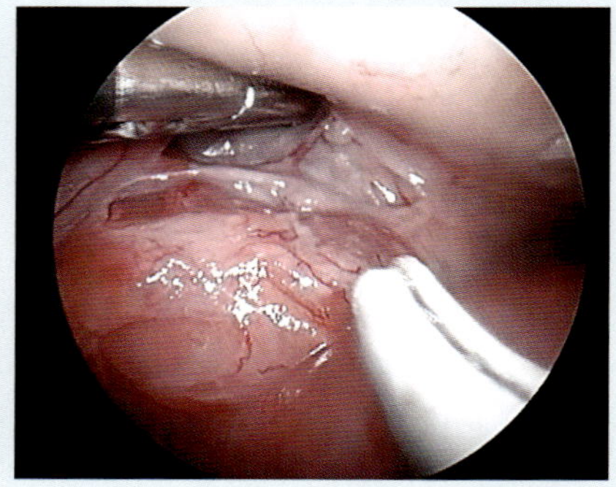

FIGURE 3. Dissection is continued to create a window for ligation and clip application. The thoracic duct or its branches may be visualized by accessing the supra-aortic space. The author typically uses fluorescence and a 2.7 mm Storz with an Olympus HD NBI mode camera, with varying degrees of success.

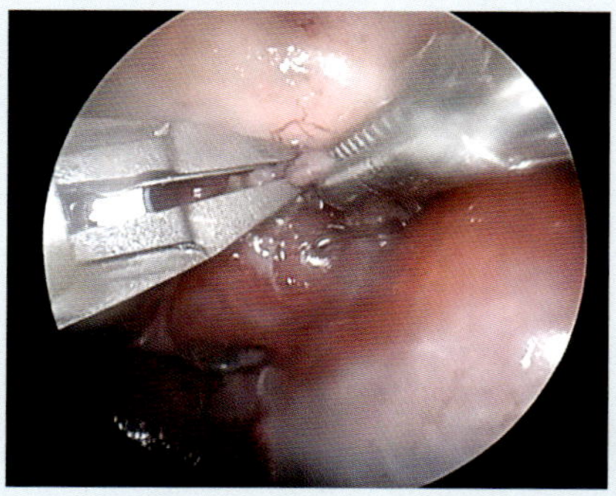

FIGURE 4. The use of the vessel-sealing device is chosen during surgery, based on the space between the clips and the amount of surrounding tissue dissected. In the image, one clip has already been applied and another is being placed.

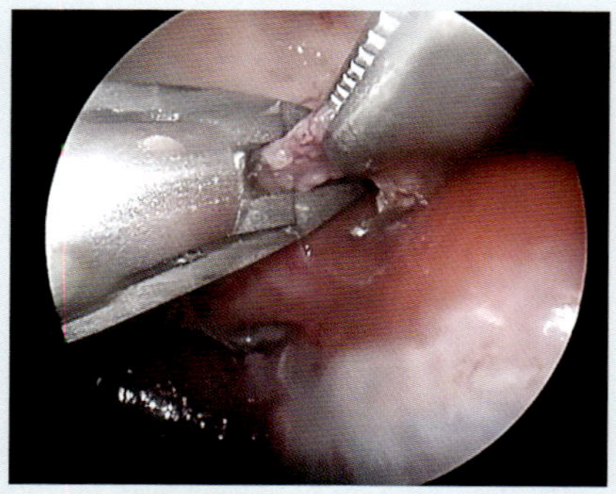

FIGURE 5. Paraxiphoid access is made with a 3 mm Ternamian cannula under visual control. The image shows a closer view of clip application. The two lateral ports are placed under visual control.

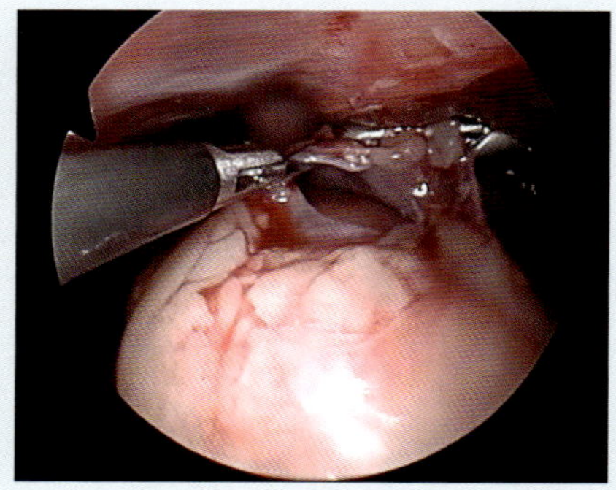

FIGURE 6. Opening made into the pericardium at the beginning of dissection.

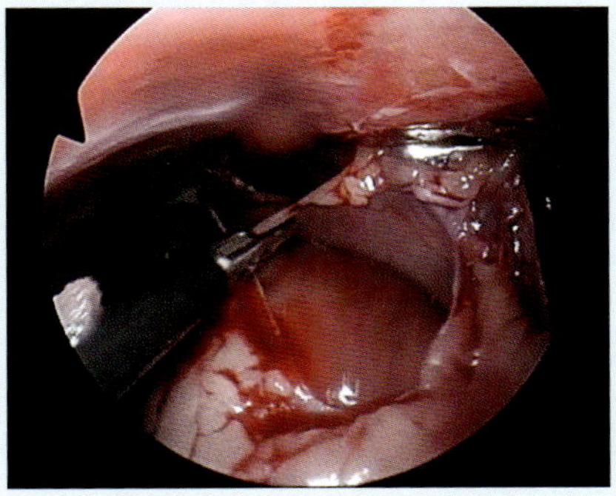

FIGURE 7. Completing dissection of the left side of the pericardium. In these cases, the pericardium is usually thicker than normal and difficult to grab with atraumatic forceps. Multiple forceps may need to be tried to achieve the best possible grasp.

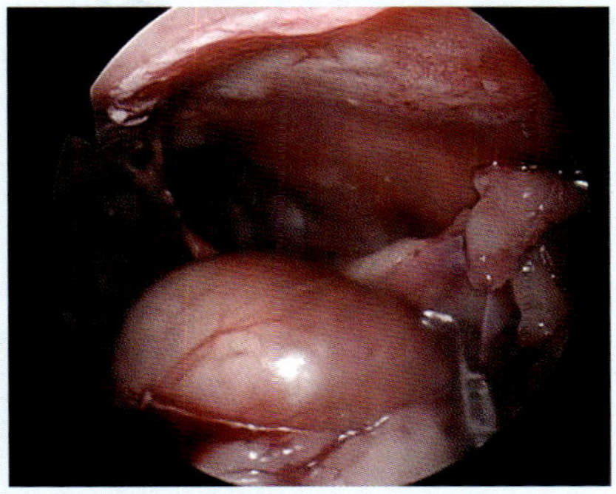

FIGURE 8. When the pericardial window is finished, the tissue is removed. Remove as much pericardium as possible, staying away from the phrenic nerve. Port accesses are closed. A double stitch can be used on the muscle/subcutaneous plane. The skin is usually glued, except on the pleural port device region.

Tips and tricks

- ✓ A 3 mm Maryland forceps helps in dissection.
- ✓ Use a 5 mm clip application device to apply three clips.
- ✓ Also use a 5 mm vessel-sealing device (LigaSure, Maryland jaw) to seal the thoracic duct between the clips.
- ✓ It is easier to finish the pericardiectomy by changing the scissor from left to right or vice versa.
- ✓ Inject indocyanine green (0.05–0.1 mg/kg) into a popliteal lymph node or the perianal region.
- ✓ Place the cat at the border on the operating table to have good range of motion with the laparoscopic instruments.

51.4 THORACOSCOPIC THORACIC DUCT LIGATION AND METHYLENE BLUE COLORATION OF MESENTERIC LYMPH NODES TO CONFIRM OCCLUSION

Leonardo Cavaliere, Flavia Catanzaro

CASE DESCRIPTION

A 10-year-old 25 kg mixed-breed dog was presented with a 3-week history of chylothorax. Idiopathic chylothorax was suspected after total body CT scan, echocardiography, and complete blood work. Before surgery, the thoracic duct was identified by CT lymphangiography to better choose the site of duct occlusion. A three-port right-sided thoracoscopic TDL was performed.

Key points

- CT lymphangiography is a great aid for surgical planning.
- If, after thoracic duct closure, contrast leakage is observed in the thorax or duct enlargement is not seen, en bloc ligation can be tried or the surgery can be converted to cisterna chyli ablation.

PORT PLACEMENT

The patient is placed in sternal recumbency, slightly tilted to the left side. The first 6 mm Endotip trocarless cannula (T1) is placed in the mid-thorax in the 10th intercostal space. The other two ports are placed in the proximal third of the thorax under scope guidance: the most cranial 6 mm port (T2) is placed in the 8th intercostal space, while the most caudal 12 mm port (T3) is placed in the 12th intercostal space. A minimally invasive paracostal right-sided 9 cm access using a wound retractor is performed to expose the mesenteric lymph nodes.

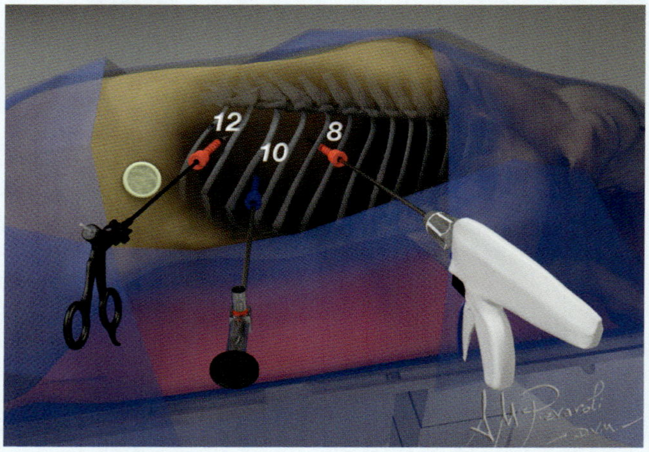

PROCEDURE

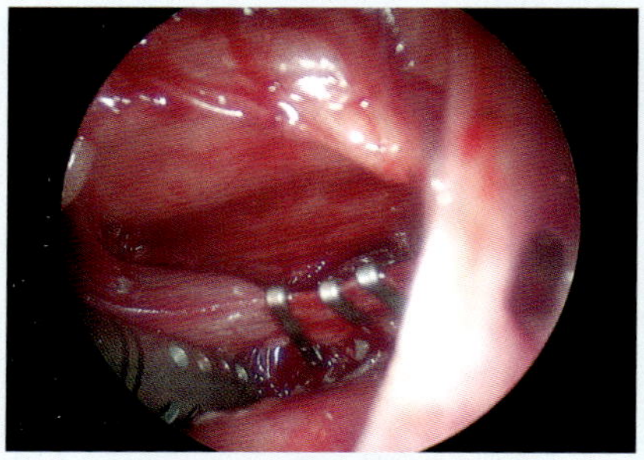

FIGURE 1. Blunt dissection of the pleura ventral to the aorta is performed immediately cranial to the diaphragm using a laparoscopic Maryland dissecting forceps between two intercostal arteries. Once visualized, the thoracic duct is occluded by applying three endoscopic clips. The duct, under lymphatic pressure, immediately enlarges caudally to the ligation site.

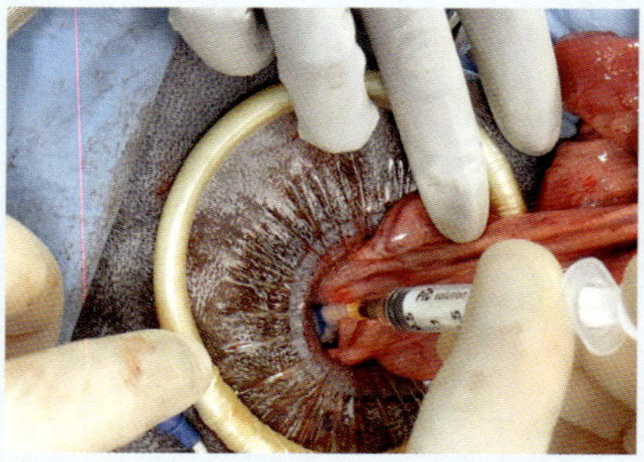

FIGURE 2. Through the wound retractor, a 1% aqueous solution of methylene blue is injected directly into the mesenteric lymph nodes at a dose 0.5 mg/kg, not exceeding 10 mg.

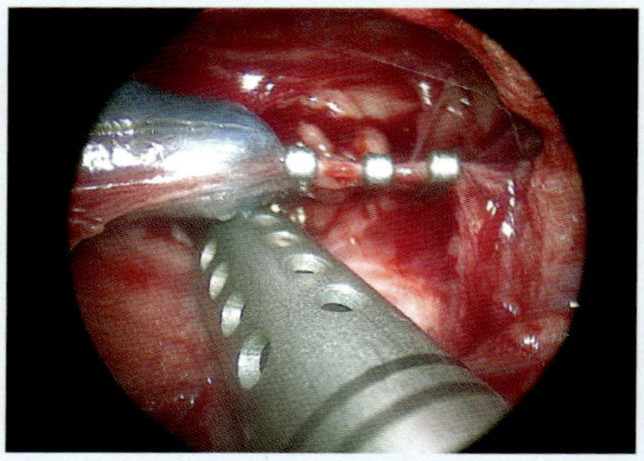

FIGURE 3. About 2 minutes after methylene blue injection, the enlarged and colored thoracic duct is visualized, thus confirming duct occlusion.

Tips and tricks

✓ Feeding the patient a fatty meal (cream or highly lipidic food) 1 hour before anesthesia helps to visualize the thoracic duct.

✓ If fluoroscopy is available and a CT lymphangiogram was not performed, consider the injection of aqueous contrast material in the mesenteric lymph nodes as described for methylene blue to better understand the anatomy of the thoracic duct.

51.5 ENDOSCOPIC-ASSISTED SURGERY FOR IDIOPATHIC CHYLOTHORAX IN A DOMESTIC SHORTHAIR CAT

Yi Fu Chang, Ming Ju Huang

CASE DESCRIPTION

A 5-year-old domestic shorthair cat was presented after repeated draining of pleural fluid for the past 6 months. The physical examination revealed a body condition score of 3/9, a respiratory rate of 60 beats per minute, a systolic blood pressure of 120 mmHg, a heart rate of 150 beats per minute, and clinical signs of mucosal cyanosis and exercise intolerance. As initial interventional treatment, a Mila chest tube was inserted and 243 mL of milky fluid was drained to relieve the signs of respiratory distress. After that, CT lymphangiography was performed to locate the thoracic duct and rule out other possible underlying causes. The tentative diagnosis was idiopathic chylothorax. On the 7th day after the first surgical procedure, the volume of pleural fluid had dropped from 150 to 70 cc/day, but on day 9 of hospitalization it suddenly increased to 150 cc/day. Therefore, a second surgery, thoracoscopic pericardiectomy and cisterna chyli ablation, was performed. Fourteen days after the second approach, the volume of pleural fluid had decreased from a high level of 37 mL/kg of body weight per day to a low value of 3 mL/kg of body weight per day, and the chest tube was removed. Two months after the second operation, ultrasound examination did not reveal the presence of pleural fluid, and the patient's body weight had increased from 3.7 to 4.25 kg. The clinical signs of exercise intolerance and respiratory distress had completely resolved.

Key points

- Bilateral thoracoscopic surgery may increase the success rate of TDL due to the variability of the duct branches. Unilateral thoracoscopic surgery may lead to incomplete ligation.
- NIR-ICG lymphangiography provides excellent images of the thoracic duct and improves the success rate of complete ligation of all duct branches.
- Thoracoscopic TDL has a high rate of complete duct occlusion. Simultaneous pericardiectomy and cisterna chyli ablation has the highest success rate to date.

PORT PLACEMENT

Five thoracoscopic ports were placed for introduction of surgical instruments, three of them on the right thoracic wall and two on the left side. A 1 cm skin incision for thoracoscope port placement (T1) was made at the mid-thorax in the right 10th intercostal space, and tissues were bluntly dissected with a Kelly forceps. A 5 mm trocar was inserted into the thoracic cavity, and a 30° rigid telescope was introduced through the port. After examination of the right hemithorax, the thoracoscope was used to facilitate placement of two additional ports in the 9th and 8th intercostal spaces: a 5 mm port (T3) for instruments and a 10 mm port (T2) for the metallic clip and absorbable vessel clip applicator, respectively. The left-side ports (T4, T5) were placed in the 9th and 10th intercostal spaces.

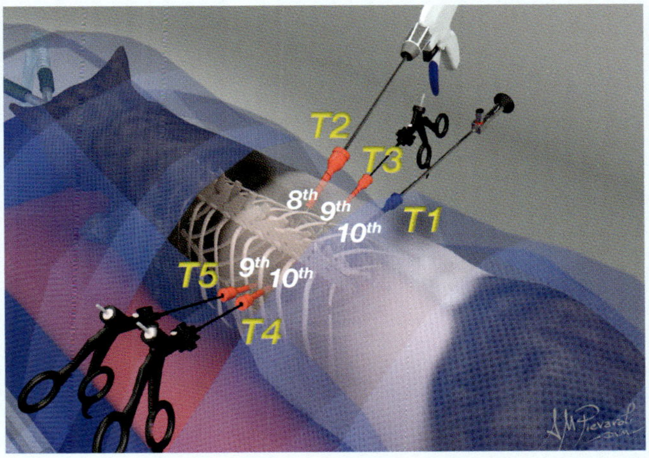

PROCEDURE

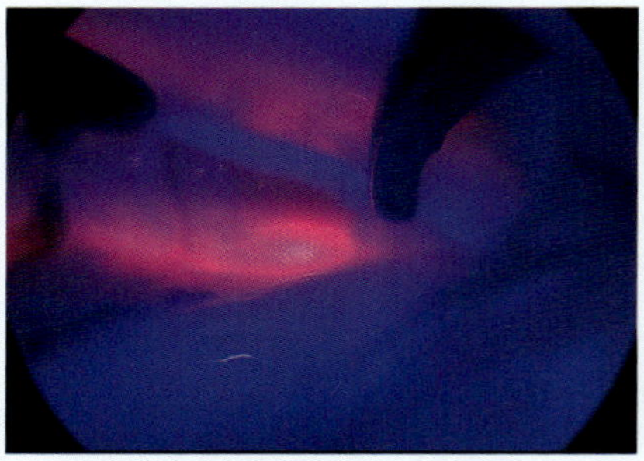

FIGURE 1. Intraoperative injection of ICG into a popliteal lymph node highlights the thoracic duct and its branches. According to the needs and interest in improving thoracic duct ligation, which is characterized by image-guided surgical strategies, NIR/ICG is receiving increased attention in veterinary medicine.

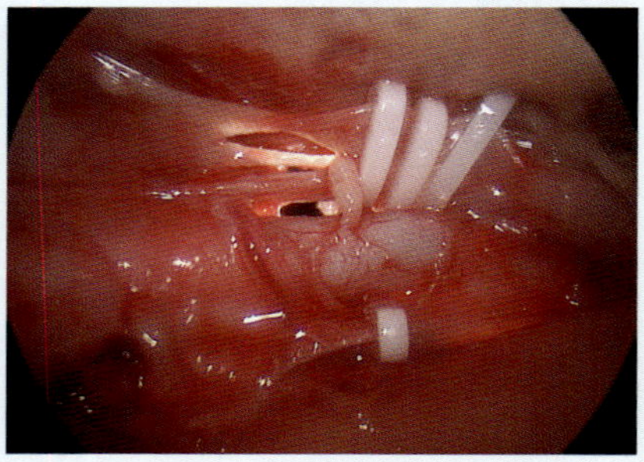

FIGURE 2. Absorbable clips can withstand a higher weight than single metal clips without slipping off of the target duct or artery. Furthermore, metal hemoclips that remain in the tissue permanently will interfere with CT or MRI scan interpretation.

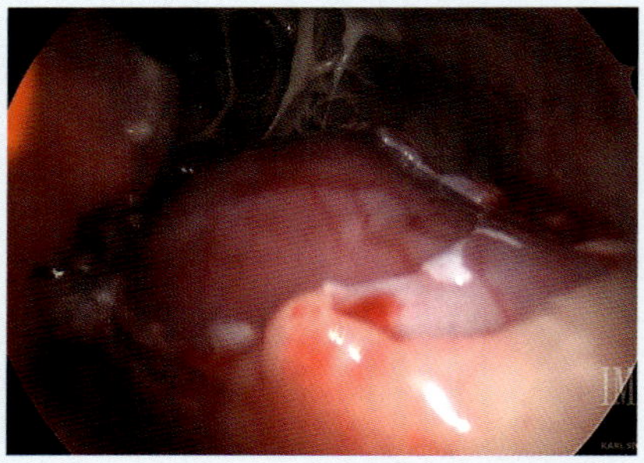

FIGURE 3. The phrenic nerve was identified to avoid damaging it. After the initial pericardial incision, dissection of the pericardium is continued with the scissors and vessel-sealing device until a 3×3 cm square window is created. Severe chronic pleuritis can be seen in the image.

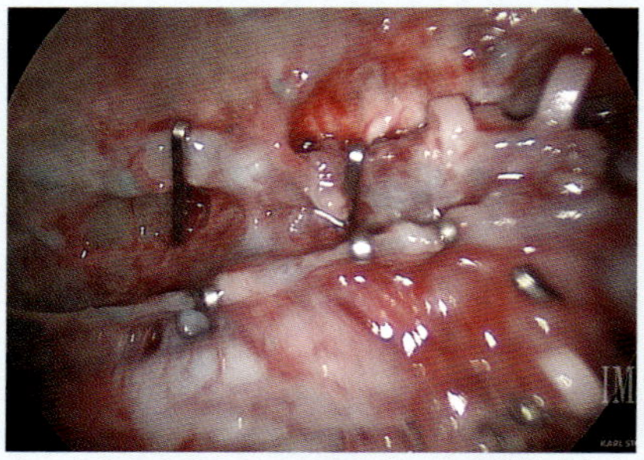

FIGURE 4. Thoracoscopic thoracic duct ligation. Fibrin development can result in restrictive pleuritis and adhesions. In these cases, the effusion is often compartmentalized and harder to dissect.

Tips and tricks

- ✓ To better visualize the thoracic duct, 1 mL of ICG was injected into the popliteal lymph node. Under NIR-ICG thoracoscopy, significant ventral retraction of the aorta using right-angle curved forceps was required to aid dissection ventrolateral to the aorta and thus ventral to the thoracic duct bilaterally.
- ✓ Curved dissecting forceps were used to dissect across the mediastinum just dorsal to the aorta. Then, four absorbable vascular clips and six metals clips were used to ligate the thoracic duct in an en bloc fashion.
- ✓ Pericardiectomy was planned in the same procedure. However, as the patient had a crisis of hypotension at minute 90 of anesthesia, the operation was suspended.

51.6 CHYLOTHORAX ASSOCIATED WITH A PERITONEOPERICARDIAL DIAPHRAGMATIC HERNIA IN A DOG

Andrea M. Pievaroli

CASE DESCRIPTION

A 5-year-old male Gordon Setter dog with chylothorax of unknown cause was referred for thoracoscopic thoracic duct occlusion. Preliminary diagnostic investigations were carried out by the referral veterinary clinic. It was not possible to obtain a CT lymphangiogram. To better identify the thoracic duct, methylene blue was injected in a popliteal lymph node. Thoracoscopy was performed to identify and occlude the duct using metallic clips plus an en bloc ligation with a silk suture. A pericardial window was also performed. In the postoperative period the pleural effusion diminished, but during a routine ultrasound check a congenital asymptomatic peritoneopericardial diaphragmatic hernia was diagnosed. The dog underwent a second surgery to close the diaphragmatic defect via a laparoscopic-assisted technique. After that, the chylothorax resolved definitively. The thoracoscopic procedure lasted about 90 minutes. During the procedure, nothing suggested the presence of a peritoneopericardial diaphragmatic hernia. The laparoscopic procedure lasted 45 minutes. It was not possible to reposition part of the left liver lobes, but this did not cause any complications. Chylothorax secondary to a peritoneopericardial diaphragmatic hernia is a rare condition. Surgery may be the method of choice to resolve the chylothorax.

Key points

- It is recommended to perform also an en bloc TDL to include all branches.
- Nonabsorbable sutures should be used.
- CT lymphangiography is useful for identifying the course of the thoracic duct and its accessory branches.

PORT PLACEMENT FOR THORACOSCOPY

- Patient in sternal recumbency
- T1, telescope, in the dorsal third of the right 11th intercostal space
- T2, in the dorsal third of the right 10th intercostal space
- T3, in the dorsal third of the right 12th intercostal space

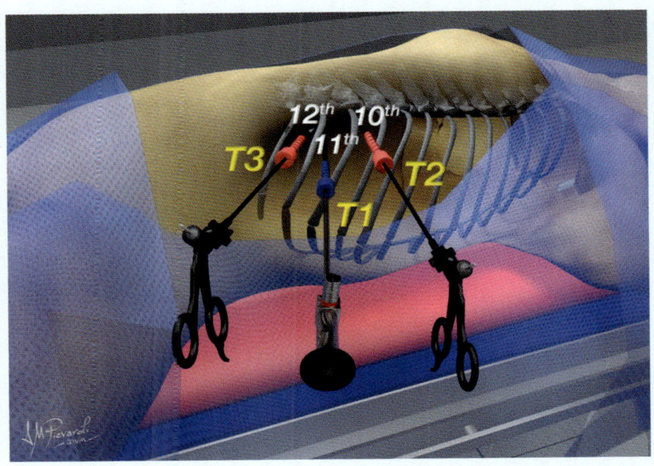

PORT PLACEMENT FOR LAPAROSCOPY

- Patient in dorsal recumbency
- T1, telescope, in the midline, 1–2 cm caudal to the umbilicus
- T2, on a left paramedian position, 3–4 cm cranial to T1
- T3, on a right paramedian position, 3–4 cm cranial to T1

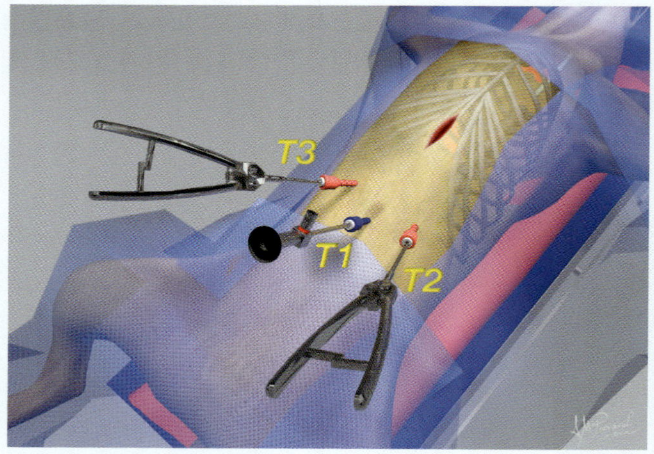

PROCEDURE

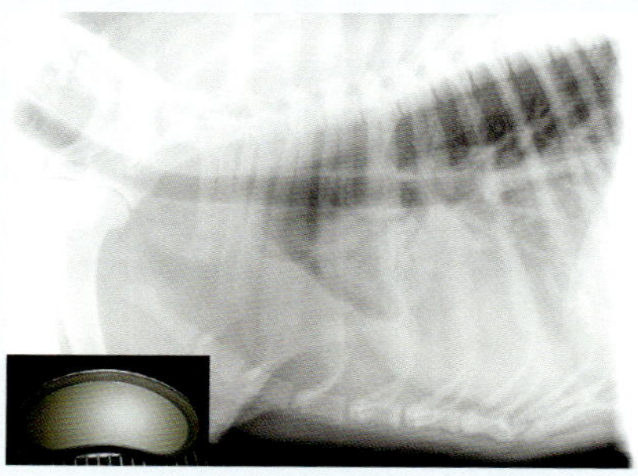

FIGURE 1. Preoperative X-ray image of the pleural effusion.

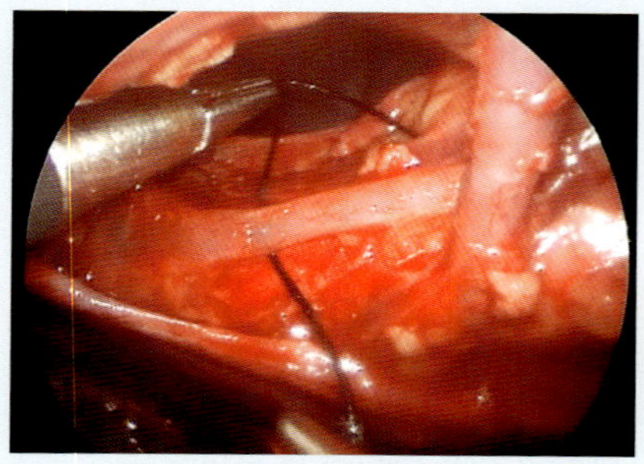

FIGURE 2. After dissection, the thoracic duct is located and an en bloc ligation is performed to ensure that all the thoracic branches are ligated.

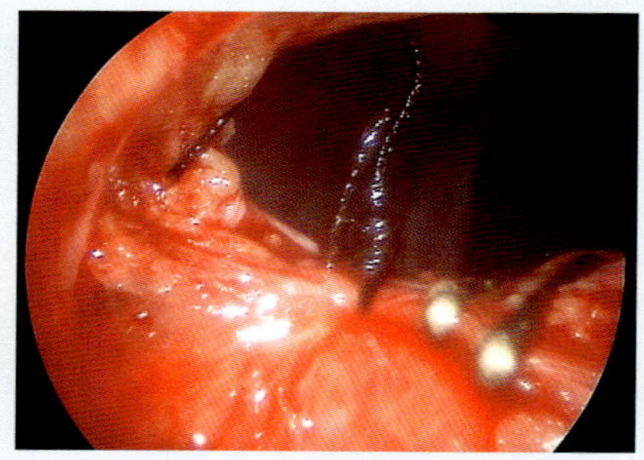

FIGURE 3. In addition to the suture, two endoscopic clips are applied.

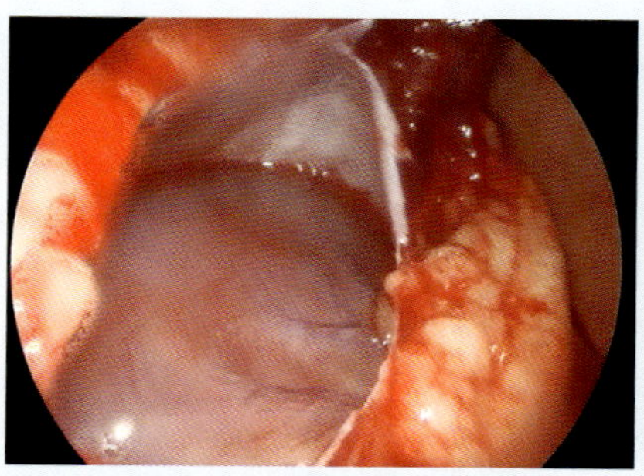

FIGURE 4. As reported in the literature, a pericardial window is also performed (with the patient in dorsal recumbency).

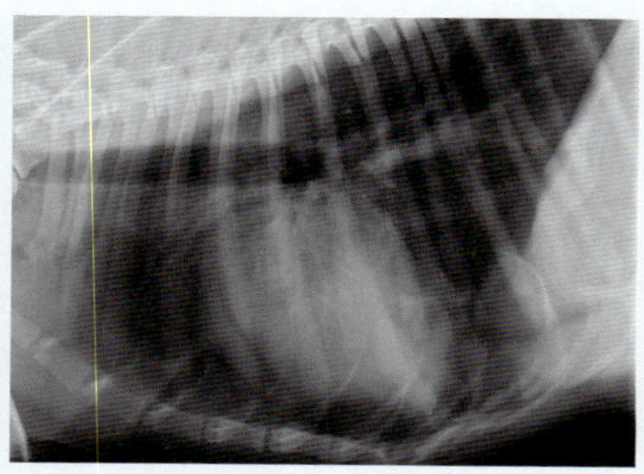

FIGURE 5. X-ray image 2 weeks after the first surgery.

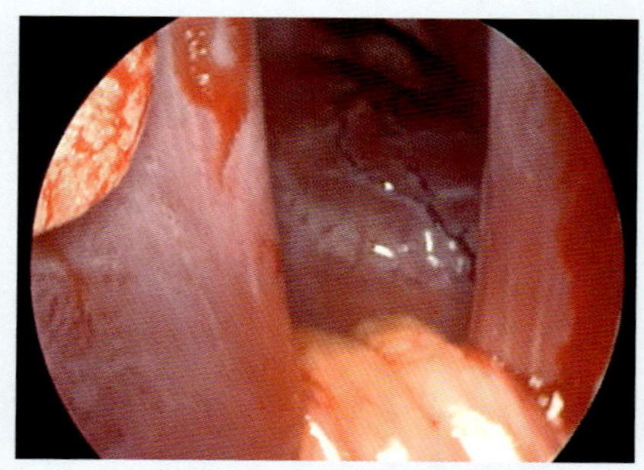

FIGURE 6. Laparoscopic-assisted surgery for the treatment of the congenital peritoneopericardial diaphragmatic hernia. Some sutures are applied laparoscopically. Then, a small incision is performed at the level of the xiphoid process to complete the closure of the hernia.

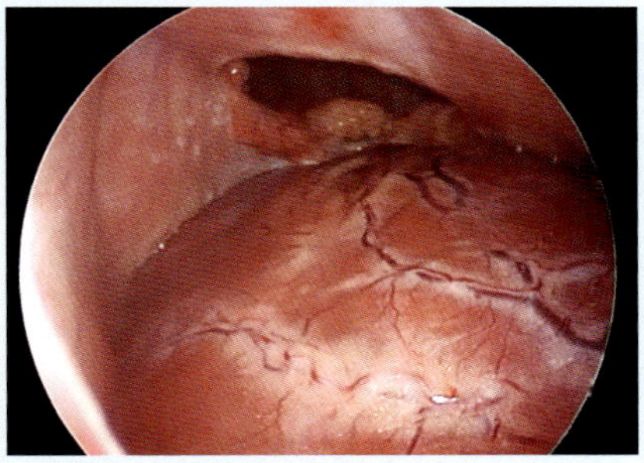

FIGURE 7. During laparoscopy, inspection of the pericardium (pericardioscopy) shows the pericardial windows previously performed in the first thoracoscopic surgery.

Tips and tricks

- ✓ In some cases, the bilateral approach of both hemithoraces may facilitate the identification and the en bloc ligation of the thoracic duct branches.
- ✓ Recently, indocyanine green has been used to better identify the thoracic duct. This modern technique requires the use of a camera and a dedicated light source.

52 THORACOSCOPIC APPROACH TO THE MANAGEMENT OF PYOTHORAX

Eric Monnet

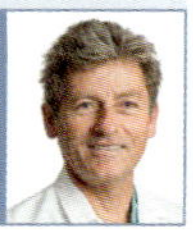

Indications

- Indications have not been clearly established in veterinary medicine. The difficulty to establish guidelines comes from the wide variety of causes for pyothorax in dogs and cats and their chronicity.
- Thoracoscopy can be used for diagnosis.
- Thoracoscopy might help to guide the treatment of pyothorax: medical vs. surgical treatment; thoracoscopy only vs. thoracotomy by visualizing the pleural space.
- Thoracoscopy aids in collecting biopsy and culture samples, in debriding the pleural space with resection of the ventral part of the mediastinum to improve drainage, and in resecting the lung lobes affected by the pyothorax. An acute pyothorax is more likely to respond better to thoracoscopy (**Fig. 1**).

Contraindications

- Thoracoscopy may not be indicated in cases of chronic pyothorax with severe adhesions and thick purulent exudate. In these patients, conversion to an open thoracotomy should be made to accomplish better debridement and lavage (**Figs. 2–4**).

Pyothorax is the accumulation of septic exudate in the pleural space. The most common cause is the migration of a foreign body from the airways to the pleural space.

A thoracoscopic approach for the treatment of pyothorax in dogs was first described by E. Monnet in 2009.

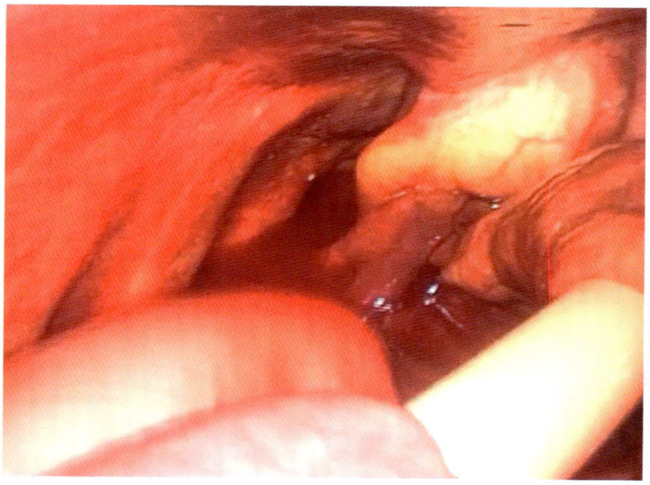

FIGURE 1. Acute pyothorax with marked accumulation of septic exudate. This case was treated by thoracoscopy followed by thoracic lavage.

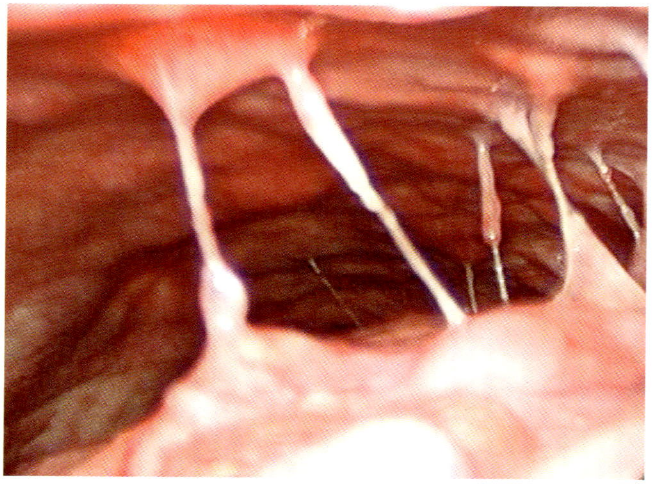

FIGURE 2. Chronic pyothorax with fibrinopurulent deposit and adhesions. This case was converted to an open thoracotomy.

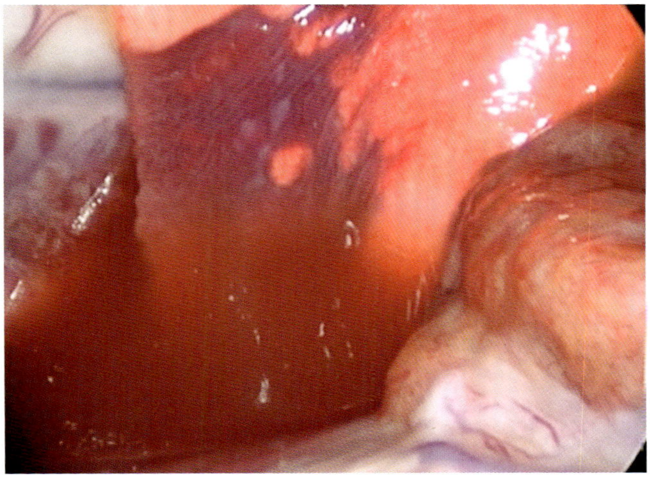

FIGURE 3. Septic exudate accumulated in the left caudodorsal recess of the diaphragm hiding the main structures in the mediastinum.

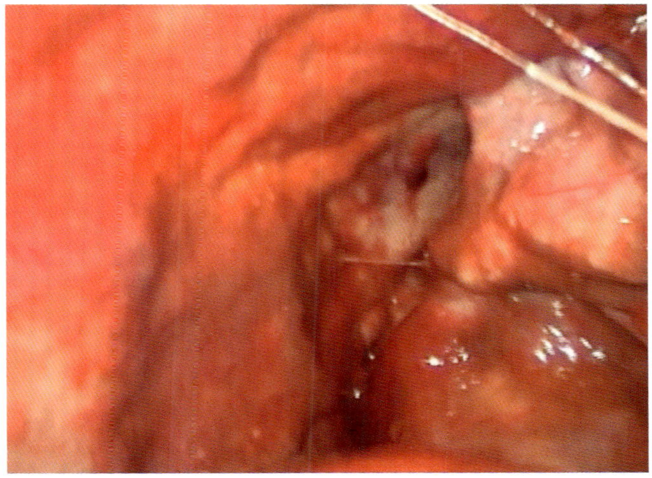

FIGURE 4. Chronic pyothorax with a fibrinopurulent deposit over the pleura interfering with the visualization of the main structures in the cranial mediastinum.

Anatomical landmarks

The main anatomical structures in the chest should be assessed upon entry into the thorax. It is important to consider the position of the internal thoracic artery in the cranial mediastinum. During the dissection and debridement of the cranial mediastinum, the internal thoracic artery is not always visible (**Fig. 5**). The phrenic and vagus nerves must be identified, especially when extensive debridement is undertaken. Accumulation of septic exudate can interfere with the visualization of major structures like the main vasculature in the cranial and caudal mediastinum (**Figs. 3 and 4**). Therefore, it is important to drain the pleural space as much as possible before starting dissection.

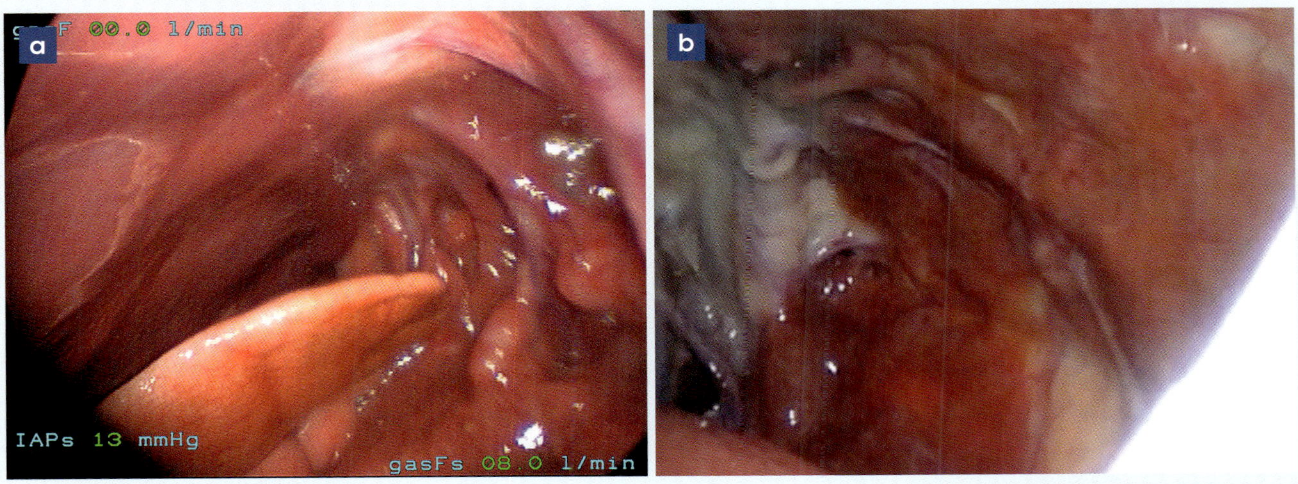

FIGURE 5. a) Chronic pyothorax with severe involvement of the mediastinum interfering with the visualization of the internal thoracic artery in the cranial mediastinum. b) Chronic pyothorax without involvement of the cranial mediastinum. The internal thoracic artery is visible.

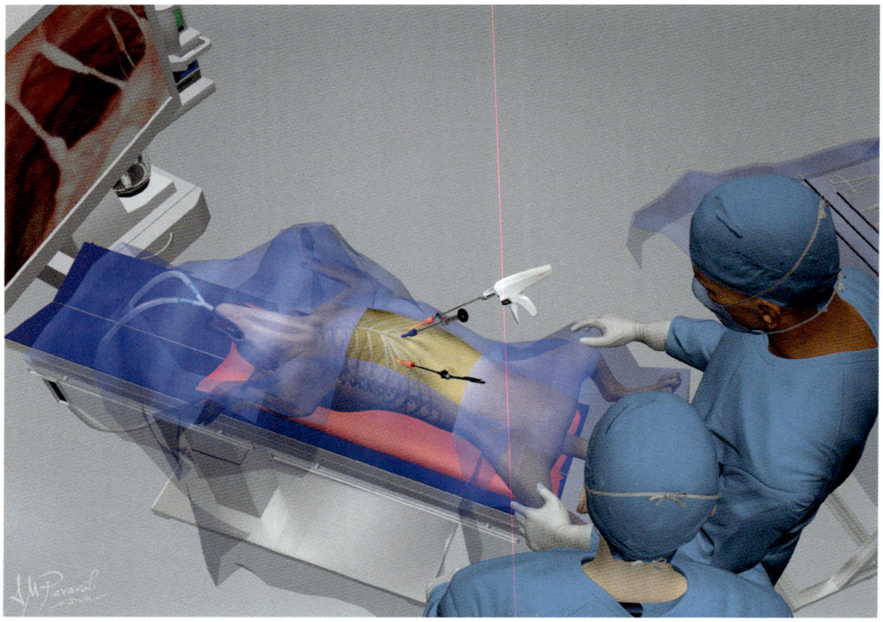

FIGURE 6. Operating room layout for the thoracoscopic management of pyothorax.

OPERATING ROOM LAYOUT

The patient is placed in dorsal recumbency at the end of the table. The surgeon positions themselves at the end of the table. The monitor and the tower are placed at the patient's head, next to the anesthesia machine. The instrument table is placed behind the surgeon. The camera assistant is on the left side of the surgeon (**Fig. 6**).

PORT PLACEMENT (FIG. 7)

- T1, transdiaphragmatic subxiphoid approach with a long 5 or 10 mm cannula for the telescope
- T2, 5 mm thoracic cannula in the left 8th–9th intercostal space close to the sternum
- T3, 12 mm thoracic cannula in the right 8th–9th intercostal space close to the sternum

PROCEDURE (VIDEO 1)

- A CT scan of the thoracic cavity should be performed before thoracoscopy to identify any lesions in the lungs or foreign bodies in the pleural space. Double-lumen endobronchial intubation might facilitate the exploration of the pleural space by alternating the side of ventilation. However, double-lumen intubation is not always feasible, depending on the patient's size and anatomy.
- Thoracoscopic exploration starts with the dissection of the sternal attachment of the mediastinum from caudal to cranial using a 10 mm vessel-sealing device (**Fig. 8**).

Instruments

- Telescope 5 mm – 0° or 30° (or a 10 mm variable-angle telescope)
- Three 5 mm thoracic cannulas + one 12 mm thoracic cannula (another 12 mm long thoracic cannula is required if an EndoCAMeleon is used)
- 5 mm palpation probe
- Two 5 mm fine-teeth grasping forceps
- 10 mm vessel-sealing device
- J-hook extension for electrocautery
- 10 mm medium/large endoclips
- 5 mm suction/irrigation device
- 10 mm retrieval pouch

VIDEO 1. Exploration and debridement of an acute pyothorax by thoracoscopy in a dog.

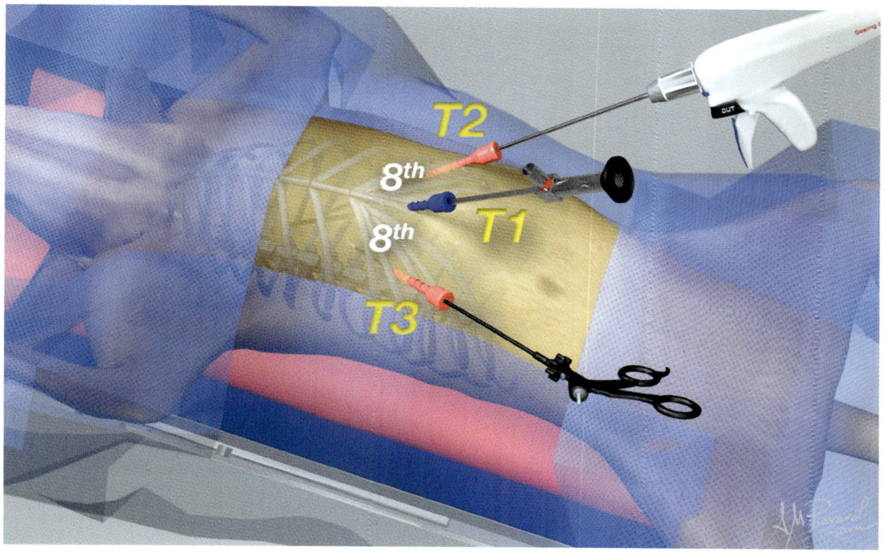

FIGURE 7. Port placement for the thoracoscopic management of pyothorax.

- The entire mediastinum should be detached from the sternum and removed from the pleural space after dissection along the pericardium and the dorsal part of the cranial mediastinum (**Fig. 9**).
- Pleural effusion should be suctioned with the suction/irrigation device to help inspect the dorsal aspect of the pleural space.
- Then, the pleural space can be evaluated from cranial to caudal on the left and right sides. It helps if the patient is tilted toward the right while evaluating the left side and vice versa. The left and right dorsocaudal recesses of the pleural space are difficult to inspect, but visualization is facilitated by using a variable-angle telescope or by moving the regular telescope to one of the cannulas on the left or right side.

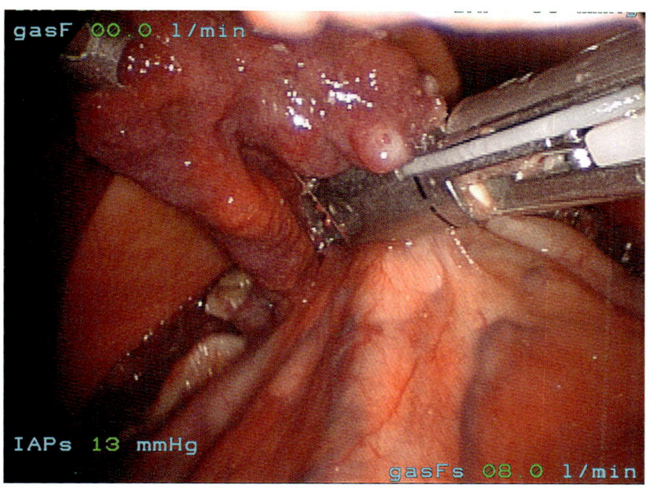

FIGURE 8. Dissection of the mediastinum from caudal to cranial with a 10 mm vessel-sealing device.

- Any tissue affected by the infection should be debrided, including lung lobectomy if lung lobes are affected or partial pericardiectomy if the infected tissue is adhered to the pericardium.
- Foreign bodies can be retrieved from the pleural space. Some dissection may be necessary to extract them from fibrous tissue (**Fig. 10**).
- Biopsy samples of the pleura, lymph nodes, or any other tissue should be submitted for histopathology and culture.
- Using the suction/irrigation device, the pleural space should be lavaged twice with at least 2 L of warm sterile saline.
- A large-bore thoracostomy tube should be placed at the end of the procedure. This tube will be used to reestablish negative pressure and perform pleural lavages in the postoperative period. The intercostal spaces used for the cannulas should be blocked with bupivacaine prior to closure.

POSTOPERATIVE MANAGEMENT

- In the postoperative period, the patient should be watched for signs of sepsis and hypoxemia.
- Supplemental oxygen should be delivered if the patient is hypoxemic.
- Pleural lavage should be performed four times a day for the next 2–3 days.
- Lidocaine and bupivacaine (1.5 mg/kg each) are administered in the pleural space through the thoracostomy tube every 6 hours. This helps to reduce the dosage of opioids.

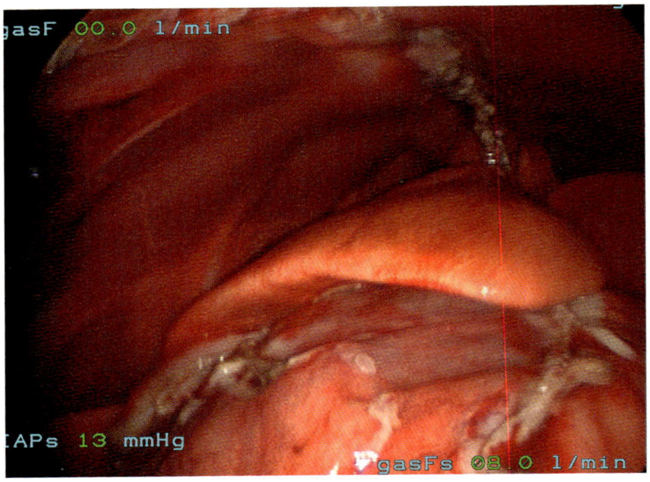

FIGURE 9. The caudal and cranial mediastinum has been debrided to better explore and lavage the pleural space.

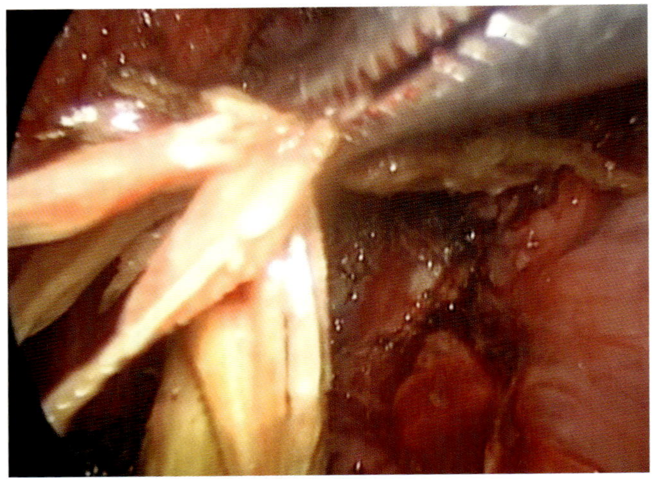

FIGURE 10. Foreign body retrieved from the cranial mediastinum and right cranial lung lobe after dissection of adhesions in the cranial mediastinum.

Complications of the thoracoscopic management of pyothorax

The complication rate mostly depends on the cause, the severity, and the chronicity of the pyothorax. In at least 50% of the cases, the cause of the pyothorax is not identified, especially if a foreign body has migrated. In a study on 14 cases treated with thoracoscopy, one dog had a recurrence 17 months after initial surgery. In humans, the outcome of pyothorax treated by thoracoscopy seems to be similar or even better than that of pyothorax treated by thoracotomy. However, it is difficult to extrapolate these data to cats and dogs because the causes of pyothorax are different in small animals compared to humans.

Conversion rate

Although the conversion rate is unknown, as this procedure is not often performed, it depends on the severity and chronicity of the pyothorax. In a study on 14 cases, the conversion rate was 14%.

Key points

- A CT scan is strongly recommended before thoracoscopic management of pyothorax.
- Double-lumen endobronchial intubation may help in exploration and debridement.
- The entire pleural space should be inspected, including the caudodorsal recesses of the diaphragm.

SUGGESTED READINGS

53 THORACOSCOPIC LUNG LOBECTOMY

Philipp D. Mayhew, Andrea Pievaroli, Roberto Properzi, Francesco Collivignarelli

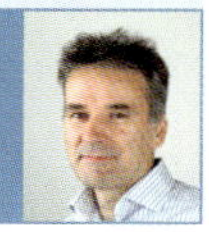

Indications

- Small mass lesions in the periphery of the lung lobes
- Most common, primary lung tumors
- Resection of single lung metastasis
- Pulmonary bullae or blebs
- Consolidated lung lobes (from pneumonia or foreign body migration)
- Lung lobe torsions

Contraindications

- Large lung mass lesions
- Large lung masses close to the hilum
- Extensive pulmonary consolidation with or without pyothorax and pulmonary adhesions

Lung lobectomies are performed in human and veterinary medicine for various conditions including neoplasia, bullae and cysts, lung lobe torsions, lung lobe consolidation or abscessation, severe bronchiectasis, trauma, and congenital anomalies. Depending on the underlying pathology, total or partial lobectomy can be performed.

In people, lung lobectomy with video-assisted thoracic surgery (VATS) is primarily recommended for small lung tumors (<2 cm). Most cases operated by VATS are non–small cell lung carcinoma stage 1a (T1N0M0). Several studies have demonstrated the short-term benefits of VATS lung lobectomy for the resection of primary lung tumors. VATS for lung lobectomy is technically demanding, and concerns about violating the principles of oncologic surgery have been raised. As only 3%–32% of lung lobectomies for primary lung tumors in people are performed by VATS, it has been suggested that this technique is still not widely accepted by all surgeons.

Thoracoscopic lung lobectomy has been reported in dogs for the removal of lung masses and pulmonary bullae. Dogs with small masses located in the periphery of the lung parenchyma have been considered better candidates for lung lobectomy via thoracoscopy. The effect of thoracoscopy on the long-term outcome after primary lung tumor resection in dogs has not been investigated.

Both VATS and thoracoscopy are minimally invasive procedures, but they do differ. During VATS, an intercostal thoracotomy is performed without retraction of the ribs to introduce standard instruments and complete the procedure. During thoracoscopy, minimally invasive surgical instruments are introduced into the thoracic cavity through cannulas. If needed, a limited intercostal thoracotomy without spreading the ribs is performed at the end of the procedure to retrieve the specimen. In people, VATS is used more often than thoracoscopy, especially for resection of primary lung tumors. However, extrapolation of data from people to dogs may not be applicable.

In dogs with lung tumors, the size and location of the mass are important criteria for patient selection. Therefore, thoracic radiographs and CT scans are important imaging modalities. For tumors in the cranial lung lobe, it can be difficult to determine if the mass is in the left or right cranial lung lobe on radiographic examination. Therefore, CT may help to further define the location of the mass and to decide the side for intercostal VATS. A CT scan also helps in the evaluation of the hilar lymph nodes. If any hilar lymph nodes look enlarged or exhibit abnormal contrast enhancement on CT scan, it is important to biopsy them during VATS. Lymph node metastasis is a strong prognostic indicator for long-term survival.

In 1992, Lewis was one of the first surgeons to report a large series of 100 consecutive patients who underwent VATS lobectomies using four ports without rib spreading.

PATIENT PREPARATION AND POSITIONING

It is mandatory to carry out an accurate preoperative diagnostic evaluation (i.e., CT, X-ray, ultrasound) to precisely locate the lesion in the affected lung lobe. This is helpful for correct port placement and triangulation. Some patients are not stable at the time of surgery, especially in case of spontaneous pneumothorax or thoracic effusion. The application of chest drainage before surgery should be considered to better control the pneumothorax or to aspirate fluids and reduce the anesthetic risks.

The patient should be fasted for 10–12 hours before surgery; water is allowed. The thorax is widely clipped, from the caudal cervical region to the cranial abdomen and from dorsal to ventral, and scrubbed according to routine protocols. Clipping the hair bilaterally in both hemithoraces is recommended. As in all thoracoscopic procedures, this is important in case of conversion to an open thoracotomy due to technical difficulties or intraoperative complications. Draping of the chest should be wide enough to include multiple intercostal spaces for proper port placement without the need for redraping if rapid conversion is needed (**Fig. 1**).

Depending on the lung lobes to be removed and anatomical location of the lesion, the patient is positioned in a lateral, sternal, or oblique position. Dorsal recumbency is most appropriate for bilateral exploration of the thoracic cavity, for biopsy of the thoracic pleura, if there are right and left lung lobe lesions, and when the location of the lesion is not precisely known. However, with this approach, hilar lymph nodes are not visible. Lateral recumbency in an oblique position is the preferred technique for lung lobectomy. In this position the thoracic organs are displaced by gravity toward the sternum, improving visualization of the hilum of the lungs and hilar lymph nodes.

Preoxygenation and all physiological parameters, such as arterial blood gas and invasive systemic pressure, must be monitored during anesthesia. The anesthetist must be skilled to manage mechanical ventilation, with good coordination between the anesthetist and the surgeons. One of the main difficulties of thoracoscopic lung lobectomy is the reduced working space in the thoracic cavity. The anesthetist must be able to reduce the tidal volume without creating failures in the patient. Alternatively, to obtain a greater working space, one-lung ventilation is recommended. This procedure, difficult to perform, is possible in medium- to large-sized dogs. Special devices (double-lumen endobronchial tube or endobronchial blocker) are used to intubate and ventilate selectively the contralateral mainstem bronchus, resulting in atelectasis of the pulmonary lobes of the hemithorax where thoracoscopy is performed.

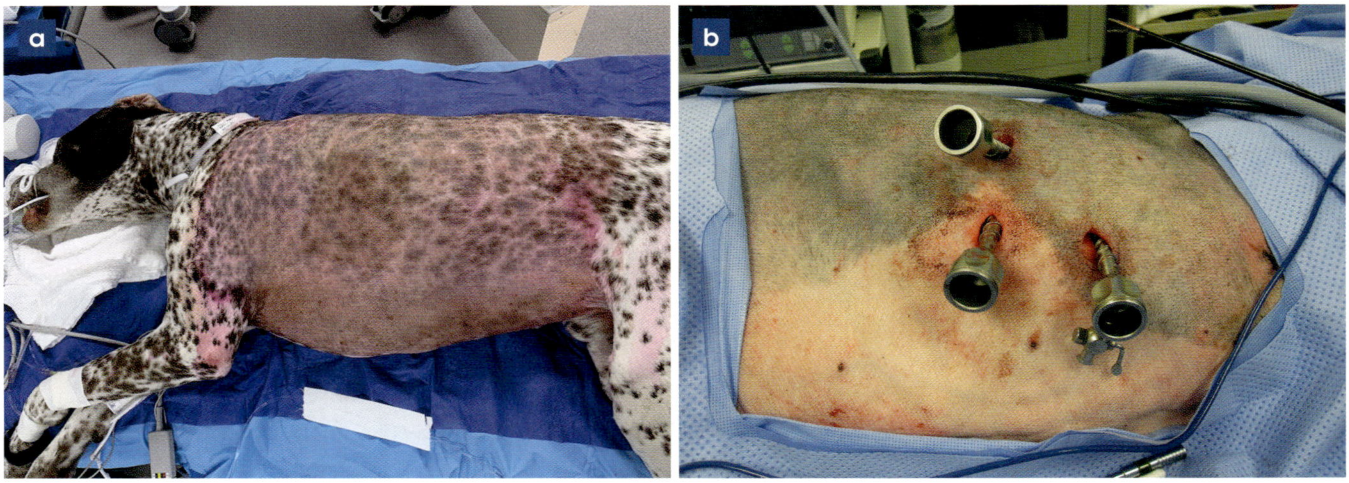

FIGURE 1. a) A wide clip and aseptic surgical scrub of the lateral thoracic wall is performed. b) After wide draping to allow access to most of the lateral thoracic wall, three thoracoscopic ports are placed in a triangulated fashion around the hilum of the lung lobe to be resected (in this case the right cranial lobe).

OPERATING ROOM LAYOUT

Thoracoscopic lung lobectomy is typically performed with the patient in lateral recumbency in an oblique position with the forelegs extended forward. The position of the operating surgeon and assistant varies depending on the lung lobe to be removed. The surgeon positions themselves towards the patient's paws. The assistant can stand on the same side of the operating table, on the opposite side, or at the caudal end of the table, depending on whether the lobectomy is caudal or cranial. The monitor is placed in front of the surgeons to facilitate appropriate triangulation and ergonomics. The anesthesia circuit and staff are positioned at the head of the operating table. The instrument table is placed near the patient's spine or laterally to the surgeon (**Fig. 2**).

The following procedures are described below:

A. Thoracoscopic lung lobectomy

B. Thoracoscopically assisted lung lobectomy

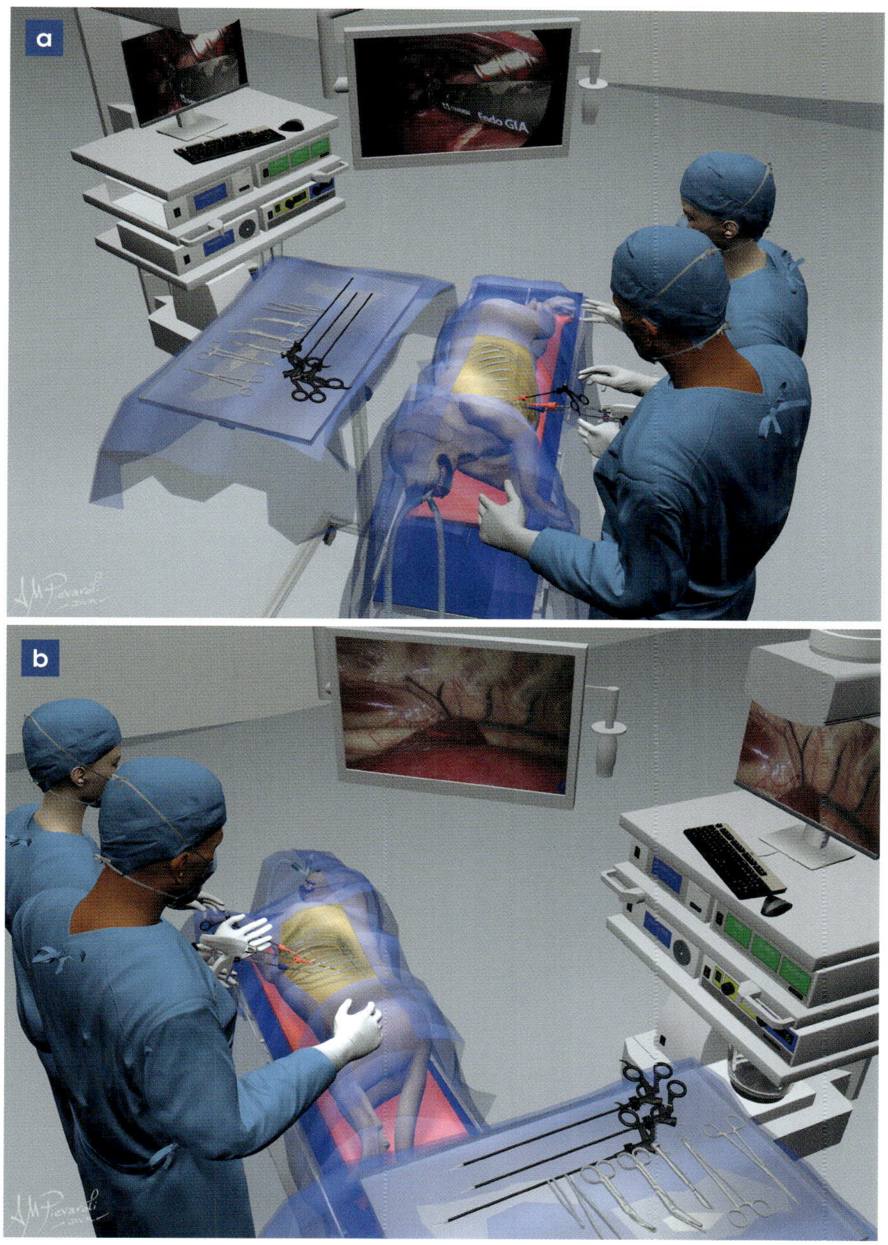

FIGURE 2. Operating room layout for thoracoscopic lung lobectomy. a) Caudal lobectomy. b) Cranial lobectomy.

Instruments

On the table:

- Standard surgical pack
- High-definition video camera
- Telescope 5 mm – 30°
- Two 5 mm threaded cannulas + one 12 mm threaded cannula
- Laparoscopic Babcock, Kelley, right-angle forceps, 5 mm
- Endoscopic stapler (EndoGIA Tri-Staple 45 and 60 mm cartridges, with different staple leg length)
- Vessel-sealing device (Enseal, LigaSure, harmonic scalpel)
- Endoscopic retrieval bag

Ready to use:

- Endoscopic cannula for aspiration/irrigation
- Laparoscopic cotton-tip blunt dissection probes, 5 mm
- L- or J-hook monopolar electrosurgical tip, 5 mm
- 3–5 cm wound retractor (e.g., Alexis wound retractor, Applied Medical)
- Fourth trocar for accessory instruments (e.g., retractor)

A THORACOSCOPIC LUNG LOBECTOMY

Thoracoscopic lung lobectomy is generally performed to remove masses up to 2–3 cm in size in dogs weighing less than 15 kg, masses up to 4–6 cm in diameter in dogs of 15–30 kg, and masses up to 8–9 cm in dogs over 30 kg.

Pulmonary bullae in any location can be resected, but care must be taken to correctly identify the leaking bullae in cases of spontaneous pneumothorax. The incidence of missed lesions may be higher with thoracoscopic treatment than with open thoracic exploration.

PORT PLACEMENT

Configuration for cranial lung lobectomy (**Fig. 3**):

- T1, telescope port (6 mm cannula if using a 5 mm telescope), in the ventral half of the 8th or 9th intercostal space
- T2, first instrument port, in the dorsal third of the same intercostal space (8th or 9th) as T1
- T3, second instrument port, usually for the endoscopic stapling device (and therefore large enough to accommodate a 12 mm instrument), in the ventral third of the 7th or 8th intercostal space

Configuration for caudal lung lobectomy (**Fig. 4**):

- T1, telescope port (6 mm cannula if using a 5 mm telescope), in the ventral third of the 3rd or 4th intercostal space

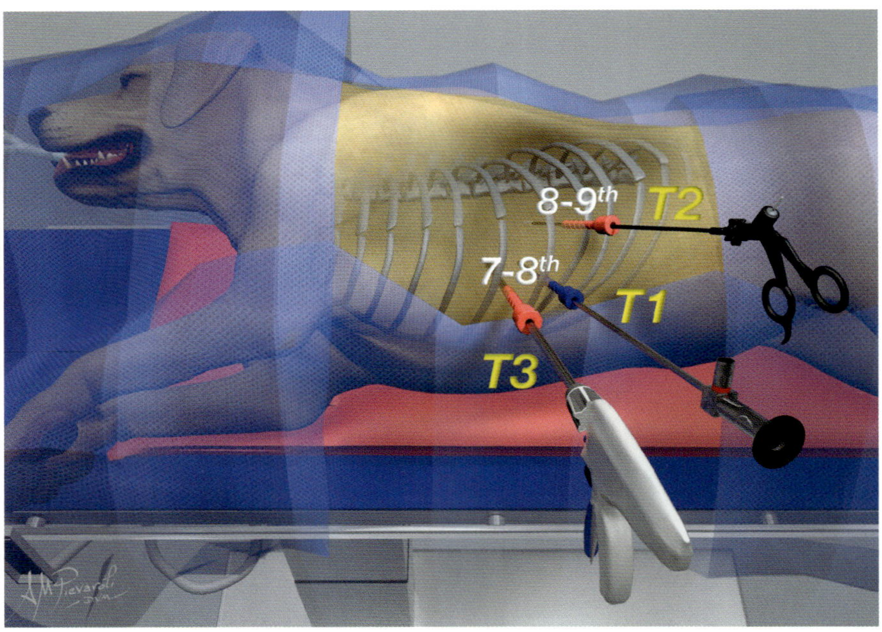

FIGURE 3. Port placement for thoracoscopic lung lobectomy of the cranial and right middle lung lobes.

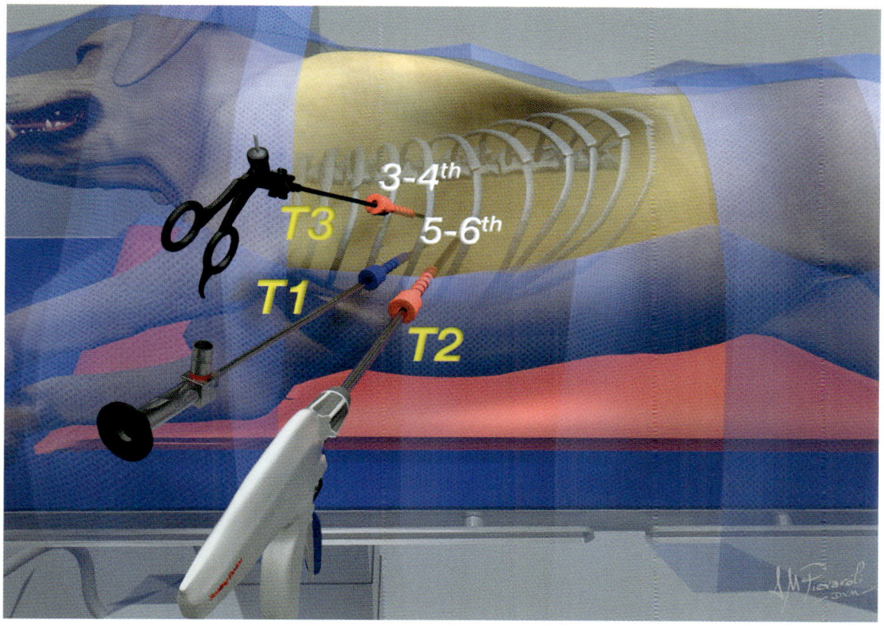

FIGURE 4. Port placement for thoracoscopic lung lobectomy of the caudal lung lobes.

- T3, first instrument port, in the dorsal third of the same intercostal space (3rd or 4th) as T1
- T2, second instrument port, usually used for the endoscopic stapling device (and therefore large enough to accommodate a 12 mm instrument), in the ventral third of the 5th or 6th intercostal space

Other configurations:

- Accessory lung lobe: same port placement as in a caudal lung lobectomy on the right side
- Right middle lung lobe: same port placement as in a cranial lung lobectomy on the right side

PROCEDURE

- After the cannulas have been placed and one-lung ventilation established, an attempt should be made to visualize the mass using the blunt probe to manipulate the affected lung lobe.
- For the caudal lung lobes and the accessory lobe, the pulmonary ligament, which attaches those lobes to the mediastinum, must be sectioned, taking care not to impinge upon the pulmonary vessels at the base of the ligament (**Fig. 5**).
- The EndoGIA stapler (Medtronic) is used to seal and divide the pulmonary artery, pulmonary vein, and bronchus. If using the traditional EndoGIA system, several cartridge lengths (30, 45, and 60 mm) and staple sizes (2.0, 2.5, 3.5, and 4.8 mm) are available. For lung lobectomy in dogs, it has been generally recommended to use 60 mm long cartridges with 3.5 mm staple leg lengths. The newer Tri-Staple technology uses graduated staple leg lengths to improve the quality of the seal. The authors usually use the purple-colored cartridge, which is available in 45 and 60 mm lengths and has staple leg lengths of 3, 3.5 and 4 mm.
- The EndoGIA is passed through the 12 mm instrument port. For a complete lung lobectomy, the cartridge is placed across the pulmonary artery, pulmonary vein, and bronchus together (**Fig. 6**). Once in the correct position, the tips are closed, the staples dispensed, and the cartridge is reopened and carefully pulled back and out of the cannula. If the

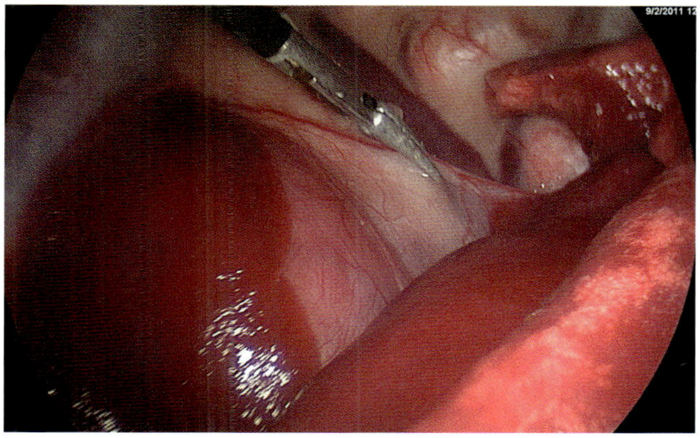

FIGURE 5. In this dog, the pulmonary ligament attaching the caudal lung lobe to the mediastinum is being sectioned with a vessel-sealing device. Note the color of the lung as a result of atelectasis due to one-lung ventilation.

EndoGIA cartridge used was not long enough to section the entire length of the lung lobe, a second cartridge can be used to complete the transection of the lung parenchyma or pulmonary hilum (**Fig. 7**).

- Once the lung lobectomy is completed, the cut surface of the pulmonary hilum is carefully examined for hemorrhage or air leakage. The resected lung lobe should be placed in a specimen retrieval bag and the bag removed through one of the port incisions (**Fig. 8**).
- At this point, inspection of the pulmonary hilum for any lymph node enlargement should be attempted. If lymphadenopathy is present, aspiration of the nodes and/or biopsy or resection may be considered. Knowledge of potential metastatic spread to lymph nodes has significant prognostic and therapeutic implications, and preoperative CT is helpful in decision-making with regard to lymph node extirpation.
- The staple line can be inked to facilitate pathological assessment of the margin of resection if a lung mass was present (**Fig. 9**).
- Once the lung lobe has been retrieved from the thorax, a chest drain is placed and port sites are closed routinely.

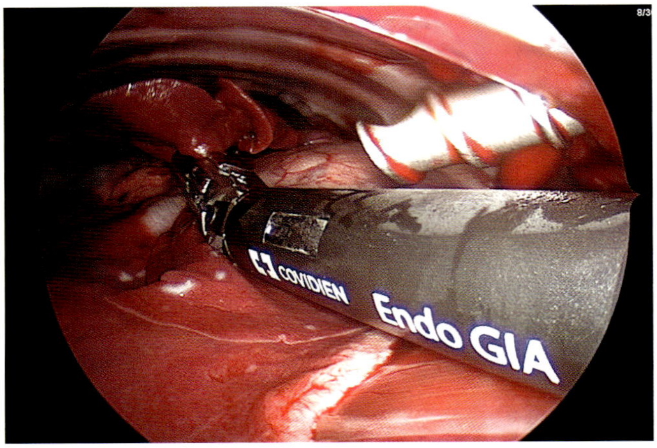

FIGURE 6. The endoscopic stapler is placed around the hilum of the cranial lung lobe.

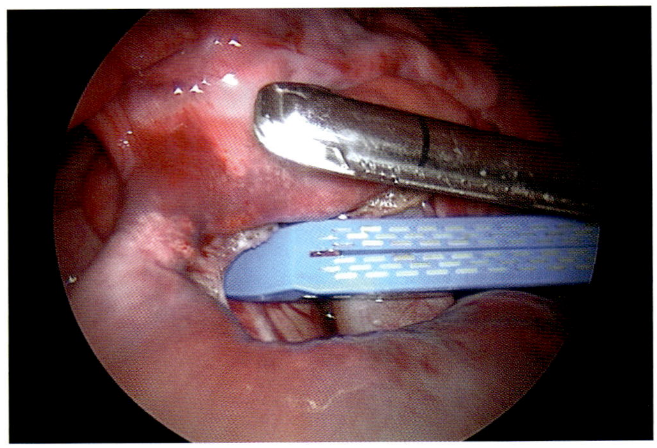
FIGURE 7. The endoscopic stapler has been fired but has resulted in incomplete separation of the pulmonary hilum in this dog. Options for completion of the resection include placement of a second stapler cartridge across the remaining tissue or use of an endoscopic loop ligature.

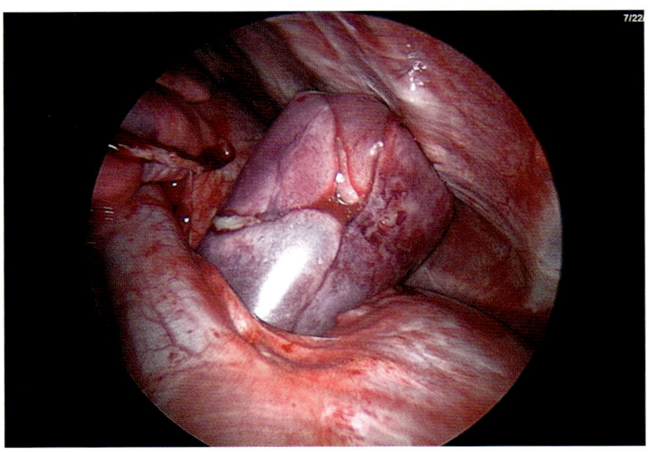
FIGURE 8. The resected lung has been placed in a specimen retrieval bag and is now ready to be withdrawn through an enlargement of the port incision.

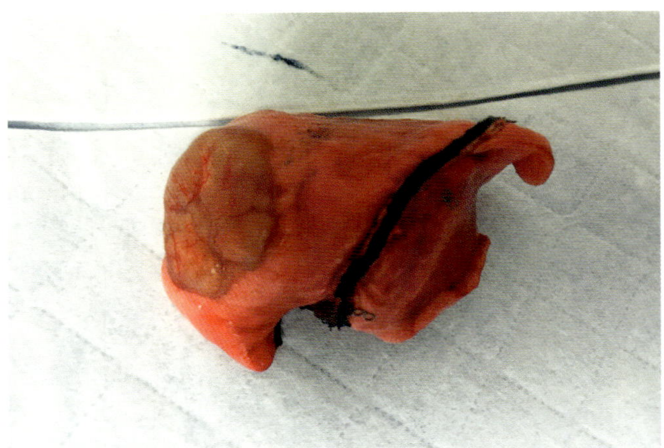
FIGURE 9. This resected lung lobe is ready to be submitted for histopathological evaluation. Note the blue surgical ink that has been placed at the surgical margin to aid in the assessment of the oncological margins.

B THORACOSCOPICALLY ASSISTED LUNG LOBECTOMY

ASSIST INCISION PLACEMENT

- The assist incision for thoracoscopically assisted lung lobectomy is best made in the 4th–6th intercostal spaces to minimize the distance from the hilum to the stapling device and to ensure optimal oncological margins for resection of mass lesions (**Fig. 10**).

PROCEDURE

- The assist incision is generally 4–6 cm long, but its length depends on the size of the lung lobe and the mass lesion to be removed. The incision edges are retracted using Army-Navy or Gelpi tissue retractors, or alternatively a wound retractor can be inserted into the incision (Alexis wound retractor, Applied Medical).
- For the caudal or accessory lung lobes, the pulmonary ligament needs to be sectioned first, as described above for totally thoracoscopic lung lobectomy. Since doing this through the assist incision can be challenging, placement of one or two additional 5–6 mm cannulas in a triangulated fashion around the caudal thorax is helpful.
- Once the mass has been identified, the affected lung lobe is exteriorized through the assist incision and the lobe is resected using a conventional or endoscopic stapling device (**Fig. 11**). If the mass is close to the hilum and placement of a thoracoabdominal stapler is challenging, an endoscopic stapling cartridge can be placed through a separate 12 mm cannula in an attempt to resect the lobe closer to the hilum, thereby achieving a potentially superior oncologic margin. If challenging to manipulate out of the incision, instruments or a finger can be used to help retract or otherwise manipulate the mass and affected lobe (**Fig. 12**).
- After the lobe has been resected, the hilum is closely inspected for hemorrhage or air leakage and the port incisions and minithoracotomy site are closed routinely.

POSTOPERATIVE MANAGEMENT

- Hospitalization time is 2–3 days.
- The thoracostomy tube can be removed 8–12 hours after surgery.
- The patient should be closely monitored for postoperative pneumothorax, which is most often caused by iatrogenic trauma to the lung parenchyma.
- Pain is controlled with a constant-rate infusion of opioids.

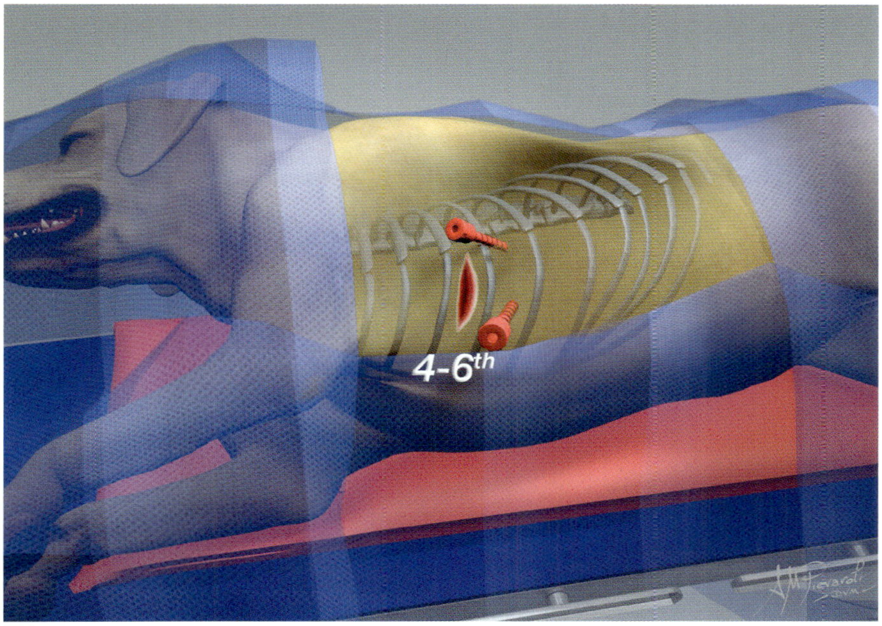

FIGURE 10. The incision for thoracoscopically assisted lung lobectomy is made in the 4th–6th intercostal spaces. Additional 5–6 mm cannulas in a triangulated fashion are often helpful.

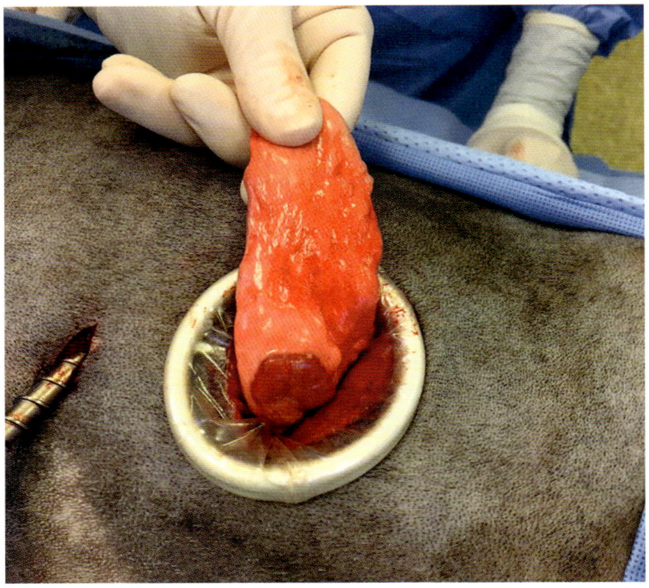

FIGURE 11. In this thoracoscopically assisted lung lobectomy, a lung mass has been exteriorized through an assist incision and is ready for resection using a stapling device.

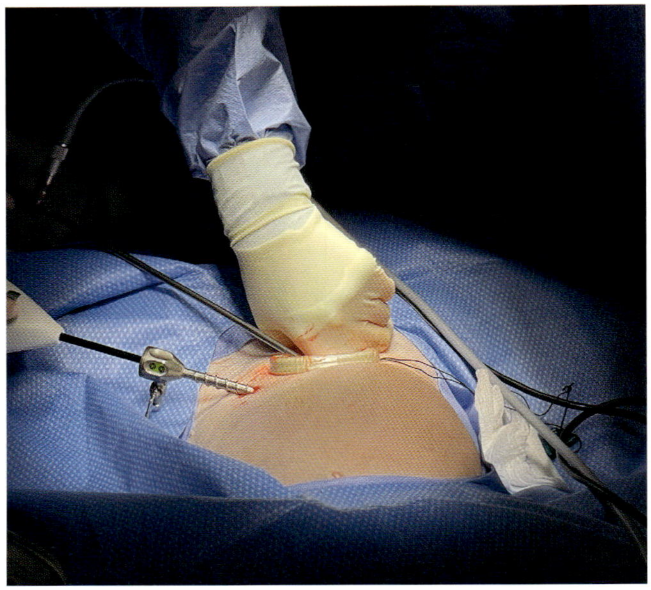

FIGURE 12. If necessary, instruments or even a surgeon's finger can be inserted through the assist incision to aid in manipulation of the pulmonary ligament or exteriorization of the affected lung lobe.

Complications of thoracoscopic lung lobectomy

- Hemorrhage from an intercostal artery.
- Seroma at incision site.
- Subcutaneous emphysema associated with the thoracostomy tube.
- Aspiration pneumonia.
- Poor oxygenation.
- Thrombocytopenia and hyperthermia.

Key points

- One-lung ventilation permits an optimal hilum visualization during thoracoscopic procedures.
- Clean margins are a good prognostic indicator after resection of primary lung tumors.
- The hilum can be difficult to visualize if the tumor is too close to the hilum or if the tumor is larger than 8 cm.
- Thoracoscopy may indirectly improve postoperative immune function by reducing the systemic inflammatory response.
- Placing the patient in slightly oblique lateral recumbency can help to visualize the hilum.
- The thoracoscopically assisted technique can be performed when one-lung ventilation or endoscopic stapling equipment are not available or in very small patients when those techniques are more challenging.

SUGGESTED READINGS

CLINICAL CASES

53.1 HILAR LUNG LOBECTOMY

Ikuya Ehara

CASE DESCRIPTION

A 1.5-year-old castrated male Toy Poodle with a body weight of 4.6 kg was presented with a 2-week history of inactiveness and productive cough and an acute onset of respiratory distress. Other than elevation of GPT (120 U/L), no significant abnormalities were observed on blood work. Radiography and CT imaging revealed a pneumothorax with right lung atelectasis as well as multiple emphysematous lesions of approximately 15.1–59.3×7.1–46.3×5.6–32.7 mm in size. The patient was scheduled for thoracoscopic lung lobectomy.

Key points

- The region was probed with Maryland forceps to reveal any adhesions to surrounding structures and the presence of any other vessels.
- The pulmonary vein was isolated with Maryland right-angle forceps.
- The pulmonary artery and bronchus were ligated en bloc due to the firm attachment between the two.
- One of the ligatures penetrated the bronchi to prevent slippage.

PORT PLACEMENT

With the patient in semilateral recumbency, ports were placed in the 3rd (T3), 5th (T1), and 7th (T2) intercostal spaces, at the level of the costochondral junction.

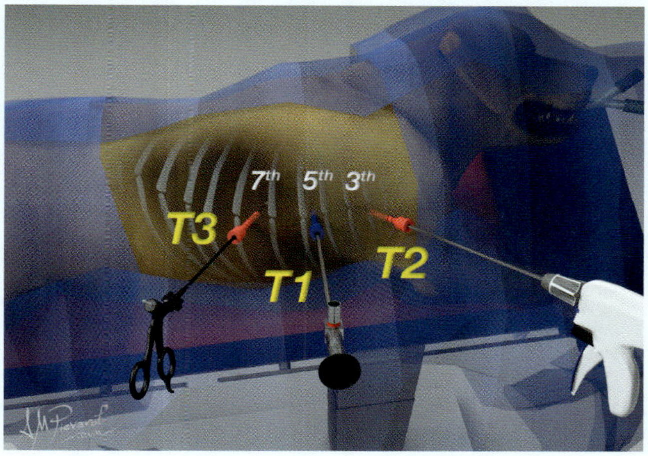

PROCEDURE

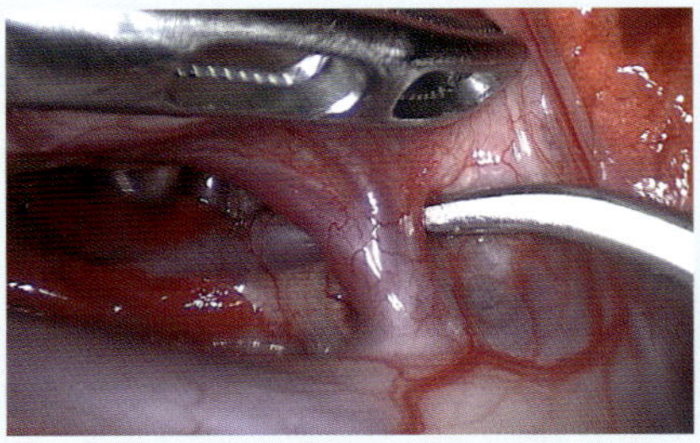

FIGURE 1. The pulmonary vein is identified.

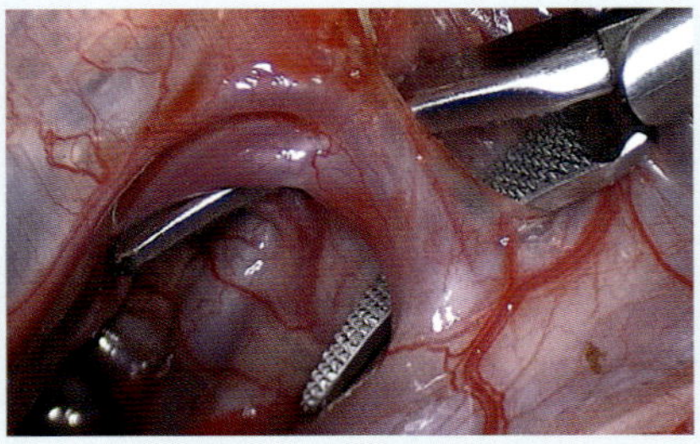

FIGURE 2. Using Maryland right-angle forceps, the pulmonary vein is isolated.

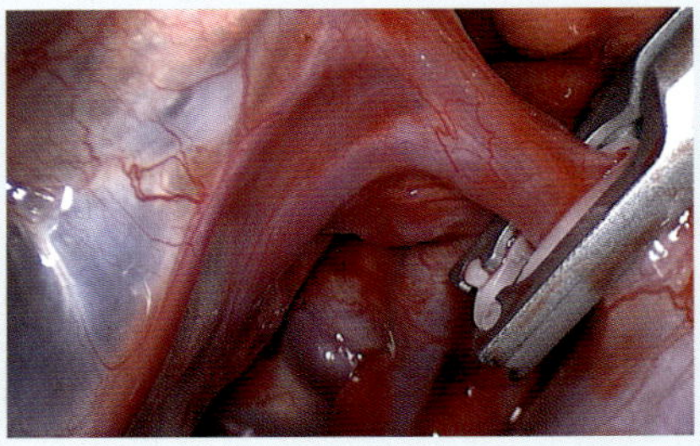

FIGURE 3. The pulmonary vein is closed with four hemoclips (5 mm Hem-o-lok, ML).

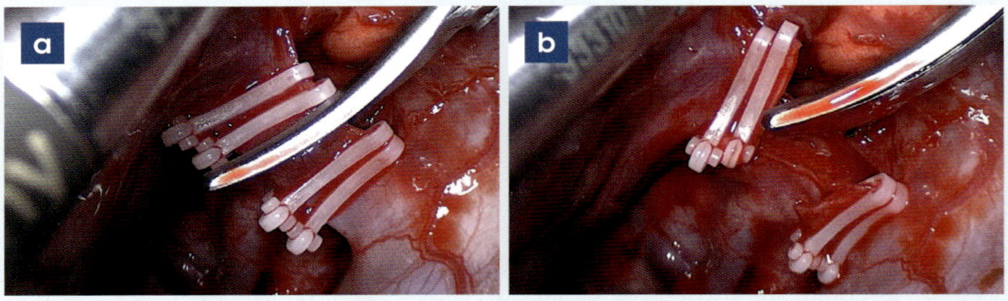

FIGURE 4. Using scissors, the pulmonary vein is transected, leaving two clips on each end.

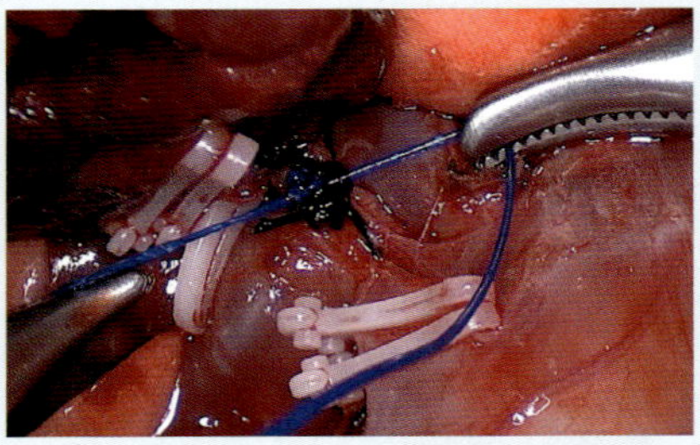

FIGURE 5. The bronchus and pulmonary artery are ligated at three sites.

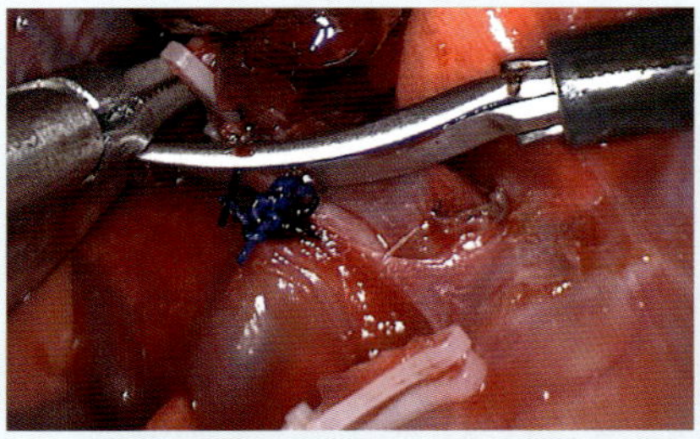

FIGURE 6. Using scissors, the bronchus and pulmonary artery are transected between the ligatures, leaving one ligature on the affected lobe and the other two intracorporeally.

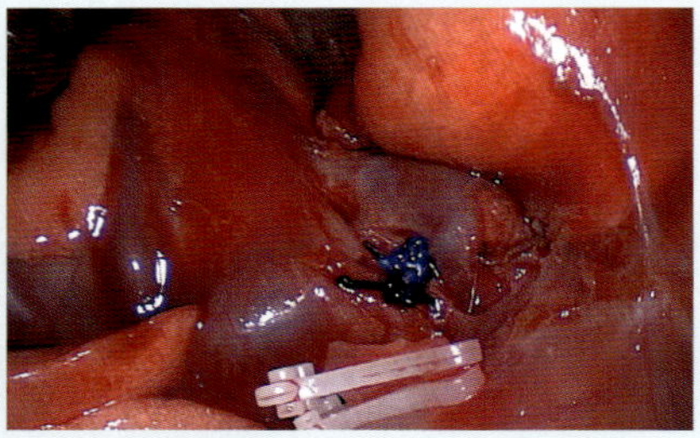

FIGURE 7. Sites of pulmonary vein as well as bronchus and pulmonary artery occlusion by the two clips and the ligature, respectively, can be seen. The right middle lung lobe was completely excised.

Tips and tricks

- ✓ Use one-lung ventilation.
- ✓ Place the patient in semilateral recumbency.
- ✓ Ligate major vessels and bronchus intracorporeally.
- ✓ Surgical staplerless procedure.
- ✓ Avoid residual lobar tissue.

53.2 VIDEO-ASSISTED THORACOSCOPIC SURGERY PULMONARY LOBECTOMY

David García Rubio

CASE DESCRIPTION

A 14-year-old mixed-breed dog was presented with an acute onset of moderate cough. Upon performing thoracic radiography, a nodular zone with increased radiodensity was seen in the dorsal pulmonary area. A CT scan showed the presence of a single mass 3 cm in diameter in the right caudal lobe and confirmed the absence of metastasis.

Key points

- A preoperative CT scan is recommended to rule out multiple masses and metastasis.
- The resected lung should be checked for bleeding or air leakage.

PORT PLACEMENT

The patient was placed in left lateral recumbency. The first trocar (T1), for the telescope, was positioned in the dorsal part of the 10th intercostal space. After establishing a pneumothorax, a second (T2) and a third (T3) trocar were placed under direct visualization in the middle area of the 10th and 5th intercostal space, respectively.

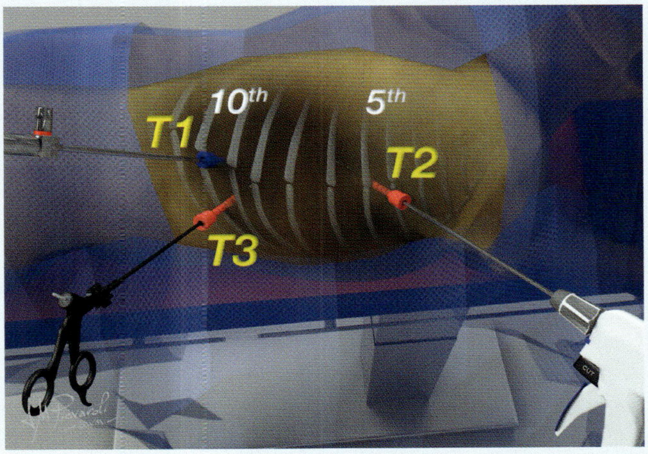

PROCEDURE

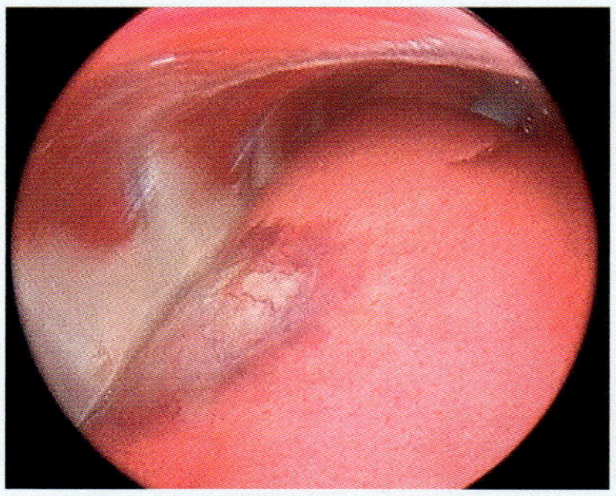

FIGURE 1. Appearance of the pulmonary neoplasia (white, sunken circular area) on the surface of the right caudal lung lobe.

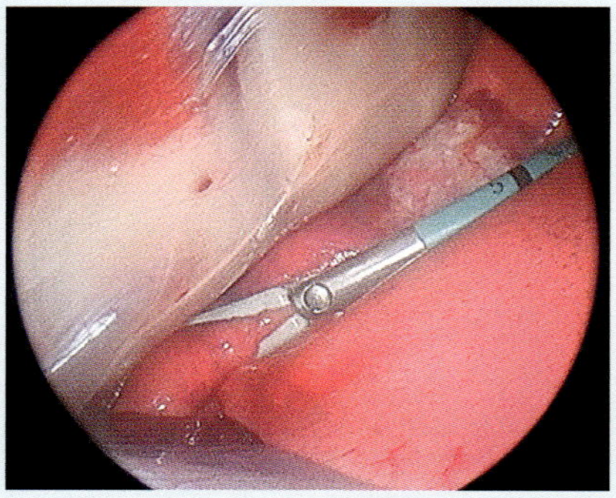

FIGURE 2. Using atraumatic forceps inserted through the 5th intercostal space port, the apex of the lung lobe is grasped and externalized.

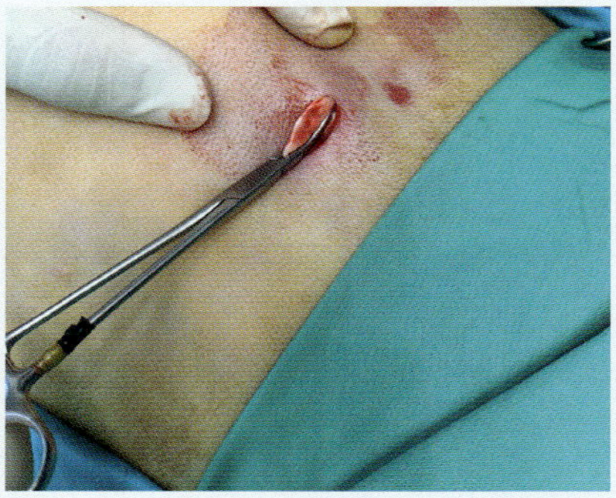

FIGURE 3. With the externalized lobe apex firmly secured, the access in the 5th intercostal space is increased until it is large enough to allow for removal of the mass.

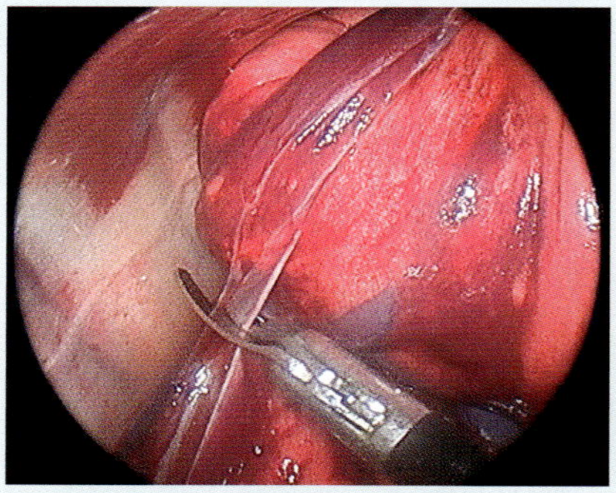

FIGURE 4. In the caudal lung lobes, the pulmonary ligament is cut to permit complete extraction of the affected lobe.

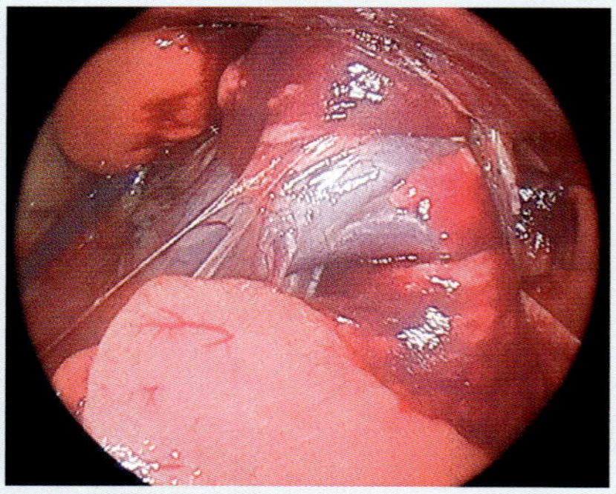

FIGURE 5. Detailed view of the pulmonary hilum following complete extraction of the lobe.

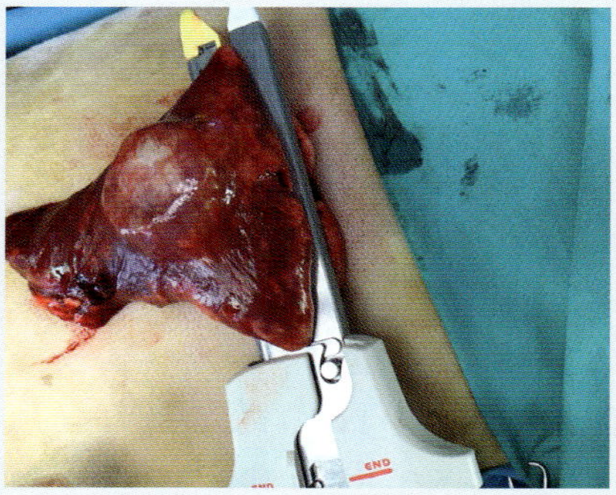

FIGURE 6. After the pulmonary mass has been completely externalized, it is closed and resected using a surgical stapler.

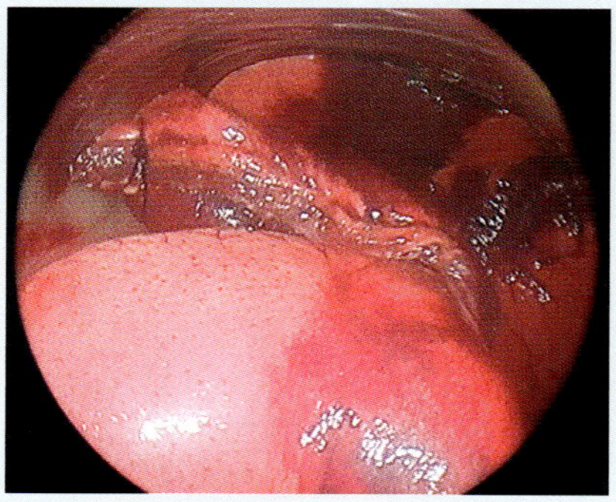

FIGURE 7. The resected lung is checked for bleeding or air leakage.

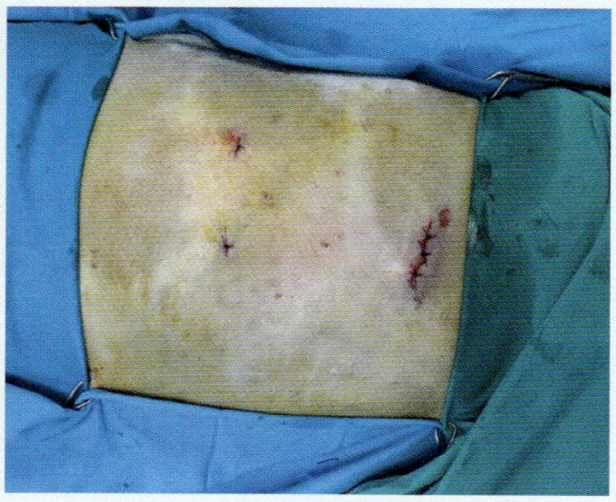

FIGURE 8. Final appearance of the surgical area after suturing and closure in layers.

Tips and tricks

- ✓ When operating on the caudal lung lobes, resect the pulmonary ligament before completely externalizing the lobe.
- ✓ Closure and sectioning of the affected lung can be completed extracorporeally for apex masses or intracorporeally (using a laparoscopic mechanical suture system) if the tumor is near the hilum of the lungs.
- ✓ Although not generally necessary, very low positive pressures of CO_2 (1–2 mmHg) may be used to improve visualization.
- ✓ Placement of the most cranial trocar depends on the lung lobe to be extirpated (see table).

Minithoracotomy site based on the lung lobe to be extirpated	
Lung lobe	**Minithoracotomy location**
Left cranial	Left 4th or 5th intercostal space, middle third
Left caudal	Left 4th or 5th intercostal space, middle third
Right cranial	Right 4th or 5th intercostal space, middle third
Right middle	Right 4th or 5th intercostal space, middle third
Right caudal	Right 5th or 6th intercostal space, middle third
Accessory	Right 6th intercostal space, middle third

53.3 THORACOSCOPIC LUNG LOBECTOMY FOR LUNG LOBE TORSION

Roberto Bussadori, Deborah De Bastiani

CASE DESCRIPTION

A 9-year-old castrated male Spanish Galgo was presented with hyperthermia, anorexia, and dyspnea for 4 days. A right middle lung lobe torsion was diagnosed after thoracic radiographs and subsequent CT scan. Totally thoracoscopic lung lobectomy was elected.

Key points

- A blunt probe was used to remove adhesions around the affected lung lobe.
- The lobe was elevated with a fan retractor to expose the pulmonary hilum.
- An EndoGIA stapler (60 mm) was used to perform the lung lobectomy.
- The resected lobe was removed with a retrieval bag.
- Thoracic drainage was utilized.

PORT PLACEMENT

The dog was placed in left lateral recumbency, in an oblique position. A three-port approach was used. To access the right medial lobe, the ports were placed as follows: 5 mm telescope port (T1) in the ventral third of the right 7th intercostal space, 12 mm instrument port (T2) in the dorsal third of the right 8th intercostal space, and 12 mm instrument port (T3) in the middle third of the right 5th intercostal space.

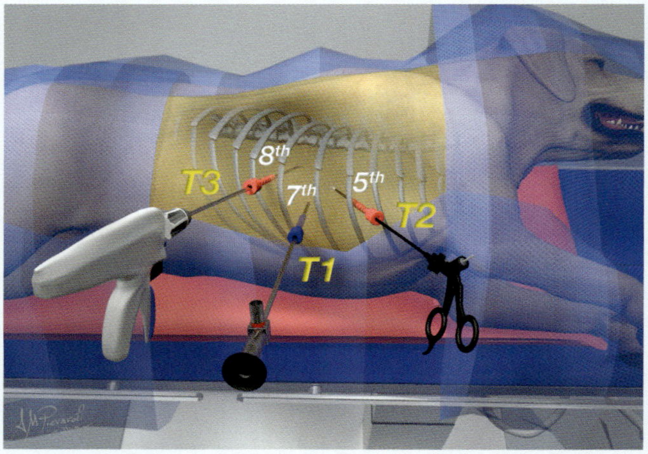

PROCEDURE

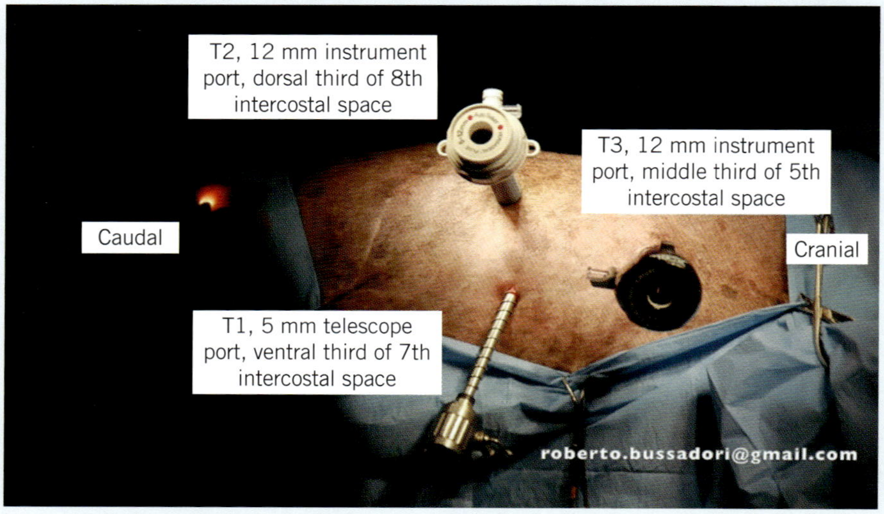

FIGURE 1. Intraoperative port placement.

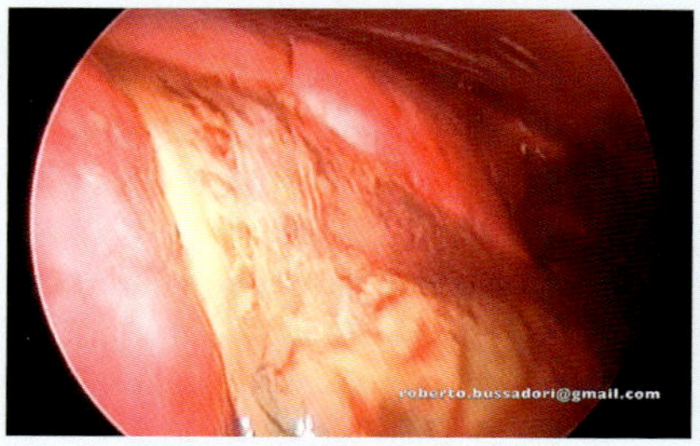

FIGURE 2. Appearance of the right medial lung lobe.

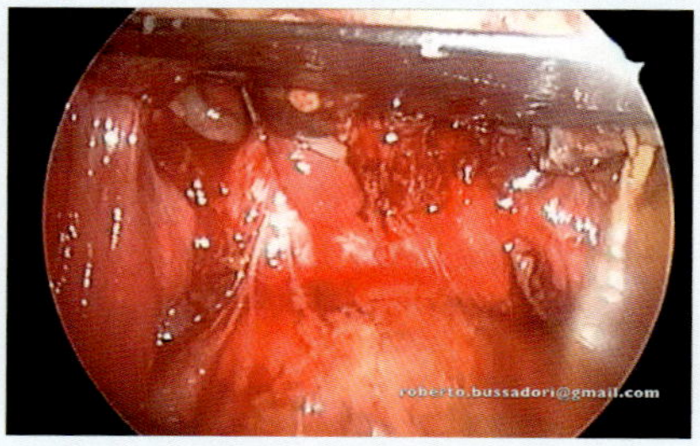

FIGURE 3. Evidence of the twisted pulmonary hilum, which is being elevated with a fan retractor.

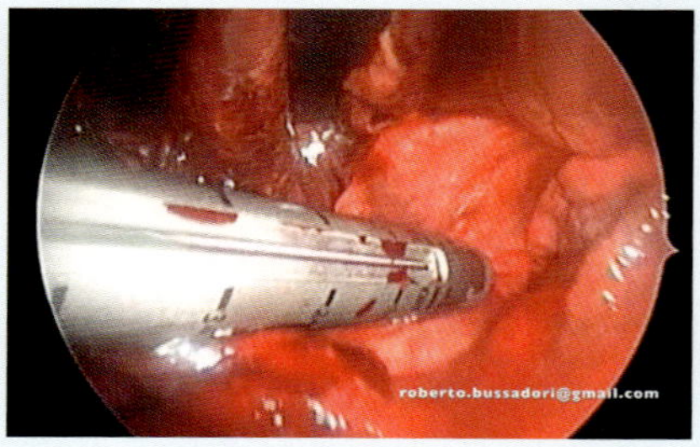

FIGURE 4. Lung lobectomy is performed using a 60 mm EndoGIA.

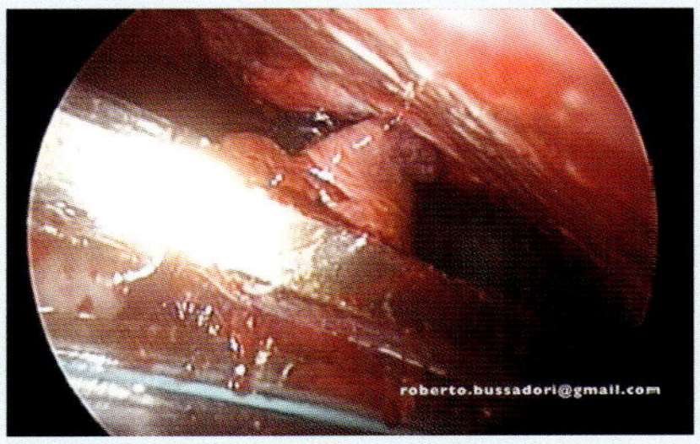

FIGURE 5. The resected lung lobe is inserted into a retrieval bag for removal.

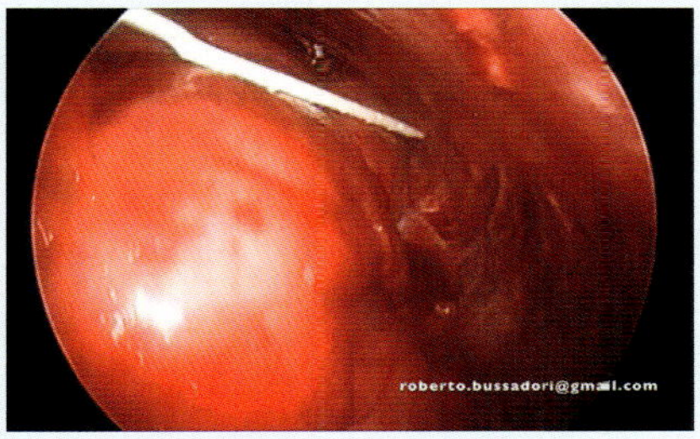

FIGURE 6. A chest drain is inserted at the end of the procedure.

Tips and tricks

- ✓ Totally thoracoscopic lung lobectomy can be performed without pulmonary exclusion.
- ✓ Place the staple line as perpendicular as possible to the hilum of the lung to optimize the use of staple length.

53.4 THORACOSCOPIC LOBECTOMY OF THE RIGHT MIDDLE LUNG LOBE IN A DOG

Li-Ren Wang, Jung-Hsien Sun, Yi-Fu Chang

CASE DESCRIPTION

A 7-year-old spayed female Maltese dog was evaluated for excision of a mass in the right thoracic cavity. The patient was presented with cough and panting for several months. On physical examination, a grade V/VI left systolic heart murmur was detected. A soft tissue mass was observed in the middle-right part of the thorax on radiographs. A CT scan revealed lung lobe torsion, and necrosis of the right middle lung lobe was suspected. The dog underwent video-assisted thoracoscopic removal of the mediastinal mass. The diagnosis was chronic, active, pyogranulomatous, necrohemorrhagic pneumonia.

Key points

- A preoperative CT angiographic scan is useful to determine the location of a mass and assess the vascular system.
- During dissection, attention should be paid to the location of the vessels and the organs such as the heart.
- It is important to seal the bronchus during lung lobectomy.

PORT PLACEMENT

The dog was placed in left recumbency, and the entire right lateral thorax was clipped. Three thoracoscopic ports were placed for the introduction of surgical instruments. A 1 cm thoracotomy incision was made in the 9th intercostal space, at mid-thorax, for placement of the first port (T1) and insertion of a 5 mm 30° telescope. After examination of the thorax, two additional ports were similarly placed under thoracoscopic visualization. The instrument port (T3) was placed in the dorsal part of the right 8th intercostal space. The vessel-sealing device port (T2) was placed in the ventral part of the right 8th intercostal space.

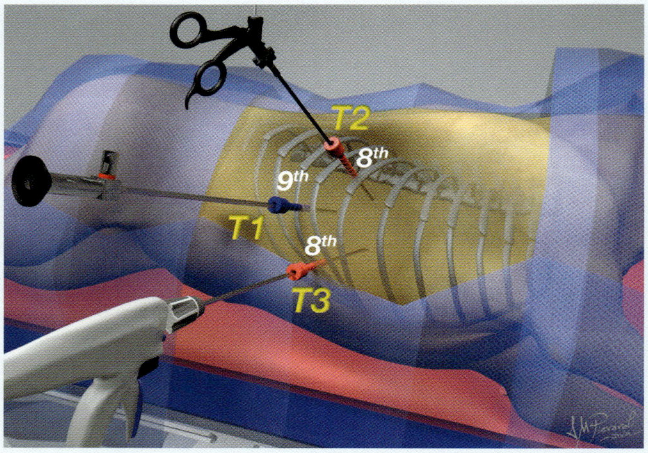

PROCEDURE

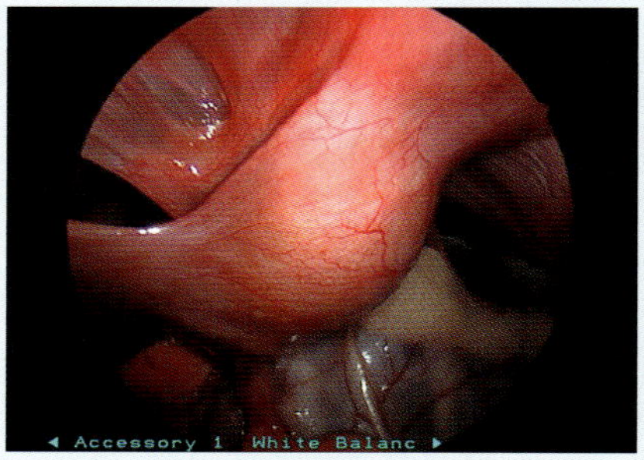

FIGURE 1. Thoracoscopic image of the mass.

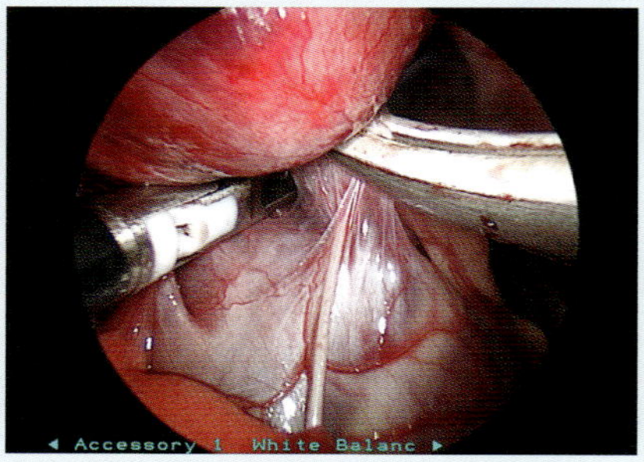

FIGURE 2. The adhesions between the lung lobe and the surrounding tissues are bluntly dissected using thoracoscopic forceps and an ultrasonic dissection device. Then, an EndoGIA stapler is used for transection of the bronchus. The resected lung lobe is placed in a sterile bag and retrieved from the thorax.

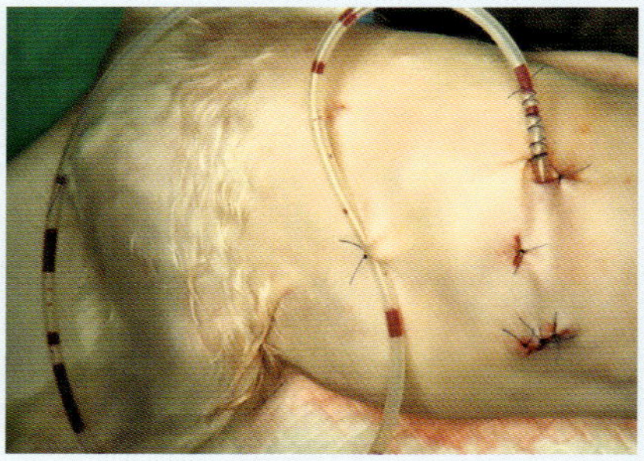

FIGURE 3. A drainage system is placed to avoid pneumothorax.

Tips and tricks

- ✓ The choice of location of the camera port is not to be underestimated.
- ✓ Create an anesthesia work team.
- ✓ Ensure clear visualization with the telescope for safe dissection.
- ✓ Before closing the thorax, place a drainage system to avoid pneumothorax.

54 THORACOSCOPIC APPROACH TO VASCULAR RING ANOMALIES

J. Brad Case

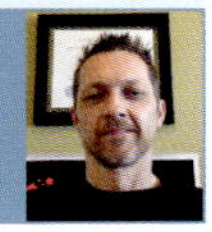

Indications

- PRAA with left ligamentum arteriosum
- PRAA with aberrant left subclavian artery

Contraindications

- Unstable or severely malnourished dogs
- Dogs with complex vascular rings (e.g., double aorta)
- Inexperience with advanced thoracoscopic surgery
- Very small patient size may be a relative contraindication

Vascular ring anomalies are developmental errors which result in complete or incomplete constriction of the esophagus and/or trachea. They result from altered involution and incorrect persistence of fetal aortic arches. In dogs, persistence of the right fourth (instead of the left fourth) aortic arch is the most common vascular ring anomaly and creates the classic persistent right aortic arch (PRAA) with left ligamentum arteriosum. The PRAA can be the sole cause of esophageal constriction or it may be present along with an aberrant left subclavian artery. In both cases, clinical signs usually appear after weaning, including regurgitation, dysphagia, and cough. Breeds commonly affected include the German Shepherd and Irish Setter, but many breeds may be affected.

Diagnostic evaluation should include survey radiography and CT of the thorax. Typical findings include a dilated esophagus cranial to the heart base, tracheal deviation to the left on ventral/dorsal projections, and ventral deviation of the trachea on lateral projections. CT is useful and is recommended to detect other concurrent vascular abnormalities such as an aberrant left subclavian artery which may require surgical ligation and division. Finally, esophagoscopy is also useful to confirm diagnosis of a PRAA and to guide thoracoscopic dissection, but it does not allow for diagnosis of other vascular malformations such as double aortic arch or a concurrent aberrant subclavian artery.

The goals of surgery are to dissect, ligate, and divide the structures responsible for constricting the esophagus. A few case series have been published in the veterinary literature describing the use of thoracoscopy to divide the left ligamentum arteriosum with or without concurrent division of aberrant left subclavian arteries. Results are generally good, with few complications reported.

> Thoracoscopic surgery of a vascular ring anomaly in a dog was first described by C. M. MacPhail in 2001.

DESCRIBED SURGICAL PROCEDURES

A three- or four-port thoracoscopic technique with 5 or 3 mm instrumentation has been described. The advantage of using a fourth port is the improvement of visualization by facilitating retraction of the left lung parenchyma. Use of one-lung ventilation and CO_2 insufflation have also been reported. However, most clinical reports describe treatment without lung manipulation, so it is unclear how beneficial additional ports or left lung collapse is.

PATIENT PREPARATION AND POSITIONING

A physical examination, complete blood count, and serum biochemistry should be performed prior to surgery. Diagnostic imaging including thoracic radiography and CT angiography are also recommended. In some cases, dogs are severely malnourished and have a poor body condition. Consideration of supportive care including elevated tube feeding beyond the esophageal constriction to improve health prior to surgery is warranted.

In general, the patient should be fasted for at least 8 hours prior to anesthesia and have an IV catheter placed for fluid and medication therapy during the procedure. Perioperative analgesia may include opioid and/or nonsteroidal medications. Local anesthesia with bupivacaine is recommended at individual port sites prior to incision. Following a 360° surgical clip including the chest and cranial abdomen, the patient is aseptically prepared according to standard techniques. Both lateral and semilateral patient positioning have been described, but the author prefers to place the patient in semilateral recumbency to facilitate ventral displacement of the lungs due to gravity. Semilateral recumbency is facilitated by placing a thin-rolled towel or sandbag under the patient's thoracic spine or by tilting the table to create approximately 15° of elevation (**Fig. 1**).

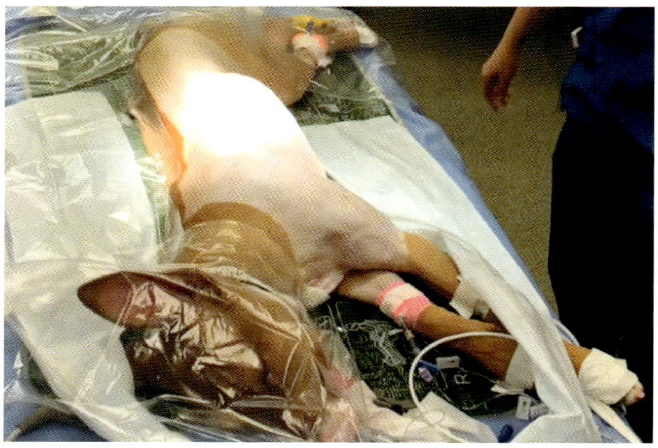

FIGURE 1. Patient positioned in semilateral recumbency for thoracoscopic division of a PRAA and left ligamentum arteriosum.

OPERATING ROOM LAYOUT

Thoracoscopic left ligamentum dissection is typically performed with the operating surgeon and the assistant standing on the same side of the operating table, towards the patient's paws. The monitors should be placed on the opposite side of the table, over the dog's spine, to facilitate appropriate triangulation. The anesthesia circuit and staff are placed at the head of the operating table. The instrument table is placed under the monitors, near the patient's spine (**Figs. 2 and 3**).

PORT PLACEMENT (FIG. 4)

- T1, in the dorsal third of the left 10th intercostal space, thoracoscope port
- T2, in the middle third of the left 11th intercostal space, dissection instrument port
- T3, in the ventral third of the left 10th or 11th intercostal space, dissection instrument port

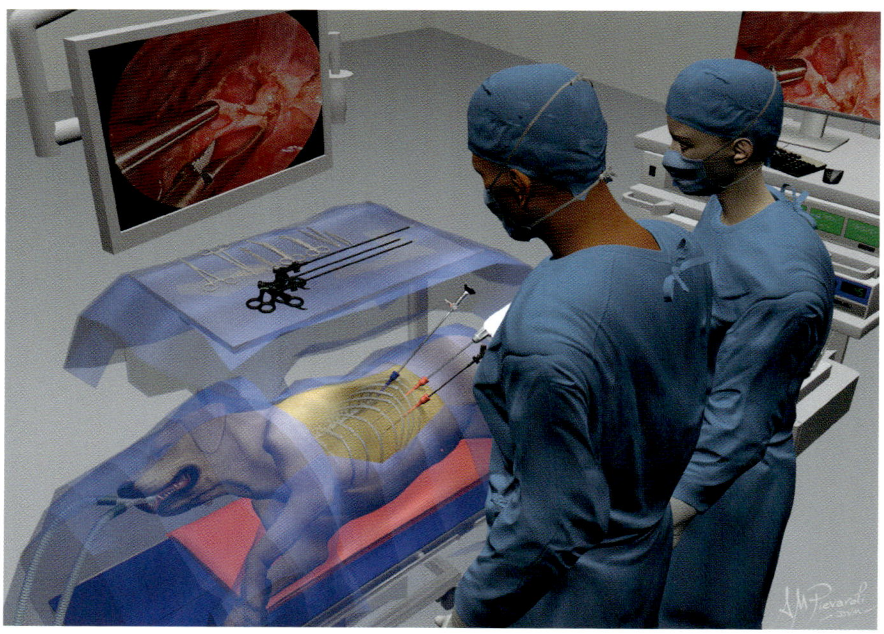

FIGURE 2. Operating room layout for thoracoscopic approach to a PRAA.

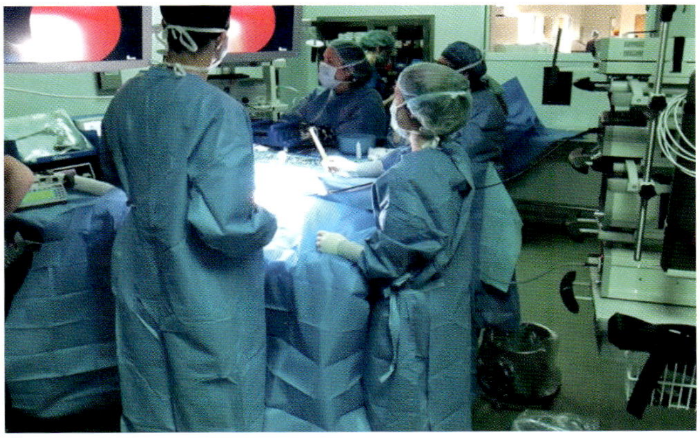

FIGURE 3. Intraoperative image of the operating room layout. Note the assistant operating the endoscope stands at the end of the operating table, while the surgeon performing the procedure stands on the side of the table.

Instruments

On the table:

- Standard surgical pack
- High-definition video camera
- Telescope 5 or 3 mm – 30°
- Three 3 or 5 mm threaded cannulas
- Laparoscopic Babcock, Kelley, right-angle forceps, 5 mm
- Laparoscopic cotton-tip, blunt dissection probes, 5 mm
- L- or J-hook monopolar electrosurgical tip, 5 mm
- Bipolar vessel-sealing device, 5 mm

PROCEDURE

- After all the ports have been placed, the left hemithorax is explored to confirm the diagnosis (**Fig. 5**). Generally, a dilated esophagus and the absence of a left descending aorta is immediately apparent. Concurrent esophagoscopy may also help to localize the site of constriction (**Fig. 6**).
- Dissection of the mediastinal pleura over the constricting ligamentum arteriosum is initiated using the bipolar vessel-sealing device. Commonly, a small pleural vein is present over the ligamentum and needs to be sealed and divided (**Figs. 7 and 8**).

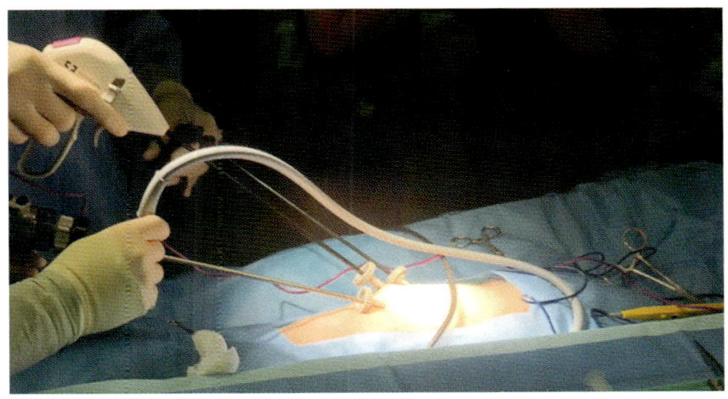

FIGURE 5. Intraoperative image of a dog with a PRAA undergoing thoracoscopic ligation and division of a left ligamentum arteriosum. Note the thoracoscope in the most dorsal port and the instruments in the middle and ventral ports. This arrangement minimizes clashing between the endoscope and instruments during the procedure.

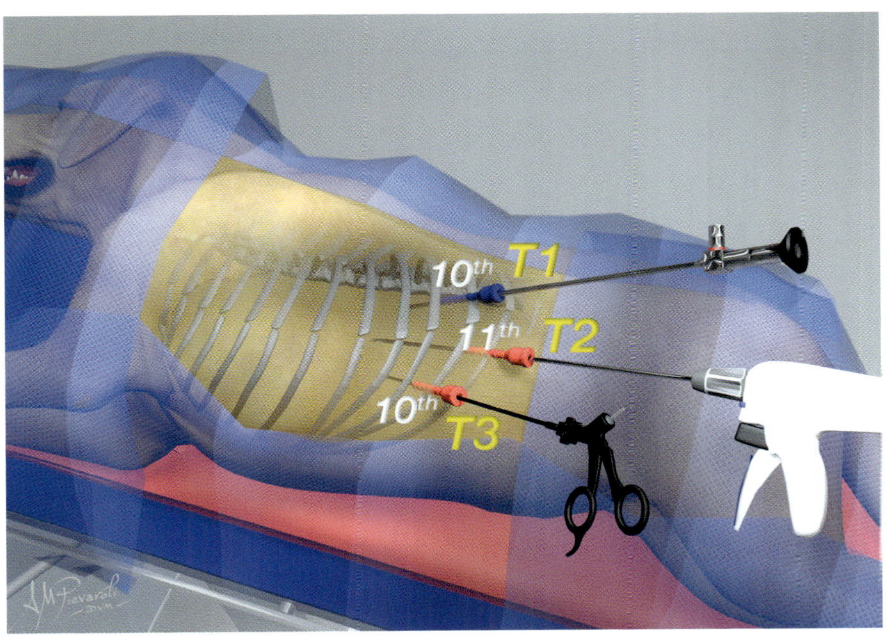

FIGURE 4. Port placement for thoracoscopic division of a PRAA and left ligamentum arteriosum. Note the caudal position of the ports, which facilitate an ergonomic approach to the ligamentum arteriosum. More cranially located ports limit the working length of the small instruments due to the close proximity to the ligamentum and make for a more challenging procedure.

- Thoracoscopic DeBakey and curved Kelly forceps are then used to dissect and undermine the ligamentum from the esophagus (**Fig. 9**). Caution should be exercised during this step to avoid accidental laceration of the esophagus. The esophagus tends to be thin and can easily get caught in the tips of the dissecting forceps and/or vessel-sealing device. The author prefers to use curved Kelly forceps for dissection and is sure to keep the forceps tips aimed away from the esophagus.
- Once a complete plane is created between the ligamentum and the esophagus, the bipolar sealing device is used to seal and divide the tissue (**Fig. 10**). Often, small residual fibers of the ligamentum will remain after division of the major ligamentous structure. Endopeanuts can be used to bluntly dissect these fibers to ensure complete disruption of any constricting tissues.
- Once the ligamentum and remaining fibers have been removed, endoscopy is repeated to confirm the patency of the esophagus. A small-gauge thoracostomy tube is then placed under thoracoscopic guidance. The author prefers a Mila 14 Fr drain for postoperative monitoring.
- Ports are removed individually under thoracoscopic observation to ensure that no hemorrhage from the intercostal vessels occurs. Port incisions are closed routinely in two layers.

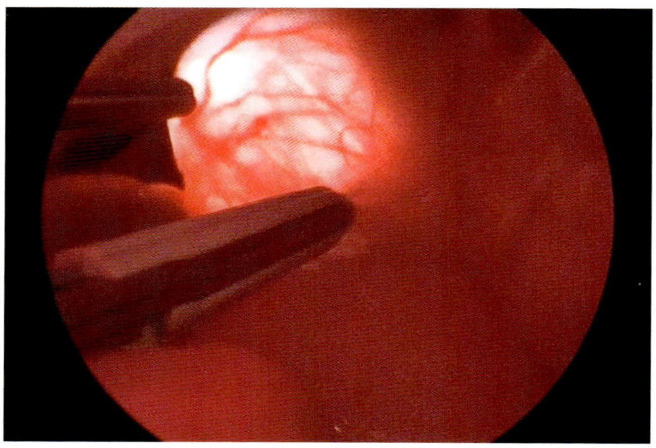

FIGURE 6. Thoracoscopic image demonstrating the use of a flexible endoscope in the esophagus to facilitate identification and division of the left ligamentum arteriosum. The white light is from the endoscope in the cranial thoracic esophagus.

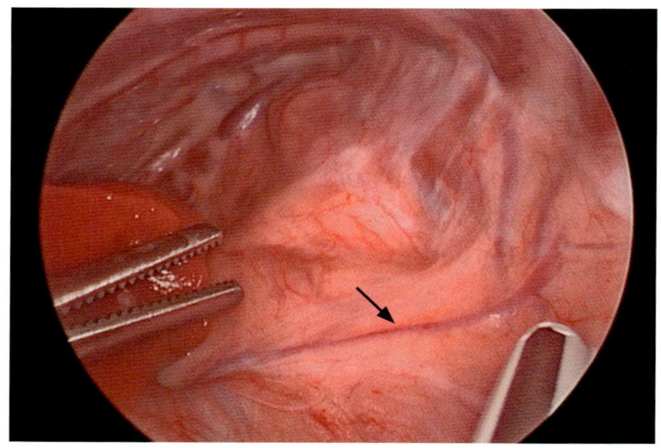

FIGURE 7. A pleural vessel (arrow) runs from dorsal to ventral. This vessel typically overlies the ligamentum arteriosum.

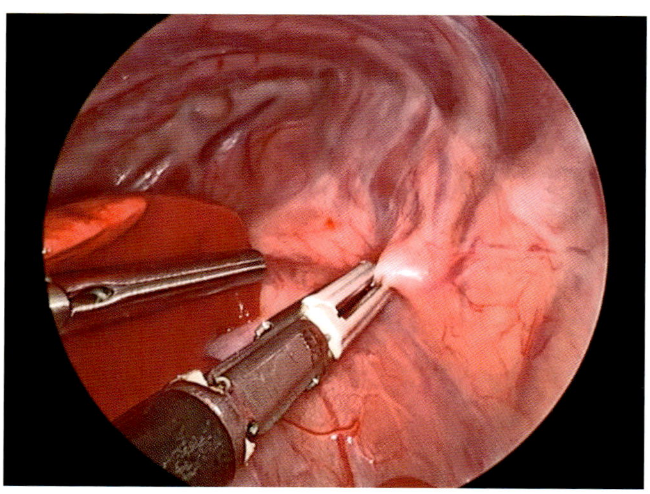

FIGURE 8. Bipolar sealing/division of the pleural vein overlying the ligamentum arteriosum.

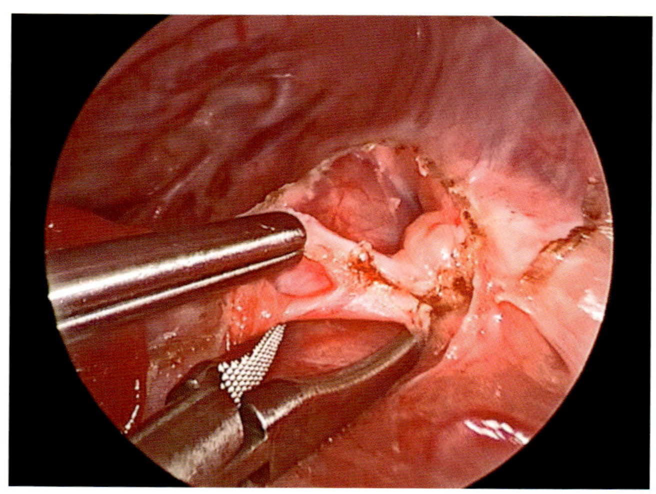

FIGURE 9. Dissection of the ligamentum arteriosum. Note that the curved dissecting forceps are utilized for blunt dissection of the ligamentum away from the esophagus.

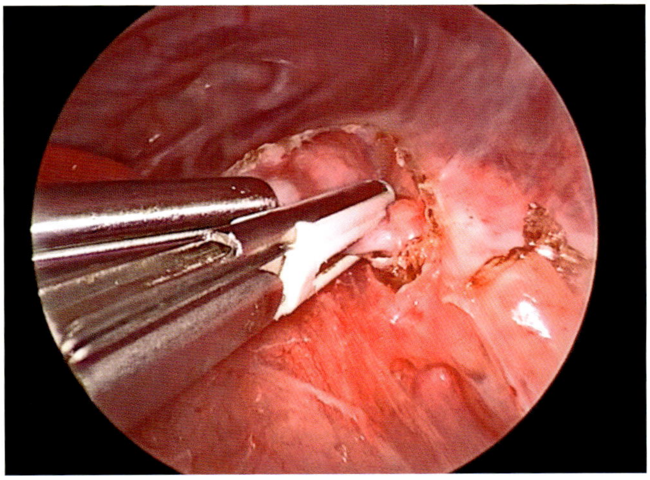

FIGURE 10. Once the ligamentum arteriosum has been dissected free from the esophagus and a plane has been created, the bipolar sealing device is used to seal and divide the ligamentum.

POSTOPERATIVE MANAGEMENT

- Intraoperative infiltration of all port sites with a local anesthetic (e.g., bupivacaine) affords 4–6 hours of analgesia postoperatively.
- The combination of nonsteroidal anti-inflammatory medication (3–5 days) and systemic opioids (12–36 hours) is generally effective for uncomplicated thoracoscopic surgery.
- Monitoring of pleural fluid production via the chest drain is recommended for 12–24 hours postoperatively.
- Recheck examination with chest radiography with or without an esophagram is recommended at 6 and 12 weeks postoperatively.

Complications of the thoracoscopic approach to vascular ring anomalies

- Esophageal laceration has been reported during thoracoscopic ligamentum arteriosum dissection. In one case, intracorporeal repair was performed, but the author recommends conversion to thoracotomy for thorough evaluation and repair of the defect.
- Port-site hemorrhage can occur after removal of an intercostal port. Hemorrhage from intercostal arteries may necessitate reoperation to locate and ligate the bleeding vessel. It is recommended that all port sites are monitored thoracoscopically during port removal. If significant hemorrhage is seen, ligation of the intercostal vessel is recommended.

Key points

- Aberrant vasculature such as a double aorta or an aberrant left subclavian artery are common and may require ligation and division.
- Preoperative CT is useful to diagnose aberrant vasculature and is recommended for surgical planning.
- Thoracoscopic dissection of the ligamentum arteriosum is challenging and requires advanced skills and precise technique to avoid complications.

SUGGESTED READINGS

CLINICAL CASES

54.1 THORACOSCOPIC APPROACH COMBINED WITH ESOPHAGOSCOPY FOR THE SURGICAL CORRECTION OF A PERSISTENT RIGHT AORTIC ARCH

F. J. Pérez Duarte, J. Gutiérrez del Sol, M. A. Sánchez Hurtado

CASE DESCRIPTION

A 4-month-old Border Collie was presented for evaluation of regurgitation and poor weight gain of 1-month duration. Radiographs and esophagoscopy revealed an extraluminal esophageal constriction at the level of the heart base. Moderate dilation of the esophagus was seen at the level of the thoracic inlet cranial to the region of constriction. A CT scan confirmed the diagnosis of PRAA. A thoracoscopic approach combined with esophagoscopy was proposed as surgical treatment. Total surgical time was 46 minutes and no complications were noted. The dog no longer regurgitated after eating.

Key points

- Very delicate dissection of the ligamentum arteriosum is required, as the esophagus wall is very thin.
- One-lung ventilation is not mandatory but can facilitate the exposition of the surgical area.
- The ligamentum arteriosum is located within the mediastinum, cranial to the heart base.
- An aspirator is used to palpate the ligamentum while a gastroscope helps to visualize it.

PORT PLACEMENT

The first 5 mm trocar (T1) is placed in the 9th intercostal space, in the middle area of the left hemithorax. Under direct vision, a 5 mm trocar (T2) and a 3 mm trocar (T3) are placed in the 9th intercostal space, thus achieving triangulation between instruments and optics. Sometimes a fourth 3 mm cannula (T4) is necessary to retract the cranial lung lobe.

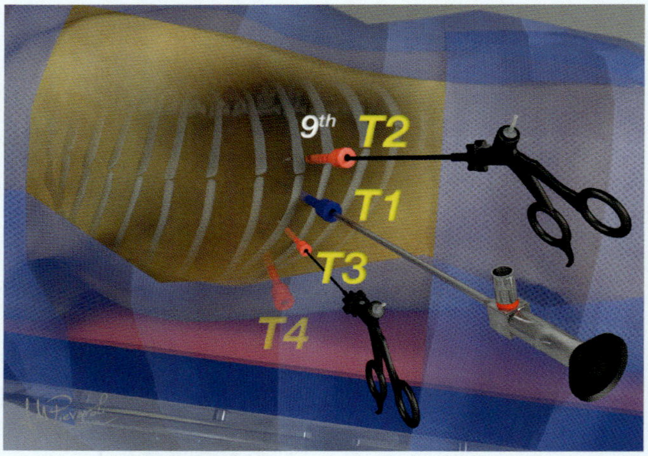

PROCEDURE

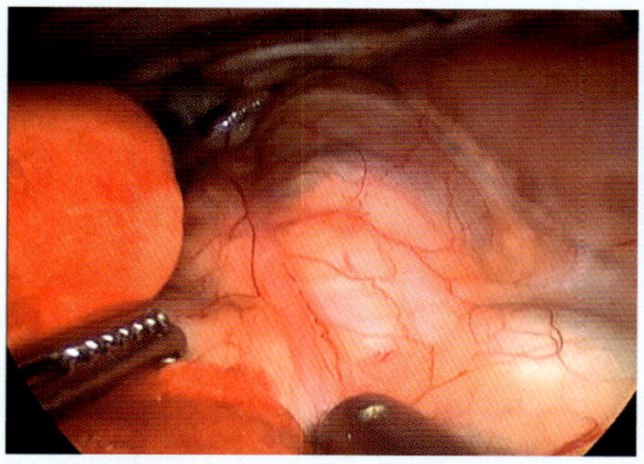

FIGURE 1. The first step of the procedure is to expose the surgical area by moving away the left cranial lung lobe.

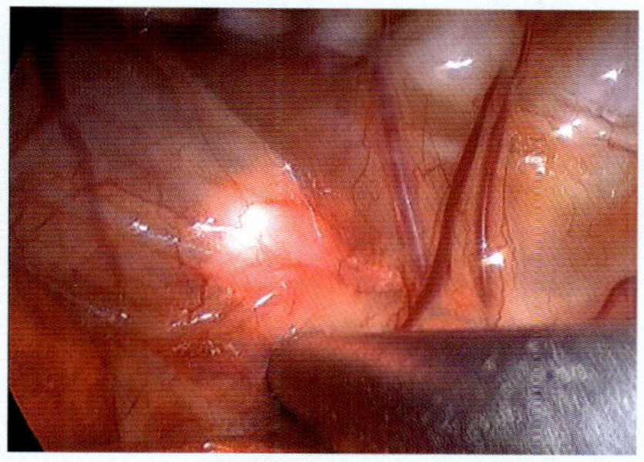

FIGURE 2. The ligamentum arteriosum is identified within the mediastinum, cranial to the heart base.

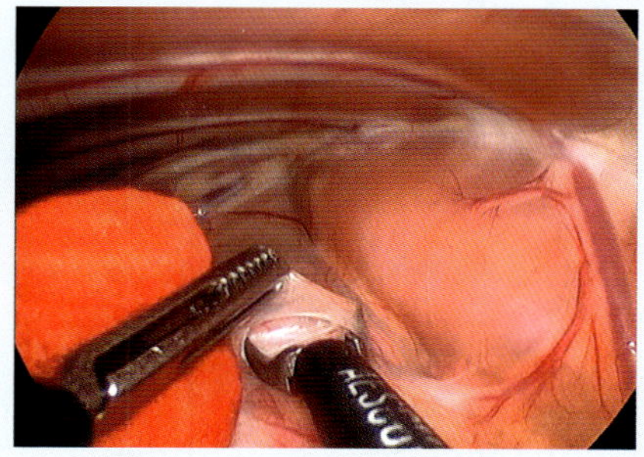

FIGURE 3. The mediastinum over the ligamentum is opened and dissected with a Maryland dissector and a vessel-sealing device.

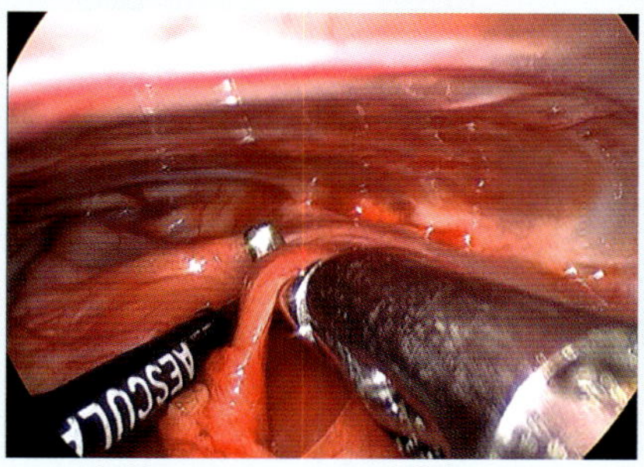

FIGURE 4. Kelly grasping forceps and a right-angle dissector are used to dissect and isolate the ligamentum.

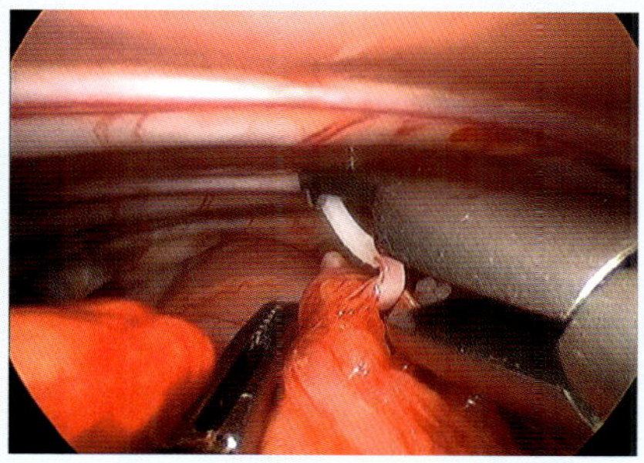

FIGURE 5. In some cases, the ligamentum arteriosum may be patent. Vascular clips are placed on the ligament to prevent bleeding. The ligamentum is then transected between the two clips.

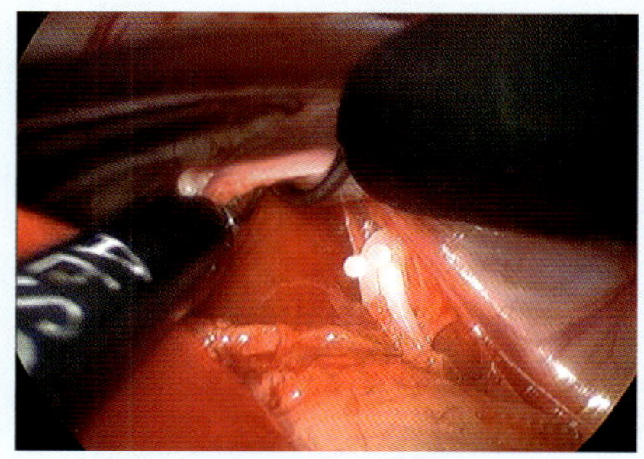

FIGURE 6. After transection of the ligamentum arteriosum, the remaining constricting fibers are dissected and the esophagus is dilated. Any remaining fiber bands limiting the expansion of the esophagus are dissected and divided.

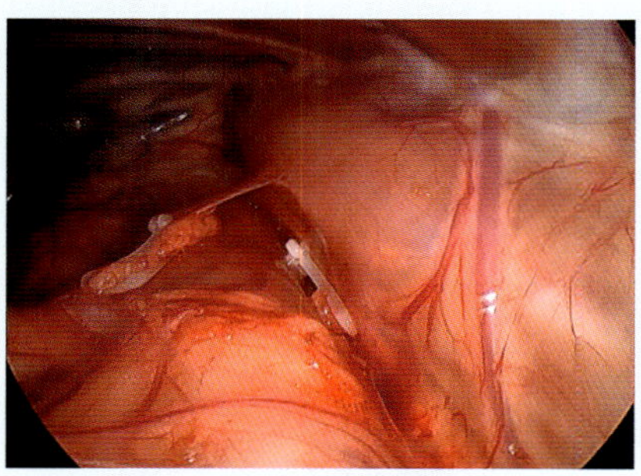

FIGURE 7. Balloon dilatation of the remaining constricting fibers is performed at the end of the procedure.

Tips and tricks

- ✓ Due to the small size of the thorax, using 3 mm instruments is recommended.
- ✓ Place the trocars caudal in the hemithorax to increase the working distance of the instruments.
- ✓ Use a gastroscope to help identify the ligamentum arteriosum.
- ✓ The light of the gastroscope is also very useful to guide the dissection of the remaining fiber bands to prevent injury to the esophagus wall.

55 THORACOSCOPIC APPROACH TO MEDIASTINAL MASS EXCISION

J. Brad Case

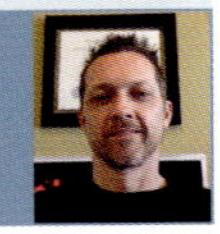

Indications

- Dogs >20 kg with noninvasive masses <7 cm in diameter
- Dogs with a thymoma but without myasthenia gravis or megaesophagus

Contraindications

- Dogs with large masses (>7 cm) or with vascular invasion
- Dogs with myasthenia gravis or megaesophagus

The cranial mediastinum contains important structures such as the esophagus, trachea, vagus and phrenic nerves, thymus, thoracic duct, and great vessels. Thus, dissection and excision of tumors in this area can be challenging. An exact understanding of the anatomy and the relationship with a mass in this area is mandatory prior to surgery regardless of the approach being considered.

The most common cranial mediastinal mass is thymoma, although lymphoma can also occur and needs to be ruled out via aspiration cytology or needle core biopsy. Thymomas can be invasive or noninvasive and may be associated with paraneoplastic syndrome. Typical paraneoplastic comorbidities are myasthenia gravis and megaesophagus. Because both of these conditions dramatically affect prognosis and treatment strategy, it is critical to test for them prior to consideration for surgery. Chest radiography and acetylcholine receptor antibody tests are sufficient for diagnosis. Additionally, because thymomas that invade vascular structures are not candidates for a thoracoscopic approach (often not for open surgery either), three-dimensional imaging (e.g., CT) is also considered mandatory for surgical planning and case selection.

> The first description of thoracoscopy for the removal of thymoma in dogs was made by P. D. Mayhew in 2008.

PATIENT PREPARATION AND POSITIONING

The dog is clipped from the cranial abdomen to the caudal cervical region and dorsally to the level of the epaxial musculature. Standard aseptic preparation is necessary prior to surgery. The patient is positioned in dorsal recumbency and the entire sternum should be accessible following draping.

OPERATING ROOM LAYOUT

The operating room should be organized in a manner that allows for an unobstructed view of the video monitor and ergonomic working conditions. Typically, the monitor is placed at the patient's right shoulder or at the head of the operating table. The instrument back table is placed at the end of the operating table. This allows for the surgeon and the assistant to work from either side of the patient and leaves room for conversion to median sternotomy should it become necessary (**Fig. 1**).

PORT PLACEMENT (FIG. 3)

- T1, 5.5 mm, on the midline, in a subxiphoid position
- T2, 12–15 mm, left 4th intercostal space
- T3, 5.5 mm, right parasternal, 7th–9th intercostal space

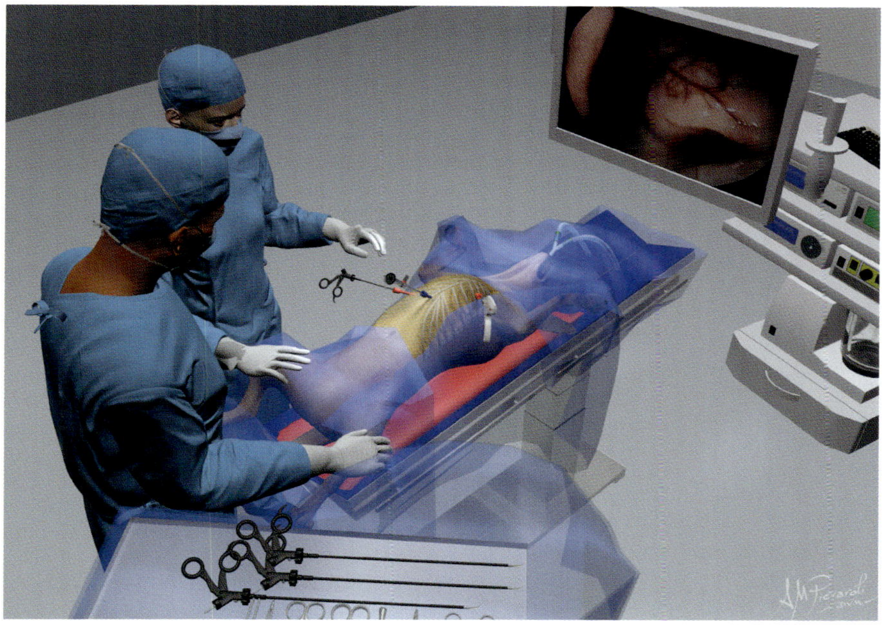

FIGURE 1. Operating room layout for thoracoscopic cranial mediastinal mass excision.

Instruments

On the table:

- Standard surgical pack
- High-definition video camera
- Telescope 5 mm – 30°
- Two 5 mm threaded cannulas + one 12 mm threaded cannula
- Laparoscopic Babcock, Kelley, right-angle forceps, 5 mm
- Laparoscopic cotton-tip, blunt dissection probes, 5 mm
- L- or J-hook monopolar electrosurgical tip, 5 mm
- Vessel-sealing device (e.g., LigaSure or harmonic shears) (**Fig. 2**)
- 3–5 cm wound retractor or specimen retrieval bag

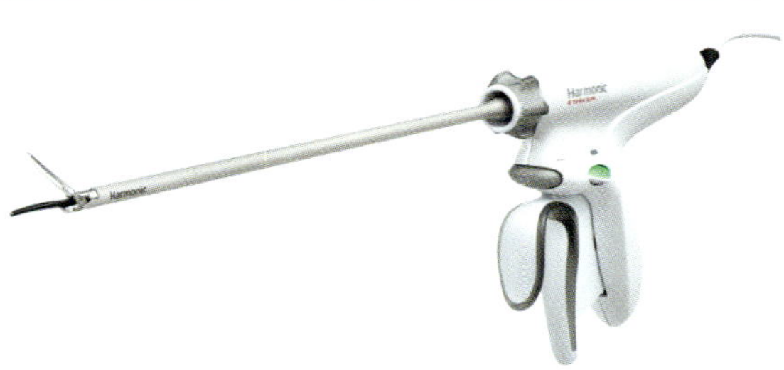

FIGURE 2. Harmonic shears.

PROCEDURE

- All the port sites are infiltrated with bupivacaine before creating the associated incision. A 5.5 mm camera/telescope port (T1) is placed in the subxiphoid region into the right hemithorax. A threaded Ternamian-style cannula is recommended. The telescope should be inserted halfway into the cannula during insertion to avoid iatrogenic pulmonary injury. A 5 mm 30° telescope is preferred, as the field of view is adequate and the angled scope allows for evaluation of all aspects of the mass during dissection.
- Once the telescope cannula is in position in the right hemithorax, a second 5.5 mm threaded blunt-end cannula (T3) is placed in an intercostal position in the ventral third of the thorax between the right 7th and 9th intercostal spaces. The port is inserted under direct video observation. Blunt-tipped cannulas are preferred in the intercostal location to minimize the chance of intercostal artery rupture.
- A bipolar vessel-sealing device is used to dissect the mediastinum to create a clear view of the contralateral hemithorax. A third cannula (11.5 mm blunt tipped) is then placed in the 4th intercostal space in the left hemithorax. This port (T2) allows for insertion of a 10 mm vessel-sealing device and specimen extraction bag.
- Dogs undergoing video-assisted thoracic surgery for cranial mediastinal mass resection first undergo mediastinal dissection (**Fig. 4**) followed by lateral and dorsal dissection of the

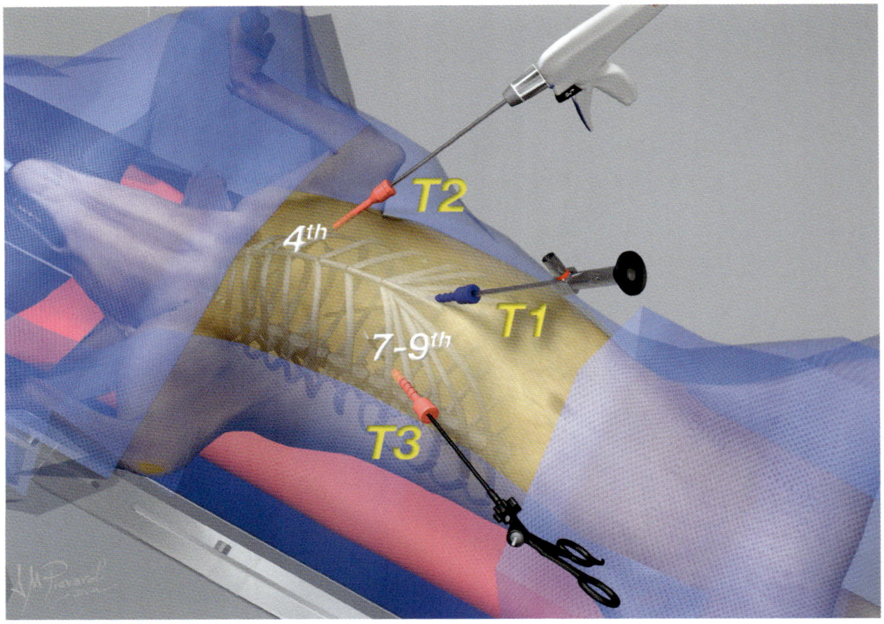

FIGURE 3. Port placement for thoracoscopic removal of thymic masses.

mass. Dissection of cranial mediastinal masses is best completed using bipolar vessel-sealing devices (e.g., LigaSure or harmonic scalpels).

- Adhesions to and/or invasion of major vessels such as the cranial vena cava, brachiocephalic artery and left subclavian artery is possible, but this is typically ruled out by preoperative CT angiography as well as initial thoracoscopic evaluation (**Fig. 5**).
- The internal thoracic vessels are usually adhered to and associated with the mass, but careful dissection allows separation of these vessels without compromising the capsule of the tumor (**Fig. 6**). Compromise of the tumor capsule may result in tumor seeding and recurrence and must be avoided during dissection of the mass.
- Perhaps the most critical aspect of the dissection is ventral retraction of the mass away from the phrenic nerves and major cardiac vessels (i.e., vena cava and brachiocephalic artery) during dissection dorsal to the mass. This is accomplished by the use of sponge forceps, Babcock forceps, fan retractors, and/or transthoracic digital retraction (**Fig. 7**).

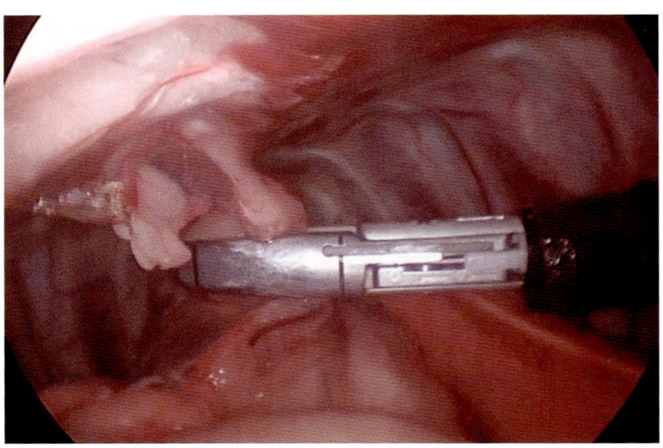

FIGURE 4. Thoracoscopic image of a dog undergoing thoracoscopic removal of a noninvasive thymoma. The first step is to dissect a window in the ventral mediastinum using a bipolar sealing device.

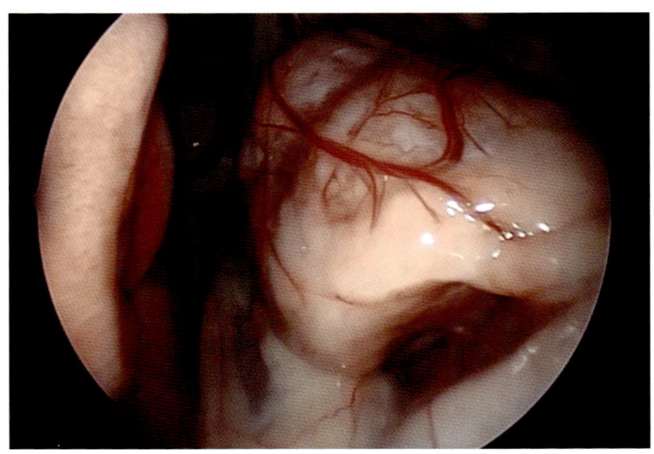

FIGURE 5. Thoracoscopic image of a dog with a noninvasive thymoma in the cranial mediastinum. Note the association with the internal thoracic vessels, which is a common feature of thymomas. The right cranial lung lobe is to the left of the image, and the cranial vena cava is to the bottom.

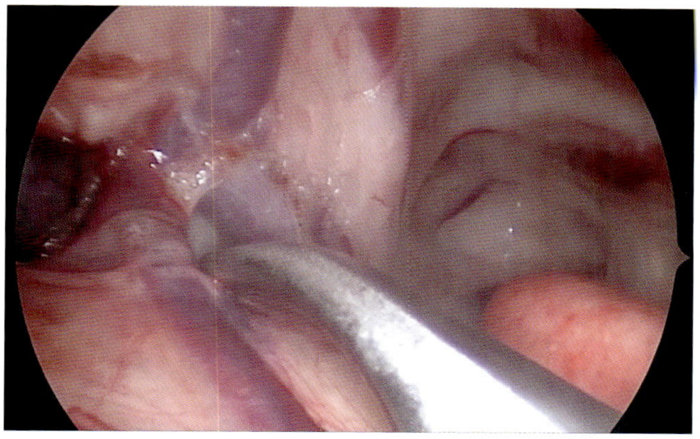

FIGURE 6. Thoracoscopic image of the dog from Figure 2. The internal thoracic vessels are dissected away from the thymoma.

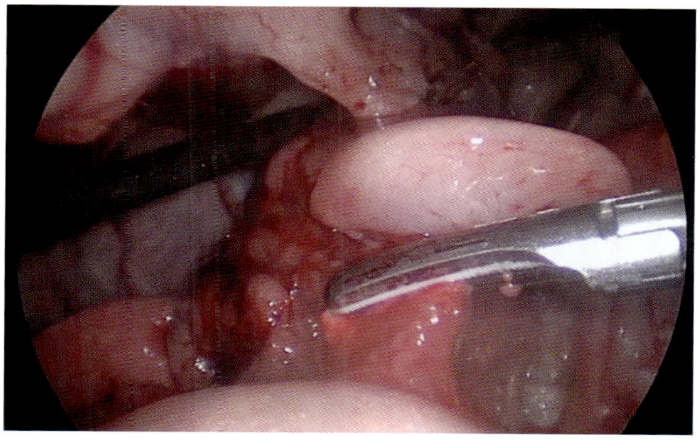

FIGURE 7. Retraction of the thymoma ventrally, away from the dorsal neurovascular structures (i.e., cranial vena cava, brachiocephalic trunk, phrenic nerves). This is critical to avoid iatrogenic laceration of these structures and to provide a visible plane of dissection dorsal to the mass. In the image, dissection is being performed between the heart and the thymoma. A harmonic scalpel is used to dissect the fat while endoscopic Babcock forceps are utilized to retract the thymic mass ventrally.

- Once the mass has been dissected free, a sterile specimen retrieval bag is used to remove the mass from the thoracic cavity (**Fig. 8**). Depending on the size of the mass, incisional enlargement may be required.
- A chest drain is placed under video observation, and the port sites are closed in two layers.

POSTOPERATIVE MANAGEMENT

- Analgesic requirements for dogs undergoing thoracoscopic mediastinal mass excision appear to be minimal.
- Intraoperative infiltration of the port sites with a local anesthetic affords 4–6 hours of analgesia postoperatively and when coupled with nonsteroidal anti-inflammatory medication (2–3 days) is generally effective for uncomplicated cases.
- If further analgesia is indicated, the addition of opioid medications postoperatively can be considered, but it is rare to require opioids beyond 48–72 hours following uncomplicated surgery.

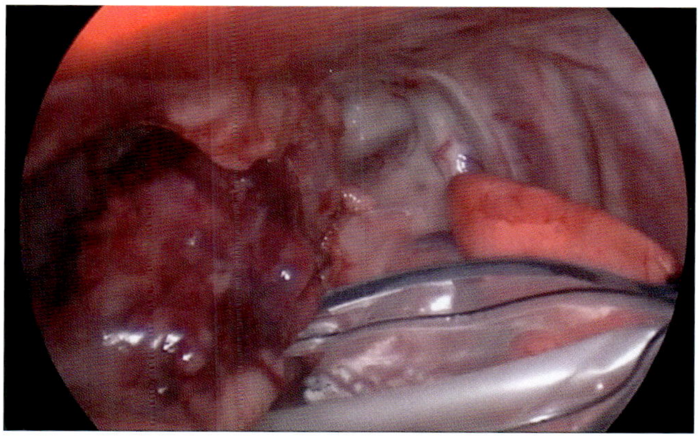

FIGURE 8. Thoracoscopic image following dissection of a thymoma just prior to placement into a specimen retrieval bag. Use of these bags prevents port-site metastasis, which has been reported following thoracoscopic thymectomy.

Complications of thoracoscopic cranial mediastinal mass excision

- Severe hemorrhage from laceration of the cranial vena cava or other great vessels is possible during dissection of cranial mediastinal masses. The surgeon should be ready to convert rapidly to median sternotomy if indicated. This complication can be avoided with careful case selection and vigilant attention to operative technique.
- Hemorrhage from the internal thoracic vessels is possible with haphazard dissection of cranial mediastinal masses and sternal lymph nodes. It is also avoided with careful technique.
- Aspiration pneumonia is common in dogs with myasthenia gravis and megaesophagus. Survival in dogs with myasthenia gravis and megaesophagus is significantly worse than in dogs with thymomas that do not have paraneoplastic syndrome.

Key points

- Retraction of cranial mediastinal masses is critical during dissection to avoid injury to large vascular structures.
- Mediastinal masses are commonly adhered to internal thoracic vessels but are typically amenable to blunt dissection away from the vessels.

SUGGESTED READINGS

CLINICAL CASES

55.1 THORACOSCOPIC MEDIASTINAL LYMPH NODE EXCISION

Justin B. Ganjei

CASE DESCRIPTION

A 7-year-old castrated male Standard Poodle was evaluated for acute onset tachypnea and lethargy. The initial diagnostic tests performed revealed a mild leukocytosis with neutrophilia and moderate to severe pleural effusion on thoracic radiographs. Thoracocentesis yielded hemorrhage effusion and the cytologic evaluation results were consistent with acute hemorrhage and mesothelial activity. A thoracic CT scan was performed and revealed marked cranial mediastinal lymphadenopathy and bilateral pleural effusion. Fine needle aspiration of the mediastinal lymph node was performed and the cytologic evaluation results were consistent with carcinoma. The patient was then referred for surgical consultation and thoracoscopic mediastinal lymph node excision and pleural port placement is recommended.

Key points

- Fine needle aspiration and cytologic evaluation of the mediastinal lymph node are crucial.
- In this case, pleural port placement is recommended.
- The use of a specimen retrieval bag to remove the dissected mediastinal lymph node out of the thoracic cavity avoids the dissemination of neoplastic cells inside the thorax.

PORT PLACEMENT

The patient was placed in dorsal recumbency. The thorax and cranial abdomen were aseptically prepared. A 1 cm incision was made in the ventral aspect of the right 7th intercostal space and a 5 mm threaded thoracoport (T3) was introduced into the thoracic cavity. Exploration of the thoracic cavity using a 5 mm 30° telescope revealed a moderate amount of hemorrhagic pleural effusion. A second port (T2) was established under direct visualization by insertion of a 5 mm threaded thoracoport into the ventral aspect of the left 7th intercostal space. A third port (T1) was established in the right paraxiphoid region under direct visualization utilizing a 5 mm threaded trocar.

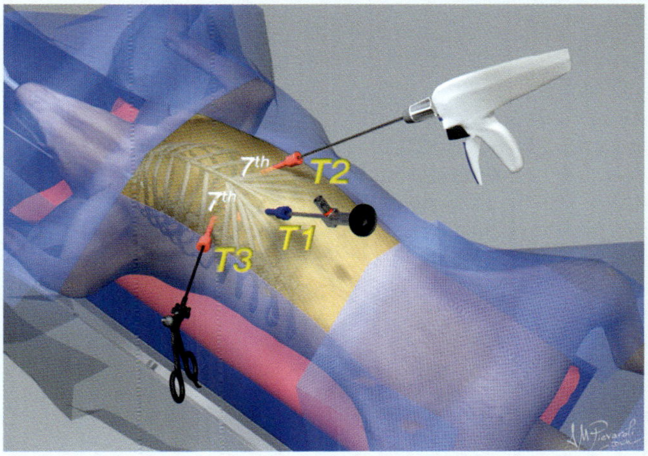

PROCEDURE

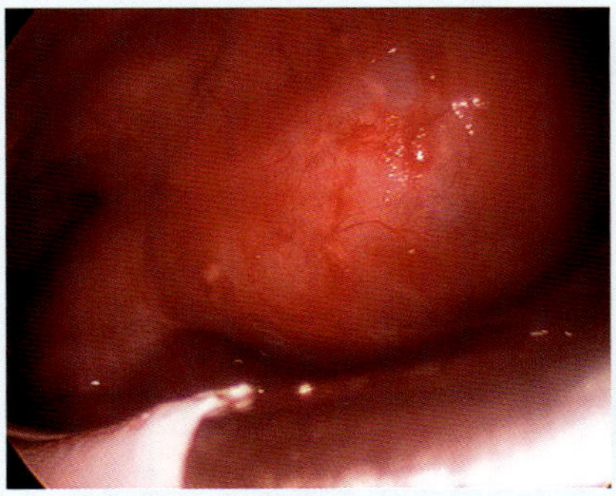

FIGURE 1. After evacuating the effusion using a laparoscopic suction/irrigation device, the mediastinum is evaluated and found to be moderately thickened. The image shows one of the two enlarged lymph nodes identified within the cranial mediastinum, measuring 2×2 cm each.

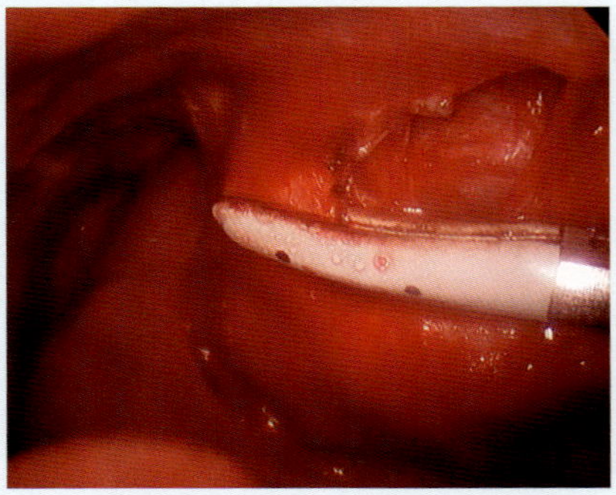

FIGURE 2. The mediastinum is partially transected using a 5 mm bipolar vessel-sealing device. The mediastinal lymph node is then dissected from the mediastinum using Mixter forceps and LigaSure.

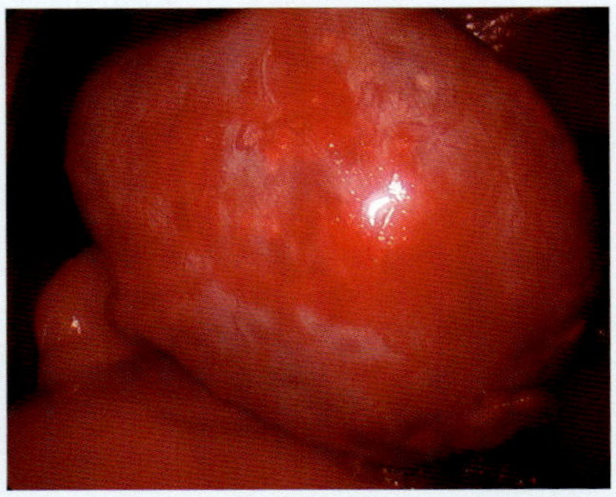

FIGURE 3. Thoracoscopic image of the completely freed cranial mediastinal lymph node. The left-sided thoracoport is then removed and the incision extended slightly to allow insertion of a 10 mm specimen retrieval bag. The lymph node is then placed in the bag and removed.

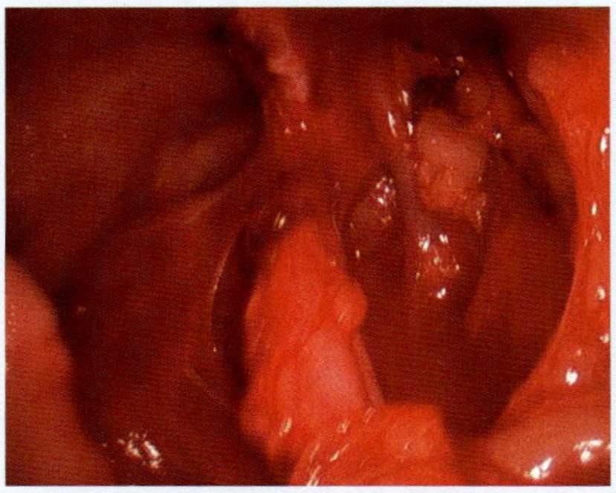

FIGURE 4. Thoracoscopic image of the cranial mediastinal region following lymph node removal. Note the left internal thoracic artery. An 18-gauge thoracostomy tube is inserted through the left 7th intercostal space. A subcutaneous vascular access port is then placed routinely. All port sites are closed in standard multilayer fashion.

Tips and tricks

- ✓ Take care to visualize the internal thoracic vessels during dissection to avoid inadvertent transection.
- ✓ Place the intercostal ports as ventral as possible to allow for easier manipulation.

55.2 THORACOSCOPIC TREATMENT IN A CAT WITH THYMOMA-ASSOCIATED EXFOLIATIVE DERMATITIS

Francesca Izzo, Luciano Borghetti

CASE DESCRIPTION

A 9-year-old spayed domestic short hair cat was referred to our clinic because of disordered eating and moderate itching throughout the body for about 15 days. The patient presented generalized alopecia, whitish scales and crusts and severe skin thickening. Dermatological evaluation showed complicated *Malassezia* dermatitis. Blood tests showed moderate normochromic normocytic anemia, neutrophilic leukocytosis, and increased lactate dehydrogenase and globulins. The patient was managed with shampoo therapy and antibiotic therapy, which only partially improved the clinical signs. Abdominal ultrasound was normal. Thoracic radiography in three projections highlighted a neoformation in the anterior mediastinum with no pleural effusion. Ultrasound-guided cytological assessment of the neoformation was compatible with thymoma. In order to assess the extent and invasiveness of the neoplasm, a total-body CT scan was performed. The study confirmed the presence of a neoformation in the cranial mediastinum, with well-defined margins of about 2.6×1.2×1 cm. The cranial vena cava was in ventral contact with the neoformation without compressive or infiltrative phenomena. Cranial mediastinal and tracheobronchial lymph nodes were morphologically normal.

The neoplasia was removed thoracoscopically. Histological examination of the neoformation confirmed the cytological suspicion of thymoma. Skin biopsy was compatible with chronic nonspecific dermatitis without obvious causative agents due to early-stage thymoma-associated paraneoplastic syndrome.

The patient was discharged 3 days after surgery. At 15 days postoperatively, dermatitis had resolved and hair had begun to grow back in the alopecic areas. At 1 month after surgery, hair had regrown all over the body. At 2 years postoperatively, the cat was in good clinical condition, with no clinical signs associated with the neoplasia.

Key points

- The criterion to define thymoma benignity or malignancy is not histological. It is defined by the biological behavior and by the possibility of surgical removal.
- A thymoma is considered benign if it is well encapsulated and noninvasive (more common in cats).
- The prognosis for cats with benign noninvasive thymomas treated with surgery is excellent, with a survival time of over 2 years.
- Surgical removal of the thymoma also results in resolution of exfoliative dermatitis.

PORT PLACEMENT

The patient was positioned in dorsal recumbency. Thoracoscopic access was achieved through placement of a 5 mm left subxiphoid cannula (T1). Once access to the chest was obtained, the thoracic cavity was insufflated with CO_2 to an intrathoracic pressure of 3 mmHg. A 5 mm 30° telescope was introduced through the 5 mm cannula to explore the thorax. Under thoracoscopic visualization, the second (T2) and the third (T3) ports were placed by inserting two 3.5 mm cannulas at the ventral third of the 6th intercostal space on the right and left side respectively.

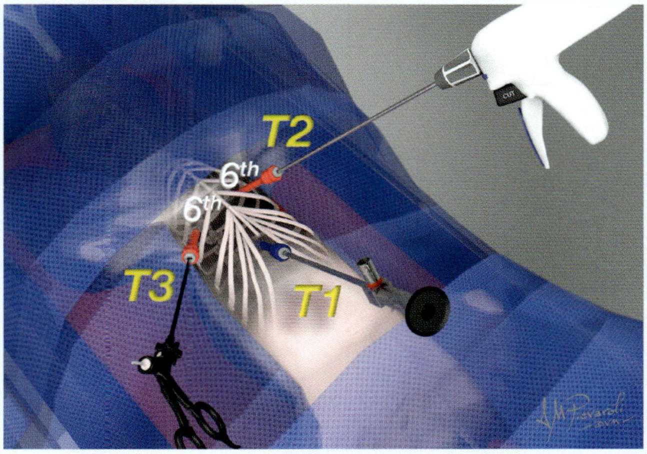

PROCEDURE

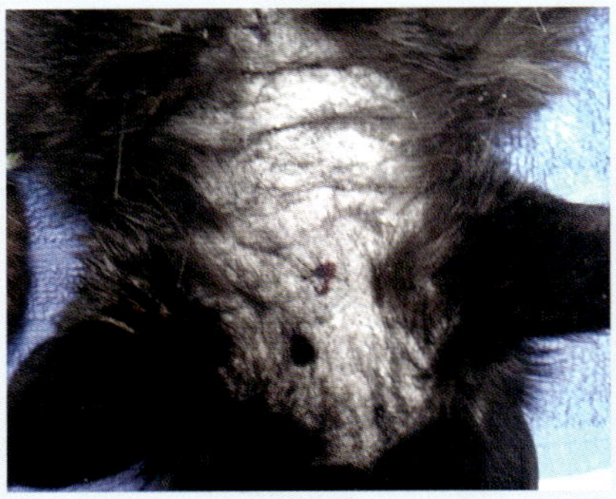

FIGURE 1. Exfoliative dermatitis (thymoma-associated paraneoplastic syndrome). Whitish scales and crusts on the patient's head.

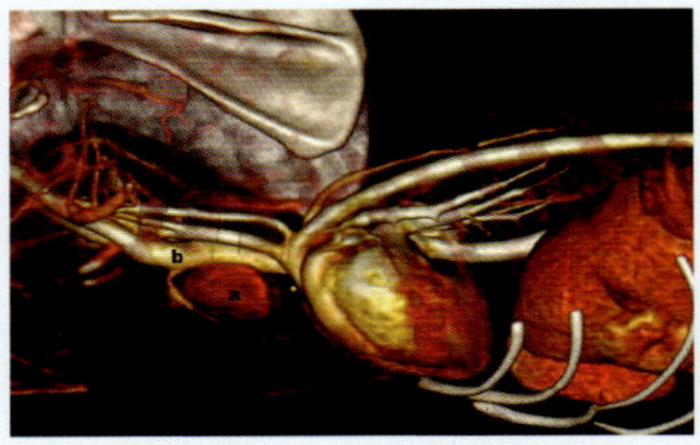

FIGURE 2. Preoperative CT scan with 3D volume rendering of the mass (a) and its relation to adjacent structures. Dorsal contact with the cranial vena cava (b) is seen.

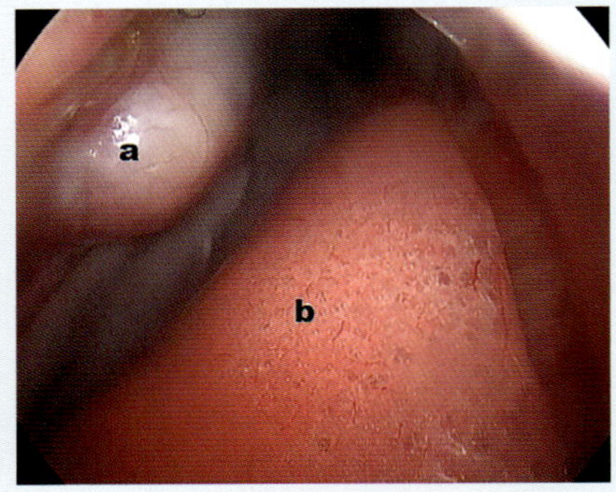

FIGURE 3. Intraoperative thoracoscopic view of the left hemithorax. Partially collapsed left lung (a). Mass (b) in the cranial mediastinum.

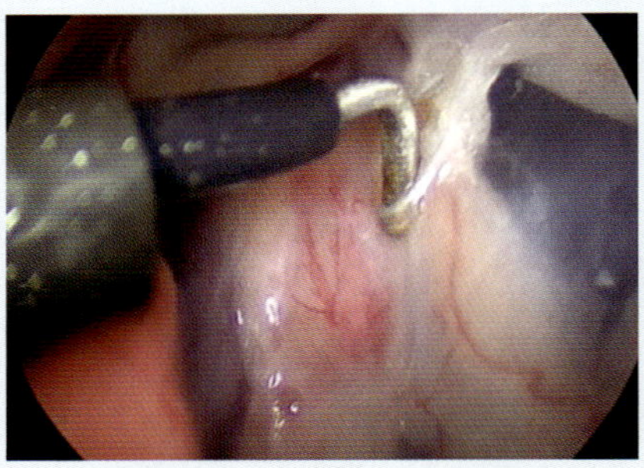

FIGURE 4. Intraoperative thoracoscopic view of the right hemithorax. The mass is dissected from the mediastinal fat using a 3.5 mm monopolar J-hook.

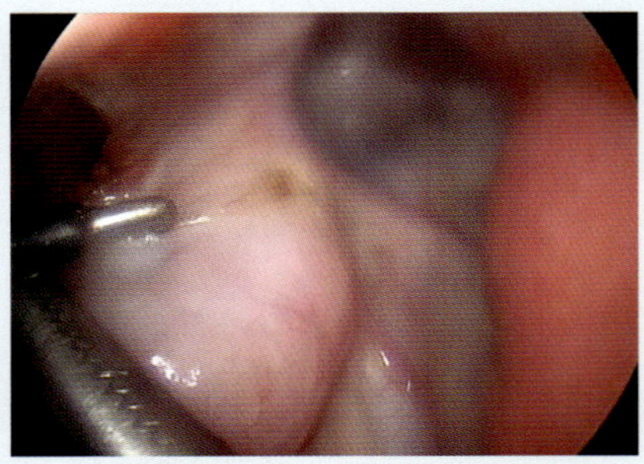

FIGURE 5. Intraoperative thoracoscopic view of the left hemithorax. The dissection of the mass is continued using the monopolar J-hook and 3.5 mm grasping forceps.

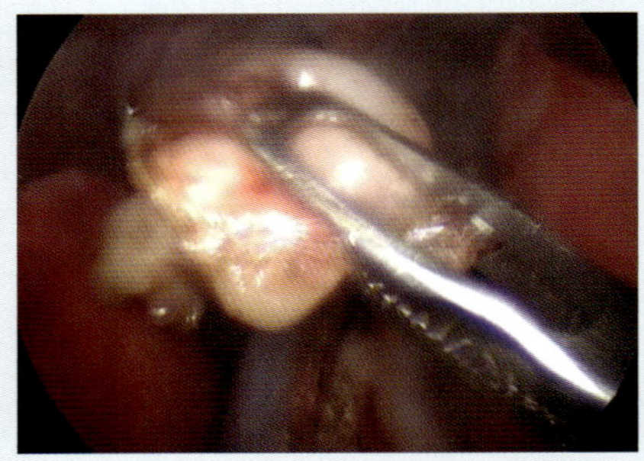

FIGURE 6. Complete excision of the mass.

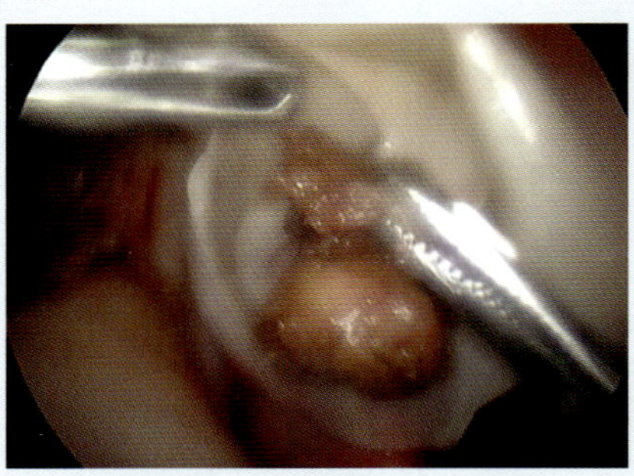

FIGURE 7. The mass is inserted into a sterile glove finger for removal from the chest.

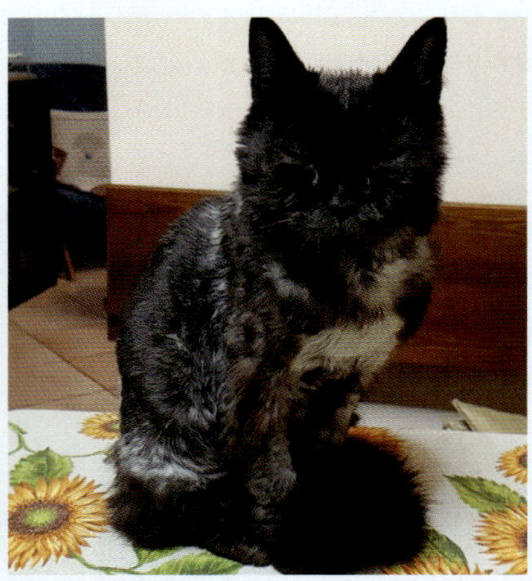

FIGURE 8. The patient 1 month after surgery. Hair has regrown all over the body.

Tips and tricks

- ✓ To obtain sufficient working space with no cardiopulmonary repercussions, it is useful to maintain an intrathoracic pressure of 3 mmHg of CO_2 during all the procedure.
- ✓ Since the lack of working space in the cat's chest does not allow the use of a specimen retrieval bag, the neoformation can be removed from the chest with the aid of a finger of a sterile surgical glove.

55.3 THORACOSCOPIC RESECTION OF A CRANIAL MEDIASTINAL MASS IN A DOG

Li-Ren Wang, Jung-Hsien Sun

CASE DESCRIPTION

A 14-year-old spayed female Maltese was evaluated for excision of a cranial mediastinal mass. The dog showed no respiratory clinical signs. On physical examination, a grade II/VI left systolic heart murmur and bilateral patellar luxation were detected. A soft tissue mass was observed in the cranioventral part of the thorax on radiographs. A CT scan revealed a 1.5×1.3×1.0 cm solid enhancing soft tissue mass in the cranial mediastinum and the intrathoracic lymph nodes were not enlarged. The patient underwent video-assisted thoracoscopic removal of the mediastinal mass. Final diagnosis was chemodectoma.

Key points

- A CT angiography scan is useful preoperatively to determine the location and vascularization of the mass.
- During dissection, the location of the aorta and soft tissue structures like the esophagus should be noted.

PORT PLACEMENT

The patient was placed in dorsal recumbency. The entire ventral thorax was clipped. Three thoracoscopic ports were established for introduction of surgical instruments. The first port (T1) was placed for subxiphoid access with the optic. After examination of the thoracic cavity, two more ports were similarly placed under thoracoscopic visualization: the instrument port (T2) was placed in the left 4th intercostal space, and the port for the vessel-sealing device (T3) was placed in the right 9th intercostal space.

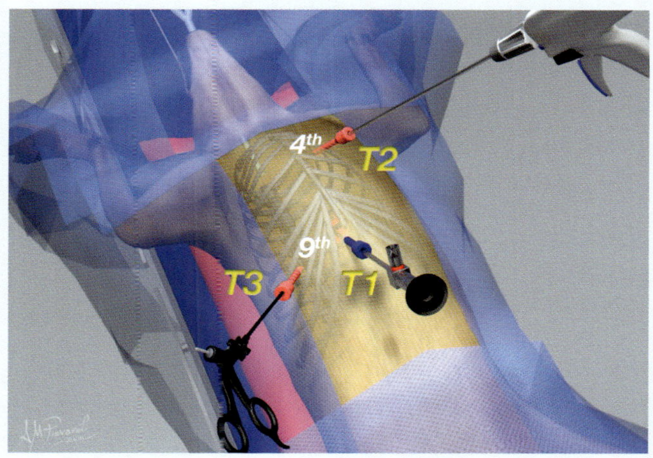

PROCEDURE

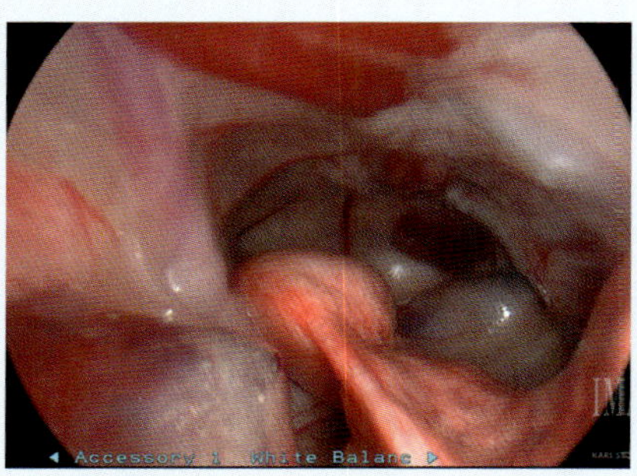

FIGURE 1. Thoracoscopic image of the mass in the cranial mediastinum.

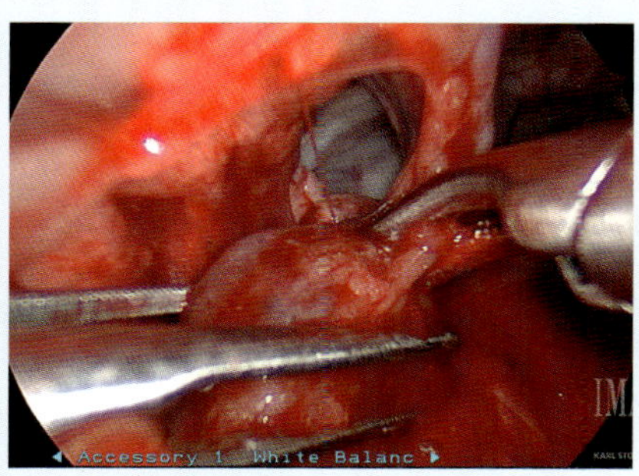

FIGURE 2. The mass and its vascular supply are bluntly dissected from surrounding retroperitoneal attachments using thoracoscopic forceps and an ultrasonic dissection device.

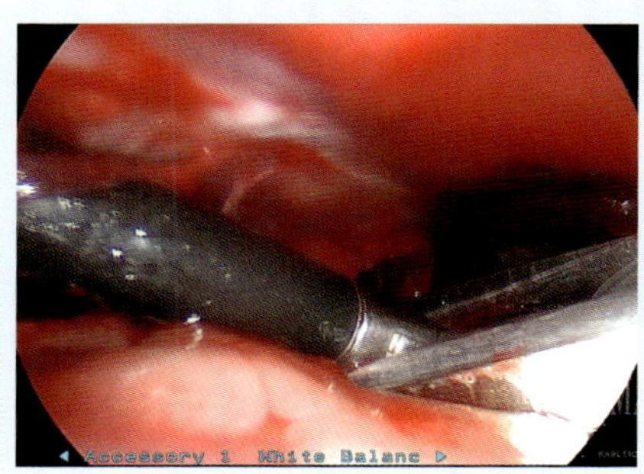

FIGURE 3. After complete dissection, the mass is removed from the chest using a sterile specimen retrieval bag.

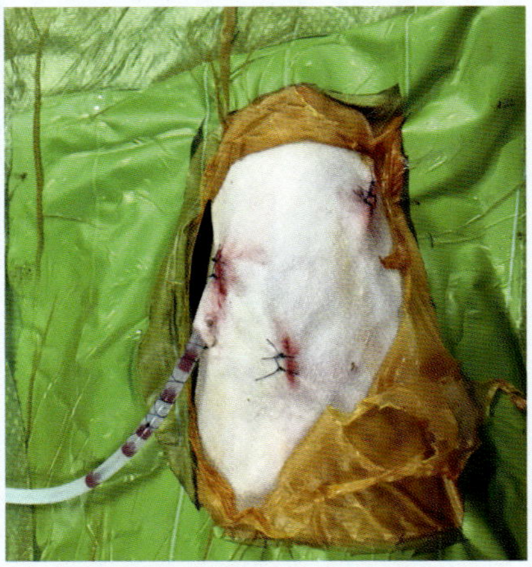

FIGURE 4. A drain tube system is placed to avoid pneumothorax.

Tips and tricks

- ✓ The choice of the location of the camera port is crucial.
- ✓ Follow the anesthesia protocol carefully to ensure patient safety.
- ✓ Make sure to achieve a clear visualization with the endoscope for safe dissection.
- ✓ Before closing the thorax, place a drain tube system to avoid pneumothorax.

55.4 THORACOSCOPIC EXCISION OF A MEDIASTINAL ECTOPIC THYROID CARCINOMA

Boris Dalpozzo

CASE DESCRIPTION

An 8-year-old mixed-breed dog weighing 7 kg was presented for investigation of recurrent cough. Radiography revealed a mass in the cranial mediastinum. An ectopic thyroid carcinoma was suspected based on CT and fine needle aspiration cytology. No invasion of main blood vessels was detected. Thoracoscopic surgical excision of the mass was performed.

Key points

- Preoperative CT is fundamental to exclude vessel and organ infiltration and to plan the surgery accurately.
- Fine needle aspiration cytology can differentiate lymphomas that are not amenable to surgical treatment.
- Good knowledge of regional anatomy is needed to avoid iatrogenic damage to vital structures.

PORT PLACEMENT

The patient was prepared for bilateral thoracic access and placed in dorsal recumbency. The telescope port (T1) was placed at the costochondral junction of the right 7th intercostal space. T2 was placed at the costochondral junction of the right 9th intercostal space. T3 was placed at the costochondral junction of the right 5th intercostal space.

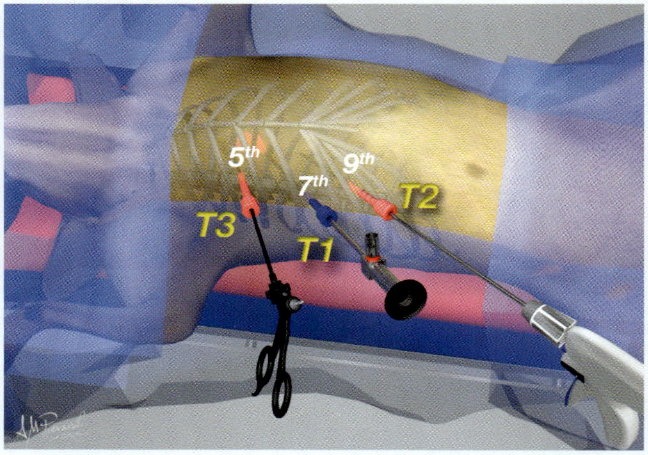

PROCEDURE

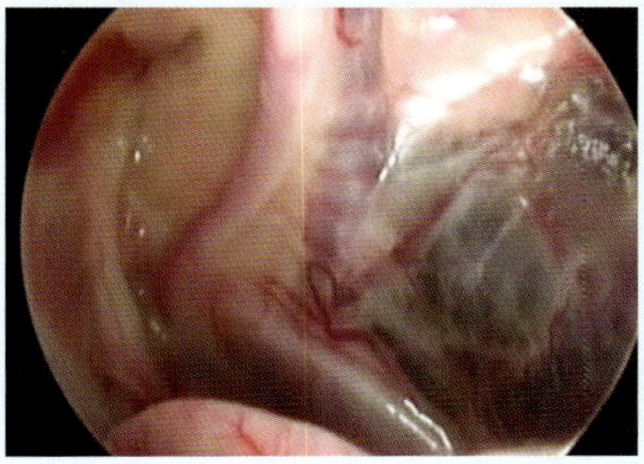

FIGURE 1. After thoracoscopic exploration to identify the regional anatomy, the ventral mediastinum is dissected first. Due to the small size of the patient, a monopolar hook is used for fine dissection. Dissection is then directed cranially.

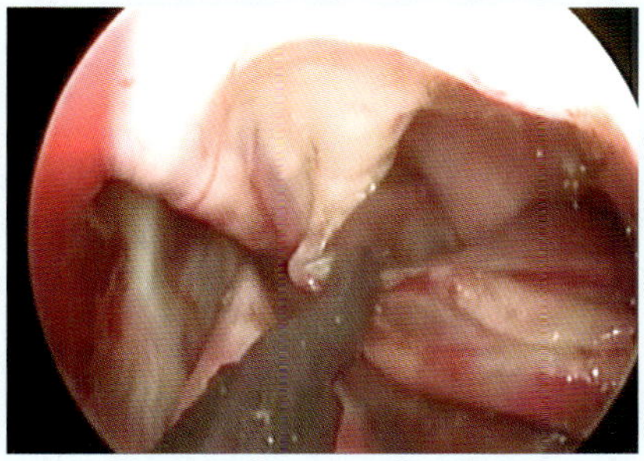

FIGURE 2. Once the ventral and cranial aspects are separated, lateral tilting is allowed and dissection from the cranial vena cava is performed. When in close proximity to large vessels and nerves, blunt dissection is preferred to avoid thermal injury.

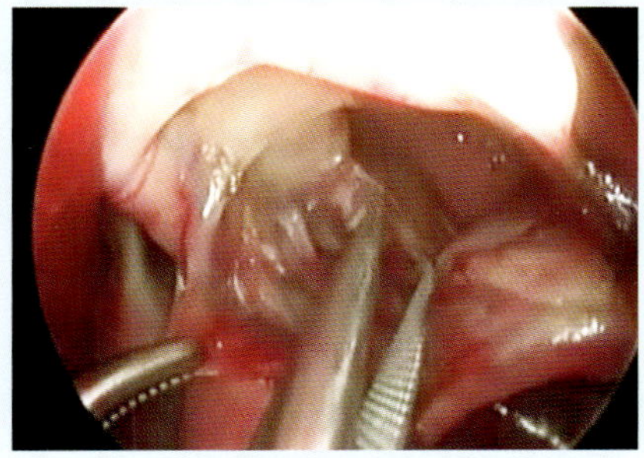

FIGURE 3. Since visualization of the caudal aspect is difficult, a finger is inserted through an enlarged port to gain tactile sense. Adhesion to the apex of the right middle lung lobe and pericardial sac is encountered.

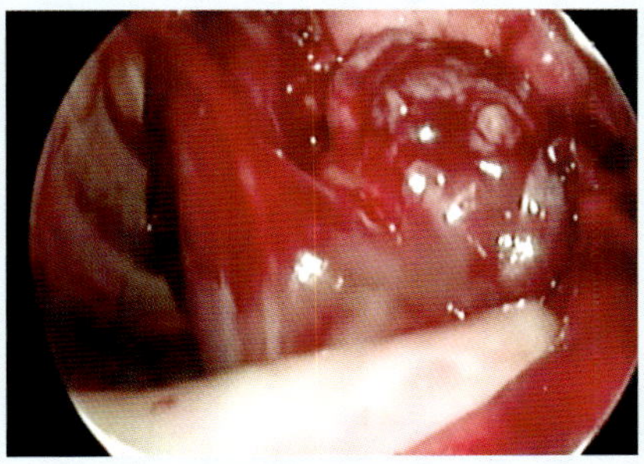

FIGURE 4. A 30 mm 3.5 EndoGIA is used to perform partial lung lobectomy.

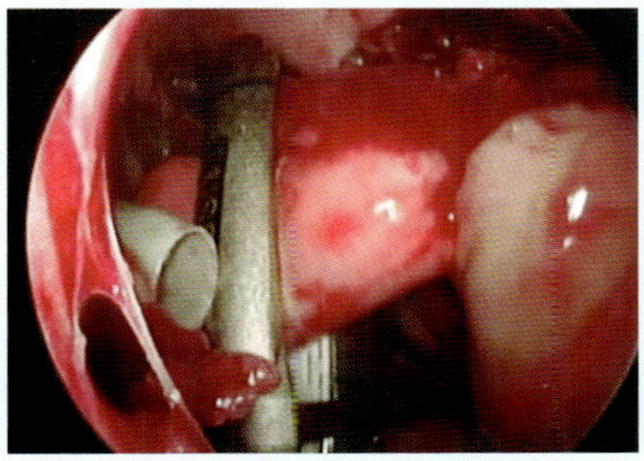

FIGURE 5. The lung stump is grasped to elevate the mass. Dorsal dissection is completed while avoiding damage to the vena cava and phrenic nerve.

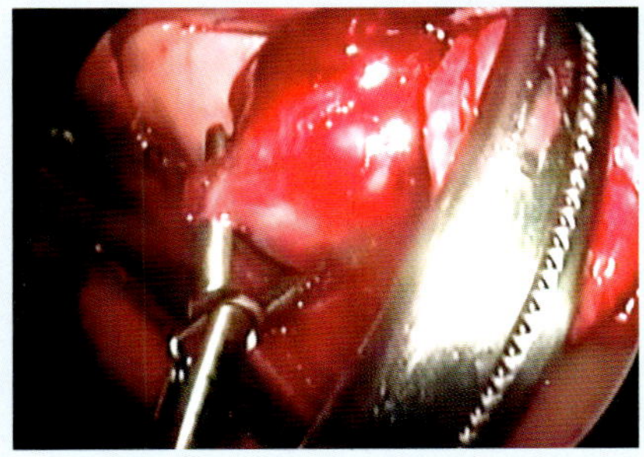

FIGURE 6. A pericardial window is needed to complete excision. The specimen is removed through an enlarged port using a retrieval bag. A chest drain is placed and ports closed routinely.

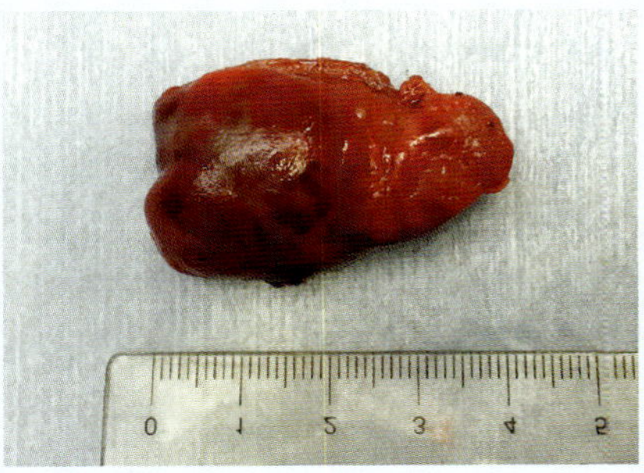

FIGURE 7. Image of the mass after removal.

Tips and tricks

- ✓ One-lung ventilation facilitates the procedure. If its use is not possible, high-rate and low-volume ventilation is helpful to improve visualization.
- ✓ Fine dissection is better performed using a monopolar hook or a blunt technique, as thermal spread to nearby main vessels and nerves can have severe consequences.
- ✓ The use of standard surgical instruments or the surgeon's fingers through an enlarged port can greatly facilitate the procedure with minimal additional trauma.

56 THORACOSCOPIC AURICULECTOMY

J. Brad Case

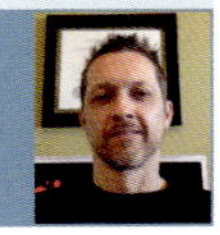

Indications

- Right auricular mass <3 cm located near the apex
- Cardiovascularly stable medium- and large-breed dogs

Contraindications

- Unstable or severely malnourished dogs
- Dogs with large auricular masses
- Lesions located at the base of the auricle
- Small patient size, due to inability to navigate an endoscopic stapler

Right atrial tumors are a common cause of pericardial effusion in dogs. Hemangiosarcoma is the most frequent right atrial tumor, while mesothelioma and heart base tumors are seen less commonly. Right atrial hemangiosarcoma has been reported most frequently in Golden Retrievers and Labrador Retrievers.

Clinical signs associated with pericardial effusion secondary to atrial mass lesions include lethargy, dyspnea, collapse, and cough. Cardiothoracic auscultation may reveal tachycardia, muffled heart sounds, and paradoxical pulse.

Diagnostic evaluation should include a complete blood count, serum biochemistry, and relevant diagnostic imaging. Thoracic radiography and echocardiography are mandatory, but CT of the thorax and abdomen should be considered for staging. Typical findings on chest X-rays include an enlarged cardiac silhouette with or without pulmonary metastasis. Echocardiography is useful to guide pericardiocentesis and is the most sensitive diagnostic test to detect right auricular mass lesions. However, it is challenging to determine the exact size and morphology of some lesions using echocardiography, which limits its utility in determining ideal candidates for thoracoscopic auriculectomy.

The vast majority of right atrial tumors (i.e., hemangiosarcomas) carry a poor prognosis. Right auricular mass resection in combination with pericardiectomy has recently been described in two studies with one and nine dogs, respectively. In the latter study, one dog died during surgery from hemorrhage, but eight dogs underwent successful resection of the atrial mass. Dogs with masses limited to the tip of the atrial appendage are considered to be good candidates for video-assisted thoracic surgery auricular resection. The benefits of performing appendage resection in conjunction with pericardiectomy are to obtain histologic diagnosis and to reduce the risk of hemorrhage from atrial rupture.

> Thoracoscopic auriculectomy was first reported in 2010 by D. M. Crumbaker et al.

DESCRIBED SURGICAL PROCEDURES

A three- or four-port thoracoscopic technique with 5 mm ports and a single 12 mm instrument port has been described. The advantage of the additional port is to improve application of the endoscopic stapler, whose positioning may vary between dogs. One-lung ventilation and CO_2 insufflation have been reported; however, as most clinical reports describe treatment without lung manipulation, it is unclear how beneficial these interventions are.

PATIENT PREPARATION AND POSITIONING

A physical examination, complete blood count, and serum biochemistry should be performed prior to surgery. A minimum hematocrit of 30% is necessary. Diagnostic imaging including thoracic radiography and echocardiography are also mandatory.

In general, the dog should be fasted for at least 8 hours prior to anesthesia and have an IV catheter placed for fluid and medication therapy during the procedure. Pericardiocentesis may be necessary if the patient has cardiac tamponade. Perioperative analgesia may include opioid and/or nonsteroidal medications. Local anesthesia with bupivacaine is recommended at individual port sites prior to incision. Following a 360° clip including the chest and cranial abdomen, the patient is aseptically prepared by standard methodology.

The dog is positioned in dorsal recumbency, but slight tilting may be beneficial in improving exposure of the auricle. The 12 mm stapler port can be placed on the left or on the right side. The exact location of the stapler may vary depending on the patient's size and morphology and on the surgeon's preference. In general, the surgeon must ensure that there is enough room to safely fit the entire length of the stapler anvil in the thorax and that the stapler can safely be articulated to the base of the auricle.

OPERATING ROOM LAYOUT

The surgeon and the assistant stand side by side at the end of the operating table. The monitors are placed on the opposite side of the table, towards the patient's head. The anesthesia circuit and staff are positioned at the head of the operating table. The instrument table is placed under the monitors, near the patient's head (**Fig. 1**).

Instruments

On the table:

- Standard surgical pack
- High-definition video camera
- Telescope 5 mm – 30°
- Three 5 mm threaded cannulas + one 12 mm threaded cannula
- Laparoscopic Babcock and/or Kelley forceps, 5 mm
- Laparoscopic cotton-tip, blunt dissection probes, 5 mm
- Endoscopic linear stapler, 45 or 60 mm
- 5 mm bipolar vessel-sealing device

PORT PLACEMENT (FIGS. 2 AND 3)

- T1, thoracoscope port, in a subxiphoid position
- T2, dissection instrument port, left parasternal at the 10th or 11th intercostal space
- T3, dissection instrument port, right parasternal at the 10th or 11th intercostal space
- T4, endoscopic stapler port, in the right hemithorax between the 4th and 8th intercostal space

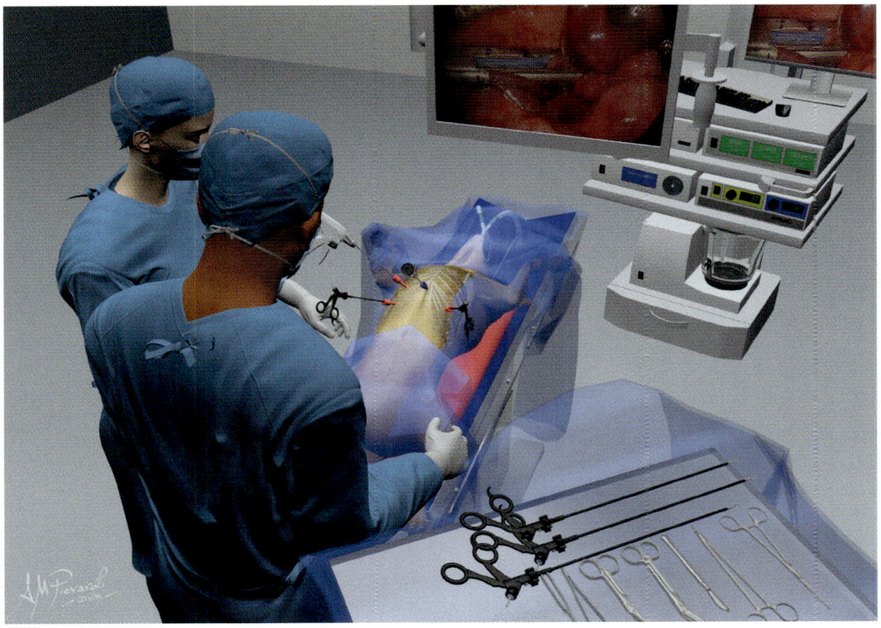

FIGURE 1. Operating room layout for thoracoscopic auriculectomy.

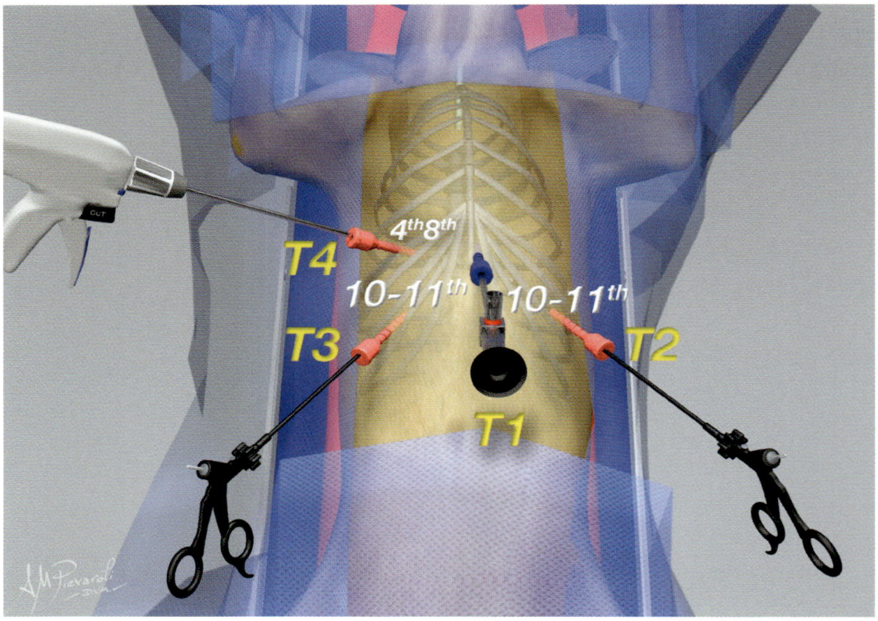

FIGURE 2. Port placement for thoracoscopic auriculectomy. An additional 12 mm port is placed in the right hemithorax cranial to T3; the position varies depending on the patient's size and morphology. It is important to ensure that there is enough room for the stapler anvil to fit within the thorax easily via this port.

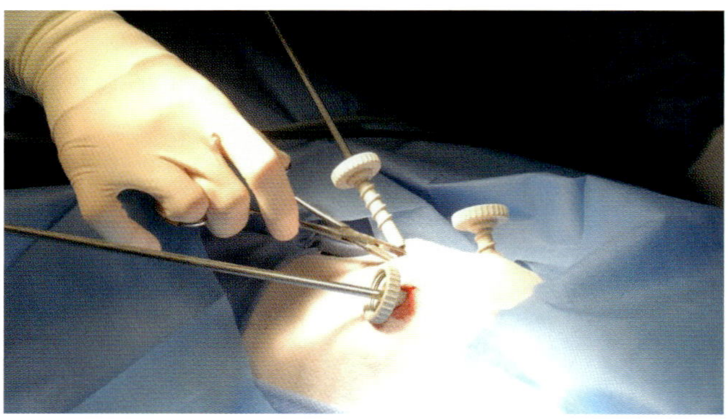

FIGURE 3. Intraoperative image of port placement for thoracoscopic pericardiectomy prior to auriculectomy. The stapler port has not been placed yet but will be added on the patient's right side between the 4th and 8th intercostal space.

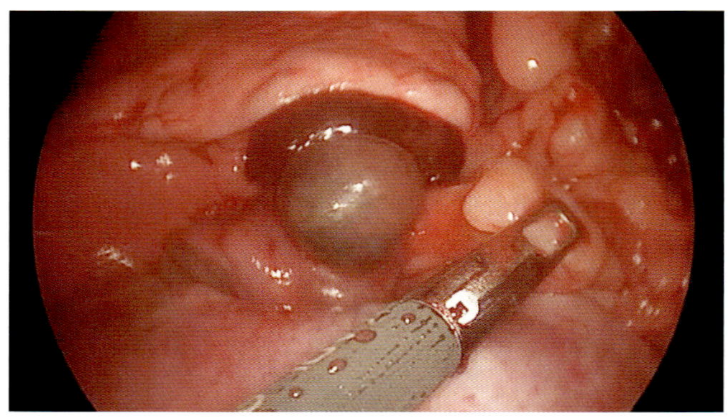

FIGURE 4. Thoracoscopic image of a modestly sized apical auricular mass following pericardiectomy. This mass is ideal for thoracoscopic auriculectomy.

PROCEDURE

- Following completion of the pericardiectomy (see Chapter 50), the right cranial region of the heart is explored. If the auricular mass is confirmed to be resectable (**Fig. 4**), an endoscopic stapler is used to isolate the base of the auricle. A blunt probe or atraumatic forceps may be needed to manipulate the auricle to facilitate cautious placement of the stapler.
- Once the stapler anvil has been closed, careful attention to ensure that no lung or pericardium was accidentally included is needed (**Fig. 5**). In small dogs, a short staple cartridge (45 mm) is necessary to maneuver safely in the thorax, and multiple staple cartridges may be required to complete the auriculectomy. In some cases, Metzenbaum scissors may be needed to separate the stapled mass from the pericardium (**Fig. 6**).
- Following complete transection of the auricular appendage, the endoscopic staple line is evaluated for proper staple closure and for any evidence of bleeding. The mass is then placed in a specimen retrieval bag for removal from the thoracic cavity.
- Once the auricular mass has been removed from the thorax in the bag, a small-gauge thoracostomy tube is placed under thoracoscopic guidance. The author prefers a Mila 14 Fr drain for monitoring postoperatively.

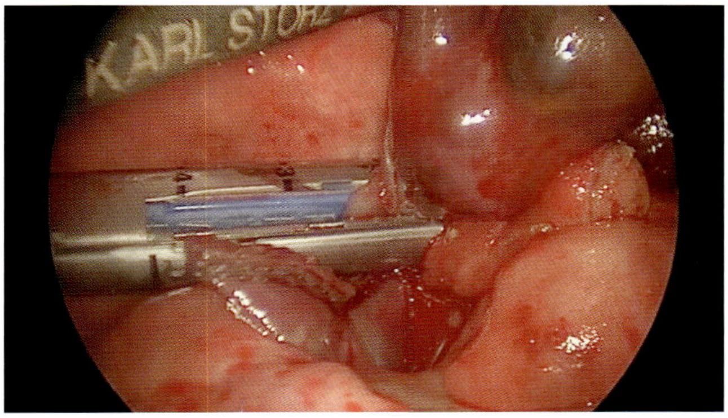

FIGURE 5. Thoracoscopic image of the auricle following positioning of the stapler anvil at the base. Note that a second 45 mm staple cartridge is being used to complete resection. Atraumatic grasping forceps are being used to retract the mass to facilitate exposure and stapler placement.

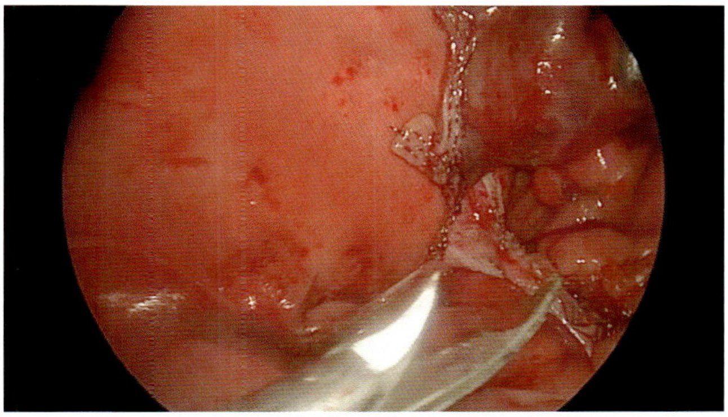

FIGURE 6. Metzenbaum scissors are used to complete the excision of the mass by cutting the stapled attachment to the edge of the pericardium.

- Port sites are removed individually under thoracoscopic observation to ensure no hemorrhage from the intercostal vessels occurs. Port wounds are closed routinely in two layers.

POSTOPERATIVE MANAGEMENT

- Intraoperative infiltration of all port sites with a local anesthetic (e.g., bupivacaine) affords 4–6 hours of analgesia postoperatively.
- The combination of nonsteroidal anti-inflammatory medication (3–5 days) and systemic opioids (12–36 hours) is generally effective for uncomplicated thoracoscopic surgery.
- Monitoring of pleural fluid production via the chest drain is recommended for 12–24 hours postoperatively.
- Recheck examination with chest X-rays is recommended at 4, 8, and 12 weeks postoperatively.

Complications of thoracoscopic auriculectomy

- Auricular masses can be friable and associated with severe hemorrhage, especially if the tissue is torn. Careful manipulation and atraumatic stapler placement are required to avoid this complication.
- Port-site hemorrhage can occur after removal of intercostal ports. In some cases, hemorrhage from intercostal arteries necessitates reoperation to locate and ligate the bleeding vessel. It is recommended that all the ports sites are monitored thoracoscopically during port removal. If significant hemorrhage is seen, the intercostal vessel should be ligated.

Key points

- The ideal lesion for thoracoscopic auriculectomy is an apical mass of a moderate size (<3 cm in diameter).
- Preoperative CT is recommended for staging of patients with auricular masses but is limited in facilitating accurate assessment of auricular mass size and characteristics.
- Thoracoscopic auriculectomy facilitates histopathologic diagnosis and may reduce the risk of sudden death from severe hemorrhage.

SUGGESTED READINGS

CLINICAL CASES

56.1 THORACOSCOPIC RIGHT AURICULAR TUMOR EXCISION USING A FOUR-PORT TECHNIQUE

Justin B. Ganjei

CASE DESCRIPTION

A 10-year-old spayed female Labrador Retriever was evaluated for acute onset collapse. She had an intramuscular hemangiosarcoma excised from her right shoulder region approximately 1 month prior. Diagnostic workup performed revealed pericardial effusion and a heterogenous, cavitated soft tissue mass arising from the right auricular appendage. Following initial stabilization and therapeutic thoracocentesis, the patient was referred for surgical consultation and subsequently taken to surgery 24 hours later for thoracoscopic pericardial window and right auricular mass excision.

Key points

- Performing a slightly larger and more ventrally/cranially situated pericardial window is helpful to allow complete visualization of the auricular appendage.
- Ease of auriculectomy is made possible by the distal location of the tumor.
- Manipulation and visualization of the entire auricular appendage to be excised within the tips of the stapling device is key to avoid severe, potentially life-threatening hemorrhage.

PORT PLACEMENT

An approximately 1 cm incision was made in the right paraxiphoid region and a 5 mm threaded trocar was inserted into the thoracic cavity to create a subxiphoid camera port (T1). A 5 mm 30° telescope was introduced. A second port (T2) was established under direct visualization by inserting a 5 mm threaded thoracoport into the ventral aspect of the left 6th intercostal space. A third port (T3) was established under direct visualization by inserting a 5 mm threaded thoracoport into the ventral aspect of the right 6th intercostal space. After pericardioscopy, a fourth port (T4) was established under direct visualization by inserting a 10 mm thoracoport into the ventral aspect of the left 9th intercostal space.

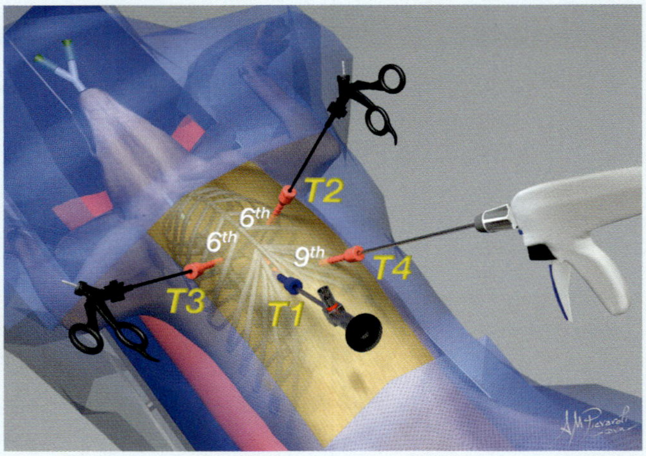

PROCEDURE

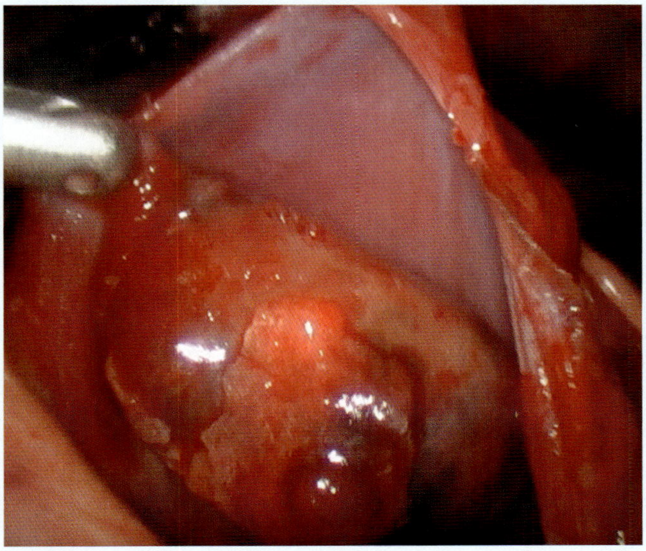

FIGURE 1. After transecting the mediastinum using a 5 mm bipolar vessel-sealing device, the pericardium apex is grasped and Metzenbaum scissors used to make a pericardial incision. A moderate volume of hemorrhagic pericardial effusion is evacuated. A 4×4 cm pericardial window is created along the ventral pericardial surface using a LigaSure. Pericardioscopy reveals a 2×2 cm mass arising from the distal aspect of the auricular appendage. Grasping forceps are used to retract the pericardium, allowing exposure of the appendage, which is grasped with Babcock forceps.

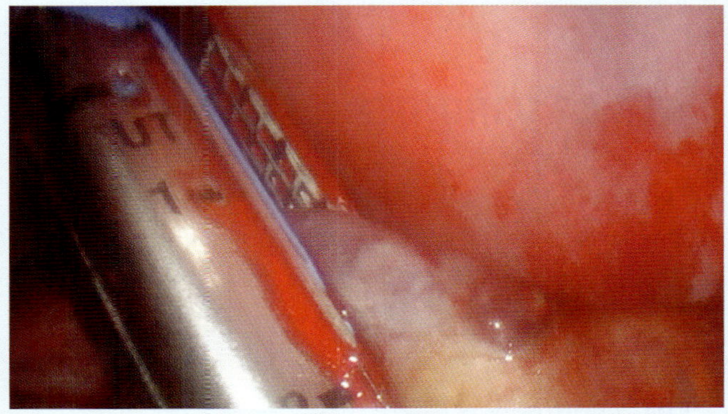

FIGURE 2. The right auricular appendage is grasped proximal to the tumor and a 10 mm EndoGIA stapling device loaded with a 60 mm 3.5 mm cartridge is placed around the appendage, proximal to the tumor. Note how the entire auricular appendage is confined within the region of the stapling device, allowing for safe transection, with extra room distally to account for movement of the auricle during compression/transection. Right auriculectomy is then performed.

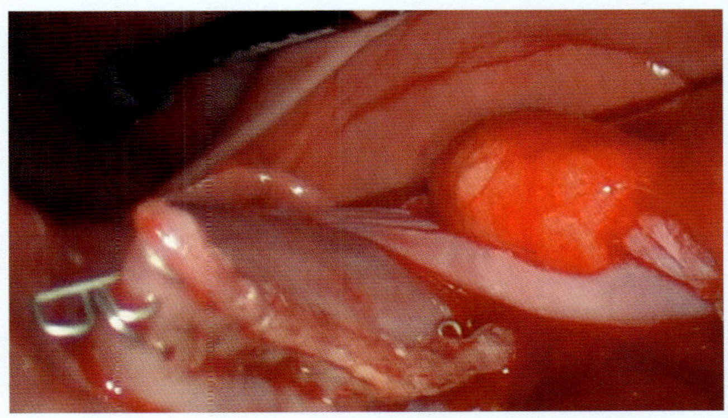

FIGURE 3. Thoracoscopic image of the staple line across the auricular appendage after transection, showing complete seal and no hemorrhage. The tumor is then removed through the 10 mm instrument port site using a specimen retrieval bag. An 18-gauge thoracostomy tube is inserted through the left 7th intercostal space. All port sites are closed in standard multilayer fashion

Tips and tricks

✓ Avoid grasping the right auricular mass. Instead, focus on manipulating the normal aspects of the auricular appendage.

56.2 SURGICAL VARIATION ON AURICULAR MASS REMOVAL TECHNIQUE

Boris Dalpozzo

CASE DESCRIPTION

A 7-year-old Australian Shepherd was presented for a recurrent hemorrhagic pericardial effusion. Echocardiography revealed a mass localized in the apex of the right auricle. Hemangiosarcoma was suspected. No metastases were identified on CT. Surgical resection was performed with a slight variation of the technique.

Key points

- When hemangiosarcoma is suspected, complete staging is highly recommended.
- Echocardiography is more sensitive than CT for detection of heart tumors and assessment of surgical resectability.
- Thoracoscopic exploration is the definitive method to evaluate surgical resectability.
- Highly specialized instrumentation is needed.

PORT PLACEMENT

The patient was prepared for bilateral thoracic access and placed in dorsal recumbency. The 5 mm telescope port (T1) was placed in a right paraxiphoid position. T2 was placed at the costochondral junction of the right 8th intercostal space. T3 was placed at the costochondral junction of the right 6th intercostal space. T4 was placed at the costochondral junction of the left 6th intercostal space.

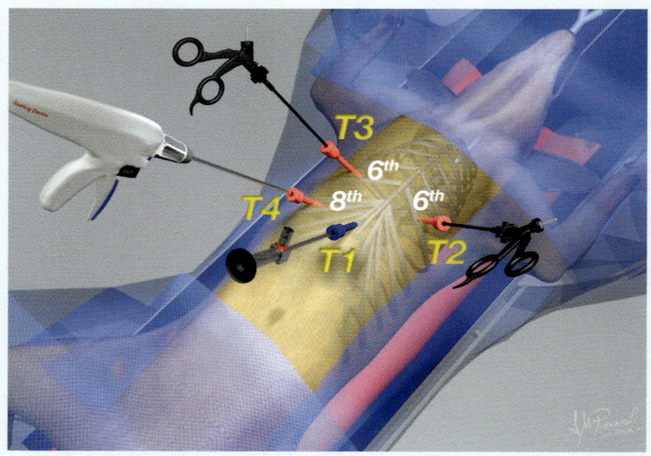

PROCEDURE

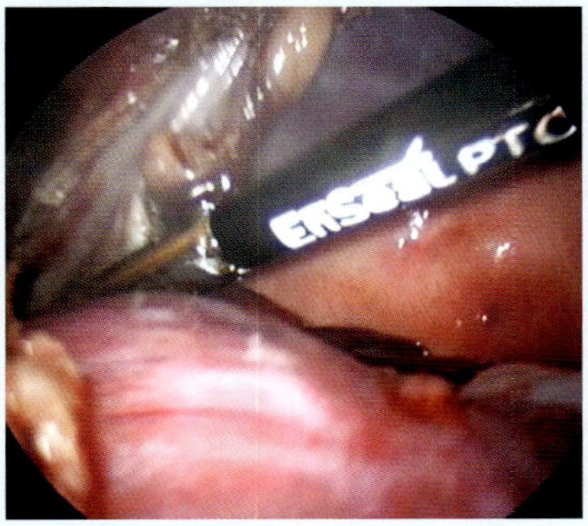

FIGURE 1. The procedure starts by performing a wide pericardial window. Potential residual blood in the pericardial sac needs to be aspirated to allow good visualization.

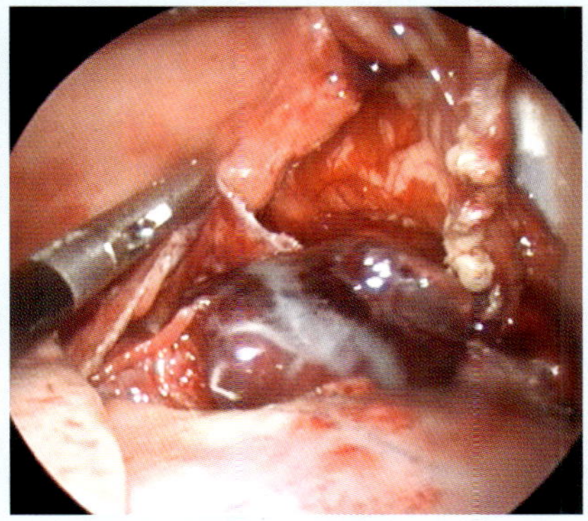

FIGURE 2. Grasping and elevating the cranial border of the pericardium and the apex of right cranial lung lobe allows exploration of the right auricle.

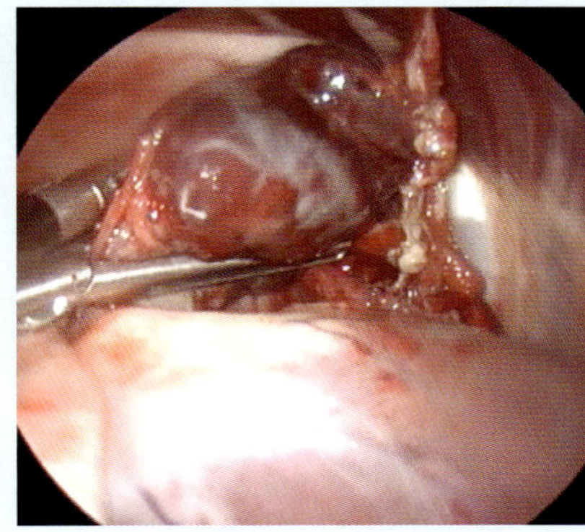

FIGURE 3. If the mass is considered surgically resectable, the right auricle is grasped with long atraumatic forceps and surgical margins are evaluated.

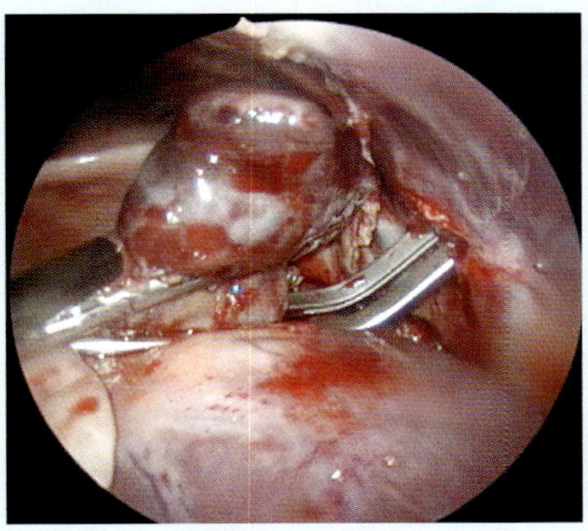

FIGURE 4. A standard aortic cross-clamp is introduced through the left-side port as far as possible and placed on the base of the auricle and proximal to the atraumatic endoscopic grasping forceps previously placed.

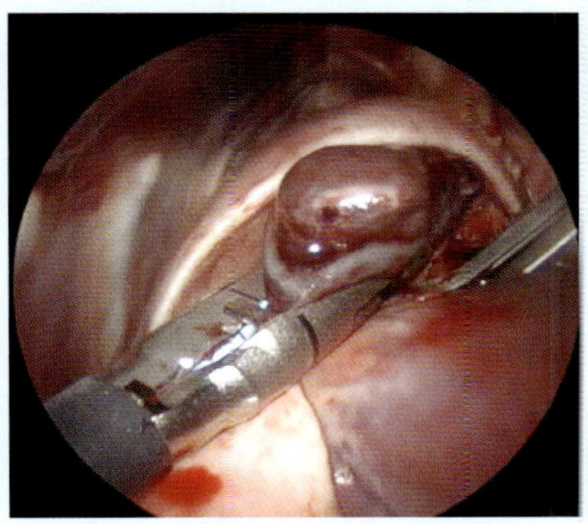

FIGURE 5. A 45 mm 3.5 EndoGIA is placed distal to the tumor. Accurate check of the right length must be made before stapling. Once fired, the stapler is opened and retracted, and the mass is grasped and removed from the thoracic cavity using a retrieval bag.

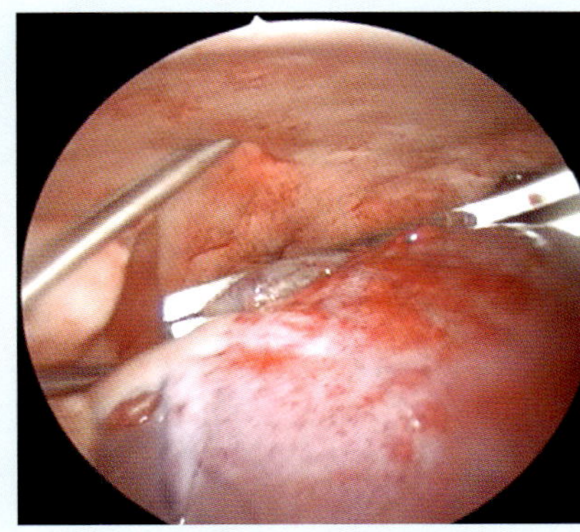

FIGURE 6. As stapler line failure can be catastrophic, the aortic clamp is slowly and progressively released under direct visualization. If signs of hemorrhage are detected, the clamp should be closed and the procedure converted to open surgery for manual oversewing.

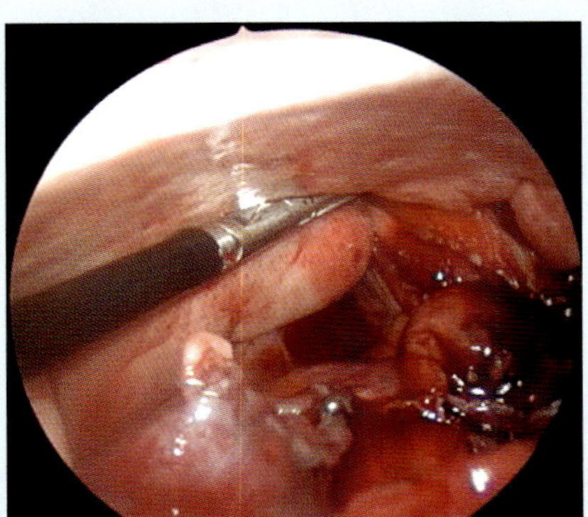

FIGURE 7. If no hemorrhage is detected, a chest drain is inserted and the ports are closed routinely.

Tips and tricks

- ✓ A large pericardial window allows better visualization and manipulation of the auricle.
- ✓ Availability of different sizes of EndoGIA is highly recommended.
- ✓ Hemorrhage can be catastrophic and difficult to control. Be prepared to prompt conversion to open surgery.

57 THORACOSCOPIC FOREIGN BODY REMOVAL

Boris Dalpozzo

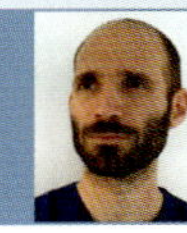

Indications

- Exploration of the thoracic cavity
- Removal of small foreign bodies
- Partial or total lung lobectomy

Contraindications

- Clinically unstable patients
- Diffuse adhesions
- Large foreign bodies
- Since the accessory lung lobe is often difficult to approach by thoracoscopy, lesions in this lobe may be a relative contraindication, especially in chronic patients

Thoracic foreign bodies (FBs) are a relatively uncommon cause of thoracic cavity and pleural disease. Presence of an intrathoracic FB can result from inhalation, ingestion, or penetrating wounds. In the author's experience, inhalation is the most frequent way of FB entrance in companion animals, especially in dogs. Vegetable seeds are the most frequently encountered FBs. Dogs living outdoors or that frequent gardens, parks, or open fields are more subject to this pathology. Once inhaled, if not expelled by sneezing or coughing, persistence of the FB in the lower airways can determine various degrees of bronchitis, pneumonia, pulmonary abscess, and/or airway perforation resulting in potential pyothorax and pneumothorax. In cases of pyothorax with no history of a penetrating wound or in cases of spontaneous pneumothorax, presence of an inhaled FB should be suspected.

Ingestion is another possible way of entrance of thoracic FBs. FBs in the thoracic esophagus are often better managed by retrieving or pushing them into the stomach via flexible endoscopy. In case of large embedded FBs or when concurrent esophageal perforation is suspected, endoscopic treatment can result in severe esophageal trauma; therefore, a surgical approach is preferred. In the majority of cases, an open surgical approach is preferred due to the potential presence adhesions and the necessity of complex esophageal suture or reconstruction.

Tips

Large FBs are often best treated by open surgery.

Penetrating wounds (e.g., gunshot wounds, stab wounds, large dog bites, severe external trauma) are a relatively uncommon cause of thoracic FB entrance. In the author's experience, hunting dogs are most frequently affected. In case of thoracic penetrating wounds, advanced imaging diagnosis or exploratory surgery are highly recommended, as damage to internal organs may be severe, even with small external wounds.

> The first mention of thoracoscopic FB removal in the dog was made by Joliffe in 2000, with right middle lung lobectomy to treat concurrent pyothorax.

DIAGNOSIS

Pneumothorax, pleural effusion, and radiopaque FBs can be identified on thoracic radiographs. Pulmonary opacity can sometimes be found as a result of pneumonia secondary to FB inhalation (**Fig. 1**), but radiographs may be normal in patients with acute intrathoracic grass awn FBs.

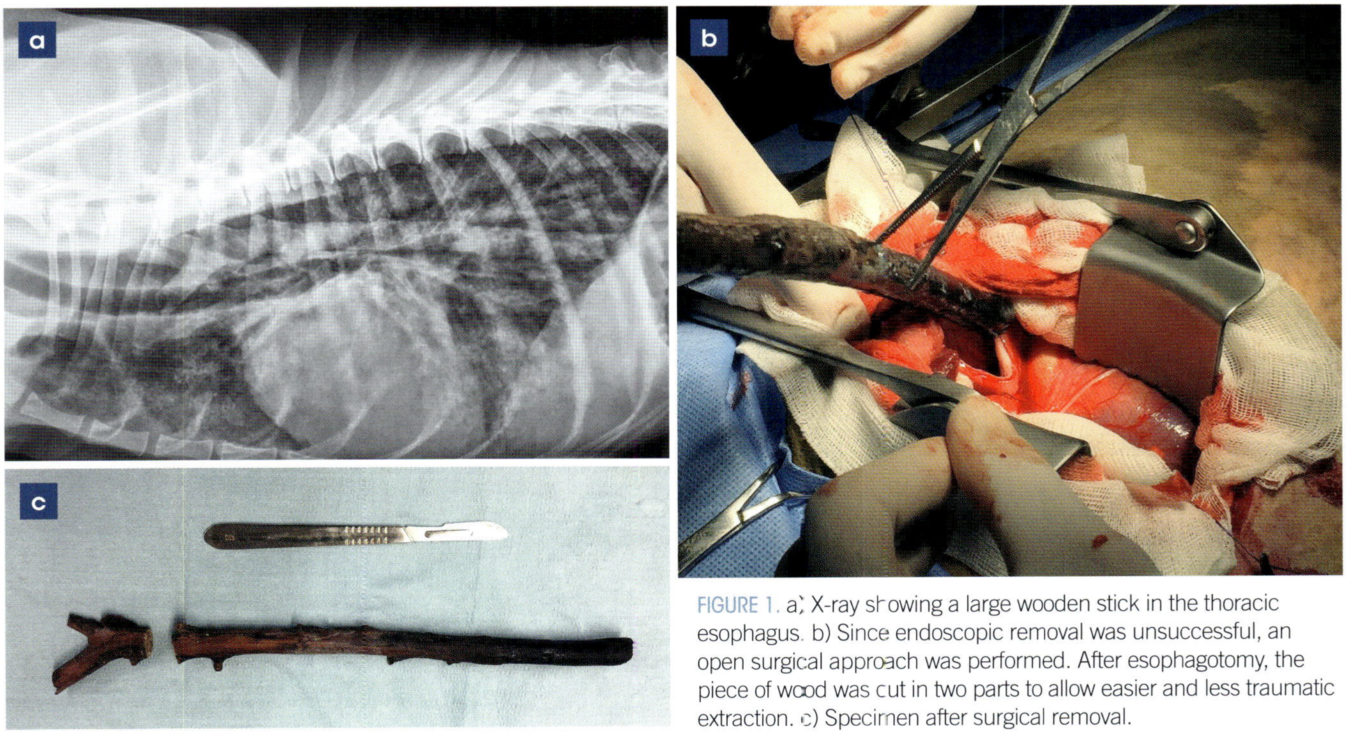

FIGURE 1. a) X-ray showing a large wooden stick in the thoracic esophagus. b) Since endoscopic removal was unsuccessful, an open surgical approach was performed. After esophagotomy, the piece of wood was cut in two parts to allow easier and less traumatic extraction. c) Specimen after surgical removal.

CT offers the best diagnostic aid because it allows to determine the precise site of abnormality to detect more lesions, and to trace the path of the FB more accurately than with radiographs. If there is a large amount of air or liquid in the pleural space, chest tube aspiration may be necessary before performing a CT scan to enhance visualization of the pulmonary parenchyma by increasing lung expansion.

In some cases, ultrasound can be used for diagnosis and guided removal of grass awn FBs and can be useful to visualize the FB within the region of the tract identified on the CT images.

PREOPERATIVE CONSIDERATIONS

Clinical management is difficult in patients with intrathoracic or sublumbar grass awns. Surgical or nonsurgical management is possible, but outcome following surgery for spontaneous pneumothorax seems to be more favorable.

Since patients with thoracic FBs often present different degrees of both pyothorax and pneumothorax, they must be considered critical patients. Adequate preoperative stabilization may be necessary prior to surgical exploration. Needle aspiration or chest tube placement allows evacuation of air or liquid to improve the patient's respiratory function and clinical status.

A sample of pleural liquid should be collected for cytological examination as soon as possible. If pyothorax is suspected, bacterial culture and antibiogram are highly recommended. Broad-spectrum antibiotic therapy should be started and then eventually corrected based on bacterial culture results.

PATIENT PREPARATION AND POSITIONING

Localization of a FB is case specific, highly variable, and not predictable. Inhaled FBs, especially grass awns, usually migrate in a straight line along the bronchial tree; therefore, the tip of the caudal lung lobes and the caudodorsal part of the thoracic cavity are more frequently involved (**Fig. 2**). In most cases, the exact location of a FB cannot be determined on CT scans, and bronchopathy or focal pneumonia are the only signs to guide surgical exploration.

The patient can be placed in sternal or lateral recumbency. Sternal recumbency provides a wider field of view and enables better exploration of the dorsal compartment. Additionally, bilateral exploration is possible without changing patient position. Placing a cushion under the sternum and the pelvis allows the abdomen to hang (**Fig. 3**), caudalizing the diaphragm and

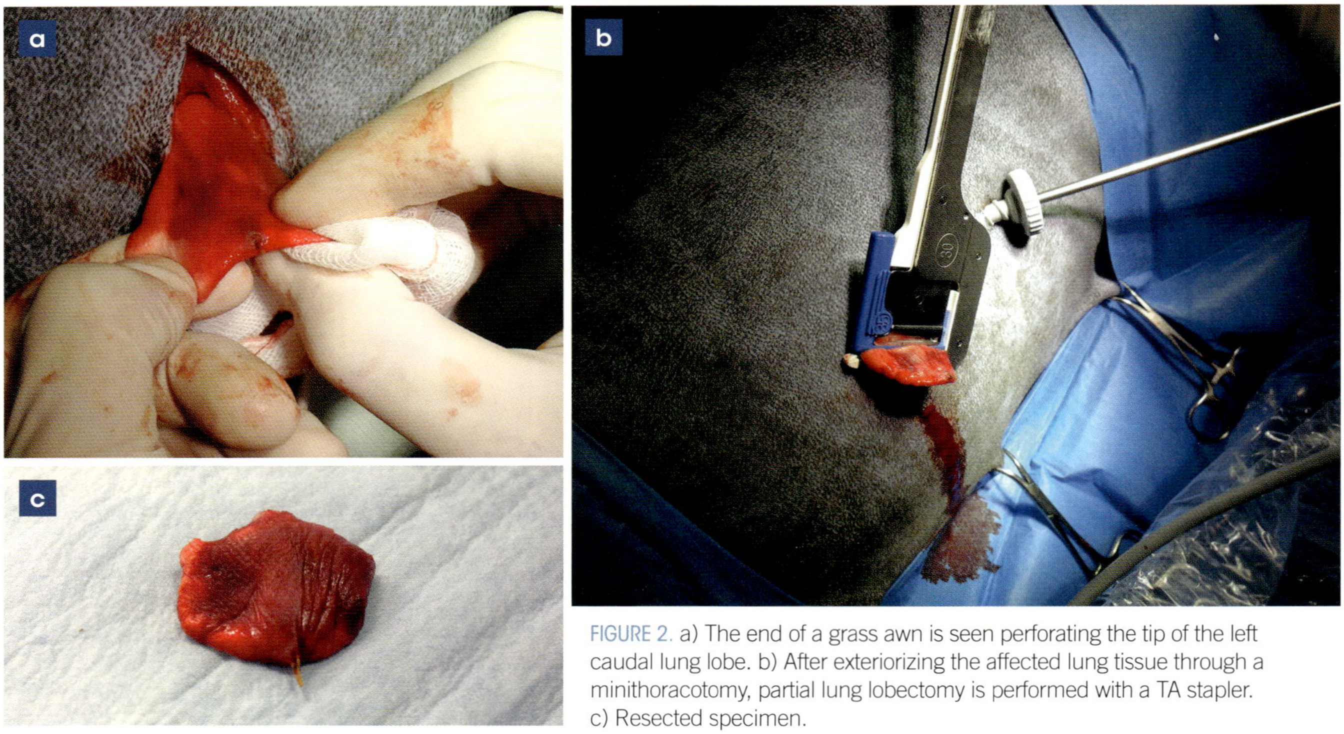

FIGURE 2. a) The end of a grass awn is seen perforating the tip of the left caudal lung lobe. b) After exteriorizing the affected lung tissue through a minithoracotomy, partial lung lobectomy is performed with a TA stapler. c) Resected specimen.

obtaining a wider view of the costodiaphragmatic recesses, where grass awns are often located. Lateral recumbency, with the affected side uppermost, is appropriate when the side of pathology is clear and if location in the middle-ventral part of the lung is suspected. Although rarely used, dorsal recumbency can be helpful in patients with involvement of the mediastinal pleura or ventral thoracic cavity.

Since a single access does not permit complete exploration of the thoracic cavity, a double approach with an intraoperative change of the patient's position may be necessary; therefore, the entire thorax should be clipped. Complications may warrant fast conversion to open surgery involving a change in patient position, and the surgical team and instruments must be prepared in advance.

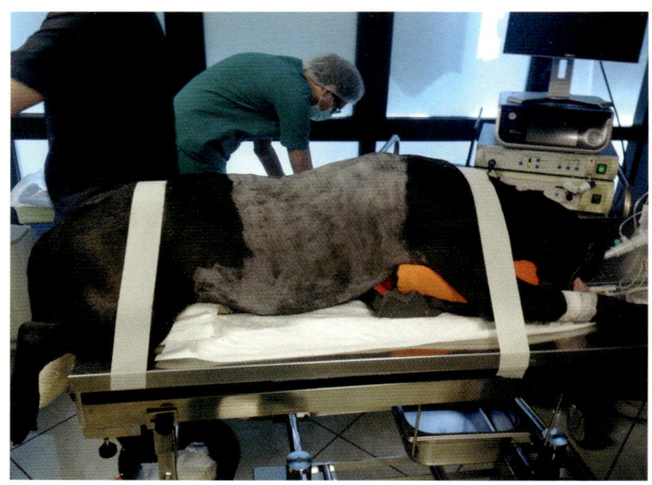

FIGURE 3. Patient in sternal recumbency. Cushions have been placed under the sternum and pubis.

OPERATING ROOM LAYOUT

With the patient in sternal recumbency, the surgeon and the assistant position themselves on the affected side of patient. The monitor is placed in front of the surgeon for unilateral exploration (**Fig. 4a**). If bilateral exploration is anticipated, the monitor should be placed caudal to the patient to avoid changing operating room layout intraoperatively.

In the lateral approach, the surgeon and the assistant stand on one side of the operating table facing the patient's ventral region. The monitor and carts are placed as described above for unilateral exploration (**Fig. 4b**).

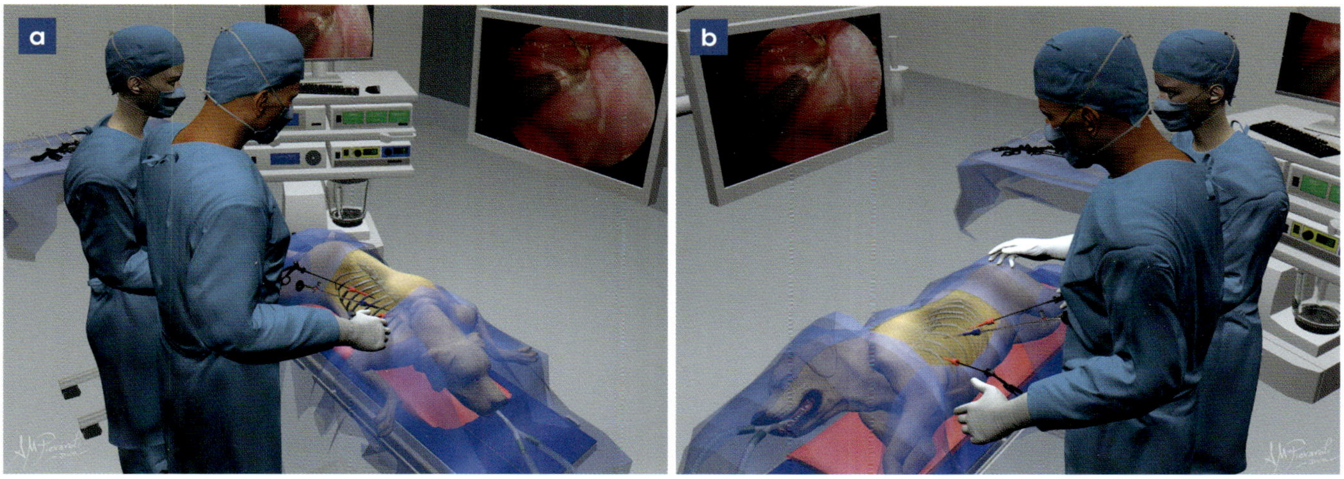

FIGURE 4. Operating room layout for thoracoscopic FB removal. a) Patient in sternal recumbency. b) Patient in lateral recumbency.

Instruments

On the table:

- Standard surgical set
- Telescope 5 mm – 30°
- Thoracic cannulas 5 and 10 mm
- Atraumatic forceps
- Maryland and Mixter dissector
- Endoscopic cannula for aspiration/irrigation

Ready to use:

- Knot pusher device or pretied suture loop
- Surgical stapling devices (e.g., TA, GIA, EndoGIA)
- Alexis wound retractor (**Fig. 5**)
- Monopolar hook
- Vessel-sealing device
- Endoscopic hemoclip applier
- Retrieval bag
- Finochietto retractor
- Thoracic instrumentation for open thoracic surgery

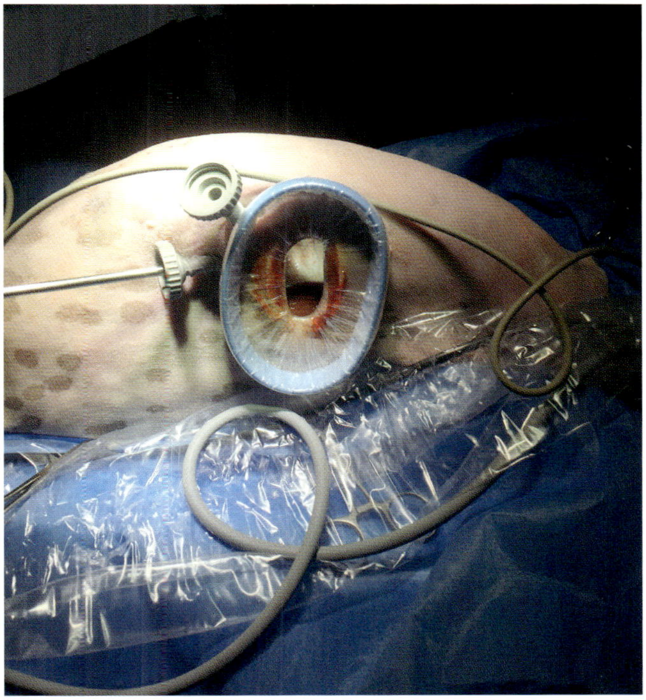

FIGURE 5. Alexis wound retractors offer great exposure even through a minithoracotomy.

PORT PLACEMENT (FIG. 6)

- T1, 7th intercostal space, middle third (lateral recumbency) or dorsal third (sternal recumbency)
- T2, based on exploration findings
- T3, based on exploration findings and triangulation

Port placement is not completely predictable, as FB location is highly variable. The procedure usually starts with exploration of the chest cavity. The first port, for scope insertion, is placed in the middle of the thorax to obtain a wide field of view; the 7th intercostal space is often a good option. The other ports are placed based on thoracoscopic exploration findings.

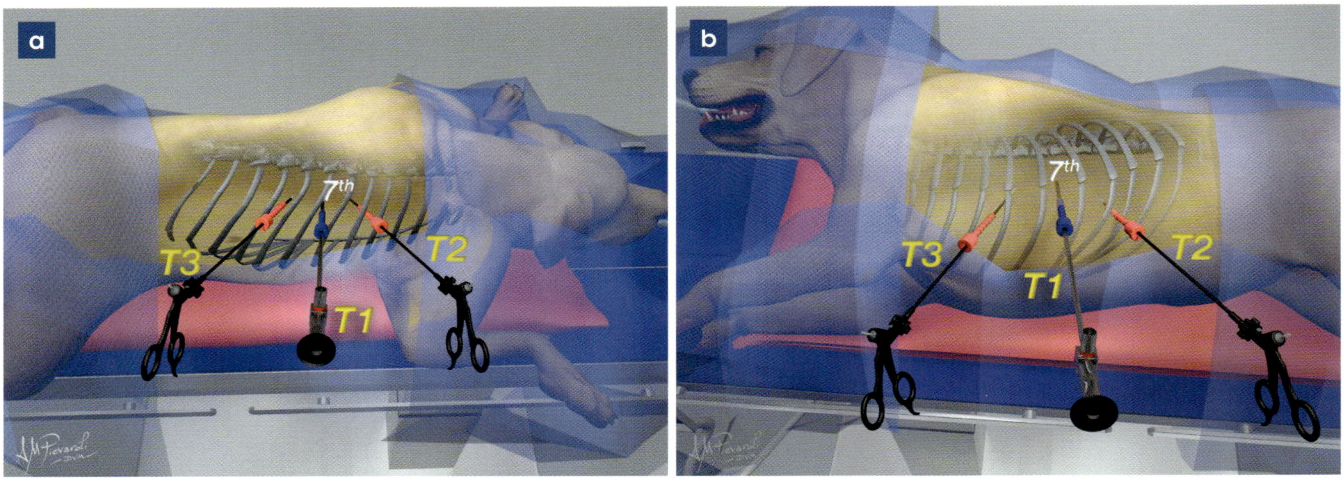

FIGURE 6. Port placement for thoracoscopic FB removal. a) Patient in sternal recumbency. b) Patient in lateral recumbency.

PROCEDURE

- After the first port has been placed, the scope is introduced and the thoracic cavity is explored. If monopulmonary ventilation is not available, ventilation is set in a low-volume, high-rate fashion to reduce lung volume and minimize lung interference, obtaining better visualization.
- The second port is eventually placed and atraumatic forceps inserted to allow lung mobilization and better exploration (**Fig. 7**). Once the area of interest has been visualized, other ports are placed or a minithoracotomy is performed. In the majority of cases with vegetable FBs, lung perforation is located at the tip of the caudal lobes (**Fig. 8**).
- If the damaged area is small, partial lobectomy can be performed with an EndoGIA. However, more often, the affected lobe is exteriorized through an enlarged port and thoracoscopic-assisted partial lobectomy is performed by hand suture or with a TA stapler (**Fig. 9**).

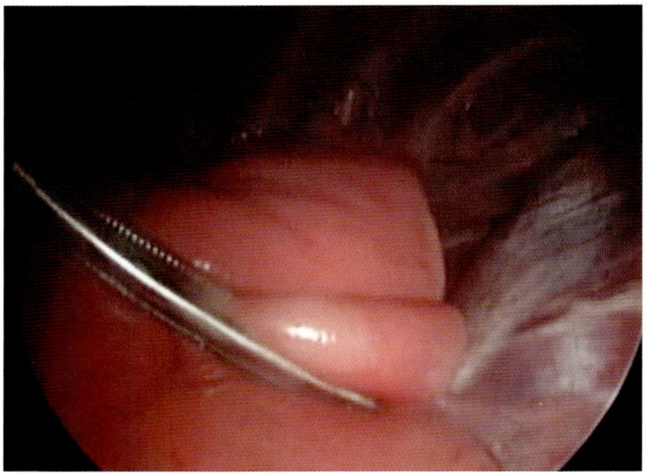

FIGURE 7. Slight patient tilting and use of long atraumatic forceps to grasp the lung parenchyma allow exploration of pulmonary and mediastinal recesses.

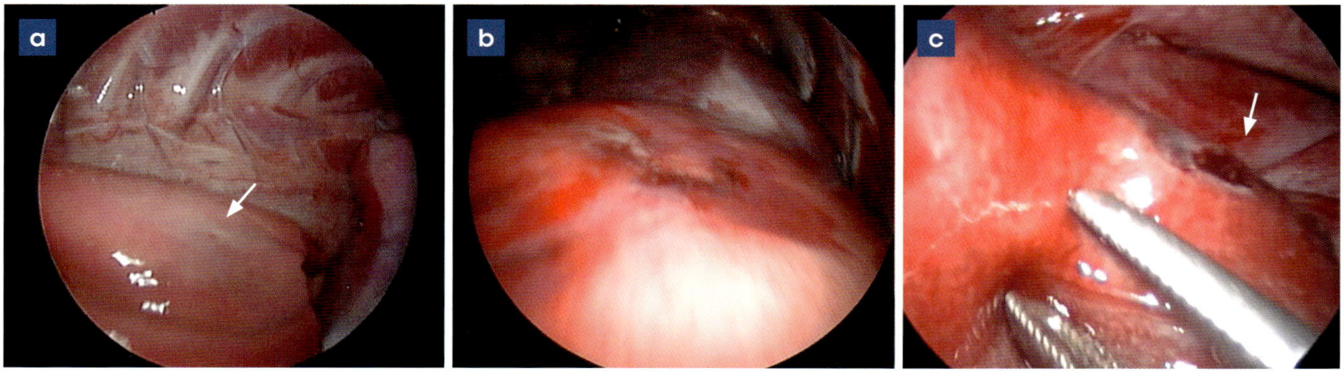

FIGURE 8. A small hole (arrow) surrounded by discolored or hemorrhagic tissue is often the sign of lung perforation by FB.

Tips

FBs located at the tip of the caudal lung lobes are usually removed by partial lobectomy with minimal loss of lung parenchyma.

- If there are no signs of lung abscess, necrosis, or severe focal pneumonia, suturing small lung perforations allows to conserve almost the entire lung parenchyma (**Fig. 10**).
- Larger lobectomies may be required for lesions not located in the tip of the lung lobes, resulting in greater lung parenchymal loss. In these cases, the pulmonary ligament can be cut with endoscopic scissors or a monopolar hook to improve mobilization and extraction of the affected lung lobe (**Fig. 11**).
- Searching for a FB can be time-consuming and frustrating. If a FB is inside the lung parenchyma, palpation or intraoperative ultrasound of the exteriorized affected lobe can help in localization (**Fig. 12**). One of the most frequent locations of migrated FBs is the costodiaphragmatic recesses, so thorough exploration of these regions is needed.
- Once identified, the FB is grasped and extracted carefully to avoid breaking it and leaving fragments inside.
- FBs may sometimes migrate far from the pulmonary exit point. In these cases, indirect signs such as pleuritis, adhesions, abscesses, or pus collections can reveal FB location (**Fig. 13**).

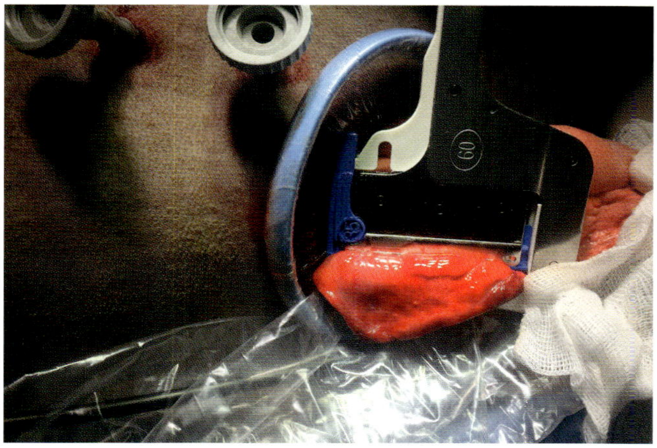

FIGURE 9. Exteriorization and stapling of the affected lobe with a TA stapler is a fast and safe technique for partial lung lobectomy.

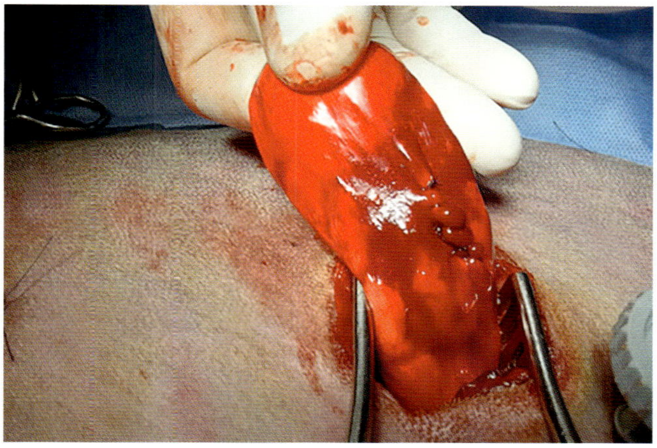

FIGURE 10. Small perforations can be treated with a mattress or double-layer pattern of 4-0 absorbable suture material.

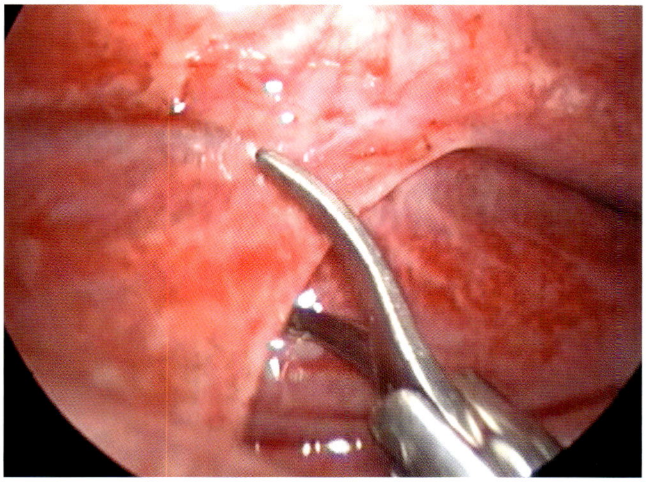

FIGURE 11. Cutting the pulmonary ligament allows better mobilization of the caudal lung lobes.

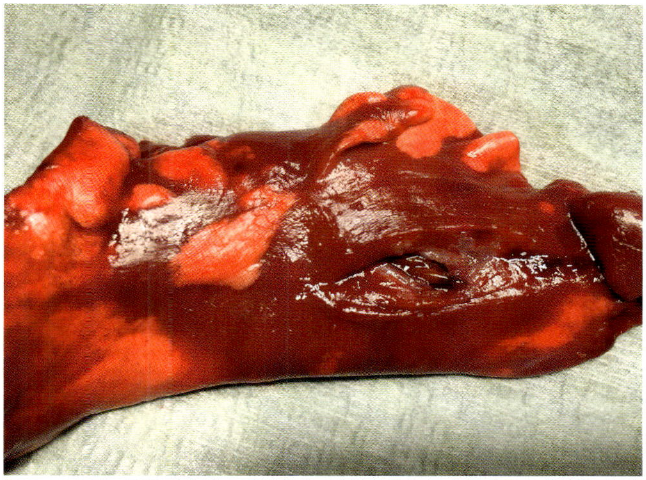

FIGURE 12. Lung specimen after resection. Exteriorization and digital palpation of the affected lobe allowed localization of a FB inside the parenchyma.

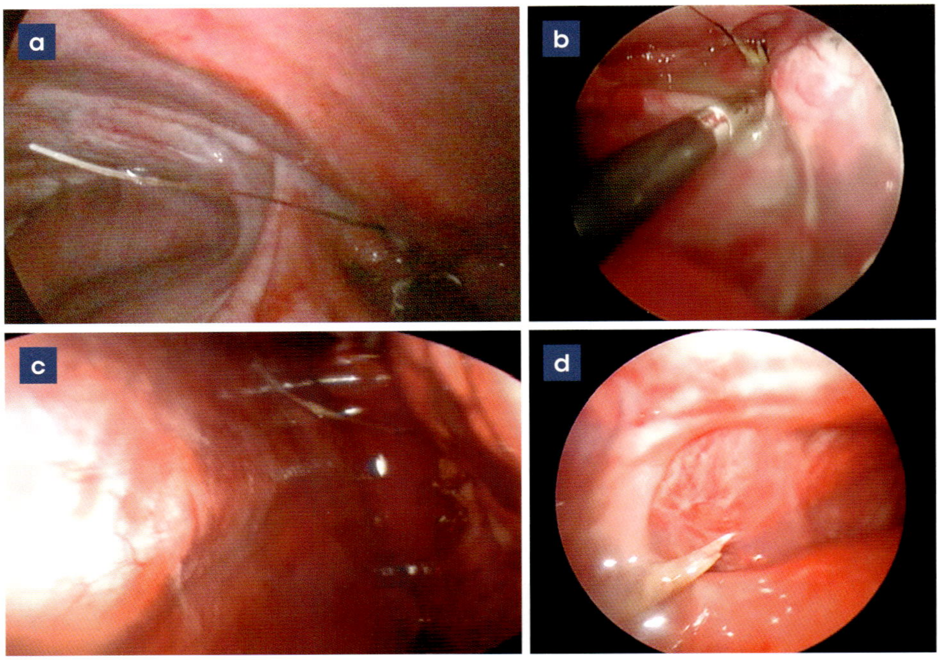

FIGURE 13. Different locations of migrated FBs. a,b) Costodiaphragmatic recess. c) A small collection of pus can reveal the presence of a FB. A grass awn fixed in the thoracic inlet was visible after gentle retraction of the thoracic artery. d) Vegetable FB located in the dorsal mediastinum between the aorta and the diaphragm.

CHRONIC FOREIGN BODIES

- Chronic cases can be challenging. Diffuse pleural adhesions are a potential contraindication to thoracoscopic surgery as they can hinder visualization and limit exploration.
- A patient was presented with a history of 5 months of cough, fever, and dyspnea. CT revealed diffuse pleural thickening, mild pneumothorax, and septic pleural effusion more evident on the left side. The patient was placed in right lateral recumbency and thoracoscopic exploration started at the 7th intercostal space.
- Due to diffuse pleuropulmonary adhesions, the working space was limited, with no room for complete insertion of the scope. A FB was immediately visible upon entrance of the scope into the pleural space (**Fig. 14**). An instrument port was placed cranial to the first port and the FB was extracted.
- Adhesions were resected with a monopolar hook (**Fig. 15**). Since lung perforation could not be identified by visual exploration, saline solution was instilled to look for the formation of bubbles indicating pneumothorax (**Fig. 16**).
- Mobilization of the affected lung lobe was not possible because it was fixed to the pleura by chronic adhesions, so there was not enough room for intracorporeal suturing. Therefore, the lung parenchyma was grasped with atraumatic forceps to overlap the edges of the perforated area and two hemoclips were applied to close the lung parenchyma (**Fig. 17**).
- The bubble test was then repeated to check for any residual air leaks and a chest drain was inserted.

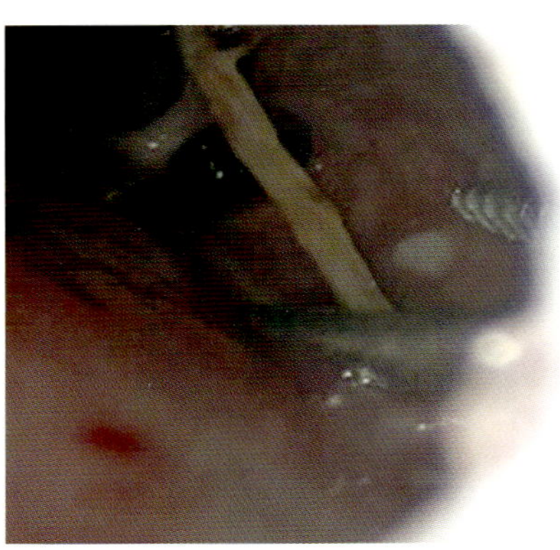

FIGURE 14. Thoracoscopic image of the FB.

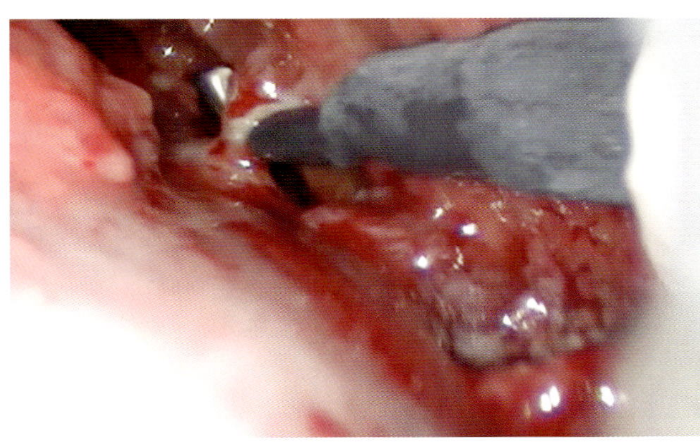

FIGURE 15. In chronic cases, adhesions may impede effective exploration. Focal adhesions can be cut with a monopolar hook to increase the working space and improve visualization.

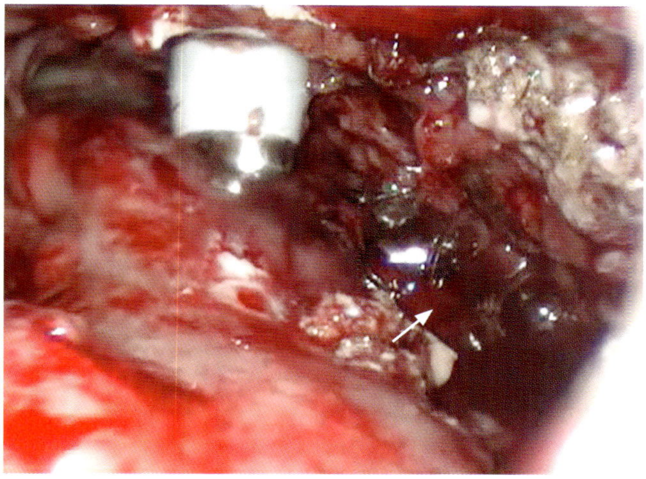

FIGURE 16. As for open surgery, air leaks can be identified by instilling saline solution and looking for bubble formation.

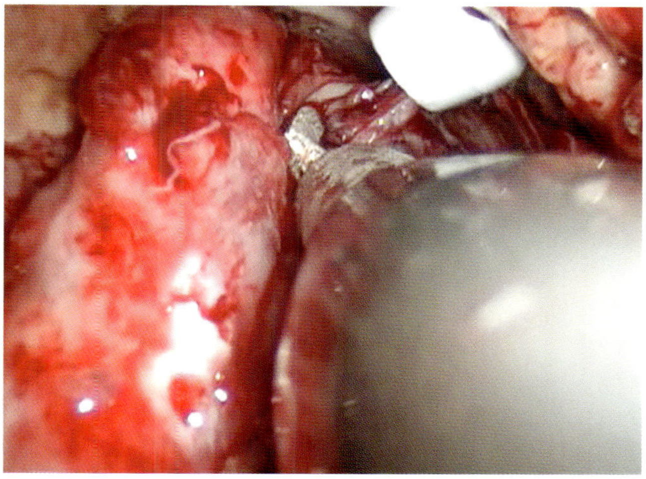

FIGURE 17. In this case, a small lung perforation was closed with two hemoclips applied to the lung parenchyma.

PENETRATING FOREIGN BODIES

- Penetrating wounds can be deceitful because even a small external wound can hide severe internal trauma. In these cases, advanced imaging and surgical exploration are highly recommended.
- A dog fell over a pile of wood during hunting and a wooden stick penetrated the left thoracic wall. The stick was extracted by the owner. The patient was subsequently presented with severe pneumothorax and hemorrhagic pleural effusion. Surgical exploration was performed with the patient in right lateral recumbency.
- After aspirating the effusion (**Fig. 18**), several wooden fragments were identified and extracted from the mediastinal pleura and lung parenchyma (**Fig. 19**).
- The left cranial lobe presented a large laceration not amenable to suturing (**Fig. 20**), so total lung lobectomy was performed with a 3.5 mm EndoGIA (**Fig. 21**).
- Thorough pleural lavage and aspiration was performed and a chest tube was placed prior to port and wound closure.

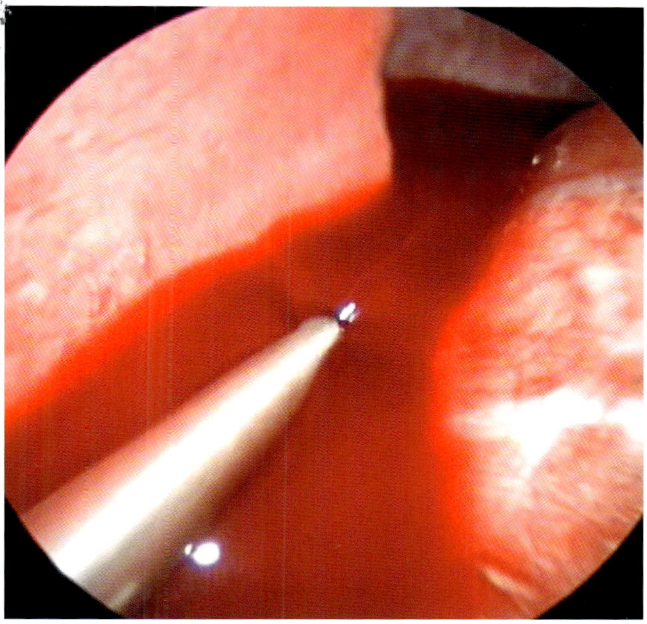

FIGURE 18. Pathological pleural fluids obscure visualization and should be aspirated before surgical exploration.

POSTOPERATIVE MANAGEMENT

- The chest tube should be left in place until resolution of pathological pleural collection, typically 24 hours after resolution of pneumothorax or when liquid drainage drops below 2 mL/kg/day and cytological examination is negative for infection. Several evacuation systems are available; closed continuous aspiration systems are preferred by the author.
- When large volumes of air or liquid are produced (especially in large patients), three-bottle or Pleur-evac systems are the best choice, but in most cases bellows drainage is sufficient. Intermittent drainage is suitable in small patients that may not tolerate bulky bellows systems.
- Oxygen supplementation is usually unnecessary but may be beneficial for initial patient stabilization or in patients with dyspnea due to severe bronchitis or pneumonia.

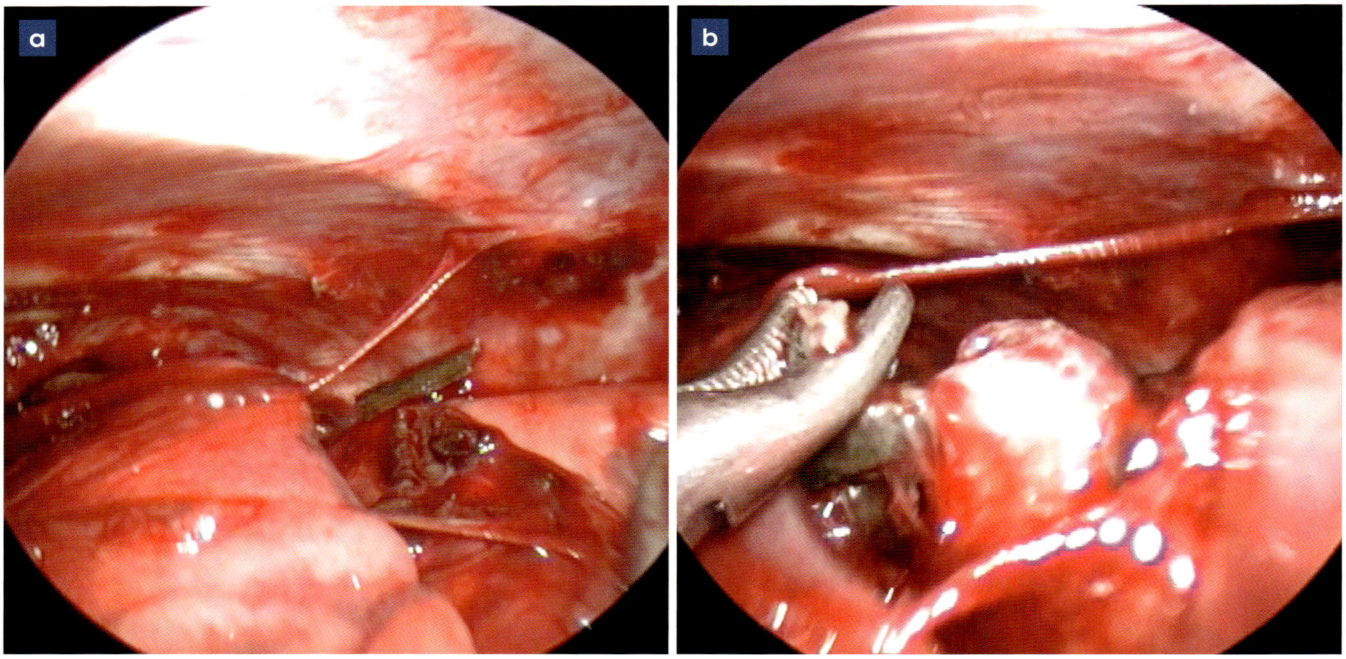

FIGURE 19. Careful exploration of the affected region revealed the presence of several wooden fragments. The FBs were extracted with grasping forceps.

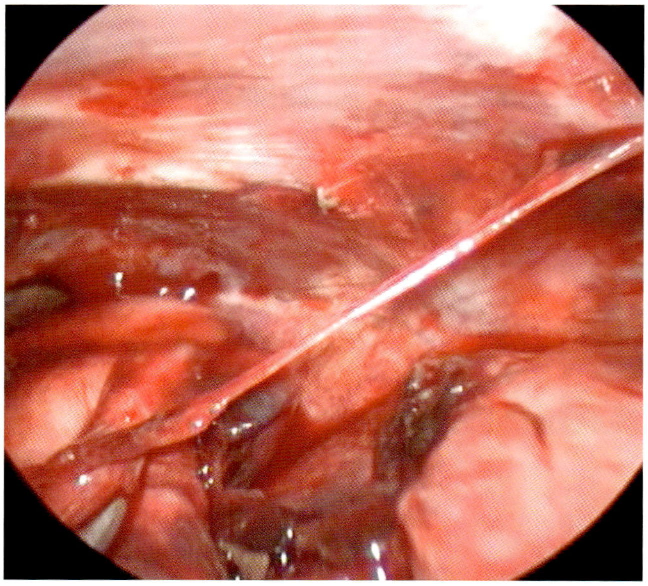

FIGURE 20. Major lung parenchyma lacerations were treated by lobectomy.

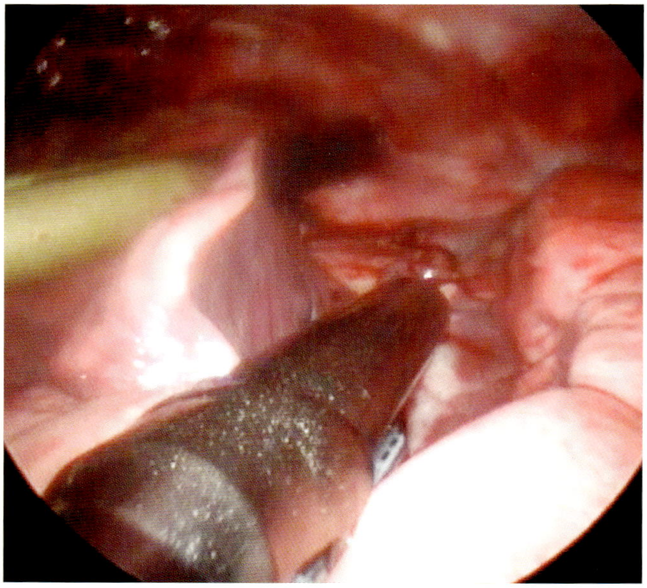

FIGURE 21. Total lobectomy of the left cranial lung lobe was performed using a 3.5 mm EndoGIA.

- If no complications occur, patients are typically discharged 2–3 days after chest tube removal if thoracic X-rays are negative for pleural effusion o pneumothorax. In case of severe septic pleuritis, antibiotic therapy should be eventually modified based on culture results and continued for 6–8 weeks. Clinical evaluation and chest X-rays are repeated 1 and 2 months after surgery.

Complications of thoracoscopic foreign body removal

- The most common complication is recurrence of pathology. Recurrent pneumothorax can result from dehiscence of the lung parenchyma suture. Since pathological tissues are often fragile and underlying infections can lead to impaired healing, in case of lung perforation the author prefers to perform a partial lung lobectomy rather than suture the lung perforation site.
- Mild persistent pneumothorax resulting from minor air leakage may heal spontaneously by leaving the chest tube in place, but severe cases may need surgical correction.
- Lack of identification of multiple FBs is the most frequent cause of recurrence. As previously mentioned, complete exploration of thoracic cavity by a single approach is not possible. Changing the patient's position intraoperatively to perform complete exploration is highly time-consuming and not justified unless multiple site pathology not manageable through a single approach is suspected on preoperative CT. Residual FBs can cause persistent pleural effusion or migrate, typically along epaxial or thoracic wall muscles, resulting in the development of abscesses and fistulas at distant sites even after a long period of time. In case of persistent septic effusion, after surgical treatment and targeted antibiotic therapy, recheck by CT and potential surgical exploration is recommended.
- Severe bacterial infection can lead to septicemia and sepsis, so careful monitoring of critically ill patient is highly recommended.

Key points

- CT imaging is highly recommended for accurate surgical planning.
- Preoperative chest tube placement can help stabilize patients with severe pneumothorax or pleural effusion and improve CT sensitivity.
- Consider oxygen supplementation in dyspneic patients.

SUGGESTED READINGS

58 THORACOSCOPIC PLACEMENT OF EPICARDIAL PACEMAKERS

Lucie Bonneau, Stéphane Libermann

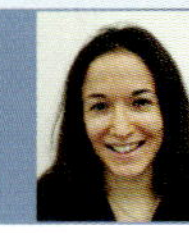

Indications

- Animals with symptomatic bradyarrhythmias (cardiac frequency <90 bpm in cats and <50 bpm in dogs) of cardiac origin: sick sinus syndrome, atrial standstill, second/third-degree atrioventricular block,
- No access or contraindications (sepsis or pyoderma in the neck, vascular anomaly, or trauma) to endovascular pacing

Contraindications

- General contraindications for thoracoscopy (see Chapter 48)
- Concomitant structural heart disease, myocarditis

Thoracoscopic epicardial pacing (TEP) has been recently described in veterinary medicine. TEP is performed with a three-port approach, thus requiring a surgical assistant. Different kinds of pacing leads are available for thoracoscopic placement, the screw-in lead being the most frequently used. However, hook leads are easier to fix to the epicardium.

Compared to other surgical techniques, TEP is a minimally invasive method to surgically implant a pacemaker. It is well tolerated by patients and the surgery is quite quick, thus reducing the anesthetic risk and the recovery period. Like other surgical techniques, TEP permits direct observation of the cardiac structures and optimizes correct lead positioning.

This technique involves few disadvantages, including the cost of the required material and the need for the surgeon to be comfortable with both procedures in case of conversion (from thoracoscopy to any open surgery cardiac pacing technique). Still, TEP is an invasive procedure when compared to transvenous techniques.

> The first pacemaker in dogs was implanted with a surgical approach in 1967. The first thoracoscopic epicardial pacing was reported in 2017.

PATIENT PREPARATION AND POSITIONING

Any patient requiring pacemaker therapy must be medically stabilized beforehand with proper therapy depending on the cardiac disease (e.g., cardiac insufficiency). For severe bradyarrhythmia, the procedure can be performed as an emergency treatment. Dogs are anesthetized with a routine protocol using an opioid to manage perioperative pain. Prophylactic antibiotic therapy is recommended. Clipping should include the entire thorax and abdomen to allow immediate conversion in case of serious impending complication following the thoracoscopic procedure. This wide clipping permits conversion to an intercostal thoracotomy or a transdiaphragmatic approach, depending on the complication. Clipping should be performed prior to anesthesia to limit anesthetic time and related complications.

Once in the operating room, the patient is placed under intermittent positive-pressure ventilation prior to surgery and positioned in dorsal recumbency with a slight tilt to the right. Cushions are used to maintain the patient in this position. The slight rotation to the right facilitates access to the left pleural space and placement of the laparoscopic cannulas and lead from the left side for ventricular implantation.

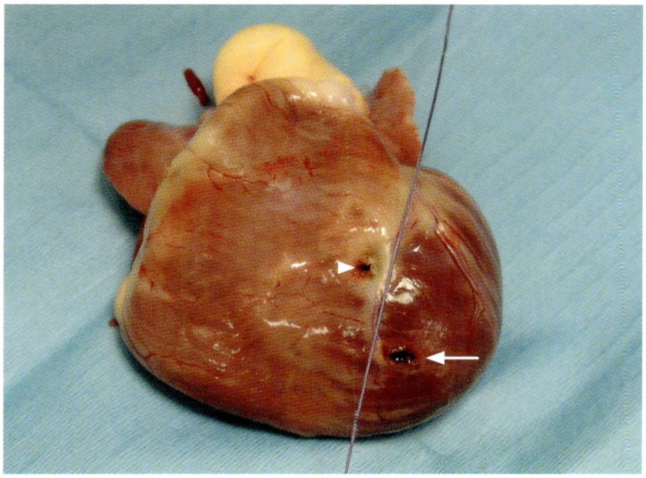

FIGURE 1. The string represents the interventricular septum; the right ventricle is on the left and the left ventricle on the right. Two holes have been made: one for TEP (arrowhead) and one for the transdiaphragmatic approach (arrow).

During TEP, cardiac structures must be identified, in particular the median septum, to pace the left ventricle instead of the right ventricle. An anatomic study showed that the TEP surgical protocol with lead implantation through the 6th intercostal space resulted in placement of the lead very close to the cardiac septum (**Fig. 1**). The surgeon should attempt to implant the lead as far on the left side as possible, close to the septum, where the myocardium is thicker, and as lateral and caudal as possible, to be far from the right ventricle. The surgeon should also keep a distance from the septum and avoid coronary vessels.

OPERATING ROOM LAYOUT

The operating room layout must be comfortable for the surgeons and the medical team. The instrument table is at the patient's head, with the endoscopy tower behind it. The monitor is to the right of the endoscopy tower. The surgeons position themselves at the caudal end of the operating table, each at one corner: the surgeon is slightly to the patient's left side, and the assistant slightly to the patient's right side (**Fig. 2**).

PORT PLACEMENT (FIG. 4)

- T1, 11 mm cannula, in a right paraxiphoid transdiaphragmatic approach to reach the right thorax. The rotating insufflation stopcock should be open to abolish the pleural void.
- T2, 15 mm cannula, at the left 6th intercostal space at the level of the chondrocostal junction. A wider cannula is used in this particular case to avoid impairing the pacemaker lead when passing through the cannula.
- T3, 6 mm cannula, at the right 6th intercostal space at the level of the chondrocostal junction.

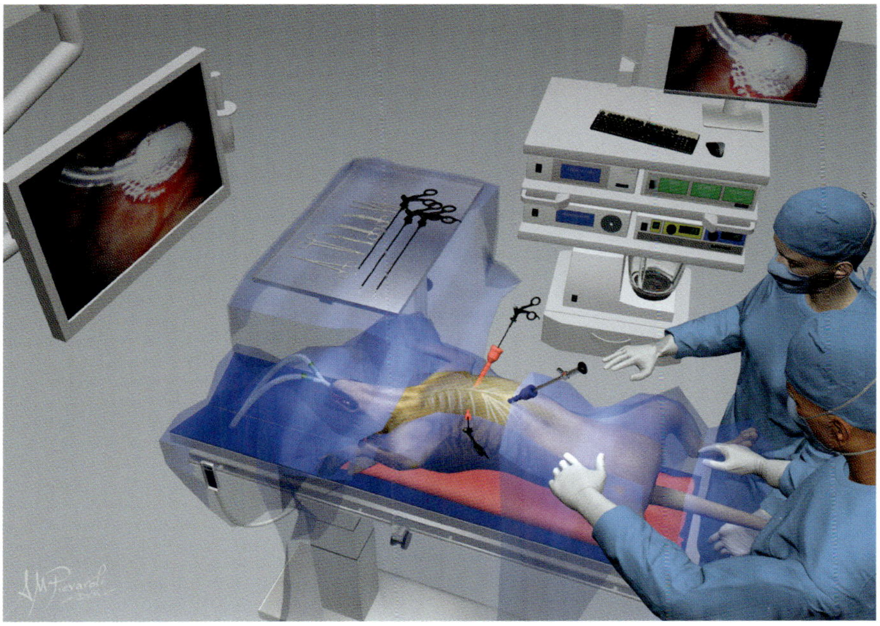

FIGURE 2. Operating room layout for thoracoscopic placement of an epicardial pacemaker.

Instruments

On the table:

- Standard surgery set
- Telescope 5 mm – 0° or 30° (depending on the surgeon's preference)
- 6 mm + 11 mm + 15 mm cannulas
- Endoscopic scissors (5 mm)
- Traumatic and atraumatic grasping forceps
- Bipolar endoscopic electrocautery or vessel-sealing device
- Thoracic tube and equipment necessary for pleural puncture

Ready to use:

- Sutureless unipolar lead with myocardial screw-in or hook fixation with its applicator and pulse generator (**Fig. 3**)

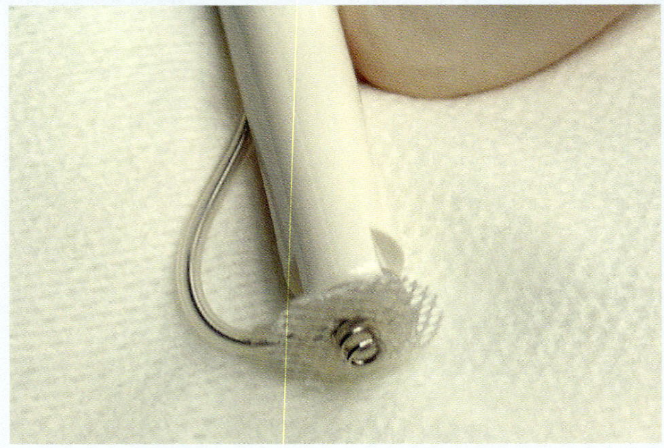

FIGURE 3. Pacemaker lead with the pigtail screw-in fixation along with the applicator (white tube). It allows for implantation and maintenance of the lead within the epicardium. Fibrosis will develop between the white patch and the epicardium and strengthen the adhesion between the two.

PROCEDURE

- After the ports have been placed, scissors are inserted through T3 to puncture the mediastinum in a nonvascular zone to extend pneumothorax to the left pleural space. The vessel-sealing device is then used (through T3) to enlarge the mediastinal incision.
- Performing a pericardial window is the next step. The pericardium is grabbed and drawn toward the sternum using grasping forceps (through T3). This step is much easier compared

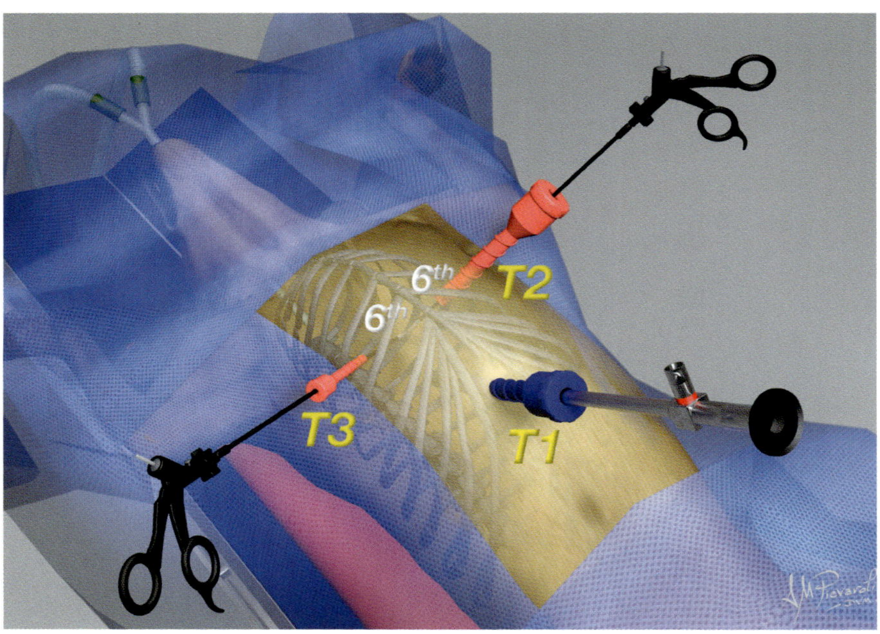

FIGURE 4. Port placement for thoracoscopic placement of an epicardial pacemaker.

to cases of pericardial effusion, in which the pericardium is thicker. Scissors are inserted through T2 and used to puncture the pericardium ventrally. This puncture should be performed a few centimeters further than the usual location of a pericardial window. Pericardiectomy is performed, obtaining a 1–2 cm^2 window. A longitudinal incision toward the left auricle is indicated to ease access to the ventricle.

- The lead applicator is then carefully inserted through the left-side cannula (**Fig. 5**). The lead should not be stretched or twisted.
- Implantation must be performed in an area that is away from the septum and free from coronary vessels. If possible, the lead should be screwed during the systole phase. During screwing, care must be taken not to perforate the myocardium, which is thin at this location. It is recommended to apply constant pressure while screwing the lead. To ensure fixation the lead must have done 1.5 turns.
- To check for proper fixation, the surgeon can gently pull the lead; it should not move and the pigtail should be invisible. The flange must be as close as possible to the epicardium (**Fig. 6**).
- In case of improper fixation, the lead can be unscrewed with the applicator and screwed again without much difficulty.
- The cable is grasped with atraumatic forceps and a large loop is created, oriented toward the ventral pleural cavity. The cable should not be twisted. This ends the thoracic phase when using a unipolar pacemaker lead.
- The lead exits the thorax by T2 and is then connected to the generator.

Tips

It should be remembered that electrocautery can be used before connection of the pacemaker generator but is completely forbidden once it is connected and working. Its use could disturb or damage the generator.

- The generator pocket is created by dissection between the intercostal and latissimus dorsi muscles a few centimeters behind T2 (**Fig. 7**). During dissection, the generator can be put in contact with any muscle to initiate cardiac stimulation in order to reduce the anesthetic risk and assistance. Once the generator is inserted in the pocket, the lead should make one 360° loop within the pocket to avoid any tension.
- ECG monitoring is checked to ensure proper cardiac stimulation. When it is functioning properly, spikes should be observed. Spikes are the typical morphology of trigger potentials. Their presence confirms the quality of the contact between the lead and the pacemaker pocket.
- When using a bipolar pacemaker, the second ventricular electrode is inserted via T2 2 cm away and cranially from the first electrode. The second cable is placed in the pleural space similarly to the first.
- A thoracic drain is placed in the right pleural space to restore the pleural void while avoiding excessive manipulation of the pacemaker cable(s).

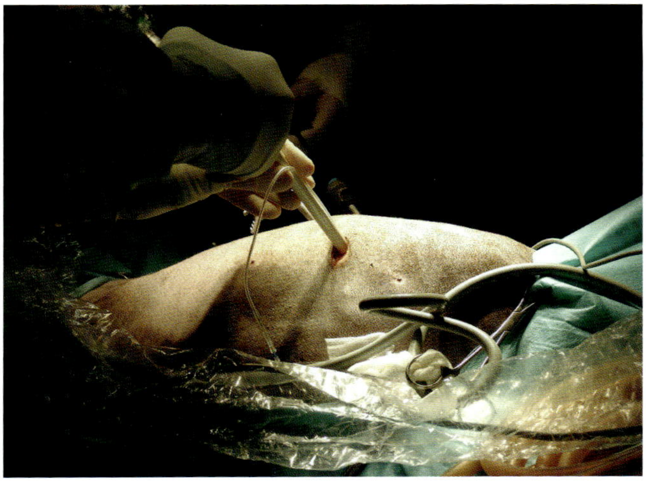

FIGURE 5. The pacemaker lead is inserted through T2.

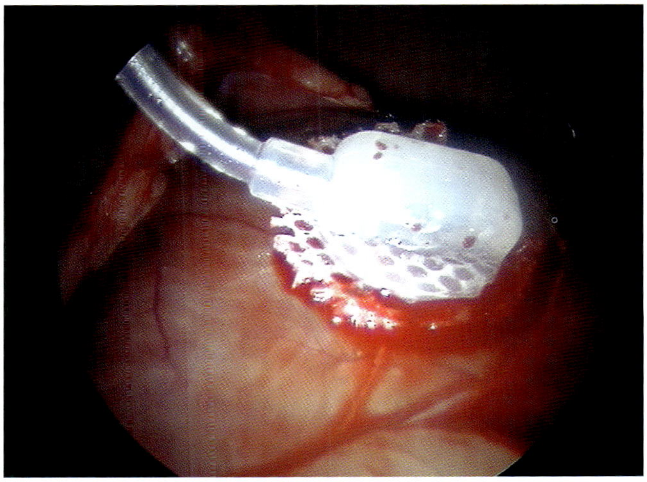

FIGURE 6. The flange should be close to the epicardium.

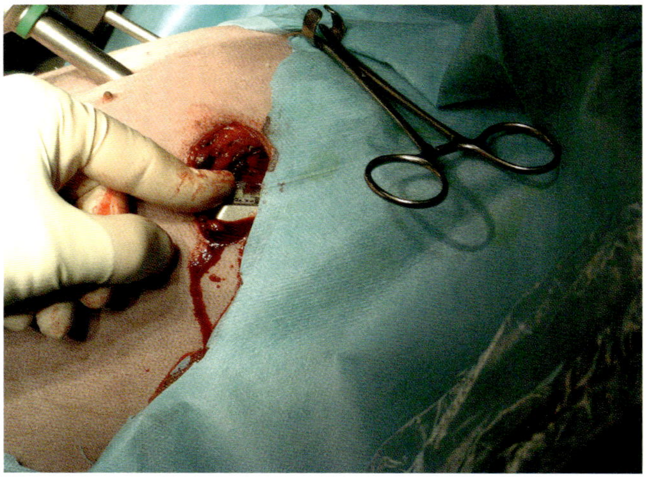

FIGURE 7. The pacemaker pocket is created. As soon as the generator is in contact with muscular tissue, the stimulation can begin prior to surgery completion.

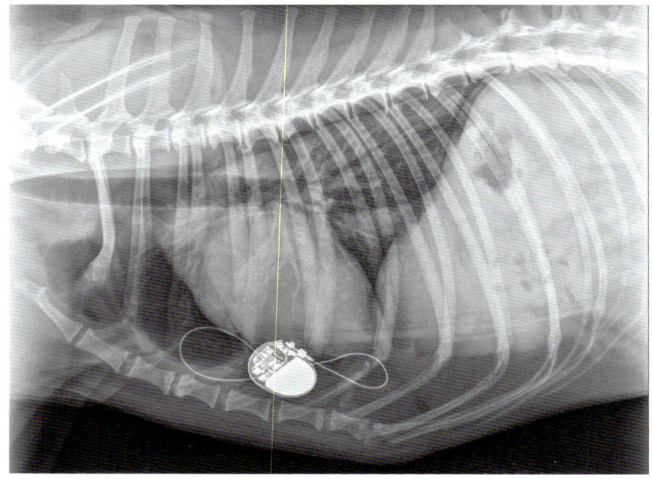

FIGURE 8. Radiograph confirming good positioning of the pacemaker.

- As with any thoracic procedure, bupivacaine (2 mg/kg) can be instilled into the wound prior to closing to help with postoperative pain management.
- The wounds are closed in a routine fashion.
- A thoracic radiograph is taken to assess the quality of the pacemaker position and the absence of pneumothorax (**Fig. 8**). The thoracic tube is then removed before waking the patient.
- Pacemaker settings are done by a veterinary cardiologist.

POSTOPERATIVE MANAGEMENT

Monitoring and follow-up after thoracoscopic implantation of an epicardial pacemaker are identical to those for standard open surgery techniques.

- Proper pacemaker configuration must be done before waking the patient. It can be performed transcutaneously in the immediate postoperative period.
- Thoracic radiographs are taken to confirm correct cable and generator positioning and the absence of pneumothorax.
- Echocardiography is generally recommended.
- ECG monitoring must be performed consistently until discharge.
- Continuous pain management is necessary (e.g., anesthetic block, opioids, nonsteroidal anti-inflammatory drugs).
- Hospitalization rarely exceeds 24 hours unless the pacemaker is misconfigured.
- Exercise restriction for 15 days is recommended.
- Medical treatment of cardiac insufficiency is pursued according to echocardiography follow-up.

Complications of thoracoscopic placement of epicardial pacemakers

There are no complications specific to TEP, so complications include those that may occur with any surgical procedure.

- Perioperative death due to right ventricular perforation or cardiac tamponade.
- Seroma at the generator pocket site.
- Infection. The pacemaker generator pocket is less exposed to wound infection or trauma in this location (deep pocket between muscles) compared to other techniques in which the generator is placed in the neck (more exposed to collar, bite wounds, etc.).
- Lead or cable defects (Twiddler's syndrome): abnormal coiling of the lead that induces lead dislodgement (**Fig. 9**).
- Dislodgement of the lead by external trauma (Reel syndrome). To avoid this, the generator pocket must be deep and in an area not exposed to trauma.
- Pacemaker syndrome: fatigue, weakness, dyspnea, dizziness, palpitations, pulsations, and chest pain secondary to misconfiguration of the pacemaker. This can lead to the development of cardiac failure.
- Lead dislodgement.
- Muscle contractions around the generator, which can lead to seroma, pain, or generator dislodgement.

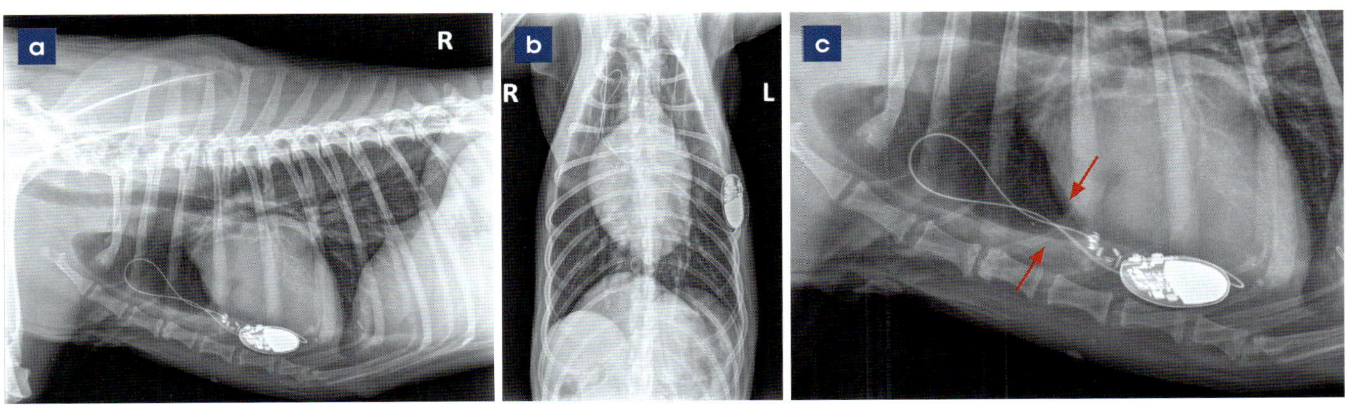

FIGURE 9. Radiographs of the same patient as in Figure 8 showing Twiddler's syndrome. Lead coiling (arrows) and dislodgement can be seen.

Key points

- Electrocoagulation must not be used once the pacemaker is connected.
- The lead should be screwed very gently to avoid perforation.
- The lead should not be twisted within the thorax. One loop is recommended within the pacemaker pocket.

SUGGESTED READINGS

59 THORACOSCOPIC-ASSISTED PLEURAL PORT PLACEMENT

Francesco Collivignarelli, Kumiko Ishigaki

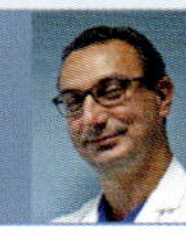

Indications

- Long-term management of refractory pleural effusion caused by idiopathic hydrothorax or chylothorax
- Intrathoracic administration of chemotherapeutic drugs in case of mesothelioma or pleural metastasis
- Drainage of pleural effusion without thoracentesis (it may reduce complications such as pneumothorax and bacterial contamination)
- Repeated administration of drugs into the thoracic cavity
- Pleural effusion secondary to metastatic disease

Contraindications

- Severe adhesions of the pleural membrane

Thoracoscopic surgery is useful for the diagnosis and treatment of thoracic diseases because the smaller incisions in the chest wall for approaching the thoracic cavity result in less pain and faster recovery compared with traditional thoracotomy. Additionally, it can be used to examine the surgical anatomy in detail by magnification of the operative field through the telescope.

The implantation of a pleural port is aimed at removing the intrathoracic fluid and/or air caused by pathological conditions. When intrathoracic fluid and/or air buildup occurs or continues after thoracoscopic surgery, pleural ports can also be helpful in the postoperative management. These ports can also be used for the control of pleural effusion and pneumothorax and the intrathoracic administration of chemotherapeutic drugs for treatment of malignant tumors.

It has been concluded that the pleural port device is a feasible option for the management of pleural effusion in dogs and cats (A. C. Brooks and R. J. Hardie).

The following procedures are described below:

A. Pleural port placement following pericardiectomy

B. Pleural port placement for the management of malignant thoracic effusion

A PLEURAL PORT PLACEMENT FOLLOWING PERICARDIECTOMY

PATIENT PREPARATION AND POSITIONING

The patient is placed in dorsal recumbency under general anesthesia. The patient should be firmly secured to the operating table, as repositioning may be necessary during the operation.

OPERATING ROOM LAYOUT

A thoracoscopic pericardial window is performed with the patient's hind end positioned at the caudal edge of the operating table. The surgeon and the assistant stand side by side at the end of the table. The monitor is placed in front of the surgeons towards the patient's head (**Fig. 1**).

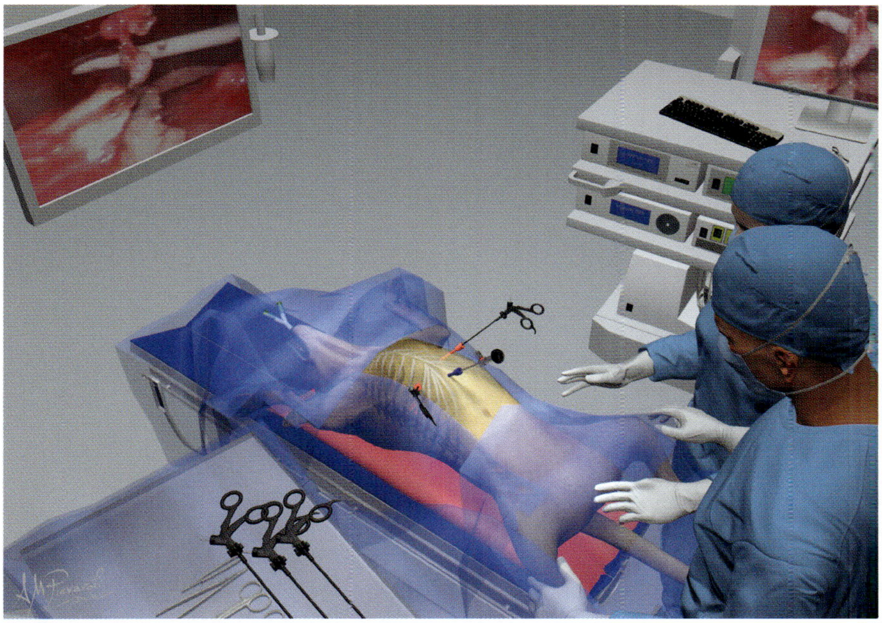

FIGURE 1. Operating room layout for pleural port placement following pericardiectomy.

Instruments

On the table:

- Pleural port device including metallic port and drainage catheter
- Standard surgery set
- Telescope 5 mm – 30°
- Two 5 mm cannulas (or one 5 mm cannula + one 10 mm cannula)
- Grasping forceps

Ready to use:

- Endoscopic cannula for aspiration/irrigation
- Endoscopic vessel-sealing system

PORT PLACEMENT (FIG. 2)

Three ports are placed for thoracoscopic pericardiectomy:

- T1, for the telescope, between the xiphoid process and the last sternocostal junction
- T2, for the grasping forceps, left or right 8th intercostal space
- T3, for the grasping forceps, contralateral 8th intercostal space

PROCEDURE

Although a pleural port can be implanted by traditional open surgery, placement is more secure under thoracoscopic guidance since the clinical applications of thoracoscopy are becoming widely spread in small animal practice. Potential advantages of the pleural port over thoracocentesis and chest tube include being minimally invasive to place, being relatively inexpensive compared with surgical options, and, since it is not exposed externally, reduced risk of ascending bacterial infection and accidental removal or destruction. The pleural port allows owners to manage pleural effusion at home, reducing the cost, the patient's stress, and the risk of pneumothorax associated with repeated thoracocentesis. In dogs with cancerous pleural effusion, chemotherapeutic drugs can be repeatedly administered into the thoracic cavity through the port similar to the technique used for vascular access ports.

- A 0.5–1 cm incision is made in a paraxiphoid or subxiphoid position and the 5 mm cannula (T1) is inserted (**Fig. 3**).
- The 5 mm telescope is then inserted and a first exploration of the thoracic cavity is performed (**Fig. 4**).
- Under direct visualization, the second port (T3 or T2) is placed (**Fig. 5**).
- The endoscopic vessel-sealing system is then inserted through T2/T3 and used for resecting the thickened mediastinum as needed, and the third port is placed in the contralateral intercostal space.

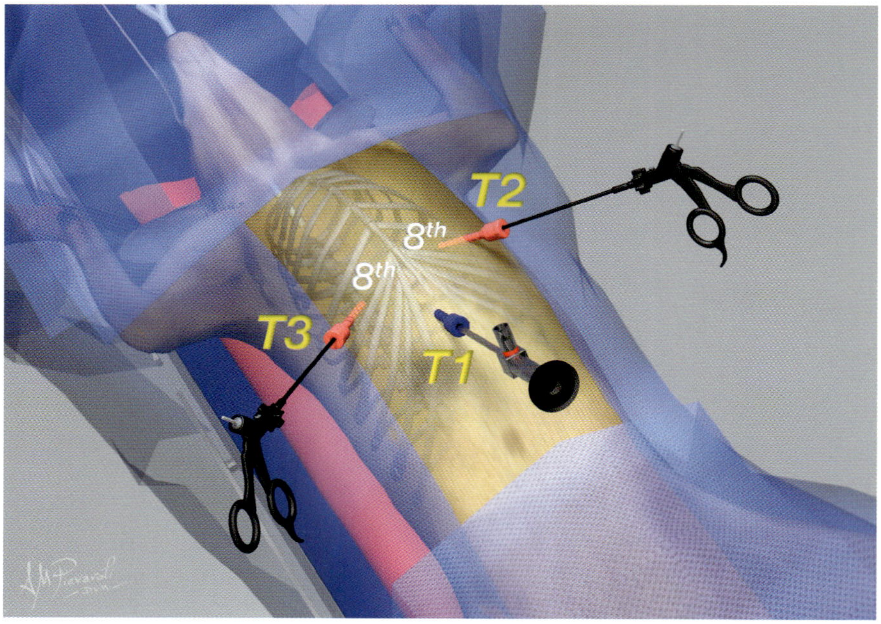

FIGURE 2. Port placement for implantation of a pleural port following pericardiectomy.

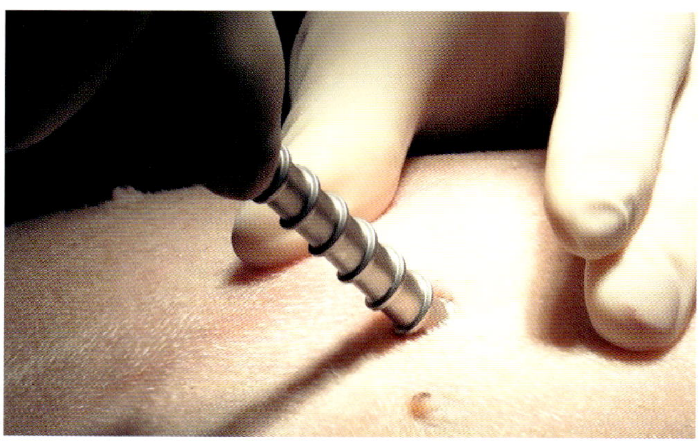

FIGURE 3. The cannula is inserted in a paraxiphoid or subxiphoid position.

- The pleural port is placed on the thoracic wall or on the abdominal wall. The chest (8th intercostal space or more caudal) is preferred for pleural port implantation because the Huber needle is easily inserted with the patient standing or in a lateral position.
- In case of thoracic placement, a semicircular incision larger than the port is made in the predetermined area of the skin (**Fig. 6**). A skin flap is then created by subcutaneous dissection with electrocautery (**Fig. 7**).
- The tip of the silicone drainage catheter is grasped using a curved or right-angled Kelly forceps, and the forceps are inserted from the base of the skin flap and advanced

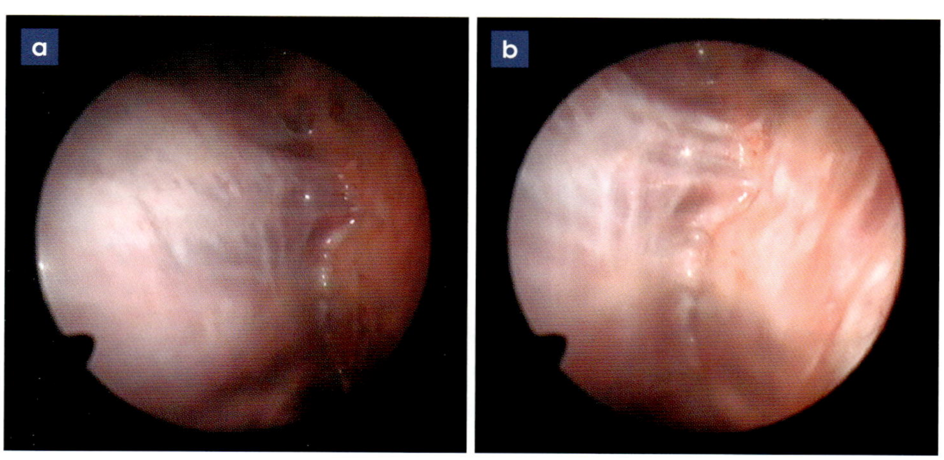

FIGURE 4. Exploration of the thoracic cavity. a) Pleural adhesions and minimal effusion. b) Intercostal arteries and veins are not visible due to chronic pleural effusion.

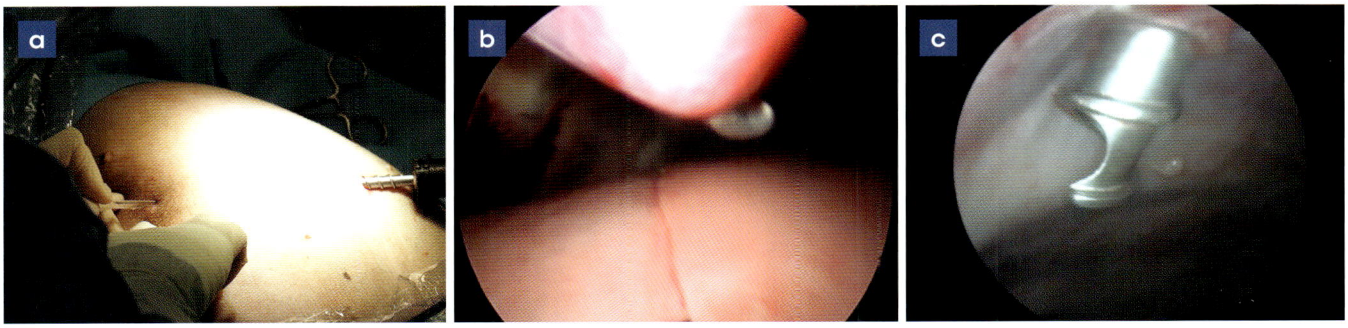

FIGURE 5. The second port is placed under direct visualization.

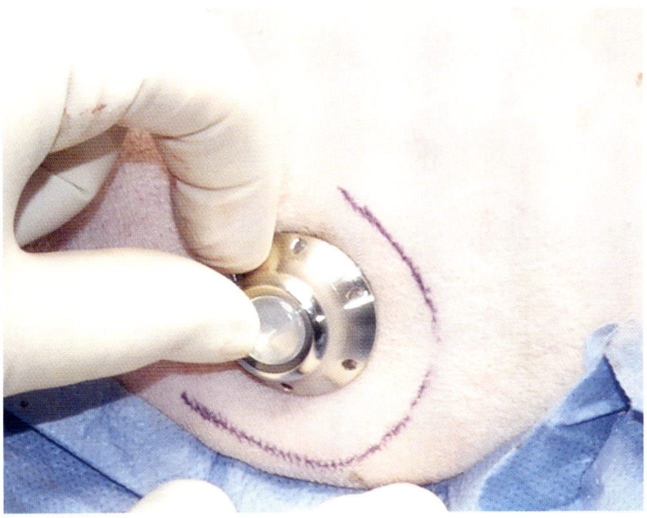

FIGURE 6. A semicircular skin incision larger than the port is made.

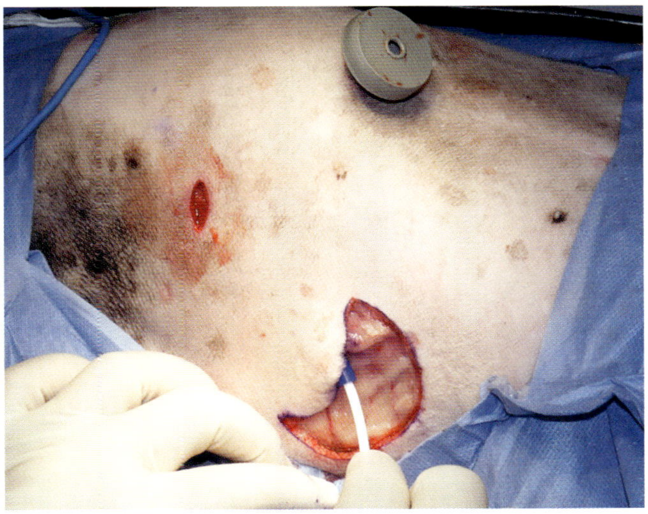

FIGURE 7. A skin flap is created.

intramuscularly in a cranioventral direction more than two intercostal spaces.

- Under direct visualization, the tip of the forceps is gently pushed and passed through the thoracic wall. The tip of the catheter is then grasped with an endoscopic grasping forceps inserted through the contralateral intercostal port, and the catheter is pulled into the thoracic cavity after removing the Kelly forceps (**Fig. 8**).
- The catheter is connected to the pleural port with a blue boot. The catheter should have the blue boot placed with the tapered end inserted proximally on the catheter away from the port. The blue boot is then advanced to cover the connection site (**Fig. 9**).
- The pleural port is gently fixed to the thoracic wall musculature with four nonabsorbable sutures (3-0 polypropylene). The port is covered with the skin flap, which is then closed routinely (**Fig. 10**).

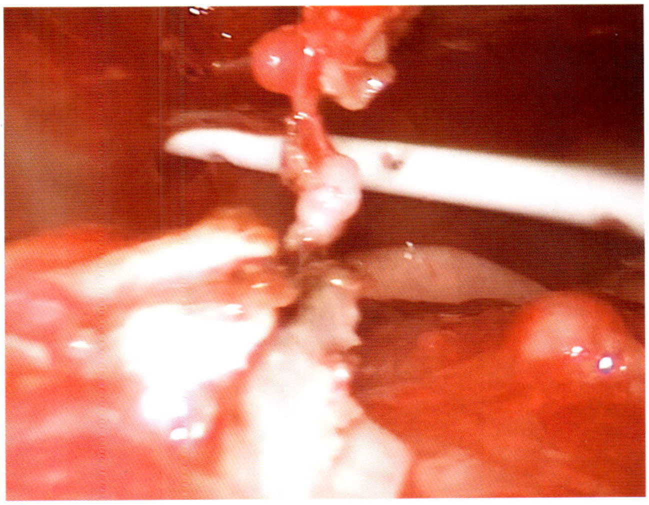

FIGURE 8. The Kelly forceps are removed and the catheter is pulled into the thoracic cavity.

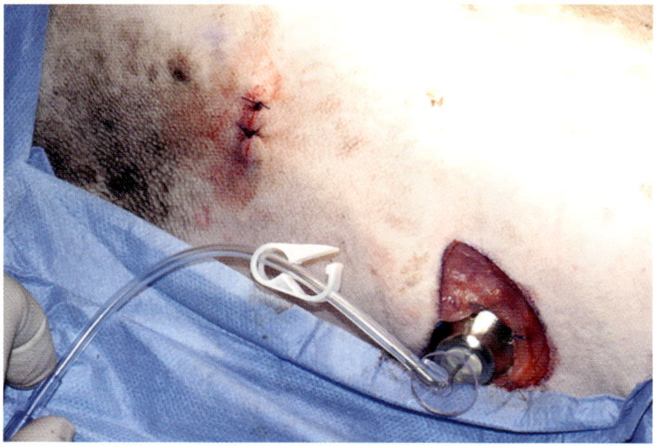

FIGURE 9. The catheter is advanced to cover the connection site.

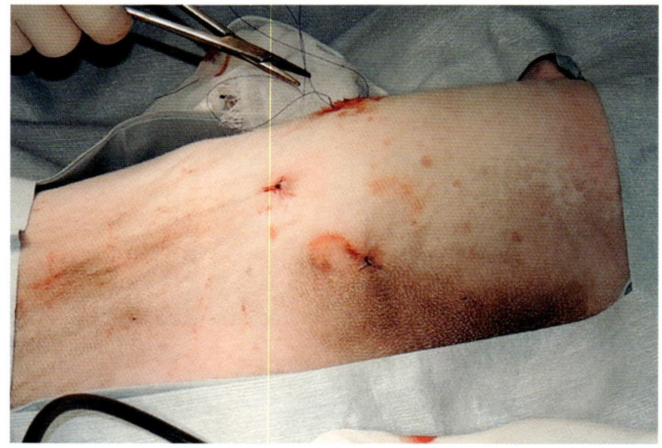

FIGURE 10. The skin flap is closed routinely.

Key points

- As the procedure is performed after partial pericardiectomy, the drainage catheter can be safely inserted under thoracoscopic guidance.

B PLEURAL PORT PLACEMENT FOR THE MANAGEMENT OF MALIGNANT THORACIC EFFUSION

PATIENT PREPARATION AND POSITIONING

The patient is placed in lateral recumbency. The entire hemithorax is clipped, from the scapular spine to the cranial abdomen and from the dorsal spine to the sternum.

OPERATING ROOM LAYOUT

The surgeon and the assistant stand at the side of the operating table facing the patient's thorax. The monitor is placed on the other side of the table (**Fig. 11**).

PORT PLACEMENT (FIG. 12)

- T1, for the thoracoscope, in the dorsal third of the 10th intercostal space
- T2, for the dissection instrument, in the middle third of the 11th intercostal space
- T3, for the dissection instrument, in the ventral third of the 10th or 11th intercostal space

Instruments

On the table:

- Pleural port device including metallic port and drainage catheter
- Standard surgery set
- Telescope 5 mm – 30°
- Two 5 mm cannulas (or one 5 mm cannula + one 10 mm cannula)
- Grasping forceps

Ready to use:

- Endoscopic cannula for aspiration/irrigation
- Endoscopic vessel-sealing system

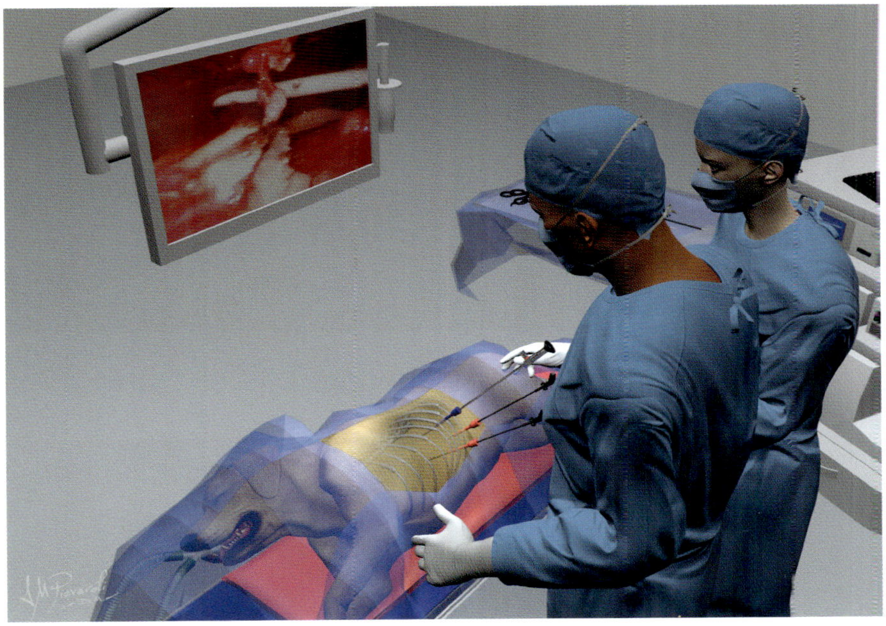

FIGURE 11. Operating room layout for pleural port placement for the management of malignant thoracic effusion.

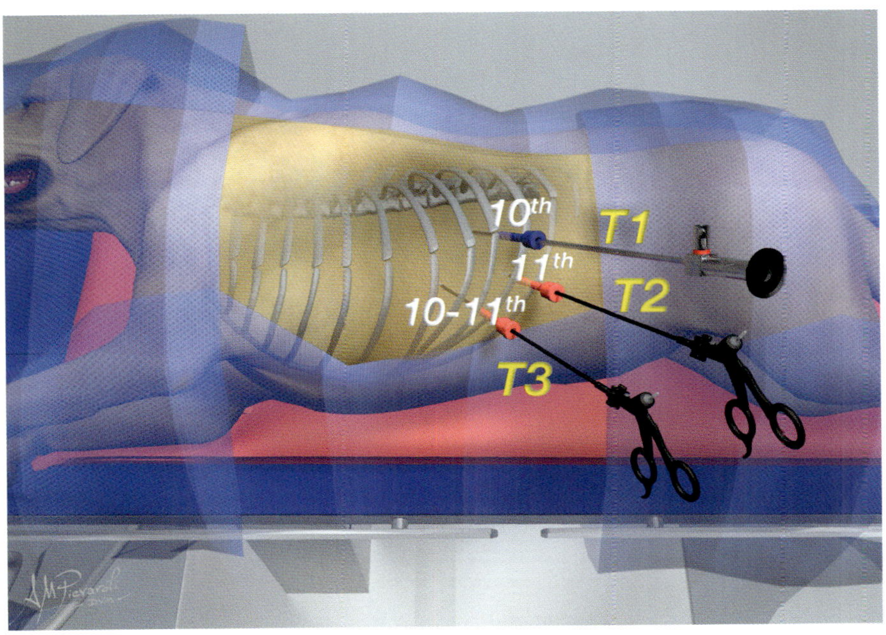

FIGURE 12. Port placement for implantation of a pleural port for the management of malignant thoracic effusion.

PROCEDURE

- After all the ports have been placed, the hemithorax is inspected to confirm the diagnosis and collect biopsy samples (**Fig. 13**).
- The tip of the drainage catheter is grasped with curved or right-angled Kelly forceps and gently pushed into the cranial thoracic cavity, taking care not to damage the lung (**Fig. 14**).
- After advancing the catheter sufficiently into the thoracic cavity, it is connected to the pleural port using a blue boot as described above (**Fig. 15**).
- The pleural port is then gently fixed to the thoracic wall musculature with four nonabsorbable sutures (3-0 polypropylene). The port is covered with the skin flap, which is then closed routinely.
- The port is tested with a Huber needle (**Fig. 16**).

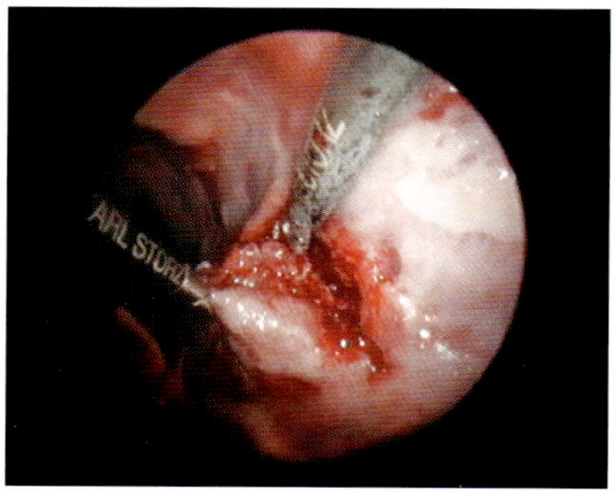
FIGURE 13. Pleural biopsy is performed.

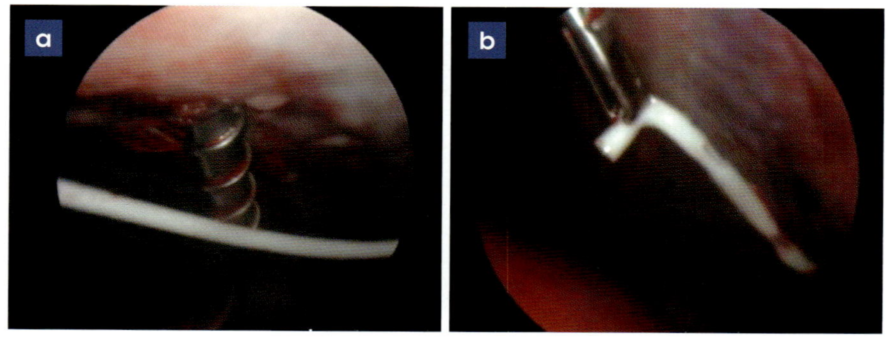

FIGURE 14. The catheter is inserted into the thoracic cavity.

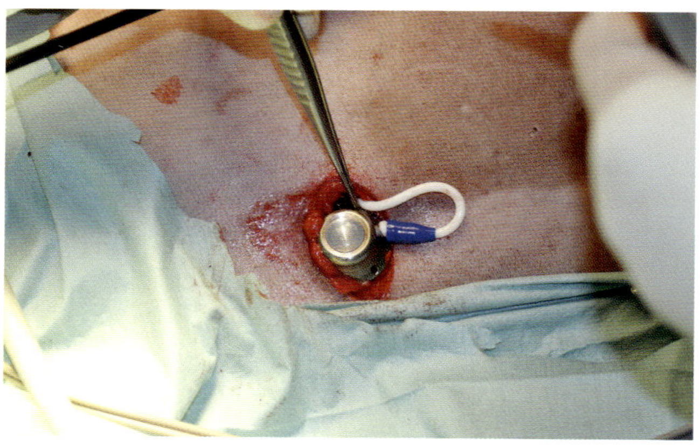
FIGURE 15. The catheter is advanced into the thoracic cavity.

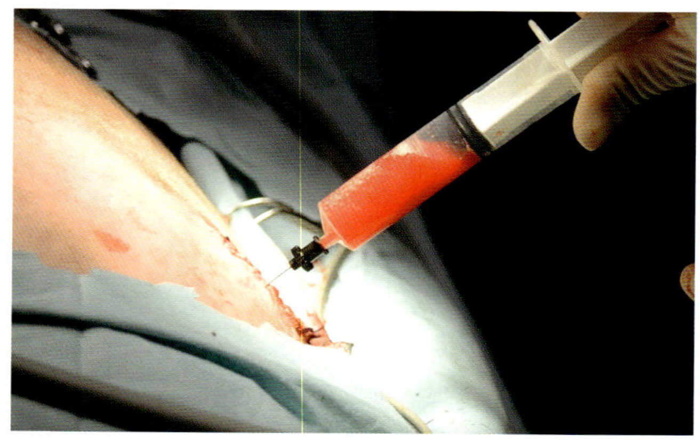
FIGURE 16. The port is tested using a Huber needle.

Key points

- Care should be taken not to damage the lung.
- Aspiration can be performed by the owners, after instruction, as there is no need for sedation. This substantially reduces the stress on patients, which usually already have compromised respiration.

POSTOPERATIVE MANAGEMENT

- Postoperative radiographs are essential to rule out the presence of residual air or fluid and to evaluate the correct placement of the pleural tube (**Fig. 17**).
- Aspiration from the chest tube can be performed every 12–24 hours.
- Although thoracoscopy is associated with less pain than thoracotomy, analgesia is warranted to control pain that may cause hypoventilation and hypoxia.
- Local anesthetics, intrapleural application of anesthetics, systemic analgesia, and the use of flexible ports contribute to pain control.

Tips

Check for pleural effusion and air leaks.

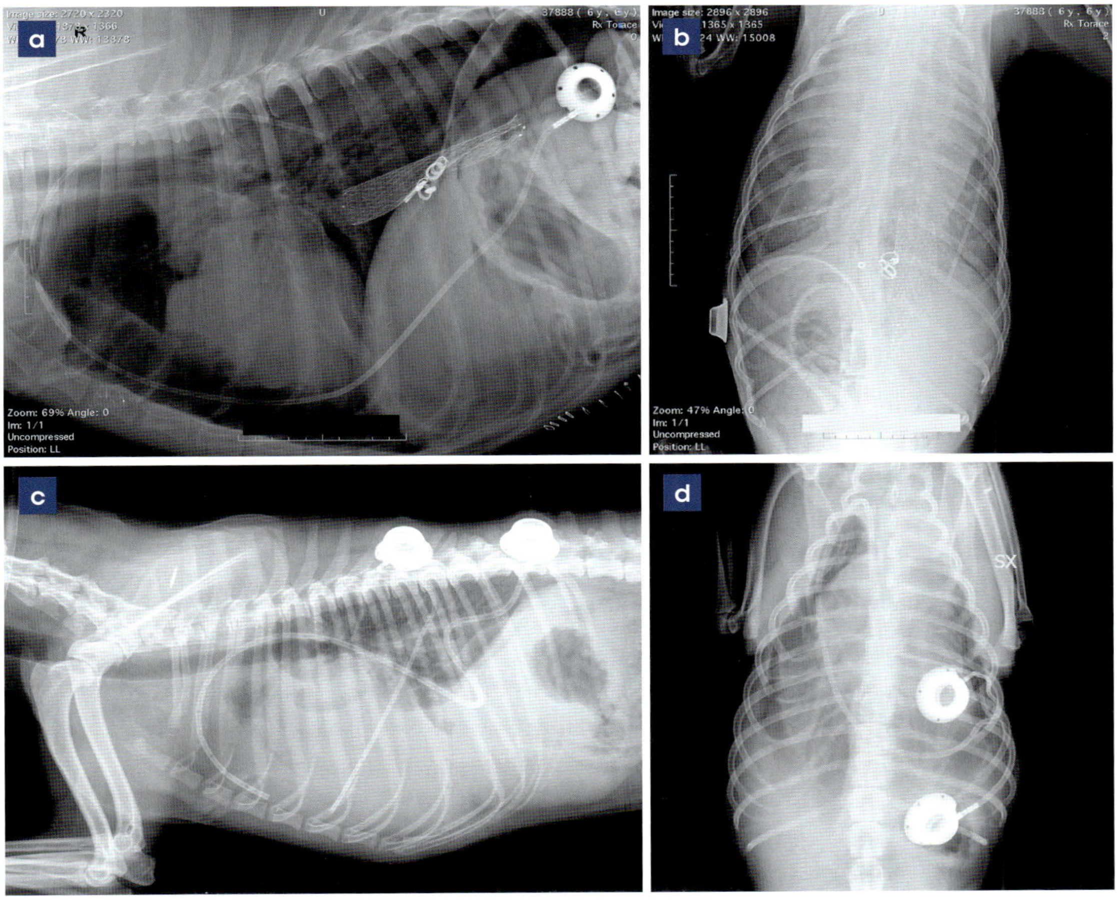

FIGURE 17. a,b) Immediate postoperative chest X-rays showing tube placement. c,d) Chest X-ray 4 weeks after pleural port placement.

Complications of thoracoscopic-assisted pleural port placement

- Bleeding.
- Pneumothorax.
- Respiratory failure due to damage to the diaphragmatic nerve.
- Obstruction of the catheter.
- Port flipped over in the subcutaneous space.
- Catheter fully moved out of the thoracic cavity.

SUGGESTED READINGS

CLINICAL CASES

59.1 PLEURAL PORT IMPLANTATION FOR THE MANAGEMENT OF MALIGNANT PLEURAL EFFUSION DUE TO METASTATIC MAMMARY CARCINOMA IN A DOG

Giulia Dolce, Flavia Catanzaro

CASE DESCRIPTION

A 16-year-old intact female Yorkshire Terrier with metastatic mammary carcinoma to the liver and lungs was evaluated for the management of malignant pleural effusion. Pleural effusion is challenging to control and can result in decreased quality of life of the animal. In this patient, pleural effusion had been drained by thoracocentesis every 48 hours for 15 days. After drainage, the patient was free from clinical signs for 36 hours. It was decided to implant a pleural port as palliative therapy to allow drainage of the effusion by the owner himself. The pleural port was inserted under thoracoscopic guidance. The owner was instructed on how to drain the effusion through the port and this was carried out at home without difficulty. At the time of this writing (3 months after port placement), the patient is alive and no major complications have been seen.

Key points

- The patient was positioned in left lateral recumbency.
- A 5 cm skin incision was made in the dorsal third of the right hemithorax in the region of the 10th intercostal space to create a subcutaneous pocket in which to place the port. A small stab incision was made between the 8th and the 7th intercostal spaces.
- The hub was sutured to the fascia with nonabsorbable monofilament suture material in a simple interrupted pattern through the prefabricated holes of the hub. The tubing was connected to the hub. The port patency was verified using a Huber-point needle.
- Surgical time was 17 minutes.
- The patient was discharged the same day of surgery.

PORT PLACEMENT

An Endotip cannula was placed at right 5th intercostal space and a 5 mm 30° rigid telescope was introduced through the port.

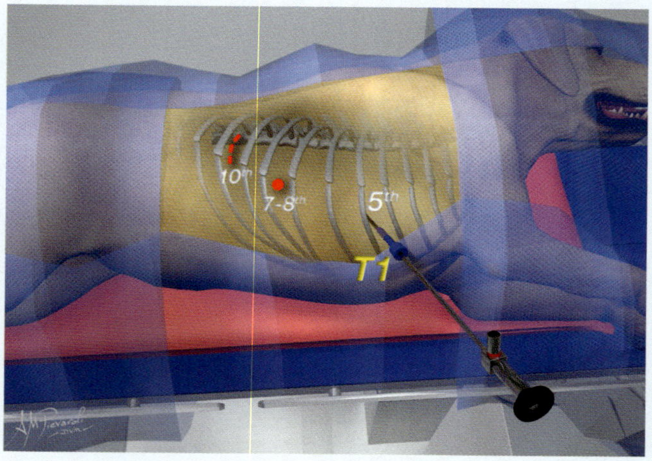

PROCEDURE

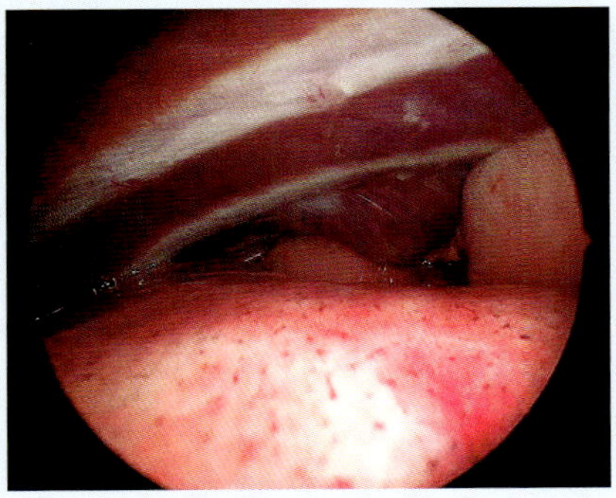

FIGURE 1. The entry point for insertion of the fenestrated tube is identified.

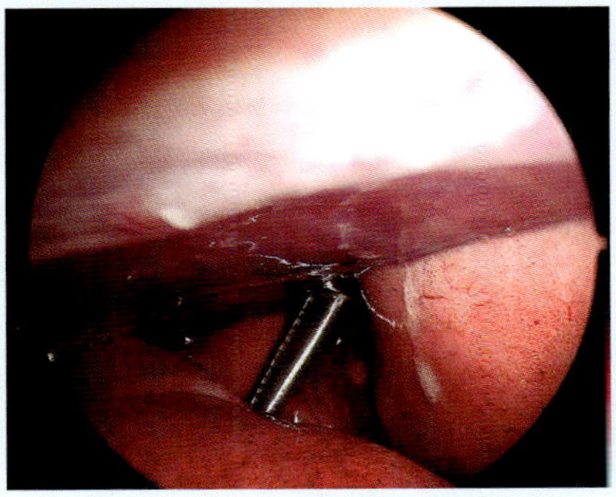

FIGURE 2. A hemostat is passed through the stab incision to facilitate tube insertion.

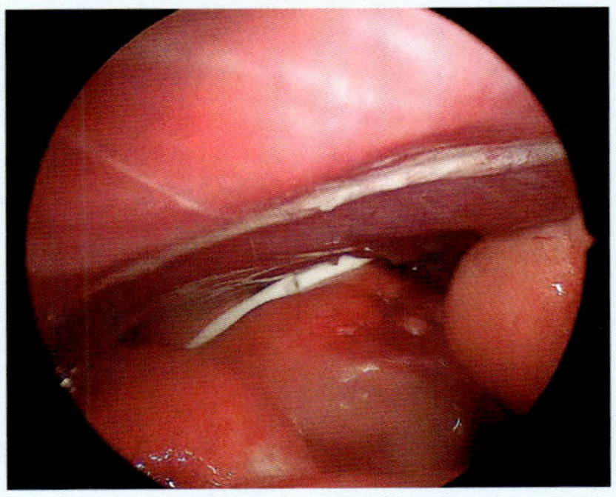

FIGURE 3. Under thoracoscopic guidance, the fenestrated tube is advanced until the marker is visualized, with all the fenestrations placed inside the thoracic cavity.

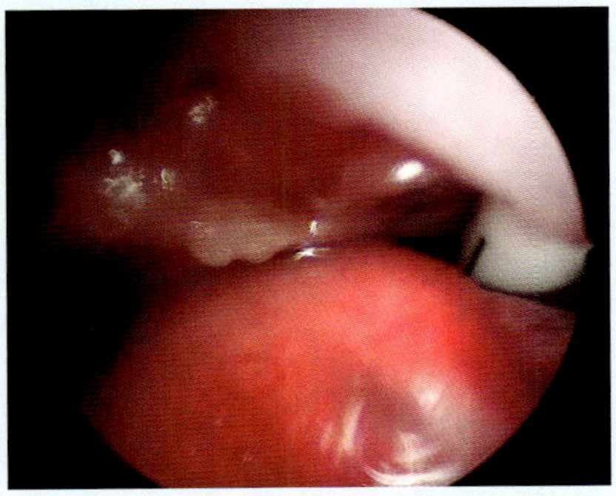

FIGURE 4. Identification of the marker to confirm correct tube positioning.

Tips and tricks

- ✓ Thoracoscopic-assisted pleural port placement allows direct visualization of the tube, minimizing the risk of iatrogenic injury and enabling confirmation of correct tube positioning.
- ✓ When necessary, biopsy can be performed during the same procedure by adding a second thoracic port.